Basic Clinical Lab Competencies for Respiratory Care

An Integrated Approach

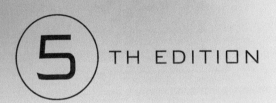

5TH EDITION

Chapter 20, 3

Basic Clinical Lab Competencies for Respiratory Care

An Integrated Approach

5 TH EDITION

Gary C. White, M.Ed., RRT, RPFT
Spokane Community College
Spokane, Washington

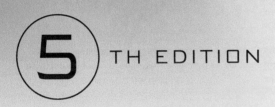

Australia • Brazil • Canada • Mexico • Singapore • United Kingdom • United States

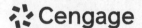

Basic Clinical Lab Competencies for Respiratory Care: An Integrated Approach,
Fifth Edition
Gary C. White

Vice President, Editorial: Dave Garza

Director of Learning Solutions: Matthew Kane

Acquisitions Editor: Tari Broderick

Managing Editor: Marah Bellegarde

Senior Product Manager: Darcy M. Scelsi

Editorial Assistant: Nicole Manikas

Vice President, Marketing: Jennifer Baker

Marketing Manager: Jonathan Sheehan

Production Director: Wendy Troeger

Production Manager: Andrew Crouth

Content Project Manager: Anne Sherman

Senior Art Director: Jack Pendleton

For product information and technology assistance, contact us at
Cengage Customer & Sales Support, 1-800-354-9706 or support.cengage.com.

For permission to use material from this text or product,
submit all requests online at **www.copyright.com.**

Library of Congress Control Number: 2011933234

ISBN-13: 978-1-4354-5365-4

ISBN-10: 1-4354-5365-4

Cengage
200 Pier 4 Boulevard
Boston, MA 02210
USA

Cengage is a leading provider of customized learning solutions with employees residing in nearly 40 different countries and sales in more than 125 countries around the world. Find your local representative at **www.cengage.com.**

To learn more about Cengage platforms and services, register or access your online learning solution, or purchase materials for your course, visit **www.cengage.com.**

Notice to the Reader

Printed at CLDPC, USA, 08-22

CONTENTS

List of Performance Evaluations

New to This Edition

CHAPTER 1

- Updated commonly used terminology: nosocomial to hospital acquired and hand washing to hand hygiene
- Revised information on contact transmission
- Updated the CDC guidelines on standard precautions and hand hygiene
- Added information on respiratory hygiene/cough etiquette

CHAPTER 5

- Added the American Thoracic Society summary of *Standardization for Spirometry*

CHAPTER 8

- Added discussion of the use of pulse oximetry to evaluate collateral circulation to the hand
- Updated the AARC Clinical Practice Guideline: Sampling for Arterial Blood Gas Analysis

CHAPTER 10

- Updated the AARC Clinical Practice Guideline: Capnography/Capnometry during Mechanical Ventilation
- Added discussion of the Masimo Rad-57™ pulse oximeter

CHAPTER 11

- Added a list of The Joint Commission abbreviations that should not be used in documentation

CHAPTER 13

- Updated the AARC Clinical Practice Guidelines for the indications, precautions, and possible complications for oxygen administration in both acute care and home care
- Added discussion of the Oxymask, Cardinal Health Hi-Ox80, and Vapotherm precision flow high-flow cannula

CHAPTER 14

- Added discussion of the following drugs: formoterol fumarate, levalbuterol, tiotropium bromide (Spiriva), budesonide, montelukast (Singulair), zafirlukast, zileuton, HandiHaler, Aerolizer, Twisthaler
- Added discussion of the following combination therapy drugs: fluticasone propionate-salmeterol, albuterol sulfate–ipratropium bromide, formoterol fumarate–budesonide
- Deleted discussion of metaproterenol, sulfate isoetharine, fluticasone propionate-salmeterol

CHAPTER 15

- Deleted discussion of the cascade humidifier
- Updated discussion of the Wick humidifier

CHAPTER 16

- Added discussion of the adjunctive devices for chest percussion
- Added discussion of the oscillating PEP therapy
- Added discussion of the Respironics Coughassist™ MI-E

CHAPTER 17

- Updated the AARC Clinical Practice Guideline: Incentive Spirometry 2011, Intermittent Positive-Pressure Breathing
- Added discussion of the Triflow incentive spirometer

CHAPTER 18

- Updated the AARC Clinical Practice Guideline: Fiberoptic Bronchoscopy Assisting

CHAPTER 20

- Updated the AARC Clinical Practice Guideline: Resuscitation and Defibrillation in the Health Care Setting 2004 Revision & Update
- Added discussion of the Combitube airway
- Added discussion of the use of end-tidal CO_2 detectors and esophageal detectors

CHAPTER 21

- Added discussion of the prevention of ventilator-associated pneumonia (VAP)
- Updated the AARC Clinical Practice Guideline: Nasotracheal Suctioning—2004 Revision and Update, Endotracheal Suctioning of Mechanically Ventilated Patients with Artificial Airways 2010
- Deleted content on the Argyle Aeroflow
- Deleted content on continuous versus intermittent suction

Former Chapter 24, Intra-Aortic Balloon Pumping, has been omitted from the fifth edition. The topic has not been incorporated into the NBRC entry-level or advanced-level examination matrices. Based on the author's clinical experience it is not a skill that the respiratory practitioner is apt to perform. IPBP is more commonly monitored and supported by nurses or cardiovascular technicians.

CHAPTER 24

- Formerly Chapter 25
- Added discussion of nasal pillows and the Total Mask™
- Added discussion of acute care ventilators

CHAPTER 25

- Formerly Chapter 26
- Updated the AARC Clinical Practice Guideline: Long-Term Invasive Mechanical Ventilation in the Home
- This chapter has been completely revamped, focusing on the differences between volume control ventilation and pressure control ventilation
- Added discussion of respiratory failure
- Added discussion of the following indications of mechanical ventilation: apnea and impending respiratory failure, acute exacerbation of COPD, acute asthma, neuromuscular disease, acute hypoxemic failure, and heart failure and cardiogenic shock
- Added discussion comparing NIV and IPPV

CHAPTER 26

- New chapter focusing on advanced modes of mechanical ventilation

CHAPTER 27

- Formerly Chapter 28

CHAPTER 28

- New chapter focusing on weaning and discontinuation of mechanical ventilation

CHAPTER 29

- Completely revised and updated chapter on neonatal and pediatric mechanical ventilation

Dedication

To my wife Carolyn, who has endured my avocation of writing for 26 of our 33 years of marriage. I would also like to acknowledge my two sons, Andrew (age 25 – Professional Pilot) and Austin (age 21 – Pharmacy Technician), who also put up with the long process of completing this edition.

Preface

Basic Clinical Lab Competencies for Respiratory Care continues to be a very popular book in respiratory care education. The integration of theoretical knowledge and psychomotor skills is unique in a text of this type. The combination has proven to be very popular and has facilitated students' learning and retention of this material. The text is more than a laboratory manual. It reinforces the rationale for therapy, typically learned in a didactic class, and applies it to the laboratory and clinical settings.

This edition continues to emphasize the important work that the American Association for Respiratory Care has undertaken with the development and publication of the Clinical Practice Guidelines. Where appropriate, these guidelines are included at the beginning of those chapters for easy reference by the students to facilitate their understanding of indications, contraindications, hazards and complications, monitoring, and outcomes assessment.

Existing chapters have been updated and revised to reflect changes in the scope of practice. The most significant changes are in the latter chapters of the text (Section IV, Ventilation). The ventilation section has been extensively revised including updates in noninvasive ventilation, pressure and volume ventilation, and advanced modes of ventilation. The neonatal pediatric ventilation chapter has been completely rewritten to reflect the common use of ventilators such as the Puritan Bennett 840, Viasys AVEA, and SERVO-i in the management of these patients. In addition, a new section on high-frequency oscillatory ventilation has been included.

The text has been divided into four major sections: Section I, Patient Assessment (Chapters 1–10); Section II: Therapeutics (Chapters 11–19); Section III: Emergency Management (Chapters 20–23); and Section IV: Ventilation (Chapters 24–29). These sections follow a logical sequence, building from simple to complex skills and tasks. The division of the text into sections also facilitates the ease of finding specific procedures related to each section.

This text is designed to provide a concise, integrated approach to laboratory and clinical instruction. Its intent is to prepare the student rapidly for entry into the clinical setting. The content provides the student with the basis required for proficient and safe practice in the clinical setting. A student who possesses a foundation in basic skills may progress very quickly in the clinical setting, focusing on problem solving and modification of therapy.

Gary C. White, MEd, RRT, RPFT

Introduction to the Text

The approach of this textbook is to integrate the theory and the psychomotor skills required to perform a therapeutic procedure safely and effectively. The theory concepts include the principles of equipment operation, troubleshooting, physiologic effects, and hazards and complications of the therapeutic modality. Only by thoroughly understanding both aspects of a therapeutic modality can the student be flexible, adapting to changes in technology and patient management.

Begin by reading the introduction to the chapter. Try to form an image in your mind, visualizing what is contained in the chapter.

Study the objectives. The objectives outline what you will be expected to know after you study the chapter. You will be held accountable for the knowledge on a written self-evaluation post test and a performance evaluation demonstrating the therapeutic modality. Refer to the objectives frequently as you study the chapter.

The American Association for Respiratory Care Clinical Practice Guidelines provide scientific evidence and expert panel consensus for the techniques and procedures employed at the bedside. The guidelines include the indications, contraindications, hazards/complications and limitations of the modality, assessment of need, monitoring, and assessment of outcomes. These guidelines provide a scientific basis and rationale for the interventions provided at the bedside. It is imperative that, as a student, you become thoroughly familiar with these guidelines, which serve as a framework of practice.

Read the theory portion of the text. If the equipment being discussed is available, keep it handy so you can refer to it as you read the text. Following the completion of the theory portion, study the theory objectives again. Ask yourself whether you understand every objective listed. If you do, take the self-evaluation post test to assess your knowledge. Review any weak areas once again.

Read the procedure portion of the text. Following completion of this section, perform the practice activities with a laboratory partner. Become familiar with all of the equipment. Understand how to set up, test, troubleshoot, and correctly apply all of the equipment discussed in the chapter.

With a laboratory partner, practice the check list for the chapter. Your partner may role-play the part of the patient while you perform the therapeutic modality. You will be expected to perform the skills on this check list during a performance evaluation conducted by your instructor. Practice the skills until they become second nature and flow smoothly from one step to the next.

Have one of your peers evaluate your skills using the performance evaluation and filling in the PEER column. When you are confident and prepared, have your instructor evaluate you.

Acknowledgments

I would like to thank all of the educators who have provided input and suggestions as to how this book could continue to be improved. Many educators have spoken to me personally, telephoned, or e-mailed me with comments, suggestions, and encouragement. The reviewers who painstakingly reviewed the fourth edition manuscript and the first draft manuscript of the fifth edition have contributed to making this book a stronger text. The reviewers are:

Diana K. Arkell, BS, RRT
Director of Clinical Education
Spokane Community College
Spokane, Washington

John L. Coldiron, BS, RRT, RCP
Program Director
American River College
Sacramento, California

Holly E. Dodds
Clinical Assistant Professor
University of Missouri—Columbia
at St. John's
St. Louis, Missouri

Marybeth Emmerth, MS, RRT, CPFT
Program Director
Wheeling Jesuit University
Wheeling, West Virginia

Marie A. Fenske, EdD, RRT
Director of Clinical Education
Gate Way Community College
Phoenix, Arizona

Lisa M. Johnson, MS, RRT-NPS
Vice Chair, Clinical Assistant
Professor
Stony Brook University
Stony Brook, New York

Lori L. Johnston, MEd, RRT
Director of Respiratory Care
Apollo College
Las Vegas, Nevada

Robert L. Joyner, PhD, RRT
Associate Professor and Chair
Salisbury University
Salisbury, Maryland

Jennifer McDaniel, RRT-NPS
Instructor
University of South Alabama
Mobile, Alabama

Michael C. McMinn, MA, RRT
Professor Emeritus
Mott Community College
Flint, Michigan

Tim Op't Holt, EdD, RRT, AE-C,
FAARC
Professor
University of South Alabama
Mobile, Alabama

Chris Russian, MEd, RRT-NPS,
RPSGT
Associate Professor
Texas State University—San Marcos
San Marcos, Texas

Edmund R. Smith, MA, RRT, RPFT
Retired Clinical Assistant Professor
St. John's Mercy Medical Center
St. Louis, Missouri

Stephen E. Swope, BA, RRT
Instructor
Idaho State University
Pocatello, Idaho

Meg Trumpp, MEd, RRT, AE-C
Program Director
Newman University
Wichita, Kansas

Mary-Rose Wiesner, BS, RRT
Director of Clinical Education
Mt. San Antonio College
Walnut, California

David Zobeck, MM, RRT, CPFT
Chair Respiratory Care Program
Lancaster General College of Nursing
and Health Science
Lancaster, Pennsylvania

I owe a special acknowledgment to the contributions made by Scott J. Mahoney, BA, RRT. Scott stepped in toward the end of this project and contributed two new chapters to the text. During 2009, illness significantly depleted my energy reserves and ability to focus on writing after my normally full teaching schedule. Scott's contribution kept this edition on track and his writing is truly remarkable. Thank you, Scott!

My wife Carolyn hasn't wavered in her support of my writing in spite of it occupying the majority of the years we have been married. Her encouragement, support, and gentle suggestions have kept me going during some very difficult times during my illness. I have a great partner in my writing and in life. Without her continued support, this edition would not have been completed.

Contributors

Scott J. Mahoney, BA, RRT
Director of Clinical Education
Seattle Central Community College
Seattle, Washington

David A. Field, RRT, RPFT
Whitman Hospital and Medical Center
Colfax, WA

Kelly P. Jones, RRT, NPS, MD
Anesthesia Associates
Spokane, WA

Stephen S. Pitts, RRT, NREMT-P
Northwest Medstar
Spokane, WA

SECTION 1
Patient Assessment

CHAPTER 1
Basics of Asepsis

INTRODUCTION

The patient who is hospitalized is at increased risk for infection. The illness or surgery that has necessitated hospitalization frequently has weakened the body's natural defense mechanisms, and the hospital setting provides the perfect setting for the growth of many "super bugs," which are resistant to standard antimicrobial agents.

Health care workers are frequently the agents for contact transmission of microorganisms between patients. There is some risk to the hospital worker as well, particularly if personal health and resistance are not carefully maintained. The respiratory practitioner may come in contact with many patients over the course of a day. It is essential for all health care workers to maintain an awareness of aseptic technique to protect themselves and the patient.

The incidence of hospital-acquired infection (HAI) is quite high. Such infections result in complications, extended hospital stays, and even death (Klevens, 2007). Through the practice of careful aseptic technique, the incidence of HAIs can be reduced.

This chapter reviews the basic principles of infection transmission and simple techniques to prevent the spread of microorganisms.

KEY TERMS

- **Airborne transmission**
- **Asepsis**
- **Contact transmission**
- **Cross-contamination**
- **Droplet transmission**
- **Fomite**
- **HEPA mask**
- **Hospital-acquired infection (HAI)**
- **Microorganism**
- **Pathogen**
- **Sterility**
- **Vector transmission**
- **Vehicle transmission**
- **Virulence**

THEORY OBJECTIVES

At the end of this chapter, the reader should be able to:

- *Define the following terms:*
  - *Asepsis*
  - *Sterility*
  - *Hospital-acquired infection (HAI)*
  - *Cross-contamination*
  - *Microorganism*
  - *Pathogen*
- *Explain the following mechanisms of microorganism transmission:*
  - *Direct contact*
  - *Airborne transmission*
  - *Droplet transmission*
  - *Vehicle transmission*
  - *Vector transmission*

- *Understand the concept and purpose of standard precautions:*
  - *Hand hygiene*
  - *Respiratory hygiene/cough etiquette*
  - *Use of personal protective equipment (PPE) such as gloves, gown, mask, eye protection, or face shield*
  - *Proper handling of equipment*
  - *Sharps precautions*
- *Explain the purpose and indication for each of the following transmission-based precautions and what procedures are required:*
  - *Contact precautions*
  - *Droplet precautions*
  - *Airborne precautions*
- *Explain what procedures may be used in the care of severely compromised patients and patients with burn injury.*

Maintaining asepsis is an essential part of the practice of respiratory care. Before learning the various techniques and skills of asepsis, it is necessary to first review some basic concepts regarding microorganisms, infection, contamination, and how microorganisms are transmitted.

Microorganisms are microscopic life forms that are present in every environment. Some of the microorganisms are beneficial and others are not. Microorganisms that are capable of causing disease in humans are termed *pathogens*. Pathogenic microorganisms vary in *virulence*, or ability to cause disease. Some are more virulent than others.

The practice of asepsis is an attitude as well as a skill. A respiratory practitioner must always remain aware of the microorganisms that exist in the environment. Transmission of microorganisms can be prevented by hand hygiene, keeping dirty equipment and supplies in plastic bags while transporting them, keeping clean and dirty equipment physically separated, and many similar practices. Only by vigilance and using aseptic techniques can the incidence of HAIs be reduced.

Asepsis

Asepsis is defined as the absence of disease-producing microorganisms. Microorganisms may include bacteria, mycoplasmas, fungi, and viruses. The concept of asepsis is generally distinguished from sterility. Total absence of disease-producing microorganisms, termed *sterility*, is difficult and expensive to sustain for a long period. Asepsis is adequate for much of the equipment and procedures in the hospital, except for so-called invasive procedures. Such procedures may adversely affect the body's natural protective defenses against infection. Respiratory care equipment is usually aseptic because it is too difficult and costly to keep sterile.

Sterility

Sterility is defined as the complete destruction of all forms of microorganisms. In the hospital environment, it is not always necessary for items to be sterile. They need only be free of pathogens, or aseptic. The operating room, however, requires sterility, owing to the invasive nature of surgery.

It is difficult to obtain and maintain sterility. Instruments or other equipment that are required to be sterile must be able to withstand the rigors of the sterilization process. Sterilization is accomplished by the use of heat or chemical agents that destroy all microorganisms.

Hospital-Acquired Infections

Hospital-acquired infection (HAI) refers to an infection a patient develops while in the hospital and did not have before hospital admission. HAIs result in countless complications, additional expenses, and deaths (Klevens, 2007).

Cross-Contamination

Cross-contamination is the transmission of microorganisms between places or persons. Pathogens can be spread from an infected patient to a noninfected patient through mutual contact with health care personnel or with clinical equipment. For example, microorganisms can build up on frequently used items such as stethoscopes. Periodic cleansing of the diaphragm and bell of the stethoscope with alcohol or other antiseptics will help to prevent cross-contamination (Cohen, 1997).

Pathogens

A *pathogen* is defined as a microorganism capable of causing disease in humans. A virulent organism is one that can produce disease very easily in many individuals. In addition to virulence, the ability of a pathogen to produce disease is dependent on the ability of the body to fight infection. Patients in the hospital are frequently infected by microorganisms not normally pathogenic to a person in good health. Many of these microorganisms are present in everyday environments but do not generally make healthy people ill because the body's defense mechanisms are adequate to prevent infection. However, these microorganisms are opportunistic; therefore, when the body's defense mechanisms are impaired due to disease processes or trauma, infection will develop.

Microorganisms may exist in great numbers in the hospital. Patients in intensive care units (ICUs) are at risk from nearly any microorganism. Burn victims, for example, have a very poor ability to resist infection; therefore, careful aseptic technique is applied such that these patients are not exposed to the potential of acquired infections. Patients receiving immunosuppressive drugs do not have the ability to resist infection and therefore are also at risk.

MICROORGANISM TRANSMISSION

Microorganisms can be transmitted in many ways. They may be transmitted by direct contact, by air currents, by vehicles, or by vectors.

Contact Transmission

Contact transmission can be divided into two subclassifications: direct contact and indirect contact transmission. Direct contact transmission occurs when microorganisms are transmitted from one person to another without an intermediate object or person. One way this can occur is by a patient's infected blood entering a respiratory practitioner's system through breaks in the skin or mucous membranes. Mucous membrane to mucous membrane contact can also result in this type of infection transmission.

Indirect contact transmission occurs when microorganisms are transmitted through an intermediate object or person. This method is the most common means of microorganism transmission and the most common cause of HAIs. Hand hygiene is an important way of minimizing this form of disease transmission. Limiting contact with potentially contaminated surfaces is also important. Do not sit on the patient's bed, lean on the bed rails, or lay a stethoscope on the bed or bedside table. Intermediate objects such as stethoscopes, otoscopes, or electronic thermometers can transmit microorganisms if not properly cleaned between patients (Siegel, 2007).

Airborne Transmission

Air currents can transport microorganisms from one area to another. Because these organisms are microscopic and very light, air currents may carry them for quite a distance. The bacterium that causes tuberculosis is commonly transmitted in this way. Patients requiring isolation should have the door closed. Laminar airflow (airflow without turbulence) in the ICU, emergency department, and surgery suite is intended to minimize *airborne transmission*.

Droplet Transmission

Droplet transmission of microorganisms is a form of contact transmission via droplets that are larger than 0.5 micrometer (μm). (This unit of measure was formerly called a micron.) Droplets of this size may be generated by coughing, sneezing, talking, or in performing procedures such as assisting with bronchoscopy, suctioning artificial airways, or changing a ventilator circuit. These droplets do not travel far or remain suspended for long; therefore, special rooms with laminar flow or negative pressure are not required. Microorganism transmission via this route is generally limited to a radius of 3 feet from the patient (Siegel, 2007).

Vehicle Transmission

Vehicle transmission is the transmission of microorganisms via inanimate objects, termed *fomites*. It may involve instruments, contaminated water or food, soil, or other objects. Vehicle transmission is important to recognize in respiratory care because some equipment may be used in the care of more than one patient. Examples of items implicated in vehicle transmission are portable respirometers, peak flowmeters, ventilators, nondisposable pulse oximeter probes, and stethoscopes.

Vector Transmission

Vector transmission is not very common in the hospital. It involves an intermediate host. The host can be an insect, an animal, or a plant. One disease transmitted in this manner is Rocky Mountain spotted fever, which is carried by a tick.

CENTERS FOR DISEASE CONTROL AND PREVENTION GUIDELINES

The Centers for Disease Control and Prevention (CDC) has revised its isolation guidelines, which are described in its publication, *Guideline for Isolation Precautions: Preventing Transmission of Infectious Agents in Healthcare Settings 2007*. The new guidelines have been divided into these major parts: *review of scientific data regarding transmission of infectious agents in health care settings, fundamental elements needed to prevent transmission of infectious agents in health care settings, and precautions to prevent transmission of infectious agents and recommendations*. These new guidelines are based on routes of transmission of microorganisms and the scientific literature.

Standard Precautions

Standard precautions combine elements of both universal precautions and body substance isolation (Siegel, 2007). Use of standard precautions is strongly recommended for all health care settings and with all patients regardless of diagnosis. Standard precautions require that the health care worker make informed decisions about the likelihood of coming into contact with moist body fluids. Based on this knowledge, the health care worker must then decide which infection control procedures are most appropriate for the immediate situation. Standard precautions include guidelines for hand hygiene; the use of gloves, mask, eye protection (or face shield), and gown; for handling of patient care equipment, patients' linens, sharps, and mask to mouth ventilation devices; and for patient placement.

Importance of Hand Hygiene

Hand hygiene includes both handwashing using soap and water and the use of alcohol-based products (foams and gels). Hand hygiene is the most important way to prevent the transmission of microorganisms via the contact route of transmission (Siegel, 2007). If one's hands are not visibly soiled, approved alcohol-based products are the preferred method for hand hygiene.

The use of alcohol-based hand hygiene products is prevalent in health care settings. When using these products, apply the product to the palm of one hand and rub the hands together, covering all surfaces of both hands and fingers, until the hands are dry. It is important that one's hands be completely dry before coming into contact with a patient or equipment following the use of these products (CDC, 2002).

The 15-second soap and water scrub is the most common hand washing protocol used in the hospital setting. It is performed between patients, before preparing medications, before and after eating, and after contact with contaminated equipment. It is also performed after use of the rest room and any other time the hands come in contact with body secretions. Even when wearing gloves, discard the gloves following patient or body fluid contact and wash the hands.

The 5-minute scrub is performed prior to surgery and before entry into specialized areas such as the newborn ICU or burn unit. It may also be required before working with particularly high-risk patients. The arms from the elbow down are scrubbed, as are the wrists and hands. In the surgery suite, sterile towels are used to dry the hands. The hands are then immediately inserted into sterile gloves.

Respiratory Hygiene/Cough Etiquette

Respiratory hygiene/cough etiquette applies to patients, visitors, and respiratory practitioners with symptoms of respiratory illness. Symptoms of a respiratory illness may include cough, rhinorrhea, or increased respiratory secretions. Respiratory hygiene/cough etiquette includes education of the facility staff, patients, and visitors; posted signage with appropriate instructions; control measures (facial tissues, masks, and appropriate disposal equipment); good hand hygiene; and physical space separation of 3 feet from the affected individual.

Cough etiquette measures include coughing into and disposal of facial tissues immediately following use. Alternatively, a surgical mask can be placed on the individual who is coughing, if tolerated. In all cases, good hand hygiene practices should be encouraged following coughing.

Personal Protective Equipment

Personal protective equipment (PPE) is a term used to describe various barrier devices to protect one's clothing, skin, or mucous membranes from contact with infectious material. PPE may include gloves, masks and goggles or face shields, gowns, and respiratory protection. The use of specific PPE devices is described below.

Use of Gloves The use of disposable gloves (latex or vinyl) is advised when procedures necessitate contact with blood, body fluids, secretions, excretions, and contaminated items. Non latex gloves, such as vinyl gloves, must be available because many patients and respiratory practitioners may have latex allergies. Gloves should also be worn before contact with mucous membranes or broken or nonintact skin. When in contact with a patient's body fluids, change gloves between tasks or procedures when working with the same patient. This measure will help to prevent the spread of microorganisms via the contact route of transmission. Prior to touching other surfaces in the room (environmental surfaces), patient care equipment, and other noncontaminated items, remove the gloves and perform hand hygiene. Always remove the gloves and properly dispose of them, performing hand hygiene between patients. For respiratory practitioners with a latex allergy, hypoallergenic gloves are available.

Use of Mask, Eye Protection, or Face Shield A health care provider who may be at risk for being splashed or sprayed by blood, body fluids, secretions, or excretions should protect his or her mouth and eyes with a mask and goggles or a face shield. The combination of a mask and eye protection (goggles with side shields) will prevent body fluids from splashing or spraying in the mouth and eyes. A face shield serves the same purpose, only it covers both the mouth and eyes as one barrier device, rather than two. In the practice of respiratory care, the risk of splashing and spraying of blood and body fluids during trauma resuscitation, airway management, ventilator circuit changes, tracheotomy care, and bronchoscopy assisting is high.

Respiratory protection is required when working with patients who are in airborne precautions. These settings require the use of National Institute for Occupational Safety and Health (NIOSH) N-95 and higher-filtration mask. These masks are individually fit tested and must be tested and certified prior to use.

Use of a Cover Gown Use of a cover gown is indicated to protect the skin and soiling of clothing during procedures or patient care situations that may produce splashes or sprays of blood, body fluids, secretions, or excretions. In some cases, a disposable paper gown is adequate for protection. Other situations (bronchoscopy assisting and trauma resuscitation) may require a waterproof gown. As soon as practicable following the procedure or patient care, properly dispose of the gown and wash the hands to prevent the spread of microorganisms via the contact transmission route.

Handling of Patient Care Equipment

Handling patient care equipment soiled with blood, body fluids, secretions, or excretions requires the same precautions as patient care situations in which the respiratory practitioner may come in contact with these secretions. The use of gloves is required, and mask/eye protection and use of a cover gown may also be required if there is a risk of splashing or spraying. All permanent equipment soiled with body fluids should be decontaminated with appropriate cleaning products prior to use in the care of another patient. All disposable equipment should be properly disposed of and handled with other contaminated waste.

Handling of Patient Linen

Linen supplies used in the care of patients that have been soiled by blood, body fluids, secretions, or excretions should be handled in a way that prevents contact with skin, mucous membranes, and clothing. This requires the use of gloves and may also require the use of a cover gown and mouth and eye protection if the linens are heavily soiled.

Sharps Precautions

The use of sharps—needles, scalpels, and other sharp instruments—requires special care and handling to prevent skin punctures following patient use. Special puncture-proof containers are provided for the disposal of these items. Do not ever attempt to recap a needle—this is the most frequent cause of needle sticks.

Do not attempt to remove discarded needles or syringes from sharps containers or attempt to force a needle or sharp instrument into an already full container. Exercising caution and common sense will prevent injury with a sharp instrument already contaminated with a patient's blood or body fluids.

Use of Mask to Mouth Ventilation Devices

Mask to mouth ventilation devices are designed to allow a rescuer to perform pulmonary resuscitation without direct contact with the patient's mucous membranes (Figure 1-1). The mask to mouth device provides a barrier between the patient and the caregiver. The availability of these devices is warranted in any area where resuscitation may be predicted or imminent.

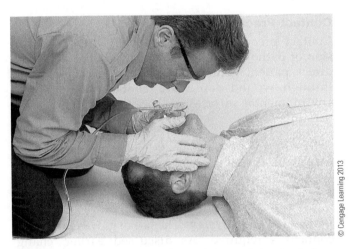

© Cengage Learning 2013

Figure 1-1 The correct use of a mask to mouth barrier device

Specific Transmission Precautions

Use of transmission precautions is recommended to address specifically the prevention of microorganism transmission via the various routes. These routes include airborne, droplet, and contact transmission. Precautions for these forms of transmission are summarized in Table 1-1.

Airborne Precautions

Airborne transmission involves microorganism transmission via small aerosolized particles of 5 μm or smaller in size. In addition to the standard precautions described previously, the following precautions are also recommended.

Patient Placement The patient should be placed in a private room with negative air pressure (relative to ambient pressure and the surrounding environment) and undergoing at least 6 to 12 air changes per hour. The door should remain closed at all times. If another patient is infected with the same microorganism and has no other infections, two patients may be placed in the same room (a practice termed *cohorting*).

This precaution is most commonly employed in the care of patients who have *Mycobacterium tuberculosis*. Other diseases placed into this category include varicella and measles.

Respiratory Protection Caregivers entering the patient's room should wear additional respiratory protection consisting of a NIOSH N-95 mask (Figure 1-2) or other respiratory filtration device approved by the Occupational Safety and Health Administration (OSHA).

TABLE 1-1: Transmission-Based Precautions			
	CONTACT	**DROPLET**	**AIRBORNE**
Private Room	Yes (cohorting is okay if patients have the same organism)	Yes (cohorting is okay if patients have the same organism)	Yes (negative pressure room with 6–12 air changes/hr)
Gloves and Gown	Gloves for patient contact; gown if anticipating becoming soiled by equipment or patient	Always glove and gown	Always glove and gown
Respiratory Precautions	None	Surgical mask	NIOSH N-95 mask
Patient Transport	Minimize and potential for contact transmission	Patient should wear a surgical mask during transport	During transport patient should wear NIOSH N-95 mask

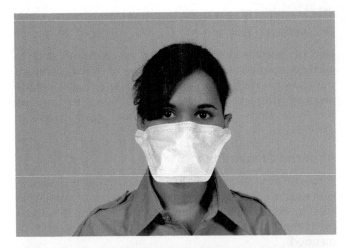

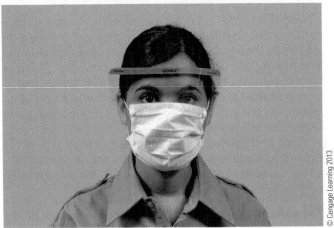

Figure 1-2 (A) A "Duckbill" N95 HEPA mask. (B) A mask and eye shield combination

Health care providers who are immune to varicella and measles may enter the hospital room without wearing HEPA protection when caring for patients infected with these conditions.

Patient Transport Avoid transporting patients who are infected with tuberculosis (TB), varicella, and measles within the hospital unless for specific essential purposes only. During transport, have the patient wear a simple surgical mask or a *HEPA mask*. This will help to prevent the transmission of droplet nuclei.

Droplet Precautions

Droplet precautions are precautions taken when transmission of microorganisms by droplets larger than 5 μm is likely. Droplets of this size can be generated by sneezing, coughing, talking, or in the performance of patient care procedures including bronchoscopy, suctioning, and ventilator circuit changes.

Patient Placement The patient should be placed in a private room. The door should remain closed at all times. If another patient is infected with the same microorganism and has no other infections, two patients may be placed in the same room (cohorting).

Respiratory Protection Caregivers who enter the patient's room should wear a mask when working within 3 feet of the patient. In some clinical facilities, all personnel who enter the patient's room may be required to wear a mask for all practical purposes, rather than strictly adhering to the 3-foot distance recommendation.

Patient Transport Avoid transporting patients who are confined with droplet precautions within the hospital unless for specific essential purposes only. During transport, have the patient wear a simple surgical mask. This is sufficient to prevent the spread of droplets.

Contact Precautions

Contact precautions are employed when transmission of pathogenic microorganisms is likely through direct patient contact. Direct contact could occur through wound care, skin contact, contact with environmental surfaces, or patient care items in the patient's room.

Patient Placement The patient should be placed in a private room. If another patient is infected with the same microorganism and has no other infections, two patients may be placed in the same room (cohorting).

Gloves and Hand Hygiene The use of gloves for patient contact is required. As discussed earlier, changing gloves between procedures on the same patient and before leaving the patient's room is required. Thorough hand washing should be performed upon entering and leaving the patient's room. The use of antimicrobial agents or a waterless antiseptic agent is advised.

Use of a Gown A cover gown is worn if clothing may have substantial contact with the patient, the patient care equipment (soiled), or other soiled environmental surfaces. The gown should be properly disposed of before leaving the patient's room.

Patient Transport Transport of the patient within the hospital should be limited to essential purposes only. During transport, exercise caution such that contact transmission is minimized to other patients or environmental surfaces.

Patient Care Equipment Permanent equipment should be dedicated to the care of patients confined by contact precautions. Avoid sharing equipment between patients. It is important to properly disinfect equipment after removing it from the patient's room and before using it for other patients.

PROFICIENCY OBJECTIVES

At the end of this chapter, the reader should be able to:

* *Demonstrate the technique used for a 5-minute hand washing protocol.*
* *Demonstrate how to glove and gown for isolation, including the following:*
  — *Wash hands.*
  — *Apply a mask, covering the mouth and nose.*
  — *Correctly apply a gown.*
  — *Demonstrate how to aseptically apply gloves.*
* *Demonstrate how to remove gloves, cap, mask, and gown when leaving isolation.*

HAND HYGIENE

As discussed in the theory portion of this chapter, hand hygiene is essential in the prevention of the transmission of microorganisms. Like other procedures in respiratory care, hand washing requires a special technique. There is a correct way to do it.

Remove Jewelry, Including Your Watch

Jewelry has small crevices that can harbor microorganisms. Sweat, dead skin, and dirt combine with a warm semimoist environment to facilitate microbial growth. Removal of jewelry and watches will allow thorough washing of the hands and wrists.

Never Contact the Sink with the Hands or Body

Moisture or water is one of the requirements for microbial growth; therefore, the sink provides an excellent area for microbial growth. In many hospitals, a variety of bacteria may be cultured from the sinks on a regular basis. *Pseudomonas aeruginosa* is a common microorganism found in the vicinity of sinks (Bert, 1998). Transmission may result from contact with hands or clothing. *P. aeruginosa* may be a virulent pathogen for debilitated patients in ICUs.

Adjust the Water Flow and Temperature

Adjust the water flow and temperature prior to actually washing the hands. Warm or cold water is better than hot water. Hot water is not hot enough to kill pathogens anyway and tends to open the pores of the skin, facilitating removal of the skin's oil. Use of hot water leads to chapped skin much more quickly than use of warm or cool water. Chapped skin, which cracks, allows for bacterial growth and infection. Adjust the flow so that it is brisk but not strong enough to cause splashing.

Wet Forearms, Wrists, and Hands

Hold the hands under the running water with the forearms more elevated than the fingertips. The fingers are considered to be the most contaminated, whereas the arms are less contaminated. Water should flow from the clean to the dirty area.

Liberally Apply Soap

Always use liquid soap from the dispenser. Special disinfectant soap is provided in the hospital. The exception is in specialty areas, such as the newborn ICU or a surgical suite, where individual disposable scrub pads are used. Never use bar soap, particularly if it is sitting in a puddle of water. Bar soap may harbor microorganisms.

Wash Palms with Strong Friction

Soap, friction, and running water are the keys to removal of microorganisms. Begin by rubbing the palms and backs of the hands, thoroughly cleaning the area.

Wash between the Fingers

Fingers may be washed individually or may be interlaced, creating sufficient friction. Be sure to clean the interdigital spaces and the knuckles.

Wash the Wrists with a Rotary Motion

The rotary motion ensures thorough cleansing due to friction.

Scrub under the Nails and around the Cuticles

Ideally, nails should be kept short and free of polish to facilitate thorough cleansing. Respiratory practitioners wearing artificial nails are more likely to harbor gram-negative pathogens; therefore, the use of artificial nails is not recommended (CDC, 2002). The nails and nailbeds provide another good environment for microbial growth. Use a nail brush to completely clean under the fingernails. The same instrument may be gently applied to the cuticle area.

Rinse Hands without Touching the Sink

Rinse the hands using the same technique used when first wetting them.

Obtain Towels Aseptically

Carefully remove the disposable paper towels from the dispenser without contacting it with the hands. Most hospital dispensers are designed so that aseptic removal is possible.

Dry Hands Using Separate Towels

Dry hands from the wrist or forearm toward the fingertips. Use a clean towel for each hand.

Turn Off the Water with a Clean, Dry Towel

Use a clean, dry towel to handle the faucet when turning off the water flow. Obtain several more towels and aseptically clean up any splashes in the vicinity.

ASEPTIC GOWNING

Gowning may be required before entering certain isolation situations. It is important to know how to apply and remove isolation clothing. Isolation attire should not be worn anywhere other than in the patient's room. Be sure to assemble all needed supplies before preparing to enter the room.

Application of a Mask

Apply the mask over the nose and mouth with the strap behind the neck. If an adjustable bridge piece is provided, adjust it to the contours of the nose by pinching the mask.

Once the mask becomes saturated with moisture from exhaled air, it is no longer effective and should be changed. Never reuse a mask.

Application of the Gown

Begin by grasping the gown by the neck and unrolling or unfolding it at arm's length or by removing it from its hanger or hook. Insert your hands into the sleeves and pull them through the cuffs without contacting the outside of the gown (Figure 1-3).

Fasten the tie at the neck. Use a bow knot to facilitate the removal of the gown later.

Close the gown completely in the back and fasten the waist tie (Figure 1-4). Again, the use of a bow knot will simplify removal later. The back is considered dirty as well as those areas below the waist.

ASEPTIC APPLICATION OF GLOVES

Examination gloves may be used for routine patient care. Choose the appropriate size (S, M, or L) and aseptically apply gloves to both hands. Use of the incorrect size will reduce dexterity or increase the risk of glove breakage or rupture.

ASEPTIC REMOVAL OF ISOLATION ATTIRE

Aseptic removal of isolation attire is just as important as aseptic application. The clothing may be removed inside or outside the room, depending on

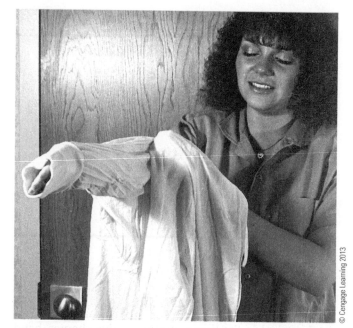

Figure 1-3 Applying an isolation gown

© Cengage Learning 2013

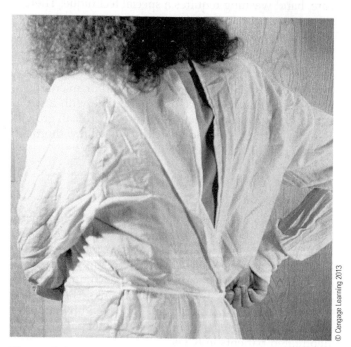

Figure 1-4 Closing the waist of an isolation gown

© Cengage Learning 2013

the type of isolation. Strict and contact isolation necessitates the removal of the attire inside of the patient's room. If removal is done improperly, contact transmission is possible. Used isolation attire should not be reused.

Remove Gloves

Gloves are easily removed by grasping the cuff and turning them inside out. Do not touch the skin when

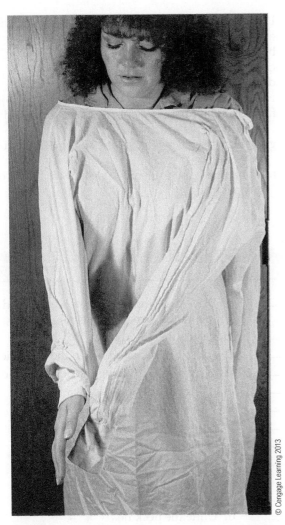

removing gloves. The second glove may be removed over the first, and then both may be discarded together.

Remove Mask

The mask is removed next (unless droplet or airborne precautions are in effect). Remove the mask without touching the hair or face with the hands.

Remove the Gown

Begin by untying the waist tie. Following this, wash the hands. The area from the waist down is considered dirty.

Untie the neck tie and shrug the shoulders forward so that the gown slips off the body down the arms. Insert one index finger between the cuff and wrist and pull the hand inside the sleeve. With the hand inside the one sleeve, remove the other sleeve (Figure 1-5).

Allow the gown to slip down so that it can be grasped inside at the neck of the gown. Fold the gown inside out and dispose of it appropriately.

Hand Hygiene

Wash the hands inside the room for 15 seconds before leaving. Outside of the room, wash the hands for 3 minutes before seeing other patients. Alternatively, if hands are not soiled, alcohol-based hand sanitizers may be used.

Figure 1-5 Removing an isolation gown aseptically

© Cengage Learning 2013

References

Bert, F. (1998). Multi-resistant *Pseudomonas aeruginosa* outbreak associated with contaminated tap water in a neurosurgery intensive care unit. *Journal of Hospital Infection, 39*(1), 53–62.

Centers for Disease Control and Prevention (CDC). (2002). Guideline for hand hygiene in health-care settings. *Morbidity and Mortality Weekly Report, 51*(RR-16).

Cohen, H. A. (1997). Stethoscopes and otoscopes—a potential vector of infection? *Family Practice, 14*(6), 446–449.

Klevens, R. M. (2007). Infections and deaths in U.S. hospitals 2002. *Public Health Reports, 122*(2).

Siegel, J. (2007). *Guidelines for isolation precautions: Preventing transmission of infectious agents in healthcare settings.* Atlanta, GA: Centers for Disease Control and Prevention.

Practice Activities: Basics of Asepsis

1. Practice washing your hands for the 5-minute scrub.
   Include the following in your practice:
   a. Remove jewelry and watch.
   b. Adjust the water flow and temperature.
   c. Wet the forearms and hands.
   d. Apply soap liberally.
   e. Wash the following with strong friction:
      (1) Palms
      (2) Between the digits
      (3) Under the fingernails and around the cuticles
   f. Wash for the appropriate length of time.
   g. Never touch the sink with your hands or body.
   h. Rinse from the forearm to the fingertips.
   i. Obtain towels aseptically.
   j. Dry hands individually using separate towels.
   k. Turn off the water using a clean, dry towel.

2. Practice applying and removing a mask, a gown, and gloves. Include the following in your practice:
   a. Wash your hands.
   b. Apply a mask, covering your nose and mouth.
   c. Apply the gown.
      (1) Pick it up by the neck.
      (2) Place the hands inside the sleeves and slip the hands through the cuffs.
      (3) Fasten the neck tie.
      (4) Close the back and fasten the waist tie.
   d. Aseptically apply examination gloves.
      (1) Choose the correct size.
      (2) Aseptically apply the gloves to both hands.

3. Practice removing the isolation attire aseptically:
   a. Remove the gloves aseptically.
   b. Remove the mask.
   c. Untie the waist tie on the gown.
   d. Untie the neck tie of the gown.
   e. Slip the gown off your shoulders.
   f. Slip a finger between cuff and your wrist and pull the sleeve partially off.
   g. Using the sleeve as protection, pull the other sleeve off.
   h. Fold the gown inside out and dispose of it properly.

Check List: Basics of Asepsis

Hand washing

_____ 1. Remove jewelry and watch.
_____ 2. Adjust the water flow and temperature.
_____ 3. Wet the forearms and hands.
_____ 4. Apply disinfectant soap liberally.
_____ 5. Wash the following with strong friction:
_____   a. Palms
_____   b. Between the digits
_____   c. Under the fingernails and around the cuticles
_____ 6. Wash for the appropriate length of time.
_____ 7. Never touch the sink with the hands or body.
_____ 8. Rinse from the forearm to the fingertips.
_____ 9. Obtain towels aseptically.
_____ 10. Dry hands individually using separate towels.
_____ 11. Turn off the water using a clean, dry towel.

Isolation Procedures

_____ 1. Perform hand hygiene.
_____ 2. Apply the gown:
_____   a. Pick it up by the neck.
_____   b. Place the hands inside the sleeves and slip the hands through the cuffs.
_____   c. Fasten the neck tie.
_____   d. Close the back and fasten the waist tie.
_____ 3. Apply a mask, covering the nose and mouth.
_____ 4. Apply the gloves aseptically:
_____   a. Choose the correct size.
_____   b. Apply the gloves aseptically.
_____ 5. Remove the isolation attire aseptically:
_____   a. Remove the gloves aseptically.
_____   b. Remove the cap and mask.
_____   c. Untie the waist tie on the gown.
_____   d. Untie the neck tie.
_____   e. Slip the gown off the shoulders.
_____   f. Slip a finger between the cuff and wrist and pull the sleeve partially off.
_____   g. Using the sleeve as protection, pull the other sleeve off.
_____   h. Fold the gown inside out and dispose of it properly.
_____ 6. Perform hand hygiene before leaving the room.
_____ 7. Perform hand hygiene again after leaving the room.

Self-Evaluation Post Test: Basics of Asepsis

1. Asepsis is defined as:
   a. the absence of all living things.
   b. the absence of disease-producing microorganisms.
   c. the absence of all forms of microorganisms.
   d. the absence of viruses.

2. Sterility is defined as:
   a. the absence of all living things.
   b. the absence of disease-producing microorganisms.
   c. the absence of all forms of microorganisms.
   d. the absence of viruses.

3. A disease may be transmitted from one patient to another by a health care practitioner. This mode of disease spread is termed:
   a. septic.
   b. contamination.
   c. vector transmission.
   d. cross-contamination.

4. A microorganism capable of producing disease in humans is termed a(n):
   a. bacterium.
   b. virus.
   c. pathogen.
   d. infection.

5. Hospital-acquired infections are _____ infections.
   a. community-acquired
   b. hospital-acquired post hospital admission
   c. nasally introduced
   d. medication-related

6. Airborne transmission precautions include which of the following?
   I.   Donning a NIOSH N-95 mask on entering the room
   II. Placement of the patient in a private room with negative pressure or laminar airflow
   III. Use of gloves
   IV. Hand washing before entering and after leaving the patient's room

   a. I
   b. I, II
   c. I, II, III
   d. I, II, III, IV

7. Microorganism transmission may occur by:
   I.   contact transmission.
   II. airborne transmission.
   III. droplet transmission.

   a. I only
   b. II only
   c. I, II only
   d. I, II, and III only

8. When working with nonisolated patients, you should wash your hands for _____ between patients.
   a. 30 seconds
   b. 1 minute
   c. 2 minutes
   d. 3 minutes

9. Standard precautions should be employed:
   a. for all health care providers working with patients.
   b. only when you are touching the patient.
   c. only by a nurse who remains in the room for extended periods.
   d. by the respiratory practitioner.

10. Droplet transmission requires:
    I.   a private room for the patient.
    II. use of a filter mask for working within 3 feet of the patient.
    II. use of gloves
    IV. use of a protective gown if soiling of clothing is likely.

    a. I
    b. I, II
    c. I, II, III
    d. I, II, III, IV

PERFORMANCE EVALUATION:
Hand washing

Date: Lab _____ Clinical _____ Agency _____

Lab: Pass _____ Fail _____ Clinical: Pass _____ Fail _____

Student name _____ Instructor name _____

No. of times observed in clinical _____

No. of times practiced in clinical _____

PASSING CRITERIA: Obtain 90% or better on the procedure. Tasks indicated by * must receive at least 1 point, or the evaluation is terminated. Procedure must be performed within the designated time, or the performance receives a failing grade.

SCORING: 2 points — Task performed satisfactorily without prompting.
1 point — Task performed satisfactorily with self-initiated correction.
0 points — Task performed incorrectly or with prompting required.
NA — Task not applicable to the patient care situation.

Tasks:	Peer	Lab	Clinical
* 1. Removes jewelry and watch	☐	☐	☐
* 2. Does not contact the sink with clothing or the body	☐	☐	☐
3. Adjusts the water flow and temperature	☐	☐	☐
4. Wets the forearms and hands thoroughly	☐	☐	☐
* 5. Applies soap liberally	☐	☐	☐
6. Washes the hands with strong friction			
* a. Palms	☐	☐	☐
* b. Wrists	☐	☐	☐
* c. Between the fingers	☐	☐	☐
* d. Under the nails and around the cuticles	☐	☐	☐
* 7. Washes for the appropriate length of time	☐	☐	☐
* 8. Does not touch the faucets, sides, or bottom of the sink with the hands or fingers	☐	☐	☐
* 9. Rinses thoroughly from the wrists to the fingertips	☐	☐	☐
* 10. Obtains paper towels without contaminating the hands	☐	☐	☐
* 11. Dries the hands and wrists thoroughly using a separate towel for each, drying from the wrists to the fingertips	☐	☐	☐
* 12. Turns off the water with a clean, dry paper towel	☐	☐	☐

SCORE: Peer   _____ points of possible 30; _____%

            Lab   _____ points of possible 30; _____%

            Clinical _____ points of possible 30; _____%

TIME: _____ out of possible 5 minutes

STUDENT SIGNATURES   **INSTRUCTOR SIGNATURES**

PEER: _____   LAB: _____

STUDENT: _____   CLINICAL: _____

PERFORMANCE EVALUATION:
Isolation Procedures

Date: Lab _____ Clinical _____ Agency _____

Lab: Pass _____ Fail _____ Clinical: Pass _____ Fail _____

Student name _____ Instructor name _____

No. of times observed in clinical _____

No. of times practiced in clinical _____

PASSING CRITERIA: Obtain 90% or better on the procedure. Tasks indicated by * must receive at least 1 point, or the evaluation is terminated. Procedure must be performed within the designated time, or the performance receives a failing grade.

SCORING: 2 points — Task performed satisfactorily without prompting.
1 point — Task performed satisfactorily with self-initiated correction.
0 points — Task performed incorrectly or with prompting required.
NA — Task not applicable to the patient care situation.

Tasks:	Peer	Lab	Clinical
* 1. Obtains the appropriate apparel	☐	☐	☐
2. Performs hand hygiene	☐	☐	☐
3. Aseptically applies the gown			
a. Picks up the gown at the neck	☐	☐	☐
b. Places the hands inside the sleeves, working the hands through the cuffs	☐	☐	☐
c. Fastens the ties at the neck	☐	☐	☐
d. Closes the gown in the back, tying the waist ties	☐	☐	☐
* 4. Applies the mask and cap, covering the hair	☐	☐	☐
5. Aseptically applies the gloves			
* a. Selects the correct size	☐	☐	☐
* b. Aseptically applies the gloves	☐	☐	☐
6. Removes the isolation attire before leaving			
* a. Removes the gloves, turning them inside out	☐	☐	☐
* b. Removes the cap and mask	☐	☐	☐
c. Removes the gown by			
(1) Untying the neck	☐	☐	☐
(2) Pulling one sleeve off by reaching inside the cuff with a finger	☐	☐	☐
(3) Using one hand inside the sleeve to pull off the second sleeve	☐	☐	☐

(4) Folding the gown inside out   ☐   ☐   ☐

(5) Disposing of the gown appropriately   ☐   ☐   ☐

* **7.** Performs hand hygiene before leaving the room   ☐   ☐   ☐

* **8.** Performs hand hygiene again outside the room   ☐   ☐   ☐

SCORE: Peer _____ points of possible 32; _____%

                    Lab _____ points of possible 32; _____%

                    Clinical _____ points of possible 32; _____%

TIME: _____ out of possible 5 minutes

STUDENT SIGNATURES   **INSTRUCTOR SIGNATURES**

PEER: _____   LAB: _____

STUDENT: _____   CLINICAL: _____

CHAPTER 2

Basic Patient Assessment: Vital Signs and Breath Sounds

INTRODUCTION

Basic patient assessment is an important aspect of respiratory care. The basic assessment skills—taking vital signs and auscultating breath sounds—provide clinical means for the examination and diagnosis of the patient. Frequently, these skills are used to measure the effects of medication or therapy being administered.

This chapter discusses the significance of the various vital signs and how to measure them, normals, and causes of abnormal findings. The theory of sound, the construction and use of the stethoscope, the various breath sounds and how they are produced, and how to auscultate the chest in a systematic way are also covered.

KEY TERMS

- **Abnormal breath sounds**
- **Apnea**
- **Auscultation**
- **Bradycardia**
- **Bradypnea**

- **Diastolic**
- **Hypertension**
- **Hyperthermia**
- **Hypotension**
- **Hypothermia**

- **Normal breath sounds**
- **Systolic**
- **Tachycardia**
- **Tachypnea**

THEORY OBJECTIVES

At the end of this chapter, the reader should be able to:

Vital Signs

- *Explain the significance of measuring body temperature.*
- *State the normal temperature range, in degrees Fahrenheit and Celsius, for adults and for children.*
- *List the causes of an abnormal body temperature.*
- *Explain the significance of the pulse and give the normal range for adults and for children.*
- *List the causes of an abnormal pulse.*
- *Explain what is meant by rhythm and strength of the pulse.*
- *Describe the significance of the respiratory rate and give the normal rate for adults and for children.*
- *Explain what is meant by the terms* tachypnea *and* bradypnea.
- *Describe the various factors that influence blood pressure:*
  - *Pumping action of the heart*
  - *Resistance in the cardiovascular system*
  - *Elasticity of the vessel walls*
  - *Viscosity of the blood*

- *Describe what is meant by the terms* systolic blood pressure *and* diastolic blood pressure.
- *State the normal ranges for blood pressure.*
- *List the following causes of abnormal blood pressure:*
  - *Hypertension*
  - *Cardiovascular disorders*
  - *Hormonal imbalance*
  - *Exercise*
  - *Stimulants*
  - *Emotional stress*
  - *Hypotension*
  - *Shock*
  - *Hormonal imbalance*
  - *Depressants*

Sound Generation

- *Define sound and identify its characteristics and physical properties.*
- *Explain how density affects sound conduction and transmission.*

Stethoscopes

- *Identify the two most common types of stethoscopes and their advantages and disadvantages:*
  - *Sprague-Rappaport stethoscope*
  - *Single tube stethoscope*
- *Discuss the importance of proper earpiece fit when using the stethoscope.*

Breath Sounds

- *Identify the following four major classifications of normal breath sounds and their characteristics, location, and relevant theory of sound production.*
  - *Vesicular*
  - *Bronchial*
  - *Bronchovesicular*
  - *Tracheal*

- *Discuss the importance of a systematic method of auscultating the chest.*
- *Describe and identify the anatomical landmarks used in auscultating the chest.*
- *Explain the importance of proper patient positioning for auscultation and under what circumstances the optimal positioning may be modified.*
- *For the following abnormal breath sounds, describe their characteristics, duration, and relevant theory of sound production:*
  - *Crackles*
  - *Wheezes*
  - *Rhonchi*
  - *Pleural rub*

BODY TEMPERATURE

The body, when in a normal state of balance between heat production and heat loss, is often referred to as being homeostatic. The normal metabolic heat-producing process is controlled primarily by the hypothalamus in the brain. The hypothalamus, when regulating temperature by controlling the sympathetic nervous system, causes vasoconstriction or dilation, sweating, shivering, and the production of epinephrine and norepinephrine.

The normal temperature range for adults is 96 to 99.5°F, equivalent to 35.5 to 37.5°C. The normal values for both temperature scales are 98.6°F and 37°C, respectively.

Children have a slightly faster metabolic rate than adults, causing their temperature to be slightly higher. The temperature in a newborn ranges from 36.1 to 37.7°C, or 97 to 99.9°F. A newborn's temperature regulation mechanism is not fully developed, allowing the temperature to fluctuate in response to the environment more than in an adult. A normal temperature of a 2-year-old should be about 37.2°C, or 98.9°F. A child's temperature will not be fully regulated until puberty, at which time it will be the same as an adult's.

Abnormal Body Temperature

An abnormally low body temperature is termed *hypothermia* and an abnormally high body temperature is termed *hyperthermia*. Abnormalities in body temperature may be caused by many different factors. Table 2-1 lists some of the causes of an abnormal body temperature.

PULSE

The pulse is a direct indicator of the heart's actions. The pulse rate is an indication of the heart rate. The pulse rhythm is an indicator of the heart's rhythm, and its contour reflects the characteristics of the heart ejecting blood, blood pressure, and the presence of aortic stenosis.

The normal heart rate for adults ranges from 60 to 90 beats per minute. Children's pulses range from 90 to 120 beats per minute.

Abnormal Heart Rates

An abnormally low heart rate is termed *bradycardia* and an abnormally high heart rate is termed *tachycardia*. Several disorders or conditions may cause an abnormal heart rate. Table 2-2 is a partial listing of the causes of bradycardia and tachycardia.

Rhythm

The rhythm is the regularity of the heartbeat. Normally, the heartbeat is regular and rhythmic. Abnormalities in the rhythm may result from cardiac arrhythmias or changes in the vascular system affecting blood flow.

Two types of altered pulse rhythms are a bounding pulse and a plateau pulse. With a bounding pulse, there are both a rapid upstroke and a rapid downstroke, with a maximum point of intensity between them (Figure 2-1). This may be caused by an abnormally high blood pressure (hypertension) or exercise.

TABLE 2-1: Causes of an Abnormal Body Temperature

CONDITION	CAUSES
Hypothermia	Exposure Increased heat loss Diaphoresis (excessive sweating) Blood loss Hypothalamus injury Hormonal imbalance
Hyperthermia	Increased environmental temperature Decreased heat loss (heavy clothing) Drug or medication reaction Hormonal imbalance Infection/illness

TABLE 2-2: Causes of Bradycardia and Tachycardia

CONDITION	CAUSES
Bradycardia	Hypothermia
	Vagal stimulation
	Heart abnormalities
	Depressant drugs
Tachycardia	Hypoxemia (decreased oxygen
	in blood)
	Fever
	Emotional stress
	Heart abnormalities
	Blood volume loss

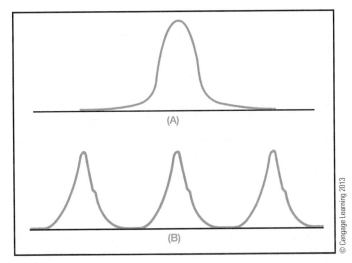

© Cengage Learning 2013

Figure 2-1 (A) A graph of a normal pulse contour. (B) A graph illustrating a bounding pulse contour

With a plateau pulse, there are both a gradual upstroke and a gradual downstroke, as illustrated in Figure 2-2. This may be caused by aortic stenosis, which is a narrowing of the aorta that causes a decrease in blood flow.

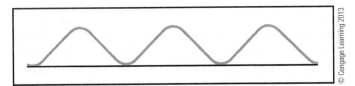

© Cengage Learning 2013

Figure 2-2 A graph illustrating a plateau pulse

RESPIRATORY RATE

The respiratory rate is the number of breaths taken by a patient in a 1-minute time interval. The respiratory rate normally varies depending on physical condition and level of activity. The normal rate for adults is between 12 and 20 and for children between 20 and 40 per minute.

It is important to determine rate as well as depth (volume of air inspired, indicated by chest wall excursion), pattern, and rhythm of respirations. Irregularities of rhythm and pattern are discussed in Chapter 3, Advanced Patient Assessment. A patient's ability to oxygenate the blood adequately may diminish when the depth becomes too shallow. This may result from the effects of depressant drugs or anxiety from pain.

Tachypnea and Bradypnea

Tachypnea and *bradypnea* refer to abnormalities in respiratory rate. *Tachypnea* is a faster than normal respiratory rate. Tachypnea can result from anxiety, exercise, fever, and hypoxemia. Frequently, tachypnea is observed as a sign of impending respiratory failure. *Bradypnea* is a lower than normal respiratory rate. Bradypnea may be caused by certain pharmacologic agents (narcotics), head injuries, or hypothermia. *Apnea* is the absence or cessation of breathing. Apnea may be caused by impaired nervous transmission from the central nervous system (injury, ischemia, or hemorrhage) or administration of drugs that block neurotransmission.

BLOOD PRESSURE

Blood pressure is the measurement of the pressure within the arterial system. Several factors influence blood pressure. These include the pumping action of the heart, resistance in the cardiovascular system, elasticity of the vessel walls, blood volume, and the viscosity of the blood.

Systolic and Diastolic Pressures

The *systolic* pressure is the pressure measured at the time the ventricles are contracting. During this period, the arteries momentarily expand to accommodate the increase in pressure from the blood volume ejected by the heart.

The *diastolic* pressure is the pressure in the arterial system when the ventricles are at rest. During this period, the aortic valve closes, causing a wave of pressure throughout the arterial system. This wave propels the blood through the arterial system. The diastolic pressure is the lowest pressure to which the arterial system and heart are subjected.

Normal Ranges

The normal range for blood pressure in adults is 90/60 to 140/90 mm Hg. The fractional representation is the systolic pressure over the diastolic pressure. Range in children will vary depending on the child's age. A neonate may have a blood pressure of 60/30 to 90/60 mm Hg. As the child becomes older, the blood pressure increases until it is equal to an adult's.

Abnormal Blood Pressure

An abnormally low blood pressure is termed *hypotension*, and an abnormally high blood pressure is termed *hypertension*. Many factors may cause a lowered or elevated blood pressure. Table 2-3 is a partial listing of some of the common causes of hypertension and hypotension.

TABLE 2-3: Causes of Hypotension and Hypertension

CAUSES	CONDITION
Hypotension	Shock
	Hormonal imbalances
	Depressant drugs
	Postural (positioning)
	Fluid loss
Hypertension	Cardiovascular imbalances
	Hormonal imbalances
	Exercise
	Stimulant drugs
	Emotional stress
	Renal failure/fluid retention

SOUND

Sound is produced by vibrations that alternately compress air into a waveform. The waveform enters the ear and causes the tympanic membrane (eardrum) to vibrate. The inner ear then conducts and converts these vibrations to nervous impulses, which we perceive as sound.

If waveforms could be perceived visually, they would be similar to the wave action observed in a pond. If a small object is dropped into a body of still water, it produces waves or ripples on the surface radiating from the point of impact. Sound waves travel in a similar way, radiating through the air in all directions from the source.

Sound has three main characteristics or properties: frequency, amplitude, and duration. Figure 2-3 illustrates these three properties using a graphic format.

A low-pitched sound is low in frequency, and a high-pitched sound is higher in frequency. Human hearing detects sounds with frequencies ranging roughly from 16 to 16,000 hertz (Hz), or vibrations per second. Although human hearing has a broad frequency range, acute hearing has a more narrow frequency band ranging from 1000 to 2000 Hz.

The amplitude of a sound wave determines its intensity. The greater the amplitude, the higher the intensity of the sound wave. If a guitarist were to pluck a string on

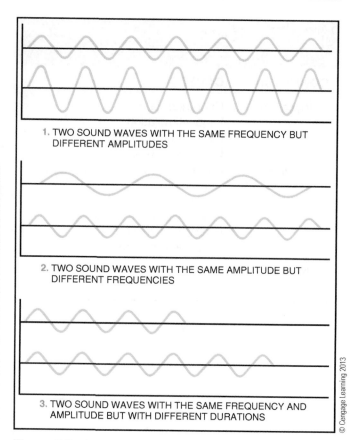

1. TWO SOUND WAVES WITH THE SAME FREQUENCY BUT DIFFERENT AMPLITUDES

2. TWO SOUND WAVES WITH THE SAME AMPLITUDE BUT DIFFERENT FREQUENCIES

3. TWO SOUND WAVES WITH THE SAME FREQUENCY AND AMPLITUDE BUT WITH DIFFERENT DURATIONS

© Cengage Learning 2013

Figure 2-3   A graph representing the properties of sound: (1) amplitude, (2) frequency, and (3) duration

an electric guitar and simultaneously increase the volume on the amplifier, the frequency would remain relatively constant while the amplitude or intensity would increase dramatically.

Duration relates to the length of time a sound continues. A sound of long duration is perceived for a longer period than one of short duration.

The Effects of Density on Sound Production and Conduction

Sound vibrations may be conducted through mediums other than air, such as solid matter or fluid. The nature of the medium may affect the distance over which a sound can be carried. The denser a material is, the more easily it can conduct sound vibrations. This concept is important from a physiologic standpoint. In our bodies, sound produced in the lungs is conducted through tissue, bone, fluid, and air. All of these structures and materials have different properties and densities. Furthermore, some disease states cause a change in the tissue density, further increasing the conduction of sound or transmitting sounds not normally heard from one location to another. *Auscultation* (listening for sounds) allows detection of changes that may indicate disease states.

STETHOSCOPES

Since its invention in 1816 the stethoscope has remained essentially the same with just a few changes and refinements. With the advances in technology, stethoscope design has been improved, resulting in greater performance, comfort, and convenience.

Parts of the Stethoscope

There are several parts that make up a stethoscope. All parts must be functioning properly for the instrument to perform well.

The chest piece is one of the more critical elements of the stethoscope. The chest piece may consist of a diaphragm, a bell, or a diaphragm-bell combination. The diaphragm is usually made from a thin semirigid polymer and has a relatively large surface area with a diameter of approximately 2 inches. The diaphragm allows the transmission of high-pitched sounds and filters out the low-pitched sounds. The diaphragm is most suited to listening to breath sounds. In general, as the diameter of the diaphragm increases, sound transmission will be improved due to increased surface area. The bell chest piece is smaller in diameter than the diaphragm and conical in shape. The bell filters high-frequency sounds and allows the transmission of low-frequency sounds. The bell is most suited to listening to heart tones and other low-pitched sounds.

The chest piece is connected to the binaurals, or earpieces, by one or two short pieces of tubing. Shorter tubing is preferred for better transmission or passage of the sounds free of artifact. Longer tubing tends to pick up external sounds and also has the tendency to rub or bump into bed frames or other objects, creating further distractions and artifact. A stethoscope with thicker tubing will generally have the best frequency response with the least amount of artifact transmission.

The binaurals should fit comfortably into the ear canals and be canted anteriorly, matching the angle of the ear canal. The binaurals should point forward toward the clavicles when inserted into the ear canals correctly. It is often helpful to have a lab partner or other clinician help fit the stethoscope precisely to the angle of the auditory canals. The earpieces must be comfortable and yet seal the canal well. Comfort is very important in reducing fatigue and allowing the maximum attenuation (lessening) of unwanted sounds.

Several major types of stethoscopes are available. Each type has its limitations and advantages for clinical use. The two common types of stethoscopes are the single tube stethoscope and the Sprague-Rappaport stethoscope.

Single Tube Stethoscope

The single tube stethoscope consists of a diaphragm or diaphragm-bell combination chest piece attached to the binaurals with a single flexible tube. Figure 2-4 shows examples of several good-quality stethoscopes. A single tube stethoscope can be a very satisfactory instrument for the respiratory practitioner. It is important to purchase the highest-quality stethoscope that is affordable.

One indicator of quality is the thickness of the tubing wall. The thicker the wall, the better it will attenuate sounds not produced by the diaphragm or bell. Stethoscopes having thin wall tubing tend to pick up sounds from the room more easily (Callahan, 2007).

The advantages of this stethoscope are its size and easy portability. Having only one piece of connecting tubing, it can easily be coiled and stuffed into a lab coat pocket.

Sprague-Rappaport Stethoscope

A Sprague-Rappaport stethoscope consists of a bell-diaphragm or diaphragm-diaphragm chest piece attached directly to the binaurals by two pieces of flexible tubing. Figure 2-5 shows a medium-quality Sprague-Rappaport stethoscope.

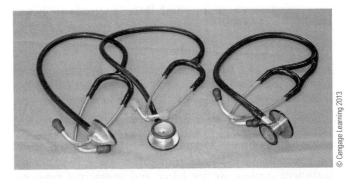

© Cengage Learning 2013

Figure 2-4   Several examples of quality single tube stethoscopes

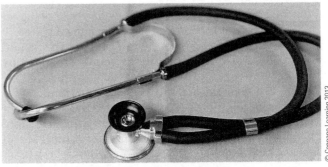

© Cengage Learning 2013

Figure 2-5   A Sprague-Rappaport stethoscope

The construction of this stethoscope is generally of more durable materials; therefore, it tends to survive the rigors of clinical practice a little better. It is also larger and a little more awkward to carry easily in the pocket compared with the single tube stethoscope.

BREATH SOUNDS

The sounds heard upon auscultating the chest have been described and classified into normal and abnormal sounds. Various descriptive terms have evolved over the years since these sounds were first described by Läennec. In the clinical setting, physicians may describe sounds using any of numerous descriptive terms or classification systems.

In recent years, the American Thoracic Society (ATS) has recommended a descriptive system to standardize the way breath sounds are described. In this chapter, the ATS system is used in the description of breath sounds.

Normal Breath Sounds

Normal breath sounds have been divided into four major classifications: vesicular, bronchial, bronchovesicular, and tracheal. Each sound has unique characteristics, and a different mechanism of sound production has been theorized for each type. Normal sounds may be heard over specific areas of the chest. If these sounds are heard elsewhere, they are then classified as abnormal.

Vesicular Breath Sounds

Vesicular breath sounds are relatively low-pitched soft sounds. They have been described as whispering or rustling in nature. The inspiratory phase is longer in duration than the expiratory phase. There is no pause between inspiration and expiration. This sound is heard over the majority of the lung periphery except over the right apex anteriorly.

Vesicular sounds are thought to be generated by turbulent airflow in the lobar and segmental bronchi. It has been theorized that the turbulent flow generates vibration in these anatomical structures, resulting in the production of sound.

Bronchial Breath Sounds

Bronchial breath sounds are loud and generally of higher pitch. The expiratory phase is longer than the inspiratory phase with a short pause between phases. This sound is often described as similar to the sound generated by blowing through a tube. It is normally heard over the upper portion of the sternum, or the manubrium.

This sound is thought to be generated by turbulent air vibrating in the trachea and right and left mainstem bronchi. This vibration ultimately produces an audible sound that can be heard when using a stethoscope.

Bronchovesicular Breath Sounds

As the name suggests, bronchovesicular sounds are characterized by the combination of bronchial and vesicular sounds. They are somewhat muted, without a pause between inspiration and expiration. The inspiratory and expiratory phases are roughly equal in length. These sounds are normally heard over the sternum at around the second intercostal space, between the scapulae and over the right apex of the lung.

Sound production is again thought to arise from turbulent airflow.

Tracheal Breath Sounds

As the name implies, tracheal sounds are characteristically heard over the trachea. Above the clavicular notch, they are very harsh and quite high pitched, with the expiratory phase lasting a little longer than the inspiratory phase.

Tracheal sounds are produced by the high-velocity, turbulent air as it passes through the trachea.

Abnormal Breath Sounds

Abnormal breath sounds are often referred to as *adventitious sounds*. Keep in mind, though, that normal breath sounds heard in an uncharacteristic location are also abnormal. The transmission of normal sounds to remote areas may be a result of consolidation or other changes affecting the transmission of that sound.

The ATS has recommended that adventitious sounds be classified as crackles, wheezes, rhonchi, and rubs.

Crackles

Crackles are abnormal sounds described as coarse or fine. The quantity (few or many) can also be noted. The phase in which such sounds occur—inspiratory or expiratory—should be indicated. It is also important to describe the location on the chest where crackles are heard. These may be almost anywhere. This finding might be charted as "coarse inspiratory crackles heard over the right middle lobe."

These sounds are thought to be produced by the sudden opening of alveoli or sections of the lung. The resultant sudden change in pressure generates the sound.

Wheezes

Wheezes are high-pitched sounds. Wheezes may also be described as continuous sounds in that they continue without interruption.

It is thought that these sounds are generated by air passing through a narrowed lumen. The passage of this air causes the lumen to vibrate much like a double reed on an oboe or bassoon.

When describing this sound, indicate its location, when it occurs with respect to inspiration or expiration, its pitch, and its intensity.

Rhonchi

Rhonchi are also continuous sounds but are quite low pitched. Rhonchi are sometimes described as similar to the sounds produced by blowing into a milkshake through a straw. Often these sounds are described as being "wet." Rhonchi are thought to be produced by fluid or secretions vibrating in the airways. They may be heard throughout the lung fields.

When describing this sound, indicate its location, pitch, and intensity. The patient can be asked to cough; rhonchi may frequently clear following a vigorous cough.

Pleural Rub

A pleural rub occurs when the two pleural layers rub together with more friction than normal. An increase in friction may be caused by irritation or inflammation. The resulting sound is often described as "creaking leather," similar to the sound produced when riding a horse using a well-worn saddle.

ANATOMICAL POSITIONS FOR AUSCULTATION

Air exchange and movement in the lungs are influenced by patient position. To optimize airflow, the patient should be sitting in an upright position to allow for good chest expansion. In the hospital, the patient who has no physical limitations should sit on the side of the bed (dangling position). In some instances, because of poor physical condition, the patient may be unable to sit unassisted in the upright position. As long as the patient will not be physically compromised, have someone assist by holding the patient in a high Fowler's position to allow auscultation of the posterior chest. Have the patient roll the shoulders forward to separate the scapulae.

Figures 2-6 and 2-7 show the anterior and posterior positions for auscultating the chest. It is important when auscultating the chest to move from one segment of the lung to the corresponding segment on the opposite side of the chest. Humans are bilateral mammals, making comparison of one side with the other a relatively informative and easy task.

When auscultating the chest, have the patient breathe slowly and a bit more deeply than normal through the mouth. Listen for one complete cycle, inspiration and expiration at each segment. Listen carefully to each segment. Compare one side with the other. Progress from the superior segments to the inferior segments when auscultating either posteriorly or anteriorly.

Environmental Considerations

During auscultation of the chest, the patient's privacy may be compromised. If possible, close the door and dismiss any visitors prior to beginning the examination. The temperature of the room should be comfortable and not too cold. Turn off any radios, televisions, or appliances that may be distracting while auscultating the chest. Lung sounds are often faint and somewhat muffled, making them difficult to hear.

The stethoscope should be used on bare skin. Contact of the stethoscope with the patient's clothing or gown may cause artificial sounds to be produced, confusing the examiner about what is real and what is not. Hair on a male patient's chest will often cause slight movement against the diaphragm of the stethoscope, producing the sound of crackles. Patients with excess adipose tissue may cause severe attenuation of breath sounds, making it very difficult to hear subtle sounds.

The female patient with large breasts presents an additional challenge in the auscultation of breath sounds. If the patient is alert and cooperative, ask her to move her breast to one side to facilitate use of the stethoscope. If the patient is unable to do so, it may be necessary for the respiratory practitioner to move the breast while preserving the patient's dignity.

The Case for a Systematic Method

Learning to recognize breath sounds requires considerable practice. The more time taken to listen to the different sounds, the sooner the respiratory practitioner will

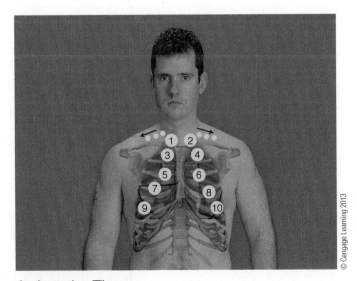

A. Anterior Thorax

© Cengage Learning 2013

Figure 2-6   Anterior positions used in auscultating the chest

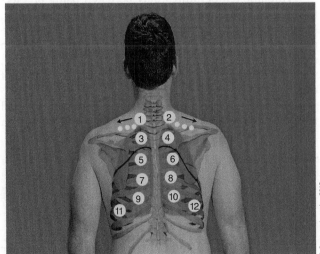

B. Posterior Thorax

© Cengage Learning 2013

Figure 2-7   Posterior positions used in auscultating the chest

be able to distinguish among them. It is important to develop a systematic method of auscultating the chest early in training. If the same technique is used consistently for all patients, the mechanics will soon become second nature. The respiratory practitioner will then be able to concentrate on recognizing the sounds. A skilled examiner is one who is able to discriminate among the sounds.

PROFICIENCY OBJECTIVES

At the end of this chapter, the reader should be able to:

VITAL SIGNS

* *Using a laboratory partner, locate the three most common sites for measuring body temperature.*
* *Using a laboratory partner, correctly measure the oral temperature.*
* *Using a laboratory partner, locate the most common sites to measure the pulse.*
* *Using a laboratory partner, measure the pulse and describe the following:*
  — *Rate*
  — *Rhythm*
  — *Normalcy*

* *Using a laboratory partner, measure the respiratory rate, determining whether the rate and rhythm are normal.*
* *Using a laboratory partner, correctly measure the blood pressure.*

BREATH SOUNDS

* *Demonstrate the proper preparation of the stethoscope for use with emphasis on aseptic technique.*
* *Demonstrate how to test the stethoscope for function and how to troubleshoot the instrument when it does not function properly.*
* *Demonstrate how to auscultate the chest in a systematic way.*

MEASURING BODY TEMPERATURE

The three most common sites used for measuring body temperature are oral, rectal, and axillary.

The oral temperature is taken by having the patient open the mouth, inserting the thermometer under the tongue, and having the patient close the mouth. The rectal temperature is taken by having the patient lie on his or her side and inserting the thermometer into the rectum.

The axillary temperature is measured by placing the thermometer within the armpit and holding the arm down snugly against the patient's side.

Tympanic temperatures may be taken using an electronic thermometer. A probe is inserted into the ear canal, sealing it. Once the temperature stabilizes, the thermometer beeps, signaling that the temperature has been measured. This thermometer is quick and accurate and, with use of disposable probe covers, minimizes the risk of cross-contamination.

The rectal temperature is 1 degree higher than the oral temperature, and the axillary temperature is 1 degree lower.

MEASURING ORAL TEMPERATURE

Equipment

An electronic thermometer and disposable probe cover are all that is required to measure a patient's temperature.

Preparation for Use

When using an electronic thermometer, aseptically apply a new disposable probe cover, per manufacturer's directions. The instrument is now ready to use.

Checking the Patient

Ask whether the patient can breathe through the nose without difficulty. Also ask whether the patient has had any food or liquids or has smoked in the past 10 minutes, as these can affect the oral temperature.

The patient should be alert and able to follow directions. If this is not the case, consider taking rectal or axillary temperatures.

Placement of the Thermometer

Ask the patient to open the mouth, and place the thermometer probe under the tongue. Ask the patient to close the mouth and not bite on the thermometer probe. Leave the thermometer probe in place long enough until a reading is made. Some instruments will emit an auditory "beep" once the temperature has stabilized.

Reading the Thermometer

Remove the thermometer. Never touch the portion of the thermometer that was inside the patient's mouth. Immediately after removing the thermometer, read and record the temperature, and properly discard the disposable probe cover.

MEASURING THE PULSE

Common Sites

The four most common sites to measure the pulse are over the radial, brachial (shown in Figure 2-8), femoral, and carotid arteries.

The femoral pulse is felt immediately lateral to the pubic bone in the pelvis. Palpate the pubic bone. In the male, the pubic bone is immediately superior to the penis, and in the female, it is immediately superior to the pudendum. On moving laterally into the area of the groin, the femoral pulse should be immediately evident.

The carotid pulse is felt lateral to the larynx on either side of the neck.

Assessment of the Pulse

The pulse should be measured for one full minute at the radial site. Measuring the pulse for a shorter time inter-

val will compromise the ability to assess for arrhythmias or irregularities.

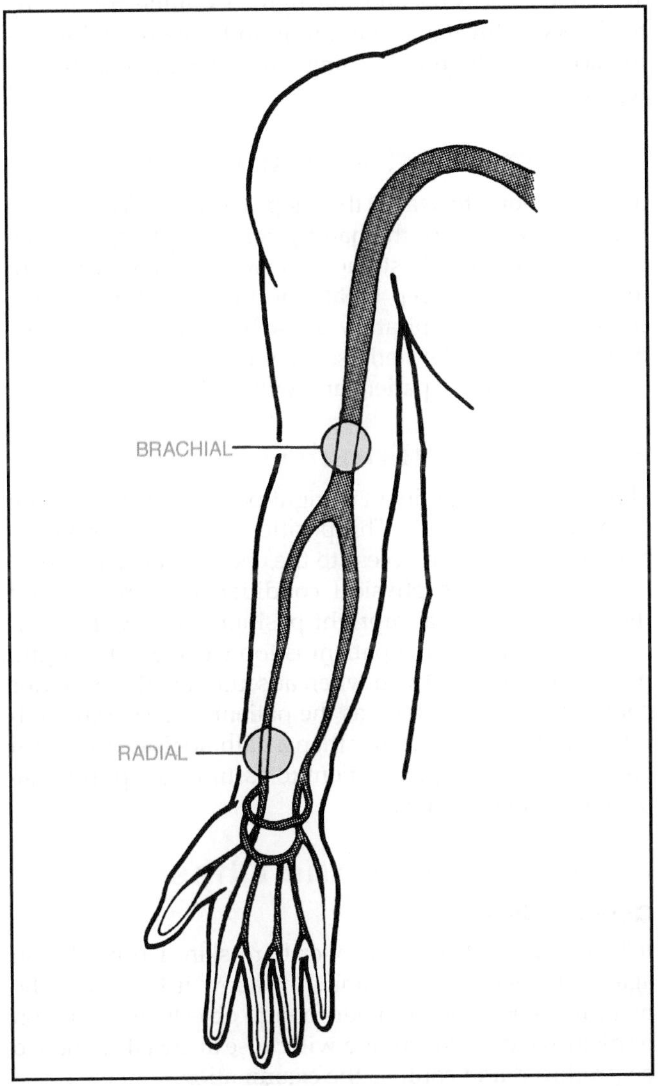

MEASURING RESPIRATORY RATE

It is often difficult to assess the respiratory rate without the patient's becoming aware of it. If the patient becomes aware that the respiratory practitioner is measuring respirations, the rate may be adversely affected. Therefore, it is beneficial not to disclose that the respiratory rate will be measured.

A way to measure the respiratory rate without the patient's awareness is to pretend to measure the pulse by palpating the radial artery while actually counting the respirations.

In some patients, the respiratory excursions are very small. It may be necessary to place a hand on the patient's abdomen in order to perceive these excursions.

ASSESSING BLOOD PRESSURE

Equipment

The equipment required for assessing blood pressure is a stethoscope and a sphygmomanometer (blood pressure cuff).

To measure blood pressure, the diaphragm of the stethoscope is used. The diaphragm is placed over the brachial artery.

Sphygmomanometer Placement

Sphygmomanometer cuff size is important in obtaining the correct reading. If a patient with a large arm size is fitted with a cuff that is too small, an erroneously high blood pressure reading will result. Table 2-4 provides a guideline for correct cuff sizing.

The sphygmomanometer is placed on the arm approximately 1 inch above the antecubital space. Palpate the brachial artery and then apply the cuff in proper position. The sphygmomanometer is commonly closed by self-fasteners (Velcro) or hooks.

Figure 2-8 The sites for assessing the radial and brachial pulses

© Cengage Learning 2013

TABLE 2-4: Guideline for Cuff Sizing

ARM CIRCUMFERENCE (MIDPOINT)	CUFF SIZE
27–34 cm	Adult
35–44 cm	Adult large
45–52 cm	Adult thigh cuff

Adapted from Perloff, D. (1993). Human Blood Pressure Determination by Sphygmomanometry, *Circulation Journal*, 88, 2460–2470.

Measuring Blood Pressure by Palpation

Palpate the brachial artery. Once the artery is located, slowly inflate the sphygmomanometer. When the artery becomes totally occluded, the pulse will no longer be felt. At this point, measure the reading on the pressure gauge. This is the systolic blood pressure. Continue to inflate the sphygmomanometer another 30 mm Hg. Immediately measure the blood pressure by auscultation.

Measuring the Blood Pressure by Auscultation

Using the stethoscope, place the diaphragm over the brachial artery. Deflate the sphygmomanometer slowly while auscultating for the blood pressure. When sound is first heard in the artery, note the reading on the pressure gauge. Continue deflating the cuff and note the reading at which all sound ceases. The point at which the sound is first heard is the systolic measurement; the point at which all sound stops is the diastolic measurement.

AUSCULTATION OF BREATH SOUNDS

Preparation of the Stethoscope

If not already done, adjust the stethoscope to your anatomy. Have a laboratory partner assist with this. Adjust the binaurals so that they fit snugly in the auditory canals but not so tight that they cause discomfort. This may be accomplished by spreading or compressing the leaf spring on which the binaurals are attached until the fit is comfortable and snug. Next, have your partner assist in adjusting the angle of the binaurals so that the tips are each pointing into the auditory canals, pointing forward toward the nose. Now the stethoscope is properly fitted to you and you alone.

Preparation and Cleaning

If the stethoscope being used is one commonly used by others, such as those found at a nurses' station, take the time to prepare the instrument for use. Using an alcohol swab, thoroughly clean the earpieces as a precaution against infection.

Whether using your own instrument or one used by others, use another alcohol swab to thoroughly clean the diaphragm and bell. The instrument should be cleaned in this manner before and after each use to help prevent the spread of communicable diseases (Cohen, 1997). Do not forget hand hygiene prior to examining the patient.

Patients in isolation will have a stethoscope in the room. Do not bring your own stethoscope into isolation. Use the one provided in the room to prevent the spread of hospital-acquired infections.

If there is occasion to lay down the stethoscope in a patient's room, do not place it on the bed. A preferable practice is to put it around the neck or return it to the pocket. The patient's bed and overbed table are places that may be colonized by bacteria and viruses. By placing a stethoscope on these surfaces, it may become a vehicle for transmitting hospital-acquired infections.

Testing

A stethoscope may be easily and quickly tested prior to use. Place the earpieces in the auditory canals and gently tap on the diaphragm and bell. It is important not to use too much force. The stethoscope greatly amplifies sound, and too forceful a tap will cause great discomfort. This is a good time to examine the diaphragm and bell for cracks or other signs of wear or abuse. If these parts need replacement, use only parts supplied by the manufacturer. X-ray film and other materials may be substituted in a pinch, but they rarely seal well and fail to provide good attenuation of sounds.

If gentle tapping fails to produce any sound, verify that the diaphragm or bell is in the proper position on the chest piece. If it is not, rotate it into proper position. If the instrument still fails to perform properly, examine the chest piece carefully and make sure that all parts are assembled correctly and are tight. Examine the tubing for kinks or breaks. If any are found, free the tubing or replace it as required, using only the manufacturer's replacement parts.

Warming of the Diaphragm

It is courteous to warm the diaphragm briefly by placing it in the palm of the hand prior to applying it to the patient's chest. A cold stethoscope will prompt the patient to initiate a very deep breath, and often there is a long pause before the expiratory phase begins. The short time it takes to warm the stethoscope will make it much more comfortable for the patient and will facilitate cooperation.

Patient Positioning

Have the patient sit in an upright position at the bedside or in a chair if possible. This position will allow for proper chest expansion and access to the chest for auscultation.

If the patient's physical condition does not permit the assumption of an upright position, modify the position as required. If the patient is too weak to sit upright, have someone assist you when auscultating the posterior chest. In general, as long as the patient's muscle strength is the limiting factor, rather than a pathological or surgical condition, assisting the patient to assume an appropriate position is permissible.

Auscultation of the Chest
General Notes

It is always best to listen over bare skin. Do not brush against the stethoscope tubing or allow it to contact the bed rail, bed frame, or other foreign objects. Any motion or disturbance of the tubing will cause artificial sounds to be produced and confuse the examination.

Turn off radios, televisions, or other noisy appliances. Make sure the room is at a comfortable temperature, and dismiss any visitors prior to the examination.

The proper hand position is important to ensure good contact between the stethoscope and the skin surface and also to minimize motion of the chest piece. The center portion of the chest piece should be placed between the first and second digits. Place the chest piece on the chest wall and hyperextend all of the digits, making contact over a broad surface area (Figure 2-9).

Close the door or use privacy drapes or screens to preserve the patient's dignity.

Anterior Chest

Beginning on the anterior chest, listen above the clavicles between the midclavicular line and the midsternal line on each side. Progress inferiorly to just below the clavicles, listening at the same lateral position. Progress inferiorly to the third intercostal space and listen on each side between the midclavicular and midsternal lines. Move inferiorly to the fourth intercostal space and listen on each side at the same lateral positions. Moving inferiorly,

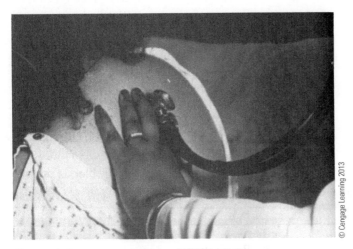

© Cengage Learning 2013

Figure 2-9   The correct way to hold the stethoscope

listen at the sixth intercostal space at the midclavicular line below the nipples.

Progress laterally to the fourth intercostal space, listening at the anterior axillary line. Move inferiorly to the fifth intercostal space and listen at the anterior axillary line. Progress inferiorly and listen at the sixth intercostal space at the posterior axillary line. Upon listening to a position on one side, be sure to compare it with the same position on the opposite side.

Posterior Chest

For auscultating the posterior chest, it is often helpful to ask the patient to shrug the shoulders forward, spreading the scapulae slightly further apart.

Begin listening at a point even with the top of the scapulae between the midscapular line and the midspinal line. Move inferiorly to the approximate midpoint of the scapulae and auscultate between the midscapular line and the midspinal line. Progress inferiorly and listen at a point even with the bottom of the scapulae between the midscapular and midspinal lines. Move inferiorly and laterally to the midscapular line and listen just below the scapulae.

As with the anterior chest, be sure to compare one side with the other before progressing inferiorly.

Postauscultation

Provide assistance as required in the reapplication of the patient's gown or any clothing removed before the examination. Help the patient to assume a comfortable and safe position prior to departing. Be courteous and thank the patient for his or her cooperation and time. Wash the hands prior to leaving the room.

Clean the diaphragm or bell, or both, with an alcohol swab.

Record the findings in the patient's chart, describing the sound and its intensity, duration, phase, and location.

References

Callahan, D. (2007). Stethoscopes: What are we hearing? *Biomedical Instrumentation & Technology, 41*(4), 318–323.

Cohen, H. A. (1997). Stethoscopes and otoscopes—a potential vector of infection? *Family Practice, 14*(6), 446–449.

Perloff, D. (1993). Human blood pressure determination by sphygmomanometry. *Circulation Journal, 88*, 2460–2470.

Additional Resources

Murphy, R. (2008). In defense of the stethoscope. *Respiratory Care, 53*(3), 355–369.

Practice Activities: Basic Patient Assessment

VITAL SIGNS

1. Using a laboratory partner, practice measuring oral body temperature. Include the following in your practice:

   a. Select the appropriate equipment.
   b. Prepare the equipment for use.
   c. Aseptically apply a probe cover and prepare the instrument for use.

d. Determine the patient's ability to breathe through the nose and determine if the patient has had anything to eat or drink or has smoked in the past 10 minutes.

e. Correctly place the thermometer probe and instruct the patient.

f. Leave the thermometer in place for an appropriate length of time.

g. Correctly read the temperature and record it.

h. Correctly dispose of the probe cover.

2. Using a laboratory partner, practice locating and measuring the heart rate at the following sites:
   a. Radial
   b. Brachial
   c. Carotid
   Include in your measurements:
   a. Rate
   b. Rhythm
   c. Normalcy

3. Using a laboratory partner, measure the respiratory rate, making sure the partner is unaware of your intentions.

4. Using a laboratory partner, practice measuring the blood pressure, including the following:
   a. Select the appropriate equipment.
   b. Correctly size the cuff.
   c. Palpate the brachial pulse.
   d. Correctly apply the cuff.

e. Measure the blood pressure by palpation during inflation of the sphygmomanometer.

f. Measure the blood pressure by auscultation during deflation of the sphygmomanometer.

g. Correctly record the blood pressure.

5. Using a laboratory partner, practice sequencing the different skills together in the following way:
   a. Perform hand hygiene.
   b. Correctly prepare and insert the thermometer for oral temperature.
   c. While waiting, measure the following:
      (1) The pulse and respirations
      (2) The blood pressure
      (3) The oral temperature (record on the chart)

BREATH SOUNDS

1. Identify all of the parts on your own stethoscope.

2. Demonstrate to your laboratory partner how to properly clean and prepare your stethoscope for use.

3. Practice auscultating the chest with a laboratory partner:
   a. Auscultate on bare skin.
   b. Instruct your laboratory partner to breathe deeply and through the mouth.
   c. Auscultate at each position bilaterally.

4. Following auscultation of your laboratory partner's chest, take a sheet of paper and chart your findings. Have your instructor critique your charting.

Check List: Vital Signs

_____ 1. Identify your patient.

_____ 2. Explain the procedure.

_____ 3. Wash your hands.

4. Prepare the thermometer for use:
   a. Electronic:
_____   (1) Apply a new cover.

5. Determine if an oral temperature is contra-indicated:
_____ a. Determine if the patient can breathe through the nose.
_____ b. Determine if the patient has had any food or drink orally in the past 10 minutes.
_____ c. Determine if the patient has smoked in the past 10 minutes.

6. Correctly place the thermometer:
_____ a. Place it under the patient's tongue.
_____ b. Instruct the patient to close the mouth and not to bite on the thermometer probe.

7. Assess pulse and respirations:
   a. Pulse:
_____   (1) Locate the site.
_____   (2) Measure the rate.
_____   (3) Assess the rhythm.

   b. Respirations:
_____   (1) Measure the rate.
_____   (2) Assess the depth.
_____   (3) Assess the rhythm.
_____   (4) Ensure that the patient is unaware of the assessment.

8. Measure the blood pressure:
_____ a. Locate the brachial pulse.
_____ b. Correctly size the cuff.
_____ c. Correctly apply the cuff.
_____ d. Measure the systolic blood pressure by palpation during cuff inflation.
_____ e. Measure the systolic and diastolic blood pressures by auscultation during cuff deflation.
_____ f. Correctly record the blood pressure.

_____ 9. Remove the thermometer and correctly measure the oral temperature.

_____ 10. Correctly care for the equipment following the procedure.

_____ 11. Thank the patient and wash your hands before leaving the room.

Check List: Breath Sounds

1. Collect and assemble the equipment:
____ a. Stethoscope
____ b. Alcohol swabs
____ c. Pen
2. Prepare and test the equipment:
____ a. Clean the earpieces if the stethoscope is not your own.
____ b. Clean the diaphragm and bell.
____ c. Test the equipment and troubleshoot.
____ 3. Wash your hands.
4. Optimize the environment:
____ a. Turn off the radio or television.
____ b. Regulate the temperature as required.
____ c. Ensure the patient's privacy.
5. Position the patient properly:
____ a. Have the patient sit in an upright position.
____ b. Ask for assistance if necessary or modify the position as required.
6. Auscultate the anterior chest:
____ a. Auscultate at each position bilaterally.
____ b. Use the stethoscope properly.
____ c. Use a systematic method.

7. Auscultate the lateral chest:
____ a. Auscultate at each position bilaterally.
____ b. Use the stethoscope properly.
____ c. Use a systematic method.
8. Auscultate the posterior chest:
____ a. Auscultate at each position bilaterally.
____ b. Use the stethoscope properly.
____ c. Use a systematic method.
9. Ensure patient safety and comfort:
____ a. Assist with clothing as required.
____ b. Help the patient back to a comfortable position.
____ c. Thank the patient.
____ 10. Wash your hands.
11. Clean your equipment:
____ a. Clean the diaphragm and bell.
____ 12. Record the findings on the patient's chart.

Self-Evaluation Post Test: Basic Patient Assessment

1. Body temperature is regulated by the:
a. hyperdermis.
b. sympathetic nervous system.
c. hypothalamus.
d. thyroid.

2. Normal temperature for an adult is:
a. 32°C. c. 98°C.
b. 35°C. d. 37°C.

3. A child's body temperature is:
a. the same as an adult's.
b. lower than an adult's.
c. higher than an adult's.
d. more precisely regulated than an adult's.

4. A decrease in body temperature below normal is termed:
a. hypotension. c. hypothermia.
b. bradypnea. d. hypertension.

5. Hypoxemia may cause:
a. bradypnea. c. hyperthermia.
b. tachycardia. d. hypertension.

6. Sound may be conducted through:
I. air.
II. fluids.
III. solids
a. I. c. I, II, III
b. I, II d. I, III

7. Which of the following determines a sound's intensity?
a. Frequency
b. Amplitude
c. Pitch
d. Duration

8. A denser material will conduct sound:
a. more easily than a less dense material.
b. more slowly than a less dense material.
c. with greater attenuation than a less dense material.
d. only in the high-frequency ranges.

9. Vesicular breath sounds:
I. are normal breath sounds.
II. are often described as quiet rustling sounds.
III. have an expiratory phase longer than the inspiratory phase.
IV. have no pause between inspiration and expiration.
a. I, II, III c. I, III, IV
b. I, II, IV d. II, III, IV

10. Bronchial breath sounds:
I. are low-pitched sounds.
II. have an inspiratory phase shorter than the expiratory phase.
III. have no pause between inspiration and expiration.
IV. are often described as hollow sounding.
a. I, III c. II, III
b. II, IV d. I, IV

CHAPTER 3
Advanced Patient Assessment: Inspection, Palpation, and Percussion

INTRODUCTION

As the scope of respiratory care has broadened over the years, the respiratory practitioner has assumed a greater responsibility for assessment of the patient and evaluation of the patient's response to therapy (Wilkins, Evans, & Specht, 2002). Physical assessment of the chest is an important tool employed in patient care. It is a quick and easy means of clinical evaluation. It places few demands on the patient, and the only equipment required is the respiratory practitioner's hands, eyes, and ears.

Like the assessment of breath sounds, physical assessment of the chest requires practice to attain proficiency. It is best to learn at the side of a skilled respiratory practitioner. As skill and confidence improves, practice will help improve abilities.

KEY TERMS

- Barrel chest
- Biot's respiration
- Cheyne-Stokes respiration
- Collarbones
- Digital clubbing
- Eupnea
- Funnel chest
- Humpback
- Hyperpnea

- Hypopnea
- Inspection
- Kussmaul's respiration
- Kyphoscoliosis
- Kyphosis
- Lordosis
- Metabolic acidosis
- Palpation
- Pectus carinatum

- Pectus excavatum
- Percussion
- Pigeon chest
- Scoliosis
- Shoulder blades
- Sternal angle
- Swayback

THEORY OBJECTIVES

At the end of this chapter, the reader should be able to:

- *Identify or locate the anatomical landmarks commonly used in assessing the chest:*
  - *Anterior Chest*
    - *Clavicles*
    - *Sternal notch*
    - *Sternal angle and second rib*
    - *Fourth rib*
    - *Midsternal line*
    - *Midclavicular line*
    - *Anterior axillary line*
  - *Lateral Chest*
    - *Anterior axillary line*
    - *Midaxillary line*
    - *Posterior axillary line*
  - *Posterior Chest*
    - *Scapulae*
    - *Seventh cervical vertebra*
    - *Thoracic spinal column*
    - *Vertebral line*
    - *Midscapular line*
- *Explain the term inspection of the chest and the purpose of the procedure.*
- *Describe the characteristics and significance of the following respiratory rates and patterns:*
  - *Eupnea*
  - *Hyperpnea*
  - *Hypopnea*
  - *Kussmaul's respiration*
  - *Cheyne-Stokes respiration*

— *Biot's respiration*
— *Paradoxical breathing*
- *Describe how the work of breathing may be assessed by inspection.*
- *Differentiate among the following abnormalities of the spine and their effects on respiratory structures and their function:*
  — *Kyphosis*
  — *Scoliosis*
  — *Lordosis*
  — *Kyphoscoliosis*
- *Compare and contrast a normal thoracic shape with that of barrel chest.*
- *Describe the appearance of digital clubbing and the significance of this change.*
- *Differentiate between the following abnormalities of the sternum:*
  — *Pectus excavatum*
  — *Pectus carinatum*

- *Describe the purpose of palpation and how it is used in detecting the following:*
  — *Areas of tenderness*
  — *Symmetry of chest excursion*
  — *Tactile fremitus*
  — *Presence of subcutaneous emphysema*
  — *Deviated position of the trachea*
- *Describe the technique of percussion:*
  — *Direct percussion*
  — *Detection of areas of tenderness*
- *Differentiate among the following percussion tones and the changes in air density versus tissue density that produce them:*
  — *Hyperresonance*
  — *Resonance*
  — *Dullness*
  — *Flatness*

CHEST LANDMARKS FOR ASSESSMENT

Abnormal findings on physical assessment or auscultation are best described in relation to anatomical landmarks and the imaginary vertical lines that divide the chest. These two location systems serve as a coordinate system, similar to that found on most road maps. For example, assessment findings might be noted as follows: "Tenderness was reported by the patient anteriorly, on the left side, at the second rib on the midclavicular line." A skilled respiratory practitioner can use the anatomical coordinates like a map to identify or describe a specific anatomical location.

Bony Structures as Anatomical Landmarks

Anterior Chest

Figure 3-1 shows the bony landmarks on the anterior chest. These include the clavicles, suprasternal notch, sternal angle, and the fourth rib. The clavicles are the prominent horizontal bones commonly called *collarbones*. The sternal notch is located where the clavicles join at the top of the sternum—the manubrium. The manubrium joins the body of the sternum at a horizontal ridge. This ridge is termed the *sternal angle*. Immediately lateral to the sternal angle is the second rib. The sternal angle is a landmark used to find the second rib. Other ribs may be easily palpated from this starting point. The fourth rib is located on the nipple line (imaginary horizontal line through the nipples). Like the second rib, it is easily located and serves as a starting point for locating other ribs.

Posterior Chest

The predominant bony landmarks on the posterior chest include the vertebrae and the scapulae (Figure 3-2).

An easy way to establish position on the vertebral column is to ask the patient to bend the neck forward.

The prominent process at the base of the neck is the seventh cervical vertebra (C7). The process immediately below it is the first thoracic vertebra (T1). Other thoracic vertebrae may be easily determined from this point.

The scapulae are the two large triangular bones below the shoulders, often referred to as the *shoulder blades*.

Vertical Division Lines

Anterior Chest

Three imaginary vertical lines are used to divide the anterior chest. These lines are the midsternal line, midclavicular line, and the anterior midaxillary line (Figure 3-3). The midsternal line is an imaginary line dividing the sternum vertically in half. Imagine a line descending from the center of the sternum to the umbilicus (navel). The midclavicular

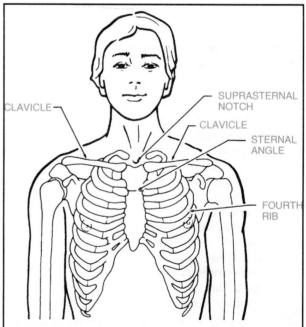

Figure 3-1 Bony landmarks on the anterior chest

CLAVICLE

SUPRASTERNAL NOTCH

CLAVICLE

STERNAL ANGLE

FOURTH RIB

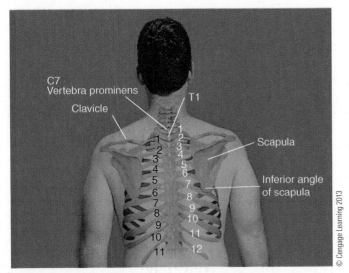

Figure 3-2   Bony landmarks on the posterior chest

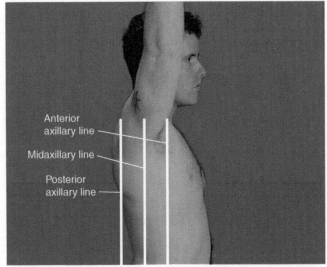

A. Right Lateral View

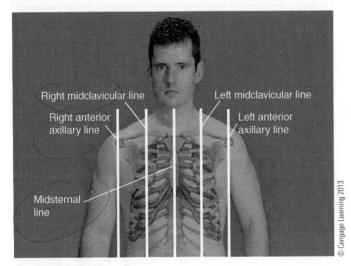

Anterior View

Figure 3-3   Anterior chest vertical division lines

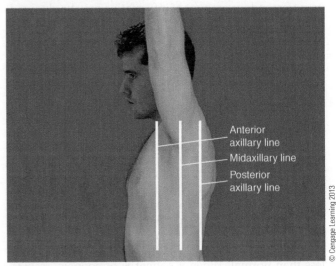

B. Left Lateral View

Figure 3-4   Lateral chest vertical division lines

lines are two vertical lines bisecting the clavicles. Each of these lines passes just medial to the nipples. The anterior axillary line is a line descending vertically from the junction of the arm and torso (at the front of the armpit).

Lateral Chest

The first division line on the lateral chest is the anterior axillary line. The two other imaginary vertical division lines are the midaxillary and posterior axillary lines (Figure 3-4). The midaxillary line is an imaginary line extending downward from the center of the armpit. The posterior axillary line is an imaginary line extending downward from the posterior junction of the arm.

Posterior Chest

There are three imaginary division lines on the posterior chest. These lines are the right and left midscapular lines and the vertebral line (Figure 3-5). The vertebral line is an imaginary line descending along the vertebral column. The left and right midscapular lines are imaginary lines bisecting the scapulae and descending vertically.

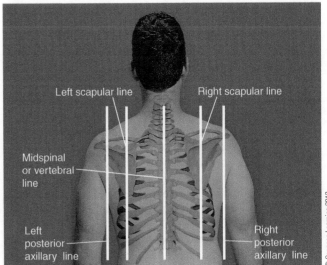

Figure 3-5   Posterior chest vertical division lines

ASSESSMENT TECHNIQUES AND ABNORMAL FINDINGS

Assessment of the chest includes inspection of the structure of the thorax, observation of patterns of movement during respiration, and percussion. For each component of the assessment, use of proper techniques and familiarity with the various types of abnormalities are essential for developing expertise in this area of respiratory care practice.

Significant Aspects of Inspection of the Chest

Inspection of the chest consists of thorough observation of the chest and its motion. By careful observation of a variety of aspects including (1) the patient's skin color, (2) the work of breathing, and (3) conformation of the digits, a tremendous amount of information may be obtained.

Respiratory Rate, Rhythm, and Pattern

Observation of respiratory rate, rhythm, and pattern is an important aspect of inspection of the chest. In an adult breathing normally at rest, the respiratory rate is between 12 and 20 breaths per minute, with an inspiratory-to-expiratory ratio (I:E) of 1:2. This normal ventilatory pattern is termed *eupnea*.

An increase in the depth of respirations to greater than normal is termed *hyperpnea*. Often hyperpnea is mistakenly called hyperventilation. Hyperventilation refers to decreased carbon dioxide (CO_2) levels in the arterial blood as a result of increased ventilation, not respiratory rate or depth. Hyperpnea may exist with or without hyperventilation, or vice versa.

Hypopnea is a decrease in the depth of respirations to less than normal. When a patient is hypopneic, respirations are very shallow. There are many causes of hypopnea; one of the more serious results from a brain stem injury, which may also be accompanied by tachycardia with a weak pulse.

Variations in the respiratory pattern may be indicators of underlying conditions. Three abnormal respiratory patterns are *Kussmaul's respiration, Cheyne-Stokes respiration,* and *Biot's respiration.* Figure 3-6 is a graphic display comparing normal, Kussmaul's, Cheyne-Stokes, and Biot's breathing patterns. Another abnormal pattern is paradoxical breathing. It is often the result of chest wall trauma or paralysis and may significantly increase the work of breathing.

Kussmaul's respiration is an increase in rate and depth. It occurs most commonly as a result of diabetic crisis. In diabetic acidosis, excessive acid is produced and circulated in the bloodstream (condition termed *metabolic acidosis*). The brain responds by increasing the respiratory rate and depth to eliminate CO_2 from the blood to correct the acidosis.

Cheyne-Stokes respiration is periodic in nature with a gradual increase in depth and respiratory rate followed by a tapering of rate and depth with periods of apnea (absence of respirations). This abnormality has been

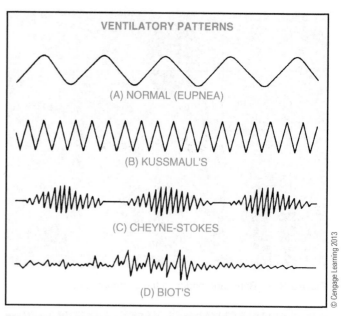

Figure 3-6 Normal or eupnea (A), Kussmaul's (B), Cheyne-Stokes (C), and Biot's (D) respiratory patterns

described as a waxing and waning of respirations. It may be associated with congestive heart failure, damage or trauma to the central nervous system (CNS), or increased cerebrospinal fluid pressure.

Biot's respiration is irregular in rate and depth. There are variable periods of apnea between respirations. This respiratory pattern is highly variable. It is frequently associated with basal encephalitis or meningitis.

Paradoxical breathing is the result of discoordinated motion of various parts of the chest wall or abdomen, or both. During normal breathing, the diaphragm descends and the ribs move up and out anteriorly and laterally. This movement increases the volume of the thoracic cavity, causing a decrease in intrathoracic pressure. Air then flows from the area of greater ambient pressure into the lungs—the area of lower pressure.

Trauma resulting in multiple rib fractures causes a loss of structural integrity of the rib cage. As the diaphragm descends, the injured section responds to the decrease in intrathoracic pressure and collapses in, rather than moving out normally. On exhalation, the increased intrathoracic pressure causes the affected area to bulge out (Figure 3-7).

Work of Breathing

A general assessment of the work of breathing may be made by careful observation. The patient's body position gives an indication of the effort being expended. A patient assuming the position shown in Figure 3-8 is trying to transfer the effort required to sit upright to the arms instead of the abdomen. This position may be termed the *tripod position*, which allows the pectoralis major accessory muscles to assist in ventilation. This position also shifts the abdominal contents away from the diaphragm, thus decreasing the work of breathing. This allows for less effort to be expended to sustain respiration. Observe the patient's use of accessory muscles while breathing.

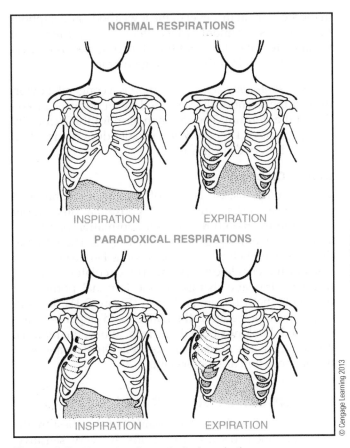

Figure 3-7 Normal and paradoxical respirations

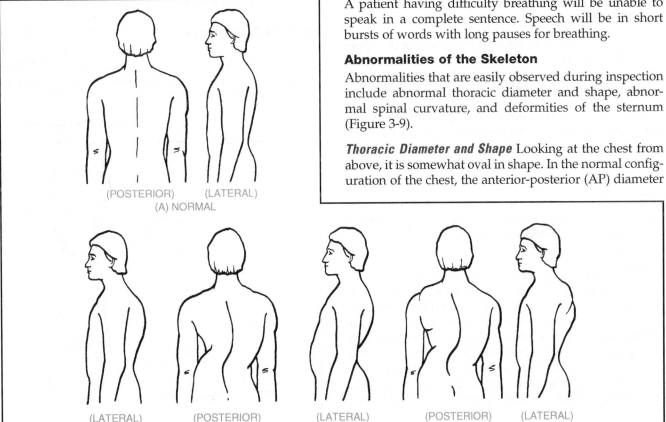

Figure 3-8 A patient assuming the tripod position, indicating an increased work of breathing position

A patient having difficulty breathing will be unable to speak in a complete sentence. Speech will be in short bursts of words with long pauses for breathing.

Abnormalities of the Skeleton

Abnormalities that are easily observed during inspection include abnormal thoracic diameter and shape, abnormal spinal curvature, and deformities of the sternum (Figure 3-9).

Thoracic Diameter and Shape Looking at the chest from above, it is somewhat oval in shape. In the normal configuration of the chest, the anterior-posterior (AP) diameter

Figure 3-9 Normal (A), kyphosis (B), scoliosis (C), lordosis (D), and kyphoscoliosis (E) spinal configurations

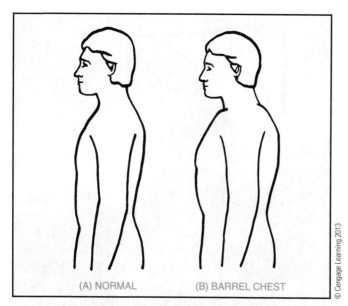

Figure 3-10   Normal (A) and barrel chest (B) configuration

(thickness) is less than the left-to-right diameter (width) (Figure 3-10).

An increase in the AP diameter to greater than normal results in a configuration termed *barrel chest*. This abnormality is commonly associated with chronic lung disease due to air trapping and a loss in lung compliance. This change in configuration is distinctive in appearance. It has the disadvantage of reducing the normal mechanical advantage of the ribs and intercostal muscles, resulting in less efficient ventilation.

Kyphosis *Kyphosis* is an abnormal curvature of the upper spine. It is an anterior-to-posterior curvature that gives the patient a *humpback* appearance. It is frequently associated with chronic lung disease.

Scoliosis *Scoliosis* is a lateral curvature of the spine. This lateral curvature causes the vertebrae in the affected area to rotate, flattening the rib cage anteriorly. Frequently, this abnormality can interfere with the mechanics of ventilation.

Lordosis *Lordosis* is an inward curvature of the lumbar spine. This curvature results in a *swayback* appearance. It is not usually associated with any pathologic respiratory condition.

Kyphoscoliosis *Kyphoscoliosis* is a combination of kyphosis and scoliosis. Assess the lateral curvature of the spine first by comparing the heights of the scapulae. Then assess the severity of the kyphosis component. This condition can profoundly affect ventilatory volume and the mechanics of respiration. It frequently results in congestive heart failure and circulatory embarrassment as well. Many patients with severe kyphoscoliosis die at an early age of acute respiratory infection or chronic respiratory insufficiency.

Pectus Excavatum *Pectus excavatum* is a congenital deformity of the sternum characterized by a depression in the sternum at the level of the lower body and xyphoid process. It is commonly called *funnel chest*, a term that visually describes the condition. If severe, pectus excavatum may result in decreased lung volumes.

Pectus Carinatum *Pectus carinatum* is a congenital deformity of the sternum characterized by an outward projection of the sternum. The common term for this deformity is *pigeon chest*. This condition usually does not result in any respiratory complications.

Digital Clubbing

Chronic lung disease is one of several conditions that may cause *digital clubbing*. Hypoxemia (insufficient oxygen in the blood) results in the formation of arterial-venous anastomoses in the terminal digits. These formations are actual circulatory connections between the two sides of the circulatory system. The circulatory changes result in dramatic changes in the terminal portions of the digits (both fingers and toes) (Figure 3-11). In clubbing, the angle between the nailbed and finger becomes increased. Looking at the digits from above, the terminal portion increases in diameter as well. Often, cyanosis of the nailbeds will also be present.

Palpation of the Chest

Palpation is the physical assessment of the chest by the sense of touch. Because the hands are very sensitive, temperature differences and vibrations may be easily perceived. The hands may also be used as indicators to assess symmetry of chest movement.

Areas of Tenderness

As a respiratory practitioner palpates the chest, the patient may complain about areas that are sore or tender to the touch. This information may provide important clues to underlying conditions.

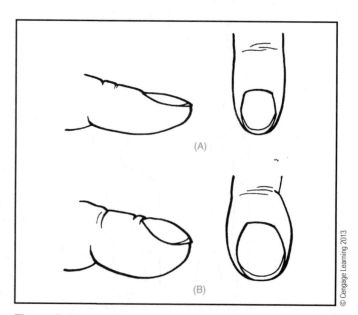

Figure 3-11   Normal digit conformation (A) and clubbing (B)

Symmetry of Excursion

Symmetry may be readily assessed by placing the hands on corresponding positions of the right and left sides of the chest and observing chest wall motion (Figures 3-12 and 3-13). As the patient inhales deeply, the respiratory practitioner's hands should move apart in a symmetrical way. If one hand moves more than the other, this may indicate consolidation (airless, fluid-filled, uncollapsed lung tissue), pleural effusion (fluid in the pleural space), atelectasis (loss of air in the lung tissue), or a pneumothorax (air in the pleural space).

Tactile Fremitus

Tactile fremitus is vibration felt on the palpation of the chest during phonation, or speech. As the patient speaks, vibrations are transmitted through the bronchi and lung parenchyma to the skin surface where they can be felt. An increase in tactile fremitus indicates an increase in density of the underlying tissue. This change may be caused by pneumonia or atelectasis.

Subcutaneous Emphysema

Subcutaneous emphysema is the presence of air beneath the skin in the subcutaneous tissues. This condition may be localized or very diffuse over a large area. Subcutaneous emphysema is sometimes a complication of tracheostomy, pneumothorax, or mechanical ventilation. The tissue changes are easily palpated; the findings are best described as feeling like a bowl of plastic beads covered with a layer of cellophane.

Tracheal Deviation

Deviation of the trachea from its normal midline position may be indicative of several underlying conditions. By depressing the index finger into the sternal notch, the respiratory practitioner can palpate the trachea. Its relative position—midline, left, or right—can be assessed (Redden, Hunton, & Kaminsky, 2003). Table 3-1 lists the direction of tracheal shift occurring as a result of different pathologic conditions.

Percussion of the Chest

Everyone has had the doctor thump on the chest as part of a routine chest or general physical examination. *Percussion* is tapping on the chest while listening for the resulting sound. There are two methods of percussing the chest: direct and indirect. The direct method involves tapping on the chest with a finger, using a short, sharp stroke. Indirect percussion involves placing a finger firmly against the chest and tapping on that finger (Figure 3-14).

Four different types of sounds may be heard during percussion of the chest: hyperresonance, resonance, dullness, and flatness.

Hyperresonance

Hyperresonance is an abnormal percussion sound heard over the chest. It occurs as a result of air trapping or from the presence of air in a closed cavity. A pneumothorax is an example of the latter category. With hyperresonance, percussion produces a loud, low-pitched sound of long

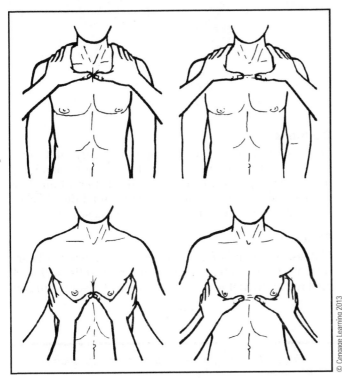

Figure 3-12   Hand positions for assessing symmetry of the anterior chest

© Cengage Learning 2013

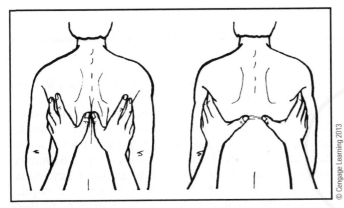

Figure 3-13   Hand positions for assessing symmetry of the posterior chest

© Cengage Learning 2013

TABLE 3-1: Causes of Change in Tracheal Position	
TRACHEAL SHIFT TOWARD AFFECTED SIDE	**TRACHEAL SHIFT AWAY FROM AFFECTED SIDE**
Atelectasis	Pleural effusion
Fibrosis	Pneumothorax
	Tension pneumothorax

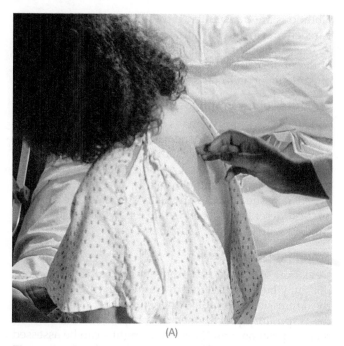

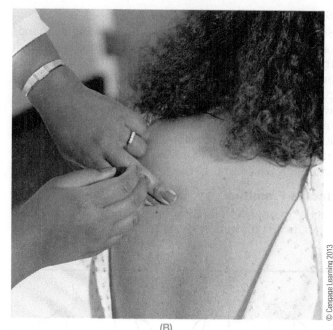

(A)   (B)

© Cengage Learning 2013

Figure 3-14   Direct (A) and indirect (B) percussion

duration. This percussion note is produced as sound passes through an area with a greater proportion of air in relation to tissue (high air-to-tissue ratio) (Redden et al., 2003). This sound can also be heard over an air-filled stomach.

Resonance

Resonance is the sound heard in percussing normal lung tissue. It is a low-pitched sound of long duration. This sound is characteristic of areas that contain equal distributions of air and tissue.

Dullness

Dullness is a sound of medium intensity and pitch with a short duration. It is heard over areas containing a greater proportion of tissue or fluid than of air. This occurs in the lungs as a result of consolidation, atelectasis, or the presence of fluid in the pleural space.

Flatness

Flatness is a sound of low amplitude and pitch. It is heard over areas containing a greater proportion of tissue than of air. Frequently, flatness is an indication of pleural effusion.

PROFICIENCY OBJECTIVES

At the end of this chapter, the reader should be able to:

- *Describe the optimal environment for the physical assessment of the chest.*
- *Using a laboratory partner, properly position and prepare the partner for physical assessment of the chest.*

- *Using a laboratory partner, demonstrate inspection of the chest.*
- *Using a laboratory partner, demonstrate palpation of the chest.*
- *Using a laboratory partner, demonstrate percussion of the chest.*

PREEXAMINATION AND OTHER CONSIDERATIONS

During physical assessment of the chest, the patient's privacy may be compromised. If possible, close the door and dismiss any visitors before beginning the examination. The temperature of the room should be comfortable and not too cold. Turn off any radios, televisions, or appliances that may be distracting. Explain to the patient what

will be done and what information it may provide about his or her condition.

Ideally, patients will be wearing hospital gowns. These gowns allow easy access to the posterior chest by unsnapping or untying them at the waist level in the back of the gown. The gown may be lifted or moved to view areas of the chest or to perform percussion or auscultation. Part of the examination will require touching the chest with the hands. A male respiratory practitioner examining a female patient should consider having a female nurse or physician present in the room when conducting the examination. Failure to do so may potentially result in litigation by the patient against the respiratory practitioner. Common sense and respect for the patient's dignity will help to prevent these complications.

INSPECTION OF THE CHEST

Inspection of the chest is a detailed observation to determine the breathing pattern, assess the work of breathing, and identify skeletal abnormalities.

Observe the patient's breathing pattern. Determine if the rate and rhythm are normal. Assess the I:E ratio; it normally is 1:2.

Assess the work of breathing. Is the patient assuming an unusual posture? Listen carefully to the patient during conversation. Is the patient able to speak in complete sentences? Observe the use of accessory muscles while the patient is breathing.

Observe the chest posteriorly with the patient sitting upright. Look at the spinal column. Check to see if it is normal in appearance. Is there evidence of kyphosis, scoliosis, lordosis, or kyphoscoliosis?

Check the AP diameter. Is the AP diameter increased, suggesting evidence of barrel chest? If the patient is barrel chested, do the digits show evidence of clubbing?

Take time to carefully observe the chest. Develop a systematic approach. Initially, it is helpful to make a brief outline of all steps to be followed in assessment. Refer to this list when practicing in the laboratory. This list will help to reinforce a mental image of the tasks being performed.

Palpation

Methodically palpate the chest posteriorly and anteriorly. Determine if there are areas of tenderness and assess the skin temperature. Palpate for subcutaneous emphysema while moving over the surface of the chest.

To evaluate chest wall motion, place the hands as shown in Figures 3-12 and 3-13. Ask the patient to take a deep breath. Observe the motion of the hands as they move apart upon the patient's inspiration. Is the motion symmetrical? Do the hands move at all? (Patients with obstructive lung disease will exhibit little or no chest excursion on inspiration.) If one area is not symmetrical in its motion, make a mental note of it. When percussing the chest, carefully assess the side that demonstrated little motion.

To evaluate tactile fremitus, place the palmar surface of the hands on the patient's chest (Figure 3-15). Alternately, the ulnar surface of the hands may be used (Figure 3-16). Ask the patient to say "ninety-nine" repeatedly. Progressively move the hands over the chest, feeling tactile fremitus. Determine if there are areas of increased fremitus (potential consolidation).

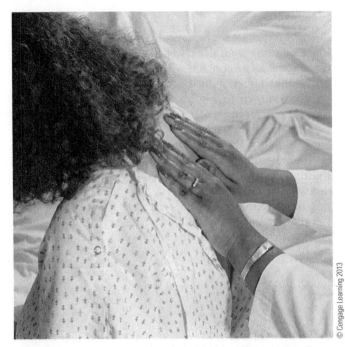

Figure 3-15   Assessment of tactile fremitus using the palmar surface of your hands

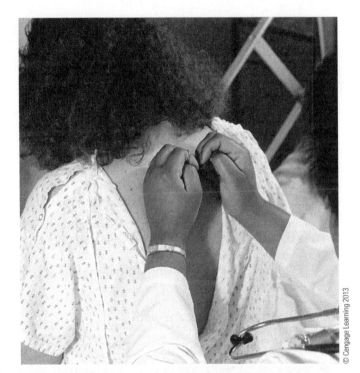

Figure 3-16   Assessment of tactile fremitus using the ulnar surface of your hands

Using an index finger, palpate at the sternal notch to assess tracheal position. Is the trachea central or deviated left or right? If it is deviated, make a mental note of which side. When percussing the chest, carefully assess the side opposite the tracheal deviation.

Percussion

Percuss the chest systematically over the entire surface. Place one finger on the chest, making sure that only the one finger is in contact with the surface of the chest. Strike that finger with the third finger on the opposite hand as shown in Figure 3-14. Progress from the top downward, comparing the tone generated by each side bilaterally. Position the finger in contact with the chest between the ribs. Do not percuss over the bone or a female patient's breast tissue. Note any changes in the tone, especially if it sounds dull (area of increased density).

The respiratory practitioner can easily assess diaphragmatic excursion on the posterior chest. Have the patient take a deep breath and hold it. Percuss down the posterior chest until dullness is heard. Now ask the patient to exhale completely and hold his or her breath. Percuss up from the mark, listening for resonance. Note this position. The distance between the two points is the diaphragmatic excursion, which may be as much as 8 centimeters in normal subjects.

Recording Your Findings

It is important to make a careful record of the findings. If abnormalities are found, note their position in relation to the imaginary vertical lines and the rib number. For example, the chart might read: "Dullness was heard on percussion anteriorly on the right side from the second to the fourth rib on the midclavicular line." Only by recording observations and serially comparing findings is physical assessment useful in following the course of a patient's progress.

References

Redden, S., Hunton, D., & Kaminsky, D. (2003). Diagnosis of a space occupying lesion by pulmonary function tests. *Respiratory Care, 48*(2), 138–141.

Wilkins, R., Evans, J., & Specht, L. (2002). A survey of physicians to identify their expectations of respiratory therapists in patient assessment. *Respiratory Care, 47*(5), 583–585.

Practice Activities: Advanced Patient Assessment

1. Using a laboratory partner, practice inspection of the chest. Include the following in your examination:
   a. Determination of respiratory rate and pattern
   b. Evaluation of the work of breathing
   c. Examination of the spine and sternum for abnormalities
   d. Comparison of the AP diameter and lateral diameter
   e. Inspection of the digits for clubbing or cyanosis

2. Using a laboratory partner, practice palpation of the chest. Assess for the following in your examination:
   a. Areas of tenderness
   b. Symmetry of movement anteriorly and posteriorly:
      (1) Upper lobes
      (2) Middle and lingular lobes
      (3) Lower lobes
   c. Tactile fremitus
   d. The presence of subcutaneous emphysema
   e. Deviation of tracheal position

3. Using a laboratory partner, practice percussing the chest. Include the following in your examination:
   a. Correct finger position and technique
   b. Systematic approach
   c. Bilateral comparison
   d. Diaphragmatic excursion

4. Describe specifically various anatomical locations in your practice using the coordinate system discussed in the theory text of this chapter.

5. Following completion of a physical examination of your laboratory partner's chest, document your findings on a piece of paper. Have your instructor critique your charting.

Check List: Advanced Patient Assessment

1. Inspect the chart:
   a. Admitting diagnosis
   b. History
   c. Laboratory tests
2. Assemble the equipment:
   a. Stethoscope
   b. Paper and pen
3. Identify the patient and introduce yourself.

4. Perform hand hygiene.
5. Optimize the environment:
   a. Turn off the radio or television.
   b. Ensure a comfortable temperature.
   c. Ensure the patient's privacy and adequate attire.
6. Explain the procedure.
7. Position the patient optimally.

8. Inspect the chest, observing the following:
_____ a. Respiratory rate and rhythm
_____ b. Work of breathing
_____ c. Spine and sternum for deformities
_____ d. AP diameter
_____ e. Appearance of the digits for clubbing or cyanosis

9. Palpate the chest, including the following:
_____ a. Identify areas of tenderness.
_____ b. Evaluate for symmetry.
_____ c. Assess for tactile fremitus.
_____ d. Determine if subcutaneous emphysema is present.
_____ e. Determine the tracheal position.

10. Percuss the chest, including the following:
_____ a. Proper technique
_____ b. Systematic method
_____ c. Diaphragmatic excursion
_____ 11. Solicit a cough for sputum examination.
_____ 12. Ensure the patient's safety and comfort.
_____ 13. Solicit and answer questions.
_____ 14. Wash your hands.
_____ 15. Record your findings on the patient's chart.

Self-Evaluation Post Test: Physical Assessment of the Chest

1. The second rib may be easily identified by:
   a. palpating the process of the seventh cervical vertebra.
   b. palpating the sternal angle.
   c. palpating the sternal notch.
   d. palpating the xyphoid process.

2. Which of the following is not a vertical division line on the anterior chest?
   a. Anterior axillary line
   b. Midsternal line
   c. Midclavicular line
   d. Vertebral line

3. Eupnea is:
   a. rapid shallow breathing.
   b. deep and rapid breathing.
   c. deep breathing with a normal respiratory rate.
   d. normal breathing.

4. The correct term for deep rapid breathing is:
   a. eupnea.   c. tachypnea.
   b. bradypnea.   d. hyperpnea.

5. A lateral curvature of the spine is termed:
   a. lordosis.   c. scoliosis.
   b. kyphosis.   d. kyphoscoliosis.

6. A lateral curvature and humpback is termed:
   a. lordosis.   c. scoliosis.
   b. kyphosis.   d. kyphoscoliosis.

7. Which of the following may be assessed by palpation?
   I. Areas of tenderness
   II. Symmetry of chest excursion
   III. Resonance
   IV. Tracheal position
   a. I, III, IV   c. I, IV
   b. II, III, IV   d. I, II, IV

8. Which of the following percussion tones is a loud, low-pitched sound of long duration?
   a. Resonance   c. Dullness
   b. Hyperresonance   d. Flatness

9. Hyperresonance may be heard:
   a. over areas of increased density.
   b. over areas containing fluid.
   c. over the trachea.
   d. over areas containing trapped air.

10. A percussion tone heard over areas of roughly equal air and tissue ratio is:
    a. hyperresonance. c. dullness.
    b. resonance.   d. flatness.

CHAPTER 4
Radiologic Assessment

INTRODUCTION

The ability to interpret and review radiographic images of the chest is important to the practice of respiratory care. A respiratory practitioner is expected to identify the presence of a pneumothorax, subcutaneous emphysema, consolidation, atelectasis, and pulmonary infiltrates. The practitioner must also be able to identify the position of endotracheal, tracheostomy, nasogastric, and chest tubes as well as pulmonary artery and central venous catheters.

A patient's disease state is often manifested by changes in the chest radiograph. These changes may include hyperinflation, accumulation of pleural fluid, development of pulmonary edema, increase in hilar markings, and mediastinal shift. The respiratory practitioner must be able to relate changes in the chest radiograph with changes in signs and symptoms presented by the patient.

Special radiographic procedures such as ventilation-perfusion scanning and angiography are used in the diagnosis of pulmonary embolism. The respiratory practitioner must be able to recognize abnormal changes associated with ventilation-perfusion mismatching and how loss of circulation to an area or segment of the lung is manifested radiographically.

Computed tomography (CT) imaging is becoming more common in the acute care setting. As a respiratory practitioner, it is essential to be able to use CT findings to aid the diagnosis and management of patients.

KEY TERMS

- Anterior-posterior
- Apical lordotic
- Atelectasis
- Computed tomography
- Consolidation
- Exposed
- Hilum
- Hyperinflation
- Lateral

- Lateral decubitus
- Lateral neck
- Left anterior oblique
- Mediastinal shift
- Pleural effusion
- Pneumomediastinum
- Pneumothorax
- Posterior-anterior
- Pulmonary angiography

- Pulmonary infiltrate
- Radiodensity
- Right anterior oblique
- Subcutaneous emphysema
- Tomogram
- Unexposed
- Ventilation-perfusion scanning

THEORY OBJECTIVES

At the end of this chapter, the reader should be able to:

- *Describe how an x-ray film of the chest is produced.*
- *Describe the differences in radiodensity of the following:*
  - *Air*
  - *Water*
  - *Fat*
  - *Bone*
  - *Plastic*
  - *Metal*
- *Differentiate among the following x-ray views of the chest:*
  - *Anterior-posterior (AP)*
  - *Posterior-anterior (PA)*
  - *Lateral*
  - *Apical lordotic*

  - *Left anterior oblique*
  - *Right anterior oblique*
  - *Lateral decubitus*
  - *Lateral neck*
- *Identify the anatomical structures and landmarks observed on normal PA and lateral chest x-ray views.*
- *Given an abnormal chest radiograph, identify the presence of extrapulmonary air:*
  - *Pneumothorax*
  - *Subcutaneous emphysema*
  - *Pneumomediastinum*
- *Given an abnormal chest radiograph, identify the following changes in lung volume:*
  - *Hyperinflation*

- *Atelectasis*
- *Mediastinal shi*
- *Consolidation*
- Given an abnorm est radiograph, identify the following fluid-related abn lities:
  - *Pleural effus*
  - *Congestive failure*
  - *Pulmonary na*
  - *Pulmonary rates*
- Given a chest ograph of a critically ill patient, identify the following:
  - *Endotrac tube*
  - *Trach y tube*
  - *Pulm artery catheter*
  - *Centra ious catheter*
  - *Naso ic tube*

- *Feeding tube*
- *Electrocardiography (ECG) leads*
- *Pacemaker wires*
- *Surgical clips or staples*
- *Foreign bodies*
- *Describe the technique of ventilation-perfusion scanning.*
- *Given a ventilation-perfusion (V/Q) scan, identify the presence and location of a ventilation-perfusion mismatch.*
- *Describe the technique of pulmonary angiography.*
- *Given an abnormal pulmonary angiogram, identify circulatory occlusion.*
- *Describe how a computed tomography (CT) scan of the chest is made.*
- *Given a CT scan of the chest, locate the cut you are viewing superiorly and inferiorly with respect to the scout image.*

PRO UCTION OF A CH T RADIOGRAPH

X-ray e a form of ionizing radiation, having a very rt wavelength of between 0.05 and 100 angstro Å). X-rays are produced by the x-ray tubes in -ray machine. A very high voltage (100 to 40 ovolts) from the x-ray machine's transformer is ducted to the x-ray tube, where it bombards a itively charged tungsten target contained in the near-vacuum of the x-ray tube (Wallace, 1995). The deflected electrons undergo physical changes after striking the tungsten target and are emitted as x-radiation (Figure 4-1). Once produced, x-rays will scatter in all directions; a narrow window channels the x-ray emissions toward the desired target. The energy not emitted by the tube is absorbed and does not escape. However, because of the x-ray's tendency to scatter, the beam will spread as distance increases from the x-ray tube. This is similar to how a flashlight beam enlarges as the distance from the bulb increases.

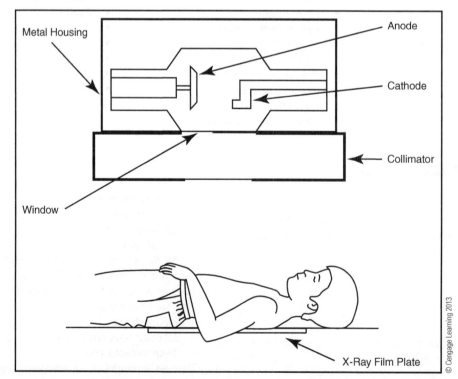

© Cengage Learning 2013

Figure 4-1 This figure illustrates how an x-ray is produced. Note the tungsten target and the window that limits the scatter of the x-ray energy

X-ray emissions, being very short wavelength electromagnetic energy, tend to penetrate objects rather than to be reflected by them as happens with energy in the visible light spectrum. The degree to which x-ray energy penetrates an object is dependent on the density of the object. If the density of the object is great, penetration is low. If the density of the object is low, penetration by x-radiation is greater. When the object of interest is placed between the x-ray tube and a sheet of photographic film, shadows are cast onto the film. The density of these shadows—light or dark—will depend on the *radiodensity* of the material between the x-ray tube and the film plane. Areas of low density will appear dark, or *exposed*, whereas areas of high density will appear white, or *unexposed*, when the film is developed. For imaging of the chest using x-rays, the patient is placed between the x-ray tube and the film plane, and shadows are cast onto the film depending on the densities of the anatomical structures the x-ray energy passes through.

RADIODENSITY OF COMMON MATERIALS

The radiodensity of anatomical structures or tissues and manmade materials is dependent on how dense the material is. An x-ray image of the chest will show many shades between black (low density) to white (high density), depending on what material the x-ray energy passes through. Common structures x-ray energy may pass through during imaging of the chest are air, water, fat, bone, plastic, and metal. All of these materials have varying radiodensities.

Air is the least radiodense of the structures x-radiation passes through during imaging of the chest. Being of low radiodensity, air is readily penetrated by the x-rays, fully exposing the x-ray film. When the film is developed, air-filled areas appear black on the x-ray image. The dark radiolucent air-filled spaces provide a good contrast to the denser tissues surrounding the air-filled alveoli and bronchi.

Water has a greater radiodensity than that of air. Some of the x-ray energy is absorbed, while the majority passes through to the x-ray film. Water, therefore, casts a gray shadow on the x-ray film when it is developed.

Fat tissue has a greater radiodensity than that of water. Fat tissue absorbs more x-ray energy than water does. The shadow produced on the developed x-ray film by fat is a lighter shade of gray than that produced by water.

Bone has the greatest density of all of the anatomical structures in the chest. The majority of x-ray energy is absorbed by bone. A bony structure, therefore, casts a white (unexposed) shadow on the developed x-ray film.

Manmade materials may also be visualized on a chest radiograph. Common materials are plastics (mostly polyvinyl chloride [PVC]) and metal. Plastics are used to make artificial airways and indwelling catheters. In its natural state, plastic has a low radiodensity, similar

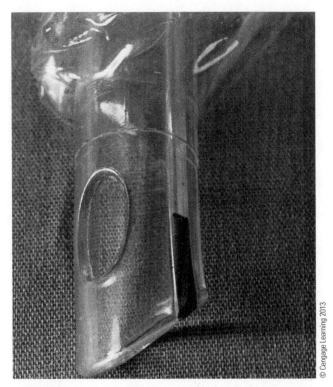

Figure 4-2 A photograph of an endotracheal tube. Notice the radiopaque line along the length of the tube extending to the distal tip

© Cengage Learning 2013

to that of fat. However, for easy visualization of these devices on an x-ray image, a radiopaque line is molded into the manufactured object (Figure 4-2). This feature allows for a more precise determination of the position of the object.

Metal is the most radiodense material viewed on a chest x-ray. Surgical clips, staples, and wire are common and are readily identified as small, thin white lines. These appear brighter than bony structures. Foreign objects made of metal that are nonsurgical may also appear on the chest film. Such objects may include bullets, coins, buckshot, or other items that have entered the thoracic cavity.

X-RAY VIEWS OF THE CHEST

Many different views of the chest can be obtained using x-ray techniques. Some views are named by the way the x-ray energy passes through the chest (anterior-posterior or posterior-anterior); others, by the way the patient is oriented (lordotic, oblique, lateral, lateral decubitus). The practitioner must know the common views of the chest, why specific views are used, and how they enhance the imaging of the chest.

The *posterior-anterior* (PA) view of the chest is one of the most common x-ray views (Figure 4-3). For the PA view, the film cassette rests on the anterior surface of the chest and the x-ray energy passes from the posterior surface through the chest, exposing the film on

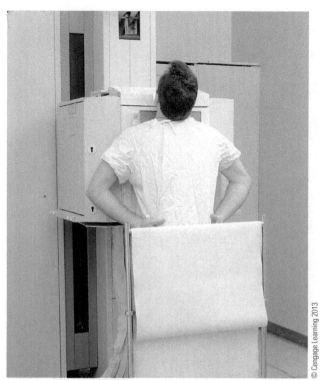

Figure 4-3   A posterior-anterior projection of the chest. Note the position of the x-ray tube, patient, and film cassette. The x-rays pass from the posterior to the anterior surface

Figure 4-4   An anterior-posterior projection of the chest. Note the position of the x-ray tube, patient, and film cassette. The x-rays pass from the anterior to the posterior surface

the anterior surface of the chest. Because the heart is more anterior than posterior within the chest, the heart shadow is smaller on a PA image than on the anterior-posterior view.

For the *anterior-posterior* (AP) view of the chest, the film cassette rests on the posterior surface of the chest and the x-ray energy passes from the anterior surface through the chest, exposing the film (Figure 4-4). The AP view is most commonly obtained by use of a "portable" technique. In the portable AP view, a mobile x-ray machine is brought to the patient's bedside, the film cassette is slid under the patient, and the x-ray picture is taken. Because the heart is more anterior, the heart shadow is magnified slightly in the AP view. Portable chest films are often used to verify tube placement (of an endotracheal, or chest tube, for example), to identify pneumothoraces, to locate foreign bodies, and so on.

For the *lateral* view, the film cassette rests on the left lateral surface of the chest, and the x-rays pass from the right side of the body through the chest, exposing the film (Figure 4-5). Because an x-ray image is a two-dimensional view or rendering, both the PA and the lateral films must be compared to locate precisely an anomaly or an object. By comparing the PA and the lateral films, a three-dimensional image may be created.

Sometimes it is necessary to focus attention on the upper lobes of the lungs. In a conventional PA view, the clavicles obscure part of the desired field of view. For the *apical lordotic* view (Figure 4-6), the patient leans backward at about 45°. This positioning moves the

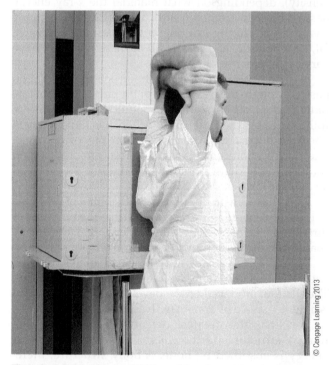

Figure 4-5   A lateral projection of the chest. Note the position of the x-ray tube, patient, and film cassette

shadow of the clavicles out of the way, allowing better imaging of the upper lobes of the lungs.

For the *lateral decubitus* view of the chest, the patient is in a side-lying position, and the film cassette rests on

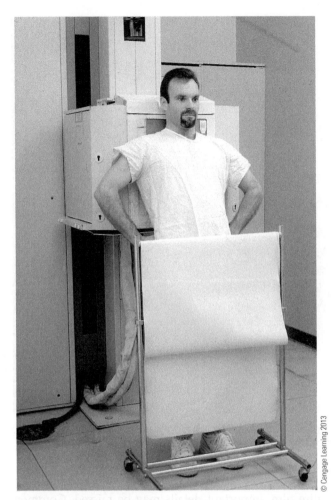

Figure 4-6 An apical lordotic projection of the chest. Note that the patient is reclined approximately 45°, moving the clavicle's shadows

the posterior surface of the chest (Figure 4-7). This view is used to identify and quantify the extent of pleural effusion (liquid in the pleural space). Because liquid is denser than air, it will travel to the dependent (inferior) portion of the lung, creating a shadow that lies along a plane parallel with the surface the patient is lying on (Figure 4-8).

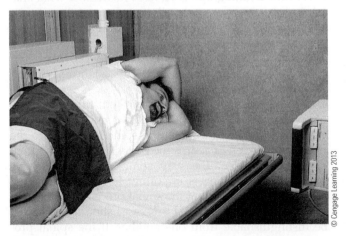

Figure 4-7 A lateral decubitus projection. Note that the patient is in a side-lying position. Any fluid present in the pleural space will migrate dependently and appear as a layer at the most inferior point

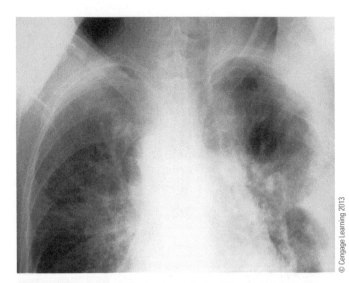

Figure 4-8 Pleural effusion is evident on the lateral decubitus view of the chest. Note the layer along the dependent portion of the chest wall

For the *left anterior oblique* view, the patient is rotated to the right (left side more forward) with the film cassette placed against the anterior surface of the chest (Figure 4-9). For the *right anterior oblique* view, the patient is rotated to the left (right side more forward) with the film cassette placed against the anterior surface of the chest (Figure 4-10). These views are used to shift the heart shadow so that the lung (left or right) is more easily visualized. These views are commonly used in ventilation-perfusion scanning, which is discussed later in the chapter.

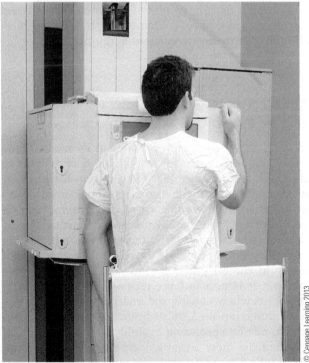

Figure 4-9 A left anterior oblique projection of the chest. Note the position of the x-ray tube, patient, and film cassette

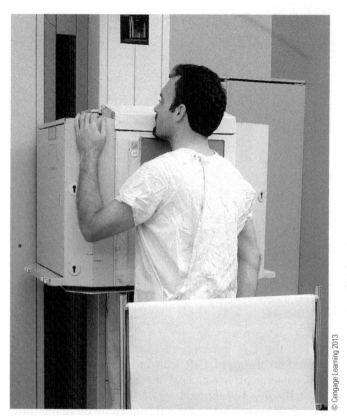

Figure 4-10 A right anterior oblique projection of the chest. Note the position of the x-ray tube, patient, and film cassette

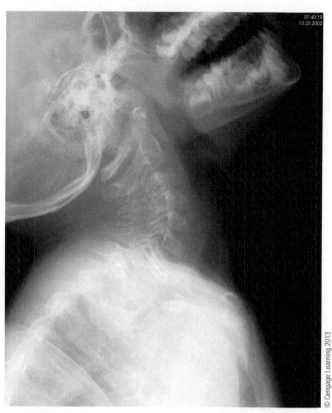

Figure 4-11 A lateral neck radiograph for soft tissue assessment. Note the swollen epiglottis almost in the shape of a finger

The *lateral neck* view is used to image the soft tissues of the upper airway. This view is commonly used in pediatrics to image the epiglottis and the larynx. In acute epiglottitis, the epiglottis becomes swollen and may obstruct the airway. Figure 4-11 is a lateral neck radiograph showing an enlarged epiglottis.

THE NORMAL CHEST RADIOGRAPH

A normal chest radiograph contains in its image many normal anatomical structures. Reading a chest film or radiograph requires the ability to distinguish those normal structures and their normal positions from others that are abnormal. Reading chest radiographs requires repeated practice, much as in auscultating breath sounds. The instructor may provide initial orientation to reading chest radiographs, providing the basics for minimal competency in clinical practice. However, to become more proficient, it is best to have repeated discussions with radiologists when viewing and interpreting patient films. Only through repeated, guided practice can the practitioner become more proficient in ability.

One of the most important aspects of reading chest radiographs is consistency. Often an abnormality stands out on the chest film, focusing attention on that feature. If the practitioner is not systematic in looking at the

entire film, important details may be missed. Common systematic approaches include the "outside-in" and the "inside-out" approaches. With the outside-in approach, the film is viewed moving from outside the chest to inside the chest. With the inside-out approach, the film is viewed moving from the heart to the structures lying on the outside of the chest wall. Some practitioners may prefer to use a technique of progressing from one level of radiodensity (high density) to the next lower density. Whatever approach adopted, be consistent, applying it every time a radiograph is viewed. Remember what anatomical structures are normally present, and do not miss evaluating each one upon viewing the film.

Figures 4-12 and 4-13 are normal PA and lateral views of the chest. On the PA film (see Figure 4-12), first determine if the patient is rotated and how well the radiograph was penetrated (exposed).

To evaluate if the patient is rotated, find the heads of both clavicles. The spine should lie right between the clavicles (see Figure 4-12). If the spine lies either to the right or to the left of center, the patient is rotated. Patient rotation can affect the way some structures appear; therefore, this finding is important to note. Penetration is evaluated by assessing the spinal processes in the center of the chest. The spinal processes should just barely be distinguishable from one another. If the spinal processes are very distinct, with dark lines separating them, the radiograph is overpenetrated (overexposed) with x-ray energy. A film that is overpenetrated will appear

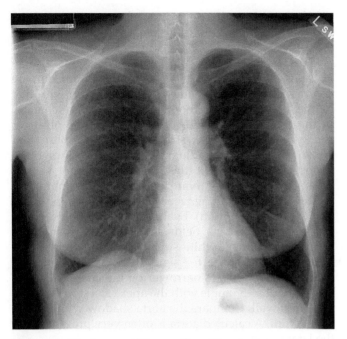

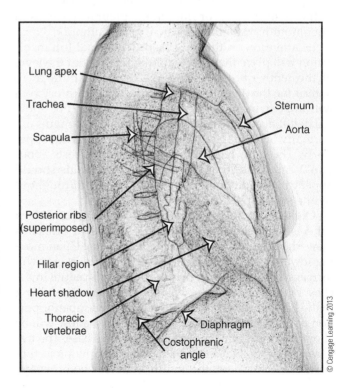

Figure 4-12   A normal PA x-ray film of the chest

darker and may be incorrectly interpreted as "normal" when the lung fields are evaluated. An underpenetrated film will appear lighter; this technical error may also lead to an incorrect interpretation.

The outer surface of the chest wall (light gray) is silhouetted against the stark dark background of air that surrounds the chest (black). Evaluate the areas outside of the chest wall, observing for dark (black) streaks against the gray tissue, indicating subcutaneous air (Figure 4-14). Air will tend to migrate upward (superiorly). Next evaluate the ribs. Trace each rib from the sternum laterally to where it joins the spine. Look for fractures (thin dark lines with or without separation), old healed fractures (increased radiodensity, making them whiter, and sometimes misshapen), and missing ribs or other anomalies. Evaluate the sternum, looking

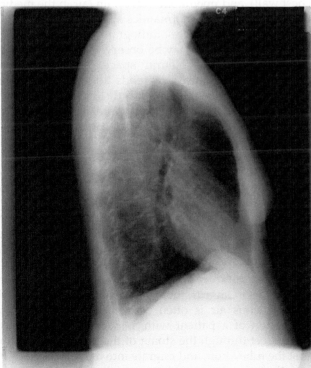

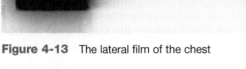

Figure 4-13   The lateral film of the chest

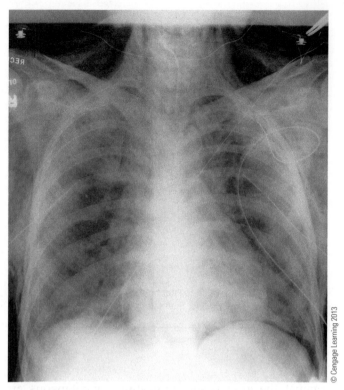

© Cengage Learning 2013

Figure 4-14 An AP projection showing subcutaneous emphysema. Note the air markings (dark streaks) that are extrapulmonary

it bifurcates into the right and left mainstem bronchi. In most films, the carina is visible and is used as a landmark for endotracheal tube placement.

The lateral chest radiograph (see Figure 4-13) may be assessed in a similar way to the PA film. Compare contrast of the tissue shadows (extrathoracic) with that of the black ambient room air. Observe for changes in the tissue density, indicating the presence of air or fluid. Evaluate the bony structures (ribs, sternum, and spine). Evaluate the radiograph for kyphosis or other abnormalities. Look at the diaphragm; there should be a slight upward curvature of the hemidiaphragms. Flattened hemidiaphragms are indicative of hyperinflation (discussed later on). Evaluate the lung fields. As on the PA view, the lung fields should appear black with vascular markings (white streaks). Look closely at the retrosternal air space for signs of hyperinflation. The heart shadow appears narrower on the lateral film and lies at about a 45° angle with the apex closest to the anterior chest wall. Compare the aorta shadow with that on the PA film. A calcified aorta is often very prominent on the lateral film.

COMMON ABNORMALITIES ON THE CHEST RADIOGRAPH

Extrapulmonary Air

Air is sometimes present outside of the lung parenchyma, which is not normal. Sources of extrapulmonary air include pneumothorax (air in the pleural space), subcutaneous emphysema (air in the soft tissues surrounding the chest wall), and pneumomediastinum (air in the mediastinal space). These abnormalities all may be identified on standard PA and AP chest radiographs.

A *pneumothorax* may be observed as a dark (black) shadow along the pleural space, usually superior (Figure 4-15) because air tends to migrate upward (superiorly). A pneumothorax is distinguished from the lung fields by the absence of vascular markings. The extent of a pneumothorax is often quantified (as 5% or 10%, for example), and its location (right or left) is identified. A pneumothorax is often caused by trauma; therefore, it is important to evaluate the bony structures of the chest and the aorta for injury. Larger pneumothoraces are treated by placement of a chest tube that is connected to a vacuum source to reexpand the affected lung. Very small pneumothoraces may not be treated but may simply be watched to ensure that they do not become larger.

Subcutaneous emphysema is presence of air in the soft tissues in an extrathoracic location (see Figure 4-14). Subcutaneous air is often associated with mechanical ventilation of a patient with a tracheostomy tube. Air can dissect through the stoma of the tracheostomy tube, past the tube's cuff, and migrate into the soft tissues. This extrathoracic air is not dangerous but should be noted

for any fractures or costochondral separations from the ribs (ribs separated from the sternum). Evaluate the spinal processes, observing for fractures, abnormal curvature (lordosis), or other changes. Evaluate the pleural space. Check for abnormal thickening (increased radiodensity), or air or fluid in the pleural space (as in pneumothorax, pleural effusion, or hemothorax). Next, focus attention on the lung fields. A normal full inspiration will place the hemidiaphragms at about the level of the tenth rib. Count the ribs to the diaphragm to determine the degree of inspiration. An expiratory film will appear more dense (cloudy) and may not show the detail needed to evaluate. The hemidiaphragms are normally arch-shaped, domed structures, arcing superiorly. The right hemidiaphragm normally rests about 1 to 2 cm higher than the left. The lung fields should appear black (air) with vascular markings throughout (white streaks).

Occasionally the practitioner will observe round black spheres surrounded by a thin white line (a bronchus viewed end on when viewing a lateral film). Upon moving toward the heart (*hilum*), the vascular markings will increase, becoming more dense. The heart is central in the chest radiograph with the major portion of the heart lying to the left and the aortic knob visible on the superior portion of the heart shadow. A normal heart shadow will be about half the diameter of the PA film at its base. The trachea can be distinguished by its dark shadow projecting downward to about the fourth vertebral body, where

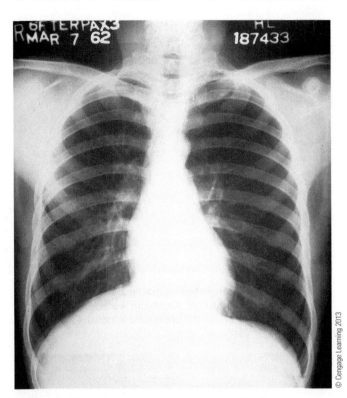

Figure 4-15   A PA projection showing a 10% left pneumothorax. Note that the pneumothorax is more evident toward the apex of the lung in this upright patient

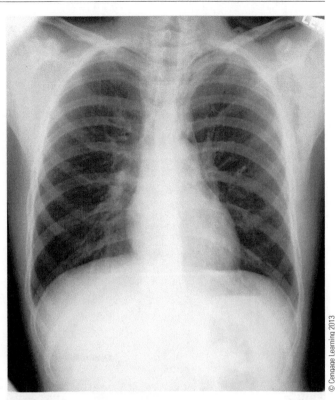

Figure 4-16   A portable chest x-ray film showing a pneumomediastinum. Note the dark thin sliver of air along the lateral heart border

and observed. Eventually, the air will be absorbed by the tissue, and the condition will resolve spontaneously (without treatment).

Pneumomediastinum occurs when air dissects into the mediastinal space (Figure 4-16). On an upright film, the dark, air-filled space may extend up into the neck. The air-filled space separates the visceral pleura from the parietal pleura of the mediastinum. In adults, pneumomediastinum may be secondary to trauma, including that affecting the large airways (Pierson & Kacmarek, 1992).

Changes in Lung Volume

Changes in lung volumes may often be observed radiographically. Changes in lung volume may occur because of hyperinflation, atelectasis, or consolidation. Sometimes, as a result of unilateral lung volume changes, the mediastinum may shift to the affected side, owing to the greater expansion of the unaffected lung. This finding is termed *mediastinal shift*.

Hyperinflation is often a finding in patients with chronic obstructive pulmonary disease (COPD). In the hyperinflated chest radiograph (Figure 4-17), the hemidiaphragms extend beyond the tenth rib space and no longer maintain their characteristic domed shape. The hemidiaphragms are flatter, being displaced downward by the overdistended lung fields. In the lateral view

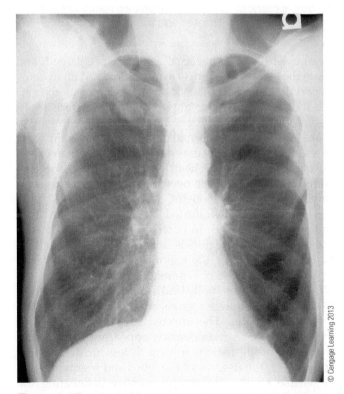

Figure 4-17   A PA projection of the chest showing hyperinflation. Note the darker appearance of the film, the diaphragm's position (around the twelfth rib), the diaphragm's flattened shape, and the increased spacing between the ribs

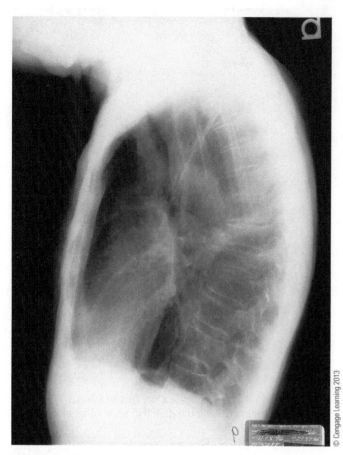

Figure 4-18 A lateral projection illustrating hyperinflation. Note the dark appearance of the film, the flattened hemidiaphragms, and the enlarged retrosternal air space

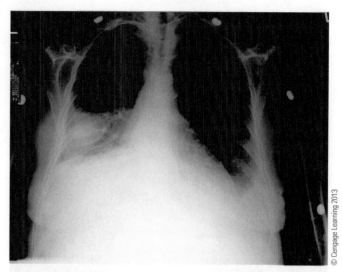

Figure 4-19 A PA projection illustrating atelectasis in the right upper lobe. Note that the right diaphragm is elevated even more than normal; the density of the upper lobe is increased

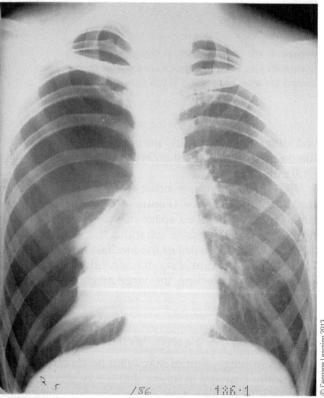

Figure 4-20 A portable chest film showing a tension pneumothorax. Note the absence of lung markings on the right and the decreased density compared with the left. Note the mediastinal shift and that the right lung has been compressed into a very small space

(Figure 4-18), the retrosternal air space is enlarged, and again the hemidiaphragms are much flatter. With extreme hyperinflation, the rib spaces become larger as the ribs are forced apart by the trapped gas. Characteristically, hyperinflated chest radiographs appear darker (owing to more air space) than normal chest radiographs. In some cases, the heart shadow may also be narrower than on the normal chest film. The heart and mediastinum become compressed between the overdistended lung fields, narrowing the cardiac silhouette.

Atelectasis is manifested by a reduction in lung volume (Figure 4-19). In obstructive atelectasis, gas in the affected lung region is absorbed by the capillary blood flow, reducing the region's volume. If the atelectasis involves a lobe or segment, the diaphragm on the affected side may actually be displaced slightly upward, as the unaffected lung regions are pulled or tethered by the affected lung. The affected area is characterized by an increase in radiodensity, appearing lighter than the surrounding regions (owing to less air density). In some cases, the fissures of the lobes and segments may be visible on the radiograph, further delineating the extent of the process (McMahon, 1999). In compressive atelectasis, pneumothorax, hemothorax, pleural effusion, or another space-occupying anomaly compresses the surrounding lung tissue, reducing its volume.

The size of the anomaly will determine the extent to which the lung is compressed. In severe cases, such as in tension pneumothorax, the mediastinum is displaced toward the unaffected side and the unaffected lung is compressed (Figure 4-20). This is a life-threatening

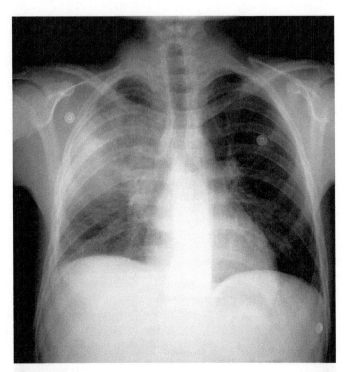

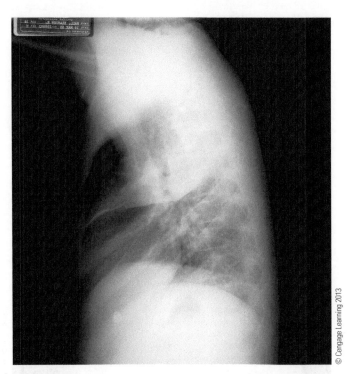

Figure 4-21 Consolidation of the right apical posterior segment (left). Compare the lateral film (right) showing the posterior nature of the consolidation

condition that requires immediate treatment (by chest tube placement).

Consolidation occurs when air-filled portions of the lung become fluid-filled, sometimes without loss of volume. Consolidation is often secondary to bacterial pneumonia. The consolidated lung region demonstrates an increased radiodensity, appearing lighter than the surrounding lung fields. Consolidation is often lobar, and when the PA projection is compared with the lateral, the lobe or segment may be easily identified (Figure 4-21).

Fluid Abnormalities

Fluid abnormalities manifested on chest radiographs may include pleural effusion, congestive failure, pulmonary edema, and pulmonary infiltrates. Any fluid abnormality will result in an increased opacity on the radiograph compared with that on a normal film. The type of abnormality will determine how it is characterized on the chest film.

Pleural effusion is the collection of fluid in the pleural space. The characteristic sign of pleural effusion on the PA projection is blunting of the costophrenic angles (Figure 4-22). Normally, the costophrenic angle is a sharply defined narrow angle at the lateral margin of the diaphragm (see Figure 4-12). The presence of pleural effusion will tend to obscure this angle, blunting it on the upright film. On a lateral decubitus film (see Figure 4-7), the fluid will form a uniform layer (at the most inferior portion of the lung), parallel to the surface the patient is lying on. In profound cases, pleural

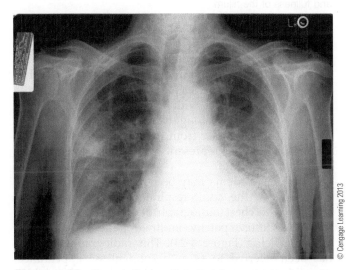

Figure 4-22 Pleural effusion. Note that the costophrenic angle is obscured

effusion may result in significant volume loss (compressive atelectasis). A thoracentesis may be performed to drain the fluid from the pleural space, reexpanding the lung.

Congestive heart failure (CHF) is often manifested on the chest radiograph. An early sign of CHF is an enlargement of the left ventricle of the heart (Pierson & Kacmarek, 1992). As the efficiency of the ventricle to pump blood declines, increasing pressure affects the lungs, causing fluid to migrate into the interstitial space (Kazerooni & Cascade, 1999). Pulmonary vascular

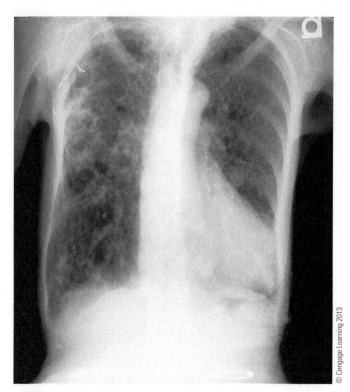

Figure 4-23   A PA projection illustrating congestive heart failure. Note the enlarged heart shadow and the increased size and fullness of the hilum

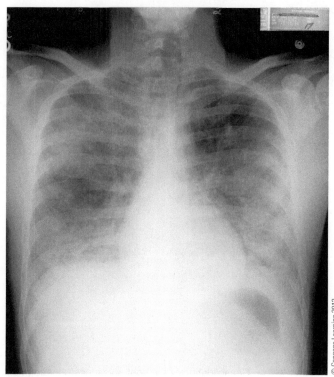

Figure 4-24   A portable film illustrating radiographic appearance in the adult respiratory distress syndrome (ARDS). Note the almost uniform patchy infiltrate pattern throughout both lung fields

consolidation occurs throughout the mediastinal area and may extend into the upper lobes (Figure 4-23). The increased fluid density results in a greater opacity of the radiograph compared with the normal film. Kerley B lines may be present along the right base of the PA film, extending horizontally from the periphery of the lung. These opaque lines represent lymphatic vessels that are engorged with fluid.

Pulmonary edema may be noncardiogenic in origin, such as with the adult respiratory distress syndrome (ARDS). The chest radiograph of a patient with ARDS shows a diffuse patchy infiltrate pattern throughout the lung fields (Figure 4-24). This radiographic pattern has been referred to as a "ground glass" appearance, describing the uniform opacity the radiograph exhibits. This infiltrate pattern represents alveolar edema and interstitial edema with regions of localized atelectasis. As the disease progresses, later chest radiographs may demonstrate changes in density from fibrosis and scarring of the tissue subsequent to the disease process.

A *pulmonary infiltrate* is visible radiographically as an area of the lung with increased opacity, appearing lighter on the chest film (Figure 4-25). Pulmonary infiltrates are often secondary to pneumonia and involve lung tissue diffusely, often in a segmental or lobar distribution. Because of the presence of fluid in these regions, the radiodensity is greater than normal. On so-called *air bronchograms*, the bronchus is seen surrounded by fluid-filled structures, creating a distinct separation between the regions of differing densities (air versus

fluid). Comparison of the lateral projection with the PA projections will help to differentiate the lobe or segment that is involved.

Foreign Objects

Besides normal anatomical structures, foreign objects may also be viewed on chest radiographs. Such objects include artificial airways, chest tubes, central catheters, feeding tubes, nasogastric tubes, and surgical clips or staples. In the critical care setting, chest radiographs are used to confirm the position and placement of these devices and to determine whether, once they have been placed, their position has changed.

Artificial airways viewed on chest radiographs include endotracheal tubes and tracheostomy tubes. The portable (AP) chest radiograph is used to confirm correct placement of the endotracheal tube following its insertion. Figure 4-26 illustrates the placement of an endotracheal tube. When the tube is placed correctly, its distal tip should be positioned 2 to 3 cm above the carina.

Tracheostomy tubes are frequently used in caring for critically ill patients and for patients requiring long-term mechanical ventilation. Figure 4-27 shows a chest radiograph of a patient with a tracheostomy tube. Occasionally, tracheostomy tubes may become displaced into the soft tissue anterior to the trachea.

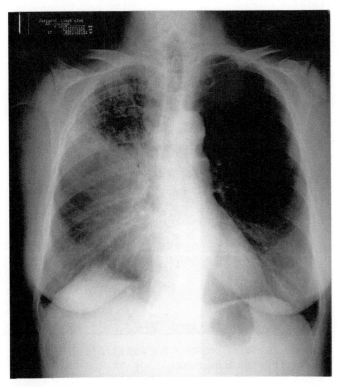

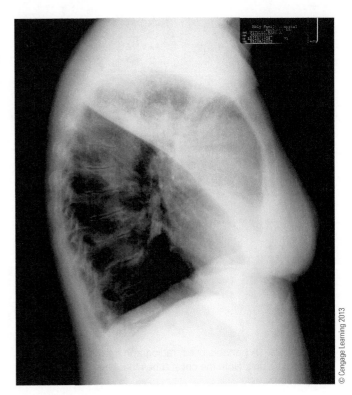

Figure 4-25 This PA projection shows a pulmonary infiltrate in the right upper lobe. Compare the PA projection with the lateral view

A lateral neck film will confirm that the tube is placed correctly in the trachea.

Chest tubes are inserted into the pleural space to evacuate air or fluid from the space to expand the lung fully. Most chest tubes are placed at about the fourth or fifth rib space laterally and are directed toward the apex of the affected lung (Figure 4-28). The proximal end of the chest tube is connected to a vacuum source, which continuously applies subambient pressure to the pleura, maintaining its position, thereby expanding the affected lung.

Central catheters used in the critical care setting include pulmonary artery catheters, central venous catheters, and intra-aortic balloon catheters. The pulmonary artery catheter passes through the right side of the heart (right atrium and right ventricle) and rests in the

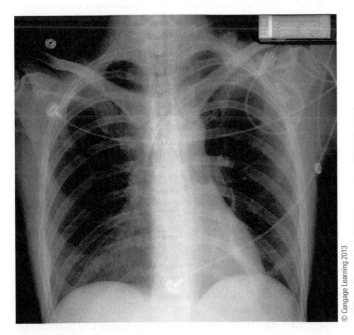

Figure 4-26 A portable film illustrating the placement of an endotracheal tube. Note the tip of the tube resting just above the carina

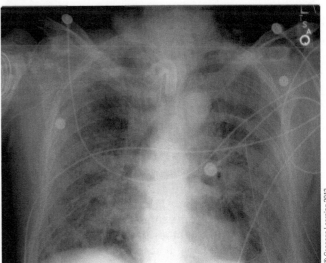

Figure 4-27 A portable film illustrating the presence of a tracheostomy tube

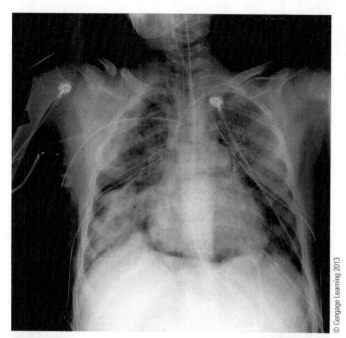

Figure 4-28 A portable chest radiograph from a patient in the intensive care unit. Note the chest tubes that have been placed in the right chest

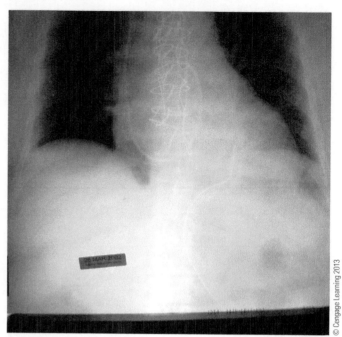

Figure 4-30 An AP projection that was taken to confirm the position of the intra-aortic balloon

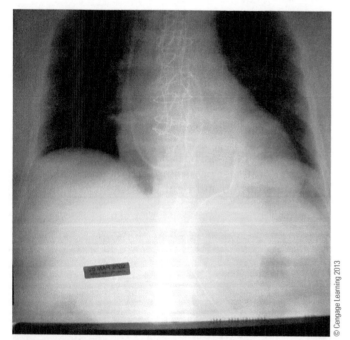

Figure 4-29 This portable film was taken to confirm the placement of a pulmonary artery catheter

pulmonary artery (Figure 4-29). The unique curve this catheter displays on the AP chest film makes it easily identifiable. The central venous catheter's tip rests in the vena cava or the right atrium. This catheter may be identified easily because it rests just inside of the cardiac silhouette. Placement of these lines may result in a pneumothorax because the venous system is accessed via the subclavian vein. Careful evaluation of the radio-

graph for a pneumothorax is part of the post–catheter placement assessment. The intra-aortic balloon pump is inserted through the femoral artery and advanced superiorly to the aorta. Figure 4-30 is a chest radiograph showing the placement of an intra-aortic balloon pump catheter.

Gastric tubes include both nasogastric tubes and feeding tubes. The nasogastric tube is passed through the esophagus, and its distal tip rests in the stomach. The nasogastric tube removes the stomach contents by application of low continuous subambient (vacuum) pressure. Figure 4-31 illustrates the placement of the nasogastric tube. Sometimes the nasogastric tube is inserted following intubation, and the nasogastric tube may follow adjacent to the endotracheal tube and be inadvertently placed into the trachea. Careful evaluation of the correct placement of this tube is important. Feeding tubes are common in the intensive care environment. Feeding tubes are inserted through the esophagus and are generally placed in the small intestine. Many tubes have small weighted tips that assist in their placement and enhance radiographic visibility. Often these tubes are placed under direct radiographic visualization, using fluoroscopy.

Cardiac leads and wires include both ECG leads for monitoring purposes and cardiac pacemaker wires. The typical patient in an intensive care unit has three ECG leads placed (right and left shoulder and left axilla). Figure 4-32 illustrates the placement of these ECG leads. Cardiac pacemakers are commonly used to correct irregular heart rhythms. Figure 4-33 illustrates the placement of the pacemaker (left shoulder) and the pacemaker wire that is threaded through the venous system into the heart.

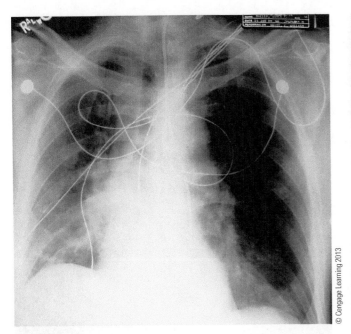

Figure 4-31 A portable film from a patient in the intensive care unit. Note the nasogastric tube

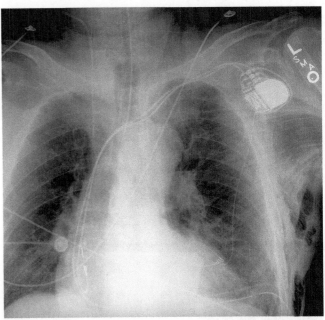

Figure 4-33 A pacemaker has been placed subcutaneously (above the left clavicle), and the pacer wire is evident

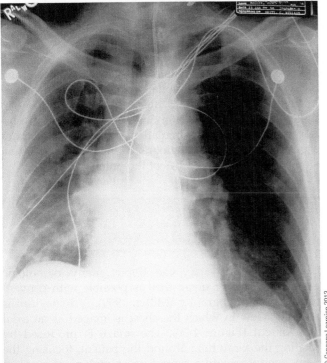

Figure 4-32 ECG leads are evident on this portable chest film

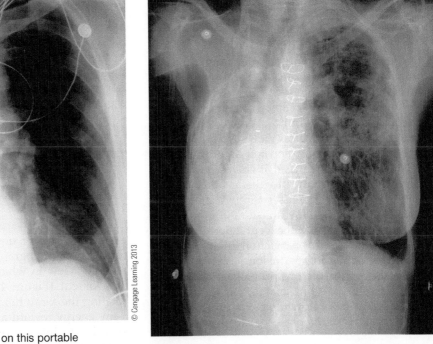

Figure 4-34 A portable chest film from a patient who had coronary artery bypass surgery. Note the wires that hold the sternum together

Surgical clips or staples and other foreign bodies are often seen on chest radiographs. Surgical clips and staples, used to hold bone and tissue together, are commonly used in thoracic surgery. Figure 4-34 is a chest radiograph from a patient following coronary artery bypass surgery. Note the wires holding the sternum together. Other foreign bodies may include bullets, knives, picks, nails, and other foreign objects. Figure 4-35 is a chest radiograph from a person who was shot by a shotgun. Note the numerous small pellets in the abdomen and lower thoracic cavity.

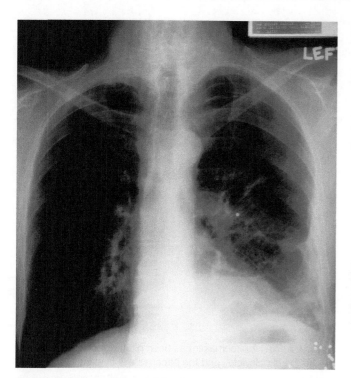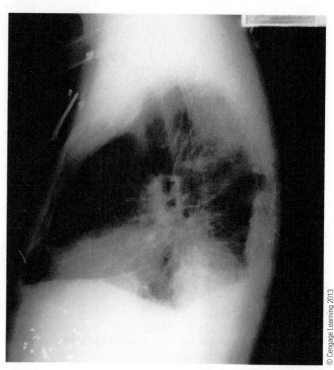

Figure 4-35   Multiple small foreign objects are evident in the abdomen and lower chest of this gunshot victim

VENTILATION-PERFUSION SCANNING

Ventilation-perfusion scanning permits comparison of lung ventilation with lung perfusion. For the ventilation scan, a radioactive gas (xenon) is inhaled while the lungs are scanned radiographically. The ventilation scan can detect defects (obstruction) to ventilation to lobes or segments of the lung. Typical views include the PA, lateral, right anterior oblique, and left anterior oblique (Figure 4-36). The perfusion scan involves injection of radioisotope-tagged albumin into the venous circulation. As the tagged albumin passes through the pulmonary vasculature, the lungs are scanned radiographically, using the same views as for the ventilation scan. The perfusion scan can detect obstruction in the pulmonary circulation. Ventilation-perfusion (V/Q) scans are used to diagnose or to rule out pulmonary embolism. Figure 4-37 illustrates V/Q mismatch; the scan is positive for pulmonary embolism (note the area showing absence of perfusion but the presence of ventilation).

PULMONARY ANGIOGRAPHY

Pulmonary angiography is another radiographic technique used to image the pulmonary vasculature. Pulmonary angiography is considered by some authorities to be more definitive in detecting pulmonary emboli. To perform a pulmonary angiogram, a pulmonary artery catheter is inserted through the venous system (via the subclavian vein) into the pulmonary artery, and radiopaque contrast material is injected into the pulmonary artery or into one of its branches. As the contrast medium passes through the pulmonary circulation, the chest is imaged radiographically. A positive angiogram is one in which the contrast medium fails to fill a branch or portion of the pulmonary circulation. Figure 4-38 illustrates a positive pulmonary angiogram. Note how circulation stops at one of the branches of the pulmonary artery.

COMPUTED TOMOGRAPHY OF THE CHEST

Computed tomography can depict many pathologic changes in greater detail than is possible with conventional chest radiography (Miller, 1999). A *tomogram* is an x-ray view in which the chest is imaged as an axial slice or cut (Figure 4-39). The image is produced by rotating the x-ray tube around the patient, focusing the x-ray energy toward a central point, making slices from superior to inferior or inferior to superior. The depth of the tomogram can vary (typically ranging from 3 to 1 cm), and as the depth becomes smaller, more detail is present. Computer systems allow much finer differentiation between shades of gray so that detection of far more subtle pathologic changes is possible (Miller, 1999). Figure 4-40 illustrates the first few cuts of a CT scan and the scout image. The scout image is a PA projection that indicates level and location of the slices or cuts made in the CT scan. One can relate the scout image to the desired level or cut (superior/inferior) of interest on the CT scan.

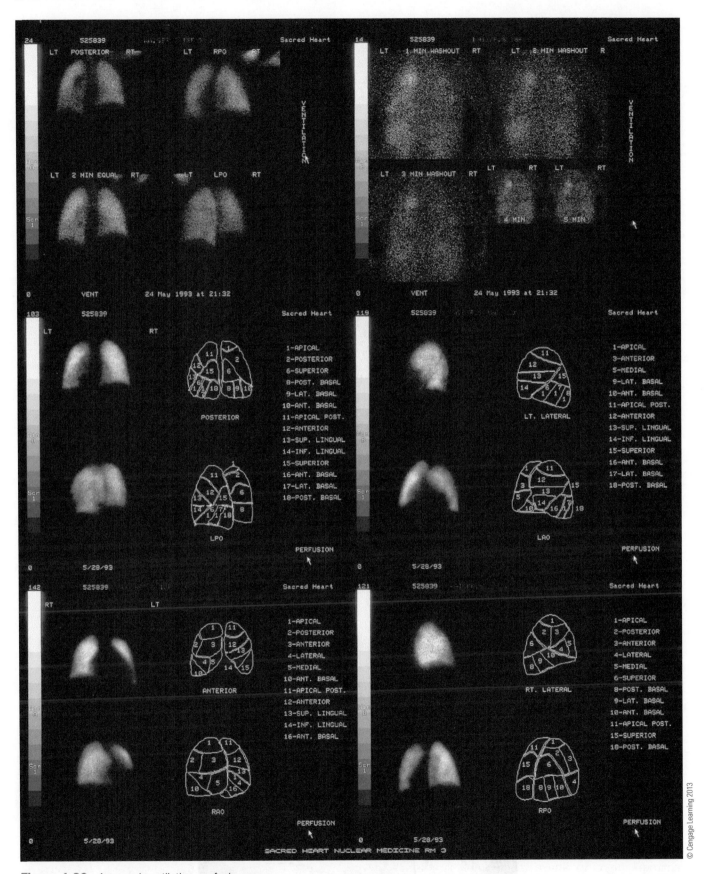

Figure 4-36   A normal ventilation-perfusion scan

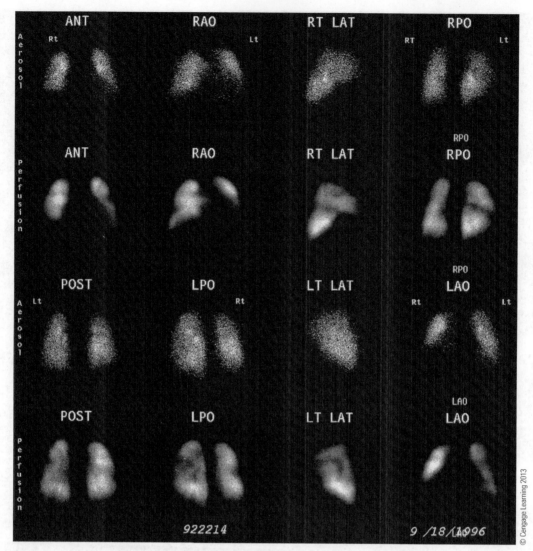

Figure 4-37 A ventilation-perfusion scan that is positive for pulmonary embolism

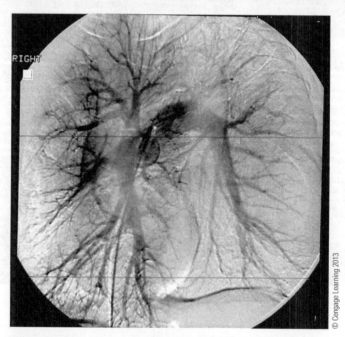

Figure 4-38 A pulmonary angiogram that is positive for pulmonary embolism. Note the area in which perfusion ceases (arrow)

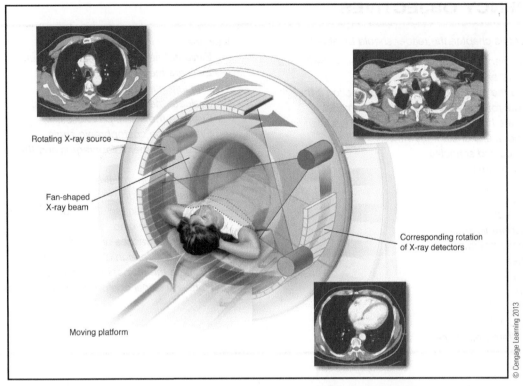

Figure 4-39 A CT scan is produced by making narrow focused cuts axially along the area of interest

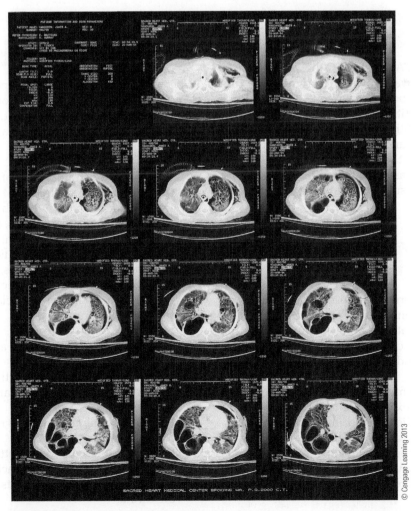

Figure 4-40 A CT scan of the chest

PROFICIENCY OBJECTIVES

At the end of this chapter, the reader should be able to:

- *Correctly orient a PA and a lateral chest radiograph on a view box for examination.*
- *Determine the penetration of the PA projection if the patient was rotated when the image was made.*
- *Demonstrate how to identify the following landmarks on the PA and lateral chest x-ray views:*
  - *Clavicles and scapulae*
  - *Spinal column*
  - *Ribs*
  - *Pleura*
  - *Lung fields*
  - *Costophrenic angle*
  - *Hemidiaphragms*
  - *Trachea*
  - *Carina*
  - *Hilum*
  - *Heart shadow*
  - *Aortic knob*
  - *Retrosternal air space*

- *View the x-ray in a systematic way:*
  - *Evaluate the extrathoracic soft tissue.*
  - *Evaluate the ribs, tracing each.*
  - *Evaluate the pleura.*
  - *Evaluate the sternum and clavicles.*
  - *Evaluate the spinal processes.*
  - *Evaluate the costophrenic angle.*
  - *Evaluate the hemidiaphragms and their relative positions.*
  - *Evaluate the lung fields.*
  - *Evaluate the hilum.*
  - *Evaluate the cardiac silhouette and estimate the cardiothoracic ratio.*
  - *Identify the trachea and carina.*
  - *Identify any foreign objects or lines.*
  - *Evaluate the retrosternal air space.*
  - *Note any spinal conformation deformities.*

CHEST FILM ORIENTATION

To correctly orient a PA chest film, the heart shadow should descend downward toward the right as the film is viewed on the view box. The patient's left should be aligned with the practitioner's right, as if the patient were facing the practitioner. Most chest radiographs will have the right (R) and left (L) marked with a radiopaque marker to assist in orientation of the film. The lateral film is oriented as if the patient is facing the PA film, with the lateral usually placed to the right of the PA film.

ROTATION AND PENETRATION

Patient rotation is determined by locating the neck of the clavicles and verifying that the spine lies equidistant between them. If the patient is rotated right or left, the spinal column will be closer to one side or the other or may even lie beyond the neck of one or the other clavicle.

Penetration is determined by examining the spinal column just above and extending into the cardiac silhouette. The vertebral bodies should just barely be distinguishable, without obvious dark spaces between them. If the vertebrae cannot be distinguished well, the film is underpenetrated. If the vertebrae are very pronounced, the film is overpenetrated and may appear unusually dark.

VIEWING THE CHEST RADIOGRAPH

When evaluating a chest radiograph, be sure to use a systematic approach each time. Through repeated practice, this approach will become habit, reducing the chance of missing important details that might otherwise go unnoticed:

1. Evaluate the extrathoracic soft tissue, observing for subcutaneous air or fluid.
2. Evaluate the ribs, tracing each, looking for fractures, healed fractures, missing ribs, or other deformities.
3. Evaluate the pleura, observing for changes in thickness and presence of air or fluid.
4. Evaluate the hemidiaphragms, noting the position of each diaphragm relative to the other.
5. Evaluate the sternum and clavicles, observing for fractures or deformities.
6. Evaluate the spinal processes.
7. Evaluate the costophrenic angles, observing for blunting.
8. Evaluate the lung fields, noting any unusual lung markings, opacities, nodular densities, or other abnormalities.
9. Evaluate the hilum, noting its relative size and extent of its fullness (radiodensity).
10. Evaluate the cardiac silhouette, noting the relative ratio of cardiac size and thoracic diameter.
11. Evaluate the trachea, noting its position, and identify the carina.

12. Identify any lines, artificial airways, ECG leads or pacemaker wires, nasogastric or feeding tubes, and chest tubes.
13. Evaluate the retrosternal air space on the lateral film.
14. Evaluate the hemidiaphragms and pleura on the lateral film.
15. Note and correlate any changes in opacity or other findings with the PA projection to form a three-dimensional image.

References

Kazerooni, E. A., & Cascade, P. (1999). Chest imaging in the cardiac intensive care unit. *Respiratory Care, 44*(9), 1033–1043.

McMahon, H. (1999). Pitfalls in portable chest radiology. *Respiratory Care, 44*(9), 1018–1032.

Miller, W. T. (1999). Uses of thoracic computed tomography in the intensive care unit. *Respiratory Care, 44*(9), 1127–1136.

Pierson, D. J., & Kacmarek, R. (1992). *Foundations of respiratory care.* New York: Churchill Livingstone.

Wallace, J. E. (1995). *Radiographic exposure principles & practice.* Philadelphia: F. A. Davis.

Practice Activities: Radiographic Evaluation

1. With a laboratory partner, practice orienting both PA and lateral chest films for viewing.
   a. Have your partner deliberately place the film incorrectly while you are not watching, and then correct it.

2. Identify the following landmarks for your laboratory partner:
   a. Clavicles, scapulae, ribs, sternum, spinal processes
   b. Pleura
   c. Costophrenic angle and hemidiaphragms
   d. Trachea and carina
   e. Hilum
   f. Heart silhouette and aortic knob; estimate the cardiothoracic ratio
   g. Retrosternal air space

3. With your laboratory partner, identify on a radiograph the presence of these manmade objects:
   a. Artificial airways (endotracheal tube or tracheostomy tube)
   b. Chest tubes
   c. Central venous catheters
   d. Nasogastric tube or feeding tube
   e. ECG leads or cardiac pacemaker and leads
   f. Intra-aortic balloon
   g. Surgical clips or staples

4. From a set of abnormal chest radiographs, identify the following abnormalities. Have your laboratory instructor critique your findings and offer suggestions for improving your skills.

a. Extrapulmonary air (as in pneumothorax, subcutaneous emphysema, or pneumomediastinum)
b. Changes in lung volume (as in hyperinflation, atelectasis, mediastinal shift, consolidation)
c. Fluid abnormalities (as in pleural effusion, CHF, pulmonary edema, pulmonary infiltrates)

5. With a laboratory partner, evaluate a lateral neck x-ray film of a pediatric patient. Identify the larynx, epiglottis, and trachea. Make a judgment about whether the epiglottis is large and if the airway is narrowed. Have your laboratory instructor confirm your findings.

6. With a laboratory partner, study a ventilation-perfusion scan, together assessing the scan for defects in ventilation or perfusion.
   a. Identify the different x-ray views: PA, right anterior oblique, left anterior oblique, lateral.
   b. Differentiate between the ventilation and perfusion scans.

7. With a laboratory partner, view a pulmonary angiogram. Carefully evaluate the study and try to identify where circulation is obstructed.

8. With a laboratory partner, evaluate a CT scan of the chest. Orient the series of images with the scout image.
   a. Identify a point on the scout image and find the same point on the CT cut.
   b. Identify as many landmarks as possible on each CT cut, and have your laboratory instructor critique your skills.

Check List: Chest X-Ray Evaluation

_____ 1. Review the patient's medical record.
_____ 2. Scan the patient's chart for any pertinent information.
_____ 3. Evaluate the extrathoracic soft tissue, observing for subcutaneous air or fluid.
_____ 4. Evaluate the ribs, tracing each and looking for fractures, healed fractures, missing ribs, and other deformities.
_____ 5. Evaluate the pleura, observing for changes in thickness and presence of air or fluid.

_____ 6. Evaluate the hemidiaphragms, noting the position of each diaphragm relative to the other.

_____ 7. Evaluate the sternum, clavicles, and scapulae, observing for fractures or deformities.

_____ 8. Evaluate the spinal processes.

_____ 9. Evaluate the costophrenic angles, observing for blunting (less acuity of the angle).

_____ 10. Evaluate the lung fields, noting any unusual lung markings, opacities, nodular densities, or other abnormalities.

_____ 11. Evaluate the hilum, noting its relative size and extent of its fullness (radiodensity).

_____ 12. Evaluate the cardiac silhouette, noting the relative ratio of cardiac size and thoracic diameter (should be less than half).

_____ 13. Evaluate the trachea, noting its position, and identify the carina.

_____ 14. Identify any lines, artificial airways, ECG leads or pacemaker wires, nasogastric or feeding tubes, and chest tubes.

_____ 15. Evaluate the retrosternal air space on the lateral film.

_____ 16. Evaluate the hemidiaphragms and pleura on the lateral film. Note any changes in opacity or other findings and correlate with the PA projection.

Self-Evaluation Post Test: Radiographic Imaging of the Chest

1. On a standard x-ray study of the chest, which of the following are the most common two views?
   I. Posterior-anterior
   II. Anterior-posterior
   III. Lateral
   IV. Apical lordotic
   a. I and III
   b. I and IV
   c. II and III
   d. II and IV

2. When the posterior-anterior (PA) view is compared with the anterior-posterior (AP) view:
   a. the heart shadow on the PA view is larger.
   b. the heart shadow on the AP view is larger.
   c. the apices are more easily visualized on the AP view.
   d. the PA view is often a portable x-ray.

3. Which of the following has the greatest radiodensity?
   a. Air
   b. Fat
   c. Water
   d. Bone

4. A possible nodular anomaly is present in the right upper lobe on a PA film but partially obscured by the clavicle. What view might show the anomaly better?
   a. AP projection
   b. Lateral projection
   c. Apical lordotic projection
   d. Left anterior oblique projection

5. During full inspiration, the hemidiaphragms on an adult chest film should be:
   a. at the C5 vertebra.
   b. at the level of the twelfth rib.
   c. at the L4 vertebra.
   d. at the level of the tenth rib.

6. When evaluating a PA film of the chest, you note that the right costophrenic angles are blunted. What does this suggest?
   a. A pneumothorax
   b. Presence of an infiltrate in the right lower lobe
   c. Presence of atelectasis in the right base
   d. Presence of a pleural effusion on the right

7. When evaluating a PA film of the chest, you note that in the left upper lobe there is a 1 cm wide sliver along the lateral margin, descending from the apex, merging with the ribs at the third rib. This narrow sliver is very black and devoid of vascular markings. This could possibly be:
   a. a pneumothorax.
   b. atelectasis.
   c. pulmonary edema.
   d. hyperinflation.

8. For evaluating the position of an endotracheal tube on an AP chest film, the tip of the endotracheal tube should rest:
   a. at the carina.
   b. at the fourth rib space.
   c. at a point 2 to 3 cm above the carina.
   d. just above the clavicles.

9. When viewing a V/Q scan, you note ventilation to be even on all views. On the perfusion scan, you note absence of perfusion in the right apical posterior segment. This finding suggests:
   a. a pulmonary infiltrate.
   b. atelectasis in the right apical posterior segment.
   c. a possible pulmonary embolus.
   d. a pneumothorax in the right apical posterior segment.

10. A pulmonary angiogram is used to:
    a. image the ventilation of the lung.
    b. image the perfusion of the lung.
    c. image the lymph system of the lung.
    d. None of the above.

PERFORMANCE EVALUATION:
Chest X-Ray Interpretation

Date: Lab _____ Clinical _____ Agency _____

Lab: Pass _____ Fail _____ Clinical: Pass _____ Fail _____

Student name _____ Instructor name _____

No. of times observed in clinical _____

No. of times practiced in clinical _____

PASSING CRITERIA: Obtain 90% or better on the procedure. Tasks indicated by * must receive at least 1 point, or the evaluation is terminated. Procedure must be performed within the designated time, or the performance receives a failing grade.

SCORING:
2 points — Task performed satisfactorily without prompting.
1 point — Task performed satisfactorily with self-initiated correction.
0 points — Task performed incorrectly or with prompting required.
NA — Task not applicable to the patient care situation.

Tasks:	Peer	Lab	Clinical
1. Reviews the patient's medical record	☐	☐	☐
2. Scans the patient's chart for any pertinent information	☐	☐	☐
* **3.** Evaluates the extrathoracic soft tissue			
a. Subcutaneous emphysema	☐	☐	☐
4. Evaluates the ribs			
a. Fractures	☐	☐	☐
b. Missing ribs	☐	☐	☐
c. Deformities	☐	☐	☐
5. Evaluates the pleura			
a. Thickness	☐	☐	☐
b. Pleural air	☐	☐	☐
c. Pleural fluid	☐	☐	☐
6. Evaluates the hemidiaphragms			
a. Position	☐	☐	☐
b. Elevation	☐	☐	☐
c. Conformation	☐	☐	☐

7. Evaluates the sternum and clavicles and scapulae

    a. Fractures ☐ ☐ ☐

    b. Deformities ☐ ☐ ☐

8. Evaluates the spinal processes

    a. Fractures ☐ ☐ ☐

    b. Deformities ☐ ☐ ☐

9. Evaluates the costophrenic angles for blunting ☐ ☐ ☐

10. Evaluates the lung fields

    a. Lung markings ☐ ☐ ☐

    b. Opacities ☐ ☐ ☐

    c. Nodular densities ☐ ☐ ☐

11. Evaluates the hilum for size and fullness ☐ ☐ ☐

12. Evaluates the cardiac silhouette

    a. Estimates the cardiothoracic ratio ☐ ☐ ☐

13. Evaluates the trachea

    a. Position ☐ ☐ ☐

    b. Identifies carina ☐ ☐ ☐

14. Identifies any lines

    a. Artificial airways ☐ ☐ ☐

    b. Chest tubes ☐ ☐ ☐

    c. ECG leads or pacemaker wires ☐ ☐ ☐

    d. Feeding tubes ☐ ☐ ☐

    e. Nasogastric tubes ☐ ☐ ☐

    f. Intra-aortic balloon ☐ ☐ ☐

15. Evaluates the retrosternal air space on the lateral film ☐ ☐ ☐

16. Evaluates the diaphragms and pleura on the lateral film ☐ ☐ ☐

17. Notes any changes in opacity or other findings and correlates with the PA projection ☐ ☐ ☐

SCORE: Peer _____ points of possible 66; _____%

        Lab _____ points of possible 66; _____%

        Clinical _____ points of possible 66; _____%

TIME: _____ out of possible 15 minutes

STUDENT SIGNATURES

PEER: _____

STUDENT: _____

INSTRUCTOR SIGNATURES

LAB: _____

CLINICAL: _____

The measurement of bedside pulmonary function parameters provides important information that may be used in a variety of ways, ranging from assessing the effectiveness of bronchodilators to evaluating the adequacy of ventilation. Minimal equipment is needed, the skills are easily learned, and the procedures are noninvasive. The respiratory practitioner will be responsible for the measurement and evaluation of a patient's lung function by performing formal pulmonary function testing. Contemporary pulmonary function testing equipment is frequently interfaced with microcomputers to eliminate the drudgery of manual calculations. Still, it is important to understand how to manually calculate pulmonary function values for assessing accuracy in the event of computer malfunction.

Basic spirometry provides volume-versus-time data. In addition, it is important to have an understanding of flow-volume loops. Flow-volume loops present the spirometry information in a way that allows easier characterization of restrictive disease and obstructive disease.

Measurement of the functional residual capacity (FRC) and residual volume (RV) is possible only through indirect methods. The respiratory practitioner must understand how gas dilution techniques allow measurement of these volumes. Additionally, body plethysmography may also be used to measure FRC and RV as well as airway resistance.

This chapter covers how to use the portable equipment for bedside monitoring as well as the techniques of routine pulmonary function testing using a water-sealed spirometer and how to calculate the results from a spirometric tracing.

KEY TERMS

- Airway resistance (R_{AW})
- Ambient temperature and pressure, saturated (ATPS)
- Anatomical dead space
- Bedside monitoring
- Body temperature and pressure, saturated (BTPS)
- Diffusion
- Expiratory reserve volume (ERV)
- $FEF_{25-75\%}$
- $FEF_{200-1200\ mL}$
- FEV_1
- Flow-volume loop
- Forced vital capacity (FVC)
- Frequency
- Functional residual capacity (FRC)
- Gas dilution technique
- Hyperventilation
- Inspiratory capacity
- Inspiratory reserve volume (IRV)
- Maximal inspiratory pressure (MIP)
- Maximum voluntary ventilation (MVV)
- Minute volume
- Nitrogen washout
- Peak expiratory flow rate (PEFR)
- Peak flowmeter
- Residual volume (RV)
- Respirometer
- Spirometer
- Tidal volume
- Total lung capacity (TLC)
- Vital capacity

THEORY OBJECTIVES

At the end of this chapter, the reader should be able to:

- *Discuss the rationale for monitoring bedside pulmonary function parameters.*
- *Compare and contrast the following spirometers and measuring devices:*
  - *Wright and Haloscale respirometers*
  - *Wright and Mini-Wright peak flowmeters*
  - *Boehringer inspiratory force manometer*
  - *Water seal spirometer*
  - *Fleisch Pneumotach spirometer*

Include:
- *(1) Principles of operation*
- *(2) Accuracy ranges*
- *(3) Limitations*
- *Select an appropriate measuring device given a specific pulmonary function parameter to measure.*
- *Discuss the significance of and normal ranges for the following respiratory function parameters:*
  - *Tidal volume*
  - *Minute volume*

- Frequency
- Peak expiratory flow
- Maximal inspiratory pressure
- Inspiratory reserve volume
- Expiratory reserve volume
- Residual volume
- Total lung capacity
- Inspiratory capacity
- Functional residual capacity

- Given a normal forced vital capacity tracing, identify and explain the clinical significance of the following forced maneuvers:
  - Forced vital capacity
  - FEV_t
  - FEV_t/FVC ratio
  - $FEF_{200-1200}$
  - $FEF_{25-75\%}$
  - PEFR

- Explain how a maximum voluntary ventilation maneuver is performed and its clinical significance.

- Explain the importance of conversion from ATPS to BTPS in the reporting of pulmonary function test results.
- Given a flow-volume loop, identify the following:
  - Inspiratory portion
  - Expiratory portion
  - Vital capacity
  - Peak inspiratory flow
  - Peak expiratory flow
- Describe how a flow-volume loop changes with restrictive and obstructive disease.
- Describe how gas dilution techniques allow the measurement of FRC and RV.
- Describe how a body plethysmograph measures V_{TG}.
- Describe how gas diffusion is measured and what the single breath diffusion test (D_LCO) is.
- Discuss the hazards of pulmonary function testing, including:
  - Hyperventilation
  - Bronchodilator side effects
  - Infection

CLINICAL PRACTICE GUIDELINES

AARC Clinical Practice Guideline Spirometry, 1996 Update

S 4.0 INDICATIONS:

The indications for spirometry (4–8) include the need to

4.1 Detect the presence or absence of lung dysfunction suggested by history or physical signs and symptoms (e.g., age, smoking history, family history of lung disease, cough, dyspnea, wheezing) and/or the presence of other abnormal diagnostic tests (e.g., chest radiograph, arterial blood gas analysis);

4.2 Quantify the severity of known lung disease;

4.3 Assess the change in lung function over time or following administration of or change in therapy;

4.4 Assess the potential effects or response to environmental or occupational exposure;

4.5 Assess the risk for surgical procedures known to affect lung function;

4.6 Assess impairment and/or disability (e.g., for rehabilitation, legal reasons, military).

S 5.0 CONTRAINDICATIONS:

The requesting physician should be made aware that the circumstances listed in this section could affect the reliability of spirometry measurements. In addition, forced expiratory maneuvers may aggravate these conditions, which may make test postponement necessary until the medical condition(s) resolve(s).

Relative contraindications (9, 10) to performing spirometry are

5.1 Hemoptysis of unknown origin (forced expiratory maneuver may aggravate the underlying condition);

5.2 Pneumothorax;

5.3 Unstable cardiovascular status (forced expiratory maneuver may worsen angina or cause changes in blood pressure) or recent myocardial infarction or pulmonary embolus;

5.4 Thoracic, abdominal, or cerebral aneurysms (danger of rupture due to increased thoracic pressure);

5.5 Recent eye surgery (e.g., cataract);

5.6 Presence of an acute disease process that might interfere with test performance (e.g., nausea, vomiting);

5.7 Recent surgery of thorax or abdomen.

S 6.0 HAZARDS/COMPLICATIONS:

Although spirometry is a safe procedure, untoward reactions may occur, and the value of the information anticipated from spirometry should be weighed against potential hazards. The following have been reported anecdotally:

6.1 Pneumothorax;

6.2 Increased intracranial pressure;

6.3 Syncope, dizziness, light-headedness;

6.4 Chest pain;

6.5 Paroxysmal coughing;

6.6 Contraction of hospital acquired infections;

6.7 Oxygen desaturation due to interruption of oxygen therapy;

6.8 Bronchospasm.

(Continued)

S 7.0 LIMITATIONS OF METHODOLOGY/ VALIDATION OF RESULTS:

7.1 Spirometry is an effort-dependent test that requires careful instruction and the cooperation of the test subject. Inability to perform acceptable maneuvers may be due to poor subject motivation or failure to understand instructions. Physical impairment and young age (e.g., <5 years of age) may also limit the subject's ability to perform spirometric maneuvers. These limitations do not preclude attempting spirometry but should be noted and taken into consideration when the results are interpreted.

7.2 The results of spirometry should meet the following criteria for number of trials, acceptability, and reproducibility. The acceptability criteria should be applied before reproducibility is checked.

7.2.1 Number of trials: A minimum of three acceptable FVC maneuvers should be performed. (3) If a subject is unable to perform a single acceptable maneuver after eight attempts, testing may be discontinued. However, after additional instruction and demonstration, more maneuvers may be performed depending on the subject's clinical condition and tolerance.

7.2.2 Acceptability: A good "start-of-test" includes:

7.2.2.1 An extrapolated volume of < or = 5% of the FVC or 150 mL, whichever is greater;

7.2.2.2 No hesitation or false start;

7.2.2.3 A rapid start to rise time.

7.2.3 Acceptability: No cough, especially during the first second of the maneuver.

7.2.4 Acceptability: No early termination of exhalation.

7.2.4.1 A minimum exhalation time of 6 seconds is recommended, unless there is an obvious plateau of reasonable duration (i.e., no volume change for at least 1 second) or the subject cannot or should not continue to exhale further. (3)

7.2.4.2 No maneuver should be eliminated solely because of early termination. The FEV_1 from such maneuvers may be valid, and the volume expired may be an estimate of the true FVC, although the FEV_1/FVC and $FEF_{25-75\%}$ may be overestimated.

7.2.5 Reproducibility:

7.2.5.1 The two largest FVCs from acceptable maneuvers should not vary by more than 0.200 L, and the two largest FEV_1s from acceptable maneuvers should not vary by more than 0.200 L.

NOTE: The ATS has changed its recommendations from those made in the 1987 ATS guideline (2) (a reproducibility criterion of 5% or 0.100 L, whichever is larger). This change is based on evidence from Hankinson and Bang suggesting that intra-subject variability is independent of body size and that individuals of short stature are less likely to meet the older criterion than are taller subjects. (11) In addition, the 0.200 L criterion is simple to apply. However, there are two concerns with this change. The first is whether the 0.200 L criterion is too permissive in shorter individuals (e.g., children). Enright and coworkers (12) reported a failure rate of only 2.1% in 21,432 testing sessions on adults using the 5% or 100 mL criterion. In addition, they found that only 0.4% of test sessions failed to meet relaxed criteria of 5% or 200 mL. These failure rates are much lower than the 5–15% failure rates reported by Hankinson and Bang. (11) Enright and coworkers did not study children, but there was some height overlap in the two studies. Thus, we are not convinced that the 5% rule is inappropriate when applied to shorter individuals. Indeed, Hankinson and Bang stated in their report, ". . . it appears that the technician appropriately responded to the lack of a reproducible or acceptable test result by obtaining more maneuvers from these subjects." The second concern is that the 0.200 L criterion may be too rigid for very tall individuals (e.g., height >75 inches). Hankinson and Bang did not study subjects taller than 190 cm (i.e., 75 inches). In order to send a consistent message, we recommend the ATS reproducibility criterion but urge therapists: (a) to use this criterion as a goal during data collection and not to reject a spirogram solely on the basis of its poor reproducibility; (b) to exceed the reproducibility criterion whenever possible because it will decrease interlaboratory and intralaboratory variability; and (c) to comment in the written report when reproducibility criteria cannot be met.

7.3 Maximum voluntary ventilation (MVV) is the volume of air exhaled in a specified period during rapid, forced breathing. (3) This measurement is sometimes referred to as the maximum breathing capacity (MBC).

7.3.1 The period of time for performing this maneuver should be at least 12 seconds but no more than 15 seconds, with the data reported as L/min at BTPS.

7.3.2 At least two trials should be obtained, and the two highest should agree within ±10%.

(Continued)

7.4 The use of a nose clip for all spirometric maneuvers is strongly encouraged.

7.5 Subjects may be studied in either the sitting or standing position. Occasionally, a subject may experience syncope or dizziness while performing the forced expiratory maneuver. Thus, the sitting position may be safer. If such a subject is standing, an appropriate chair (i.e., with arms and not on rollers) should be placed behind the subject in the event that he or she needs to be seated quickly. When the maneuver is performed from a seated position, the subject should sit erect with both feet on the floor, and be positioned correctly in relation to the equipment. Test position should be noted on the report.

7.6 Spirometry is often performed before and after inhalation of a bronchodilator.

7.6.1 The drug, dose, and mode of delivery should be specifically ordered by the managing physician or determined by the laboratory and should be noted in the report.

7.6.2 The length of the interval between administration of the bronchodilator and postbronchodilator testing varies among laboratories, (13–17) but there appears to be more support for a minimum interval of 15 minutes for most short- and intermediate-acting beta-2 agonists. (14–17) This does not guarantee that peak response will be determined, and underestimation of peak bronchodilator response can occur.

7.6.3 Subjects who use inhaled short-acting bronchodilators should be tested at least four to six hours after the last use of their inhaled bronchodilator to allow proper assessment of acute bronchodilator response. Long-acting inhaled bronchodilators may need to be withheld for a more extended period. Subjects should understand that if they need to administer their bronchodilator prior to the test because of breathing problems, they should do so. Bronchodilators taken on the day of testing should be noted in the report. Table 5-1 lists commonly used drugs that may confound assessment of acute bronchodilator response and the recommended times for withholding.

7.6.4 Interpretation of response to a bronchodilator should take into account both magnitude and consistency of change in the pulmonary function data. The recommended criterion for response to a bronchodilator in adults for FEV_1 and FVC is a 12% improvement from baseline and an absolute change of 0.200 L. (18) However, because the peak effect of the drug may not always be determined, the inability to meet this response criterion does not exclude a response. In addition, dynamic compression of the airways during the forced expiratory maneuver may mask bronchodilator response in some subjects, and the additional measurement of

TABLE 5-1: Recommended Times for Withholding Commonly Used Bronchodilators When Bronchodilator Response Is to Be Assessed*	
DRUG	**WITHHOLDING TIME (hours)**
Salmeterol	12
Ipratropium	6
Terbutaline	4–8
Albuterol	4–6
Metaproterenol	4
Isoetharine	3

Based on consensus of committee and known duration of action.

airway resistance and calculation of specific conductance and resistance may provide documentation of airway responsiveness. (19)

7.7 Reporting of results:

7.7.1 The largest FVC and FEV_1 (at BTPS) should be reported even if they do not come from the same curve.

7.7.2 Other reported measures (e.g., $FEF_{25-75\%}$ and instantaneous expiratory flow rates, such as FEF_{max} and $FEF_{50\%}$) should be obtained from the single acceptable "best-test" curve (i.e., largest sum of FVC and FEV_1) and reported at BTPS.

7.7.3 All values should be recorded and stored so that comparison for reproducibility and the ability to detect spirometry-induced bronchospasm (as evidenced by a worsening in spirometric values with successive attempts — and not related to fatigue) are simplified.

7.7.4 The highest MVV trial should be reported.

7.8 Subject demographics and related information:

7.8.1 Age: The age on day of test should be used.

7.8.2 Height: The subject should stand fully erect with eyes looking straight ahead and be measured with the feet together without shoes. An accurate measuring device should be used. For subjects who cannot stand or who have a spinal deformity (e.g., kyphoscoliosis), the arm span from finger tip to finger tip with arms stretched in opposite directions can be used as an estimate of height. (20)

7.8.3 Weight: An accurate scale should be used to determine the subject's weight while wearing indoor clothes but without shoes.

7.8.4 Race: The race or ethnic background of the subject should be determined and reported to help ensure the use of appropriate reference values and appropriate interpretation of data.

(Continued)

7.8.5 The time of day, equipment or instrumentation used, and name of the technician administering the test should be recorded.

7.9 Open- and closed-circuit testing:

7.9.1 Open circuit: The subject takes a maximal inspiration from the room, inserts the mouthpiece into the mouth, and then blows out either slowly (SVC) or rapidly (FVC) until the end-of-test criterion is met. Although the open-circuit technique works well for some subjects, others have difficulty maintaining a maximum inspiration while trying to position the mouthpiece correctly in the mouth. These subjects may lose some of their vital capacity due to leakage prior to the expiratory maneuver. (11)

7.9.2 Closed-circuit: The subject inserts the mouthpiece into the mouth and breathes quietly for no more than five tidal breaths, takes a maximal inspiration from the reservoir, and then blows out either slowly (SVC) or rapidly (FVC) until the end-of-test criterion is met. This rebreathing technique is preferred if the spirometer system permits because it (1) allows the subject to obtain a tight seal with the mouthpiece prior to inspiration and (2) allows evaluation of the volume inspired.

S 8.0 ASSESSMENT OF NEED:

Need is assessed by determining that valid indications are present.

S 9.0 ASSESSMENT OF TEST QUALITY:

Spirometry performed for the listed indications is valid only if the spirometer functions acceptably and the subject is able to perform the maneuvers in an acceptable and reproducible fashion. All reports should contain a statement about the technician's assessment of test quality and specify which acceptability criteria were not met.

9.1 Quality control: (21)

9.1.1 Volume verification (i.e., calibration): at least daily prior to testing, use a calibrated known-volume syringe with a volume of at least 3 L to ascertain that the spirometer reads a known volume accurately. The known volume should be injected and/or withdrawn at least three times, at flows that vary between 2 and 12 L/s (3 L injection times of approximately 1 second, 6 seconds, and somewhere between 1 and 6 seconds). The tolerance limits for an acceptable calibration are ±3% of the known volume. Thus, for a 3 L calibration syringe, the acceptable recovered range is 2.91–3.09 L. We encourage the therapist to exceed this guideline whenever possible (i.e., reduce the tolerance limits to <±3%).

9.1.2 Leak test: Volume-displacement spirometers must be evaluated for leaks daily. One recommendation is that any volume change of more than 10 mL/min while the spirometer is under at least 3-cm-H_2O pressure be considered excessive. (22)

9.1.3 A spirometry procedure manual should be maintained.

9.1.4 A log that documents daily instrument calibration, problems encountered, corrective action required, and system hardware and/or software changes should be maintained.

9.1.5 Computer software for measurement and computer calculations should be checked against manual calculations if possible. In addition, biologic laboratory standards (i.e., healthy, nonsmoking individuals) can be tested periodically to ensure historic reproducibility, to verify software upgrades, and to evaluate new or replacement spirometers.

9.1.6 The known-volume syringe should be checked for accuracy at least quarterly using a second known-volume syringe, with the spirometer in the patient-test mode. This validates the calibration and ensures that the patient-test mode operates properly.

9.1.7 For water-seal spirometers, water level and paper tracing speed should be checked daily. The entire range of volume displacement should be checked quarterly. (21)

9.2 Quality Assurance: Each laboratory or testing site should develop, establish, and implement quality assurance indicators for equipment calibration and maintenance and patient preparation. In addition, methods should be devised and implemented to monitor technician performance (with appropriate feedback) while obtaining, recognizing, and documenting acceptability criteria.

S 11.0 MONITORING:

The following should be evaluated during the performance of spirometric measurements to ascertain the validity of the results: (3, 24)

11.1 Acceptability of maneuver and reproducibility of FVC, FEV_1 (25)

11.2 Level of effort and cooperation by the subject

11.3 Equipment function or malfunction (e.g., calibration)

11.4 The final report should contain a statement about test quality.

11.5 Spirometry results should be subject to ongoing review by a supervisor, with feedback to the technologist. (12) Quality assurance and/or quality improvement programs should be designed to monitor technician competency, both initially and on an ongoing basis.

Reprinted with permission from *Respiratory Care* 1996; 41: 629–636. The complete AARC Clinical Practice Guidelines are available from the AARC Web site (http://www.aarc.org), the AARC Executive Office, or from the *Respiratory Care* journal.

AMERICAN THORACIC SOCIETY INDICATIONS

The American Thoracic Society has published a document, *Standardization of Spirometry* (Miller, 2005), which is a guide toward making spirometry measurements more uniform on a worldwide basis. Included in this document are the indications for spirometry, which are summarized in Figure 5-1.

RATIONALE FOR BEDSIDE MONITORING

Bedside monitoring is an effective tool for rapidly assessing the mechanics of ventilation. The information obtained may be useful in assessing the patient's ability to reverse atelectasis, overcome airway obstruction, mobilize secretions, and maintain ventilation as well as to evaluate the effectiveness of bronchodilator or other therapy. Some of the bedside parameters monitored require patient cooperation. In the comatose patient, the respiratory practitioner may be able to assess only a portion of the parameters discussed in this chapter. However, those parameters that will be monitored are very useful and generally provide an adequate indication of the mechanics of ventilation.

- Diagnostic Indications
  - Evaluate symptoms, signs or abnormal laboratory tests
  - Measure the effect of disease on pulmonary function
  - Screen individuals at risk of having pulmonary disease
  - Assess pre-operative risk
  - Assess prognosis
  - Assess health status before beginning strenuous physical activity programs

- Monitoring Indications
  - Assess therapeutic intervention
  - Describe the course of diseases that affect lung function
  - Monitor people exposed to injurious agents
  - Monitor for adverse reactions to drugs with known pulmonary toxicity

- Disability Determination
  - Assess patients as part of a rehabilitation program
  - Assess risks as part of an insurance evaluation
  - Assess individuals for legal reasons

- Public Health Indications
  - Epidemiologic surveys
  - Derivation of reference equations
  - Clinical research

Figure 5-1 American Thoracic Society, indications for spirometry. Reproduced with permission of the European Respiratory Society ©

Frequently, some of these bedside parameters are monitored to assess pending respiratory failure such as patients with Guillain-Barré or other progressive neuromuscular diseases. Depending on circumstances, a patient may be monitored as frequently as every 2 hours.

EQUIPMENT USED IN MEASURING BEDSIDE PARAMETERS

Respirometers

A *respirometer* is a device used to measure ventilatory volumes. The Wright and Haloscale respirometers are small portable respirometers (Figure 5-2).

These instruments work by rotation of a thin vane with gas flow. As the vane rotates, it turns a series of gears, rotating the hands on the dial indicating the volume. The inner workings look much like those of a watch. Slots or channels surround the vane, directing the flow of gas through it in only one direction. Figure 5-3 shows an internal schematic of the respirometers.

These respirometers are designed to operate between 3 and 300 liters per minute. Flows in excess of 300 liters per

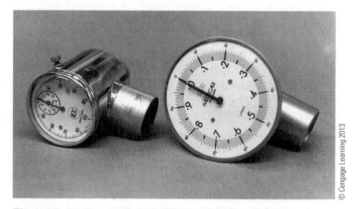

Figure 5-2 The Wright and Haloscale respirometers

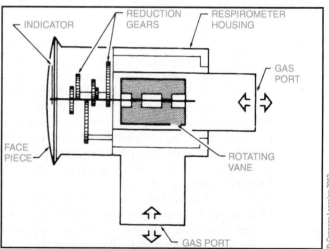

Figure 5-3 An internal schematic of the Wright and Haloscale respirometer

minute may cause internal damage to the delicate vane as well as affect its accuracy. Therefore, using these devices is not recommended for forced maneuvers such as that needed to measure the forced vital capacity (FVC). Accuracy is between 5% and 10% at 60 liters per minute. These devices are susceptible to inertia. The vane can be spun up so that the measurement is taken after the flow has stopped. This can be observed by gently puffing into the respirometer and observing the dial motion.

These respirometers are very delicate and do not tolerate being dropped. To prevent damage, a neck strap should be worn to prevent inadvertently dropping the instrument.

Peak Flowmeters

A *peak flowmeter* is a device that measures ventilatory flow rates. The Wright and Mini-Wright peak flowmeters are two devices that measure expiratory flow rates. Figure 5-4 shows both the Wright and Mini-Wright peak flowmeters.

Expired gas pushes against a spring-loaded vane or diaphragm (as in the Mini-Wright device). As the vane or diaphragm is displaced, holes or a slot (as in the Mini-Wright) is exposed, allowing gas to escape. As more holes or more of the slot is exposed, additional flow must be generated to move the vane or diaphragm. Figure 5-5 shows a schematic of the Mini-Wright device. The scale is calibrated in liters per minute.

Both of the devices are delicate. Dropping them may result in their failure to operate properly.

The Wright peak flowmeter is calibrated from 50 to 1000 liters per minute. The Mini-Wright peak flowmeter is calibrated from 60 to 800 liters per minute.

The Boehringer inspiratory force manometer device is used to measure negative pressure generated on inspiration.

The inspiratory force manometer operates by transmittal of pressure to a sealed diaphragm and pivot assembly, as in an aneroid barometer. As more negative pressure is generated by the patient, the pivot deflects the needle further, indicating more negative pressure on the dial.

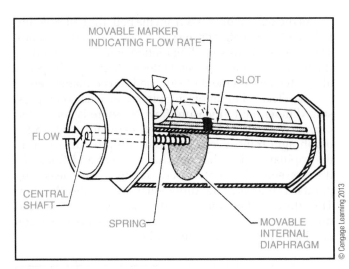

Figure 5-5 An internal schematic of the Mini-Wright peak flowmeter

This device is delicate, and dropping or abusing it will render it inoperative.

Types of Spirometers

A *spirometer* is a device that measures ventilatory volumes and airflow.

The water seal spirometer is the most common pulmonary function measuring device. As the name implies, this spirometer relies on a water seal to separate the spirometer bell from the atmosphere. The Warren E. Collins Company (Braintree, Massachusetts) manufactures several spirometers that employ this principle. Figure 5-6 shows a cross section of this type of spirometer.

A rotating drum (kymograph) and pen is incorporated with the bell, tracing the bell's motion. This pen mechanism may be suspended by a chain and pulley or attached directly to the bell itself.

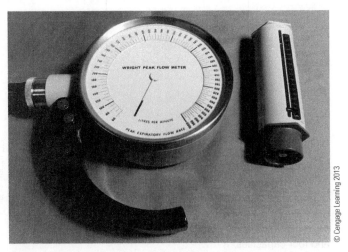

Figure 5-4 The Wright and Mini-Wright peak flowmeters

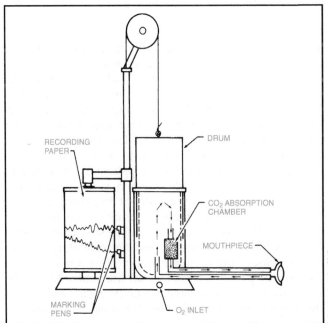

Figure 5-6 A cross section of a Collins water seal spirometer

As the patient breathes from the bell, the bell rises and falls with the patient's inspired and expired volumes. These cause a corresponding motion of the pen, recording the tracing on graph paper. Different kymograph speeds allow the measurement of slow and forced maneuvers.

The Fleisch Pneumotach Spirometer relies on a pressure differential to measure flow. Pressure is conducted proximal and distal to a heated capillary grid and a diaphragm transducer. A pressure drop occurs distal to the capillary grid. The transducer senses and transmits the pressure differential between the two measuring points. The greater the differential, the greater the flow. This flow is then interpreted as a volume or is read directly from the device. Figure 5-7 shows a cross section of a Fleisch pneumotachometer head.

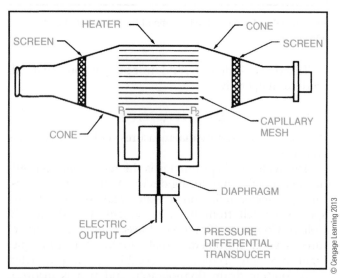

Figure 5-7   A cross section of the Fleisch pneumotachometer

BEDSIDE MEASUREMENTS

Minute Volume

The *minute volume* is the volume of air inhaled or exhaled during 1 minute. In the normal adult at rest, minute volume ranges between 5 and 7 liters per minute. As minute volume increases, so does the work of breathing. When minute volume decreases, hypoxemia and hypercapnia may result from less gas exchange at the alveolar level. An increase in minute ventilation may occur as a result of hypercapnia, exercise, increased dead space, or alveolar hypoventilation. A patient with sufficient muscle strength may be able to sustain an increased minute ventilation for some time without becoming severely fatigued. However, an increase in minute ventilation in excess of 10 liters per minute cannot be sustained for long and may be an indication of pending respiratory failure.

To measure the minute volume, place a pair of nose clips on the patient's nose. Instruct the patient to breathe normally into the respirometer. Observing a watch, count the respiratory rate and, after 1 minute, terminate the measurement. The exhaled volume is the minute volume.

Tidal Volume

The *tidal volume* is the amount of air moved into or out of a resting patient's lungs with each normal breath. The tidal volume can be calculated by dividing the minute volume by the respiratory rate. It is to measure this volume during inspiration or expiration, but not during both. Normal tidal volume may be estimated by multiplying the normal body weight (in kilograms) by 5 to 7 mL/kg. For instance, for a 75 kg man, we could estimate a tidal volume of 450 mL (75 kg × 6 mL/kg = 450 mL). To convert a patient's weight from pounds to kilograms, divide the weight in pounds by 2.2 pounds/ kilogram.

$$kg = \frac{weight(lb)}{2.2 lb/kg}$$

For example, a patient weighs 270 lb. What is the patient's weight in kilograms?

$$kg = \frac{270 lb}{2.2 lb/kg} = 122.7 \text{ kg}$$

Figure 5-8 shows how the tidal volume appears on a slow vital capacity tracing.

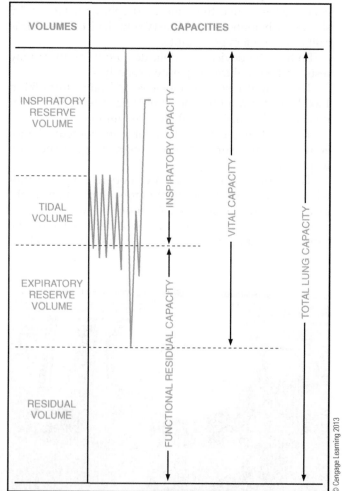

Figure 5-8   A slow vital capacity tracing showing four volumes and four capacities

A portion of the tidal volume does not participate in respiration (actual gas exchange). This portion of the tidal volume is termed *anatomical dead space*. This volume may be estimated by multiplying the normal body weight based on height (in kilograms) by 2.2 mL/kg. For instance, a 75 kg man would have an anatomical dead space of approximatel 165 mL (75 kg × 2.2 mL/kg = 165 mL).

As tidal volume decreases, the anatomical dead space does not decrease with it. Assume that our 75 kg male patient's tidal volume drops to 300 mL. By subtracting the anatomical dead space (165 mL), only 135 mL is potentially participating in respiration or gas exchange. This is significant because such a small volume will not sustain a person for very long before respiratory failure occurs.

Excessive oxygenation and hyperventilation may also cause a decrease in tidal volume and respiratory rate. This is the result of an increase in the partial pressure of oxygen (PaO_2) and a decrease in the partial pressure of carbon dioxide ($PaCO_2$). The brain normally responds to these two conditions by decreasing ventilation.

Frequency

Respiratory *frequency* is the number of breaths per minute. Normal respiratory frequency for the adult is 12 to 20 breaths per minute. An increased respiratory rate may indicate increased hypoxemia, fear, pain, anxiety, or hypercapnia. A rate in excess of 35 breaths per minute may be an indication of pending respiratory failure.

Conversely, a low respiratory rate may result from central nervous system (CNS) depression caused by drugs, hypercapnia, or nervous system disorders. Bradypnea can lead to hypoxemia and hypercapnia.

Vital Capacity

Vital capacity is the maximum volume of air that can be exhaled after a maximal inspiration. A capacity by definition is two or more volumes. The vital capacity is made up of the *expiratory reserve volume (ERV)*, tidal volume, and the *inspiratory reserve volume (IRV)*. Figure 5-8 illustrates the relationship of the three volumes that in combination equal the vital capacity.

To measure the vital capacity, place a pair of nose clips on the patient's nose. Instruct the patient to inhale as deeply as possible and then exhale through the respirometer. This test requires cooperation and effort. Coach and encourage the patient while performing this measurement.

The vital capacity is an indicator of ventilatory reserve. A patient with a large vital capacity has a large reserve and sufficient muscle strength to sustain ventilation. A patient with a low vital capacity does not have much ventilatory reserve to sustain ventilation. Normal vital capacity may be estimated by multiplying the normal body weight (in kilograms) by 65 to 75 mL/kg. Our 75 kg male patient would have an estimated vital capacity of 5.25 liters (75 kg × 70 mL/kg = 5.25 liters).

A vital capacity of less than 10 mL/kg of normal body weight may be a sign that respiratory failure is imminent. This volume/weight provides little reserve to reverse atelectasis, cough, or mobilize secretions and to sustain ventilation. Fatigue may soon occur, resulting in a decrease in minute volume and worsening of hypoxemia and hypercapnia.

Peak Expiratory Flow Rate

The *peak expiratory flow rate (PEFR)* is the maximum flow rate attained during a forced expiration after a maximal inspiration. It requires patient cooperation to measure and is a good indicator of airway obstruction and muscle strength. This measurement is commonly used to assess the effectiveness of bronchodilators and the reversibility of an obstruction. A normal PEFR for an adult is greater than 500 L/min.

To measure the peak expiratory flow (PEF), instruct the patient to inhale as deeply as possible and then exhale as forcefully as possible through the peak flowmeter. The PEF usually occurs in the first second or two of expiration.

Maximal Inspiratory Pressure

Maximal inspiratory pressure (MIP) is the amount of negative pressure a patient is able to generate when trying to inhale. It is an indicator of muscle strength and ventilatory reserve. This relates to the patient's ability to reverse atelectasis, cough effectively, and manage airway secretions. Patient cooperation is not necessary to measure this component of pulmonary function. It can be performed on the comatose patient. MIP is measured using an inspiratory force manometer calibrated in cm H_2O (refer to Figure 5-23). A normal patient should be able to generate a MIP of −60 cm H_2O or greater. An MIP of less than −20 cm H_2O is a sign of impending respiratory failure. A patient with an MIP value this low may not have the muscle strength to reverse atelectasis or to sustain normal ventilation before fatigue occurs, exacerbating the situation.

To measure the MIP, inform the patient that for a brief moment, inspiration of air will not be possible. Use of nose clips for the patient without an artificial airway is required. Have the patient breathe normally through the special 15 mm adapter on the inspiratory force manometer. Occlude the side port and instruct the patient to inhale as deeply as possible. The needle will deflect into the negative range, indicating the MIP generated. In the comatose patient, occlude the side port for 15 to 30 seconds and record the highest negative pressure generated along with the time interval.

BASIC SPIROMETRY

Determination of a slow vital capacity is often used to measure lung volumes and capacities. A complete inspiration slowly exhaled will often produce greater volumes than a forced maneuver, owing to airway closure causing air trapping with the latter. Figure 5-8 shows a typical slow vital capacity tracing. From this spirogram, four volumes and four capacities may be measured. A capacity by definition is two or more combined volumes.

Volumes

Tidal Volume

The tidal volume is defined as the amount of air moved into or out of a resting patient's lungs with each normal breath (see Figure 5-8).

Inspiratory Reserve Volume

Inspiratory reserve volume is defined as the maximum volume that can be inhaled after a normal inspiration (refer to Figure 5-8).

Expiratory Reserve Volume

Expiratory reserve volume is defined as the maximum amount of air that can be expired after a normal expiration (refer to Figure 5-8).

Residual Volume

The *residual volume (RV)* is the volume of gas left in the lungs following a maximal expiration. This volume cannot be measured directly but must be measured indirectly using nitrogen washout, helium dilution, or carbon monoxide methods.

CAPACITIES AND THEIR SIGNIFICANCE

Inspiratory Capacity

The *inspiratory capacity* is a combination of the tidal volume and the inspiratory reserve volume. This is the maximum volume that can be inspired from a resting expiratory level.

Normally, the inspiratory capacity approximates 75% of the vital capacity. Any increase or decrease in the inspiratory capacity will usually also be seen in the vital capacity.

Vital Capacity

The vital capacity is defined as the amount of air that can be exhaled following a maximal inspiration (see Figure 5-8). The vital capacity is a combination of the inspiratory reserve volume, tidal volume, and expiratory reserve volume.

Functional Residual Capacity

The *functional residual capacity (FRC)* is a combination of the ERV and the RV.

An increase in the FRC is considered pathologic. This change reflects hyperinflation and air trapping.

Total Lung Capacity

The *total lung capacity (TLC)* is a combination of all lung volumes. An increase or decrease in TLC may signify pulmonary disease. Typically, the TLC is compared with the vital capacity in determining the underlying cause of the reduction or increase in volume. The TLC cannot be measured at the bedside.

THE FORCED VITAL CAPACITY TRACING

Figure 5-9 illustrates a typical *forced vital capacity (FVC)* tracing. From this tracing, the FVC, timed forced expired volume (FEV_1), forced expired flow between 200 and 1200 mL ($FEF_{200-1200}$), midexpiratory forced expired flow ($FEF_{25-75\%}$), and PEFR can be measured. The FVC is measured by having the patient inhale maximally and then exhale maximally into a spirometer.

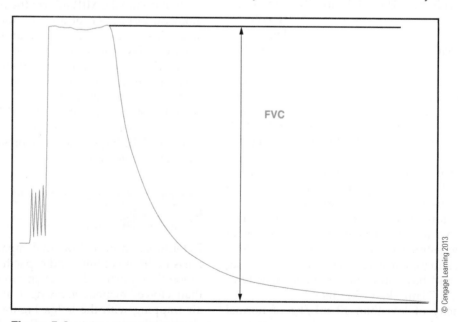

FVC

© Cengage Learning 2013

Figure 5-9   A forced vital capacity tracing

This exhalation is a forced maneuver accomplished by encouraging the patient to blow the air out of the lungs as quickly as possible.

Timed Forced Expired Volume

The FEV_t is the forced expired volume over a given time interval. The common time intervals over which the volume is measured are 0.5, 1, and 3 seconds. The most common measurement is performed after 1 second. Figure 5-10 shows the FEV_1 measurement. Note the starting point of the FVC maneuver in the figure. The kymograph is rotating at 1920 mm/min or 32 mm/sec. Therefore, a 32 mm horizontal distance from the beginning of the maneuver corresponds to a 1-second time interval.

This measurement can provide an indication of obstruction. However, the test validity depends on the effort and cooperation of the patient. A decreased FEV_t may indicate obstruction and restriction. The FEV_1 is often compared to the FVC as the ratio FEV_1/FVC, or FEV%. Generally, patients with obstruction show a reduction in FVC%, whereas patients with restriction show a normal FEV_1% (Pellegrino, 2005).

Forced Expired Flow between 200 and 1200

$FEF_{200-1200\ mL}$ is a measurement of the flow rate between 200 and 1200 mL on the FVC curve. Figure 5-11 is a measurement of this flow. Two points on the FVC curve are marked, indicating the exhalation of 200 mL and of 1200 mL. A line is drawn intersecting these points and extending over a 1-second interval. The corresponding flow may then be measured in liters per second.

The $FEF_{200-1200}$ generally indicates the airflow characteristics of the large airways. Obstructive disease processes will cause a decrease in the $FEF_{200-1200}$. A decrease in this flow rate normally occurs with aging.

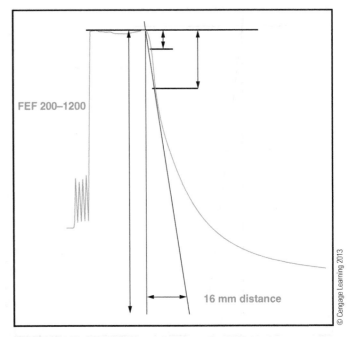

Figure 5-11 The $FEF_{200-1200}$ shown on the FVC tracing

Midexpiratory Forced Expired Flow

$FEF_{25-75\%}$ is the flow rate over the middle portion of the FVC maneuver. The FVC tracing is divided into four parts, and the flow rate over the middle two parts (middle 50%) is calculated (Figure 5-12).

The $FEF_{25-75\%}$ is indicative of the flow characteristics of small-size airways (Pellegrino, 2005). A decrease in the $FEF_{25-75\%}$ may signify obstruction. Because the test detects the airflow characteristics of the smaller airways, it is less dependent on effort and is often used for the early detection of obstructive disease. This flow rate decreases normally with advancing age.

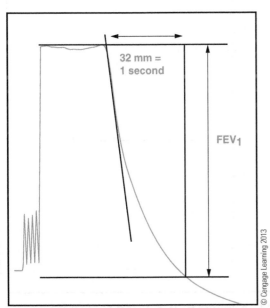

Figure 5-10 The FEV_1 shown on the FVC tracing

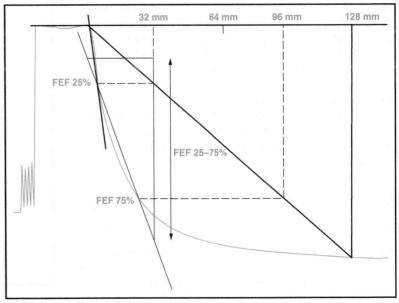

Figure 5-12 The $FEF_{25-75\%}$ shown on the FVC tracing

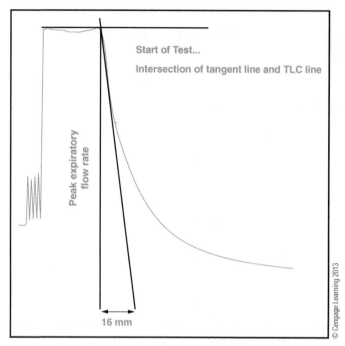

Figure 5-13 The peak expiratory flow rate calculated from the FVC

Peak Expiratory Flow Rate

The PEFR may be measured by extrapolating the steepest portion of the FVC tracing over a 1-second time interval (Figure 5-13). The flow may then be calculated in liters per second.

The PEFR is of little clinical significance. A patient with obstructive disease may have an initially high PEFR that rapidly decreases over time.

MAXIMUM VOLUNTARY VENTILATION

The *maximum voluntary ventilation (MVV)* is measured by having the patient stand (if possible) and breathe as deeply and rapidly as possible over a 10-, 12-, or 15-second interval. The volumes may be added individually, or if the spirometer has an accumulator pen, the volumes are added automatically. The volume is then extrapolated and measured in liters per minute.

The MVV is very effort-dependent and is therefore more of a reflection of muscle strength, airway resistance, and compliance. Patients with obstructive disease have a reduced MVV volume.

ATPS TO BTPS CONVERSION

All pulmonary function testing is performed at *ambient temperature and pressure, saturated (ATPS)*. Volumes and flows must be converted to reflect conditions of *body temperature and pressure, saturated (BTPS)*. This conversion is important because the volumes are larger under BTPS conditions. As the temperature of a gas increases,

it expands. The difference between ambient temperature and body temperature is typically 13°C. If the measurements were not converted, the difference would represent a significant error.

FLOW-VOLUME LOOPS

Flow-volume loops present spirometry information in a way different from that used with the volume-time curves discussed so far. A flow-volume loop plots flow along the vertical axis and volume along the horizontal axis (Figure 5-14). The expiratory portion of the curve is above the volume axis line—the *iso flow line*. The inspiratory portion of the curve is below the iso flow line.

The FVC is determined by measuring along the horizontal axis using the volume scale provided from point *A* to point *B* on Figure 5-15. This horizontal distance (volume), as in volume-versus-time spirometry, is measured at ATPS and therefore must be converted to reflect BTPS conditions.

Flows on the flow-volume loop are determined by evaluating the tracing in relation to the vertical axis. The PEF is determined by finding the highest point the curve reaches above the iso flow line. Once this point has been determined, the flow is read directly from the flow scale (Figure 5-16). An advantage of the flow-volume loop over volume-versus-time spirometry is the capability to directly measure flow at any point on the curve. The peak inspiratory flow is determined in a similar way to the PEF. Simply identify the lowest point on the inspiratory portion of the tracing and measure the flow directly from the flow axis at that point (Figure 5-16). As with volume determination, the flows should also be converted from ATPS to BTPS and reported in BTPS.

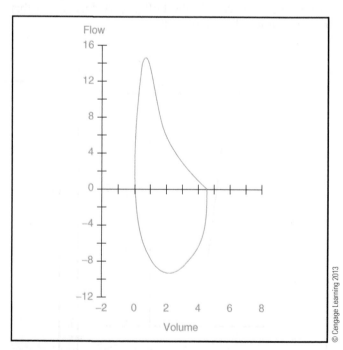

Figure 5-14 A flow volume loop. Note the vertical axis is scaled in L/sec and the horizontal axis is scaled in L. Expiration is above the iso-flow line and inspiration is below it

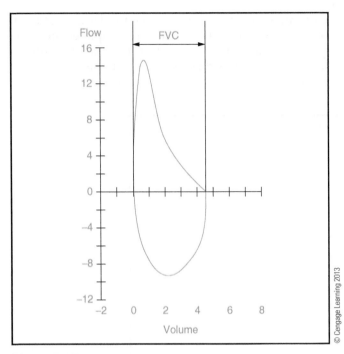

Figure 5-15 Calculation of the FVC. Note that the FVC is the volume between points *A* and *B*

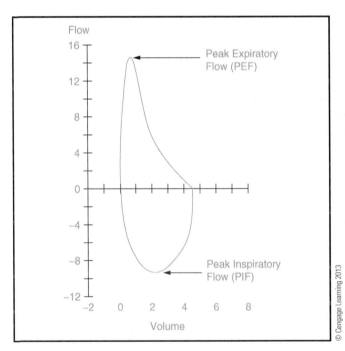

Figure 5-16 Determination of peak inspiratory and peak expiratory flows. Peak inspiratory flow corresponds to (A), whereas peak expiratory flow corresponds to (B)

With obstructive and restrictive pulmonary disease, the shape (morphology) of the flow-volume loop is altered. In obstructive disease, note that the expiratory portion of the curve is not as linear, as seen in Figure 5-17. Sometimes this characteristic is termed "scooping." A patient with obstructive disease is unable to generate sufficient expiratory flows; therefore, the shape of the expiratory curve changes (Fitzgerald, Speir, & Callahan, 1996). In restrictive disease, the patient is unable to inspire as fully as a normal person can. Also, because of a general

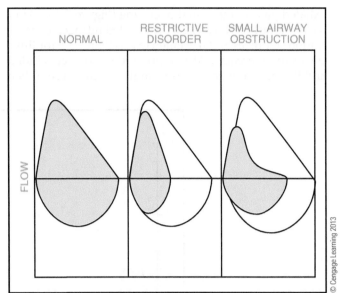

Figure 5-17 An obstructive and restrictive patient's flow-volume loop. Note how the expiratory portion is not as linear as the normal tracing (dashed line). In the restrictive tracing, note how it appears "tall and skinny."

decrease in pulmonary compliance, there is a greater elastic recoil of the lungs. These pathophysiologic changes result in a tall, skinny flow-volume loop (Figure 5-17). The volume is decreased (horizontal axis), whereas flows are normal or greater than normal (vertical axis).

MEASUREMENT OF FUNCTIONAL RESIDUAL CAPACITY AND RESIDUAL VOLUME

Both the FRC and RV cannot be measured by using direct spirometry. Both volumes, however, contribute to the TLC and are often helpful in the diagnosis of both obstructive and restrictive lung disease. Two common techniques are used to determine the FRC and RV: gas dilution techniques and body plethysmography.

Gas Dilution Techniques

Gas dilution techniques include nitrogen washout and helium dilution techniques. Because both techniques measure FRC and RV using a similar method, only one, *nitrogen washout*, is discussed here. Both methods are based on the following formula:

$$C_1V_1 = C_2V_2$$

where the initial concentration and volume (C_1 and V_1) and the final concentration (C_2) are known and the final volume (lung volume V_2) is unknown. For measuring FRC using the nitrogen washout technique, the patient breathes in oxygen (100%) and exhales into the spirometer system. During the test, nitrogen (from room air) in the lungs is replaced by the oxygen as it is diluted. The exhaled volume and nitrogen concentration of the exhaled gas are measured over time (Figure 5-18). After 3 to 8 minutes (typically 7), the exhaled nitrogen concentration stabilizes and has fallen to less than 1.5% for three consecutive breaths. At that point, the test is concluded and the patient is removed from the mouthpiece. When performing this test, it is important to keep a tight seal on the mouthpiece (scuba-type mouthpieces are often used) and also to use nose clips. If a leak develops so that the patient breathes room air, a sudden spike in the exhaled nitrogen concentration will occur (Figure 5-19).

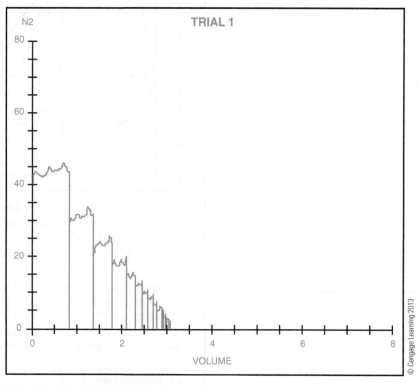

© Cengage Learning 2013

Figure 5-18 The exhaled nitrogen tracing from a nitrogen washout determination of FRC. Note how the nitrogen concentration falls over time

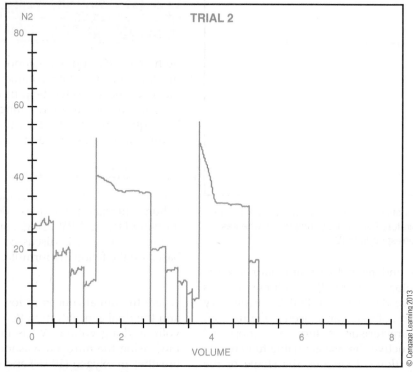

© Cengage Learning 2013

Figure 5-19 A leak occurred during this N_2 washout study. Note the sudden spike (increase) in exhaled nitrogen concentration

Computer-based pulmonary function systems automatically measure the final nitrogen concentration and exhaled volume, calculating the FRC, RV, and TLC. This technique can only measure gas that is in communication with the mouth. Any trapped gas distal to airway obstruction will not be measured (nitrogen will not be washed out). Therefore, this technique will underestimate RV and FRC in patients with obstructive disease (Brown, 1997).

Body Plethysmography

A body plethysmograph is a closed chamber that uses the principle of Boyle's law to measure lung volumes (Figure 5-20).

A patient is seated in the plethysmograph and the door is closed. After a minute or two, temperature stabilizes (the patient's body warms the interior of the plethysmograph). Once the temperature is stable, the patient splints the cheeks with the hands and gently pants (about 50 mL of volume at 1 pant per second [1 Hz]), as shown in Figure 5-20. A shutter closes, and mouth pressure is measured before and after shutter closure. The computer knows mouth pressure (before and after shutter closure) and plethysmograph volume. The unknown volume (thoracic gas volume, V_{TG}) of the lungs is then calculated. This technique is more accurate for RV and TLC determination in patients who have obstructive disease (Brown, 1997).

A body plethysmograph may also be used to measure *airway resistance*. The patient splints the cheeks with the hands and gently pants (about 50 mL of volume) but at a pant frequency of 90 to 150 per minute, which is faster than the V_{TG} pant frequency. Mouth (alveolar) and

plethysmograph pressures are recorded before and after shutter closure. The relationship between airflow and the pressure changes in the plethysmograph during panting determines airway resistance (R_{AW}). Normal airway resistance is between 0.6 and 2.4 cm $H_2O/L/sec$.

DIFFUSION: SINGLE BREATH CARBON MONOXIDE TEST

Clinically, it would be very useful to know how well oxygen and carbon dioxide diffuse across the alveolar capillary membranes between the blood and the ambient air. However, owing to the presence of these gases both dissolved in the blood and in the air, it is not possible to measure their diffusion directly. Carbon monoxide (CO), however, is not normally present in the blood and may be present only in trace quantities in the ambient air (under normal circumstances). In addition, CO has an affinity for hemoglobin that is 210 times greater than that of oxygen (MacIntyre et al., 2005). Once CO is present in the lungs, it rapidly diffuses across the alveolar-capillary membranes and binds with hemoglobin. Therefore, CO is an ideal gas to use for measuring how well *diffusion* occurs.

For the single breath CO diffusion test (single breath D_LCO test, where *L* refers to "lung"), the patient inspires CO, helium or neon, and oxygen in known concentrations. The CO is used to measure diffusion, whereas the helium or neon is used to measure alveolar volume (TLC) using a dilutional (washout) method. The patient inhales this mixture from RV to TLC and holds the breath at TLC for 10 seconds. Once the breath hold is met, the patient exhales back to RV. The first 750 to 1000 mL of gas is discarded. The sample volume of between 500 and 1000 mL is then collected and measured (MacIntyre, 2005). The computer system knows the inspired gas concentrations, measures the expired concentrations and exhaled volume, and calculates alveolar volume (V_A) and D_LCO. Figure 5-21 illustrates the inspiration from RV to TLC, the breath hold, and the exhaled gas tracings (concentrations).

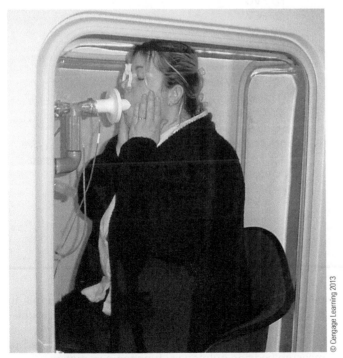

Figure 5-20 A patient seated in a body plethysmograph ready for V_{TG} determination. Note how the hands are splinting the cheeks and the elbows are at the patient's side

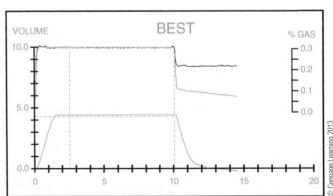

Figure 5-21 The tracing produced from a single breath carbon monoxide study (D_LCO). Note the inspiratory capacity and exhaled gas tracings

HAZARDS OF PULMONARY FUNCTION TESTING

Hyperventilation

The majority of the pulmonary function maneuvers involve greater than normal volumes and effort. Therefore, it is not uncommon for patients to become lightheaded or dizzy from the corresponding decrease in $PaCO_2$. With continued effort, *hyperventilation* may result.

Careful patient monitoring is essential for the prevention of this complication. Allow frequent rest periods. The rest periods allow the patient to recover to a normal ventilatory state and also help to ensure maximal efforts for all maneuvers. Patients who are very ill may easily overextend themselves and become compromised.

Cardiac Stimulation from Bronchodilators

The most common bronchodilators are sympathomimetic agents with $beta_1$-adrenergic side effects. Bronchodilators are administered during pulmonary function testing to assess the reversibility of lung dysfunction. A potential side effect is tachycardia, although newer medications have fewer side effects compared with earlier generations of $beta_1$-adrenergic drugs. Careful patient monitoring will ensure early detection of this complication.

Infection

Cross-contamination from the pulmonary function circuitry is not uncommon in patients undergoing pulmonary function testing. Patients with undiagnosed contagious pulmonary disease may be sent for testing. If permanent reusable circuitry is used, ensure that a clean, disinfected circuit is used for each patient. Disposable circuitry has recently become available, helping to minimize this potential hazard.

PROFICIENCY OBJECTIVES

At the end of this chapter, you should be able to:

* *Assemble and test the equipment required for bedside monitoring and basic spirometry:*
  — *Respirometer*
  — *Peak flowmeter*
  — *Inspiratory force manometer*
  — *Flow or self-inflating manual resuscitator*
  — *Collins spirometer*
* *Using a laboratory partner, demonstrate the proper position for bedside monitoring.*
* *Discuss the importance of coaching and solicitation to a maximal patient effort.*
* *Explain the rationale for obtaining multiple tracings for pulmonary function testing.*
* *Using a laboratory partner, demonstrate how to measure the following bedside pulmonary function parameters:*
  — *Minute volume*
  — *Frequency*
  — *Tidal volume*
  — *Vital capacity*
  — *Maximal inspiratory force*
  — *Peak expiratory flow*
* *Using a laboratory partner, demonstrate how to perform the following tests using the Collins spirometer:*
  — *Slow vital capacity*
  — *Forced vital capacity*

— *Maximum minute ventilation*
— *From these tracings, measure and calculate the following:*

Slow Vital Capacity
(1) IRV
(2) Tidal volume
(3) ERV
(4) VC

Forced Vital Capacity
(1) FVC
(2) FEV_1
(3) $FEF_{200-1200}$
(4) $FEF_{25-75\%}$
(5) PEFR

Maximum Voluntary Ventilation
(1) Respiratory rate
(2) Minute volume
— *Using the foregoing measurements, calculate the predicted values for your laboratory partner and give each measured value as a percent of the predicted.*
— *Interpret the results of the tracings as normal, restricted, or obstructed.*

BEDSIDE MONITORING: EQUIPMENT ASSEMBLY AND TESTING

A few pieces of specialized equipment and a watch are all that is required to measure bedside pulmonary function parameters. The equipment is generally quite simple in its design and operation; therefore, problems and troubleshooting are minimal.

Figure 5-22 is a listing of the equipment required to measure bedside pulmonary function parameters.

These simple instruments require little in the way of preparation. Preparation and testing of the various instruments are discussed in the following paragraphs.

- Respirometer
- Inspiratory force manometer
- Peak flowmeter
- Watch (with a sweep second hand)

Figure 5-22 Equipment required for bedside monitoring

Respirometers

Wright and Haloscale Respirometers may be tested by sliding the on/off switch to the on position and gently blowing into the base of the respirometer. The dial should indicate the volume exhaled. If no reading is indicated, verify that the switch is in the on position and that the flow is directed into the spirometer through the port at the 6 o'clock position as the dial is read. If no recording is made, the unit is probably inoperative.

Attach a mouthpiece, using a short piece of large-bore aerosol tubing and the 22 mm adapter supplied with the respirometer. This respirometer is now ready for use.

Peak Flowmeters

Proper operation of Wright and Mini-Wright peak flowmeters can be verified by blowing into the units and observing if flow is registered. The mouthpieces provided by the manufacturer may be used, or cardboard mouthpieces commonly used for pulmonary function testing may be substituted.

The operation of the Boehringer inspiratory force manometer may be tested by attaching a short piece of tubing to the 15 mm adapter and inhaling, generating a negative pressure. If pressure is recorded, the unit is functional. This device has a second indication hand that may be positioned over the measuring hand on the dial. The second indication hand indicates the maximum negative pressure generated. Figure 5-23 shows the correct positioning of the two hands for inspiratory force measurement.

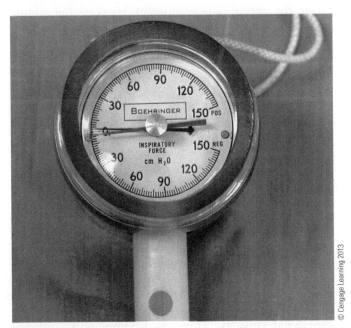

Figure 5-23 The Boehringer inspiratory force manometer prepared for use

PREPARATION OF THE COLLINS WATER SEAL SPIROMETER

The Collins water seal spirometer is one of the most frequently used spirometers in clinical practice today. Contemporary spirometers are often interfaced with a computer that hastens the process of calculating values for the pulmonary function measures. However, when a computer fails, a backup Collins water seal spirometer is frequently used, and all results are calculated manually.

It is very easy to learn pulmonary function testing on a computerized spirometer. However, the process and concepts are more thoroughly learned when the pulmonary function study values are manually calculated. It is important to understand the concepts and to visualize the process. Learning how to calculate pulmonary function testing values manually, without the aid of computers, will help the respiratory practitioner to understand how these values are derived.

Level the Spirometer and Fill with Water

Level the spirometer by using the leveling screws at the four corners of the spirometer. When the spirometer is level, check the water level using the glass sight gauge.

If required, fill the spirometer by raising the bell halfway and pouring water against the side of the bell. The water will run down into the reservoir surrounding the bell. Fill the spirometer with water until the water level is midway up the sight gauge.

Check for Excessive Resistance

Raise the spirometer bell and remove it. Remove the CO_2 absorber in the center of the spirometer and replace the bell. If resistance is improved, repack the CO_2 absorber with Collins soda lime CO_2 absorbent (the indicator turns violet when it has been used), and replace the CO_2 absorber.

Adjust the Bell and Pulley System

Adjust the angle of the pulley system so that the bell is suspended without contacting the sides of the spirometer. This will ensure that the bell is free to move without excessive resistance.

Attach the Pens to the Recorder

Place fresh pens into their holders on the recorder. Black is traditionally used for the spirometry tracing, and red is used for the accumulator pen. The spirometer pen has the greater motion of the two recorders. Keep caps on the pens at all times unless performing a study. This precaution will help to minimize extraneous lines due to inadvertent pen contact with the paper.

Attach the Paper to the Kymograph

Turn the kymograph to its highest speed and note the direction of rotation. When attaching the paper, position it so that the overlap does not catch on rotation of the drum. Attach the paper with masking tape and ensure that it is straight and square to the kymograph drum.

Flush the Spirometer

Flush the spirometer by raising and lowering the bell several times to expel any stale air that may be in the bell. This will facilitate patient cooperation and hygiene.

Attach Clean Tubing, Valve, and Mouthpiece

When attaching clean tubing to the inlet and outlet sides of the spirometer, it is imperative to avoid accidental flow restriction; be sure to use tubing of the proper diameter. Attach clean tubing to the inlet and the outlet of the spirometer. Attach a clean valve with mouthpiece to the tubing and secure it to the support arm. The spirometer is now ready to be used for testing.

PATIENT FACTORS IN SPIROMETRY

Patient Positioning

The correct patient position for measuring these parameters is an upright position. Position the patient upright without causing undue harm. This will allow the lungs to expand freely without interference.

The Importance of Coaching

The success and validity of pulmonary function tests are largely dependent on patient response and cooperation. Therefore, it is to the practitioner's advantage to elicit the maximum patient response and cooperation. This may be facilitated in several ways. Treat the patient as a respected individual. Thoroughly explain the maneuvers to the patient, and encourage and coach the patient throughout the testing.

Patient instruction is very important. These measurements are very effort-dependent. Take time to explain in detail what is required for each test. Have the patient practice the maneuver quietly and without a great deal of effort. This rehearsal may ease any anxieties the patient has and help to obtain good results when the actual tracing is measured.

During the testing, coach and encourage the patient. If more effort is required to obtain a good tracing, raise the voice when coaching. Pulmonary function testing is somewhat like cheerleading: it takes effort to elicit a good response.

Why Multiple Tests or Tracings?

Multiple tracings are frequently obtained from the same patient. The respiratory practitioner will often be assessing patients for disability payments. There is a monetary reward for poor performance on the tests in such cases. A patient may be deliberately malingering. If this is suspected, be very firm and insistent on obtaining the patient's best effort. Remember that results will determine payment or nonpayment. Take more than one measurement of each tracing, preferably making three. Results for all tracings should be within 5% of each other to establish reproducibility. The best tracing is one with the greatest sum of the FVC and FEV_1.

MEASURING THE BEDSIDE PULMONARY FUNCTION PARAMETERS

Aseptic Technique

Strict adherence to aseptic technique is important to prevent the spread of hospital-acquired infections. A separate mouthpiece should be used for each patient. Some facilities provide a plastic bag to store mouthpieces and other equipment in a patient's room. Avoid handling the portion of the mouthpiece in contact with the patient. The possibility of acquiring and spreading bacteria by this means is obvious.

Do not lay the equipment (spirometer, peak flowmeter, MIP manometer) on the patient's bed or bedside table. These areas harbor bacteria, and the measuring devices can be the vehicle for spreading them to other areas.

Measurements

Using the appropriate equipment, measure the minute volume, frequency, tidal volume, vital capacity (VC), PEFR, and MIP.

BASIC SPIROMETRY: USING THE COLLINS WATER SEAL SPIROMETER

Kymograph Speeds

There are several kymograph speeds available, depending on the individual manufacturer. Two speeds, low and high, are fairly standard. These speeds are 32 mm/min on the low speed and 1920 mm/min on the high speed. The variation in speeds among kymographs is commonly found in the middle or medium speed. The two most common speeds are 160 mm/min and 480 mm/min, depending on the spirometer.

The slow speed allows a better measurement of the slow vital capacity. This speed provides a complete tracing in a relatively small area of paper. All volumes are easily seen and read.

The medium speed is used for the MVV maneuver. At the slower speed, it becomes difficult to measure the individual volumes and count the respiratory rate. At the highest speed, the tracing would wrap itself more than once as the drum rotated. The fastest speed is used to perform the FVC tracing. This is considered to be the universally acceptable kymograph speed for FVC measurement. The tracing is relatively compact and yet easy to read.

If careful with paper usage, the respiratory practitioner can obtain a slow VC, FVC, and MVV tracing all on one sheet of paper.

Alignment of the Pen Mechanism to the Paper

Remove the cap from the black tracing pen and position it against the paper. Draw a vertical line by moving the bell up and down. The line will serve as a reference for measuring the values; it is a true vertical line. Recap the pen.

Measuring Testing Conditions

Note on the graph paper the conditions of the testing environment such as spirometer temperature (ambient temperature may be substituted in the absence of a spirometer thermometer) and barometric pressure in millimeters of mercury (mm Hg).

Bell Factor

The *bell factor* is used to calculate the volumes and flows from tracings. This bell factor is specific for the spirometer that is being used. The bell factor is expressed in milliliters per millimeter (mL/mm). Typical bell factors are 20.73 mL/mm and 41.27 mL/mm. Record the bell factor on the graph paper for the spirometer in use. It is usually indicated on a plate attached to the spirometer.

PULMONARY FUNCTION TESTS

Slow Vital Capacity

Turn the valve to the off position (so that the patient is breathing room air and not into the spirometer). Remove the pen cap and position it on the paper. Explain what the patient needs to do and what to expect. Have the patient breathe quietly through the mouthpiece with the value in the off position to become accustomed to the device. Place nose clips on the patient's nose and allow a few breaths for the patient to become accustomed to this way of breathing.

Turn the kymograph to the lowest speed (32 mm/min) and check to be certain that the kymograph drum is moving because it is difficult to detect motion at this speed. Upon opening the valve to the spirometer, the pen will begin to move, recording the patient's volumes. Have the patient breathe normally for approximately 5 breaths. Instruct the patient to inhale as deeply as possible and then to slowly blow out all the air in the lungs. Coach the patient by encouraging a maximal effort and volume. Allow the patient to relax by breathing at a "resting" tidal volume level.

Turn off the valve to the spirometer and allow the patient to rest a minute or two. Check the tracing and do a rough measurement to see if it approximates a normal value for that patient. If the practitioner suspects that the patient was malingering or that the effort was not maximal, the test should be repeated.

Forced Vital Capacity

Remove the CO_2 absorber from the spirometer bell. The absorber creates a resistance to air as the patient's volumes move through the spirometer circuit. Leaving the absorber in place during forced maneuvers will simulate an obstructive condition.

This test requires some timing and coordination between the practitioner and the patient. Read through this section thoroughly before attempting this test.

Turn the valve to the off position (so that the patient is breathing room air and not into the spirometer). Remove the pen cap and position it on the paper.

Explain what the patient needs to do and what to expect. Have the patient breathe quietly through the mouthpiece in the off position for a few breaths to become accustomed to the device. Place nose clips on the patient's nose and allow a few breaths for the patient to become accustomed to this way of breathing.

Remove the cap from the pen and turn the kymograph on to its lowest speed (32 mm/min). Turn the valve on so that the patient is breathing through the spirometer. Have the patient inhale as deeply as possible and instruct the patient to hold up a hand when further inhaling is impossible. Be sure to coach the patient. When the patient's lungs are full, ask the patient to hold his or her breath. Immediately turn the kymograph to its fastest speed (1920 mm/min) and tell the patient to exhale as forcefully and as quickly as possible. Coach the patient to produce a maximal effort. After the patient has exhaled as much as possible, turn off the kymograph and recap the pen.

Allow the patient to rest. Take this opportunity to quickly measure the tracing to see if it is close to what is expected. If the practitioner suspects that the patient was malingering or that the effort was not maximal, the test should be repeated. The test should be repeated a minimum of three times. Results for three tests should be within 5% of one another. The best result is defined as the one with the greatest sum of the FVC and FEV_1.

Measuring Maximal Voluntary Ventilation (MVV) with a Spirometer and Accumulator Pen

Turn the valve to the off position (so that the patient is breathing room air and not into the spirometer). Remove the pen cap and position the pen on the paper. Explain what the patient needs to do and what to expect. Have the patient breathe quietly through the mouthpiece with the valve in the off position for a few breaths to become accustomed to the device. Place nose clips on the patient's nose and allow the patient a few breaths to become accustomed to this way of breathing.

Start the accumulator pen by engaging the plate/gear mechanism of the Reicher Ventilometer. Pushing the clutch plate in engages it; pulling it out disengages it. Remove the caps from the red and black recording pens and position them on the paper. Turn the kymograph to the medium speed and turn on the valve so that the patient is breathing through the spirometer. Instruct the patient to breathe as deeply and as quickly as possible. This is similar to panting. Coach the patient to obtain the best effort. Time the maneuver for 15 seconds; then turn off the kymograph and valve. Allow the patient to rest. If the practitioner suspects that the patient was malingering or that the effort was not maximal, the test should be repeated. Recap the pens. This concludes the maneuvers performed for basic spirometry.

If the spirometer in use does not have an accumulator pen, measure the MVV using the following method. Allow the patient to become accustomed to the spirometer with the valve in the off position. Turn the kymograph to medium speed and turn the valve to the on position and have the patient breathe as deeply and quickly as possible. Time the maneuver for 15 seconds. Turn off the kymograph and allow the patient to rest.

MEASURING AND CALCULATING COMPONENTS OF A PULMONARY FUNCTION TESTING TRACING

Tidal Volume

The tidal volume is the smallest tracing on the slow VC tracing (Figure 5-24). Draw horizontal lines across the top and bottom of the tracing, as shown in Figure 5-24. These lines should be at right angles to the reference line drawn by the pen before beginning the testing. Perform the following steps to measure and calculate the tidal volume:

1. Measure the distance between the two lines, represented in Figure 5-24 as *A*.
2. Take this distance in millimeters and multiply it by the bell factor. This is the tidal volume.

Tidal volume = distance (mm) × bell factor (mL/mm)

Inspiratory Reserve Volume

The inspiratory reserve volume (IRV) is the maximum volume that can be inhaled after a normal inhalation. Draw a horizontal line (at a right angle to the reference line) across the point of maximal inspiration, as shown in Figure 5-24.

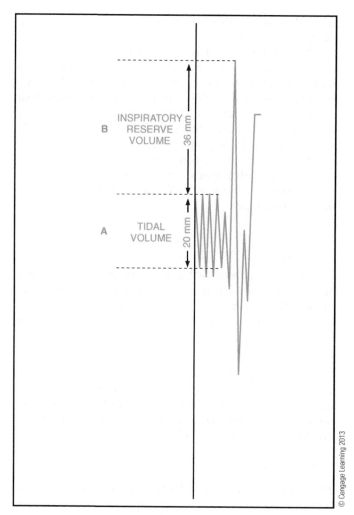

Figure 5-24 Calculating the tidal volume and the inspiratory reserve volume

The IRV is the distance *B* in the figure. To measure and calculate the IRV, complete the following steps:

1. Measure the distance between the point of maximum inspiration and the upper limit of a normal tidal volume (refer to Figure 5-24).
2. Multiply this distance in millimeters by the bell factor.

Inspiratory reserve volume = distance (mm) × bell factor (mL/mm)

Expiratory Reserve Volume

The expiratory reserve volume (ERV) is the maximum amount of air that can be exhaled from a resting expiratory level. Draw a horizontal line through the point of maximal exhalation (at a right angle to the reference line). Measure the distance between this line and the resting expiratory level. This is represented by distance *C* in Figure 5-25. To calculate the ERV, use the following steps:

1. Measure the distance between the point of maximal exhalation and the resting expiratory level in millimeters.

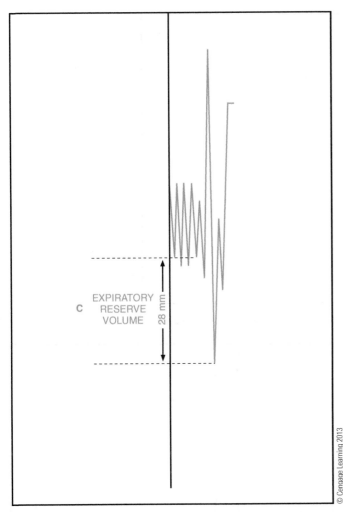

Figure 5-25   Calculating the expiratory reserve volume

2. Multiply the measurement by the bell factor.

$$ERV = distance\ (mm) \times bell\ factor\ (mL/mm)$$

Residual Volume

The RV requires a nitrogen washout test to determine the volume. It also requires special equipment to measure the nitrogen concentration. Not all schools or facilities have this equipment. If the practitioner has access to this equipment and wishes to perform this test, he or she should consult the *Manual of Pulmonary Function Testing* by Gregg Ruppel (see Additional Resources at the end of the chapter) for instructions.

MEASURING AND CALCULATING THE FORCED VITAL CAPACITY

Forced Vital Capacity (FVC)

The FVC is the maximum volume forcefully expired after a maximal inspiration. This can be identified as between the highest and lowest volumes on the curve. This volume

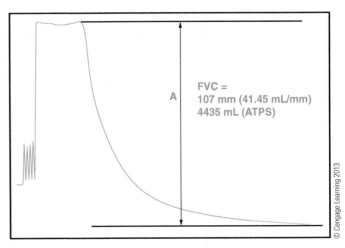

Figure 5-26   Calculating the forced vital capacity

is represented by distance *A* in Figure 5-26. Draw a horizontal line (at a right angle to the reference line) across the point of maximal inspiration and expiration as shown in Figure 5-26. To calculate the FVC, complete the following steps:

1. Measure the distance in millimeters from the point of maximal inspiration to maximal expiration.
2. Multiply this distance by the bell factor.

$$FVC = distance\ (mm) \times bell\ factor\ (mL/mm)$$

Forced Expired Volume in 1 Second (FEV$_1$)

This is the portion of the FVC that was expired in the first second of the maneuver.

To measure this, first establish the starting point of the maneuver. On some tracings this is very clearly defined as shown in Figure 5-27, graph *A*. Note the clear, sharp transition between the point at which the patient was holding the breath (level plateau) and the FVC maneuver. This starting point is not always clear, owing to hesitation on the part of the patient. The starting point may then be extrapolated.

To extrapolate the starting point, identify the steepest portion of the FVC tracing (maximal flow). Draw a line tangent to this portion of the FVC tracing. Intersect this line with a horizontal line (at a right angle to the reference line) even with the point of maximal inspiration, as shown in Figure 5-27, graph *B*.

From this starting point, measure a 32 mm horizontal distance from the starting point. A distance of 32 mm represents 1 second (1920 mm/min for 60 seconds = 32 mm). Draw a vertical line from this point until it intersects the FVC tracing. Make certain that this line is parallel to the reference line. Measure this distance, represented by distance *B* in Figure 5-28. To calculate the FEV$_1$, complete the following steps:

1. Measure a 32 mm horizontal distance from the start of the FVC tracing.
2. Draw a vertical line down from this point until it intersects the FVC tracing.

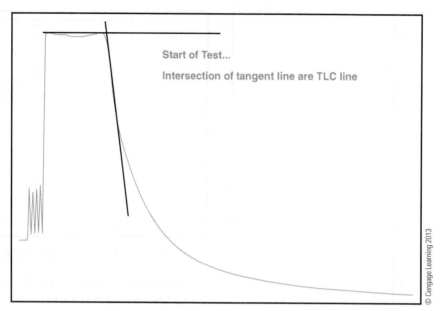

Figure 5-27   Identifying the starting point of the forced vital capacity maneuver

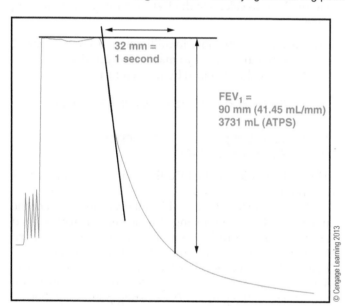

32 mm =
1 second

$FEV_1 =$
90 mm (41.45 mL/mm)
3731 mL (ATPS)

Figure 5-28   Calculating the FEV_1

3. Measure the distance of this vertical line in millimeters.
4. Multiply this distance by the bell factor.

$$FEV_1 = \text{distance (mm)} \times \text{bell factor (mL/mm)}$$

Forced Expired Flow between 200 and 1200 mL

The $FEF_{200-1200}$ is the flow rate between 200 and 1200 mL on the FVC tracing. To calculate this, first establish the points on the FVC tracing that correspond to 200 mL and to 1200 mL.

To find these points, divide the desired volumes by the bell factor, as shown next:

$$200\ mL = 200\ mL/41.27\ mm/mL$$
$$= 4.8\ mm$$
$$1200\ mL = 1200\ mL/41.27\ mm/mL$$
$$= 29\ mm$$

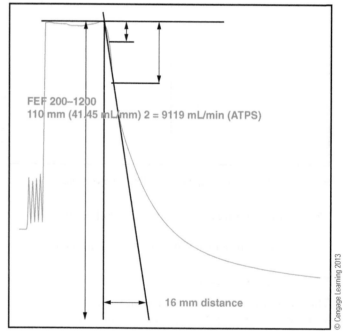

FEF 200–1200
110 mm (41.45 mL/mm) 2 = 9119 mL/min (ATPS)

16 mm distance

Figure 5-29   Calculating the $FEF_{200-1200}$

Note that these distances were calculated using the bell factor for the spirometer used in the figures in this chapter. Be certain to use the bell factor for the spirometer in use.

Once the distances for 200 and 1200 mL represented on the FVC tracing have been calculated, measure these distances from the point of maximal inspiration, as shown in Figure 5-29. It is convenient to use the vertical line when measuring the FEV_1 to establish these points. Transfer these points onto the FVC tracing.

Draw a line intersecting these two points, and extend that line so that a 32 mm horizontal distance is covered, as shown in Figure 5-29. Measure the vertical distance A as shown in Figure 5-29. Multiply this distance by the bell factor. This is the $FEF_{200-1200}$ in milliliters per second.

Midexpiratory Forced Expired Flow

The $FEF_{25-75\%}$ is the flow rate over the middle portion of the FVC tracing. To calculate the $FEF_{25-75\%}$, first divide the FVC tracing into four parts.

To divide the tracing into four parts, measure a 128 mm horizontal distance from the beginning of the FVC tracing. Mark this horizontal line into four 32 mm segments. Draw a horizontal line extending toward the beginning of the FVC curve even with the point of maximal expiration. Intersect this line with a vertical line from the 128 mm distance previously measured. Extend two more vertical lines extending from the 32 mm mark (25%) and the 96 mm point (75%) that intersect the FVC

tracing. When this is completed, the divisions should appear as they are in Figure 5-30. The tracing should now be divided into four equal parts.

The practitioner may also find the 25% and 75% points on the FVC tracing using the following method. Multiply the distance of the FVC in millimeters by 0.25 and 0.75.

$$25\% \text{ of FVC} = \text{FVC (mm distance)} \times 0.25$$
$$75\% \text{ of FVC} = \text{FVC (mm distance)} \times 0.75$$

Once these distances have been calculated, subtract them from the beginning of the FVC tracing along a vertical line (the FEV_1 is convenient) and mark the corresponding points on the FVC tracing, as shown in Figure 5-31.

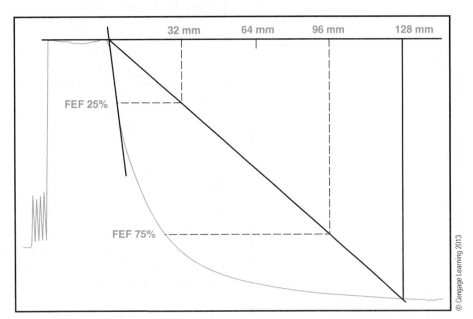

Figure 5-30   Dividing the FVC tracing into four equal parts and marking the points on the FVC tracing

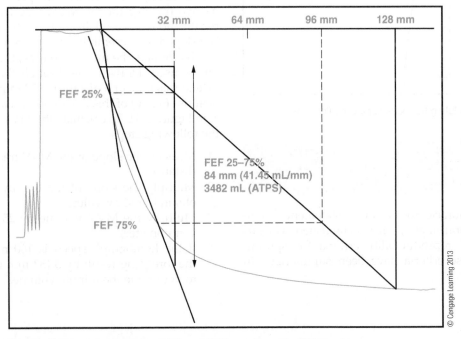

Figure 5-31   Measuring the 25% and 75% points on the FVC tracing

Once the $FEF_{25\%}$ and $FEF_{75\%}$ points are established, draw an intersecting line through them and extend the line so that a 32 mm horizontal distance is covered. Measure the vertical distance *A* as shown in Figure 5-31. Multiply this distance by the bell factor. This is the $FEF_{25-75\%}$ in milliliters per second.

Peak Expiratory Flow Rate

The PEFR may be calculated by identifying the steepest portion of the FVC tracing and drawing a line tangent to the tracing. Extend this line over a 32 mm horizontal distance. Measure the vertical distance in millimeters. Multiply this distance by the bell factor, as shown in Figure 5-32. This is the PEFR in milliliters per second.

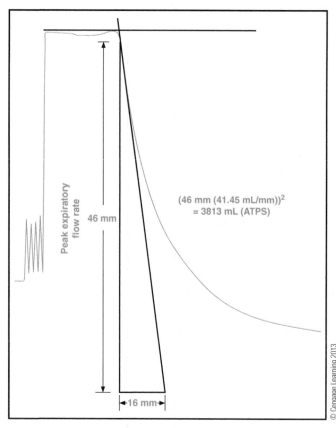

Figure 5-32 Calculating the peak expiratory flow rate

ACCEPTABILITY AND REPRODUCIBILITY CRITERIA

The American Thoracic Society in its statement, "Standardization of Spirometry," has established various acceptability and reproducibility criteria for spirometry studies. These criteria have been summarized in Figure 5-33.

Acceptability Criteria

- No coughing during the first second of the forced maneuver
- No early glottis closure
- Smooth continuous exhalation
- No leaks at the mouthpiece
- No obstruction of the mouthpiece with tongue or dentures
- Back extrapolation is ≤0.150 L or 5% whichever is greater
- Exhalation time is at least 6 seconds
- No change in volume (≤0.125 L) for ≥1 second at RV

Reproducibility Criteria

- At least three acceptable efforts (meet acceptability criteria)
- The two largest FVC and FEV_1 are + 150 mL
- Up to eight maneuvers may be performed to obtain three acceptable maneuvers

Figure 5-33 American Thoracic Society acceptability and reproducibility criteria

MAXIMUM VOLUNTARY VENTILATION

The MVV is the maximum amount of air that a patient can breathe in an interval of 1 minute. The test is measured over a 10-, 12-, or 15-second interval, and the measurement is extrapolated to 1 minute.

Measurement Using an Accumulator Pen (Ventilometer)

When using the accumulator pen feature, there will be two tracings for the MVV. One tracing records each breath and is sawtooth in configuration. The other tracing is a sloped line resembling a stair step pattern.

To calculate the minute volume, the stair step sloping line is used. Draw a line through the sloping line and extend this line for a distance of 32 mm. Measure the vertical rise (slope) of this line in millimeters, represented by *A* in Figure 5-34. To calculate the MVV volume, complete the following steps:

1. Measure the slope of the MVV tracing over a 32 mm distance.
2. Multiply the slope of the line by the bell factor to obtain the MVV volume.
3. Multiply the MVV volume by 25 (gear ratio of the ventilometer).
4. If the kymograph speed is 160 mm/min, multiply the foregoing result by 5 (32 mm distance = 12 sec) to determine the minute volume.

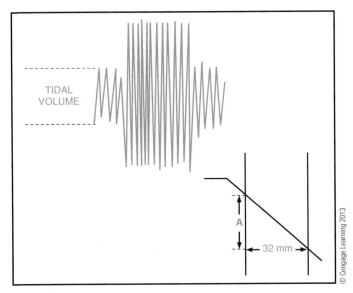

Figure 5-34 Calculating the MVV from the accumulator pen tracing

Calculating the MVV Manually

To calculate the MVV manually, mark off a 32 mm length along the sawtooth tracing. Each volume recorded on the sawtooth tracing must be individually measured. Add all of the measurements together. Multiply that measurement by the bell factor. Multiply this volume by 5 (12 sec = 32 mm at a kymograph speed of 160 mm/min). This is the minute volume.

Calculating the Respiratory Rate

Using the sawtooth-shaped tracing, count the number of breaths over a 32 mm horizontal interval. Multiply this number by 5 (32 mm horizontal distance = 7–12 sec at a kymograph speed of 480 mm/min).

CONVERSION FROM ATPS TO BTPS

All of the measurements that were made in the pulmonary function study were recorded at ambient temperature and pressure, saturated (ATPS). These values need to be converted to reflect body temperature and pressure, saturated (BTPS) conditions to be reported accurately. To convert these values, use the following formula:

$$\text{Volume (BTPS)} = \text{volume (ATPS)} \times \frac{P_B - P_{H_2O}}{P_B - 47} \times \frac{310}{273 + T}$$

where

P_B = barometric pressure
P_{H_2O} = partial pressure of H_2O at ATPS
273 = absolute temperature conversion factor
310 = absolute body temperature
47 = partial pressure of H_2O at BTPS

The partial pressure of H_2O at ATPS may be found by consulting tables in other references (White, 2005). After completing this formula, the practitioner will have a factor enabling conversion of ATPS volume to BTPS volume by multiplying by this factor: BTPS volume = ATPS volume × factor.

CALCULATING PREDICTED VALUES

Predicted values can be determined by using nomograms. These nomograms are available in many textbooks.

A complete set of nomograms is available through the Intermountain Thoracic Society (Salt Lake City, Utah). Figure 5-35 presents two of the more common nomograms used in calculating pulmonary function tests. To use the nomograms to calculate a patient's normal values, it is essential to know the patient's age and height. Lay a straightedge between the patient's height as read on the height scale and the patient's age as it appears on the age scale.

Once the normal values for the patient are known, all measured BTPS volumes should be divided by the predicted values to obtain a value reported as a percentage of predicted values.

Measured BTPS	Predicted BTPS	% Predicted
VC = 3.4 liters	VC = 4.2 liters	80.9%

INTERPRETATION OF THE RESULTS

Once the pulmonary function parameters have been measured and calculated, interpretation of the results is the last step. The respiratory practitioner must be able to recognize the significance of study findings. However, the physician is the person who reports the final results of any pulmonary function study.

Using Tables-5-2 and 5-3, determine the interpretation of the pulmonary function study results.

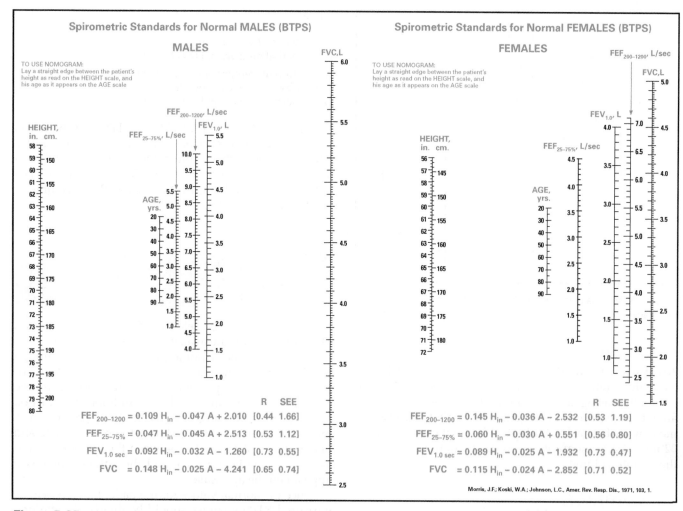

Figure 5-35 Nomograms used to find the predicted values for male and female patients (Courtesy of *American Review of Respiratory Disease*)

TABLE 5-2: Restriction and Obstruction		
TEST	**RESTRICTION**	**OBSTRUCTION**
Tidal volume	Decreased	Normal
IC	Decreased	Decreased
ERV	Decreased	Decreased
FVC	Decreased	Decreased
FEV₁	Normal	Decreased
$FEF_{25-75\%}$	Normal	Decreased
$FEF_{200-1200}$	Somewhat decreased	Decreased
MVV	Decreased	Decreased

TABLE 5-3: Severity of Abnormality	
Normal	>80%
Mild	70–80%
Moderate	60–70%
Moderately severe	50–60%
Severe	34–50%
Very severe	<34%

References

American Association for Respiratory Care. (1996). AARC clinical practice guideline: Spirometry, 1996 update. *Respiratory Care, 41*(7), 629–636.

American Thoracic Society. (2005). AU NOTE: Same reference as MacIntyre below. (GW 8/18/11)

Brown, R. A. (1997). Derivation, application, and utility of static lung volume measurements. *Respiratory Care Clinics of North America, 3*(2), 183–220.

Fitzgerald, D. J., Speir, W. A., & Callahan, L. A. (1996). Office evaluation of pulmonary function: Beyond the numbers. *American Family Physician, 54*(2), 525–534.

MacIntyre, N., Crapo, R. O., Viegi, G., Johnson, D. C., van der Grinten, C. P. M., Brusasco, V., et al. (2005), Standardization of the single-breath determination of carbon monoxide uptake in the lung. *European Respiratory Journal, 26*, 720–735.

Miller, M. R., et al. (2005). Standardization of spirometry, American Thoracic Society. *European Respiratory Journal, 26*, 319–339.

Pellegrino, R., Viegi, G., Brusasco, V., Crapo, R. O., Burgos, F., Casaburi, R., et al. (2005). Interpretive strategies for lung function tests. *European Respiratory Journal, 26*, 948–968.

White, G. C. (2005). *Equipment theory for respiratory care.* Clifton Park, NY: Delmar Cengage Learning.

Additional Resource

Ruppel, G. (2008). *Manual of pulmonary function testing* (9th ed.). St. Louis, MO: Elsevier.

Practice Activities: Pulmonary Function Testing: Bedside Monitoring and Basic Spirometry

Bedside Monitoring

1. Assemble the equipment needed for monitoring bedside pulmonary function parameters:
   a. Respirometer
   b. Peak flowmeter
   c. Inspiratory force manometer
   d. Flow or self-inflating manual resuscitator
   e. Watch

2. Demonstrate the following for the listed respirometers:
   a. Assemble the spirometer.
      (1) For a spontaneously breathing patient
   b. Test the spirometer for proper operation.
      (1) Wright respirometer
      (2) Haloscale respirometer

3. Practice measuring a vital capacity on a laboratory partner, taking several determinations. Ask your laboratory instructor to confirm your measurements.
   a. Coach your laboratory partner during the procedure.
   b. Ensure that flow rates are slow to avoid respirometer damage.

4. Using a laboratory partner, practice positioning for the measurement of bedside pulmonary function parameters.
   a. Place your laboratory partner in an upright position.
   b. Simulate clinical conditions that would require modification of this position.

5. Using a laboratory partner, measure all of the bedside pulmonary function parameters:
   a. Minute volume
   b. Frequency
   c. Tidal volume
   d. Vital capacity
   e. Maximal inspiratory pressure
   f. Peak expiratory flow rate
   Demonstrate the following while performing the procedure:
      (1) Instruct the patient in a clear, concise manner.
      (2) Accurately measure and record each measurement.
      (3) Use nose clips.
      (4) Allow sufficient rest periods between each measurement.

6. Following completion of your bedside pulmonary function assessment, document your findings on a blank sheet of paper. Have your instructor critique your charting.

Basic Spirometry

7. Prepare the Collins spirometer for use.

8. Turn on the kymograph to the various speeds to become accustomed to the different speeds.

9. Practice breathing through the spirometer.
   a. Note the direction of the pen motion
      (1) During inspiration
      (2) During expiration
   b. Breathe normally.
   c. Take an extra deep breath.
   d. Observe what effect different kymograph speeds have on the tracing.

10. Using a laboratory partner, practice giving instructions for the following maneuvers:
    a. Slow vital capacity
    b. Forced vital capacity
    c. Maximum voluntary ventilation

11. Using a laboratory partner, perform pulmonary function testing, including the following:
    a. Slow vital capacity
    b. FVC
    c. MVV

12. Calculate the following from the pulmonary function tracing you recorded.
    a. Slow vital capacity
       (1) IRV
       (2) Tidal volume
       (3) ERV

   b. FVC
      (1) FVC
      (2) FEV_1
      (3) $FEF_{200-1200}$
      (4) $FEF_{25-75\%}$
      (5) PEF
   c. MVV
      (1) Minute volume
      (2) Respiratory rate

13. Using a laboratory partner, simulate the following conditions:
    a. Restrictive
       (1) Use a Scultetus bandage or abdominal binder to restrict motion of the chest.
    b. Obstructive
       (2) Partially occlude the mouthpiece.
    c. Calculate the results and compare them with the results in Practice Activity 6.

Check List: Pulmonary Function Testing: Bedside Monitoring and Basic Spirometry

Bedside Monitoring

_____ 1. Assemble and test all of the equipment required:
_____   a. Respirometer
_____   b. Peak flowmeter
_____   c. Maximal inspiratory force manometer
_____   d. Watch
_____ 2. Position the patient for the procedure.
_____ 3. Measure all bedside pulmonary function parameters:
_____   a. Minute volume
_____   b. Frequency
_____   c. Tidal volume
_____   d. Vital capacity
_____   e. Maximal inspiratory force
_____   f. Peak expiratory flow rate
     4. Demonstrate the following while measuring the parameters:
_____   a. Instruct the patient clearly and concisely.
_____   b. Use nose clips.
_____   c. Accurately record each measurement.
_____   d. Allow sufficient rest periods between measurements.

_____ 5. Reposition the patient, and return to previous O_2 therapy.
_____ 6. Record the results on the patient's chart.

BASIC SPIROMETRY

_____ 1. Prepare the spirometer for use.
_____ 2. Record ambient conditions.
_____ 3. Explain the procedure to the patient.
     4. Perform the testing:
_____   a. Slow vital capacity
_____   b. FVC
_____   c. MVV
_____ 5. If you suspect the patient is not providing an optimal effort, be encouraging and more forceful in your coaching to obtain a maximal effort. If you suspect that the patient was unable to provide a good effort, make a note in your comments, describing the situation.
_____ 6. Thank the patient for his or her time and cooperation.
_____ 7. Calculate the results of the pulmonary function study.
_____ 8. Interpret the results.

Self-Evaluation Post Test: Pulmonary Function Testing: Bedside Monitoring and Basic Spirometry

1. Normal tidal volume may be estimated at:
   a. 2 to 3 mL/kg of body weight.
   b. 3 to 5 mL/kg of normal body weight.
   c. 3 to 7 mL/kg of normal body weight.
   d. 5 to 7 mL/kg of normal body weight.

2. Which of the following respirometers operate using a rotating vane?
   a. Collins spirometer
   b. Wright peak flowmeter
   c. Wright respirometer
   d. Boehringer inspiratory force manometer

3. It would be appropriate to use the Wright respirometer to measure which of the following parameters?
   I. Tidal volume
   II. Vital capacity
   III. Forced vital capacity
   IV. Peak expiratory flow rate
   V. Minute volume
   a. I, II, III   c. I, II, IV
   b. I, III, IV   d. I, II, V

4. Which one of the following maximal inspiratory forces indicates a reduced ventilatory reserve or possible muscle weakness?
   a. -60 cm H_2O c. -30 cm H_2O
   b. -50 psi   d. -20 cm H_2O

5. Which of the following is used to assess the effectiveness of a bronchodilator?
   a. Maximal inspiratory pressure
   b. Vital capacity
   c. Tidal volume
   d. Peak expiratory flow

6. The volumes measured during a PFT are measured at:
   a. BTPS.   c. BTPD.
   b. ATPS.   d. STPD.

7. The vital capacity includes:
   I. tidal volume.
   II. inspiratory reserve volume.
   III. expiratory reserve volume.
   IV. residual volume.
   a. I, II   c. I, II, III
   b. II, III   d. I, II, IV

8. Which of the following are derived from an FVC tracing?
   I. Tidal volume
   II. Forced vital capacity
   III. FEV_1
   IV. $FEF_{200-1200}$
   V. $FEF_{25-75\%}$
   VI. MVV
   a. I, II, III, V   c. II, III, IV, VI
   b. I, III, IV, V   d. II, III, IV, V

9. A subject's MVV tracing shows 15 breaths for a 32 mm horizontal distance; the patient's actual rate in breaths per minute is (assuming a kymograph speed of 160 mm/min):
   a. 15 breaths/min.   c. 50 breaths/min.
   b. 30 breaths/min.   d. 75 breaths/min.

10. A subject performs an MVV maneuver for 12 seconds; the total volume expired in this interval is 32 liters. What is the MVV volume in liters per minute?
    a. 32 liters/min   c. 160 liters/min
    b. 64 liters/min   d. 128 liters/min

PERFORMANCE EVALUATION:
Bedside Pulmonary Function Testing

Date: Lab _____ Clinical _____ Agency _____

Lab: Pass _____ Fail _____ Clinical: Pass _____ Fail _____

Student name _____ Instructor name _____

No. of times observed in clinical _____

No. of times practiced in clinical _____

PASSING CRITERIA: Obtain 90% or better on the procedure. Tasks indicated by * must receive at least 1 point, or the evaluation is terminated. Procedure must be performed within the designated time, or the performance receives a failing grade.

SCORING:
2 points — Task performed satisfactorily without prompting.
1 point — Task performed satisfactorily with self-initiated correction.
0 points — Task performed incorrectly or with prompting required.
NA — Task not applicable to the patient care situation.

Tasks:	Peer	Lab	Clinical
* 1. Verifies the physician's order	☐	☐	☐
2. Gathers the equipment	☐	☐	☐
* a. Respirometer	☐	☐	☐
* b. Maximal inspiratory force manometer	☐	☐	☐
* c. Peak flowmeter	☐	☐	☐
* d. Watch	☐	☐	☐
3. Assembles and tests the equipment	☐	☐	☐
* 4. Explains the procedure	☐	☐	☐
* 5. Performs hand hygiene	☐	☐	☐
* 6. Positions the patient	☐	☐	☐
* 7. Measures minute volume and frequency	☐	☐	☐
* 8. Calculates the tidal volume	☐	☐	☐
* 9. Measures the vital capacity	☐	☐	☐
* 10. Measures the maximal inspiratory pressure	☐	☐	☐
* 11. Measures the peak expiratory flow	☐	☐	☐
* 12. Allows the patient to rest as required	☐	☐	☐
* 13. Practices aseptic techniques	☐	☐	☐
* 14. Records all measurements on the patient's chart	☐	☐	☐

SCORE: Peer   _____ points of possible 34; _____%

Lab   _____ points of possible 34; _____%

Clinical _____ points of possible 34; _____%

TIME: _____ out of possible 15 minutes

STUDENT SIGNATURES

PEER: _____

STUDENT: _____

INSTRUCTOR SIGNATURES

LAB: _____

CLINICAL: _____

PERFORMANCE EVALUATION:
Basic Spirometry

Date: Lab _____ Clinical _____ Agency _____

Lab: Pass _____ Fail _____ Clinical: Pass _____ Fail _____

Student name _____ Instructor name _____

No. of times observed in clinical _____

No. of times practiced in clinical _____

PASSING CRITERIA: Obtain 90% or better on the procedure. Tasks indicated by * must receive at least 1 point, or the evaluation is terminated. Procedure must be performed within the designated time, or the performance receives a failing grade.

SCORING: 2 points — Task performed satisfactorily without prompting.
1 point — Task performed satisfactorily with self-initiated correction.
0 points — Task performed incorrectly or with prompting required.
NA — Task not applicable to the patient care situation.

Tasks:	Peer	Lab	Clinical
* 1. Verifies the order	☐	☐	☐
2. Scans the chart for pertinent information	☐	☐	☐
3. Gathers the appropriate equipment	☐	☐	☐
* 4. Observes standard precautions, including washing hands	☐	☐	☐
* 5. Prepares the spirometer for use	☐	☐	☐
* 6. Introduces self and explains the procedure to the patient	☐	☐	☐
7. Performs the following tests			
* a. Slow vital capacity	☐	☐	☐
* b. FVC	☐	☐	☐
* c. MVV	☐	☐	☐
* 8. Coaches the patient for optimal performance	☐	☐	☐
* 9. Repeats the test if the patient is malingering	☐	☐	☐
10. Thanks the patient for cooperating	☐	☐	☐
11. Correctly calculates			
* a. IRV	☐	☐	☐
* b. Tidal volume	☐	☐	☐
* c. ERV	☐	☐	☐
* d. FVC and FEV_1	☐	☐	☐

*   e. $FEF_{200-1200}$ and $FEF_{25-75\%}$ ☐ ☐ ☐

*   f. PEFR   ☐ ☐ ☐

*   g. MVV   ☐ ☐ ☐

* **12.** Converts values to reflect BTPS conditions and reports the results   ☐ ☐ ☐
as percent of the predicted result

* **13.** Interprets the results   ☐ ☐ ☐

* **14.** Reports the results to the appropriate personnel   ☐ ☐ ☐

SCORE: Peer _____ points of possible 44; _____%

Lab _____ points of possible 44; _____%

Clinical _____ points of possible 44; _____%

TIME: _____ out of possible 60 minutes

STUDENT SIGNATURES   **INSTRUCTOR SIGNATURES**

PEER: _____   LAB: _____

STUDENT: _____   CLINICAL: _____

CHAPTER 6
Electrocardiography

The electrocardiogram (ECG) is one of the most important diagnostic tools used in medicine. The information obtained noninvasively from the ECG tells the diagnostician about the electrical activity of the heart. From this information appropriate treatment can be prescribed to correct some of the abnormalities diagnosed using the ECG.

Because respiratory care involves the diagnosis and treatment of cardiopulmonary disorders, many respiratory care departments routinely perform electrocardiography as a part of their daily responsibilities. It is important for a respiratory practitioner to understand what an ECG is, how to recognize normal and abnormal ECG rhythms, and how to perform an ECG using an electrocardiograph machine.

This chapter explains how ECG signals originate and what normal and abnormal ECG tracings look like. It also covers how to recognize artifact (abnormal signal generated from sources other than the heart) and how to operate an electrocardiograph to obtain an ECG tracing.

KEY TERMS

- Atrial fibrillation
- Atrioventricular node
- Bundle of His
- Depolarization
- P wave
- Premature ventricular complexes
- Purkinje fibers
- QRS complex
- Repolarization
- Right and left bundle branches
- Sinoatrial node
- T wave
- Ventricular asystole
- Ventricular fibrillation
- Ventricular tachycardia
- Wandering baseline

THEORY OBJECTIVES

At the end of this chapter, the reader should be able to:

- *Understand the origin of the electrical signals recorded on an ECG:*
  - *Describe how electrical signals are generated.*
  - *Describe the conduction system of the heart.*
- *Correlate the features of a normal ECG with the electrical activity of the heart.*
- *Understand why 12 leads (electrodes) are used for performing an ECG and describe the following:*
  - *The concept of views of the heart*
  - *Einthoven's triangle*
  - *Augmented limb leads*
  - *Precordial leads*
- *Demonstrate how to recognize the following dangerous and life-threatening arrhythmias:*
  - *Sinus bradycardia*
  - *Sinus tachycardia*
  - *Atrial fibrillation*
  - *Premature ventricular complexes*
  - *Ventricular tachycardia*
  - *Ventricular fibrillation*
  - *Ventricular asystole*
- *Demonstrate how to recognize the following artifacts on an ECG tracing:*
  - *Motion artifact*
  - *Wandering baseline*
  - *60 Hz artifact*
- *Understand how an electrocardiograph operates and how an ECG tracing is obtained, including:*
  - *How the electrocardiograph makes the tracing*
  - *How time and voltage are read from an ECG*

ELECTRICAL PHYSIOLOGY OF THE HEART

Production of Electrical Current in the Heart

The heart is a four-chambered muscle that functions as a pump to move blood through the circulatory system (Figure 6-1). This hollow muscle is composed of cardiac muscle cells. When the muscle cells are stimulated and contract, the cells undergo *depolarization* (exchanging potassium for sodium)—they become negatively charged on their outside surface (Figure 6-2). After contraction (depolarization), the muscle cells undergo *repolarization* (exchanging sodium for potassium)—they become positive on their outside surface. When this ion exchange occurs, an electrical potential (charge) of very small voltage is produced; this is conducted through the body to the surface of the skin. The resulting electrical signals (voltage changes) are what the electrocardiograph records, and the signals form an ECG tracing.

Cardiac Conduction System

The heart is really two parallel pumps—the atria and the ventricles. Therefore, an organized conduction system must exist for it to function properly. This conduction system consists of the *sinoatrial node* (SA node), *atrioventricular node* (AV node), *bundle of His, right and left bundle branches*, and the *Purkinje fibers* (Figure 6-3).

The SA node functions as the heart's pacemaker. It ensures that the heart will beat rhythmically without any external sources of stimulation. The cardiac conduction cycle begins at the SA node. The electrical impulse from the SA node causes the muscle cells in the atria to contract simultaneously as the impulse is conducted through the atria. When the electrical impulse from the atria is conducted to the AV node, it transmits the electrical impulse to the bundle of His and the right and left bundle branches.

The right and left bundle branches conduct the electrical impulse to the apex (base) of the heart, where it is transmitted to the ventricles through the Purkinje fibers. As the impulse travels up the Purkinje fibers, the muscle cells of the ventricles contract simultaneously.

During the contraction of the ventricles, the muscle cells in the atria repolarize, bringing them to the polarized resting state. Following ventricular contraction, the ventricles repolarize, like the atria.

THE NORMAL ECG AND THE ELECTRICAL ACTIVITY OF THE HEART

Figure 6-4 represents a normal ECG tracing. The ECG tracing is divided into five waves: P, Q, R, S, T, and sometimes U. Each wave represents a portion of the heart's electrical activity.

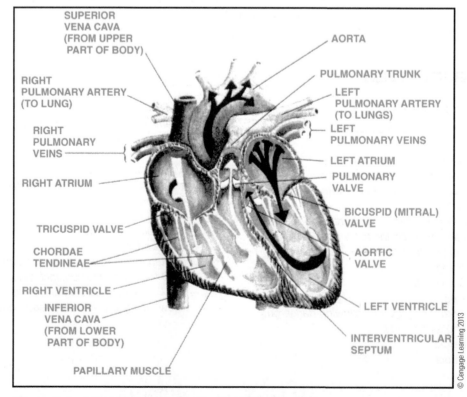

Figure 6-1   A line drawing showing the chambers of the heart

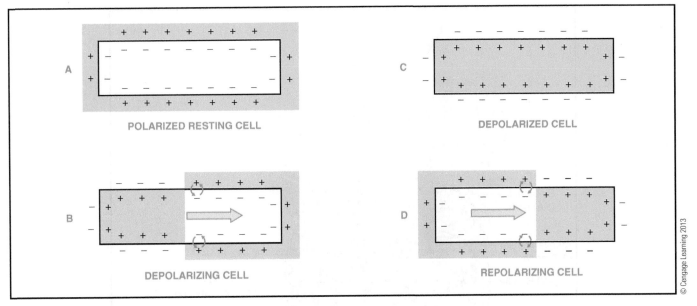

Figure 6-2 Depolarization and repolarization of the cell

A. Polarized resting cell. The heart muscle is in the resting, or polarized state; that is, the cell carries an electrical charge, with the inside negatively charged with sodium

B. Depolarizing cell. When the muscle cell is stimulated, the cell begins to depolarize; that is, the positively charged ions flow into the cell, and the negatively charged ions flow out of the cell

C. Depolarized cell. During the period that the cell is depolarized, all the positively charged ions are on the inside of the cell, and all the negatively charged ions are on the outside of the cell

D. Repolarizing cell. After the muscle cell has depolarized, it begins to return to the resting state; that is, the negatively charged ions flow into the cell, and the positively charged ions flow out of the cell

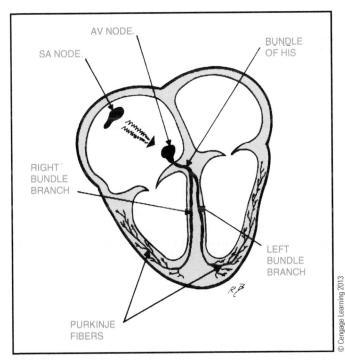

Figure 6-3 The cardiac conduction system

The *P wave* is the voltage rise that occurs when the atria depolarize. As discussed earlier, depolarization results in transmission of an electrical signal to the surface of the skin.

The *QRS complex*—composed of the Q, R, and S waves—represents the depolarization of the ventricles. During ventricular depolarization, the atria repolarize. Owing to the larger number of muscle fibers in the ventricles than in the atria, the voltage generated is much larger than the voltage generated during depolarization of the atria. As a result, the repolarization of the atria is "lost" or not seen in the QRS complex. The *T wave* is a voltage that is generated as the ventricles repolarize.

The ECG tracing presents a two-dimensional view of the heart's electrical activity. Think of it as an electrical "snapshot" of a cardiac cycle. The heart, however, is a three-dimensional object. To adequately describe the electrical activity of the heart, more than one view is needed.

THE TWELVE LEADS OF AN ECG

When an engineer designs a part for a ventilator, at least three views must be drawn to describe it fully (length, width, and depth). Like an engineering drawing, an ECG must contain more than one "view" to adequately describe the electrical activity of the heart. Twelve standard leads are used to obtain these views.

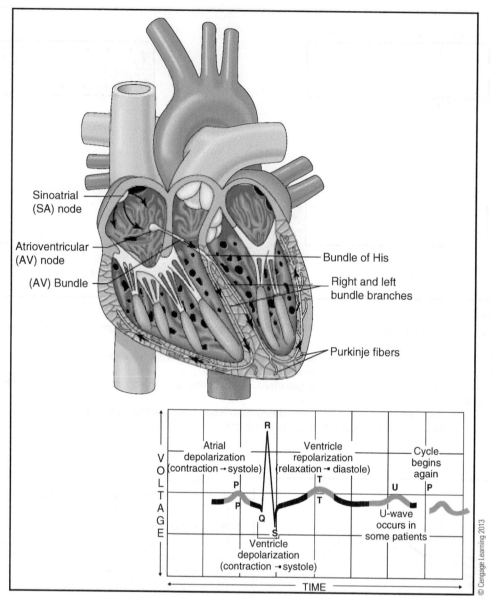

Figure 6-4   A normal ECG tracing

Einthoven's Triangle

Einthoven's triangle is named for an early pioneer of electrocardiography, Willem Einthoven. Einthoven connected positive and negative electrodes to the limbs of the body in three specific patterns—leads I through III—to generate standard ECG tracings (Barold, 2003). (More formally, "leads" are the wires connecting the patient to the electrocardiograph machine, but they also name the tracings obtained with each pattern of electrode placement.) For lead I, the left arm is positive and the right arm is negative. For lead II, the right arm is negative and the left leg is positive. For lead III, the left arm is negative and the left leg is positive (Figure 6-5). The electrical current measured and recorded represents a vector, having a length (voltage) and a direction

(orientation) (Figure 6-6). These vector orientations then represent a given view, or electrical "snapshot," of the heart. These three leads and the augmented leads are bipolar (containing both a positive and a negative electrode).

Augmented Leads

With augmented leads, the electrodes are positioned to make a single limb positive and all other limbs negative. They are termed *augmented leads* because the electrocardiograph machine must amplify or augment the weak signal more than is needed for the other leads to generate a useful tracing. Figure 6-7 shows electrode polarity for augmented leads and their associated ECG tracings. Like those for the leads in Einthoven's triangle, the tracings

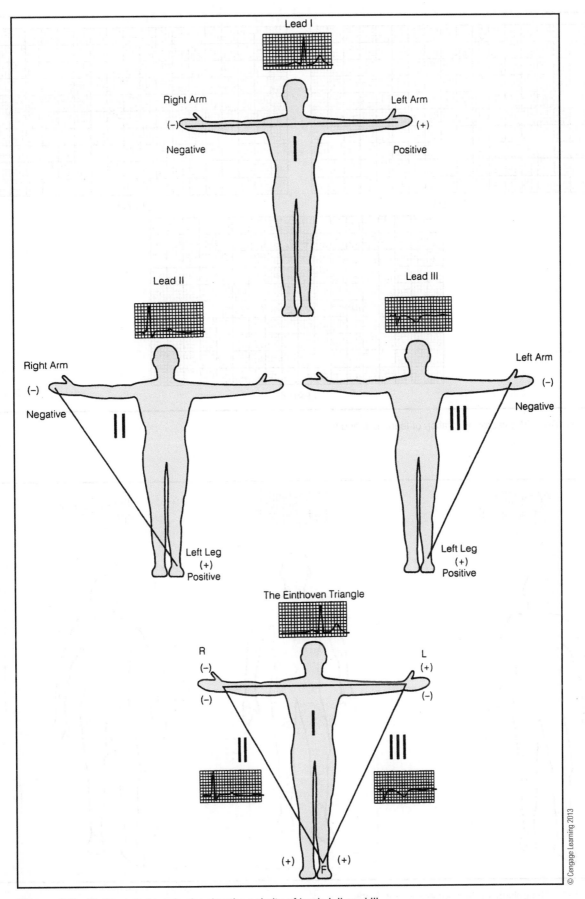

Figure 6-5 Einthoven's triangle showing the polarity of leads I, II, and III

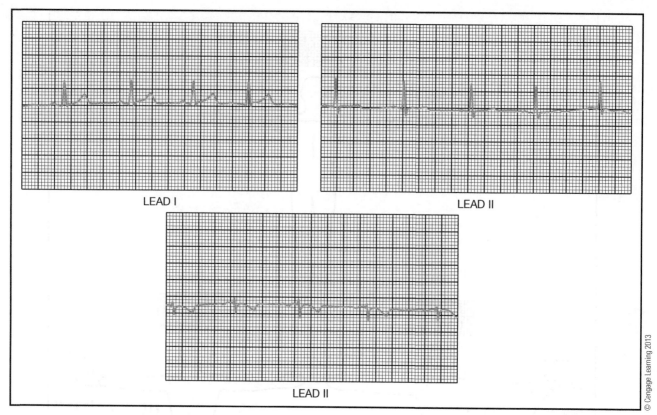

Figure 6-6 The vector orientation of leads I, II, and III

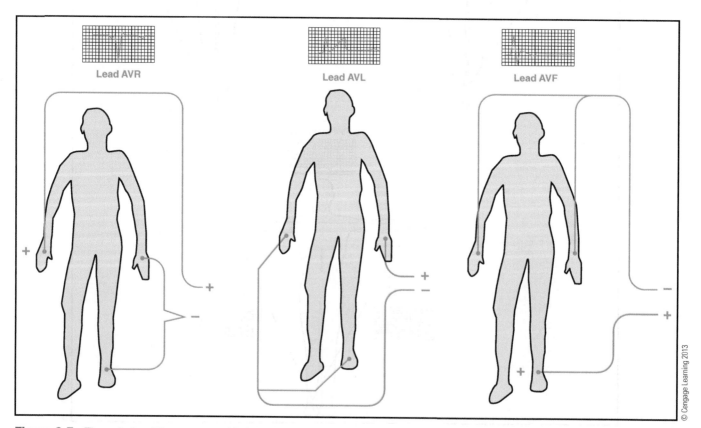

Figure 6-7 The polarity of the augmented limb leads

for augmented leads also represent vectors or views of the heart.

Precordial Leads

The *precordial leads* are unipolar. The tracings obtained with these leads represent horizontal views of the heart. These unipolar leads record the electrical activity that occurs directly under each lead. Precordial leads provide an electrical image of the heart in the horizontal plane (Figure 6-8). The precordial leads are helpful in the diagnosis of the location of a myocardial infarction.

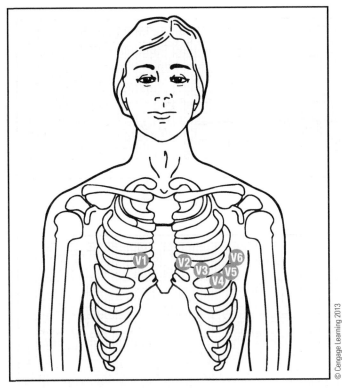

Figure 6-8   Positions of the precordial leads

NORMAL SINUS RHYTHM

A normal sinus rhythm consists of four distinct waves, or changes in voltage potential. These four waves are identified as the P, Q, R, S (or QRS complex) and T waves (Figure 6-9). Each P wave is followed by a QRS complex. The PR interval should be between 0.11 and 0.2 (3 to 5 small squares) second, the QRS complex less than 0.12 second (3 small squares), and the QT interval should be 0.42 second. A normal rate is between 60 and 100 beats per minute.

The normal paper speed on an ECG is 25 mm per second. Each large box on the ECG paper is 5 mm. At the normal paper speed, 5 boxes are recorded each second, making each large box 0.2 second (5 × 0.2 second = 1 second). If the heart rate was 300 beats per minute (tachycardia), a QRS complex would occur every 5 mm (one large box). To determine any heart rate, count the large boxes between the QRS interval, including any fraction of a large box. Divide 300 by the number of boxes between the QRS complexes. If the rate is irregular, several QRS complexes must be counted and averaged to arrive at the correct heart rate.

DANGEROUS AND LIFE-THREATENING ARRHYTHMIAS

As a respiratory practitioner performing ECGs, life-threatening conditions during procedures may be observed. It is important to be able to recognize these conditions and to summon qualified help for that patient. In addition to the arrhythmias that may be observed, it is also important to assess and monitor the patient during the procedure. The patient's signs, symptoms, and complaints are just as useful to a physician as the ECG tracing is during the abnormal event. The respiratory practitioner's ability to recognize these abnormalities as they occur may help save a patient's life.

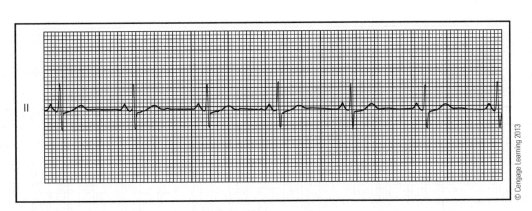

Figure 6-9   An ECG showing a normal sinus rhythm

Sinus Bradycardia

Sinus bradycardia is a normal sinus rhythm at a lower than normal heart rate (Figure 6-10). Bradycardia is defined as a heart rate of less than 60 beats per minute (White, 2008). Notice that the rhythm is normal but the rate is low. Sinus bradycardia may indicate sinus node disease or increased parasympathetic tone or may be caused by drugs (digitalis).

Sinus Tachycardia

Sinus tachycardia is a normal sinus rhythm at higher than normal rate (Figure 6-11). Sinus tachycardia is defined as a heart rate of greater than 100 beats per minute. The range for sinus tachycardia is between 100 and 160 beats per minute. Sinus tachycardia is a normal response to exercise, stress, or fright. Other causes for sinus tachycardia may include fever, anxiety, sepsis, or pulmonary embolism.

Atrial Fibrillation

With *atrial fibrillation*, there is not an organized stimulation of the atria from the SA node. Multiple stimuli occur from many different sources. As a result, each stimulus only causes a small portion of the atria to contract. The result is an unorganized pattern with a very fast heart rate (400 to 700 beats per minute) observed on the ECG tracing (Figure 6-12). Because atrial depolarization does not occur, there is no P wave.

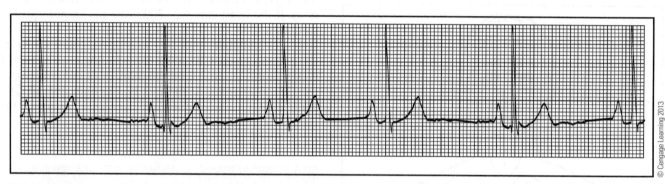

© Cengage Learning 2013

Figure 6-10   An ECG showing sinus bradycardia

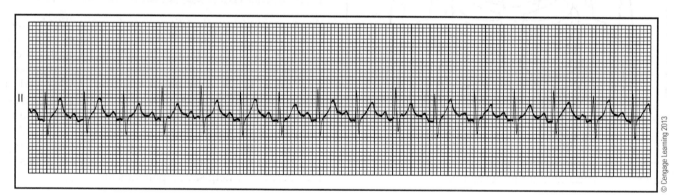

© Cengage Learning 2013

Figure 6-11   An ECG showing sinus tachycardia

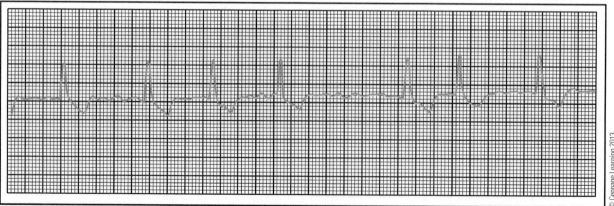

© Cengage Learning 2013

Figure 6-12   An ECG showing atrial fibrillation

Because of the unorganized nature of the stimuli in atrial fibrillation, the atria never fully contract. This impedes the filling of the ventricles and reduces the cardiac output. Furthermore, because the electrical activity is disorganized, ventricular rate is also irregular.

Atrial fibrillation may be caused by underlying heart disease, hyperthyroidism, mitral valve disease, or even pulmonary emboli.

Premature Ventricular Complexes

Premature ventricular complexes (PVCs) occur when the ventricles are stimulated prematurely. This premature stimulation results in an unusually wide QRS complex (Figure 6-13). This widening occurs because one ventricle depolarizes before the other out of sequence.

PVCs are usually followed by a long pause before the next beat occurs. PVCs are common when patients are hypoxemic and may be observed during endotracheal suctioning.

PVCs occur randomly in normal persons; however, if they occur in runs (more than 3), or if they fall on a T wave, they are cause for concern. *Bigeminy* refers to the occurrence of PVCs every other beat (every second beat); *trigeminy* describes their occurrence every third beat (Figure 6-14).

Ventricular Tachycardia

With *ventricular tachycardia*, the ventricles are stimulated at a faster than normal rate (greater than 100 beats per minute). The ECG rhythm may be regular or irregular in appearance (Figure 6-15). Sometimes P waves between

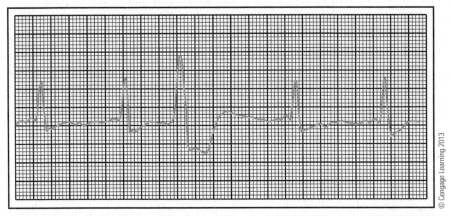

Figure 6-13   An ECG showing a premature ventricular complex

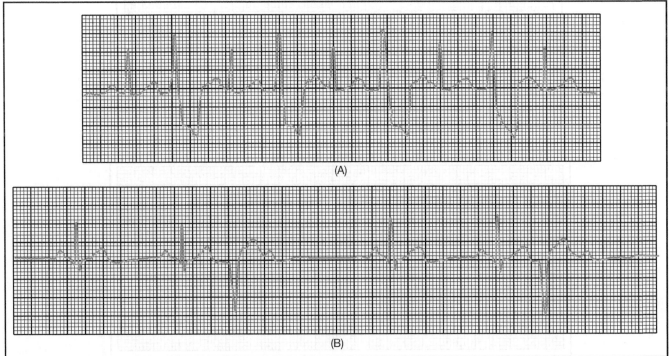

(A)

(B)

Figure 6-14   An ECG showing bigeminy (A) and trigeminy (B)

the QRS complexes are observed, and at other times they may not be.

Ventricular tachycardia may represent a grave condition for the patient, especially if there is underlying heart disease. This condition should be promptly identified and appropriate treatment should be initiated.

Ventricular Fibrillation

Ventricular fibrillation, like atrial fibrillation, results from unorganized stimulation. The unorganized stimulation of the ventricles results in depolarization of only a small part of the ventricle with each stimulus. Ventricular fibrillation has a very irregular, disorganized pattern (Figure 6-16).

Ventricular fibrillation is a life-threatening condition. It requires immediate attention and treatment.

Ventricular Asystole

Ventricular asystole is the total absence of any cardiac electrical activity (Figure 6-17). It is sometimes termed

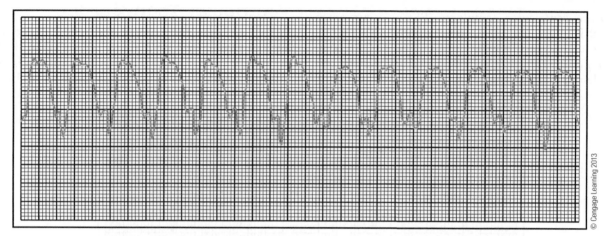

Figure 6-15 An ECG showing ventricular tachycardia

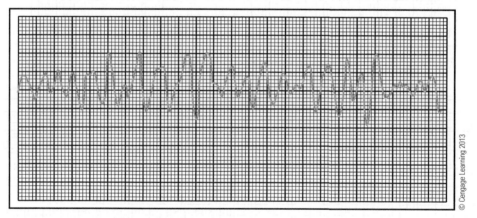

Figure 6-16 An ECG showing ventricular fibrillation

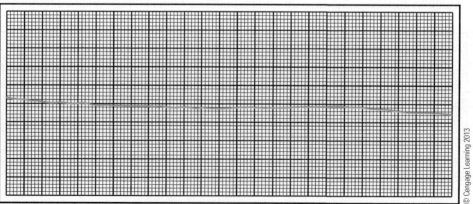

Figure 6-17 An ECG showing ventricular asystole

cardiac standstill, observed as a "flat line" on the ECG tracing. Ventricular asystole is always life threatening and requires immediate intervention.

ECG ARTIFACT

An ECG tracing represents the electrical activity of the heart. Because very small voltages (as low as 1 millivolt or less) are being amplified and recorded, artifact, or nonphysiologic (artificial) electrical current, may also be picked up. Such extraneous signal can ruin an otherwise good ECG tracing. Artifact may be patient generated or may even be from a source external to the patient. The three most common types of artifact are patient motion artifact, wandering baseline, and 60 Hz artifact.

Patient Motion

Patient motion artifact occurs when the patient is restless or moves the limbs during the ECG. Sometimes patient motion cannot be avoided, especially if the patient is in severe distress or pain. Motion artifact usually causes an irregular appearance of the tracing. Figure 6-18 illustrates an example of motion artifact in an ECG. Sometimes an inexperienced respiratory practitioner will confuse motion artifact with an atrial arrhythmia.

Wandering Baseline

A *wandering baseline* is caused by poor electrical contact between the patient and the electrodes placed on the patient to record the ECG. The baseline rises and falls, as shown in Figure 6-19.

Electrical contact may be improved by cleaning the patient's skin with isopropyl alcohol, using more electrode cream, or cleaning the electrode contacts and connections. Male patients with abundant chest hair may require that their chest be shaved in the locations where ECG leads will be placed. Chest hair can interfere with the ability of the electrode and gel to make good skin contact.

60 Hz Artifact

Artifact may also occur from electrical interference external to the patient (Figure 6-20). The cause may be a faulty ground on the electrocardiograph or current leakage from adjacent equipment. This type of artifact is called 60 Hz artifact because in the United States and Canada, electricity is supplied as alternating current at 110 volts and 60 Hz.

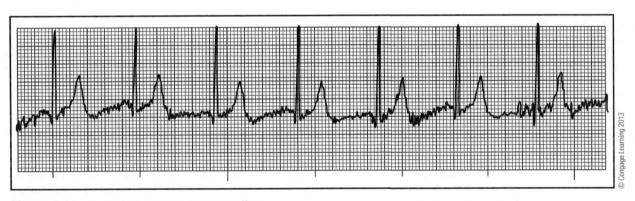

Figure 6-18 An ECG showing movement artifact

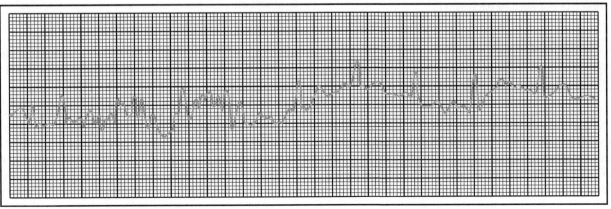

Figure 6-19 An ECG showing a wandering baseline

PROFICIENCY OBJECTIVES

At the end of this chapter, the reader should be able to:

* *Collect and assemble the supplies necessary for an electrocardiogram.*
* *Demonstrate how to position the patient correctly for an electrocardiogram.*
* *Correctly identify anatomical landmarks and correctly place all ECG leads.*

* *Demonstrate how to operate the electrocardiograph machine correctly to obtain a 12-lead ECG.*
* *Describe how to recognize any life-threatening arrhythmias.*
* *Demonstrate how to recognize any artifact and correct it.*
* *Demonstrate what to do with the ECG tracing after it is obtained, ensuring that the appropriate personnel see the tracing.*

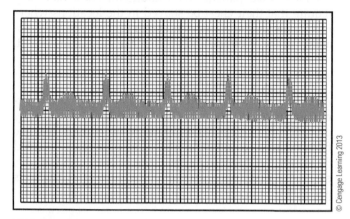

© Cengage Learning 2013

Figure 6-20   An ECG showing 60 Hz artifact

ELECTROCARDIOGRAPH EQUIPMENT

The electrocardiograph is a very sensitive voltmeter that records the extremely small voltages generated by the heart's electrical activity. These signals are filtered and amplified and then recorded on a moving graph.

Length on the graph represents time. One small square is 0.04 second. One of the larger squares represents 0.20 second (5 small squares). If the time interval between squares is known, the heart rate may be calculated by measuring between R waves.

Height (vertical distance) on the graph paper is representative of voltage. A 1-millivolt standard is used to determine the voltages of each wave.

EQUIPMENT REQUIRED FOR AN ELECTROCARDIOGRAM

Several pieces of equipment are required to perform an ECG. Many contemporary electrocardiograph machines are secured to a portable cart with wheels. Many of these carts have cupboards or pockets for storage of this equipment. Check the electrocardiograph machine's cart before searching for the following supplies:

* The electrical wires (leads) that will be attached to the cable providing the input to the electrocardiograph. Some machines have five wires (necessitating separate measurement of the precordial leads), whereas others have 12 wires and can record the precordial leads without moving an electrode.
* Isopropyl alcohol and a clean towel or washcloth to clean the patient's skin before performing the ECG. If the patient has been brought into the emergency setting from the field and is obviously dirty, quickly clean the skin to prevent artifact before beginning the ECG. Male patients with abundant chest hair may need to be shaved prior to placing the ECG electrodes.
* Having a second clean towel or washcloth available is helpful for removal of any electrode jelly left by the electrode patches after the ECG is completed.

PATIENT POSITIONING

The patient must always be placed supine for an electrocardiogram. Patient position can alter the contour of ECG tracings. The patient should be instructed to uncross the ankles during the ECG recording. If a patient cannot lie flat AU NOTE: Suggest using "because of". (GW 8/18/11) shortness of breath, the ECG can still be performed while the patient is in a semi-Fowler's position. The supine position is considered to be the standard ECG position.

LEAD PLACEMENT

Correct lead placement for an ECG is essential to obtain consistent results. An error of only a quarter of an inch may affect the ECG tracing (White, 2008).

The limb leads are placed on the right and left arms and on the right and left feet. The limb leads may be modified by using the right and left shoulder, right and left ankle or inner calf or hips. The precordial leads are positioned at precise locations around the anterior chest.

The precordial leads are placed as shown in Figure 6-21. V_1 and V_2 are placed at the fourth intercostal

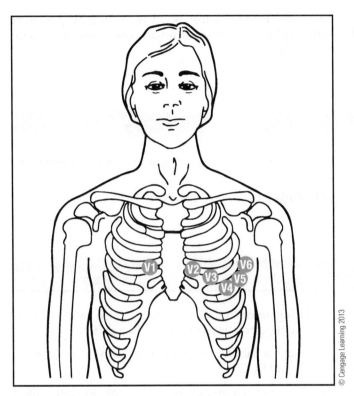

Figure 6-21 Correct precordial lead placement

space adjacent to the sternum. V_1 is to the right of the sternum and V_2 is at the left sternal border. Sometimes respiratory practitioners have a difficult time identifying the fourth intercostal space. By palpating the manubrium sternal junction, or *sternal angle* (where the manubrium and body join), the practitioner can identify the second intercostal space. By palpating two ribs inferiorly from this point, the practitioner can identify the fourth intercostal space. V_4 is placed at the fifth intercostal space along the midclavicular line. V_3 is placed directly between V_2 and V_4. V_5 is placed at the anterior axillary line even with V_4. V_6 is placed at the midaxillary line, in line with V_4 and V_5.

ARRHYTHMIA RECOGNITION

As stated earlier, life-threatening arrhythmias may occur during an ECG. The respiratory practitioner's ability to recognize these events and obtain appropriate treatment may save a patient's life. Review the arrhythmias discussed in the theory portion of this chapter at this time. During clinical rotation, spend some time in the coronary care unit at the assigned hospital. Ask the nursing staff to help learn to recognize these arrhythmias on an ECG tracing. Many nurses are more than willing to run strips to use of practice.

OPERATING THE ELECTRO-CARDIOGRAPH MACHINE

Many types of electrocardiographs are in use today. Some are manual, single-channel machines (requiring the operator to switch leads manually), whereas others are multichannel and automatic (recording all 12 leads automatically). Some instruments have arrhythmia recognition and interpretation built into their electronics by the manufacturers. Experienced cardiologists will agree with a machine interpretation greater than 90% of the time.

It is important for the respiratory practitioner to learn about the machine in use. It is not practical in this text to cover every available machine. Read the owner's manual on how to operate the machine in use. Observe a skilled respiratory practitioner obtain an ECG on several patients. After observation, have the same practitioner observe you in the use of the equipment. Through practice the respiratory practitioner will become proficient.

ARTIFACT RECOGNITION

Like many other aspects of respiratory care practice, proficiency in artifact recognition requires time and exposure. Careful patient preparation (clean skin, good electrode contact, shaving of chest hair, and sufficient electrode jelly) will eliminate wandering baselines. Patient motion is often difficult to control.

Provide instructions to the patient to lie still and emphasize how important absence of motion may help. As discussed earlier, pain, anxiety, and restlessness are difficult to control. Sometimes it is necessary to just do the best to obtain the best tracing.

In some cases, 60 Hz artifact may be eliminated by changing electrical outlets that power the electrocardiograph or by turning off unneeded electrical equipment near the patient. Fans, vacuums, or other motor-driven equipment may generate this type of artifact.

PROPER HANDLING OF AN ELECTROCARDIO-GRAPHIC TRACING

Once an ECG tracing is obtained, it is usually interpreted by a physician or a cardiology specialist. In the emergency setting, the attending physician or emergency department physician will want to see the ECG as soon as it is obtained. In other parts of the hospital, ECGs may be returned to the respiratory care department and placed into a file for interpretation or delivered to the cardiology department.

As always, it is important to record the patient's name and hospital number and the date and time of the ECG tracing. The newer machines have a computer keyboard for use in recording all pertinent information, which is automatically transferred onto the tracing.

References

Barold, S. S. (2003). Willem Einthoven and the birth of clinical electrocardiography a hundred years ago. *Cardiac and Electrophysilogy Review, 1,* 99–104.

White, G. (2008). *Respiratory notes respiratory therapists pocket guide.* Philadelphia: F. A. Davis.

Practice Activities: Electrocardiography

1. Obtain a 12-lead ECG and identify tracings for the following leads:
   a. Lead I
   b. Lead II
   c. Lead III
   d. AVR
   e. AVL
   f. AVF
   g. The six precordial leads

2. Using an arrhythmia generator, flash cards, or ECG tracings, practice arrhythmia recognition.

3. Using a laboratory partner, practice performing a 12-lead ECG.

4. With your laboratory partner, create motion artifact and a wandering baseline and then identify these common artifacts.

Check List: Performing an ECG

_____ 1. Check the patient's chart for a physician's order.

_____ 2. Wash your hands.

_____ 3. Obtain all of the appropriate equipment, as required, including:
_____ a. Electrocardiograph machine
_____ b. All leads (wires)
_____ c. Suction cups or disposable electrode pads
_____ d. Isopropyl alcohol
_____ e. Clean towels or washcloths

_____ 4. Assemble and check the equipment to ensure that it functions properly.

_____ 5. Identify the patient using the arm band.

_____ 6. Explain the procedure to the patient and emphasize the importance of being still during the procedure.

_____ 7. Place the patient in the supine position with the patient's ankles uncrossed.

_____ 8. Correctly place all limb leads.

_____ 9. Identify the anatomical landmarks on the anterior chest and place the precordial leads correctly.

_____ 10. Correctly operate the electrocardiograph machine to obtain an ECG tracing.

_____ 11. Identify any life-threatening arrhythmias.

_____ 12. Recognize and, if possible, correct an artifact.

_____ 13. Clean up following the procedure by discarding any disposable items. Clean up the patient by wiping off any excess conductive jelly.

14. Ensure that the ECG tracing is labeled with the following information:
_____ a. Patient's name
_____ b. Patient's hospital number
_____ c. Date and time of the tracing

_____ 15. Ensure the patient's safety and comfort.

_____ 16. Wash your hands.

_____ 17. Ensure that the ECG tracing is given to the appropriate physician or is correctly filed for interpretation.

_____ 18. Document in the patient's chart the date and time of the tracing and the fact that it was performed.

Self-Evaluation Post Test: Electrocardiograms (ECGs)

1. Depolarization of the myocardium causes:
   I. ion transfer.
   II. exchange of potassium and sodium.
   III. a voltage to be produced.
   IV. the outside of the cell to become negatively charged.
   a. I
   b. I, II
   c. I, II, III
   d. I, II, III, IV

2. Atrial depolarization is represented on the ECG by the:
   a. P wave.
   b. Q wave.
   c. R wave.
   d. T wave.

3. Depolarization of the ventricles is represented on the ECG by the:
   a. P wave.
   b. R wave.
   c. QRS complex.
   d. T wave.

4. Repolarization of the ventricles is represented by the:
   a. P wave.
   b. Q wave.
   c. QRS complex.
   d. T wave.

5. Which of the following are bipolar leads?
   I. Leads I, II, and III
   II. Leads AVR, AVL, and AVF
   III. The precordial leads
   a. I
   b. I, II
   c. I, III
   d. II, III

6. Identify the following arrhythmia:

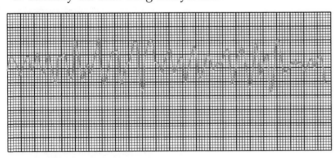

   a. Atrial fibrillation
   b. Premature ventricular complexes (PVCs)
   c. Ventricular fibrillation
   d. Ventricular tachycardia

7. Identify the following arrhythmia:

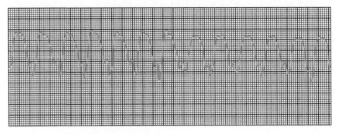

   a. Atrial fibrillation
   b. Premature ventricular complexes (PVCs)
   c. Ventricular fibrillation
   d. Ventricular tachycardia

8. Identify the following arrhythmia:

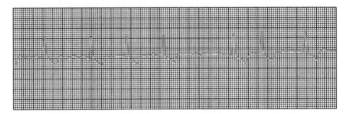

   a. Sinus bradycardia
   b. Atrial fibrillation
   c. Premature ventricular complexes (PVCs)
   d. Ventricular fibrillation

9. An anatomical landmark used to help identify the second intercostal space is the:
   a. xiphoid process.
   b. manubrium.
   c. sternal angle.
   d. clavicle.

10. Common artifact on an ECG may include:
    I. motion artifact.
    II. wandering baseline.
    III. inductance interference.
    IV. 60 Hz artifact.
    a. I, II
    b. I, II, IV
    c. II, III
    d. II, III, IV

Chapter Post-Test

1. Repolarization of the myocardium causes:
   I. ion transfer.
   II. exchange of potassium and sodium.
   III. a voltage to be produced.
   IV. the outside of the cell to become negatively charged.

   a. I
   b. I, III
   c. I, II, III
   d. I, II, III, IV

2. Atrial depolarization is represented on the ... by the
   a. P wave
   b. Q wave
   c. R wave
   d. T wave

3. Depolarization of the ventricles is represented on the ECG by the
   a. P wave
   b. R wave
   c. QRS complex
   d. T wave

4. Repolarization of the ventricles is represented by the
   a. P wave
   b. Q wave
   c. ...
   d. T wave

5. Which of the following are Einthoven's leads?
   I. Leads I, II, and III
   II. Leads AVR, AVL, and AVF
   III. The precordial leads

   a. I
   b. II
   c. I, II
   d. II, III

6. Identify the following activities:

PERFORMANCE EVALUATION:
Electrocardiograms (ECGS)

Date: Lab _____ Clinical _____ Agency _____

Lab: Pass _____ Fail _____ Clinical: Pass _____ Fail _____

Student name _____ Instructor name _____

No. of times observed in clinical _____

No. of times practiced in clinical _____

PASSING CRITERIA: Obtain 90% or better on the procedure. Tasks indicated by * must receive at least 1 point, or the evaluation is terminated. Procedure must be performed within the designated time, or the performance receives a failing grade.

SCORING:
2 points — Task performed satisfactorily without prompting.
1 point — Task performed satisfactorily with self-initiated correction.
0 points — Task performed incorrectly or with prompting required.
NA — Task not applicable to the patient care situation.

Tasks:		Peer	Lab	Clinical
*	1. Verifies the physician's order	☐	☐	☐
*	2. Performs hand hygiene	☐	☐	☐
*	3. Obtains the required equipment			
	a. Electrocardiograph	☐	☐	☐
	b. All leads	☐	☐	☐
	c. Suction cups or disposable pads	☐	☐	☐
	d. Isopropyl alcohol	☐	☐	☐
	e. Clean towels	☐	☐	☐
*	4. Assembles and checks all equipment for function	☐	☐	☐
	5. Identifies the patient	☐	☐	☐
	6. Explains the procedure to the patient	☐	☐	☐
*	7. Positions the patient	☐	☐	☐
*	8. Places the leads correctly	☐	☐	☐
*	9. Correctly operates the electrocardiograph	☐	☐	☐
*	10. Identifies any life-threatening arrhythmias	☐	☐	☐
*	11. Recognizes and corrects artifact	☐	☐	☐
*	12. Cleans the patient and cleans up the area afterward	☐	☐	☐

* **13.** Ensures that the ECG tracing is filed or that appropriate physicians receive it

☐ ☐ ☐
☐ ☐ ☐

* **14.** Documents the procedure in the patient's chart

SCORE: Peer _____ points of possible 36; _____%

                          Lab _____ points of possible 36; _____%

                          Clinical _____ points of possible 36; _____%

TIME: _____ out of possible 30 minutes

STUDENT SIGNATURES

PEER: _____

STUDENT: _____

INSTRUCTOR SIGNATURES

LAB: _____

CLINICAL: _____

CHAPTER 7
Phlebotomy
Kelly P. Jones

INTRODUCTION

As hospitals restructure staff responsibilities to control costs, the role of respiratory practitioners will expand to include tasks normally assigned to other staff specialists. One specialized task the respiratory practitioner can perform proficiently is phlebotomy. *Phlebotomy* is the invasive puncturing of a vein for the purpose of collecting blood.

Phlebotomy is a routine task, one that can be easily learned with proper preparation and supervised practice. Respiratory practitioners traditionally have been flexible, well-rounded clinicians who can quickly learn and absorb new skills and techniques.

This chapter presents a step-by-step procedure for drawing blood specimens. The procedure includes patient preparation, blood drawing, and follow-up actions. The chapter also discusses exposure control policies and your obligation to maintain a safe working environment.

KEY TERMS

- **Butterfly needle**
- **Exposure control policy**
- **Phlebotomy**
- **Vacuum collection tubes**

THEORY OBJECTIVES

At the end of this chapter, the reader should be able to:

- *Identify obligations in collection of blood specimens from a patient:*
  - *Obligation to the patient*
  - *Obligation to the laboratory*
  - *Obligation to self*
- *Know how to maintain a safe environment:*
  - *Describe the purpose of exposure control policy*
  - *Identify the appropriate steps to take if blood exposure occurs*
  - *Identify the steps to take if blood spill occurs*
  - *Identify proper waste disposal*
- *Demonstrate working knowledge of equipment used in venous blood collection:*
  - *Basic equipment*
  - *Needle types*
  - *Vacuum tubes*

- *Describe appropriate venipuncture technique:*
  - *Patient identification*
  - *Verification of test ordered*
  - *Patient preparation*
  - *Venipuncture site selection*
  - *Site decontamination*
  - *Needle placement*
  - *Blood collection*
  - *Removal of tourniquet*
  - *Needle removal and site pressure*
  - *Specimen labeling*
  - *Disposal of supplies*
  - *Hazards and complications*
  - *Delivery of samples to laboratory*

OBLIGATIONS RELATED TO PERFORMANCE OF PHLEBOTOMY

A respiratory practitioner may be called upon to perform any number of tasks when a patient blood specimen is required. The practitioner may act as the support person who helps hold a combative patient in the emergency department or intensive care unit. The practitioner may also be asked to transport blood samples to the laboratory. Once trained, however, the practitioner can be the person responsible for drawing blood specimens. No matter the role, the practitioner has obligations to the patient, to the laboratory receiving the specimen, and to him or herself.

The first obligation is always to the patient. Make sure the patient understands the procedure to be performed. Check the blood drawing order and patient identification; make sure the proper procedure is being performed on the correct patient. Then, identify yourself to the patient and explain the procedure. Many patients are afraid of hospitals and do not like needles. Put the patient at ease; tell the patient what is going to be done. Perform the procedure quickly and safely. Protect the patient by using proper aseptic technique when preparing the skin for venipuncture. Finally, properly dress the site afterward.

The obligation to the laboratory is simple. Always use aseptic techniques to prevent contamination of the specimen. Label each blood sample correctly with the patient's identification.

The respiratory practitioner is obligated to protect him or herself from inadvertent exposure to blood specimens. This obligation may be satisfied through knowledge, preparation, and procedure. The practitioner protects him or herself by knowing what is to be done, preparing for the procedure by assembling the correct materials, and performing the procedure step by step.

MAINTAINING A SAFE ENVIRONMENT

This last obligation is a small part of a larger objective—maintaining a safe environment. Every place in which the respiratory practitioner works will have an *exposure control policy*. This policy is the key to maintaining a safe environment.

Exposure control policy is put into place to protect health care providers as well as patients and support staff. The policy may differ slightly from workplace to workplace, so the respiratory practitioner should be sure to read and understand the policy instructions for each facility. Policy instructions describe what to do if exposed to body fluids or specimens. Exposure can come from a needle stick, a splash of secretions in the eye, or any other form of accidental exposure to patient body fluids. Along with knowing where to find this set of instructions, the respiratory practitioner should have absolute knowledge of all equipment available to treat exposure, such as eyewash stations, handwashing areas, the content of first aid kits, and the location of ointment and adhesive strips or tape.

Although exposure control policy may differ slightly from institution to institution, some general rules apply if exposure occurs. First, if an accidental needle stick occurs, notify the supervisor as soon as possible. Do not press the injured area hard enough to increase perfusion. Just gently press around the site until a droplet or two of blood seeps out. Next go to a handwashing area and perform a 2-minute scrub with antimicrobial soap. Once the scrub is completed, apply an ointment such as polymixin-bacitracin to the area and cover the stick with an adhesive strip.

In the case of a needle stick, the supervisor will ask the patient to allow a blood draw to test for hepatitis and to screen for human immunodeficiency virus (HIV). If the patient agrees, these blood tests will be performed, and the practitioner will be notified if results are positive. If the patient denies the request for tests, then the practitioner's blood will be drawn and tested immediately. Blood will be tested again at 1, 3, 6, and 12 months after the accidental needle stick.

If a blood spill occurs, contain the spill by blocking off the area. Always report any blood spill or exposure to the supervisor. If the health care facility has a housekeeping or environmental service, contain the spill safely and notify the service. If the service is not available, begin by saturating the spill with an appropriate cleaning agent. Allow the saturated spill to sit for the time allotted in the exposure control policy instructions. Then clean up thoroughly with a mop or towels.

Contaminated material generated by cleaning the spill, such as towels, blankets, or mops, must be disposed of using a red biohazard bag (Figure 7-1). The exposure control policy instructions should explain where the bags are stored. Put the contaminated material in the bag and tie it off. All other contaminated items that could cause injury should go into a sharps container (see Figure 7-12 later in the book).

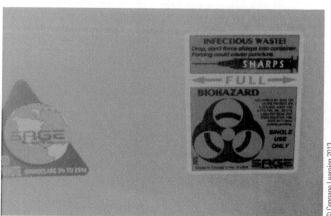

Figure 7-1 A photograph showing a biohazard bag and the universal biohazard label

EQUIPMENT

Blood is drawn for hundreds of different tests; some of the most common tests are emergency department panels, complete blood count (CBC), hematocrit determination (such as with Autoheme), and cardiac enzymes. If a blood test is ordered and it does not require an arterial sample or a specimen for a blood culture, then simple blood drawing equipment will suffice.

Once an order for the blood test is obtained, gather the equipment necessary for the job. For any test, gather the following basic equipment (Figure 7-2):

- A set of gloves
- An alcohol and iodine swab
- Two 2 × 2-inch gauze pads
- Tourniquet
- Tape or adhesive strip
- Vacuum collection tubes

Figure 7-2 also shows one of the many types of needle and holder combinations available. The sterile packaging that contains the needle is opened, and the needle is attached to the holder. The needle size is indicated by a number on the packaging. The larger the number, the smaller the needle. For patient comfort, always use the smallest needle that will do the job.

Blood specimens are collected in "vacuum tubes" (Figure 7-3). Attach the tubes to the portion of the needle projecting through the holder after it is inserted in the patient's vein. The vacuum in the tube then draws the blood from the vein. Never attach the tube to the needle before inserting the needle in the vein; the vacuum will be lost and be unable to draw the blood. *Vacuum collection tubes* come in many different sizes and colors. Only a few are illustrated in Figure 7-3. The respiratory practitioner will need to learn the types and colors used by the medical facility. Each color indicates a different medium. The respiratory practitioner must use the correct vacuum tube, or the laboratory will not be able to perform the test on the physician's order.

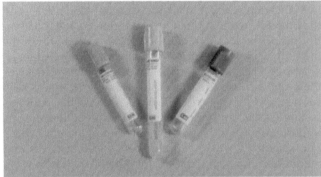

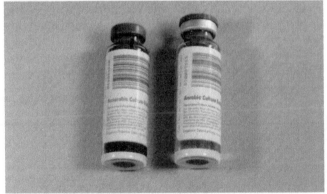

Figure 7-3   Common vacuum tubes used to withdraw blood samples

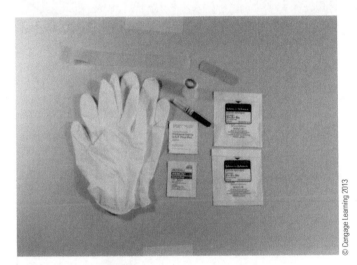

Figure 7-2   Equipment required for phlebotomy, including gloves, alcohol and iodine swabs, 2× 2-inch gauze pads, tourniquet, and tape or adhesive strips

© Cengage Learning 2013

PROFICIENCY OBJECTIVES

At the end of this chapter, the reader should be able to:

- *Identify the roles and obligations of the phlebotomist.*
- *Describe how to maintain a safe environment, including institutional protocols for:*
  - *— Exposure control policies*
  - *— Blood exposure and spills*
  - *— Waste disposal*
- *Demonstrate working knowledge of equipment used in blood drawing.*
- *Demonstrate how to verify properly both the test ordered and patient identification.*

- *Demonstrate how to prepare the patient while selecting a venipuncture site.*
- *Demonstrate a venipuncture, including:*
  - *— Site decontamination*
  - *— Needle placement*
  - *— Blood collection*
  - *— Specimen labeling*
  - *— Waste disposal*
- *Describe the possible complications and hazards of venipuncture.*

VENIPUNCTURE TECHNIQUE

Once all necessary equipment is assembled, perform the steps that follow to collect the specimen safely.

First, verify the blood drawing order and patient information. Always verify the written order to draw a blood specimen. Although there are exceptions for emergency treatment, and although some institutions allow telephone orders, an order to collect a specimen should normally be written in the patient's chart.

Once the order is verified, identify the patient. The simplest and safest way to do this is to look at the patient's identification band, if available. Often patients who are confused or who cannot hear well will answer to any name. Therefore, do not address a patient by name to confirm the patient's identity. Ask the patient to state his or her name. Confirm the reply by checking the patient's identification band, if available. Compare the name with the blood drawing order. Never assume a patient's identity simply by location. Patients can be moved within the medical facility without the practitioner's knowledge.

While verifying the patient's identification, look for the best venipuncture site. At the same time, assess how cooperative the patient will be as well as the patient's fasting status and medications. If the patient seems uncooperative, get help before attempting venipuncture. The laboratory will need the patient's fasting status and medications for some tests. It is also helpful to know if the patient is taking blood-thinning medication. In patients receiving such medication, the practitioner will need to apply pressure at the venipuncture site, after removing the needle, for a longer time than is usual.

There are many veins suitable as venipuncture sites. Figure 7-4 illustrates some acceptable sites. Antecubital veins, which are found anterior to the elbow joint, are usually the largest veins and easiest to use. Often it is necessary to put the patient's extremity in a dependent position, as shown in Figure 7-5. Figure 7-5 also shows the patient's clenched fist. Holding the fist clenched will increase venous distention and make the vein easier to locate. If the patient does not have easily accessible veins, a tourniquet can be applied 8 to 10 cm above the venipuncture site (Figure 7-6).

Once a suitable vein is located for venipuncture, put on a pair of disposable gloves. Open the packaging on all supplies: 2 × 2-inch gauze pads, alcohol,

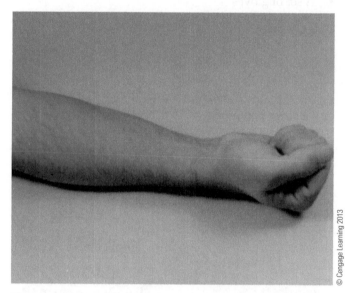

Figure 7-5   A patient with the arm in a dependent position with a clenched fist

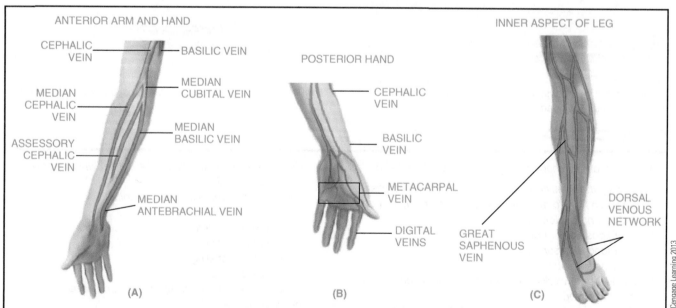

Figure 7-4   Sites for phlebotomy on the arm (A), the hand (B), and the leg (C)

iodine, and adhesive strip. Prepare the site by wiping the skin with iodine, starting in the middle of the site and working outward in a circle (Figure 7-7). Never go over the same spot twice. This maintains a sterile field. Repeat this same procedure using the alcohol prep pad (Figure 7-8). After applying the alcohol and iodine to the site, wipe the area from superior to inferior with one of the 2 × 2-inch gauze pads.

The site is now sterile and ready for venipuncture. Warn the patient before inserting the needle. A reminder such as "You may feel a small stick" can prevent a reflex action that could cause pain. Take the needle and holder and position the point at a 25° to 30° angle (Figure 7-9). Place a vacuum tube loosely inside the holder but do not push it onto the needle yet. If the vacuum tube is pushed in too soon, the negative pressure stored in the tube will be lost.

Insert the needle until it is felt in the vein. Once the needle is in the vein, advance the vacuum tube onto the needle and look for blood to begin flowing into the tube. If no blood flows into the tube, advance the needle, slowly, further into the vein. If no blood flows into the tube after this second advance into the vein, remove the needle slowly. If the blood does not flow into the tube, it is likely that the vein was missed. Remove the needle, obtain a new vacuum tube, and start over. It is also possible to insert the needle completely through the vein. This is characterized by a quick flash of blood into the tube; then the blood flow stops.

Besides missing the vein or advancing the needle completely through the vein, other problems can occur. The vein may collapse or the blood may clot before it can flow into the tube. If the tube begins to fill but stops halfway through, this may be an indication that the

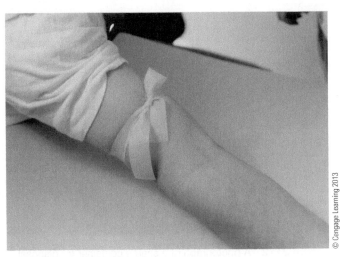

Figure 7-6   A photograph showing the application of a tourniquet

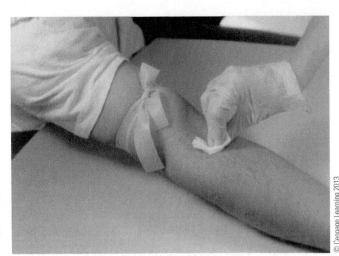

Figure 7-8   Prepping the puncture site using an alcohol prep pad

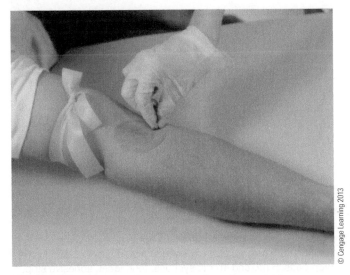

Figure 7-7   Prepping the puncture site using an iodine prep pad

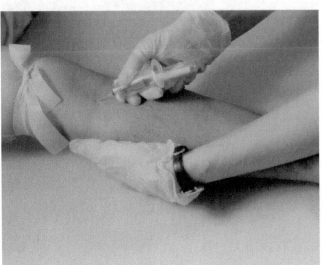

Figure 7-9   The correct technique of puncturing the skin at a 25° to 30° angle

vacuum tube has caused the vein to collapse. By removing the tube from the needle and releasing the tourniquet while leaving the needle in the vein, the blood flow may begin again in 30 to 40 seconds. Reconnect the tube and finish drawing blood. If blood does not enter the tube, start over. If the blood clots in the tube or needle, the only option is to start over.

Once tubes have been filled, release the tourniquet and pull the last tube off the needle and holder. Take the remaining 2 × 2-inch gauze pad and apply gentle pressure to the venipuncture site as the needle is withdrawn. Apply pressure for 1 minute if the patient has no history of bleeding or is not taking blood-thinning medication. If the patient has a history of bleeding or is taking blood-thinning medication, apply pressure for 2 to 5 minutes, or until bleeding stops (Figure 7-10). Once bleeding has stopped, cover the venipuncture site with an adhesive

strip or tape (Figure 7-11). Dispose of the needle by placing it in a sharps container with the appropriate biohazard markings (Figure 7-12).

When using a *butterfly needle* for blood cultures or difficult blood draws, the same equipment is needed, minus the needle and holder. A butterfly needle and syringes are needed to draw the specimen (Figure 7-13).

Follow the same steps, starting with the alcohol swab followed by the povidone-iodine swab. Wipe the area dry with one sterile 2 × 2-inch gauze pad. Insert the butterfly needle at a 25° to 30° angle (Figure 7-14). Once the needle is in place and blood enters the line, place a piece of tape on the butterfly (Figure 7-15). Attach either a 5 mL or a 10 mL syringe to the line. Gently pull the syringe plunger back to draw blood into the syringe (see Figure 7-15). If blood is in the line but does not enter the syringe, reposition the butterfly. If no blood

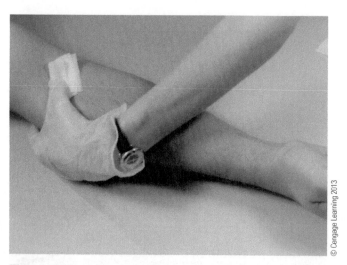

Figure 7-10 Application of firm pressure using a 2 × 2-inch gauze pad following venous access

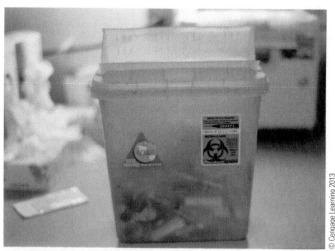

Figure 7-12 A photograph of a sharps container for disposal of the needle used for venous access

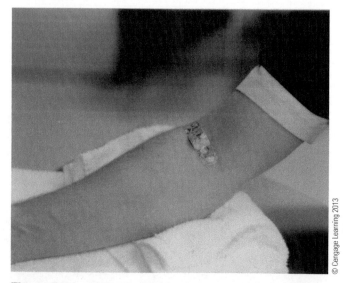

Figure 7-11 Application of adhesive tape or strip following venous puncture

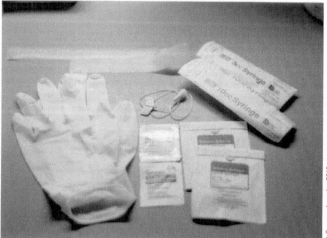

Figure 7-13 A photograph of the equipment required for venipuncture using a butterfly needle: gloves, alcohol, and iodine prep pads, 5 mL and 10 mL syringes, tourniquet, adhesive strip, and a butterfly needle

© Cengage Learning 2013

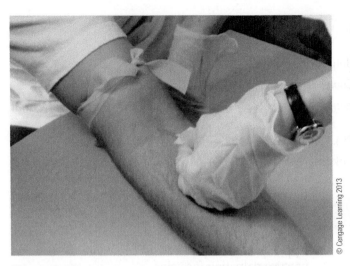

Figure 7-14 Insertion of a butterfly needle at a shallow (a 25° to 30°) angle

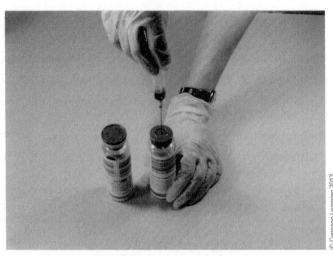

Figure 7-16 A photograph showing injection of the blood sample into the vacuum (blood culture) bottle

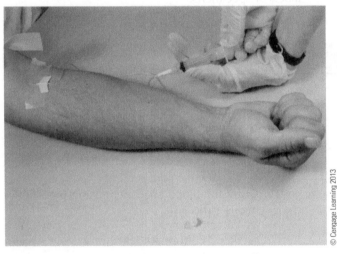

Figure 7-15 A photograph showing the butterfly needle taped in position and a syringe being used to withdraw the blood from the vein

enters the syringe after moving the butterfly, change syringes and try again. If this fails, remove the butterfly and restart. When the syringe is full, remove it from the line and attach a sterile needle to the end of the syringe. Then break the seal on top of the blood culture bottles. Clean the top of the blood culture bottles to prevent contamination. Insert the needle on the syringe into the blood culture bottle (Figure 7-16). The vacuum in the bottles will automatically draw an exact amount of blood out of the syringe.

Upon completion of drawing blood cultures, use gentle pressure to apply a 2 × 2-inch gauze pad at the venipuncture site while slowly removing the needle. Apply pressure to the site for 1 minute, or until bleeding has stopped. Place a piece of tape or an adhesive strip over the site.

There are several complications and hazards associated with venipuncture. Complications can range from slight bruising to large hematomas at the venipuncture site. The extent of bruising or bleeding can be aggravated by blood thinners. Always apply pressure at the site after needle removal. If the needle is inserted too deeply or moved from side to side while under the skin, nerve damage is possible, though extremely rare. Infection is a technique-dependent complication. Venipuncture invades the patient's body, breaking down the defense system by puncturing the skin. Good aseptic technique before venipuncture and proper cover over the site afterward will greatly reduce the probability of infection.

Upon completion of the blood draw, label the tubes. After completing all blood draws, transport them to the laboratory. Most institutions require the label to include the patient's identification number and name. The label may also include the patient's date of birth, the time and date the sample was drawn, the name of the person who drew the sample, and that person's initials. This is all that is usually required, but check the employer's policy requirements.

Transporting is accomplished through several ways. The practitioner may carry the blood to the laboratory him or herself, or the laboratory may pick up the samples at some collection point. Some institutions use pneumatic tubes that run throughout the facility. Pneumatic tubes can sometimes be unreliable and samples may be lost. Keep this possibility in mind for code situations or difficult patients. Also, transport through these tubes is rough going, so for very fragile samples, like blood culture specimens, walk them to the laboratory.

The skills needed to become proficient at venipuncture are not demanding. By studying the procedure outlined here and practicing under supervision, the respiratory practitioner can add phlebotomy to the list of skills as a respiratory practitioner.

Additional Resources

Black, J. M. (1997). *Medical surgical nursing* (5th ed.). Philadelphia: Saunders.

Dantzker, D. R., MacIntyre, N. R., & Bakow, E. D. (1995). *Comprehensive respiratory care*. Philadelphia: Saunders.

DeLaune, S. C., & Ladner, P. K. (2006). *Fundamentals of nursing: Standards & practice* (3rd ed.). Clifton Park, NY: Delmar Cengage Learning.

Delmar's nursing image library [Computer software]. (1999). Clifton Park, NY: Delmar Cengage Learning.

Holy Family Hospital policy and procedure manuals. (1995). Spokane, WA.

Practice Activities: Phlebotomy

1. Collect, identify, and describe the function of all materials needed for venipuncture:
   a. Gloves
   b. Alcohol and iodine swabs
   c. Two 2 × 2-inch gauze pads
   d. Tourniquet
   e. Tape or bandage
   f. Needle and vacuum tubes

2. Apply the tourniquet 8 to 10 cm above the site and practice palpating for veins.

3. Practice removing the tourniquet and applying gentle pressure to the site.

4. Describe what information should be included on all labels of specimens.

Check List: Venipuncture

_____ 1. Review obligations to the patient, laboratory, and self.

_____ 2. Review the exposure control policy.

_____ 3. Identify the steps to take if accidental needle stick occurs.

_____ 4. Identify and locate proper waste disposal.

5. Obtain all the equipment necessary for venipuncture:
   _____ a. Pair of gloves
   _____ b. Alcohol and iodine swabs
   _____ c. Two 2 × 2-inch gauze pads
   _____ d. Tourniquet
   _____ e. Tape or bandage
   _____ f. Needle or butterfly

6. Verify the physician orders:
   _____ a. Refer to the physician order sheet.

7. Verify patient identification:
   _____ a. Check the identification band.
   _____ b. Ask the patient's name.

8. Prepare the patient:
   _____ a. Assess patient attitude.
   _____ b. Check fasting status/medications.
   _____ c. Apply one pair of gloves.

9. Select the venipuncture site and instruct the patient:
   _____ a. Place the extremity in dependent position.
   _____ b. Have the patient clench the fist and hold.
   _____ c. Use the tourniquet if needed.

10. Decontaminate the site:
    _____ a. Alcohol
    _____ b. Povidone-iodine
    _____ c. 2 × 2-inch gauze pad

11. Use correct needle placement:
    _____ a. 25° to 30° angle

12. Draw the blood specimen, using the following as indicated:
    _____ a. Vacuum tubes
    _____ b. Blood culture bottles

_____ 13. Remove the tourniquet.

_____ 14. Pull the vacuum tube off the needle and holder.

15. Remove the needle and attend to the puncture site:
    _____ a. Apply pressure to the site.
    _____ b. Apply bandage or tape.

_____ 16. Properly dispose of materials.

17. Label the specimen:
    _____ a. Patient identification
    _____ b. Time
    _____ c. Date
    _____ d. Your initials

_____ 18. Transport the specimen.

Self-Evaluation Post Test: Phlebotomy

1. In which role might you find a respiratory practitioner?
   a. Support staff
   b. Transport staff
   c. Staff responsible for actual blood draw
   d. All of the above

2. Why is the exposure control policy put into place?
   a. To protect patients and staff
   b. To maintain a safe environment
   c. To give employees something to read during slow times
   d. Both a and b

3. If an accidental needle stick occurs, what should you do?
   a. Squeeze your finger and hold it.
   b. Gently milk the area.
   c. Apply a tourniquet to your arm.
   d. Lance the wound to promote increased blood flow.

4. Which of these materials will *not* be needed for a blood draw?
   a. Gloves
   b. Syringe and needle
   c. Alcohol and iodine
   d. Antibiotic ointment

5. It is acceptable *not* to check the patient's identification band if the patient can state his or her name.
   a. True   b. False

6. It is acceptable to move the needle side to side once under the skin.
   a. True   b. False

7. What are some hazards and complications of venipuncture?
   I. Slight bruising
   II. Hematomas at the site
   III. Infection
   IV. Nerve damage
   a. I and II   c. I, II, and III
   b. I and III   d. I, II, III and IV

8. At which angle do you insert the needle for blood draws?
   a. $10°$ to $20°$ angle   c. $45°$ to $50°$ angle
   b. $25°$ to $30°$ angle   d. $90°$ angle

9. If a patient has a bleeding history or is taking blood thinners, how long must pressure be applied to the venipuncture site?
   a. For 2 to 5 minutes   c. For 30 seconds
   b. For 1 minute   d. For 10 minutes

10. Gloves are not required if you believe that the patient does not have HIV infection.
    a. True   b. False

PERFORMANCE EVALUATION:
Venipuncture

Date: Lab _____ Clinical _____ Agency _____

Lab: Pass _____ Fail _____ Clinical: Pass _____ Fail _____

Student name _____ Instructor name _____

No. of times observed in clinical _____

No. of times practiced in clinical _____

PASSING CRITERIA: Obtain 90% or better on the procedure. Tasks indicated by * must receive at least 1 point, or the evaluation is terminated. Procedure must be performed within the designated time, or the performance receives a failing grade.

SCORING:
2 points — Task performed satisfactorily without prompting.
1 point — Task performed satisfactorily with self-initiated correction.
0 points — Task performed incorrectly or with prompting required.
NA — Task not applicable to the patient care situation.

Tasks:	Peer	Lab	Clinical
* 1. Reviews obligation to patient, self, and laboratory	☐	☐	☐
* 2. Reviews the exposure control policy	☐	☐	☐
* 3. Identifies the steps to be taken if accidental needle stick occurs	☐	☐	☐
* 4. Identifies and locates proper waste disposal	☐	☐	☐
* 5. Obtains all necessary equipment			
a. Pair of gloves	☐	☐	☐
b. Alcohol and iodine swabs	☐	☐	☐
c. Two 2 × 2-inch gauze pads	☐	☐	☐
d. Tape or bandage	☐	☐	☐
e. Tourniquet	☐	☐	☐
f. Needle or butterfly	☐	☐	☐
* 6. Verifies the physician orders	☐	☐	☐
* 7. Verifies the patient's identification band	☐	☐	☐
* 8. Prepares the patient for venipuncture			
a. Assesses the patient's cooperativeness	☐	☐	☐
b. Explains the procedure to the patient	☐	☐	☐
c. Checks the patient's fasting status and medications	☐	☐	☐
* 9. Performs hand hygiene	☐	☐	☐

* **10.** Applies gloves ☐ ☐ ☐

* **11.** Selects a venipuncture site

    a. Extremity in dependent position ☐ ☐ ☐

    b. Fist clenched and held ☐ ☐ ☐

    c. Applies the tourniquet 8 to 10 cm above the site ☐ ☐ ☐

* **12.** Properly decontaminates the site

    a. Alcohol swab in circular motion ☐ ☐ ☐

    b. Iodine swab in circular motion ☐ ☐ ☐

    c. Swipes area with a 2 × 2-inch gauze pad one time ☐ ☐ ☐

* **13.** Places the needle at a 25° to 30° angle ☐ ☐ ☐

* **14.** Applies proper blood collection tubes ☐ ☐ ☐

* **15.** Removes the collection tubes from the needle ☐ ☐ ☐

* **16.** Removes the tourniquet ☐ ☐ ☐

* **17.** Removes the needle and applies pressure and a bandage ☐ ☐ ☐

* **18.** Disposes of all sharps and biohazard material in the proper waste disposal container ☐ ☐ ☐

* **19.** Properly labels the blood samples

    a. Patient identification number ☐ ☐ ☐

    b. Date and time blood was drawn ☐ ☐ ☐

    c. Initials of the person who drew blood ☐ ☐ ☐

20. Transports the blood tubes to the laboratory via appropriate means ☐ ☐ ☐

SCORE: Peer _____ points of possible 66; _____%

               Lab _____ points of possible 66; _____%

               Clinical _____ points of possible 66; _____%

TIME: _____ out of possible 20 minutes

STUDENT SIGNATURES

PEER: _____

STUDENT: _____

INSTRUCTOR SIGNATURES

LAB: _____

CLINICAL: _____

CHAPTER 8
Arterial Blood Gas Sampling

INTRODUCTION

Arterial blood gas (ABG) analysis is an extremely useful diagnostic test for the clinical assessment of ventilation, acid-base status, and oxygenation. Collection of an arterial sample may be done quickly, and it provides important information for decision making in the management of the patient requiring oxygen or ventilatory assistance.

Collection of an arterial blood sample is commonly done by arterial puncture or, in the intensive care unit, by drawing a sample from an indwelling arterial catheter. In an infant weighing less than 30 pounds, arterialized blood may be obtained from a capillary stick, or in a newborn, from an umbilical artery catheter.

Arterial puncture is a skill that is easily learned. However, it is not without hazards and potential complications because it disrupts the integrity of a large high-pressure vessel of the arterial system. Possible complications of arterial puncture at any site are vessel trauma and occlusion, embolization, infection, and vessel spasm. If properly done by a skilled practitioner, arterial puncture provides safe, reliable information for patient management.

This chapter discusses the three common sites for arterial puncture, how to perform an arterial puncture, and the advantages and disadvantages of each site. The respiratory care practitioner will also learn how to perform arterial line sampling and the hazards and complications of this procedure.

KEY TERMS

- **Arterialization**
- **Arterial line sampling**
- **Capillary blood gas sampling**
- **Flash**
- **Modified Allen's test**
- **Oximetry**

THEORY OBJECTIVES

At the end of this chapter, the reader should be able to:

- *Identify the three common anatomical locations for arterial puncture:*
  - *Radial*
  - *Brachial*
  - *Femoral*
  State the advantages and disadvantages of each site.
- *Explain the complications associated with arterial puncture.*
- *Explain the rationale for the modified Allen's test for evaluation of collateral circulation.*
- *Describe the use of pulse oximetry to evaluate collateral circulation to the hand.*
- *Discuss the use of a glass syringe versus a specialized plastic syringe for arterial sampling.*
- *Describe the six most common technical causes of blood gas sampling errors and their prevention:*
  - *Room air mixed with the sample*
  - *Delay in analyzing the sample*
  - *Drawing a venous sample by mistake*
  - *Heparin contamination*
  - *Patient anxiety causing hyperventilation*
  - *Plastic syringes*
- *State the appropriate anticoagulant to use when drawing an arterial sample for blood gas analysis.*
- *Explain the advantages, disadvantages, and hazards of drawing blood from an arterial line.*
- *Describe the rationale for capillary blood sampling in infants.*
- *Describe the three most common errors in capillary blood sampling:*
  - *Poor blood flow during sampling*
  - *Introduction of air into the capillary sample*
  - *Inadequate mixing of heparin in the sample*

CLINICAL PRACTICE GUIDELINES

AARC Clinical Practice Guideline Sampling for Arterial Blood Gas Analysis

BGA 4.0 INDICATIONS:

Indications for blood gas and pH analysis and hemoximetry include:

4.1 the need to evaluate the adequacy of a patient's ventilatory ($PaCO_2$), acid-base (pH and $PaCO_2$), and/or oxygenation (PaO_2 and O_2Hb) status, the oxygen-carrying capacity (PaO_2, O_2Hb, tHb, and dyshemoglobin saturations)[1,2,4] and intrapulmonary shunt (Q_{sp}/Q_t);

4.2 the need to quantitate the response to therapeutic intervention (eg, supplemental oxygen administration, mechanical ventilation) and/or diagnostic evaluation (eg, exercise desaturation);[1-3]

4.3 the need to monitor severity and progression of documented disease processes.[1,2]

BGA 5.0 CONTRAINDICATIONS:

Contraindications to performing pH-blood gas analysis and hemoximetry include:

5.1 an improperly functioning analyzer;

5.2 an analyzer that has not had functional status validated by analysis of commercially prepared quality control products or tonometered whole blood[5,8-10] or has not been validated through participation in a proficiency testing program(s);[5,8,10-13]

5.3 a specimen that has not been properly anticoagulated;[4,5,14]

5.4 a specimen containing visible air bubbles;[1,4]

5.5 a specimen stored in a plastic syringe at room temperature for longer than 30 minutes, stored at room temperature for longer than 5 minutes for a shunt study, or stored at room temperature in the presence of an elevated leukocyte or platelet count (PaO_2 in samples drawn from subjects with very high leukocyte counts can decrease rapidly. Immediate chilling and analysis is necessary).[4,15-20]

5.6 an incomplete requisition that precludes adequate interpretation and documentation of results and for which attempts to obtain additional information have been unsuccessful. Requisitions should contain

    5.6.1 patient's name or other unique identifier, such as medical record number; birth date or age, date and time of sampling;

    5.6.2 location of patient;

    5.6.3 name of requesting physician or authorized individual;

    5.6.4 clinical indication and tests to be performed;

    5.6.5 sample source (arterial line, central venous catheter, peripheral artery);

    5.6.6 respiratory rate and for the patient on supplemental oxygen fractional concentration of inspired oxygen (FIO_2) or oxygen flow;

    5.6.7 ventilator settings for mechanically ventilated patients (tidal volume, respiratory rate, FIO_2, mode);

    5.6.8 signature of person who obtained sample.[4,6]

It may also be useful to note body temperature, activity level, and working diagnosis. Test requisition should be electronically generated or handwritten and must be signed by the person ordering the test. Oral requests must be supported by written authorization within 30 days.[6]

5.7 an inadequately labeled specimen lacking the patient's full name or other unique identifier (eg, medical record number), date, and time of sampling.[4,5]

BGA 6.0 HAZARDS/COMPLICATIONS:

Possible hazards or complications include:

6.1 infection of specimen handler from blood carrying the human immunodeficiency virus, or HIV, hepatitis B, other blood-borne pathogens;[5,7,9,21]

6.2 inappropriate patient medical treatment based on improperly analyzed blood specimen or from analysis of an unacceptable specimen or from incorrect reporting of results.

BGA 8.0 ASSESSMENT OF NEED:

THE PRESENCE OF A VALID INDICATION (BGA 4.0) IN THE SUBJECT TO BE TESTED SUPPORTS THE NEED FOR SAMPLING AND ANALYSIS.

BGA 11.0 MONITORING:

Monitoring of personnel, sample handling, and analyzer performance to assure proper handling, analysis, and reporting should be ongoing, during the process.

AARC Clinical Practice Guideline Capillary Blood Gas Sampling for Neonatal and Pediatric Patients

CBGS 4.0 INDICATIONS:

Capillary blood gas sampling is indicated when:

4.1 Arterial blood gas analysis is indicated but arterial access is not available.

Reprinted with permission from *Respiratory Care* 2001; 46: 498–505. The complete AARC Clinical Practice Guidelines are available from the AARC Web site (http://www.aarc.org), from the AARC Executive Office, or from *Respiratory Care* journal.

(Continued)

4.2 Noninvasive monitor readings are abnormal: transcutaneous values, end-tidal CO_2, pulse oximetry.

4.3 Assessment of initiation, administration, or change in therapeutic modalities (i.e., mechanical ventilation) is indicated.

4.4 A change in patient status is detected by history or physical assessment.

4.5 Monitoring the severity and progression of a documented disease process is desirable.

CBGS 5.0 CONTRAINDICATIONS:

5.1 Capillary punctures should not be performed:

   5.1.1 At or through the following sites (10):

      5.1.1.1 Posterior curvature of the heel, as the device may puncture the bone (11)

      5.1.1.2 The heel of a patient who has begun walking and has callus development (12)

      5.1.1.3 The fingers of neonates (to avoid nerve damage) (13)

      5.1.1.4 Previous puncture sites (14,15)

      5.1.1.5 Inflamed, swollen, or edematous tissues (14,15)

      5.1.1.6 Cyanotic or poorly perfused tissues (14,15)

      5.1.1.7 Localized areas of infection (14,15)

      5.1.1.8 Peripheral arteries

   5.1.2 On patients less than 24 hours old, due to poor peripheral perfusion (1)

   5.1.3 When there is need for direct analysis of oxygenation (1–3)

   5.1.4 When there is need for direct analysis of arterial blood

5.2 Relative contraindications include:

   5.2.1 Peripheral vasoconstriction (1)

   5.2.2 Polycythemia (due to shorter clotting times) (1)

   5.2.3 Hypotension may be a relative contraindication (1)

CBGS 6.0 HAZARDS/COMPLICATIONS:

6.1 Infection

   6.1.1 Introduction of contagion at sampling site and consequent infection in patient, including calcaneus osteomyelitis (9,16) and cellulitis

   6.1.2 Inadvertent puncture or incision and consequent infection in sampler

6.2 Burns

6.3 Hematoma

6.4 Bone calcification (14)

6.5 Nerve damage (9)

6.6 Bruising

6.7 Scarring (12)

6.8 Puncture of posterior medial aspect of heel may result in tibial artery laceration (11)

6.9 Pain

6.10 Bleeding

6.11 Inappropriate patient management may result from reliance on capillary PO_2 values (17,18)

CBGS 8.0 ASSESSMENT OF NEED:

Capillary blood gas sampling is an intermittent procedure and should be performed when a documented need exists. Routine or standing orders for capillary puncture are not recommended. The following may assist the clinician in assessing the need for capillary blood gas sampling:

8.1 History and physical assessment (23)

8.2 Noninvasive respiratory monitoring values

   8.2.1 Pulse oximetry (23)

   8.2.2 Transcutaneous values

   8.2.3 End-tidal CO_2 values

8.3 Patient response to initiation, administration, or change in therapeutic modalities (23–25)

8.4 Lack of arterial access for blood gas sampling (1–3)

CBGS 11.0 MONITORING:

11.1 FIO_2 or prescribed oxygen flow (10,23,28,29)

11.2 Oxygen administration device or ventilator settings (10,23,27,28)

11.3 Free flow of blood without the necessity for "milking" the foot or finger to obtain a sample (10,14)

11.4 Presence/absence of air or clot in sample (10,26,27)

11.5 Patient temperature, respiratory rate, position or level of activity, and clinical appearance (10,27)

11.6 Ease or difficulty of obtaining sample (10,27,28)

11.7 Appearance of puncture site (14,15)

11.8 Complications or adverse reactions to the procedure

11.9 Date, time, and sampling site (10)

11.10 Noninvasive monitoring values: transcutaneous O_2 & CO_2, end-tidal CO_2, and/or pulse oximetry (23)

11.11 Results of the blood gas analysis

Reprinted with permission from *Respiratory Care*. 46(5): 506–513. The complete AARC Clinical Practice Guidelines are available from the AARC Web site (http://www.aarc .org), from the AARC Executive Office, or from *Respiratory Care* journal.

ANATOMICAL LOCATIONS FOR ARTERIAL PUNCTURE

Radial Artery

The radial artery's location makes it easily accessible. It is located in the wrist on the radial side (thumb side), close to the surface of the skin. It is the site most commonly used for taking a patient's pulse. Figure 8-1 shows the location of the radial artery where it is most accessible for puncture.

A big advantage of performing arterial puncture at the radial site is the safety afforded by the presence of collateral circulation. The hand is supplied with blood by both the radial and ulnar arteries. Because repeated punctures may result in vessel damage, swelling with partial or complete occlusion of the vessel may occur. If circulation is inadvertently interrupted resulting from radial artery puncture, the ulnar artery will continue to supply the circulatory needs of the hand. There are no veins or nerves immediately adjacent to the radial artery; consequently, arterial sampling at this site is facilitated by a reduced chance of inadvertent venous puncture or nerve damage.

The disadvantage of radial artery puncture is the small size of this artery. The radial artery is a small target. But through careful observation, palpation, and considerable practice, the radial artery can be punctured easily. However, in case of hypotensive and hypovolemic states or low cardiac output, puncture at this site may be particularly difficult.

Brachial Artery

The site where the brachial artery is commonly punctured is at the elbow in the antecubital fossa. Figure 8-2 shows its location. It is located on the medial side of the fossa near the insertion of the biceps muscle at the radial tuberosity.

An advantage of the brachial artery puncture site is its size. It is large and easily palpated.

There are several disadvantages to using the brachial artery. It is close to both a large vein and a nerve. Inadvertent venous sampling is common at this site. Accidental contact with the nerves at this site may cause extreme discomfort. Also, this site does not have the advantage of collateral circulation. Inadvertent injury leading to stoppage of circulation may result in the loss of the limb.

Femoral Artery

The femoral artery is accessible for arterial sampling in the groin. It may be palpated laterally from the pubis bone. Figure 8-3 shows the location for arterial puncture at this site.

The femoral artery is very large. It is easily palpated and presents a large target. The femoral artery may be the only site where arterial sampling is possible in cases of hypovolemia or hypotension, during cardiopulmonary resuscitation (CPR), or with low cardiac output.

There are several disadvantages to arterial puncture at this site, including the proximity of a major vein and a lack of collateral circulation. The artery may also be deep and difficult to locate. Atherosclerotic plaques commonly

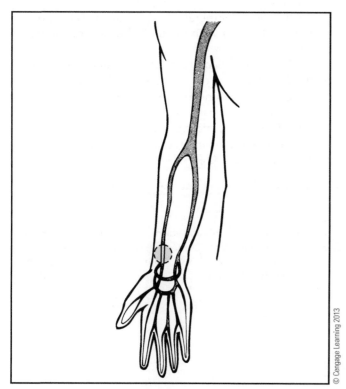

Figure 8-1   The radial puncture site

© Cengage Learning 2013

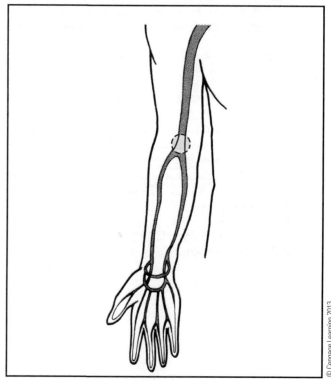

Figure 8-2   The brachial puncture site

© Cengage Learning 2013

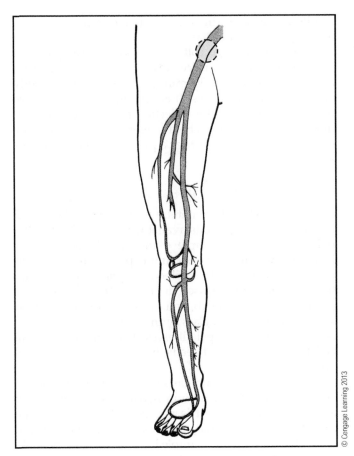

Figure 8-3   The femoral puncture site

form in the femoral artery. If a plaque is dislodged as a result of arterial puncture, circulation to the entire leg may be compromised by formation of emboli. In addition, the close proximity of the femoral vein makes the certainty of arterial sampling questionable.

COMPLICATIONS OF ARTERIAL PUNCTURE

There are several potential complications and hazards of arterial puncture, including vessel spasm and formation of thrombi or emboli, infection, and loss of blood flow and circulation. When an artery is punctured, arteriospasm may result. The artery is surrounded by a layer of muscle. The irritation caused by the penetration of the hypodermic needle may induce the muscle to spasm. There is a possibility of dislodging an atherosclerotic plaque or thrombus as a result of arterial puncture. If this happens, circulation to that limb or area may be seriously compromised. It could be severe enough that the circulation would be totally interrupted. Air emboli may also be inadvertently introduced into the vessel by improper technique. These emboli may result in serious consequences. Repeated punctures may compromise the vessel's integrity and circulation.

The Modified Allen's Test for Collateral Circulation

An advantage of performing an arterial puncture at the radial site is that the vascular anatomy allows testing for collateral circulation. The *modified Allen's test* should be done before arterial puncture to determine the adequacy of circulation supplied by the ulnar artery.

To perform the modified Allen's test, elevate the patient's hand higher than the level of the heart. Have the patient make a fist for approximately 30 seconds. Apply pressure to both the radial and ulnar arteries occluding them. Have the patient open his or her hand (it should appear blanched). Release pressure on the ulnar artery. Color should return to the hand within 7 to 10 seconds. Figure 8-4 shows the correct hand position for the modified Allen's test.

If the hand does not flush pink, it is likely that blood flow through the ulnar artery is insufficient to provide circulation if the radial artery loses patency. If this happens, try the other hand. If this also fails, choose the brachial site for puncture.

This test may be done on an unconscious patient by holding the hand above the heart for 30 to 60 seconds before releasing pressure on the ulnar artery.

Use of Pulse Oximetry to Assess Collateral Circulation of the Hand

Pulse oximetry may be used to assess collateral circulation of the hand and may actually be more sensitive than the modified Allen's test (Barbeau, 2004). *Pulse oximetry* is the measurement of oxygen saturation noninvasively using multiple wavelengths of light. A finger probe from a pulse oximeter is placed on the hand where collateral circulation is to be assessed. The baseline SpO_2 is measured as well as the signal quality (plethysmographic waveform). Both radial and ulnar arteries are occluded using a firm grip. Oxygen desaturation and loss of signal quality are then noted. Once the ulnar artery pressure is released, the SpO_2 will return to the baseline value and signal strength within 15 seconds if collateral circulation is good.

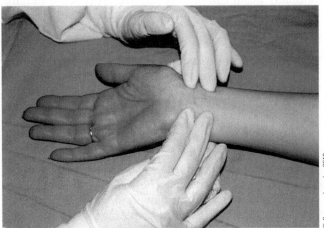

Figure 8-4   Performing the modified Allen's test

Sampling Syringes

Recent advances in plastics technology have eliminated accuracy errors that result from diffusion of gases through the plastic of the syringe. Many specialized plastic syringes are commercially available for arterial sampling. If these syringes are used according to the manufacturer's directions, little or no error will be introduced.

ABG sampling kits are commonly available. These kits contain a syringe, needle, alcohol and/or iodine-based prep pads, label, rubber stopper or cap, and a bag or container for transport of the specimen.

BLOOD GAS SAMPLING ERRORS

The reliability of blood gas analysis is very technique dependent. Every step of the process, from preparation of equipment through reporting the data, has potential problems that affect data reliability. That is, knowledge and skill as a respiratory care practitioner will often determine the accuracy of the procedure. Knowledge of the factors that contribute to sampling errors will help to prevent their occurrence in clinical practice. If a sample is questionable, the relevant facts should be noted with the results of analysis. Clinical decisions are frequently based on data assumed to be entirely accurate.

Bubbles

Particularly if the sample is aspirated, air bubbles are often present in the collected blood sample. These bubbles must be expelled immediately upon collection. Room air contains enough oxygen that it can diffuse into the sample, increasing the arterial oxygen tension (PaO_2), or if the PaO_2 is greater than 160 mm Hg, it can decrease the PaO_2. This diffusion problem is especially true in patients with hypoxemia. Carbon dioxide is present in the atmosphere in a concentration of only 0.003%, or around 2 mm Hg at sea level. Because arterial blood normally has a carbon dioxide tension ($PaCO_2$) ranging from 35 to 45 mm Hg, CO_2 dissolved in blood will tend to diffuse into the bubbles in the sample, lowering the measured value.

Ideally, if a large quantity of bubbles is present in the sample, it is best to discard it and draw another sample, being more attentive with the technique. However, this may not be practical in the clinical setting.

Delay in Sample Analysis

Blood contains living cells with their own metabolism and metabolic needs. These cells will continue to consume oxygen and nutrients and produce acids and CO_2 even after being withdrawn from the body. Thus, if 15 minutes elapses before the sample is analyzed, the results can change dramatically (American Association for Respiratory Care, 2001).

Immediately after collection, cool the sample in a slush of ice and water. Ice slows the cells' metabolism, and even a delay of 30 minutes will not significantly affect the analysis results. It is best, however, to analyze the sample as soon after collection as possible. Ten minutes is optimal. Samples held longer than this may show lower PaO_2, higher $PaCO_2$, or a pH less than the patient's actual pH.

Use of the Proper Anticoagulant

Oxalates, ethylenediaminetetra-acetic acid (EDTA), and the citrate anticoagulants available for use will alter the pH of the arterial sample (American Association for Respiratory Care, 2001). Sodium heparin is the best anticoagulant to use in arterial blood sampling. Even sodium heparin, if too much is used (more than 0.1 mL of heparin per 1 mL of whole blood), will cause acidosis in the blood sample. If preparing a glass syringe for use, a safe general rule to follow is to expel all excess heparin. Heparin will be left in the needle and needle hub, occupying a minimal volume.

The syringes in blood gas sampling kits often contain crystalline heparin or lithium heparin. No aspiration of additional anticoagulant is necessary. Simply draw the sample, and the anticoagulant will dissolve. However, it is important to mix the sample by gently rolling or shaking the syringe after collection.

Venous Sampling

In a sample drawn from a patient with hypoxemia, it is difficult to distinguish arterial blood from venous blood by color. When an arterial sample is drawn, the plunger of the syringe tends to pulsate as the sample fills the barrel. If the syringe does not fill without assistance, be suspicious of the sample site.

Patients in cardiopulmonary arrest, hypovolemia, hypotension, or low cardiac output often have low blood pressure. Samples from these patients must usually be aspirated. Drawing from the brachial or femoral site will help to ensure obtaining an arterial sample.

In the event of collection of a venous sample, draw another sample for analysis. If this is not possible, note with the sample results that it may be a venous sample.

Under some circumstances, a venous sample may be intentionally drawn as well as an arterial sample. The technique for venipuncture is different from that for arterial puncture and is discussed in Chapter 7.

Patient Anxiety

It is a rare person who enjoys having blood drawn. It is natural to be a little apprehensive before the skin is punctured by a needle. However, if extreme, this anxiety may lead to hyperventilation and consequent altering of the $PaCO_2$.

Anxiety can be minimized by doing the procedure quickly and being prepared before reaching the bedside. Do not stress the pain and discomfort a patient may experience with arterial puncture. There is a difference between informed consent and scaring the patient. A statement such as "You will feel a little poke" is sufficient. If an arterial puncture is performed properly by a skilled practitioner, the blood sample can be drawn with minimal pain and discomfort.

CAPILLARY BLOOD GAS SAMPLING

In infants, *capillary blood gas sampling* is frequently performed in lieu of arterial puncture. Performing arterial puncture in an infant requires a large degree of skill and good technique for best results. The infant's vessels are very small and are difficult to palpate and puncture.

Technique

Capillary samples are usually obtained from the infant's heel but may also be obtained from the finger. When capillary blood is drawn from the heel, this sampling technique is sometimes referred to as a *heel stick*. *Arterialization* (warming to maximize blood flow) of the infant's heel is done before sampling, and then a lancet is used to puncture the skin surface. A sample from an adequately arterialized limb will yield reliable pH and

PaCO$_2$ values, whereas PaO$_2$ values will vary from those determined using blood drawn by arterial puncture.

Capillary Sampling Errors

Poor Blood Flow

In performing capillary blood sampling, it is important to obtain a free-flowing sample. Do not squeeze the infant's foot when drawing the sample into a capillary tube. Squeezing the foot excessively could result in injury to the foot, leading to altered blood gas values. If blood at the puncture site does not flow freely, repeat the puncture to obtain a freely flowing blood sample.

Introduction of Air into the Sample

As with arterial puncture techniques, it is important to minimize the blood sample's exposure to air. Air may be introduced when it is drawn into the capillary tube, causing bubbles. The presence of air bubbles will alter the blood gas results; therefore, introduction of air should be avoided. If the sample contains visible bubbles, discard it and draw another (or remove the air bubbles as they enter the capillary tube).

Inadequate Mixing of Heparin

Once the sample has been drawn into the capillary tube, one end may be sealed with clay or a rubber stopper. A small metal rod is inserted into the capillary tube, and a magnet is passed back and forth along the length of the tube to mix the heparin in the capillary tube with the blood sample. It is important to mix the heparin well to avoid clotting prior to sampling.

PROFICIENCY OBJECTIVES

At the end of this chapter, the reader should be able to:

ARTERIAL PUNCTURE

- *Collect and properly assemble the supplies needed for arterial puncture.*
- *Demonstrate how to prepare a syringe properly for arterial puncture.*
- *Locate the three sites for arterial puncture:*
  — *Radial*
  — *Brachial*
  — *Femoral*
- *Using a laboratory partner, demonstrate the modified Allen's test for collateral circulation.*
- *Using an arterial arm simulator or the arm of a laboratory partner, demonstrate:*
  — *Radial artery puncture*
  — *Brachial artery puncture*
- *Demonstrate how to properly label and prepare the sample for transport.*

- *Demonstrate how to draw an arterial sample from an indwelling radial artery catheter.*

CAPILLARY SAMPLING

- *Collect and properly assemble the supplies needed for capillary blood sampling.*
- *Using a resuscitation mannequin or an infant, correctly demonstrate how to arterialize an infant's heel prior to puncture.*
- *Using a resuscitation mannequin or an infant, demonstrate correct techniques for obtaining a capillary blood sample:*
  — *Site preparation*
  — *Use of the lancet*
  — *Drawing the capillary sample*
  — *Mixing the heparin*
  — *Care of the puncture site following the procedure*

SUPPLIES NEEDED FOR ARTERIAL PUNCTURE

The supplies needed for arterial puncture are usually contained in an ABG kit. If the practitioner needs to assemble supplies separately, the supplies needed are listed in Figure 8-5.

PUNCTURE TECHNIQUES

Standard Precautions

As discussed in Chapter 1, blood and blood products are body fluids that come under the classification of biohazards. As such, it is important to adhere to the guidelines provided by the Centers for Disease Control and Prevention (CDC) and comply with all standard precautions.

To perform arterial puncture, arterial line sampling, or capillary blood sampling (heel sticks), the practitioner should wear personal protective equipment. As a minimum, wear disposable gloves and eye protection (either goggles or a face shield). Always exercise caution when using sharps (needles or lancet) to prevent sticks or punctures of your own skin. Always handle sharps carefully, and properly dispose of them into an approved biohazard sharps container.

Patient-Related Considerations

A physician's order is required before performing this or any other procedure. It is important to check the patient's chart for a physician's order for anticoagulant therapy or oxygen therapy before arterial sampling.

Anticoagulant therapy may necessitate putting pressure on the site for up to 15 minutes to stop the bleeding following arterial puncture.

It is important to assess if the patient is receiving the proper oxygen therapy (or to identify the lack of therapy) before doing the puncture. ABG analysis is a useful tool for judging the adequacy of oxygen therapy. If blood is drawn while the patient is receiving the wrong oxygen regimen, however, a repeat arterial puncture is necessary. Mistakes can be avoided by checking the chart and the patient first. Usually, 10 to 30 minutes are needed before arterial puncture after any oxygen concentration change.

5-mL preheparinized disposable sampling syringe
Needles (20 to 25 gauge, in various lengths)
Rubber stopper or rubber syringe cap
Adhesive strip or Elastoplast tape
Iodine and alcohol prep pads
Plastic bag or other container to transport sample
Ice slush
Lidocaine anesthetic 2% solution (if ordered)
—Disposable latex gloves
—Eye protection (goggles or face shield)

© Cengage Learning 2013

Figure 8-5 Supplies needed for arterial puncture

The patient should be reassessed 20 to 30 minutes following arterial puncture. Check the circulation distal to the puncture site and for any bleeding at the site.

Use of an Anesthetic

The use of an anesthetic prior to arterial puncture requires a physician's order and a specific protocol. The puncture site should be prepared as though an arterial puncture is being performed. Draw up 0.1 to 0.2 mL of 2% lidocaine into a tuberculin syringe with a 25-gauge needle. Puncture the skin near the artery and draw back on the plunger. If blood appears in the syringe, the needle is in a vessel. Withdraw the syringe and redirect the needle. Repeat the aspiration step. If there is no blood return, make a small wheal by injecting part of the anesthetic. Try to surround the artery with anesthetic. Allow 2 to 3 minutes to lapse before performing the arterial puncture.

Puncture Preparation

Prepare the syringe as outlined in the previous section. If using a preheparinized syringe, follow the manufacturer's instructions for preparation. It is best to arrange all of the supplies needed within easy reach. The rubber stopper, 2 × 2-inch gauze pads, container with ice slush, and adhesive strip should be arranged so that immediate retrieval is possible.

If doing a radial puncture, perform the modified Allen's test. Carefully palpate the puncture site. Try to form a mental image of the course and direction of the artery. Note the strength of the pulse and try to estimate the depth of the artery below the skin.

Using an iodine-based prep pad, cleanse the site. Use firm pressure, scribing a circle from the puncture site out. Follow the iodine-based preparation with an alcohol prep pad, using the same technique.

Obtaining the Specimen

Radial and Brachial Sites

Hold the syringe like a pencil. Palpate the pulse and visualize the artery location.

For sampling at the radial site, with the needle bevel up, puncture the skin at a 45° angle. Once the needle is below the skin surface, visualize the artery location and slowly advance the needle toward the artery. Observe the hub of the needle. When the artery is punctured, blood will quickly appear in the needle hub. This is termed a *flash*. Upon seeing the flash, do not move. Allow the syringe to fill.

For sampling at the brachial site, with the needle bevel up, puncture the skin at a 45° to 90° angle. Advance the needle slowly toward the artery, watching for the flash. When the flash is observed, do not move. Allow the syringe to fill.

Femoral Site

The femoral artery is deep and may require a longer needle for successful puncture. With the bevel of the needle facing the patient's head and perpendicular to the skin's surface, puncture the skin. Watch for the flash and allow the syringe to fill.

Postpuncture Care

After the sample is collected, withdraw the needle and apply firm pressure with a 2 × 2-inch gauze pad. Expel any air and insert the needle into a rubber stopper to seal it. Many disposable blood gas collection kits come with one-handed safety caps. Use of these devices minimizes the risk of inadvertent needle sticks by elimination of recapping the syringe. Continue to apply firm pressure to the puncture site for a minimum of 5 minutes.

While holding firm pressure to the puncture site, mix the sample in the syringe. The sample may be mixed by gently rolling the syringe between the thumb and fore-finger. Rolling the syringe will mix the heparin with the blood and prevent clotting.

Ice the sample after mixing by placing it into the container of ice slush.

Check the puncture site after 5 minutes has passed. Observe the color of the skin distal to the puncture. Check for circulation by palpating the artery distal to the puncture site. The skin should be warm to the touch, and when the tissue is firmly pressed and released, capillary refill should be evident. An adhesive strip may be applied now.

Label the sample with the patient's name and room number, time of collection, and the fraction of inspired oxygen (FIO_2) inhaled by the patient, respiratory rate, or ventilator settings as appropriate. Transport the sample to the laboratory for analysis.

After 20 minutes, check the puncture site again, using the same criteria described earlier.

INDWELLING ARTERIAL CATHETER SAMPLING

The placement of an indwelling arterial catheter is common in critically ill patients. The catheter supplies moment-by-moment pressure monitoring and allows repeated arterial sampling with minimal trauma to the patient. However, *arterial line sampling* poses certain hazards, including the introduction of air emboli, infection, and inadvertent loss of the line by decannulation.

To prevent the blood in the catheter from clotting, a continuous drip of sodium heparin at a pressure greater than arterial pressure is maintained. If a sample is drawn without first flushing the line, the sample would be severely diluted with heparin.

To flush the line, remove the cap from the sampling port. Clean the port with an alcohol prep pad. Attach a sterile 3 mL syringe, and rotate the stopcock so that blood flows to the sampling port. Withdraw 3 to 5 mL of blood so that undiluted blood flows freely into the syringe. Close the stopcock and discard the syringe.

Attach a new 5 mL syringe, properly prepared, for arterial sampling and draw 3 to 5 mL of undiluted arterial blood. Close the stopcock at the sampling port. Cap the syringe to maintain anaerobic conditions and ice the sample.

Flush the catheter by opening the stopcock to the heparin reservoir bag and allowing heparin to flow through

the catheter. Continue flushing the line until it is clear. Figure 8-6 shows the sequence of arterial sampling from an indwelling arterial catheter.

SUPPLIES FOR CAPILLARY SAMPLING

The supplies needed for capillary sampling are listed in Figure 8-7. It is important to have all of the supplies required for this procedure on hand and ready to use. Infants are very active, and it is difficult to obtain equipment when needed under the best of circumstances.

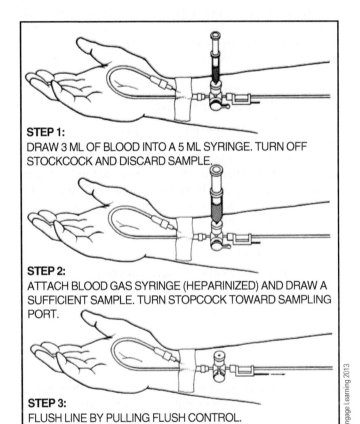

STEP 1:
DRAW 3 ML OF BLOOD INTO A 5 ML SYRINGE. TURN OFF STOCKCOCK AND DISCARD SAMPLE.

STEP 2:
ATTACH BLOOD GAS SYRINGE (HEPARINIZED) AND DRAW A SUFFICIENT SAMPLE. TURN STOPCOCK TOWARD SAMPLING PORT.

STEP 3:
FLUSH LINE BY PULLING FLUSH CONTROL.

© Cengage Learning 2013

Figure 8-6 The sequence for obtaining a sample from an arterial line

Latex gloves
Eye protection
Heparinized capillary tubes
Metal rod
Hot packs or towels saoked in hot water
Clay or rubber caps for capillary sample tubes
Lancets
Povidone-iodine, alcohol prep pads, and 2 × 2-inch gauze pads
Adhesive strip
Paper cup filled with an ice slush

© Cengage Learning 2013

Figure 8-7 Supplies needed for capillary sampling

CAPILLARY SAMPLING TECHNIQUES

Standard Precautions

As discussed in Chapter 1, blood and blood products are body fluids that come under the classification of biohazards. As such, it is important to adhere to the CDC guidelines and comply with all standard precautions.

To perform arterial puncture, arterial line sampling, or capillary blood sampling (heel sticks), the practitioner should wear personal protective equipment. As a minimum the practitioner should wear disposable gloves and eye protection (either goggles or a face shield). Always exercise caution when using sharps (needles or lancet) to prevent sticks or punctures of your own skin. Always handle sharps carefully, and properly dispose of them into an approved biohazard sharps container.

Arterialization of the Puncture Site

It is important to arterialize the puncture site before obtaining the sample to increase blood flow to the area. A hot (45°C) pack or towels soaked in warm water should be applied to the heel for at least 5 minutes prior to performing the puncture. The site should be very pink or red following the application of heat, indicating an increase in capillary circulation.

Site Preparation

The site should be cleansed with an alcohol prep pad followed by a povidone-iodine prep pad. It is important to use aseptic technique to avoid exposing the patient to the risks of infection.

Obtaining the Sample

Using the lancet, quickly puncture the skin on the lateral surface of the heel. The lancet should penetrate approximately 3 mm to ensure adequate blood flow. The blood should flow freely from the puncture site without having to squeeze the infant's heel to augment blood flow.

The initial blood should be discarded and not obtained as part of the sample. Once the blood is flowing freely, use the heparinized capillary tube to draw the sample. Be careful not to introduce air or bubbles into the sample.

Care of the Sample

Once the capillary sample has been obtained, seal one end of the tube with clay or a rubber stopper. Introduce a metal rod into the open end, and using a magnet, move the rod back and forth through the tube, mixing the heparin.

Ice the sample and analyze it as quickly as possible. An ice slush promotes good heat transfer and will cool the sample more quickly than ice alone.

Care of the Puncture Site

Using a sterile 2 × 2-inch gauze pad, apply pressure to the site if blood is continuing to flow. Once blood flow has stopped, apply an adhesive strip or another dry dressing to protect the site.

References

American Association for Respiratory Care. (1994). AARC clinical practice guideline: Capillary blood gas sampling for neonatal and pediatric patients. *Respiratory Care, 39*(12), 1180–1183.

American Association for Respiratory Care. (2001). AARC clinical practice guideline: Blood gas analysis and hemoximetry: 2001 revision & update. *Respiratory Care, 46*(5), 498–505.

Barbeau, G. R. (2004). Evaluation of the ulnopalmar arterial arches with pulse oximetry and plethysmography: Comparison with the Allen's test in 1010 patients. *American Heart Journal, 147*(3), 489–493.

Practice Activities: Arterial Blood Gas Sampling

1. Using a laboratory partner, perform the following for the listed arterial puncture sites:
   a. Properly position the patient.
   b. Locate the site.
   c. Palpate the site.
      (1) Radial site
      (2) Brachial site

2. Properly prepare a glass syringe or ABG kit for arterial puncture.
   a. Use aseptic technique.
   b. Lubricate the barrel with sodium heparin or prepare a disposable syringe.
   c. Expel excess heparin.
   d. Handle the syringe without introducing room air.

3. Using a laboratory partner, perform the modified Allen's test for collateral circulation.

4. Using a laboratory partner, assess collateral circulation using a pulse oximeter.

5. Using an arterial arm simulator:
   a. Practice correct technique for radial artery puncture.
   b. Practice correct technique for brachial artery puncture.

Incorporate the following:
   (1) Practice using standard precautions.
   (2) Practice aseptic technique.
   (3) Practice puncture skills.
   (4) Practice correct sample-handling skills.

6. Using an arterial arm simulator, draw an arterial sample from an indwelling radial artery catheter.

Check List: Arterial Blood Gas Sampling

_____ 1. Verify the physician's order.

2. Check the patient's chart:
_____ a. Anticoagulant therapy
_____ b. Oxygen therapy

3. Gather the required supplies.
_____ a. Disposable gloves
_____ b. Eye protection
_____ c. 5 mL syringe
_____ d. 20 to 25 gauge needle
_____ e. Sodium heparin
_____ f. Syringe cap and rubber stopper
_____ g. Adhesive strip
_____ h. Elastoplast tape
_____ i. Iodine-based prep pad
_____ j. Alcohol-based prep pad
_____ k. Lidocaine anesthetic, if ordered
_____ l. Ice

_____ 4. Wash your hands.

_____ 5. Don disposable gloves prior to patient contact.

_____ 6. Explain the procedure to the patient.

7. Position the patient:
   a. Radial site
_____   (1) Hyperextend the wrist and support it slightly with a towel or washcloth.
   b. Brachial site
_____   (1) Lay the arm flat, palm side up.
   c. Femoral site
_____   (1) Lay the patient in a supine position with access to the groin.

8. Palpate the puncture site:
_____ a. Visualize the course of the artery.
_____ b. Estimate the depth.

_____ 9. For a radial artery puncture, perform the modified Allen's test for collateral circulation or assess collateral circulation using a pulse oximeter.

10. Prepare the site:
_____ a. Use iodine first.
_____ b. Cleanse with alcohol.

11. If one has been ordered, administer the anesthetic:
_____ a. Do not use more than 0.2 mL.
_____ b. Use a small-gauge needle (25 gauge recommended).
_____ c. Surround the puncture site and artery.

12. Properly perform the puncture:
_____ a. Use the correct angle and bevel position.
_____ b. Penetrate the skin quickly.
_____ c. Advance the needle, watching for the flash in the hub of the needle.

13. Collect the sample:
_____ a. 3 to 5 mL

_____ 14. Withdraw the needle and apply firm pressure to the area.

15. Insert the needle into the stopper or safety cap and ice the sample:
_____ a. Expel any air bubbles.
_____ b. Insert the needle into the stopper or safety cap.
_____ c. Ice the sample.
_____ d. Label the sample.

16. Check for circulation distal to the puncture site.
_____ a. Color
_____ b. Pulse

17. Make the patient comfortable:
_____ a. Apply an adhesive strip.
_____ b. Help the patient to a comfortable position.

18. Transport the sample to the laboratory:
_____ a. Label the sample.
_____ b. Prepare the required laboratory slips and paperwork.

19. Check the puncture site after 20 minutes:
_____ a. Check the circulation.
_____ b. Check for bleeding.

_____ 20. Correctly record the procedure on the chart.

Check List: Arterial Line Sampling

_____ 1. Verify the physician's order for therapy.
_____ 2. Verify the oxygen concentration.
3. Gather the appropriate equipment:
_____ a. Disposable gloves
_____ b. Eye protection
_____ c. 5 mL syringe
_____ d. Blood gas syringe
_____ e. Sodium heparin
_____ f. Syringe cap or stopper
_____ g. Ice slush
_____ 4. Wash your hands.
_____ 5. Don disposable gloves prior to patient contact.
_____ 6. Explain the procedure and position the patient.
_____ 7. Assemble and prepare the equipment.
_____ 8. Turn off the monitoring alarms.
_____ 9. Open the sampling port, removing the cap aseptically.
_____ 10. Attach a disposable syringe.
_____ 11. Turn the stopcock to fill the syringe and draw 3 mL of blood.
_____ 12. Turn off the stopcock and remove the syringe.
_____ 13. Attach the heparinized blood gas syringe.
_____ 14. Open the stopcock and draw a sufficient sample.
_____ 15. Close the stopcock and remove the syringe.
_____ 16. Expel any air from the sample.
_____ 17. Cap and ice the sample.
_____ 18. Flush the sampling port with heparin using the flush control.
_____ 19. Clean up the area and dispose of the 3 mL blood sample collected before the blood gas.
_____ 20. Reset the alarm and observe the monitor for the correct waveform.
_____ 21. Label and transport the sample.
_____ 22. Record the procedure on the chart.

Check List: Capillary Sampling

_____ 1. Verify the physician's order for therapy.
_____ 2. Wash your hands.
3. Obtain the required supplies for the procedure:
_____ a. Disposable gloves
_____ b. Eye protection
_____ c. Heparinized capillary tubes
_____ d. Clay or rubber stopper
_____ e. Povidone-iodine and alcohol prep pads
_____ f. Hot pack or hot towels
_____ g. Metal rod and magnet
_____ h. 2 × 2-inch gauze pads and adhesive strips
_____ i. Cup filled with an ice slush
_____ 4. Wash your hands before the procedure.
_____ 5. Apply disposable gloves prior to patient contact.
_____ 6. Position the patient and interact with the patient and the patient's family appropriately.
_____ 7. Apply the hot pack or hot towels for 5 minutes to arterialize the sample site.
_____ 8. Prepare the puncture site using alcohol and a povidone-iodine prep pad.
_____ 9. Using the lancet, quickly puncture the lateral surface of the heel. Pierce the skin to a depth of 3 mm to ensure adequate blood flow.
_____ 10. Obtain a blood sample using the capillary tubes.
11. Correctly care for the sample:
_____ a. Cap one end of the capillary tube with clay or a rubber stopper.
_____ b. Insert the metal rod, and using the magnet, mix the heparin with the blood sample.
_____ c. Ice the sample.
_____ 12. Using a 2 × 2-inch gauze pad, apply pressure to the puncture site until bleeding has stopped.
_____ 13. Apply another 2 × 2-inch gauze pad as a dressing or use an adhesive strip to protect the puncture site.
_____ 14. Clean up the area following the procedure.
_____ 15. Label and transport the sample to the laboratory for analysis.
_____ 16. Record the procedure in the patient's chart.

Self-Evaluation Post Test: Arterial Blood Gas Sampling

1. The modified Allen's test is a test for:
   a. adequate blood pressure.
   b. collateral circulation.
   c. ulnar pulse.
   d. muscle tone of the hand.

2. The radial artery is a preferred arterial site because:
   a. it is near the surface.
   b. the ulnar artery can provide collateral circulation to the hand.
   c. no major veins are nearby.
   d. it is the largest vessel accessible.

3. Air bubbles that are present in an arterial blood sample after collection:
   a. have no significant effect.
   b. will be compensated for by the blood gas analyzer.
   c. should be expelled immediately.
   d. should be forced into solution immediately.

4. If an arterial blood sample contains large amounts of air bubbles after collection:
   a. it should be iced immediately.
   b. discard it and draw another sample.
   c. the bubbles should be forced into solution.
   d. they will have no effect on the sample.

5. Air bubbles, if present in an arterial blood sample, will:
   I.   increase PaO_2.
   II. decrease PaO_2.
   III. increase $PaCO_2$.
   IV. decrease $PaCO_2$.
   V.   increase pH.

   a. I, IV
   b. I, III
   c. II, III
   d. II, IV

6. If the patient is on oxygen therapy, you should do the following before collecting ABG samples:
   a. Verify the physician's order.
   b. Verify that the patient is receiving the correct oxygen therapy.
   c. Remove the oxygen because it adversely affects results.
   d. Both a and b.

7. If the patient is very hypotensive, the best site(s) for arterial blood sampling is (are):
   a. the radial site.
   b. the brachial site.
   c. the femoral site.
   d. a and b.

8. The site for arterial blood sampling that is associated with the highest likelihood of obtaining a venous sample is:
   a. the radial site.
   b. the brachial site.
   c. the femoral site.
   d. the carotid.

9. If the modified Allen's test is negative, you should:
   a. go ahead and use the radial artery.
   b. call the physician.
   c. perform an Allen's test on the other arm.
   d. use the brachial site.

10. The site for arterial blood sampling with the greatest risk of complications resulting from arterial puncture is:
    a. the radial site.
    b. the femoral site.
    c. the brachial site.
    d. the saphenous vein.

PERFORMANCE EVALUATION:
Arterial Puncture

Date: Lab _____ Clinical _____ Agency _____

Lab: Pass _____ Fail _____ Clinical: Pass _____ Fail _____

Student name _____ Instructor name _____

No. of times observed in clinical _____

No. of times practiced in clinical _____

PASSING CRITERIA: Obtain 90% or better on the procedure. Tasks indicated by * must receive at least 1 point, or the evaluation is terminated. Procedure must be performed within the designated time, or the performance receives a failing grade.

SCORING: 2 points — Task performed satisfactorily without prompting.
1 point — Task performed satisfactorily with self-initiated correction.
0 points — Task performed incorrectly or with prompting required.
NA — Task not applicable to the patient care situation.

Tasks:	Peer	Lab	Clinical
* 1. Verifies the physician's order	☐	☐	☐
2. Scans the chart	☐	☐	☐
* 3. Verifies the oxygen concentration	☐	☐	☐
4. Gathers the required equipment			
* a. Disposable gloves	☐	☐	☐
* b. Eye protection	☐	☐	☐
* c. 5 mL syringe and needles	☐	☐	☐
* d. Rubber stopper or cap	☐	☐	☐
* e. Adhesive strip	☐	☐	☐
* f. Iodine and alcohol prep pads	☐	☐	☐
* g. Lidocaine anesthetic	☐	☐	☐
* h. Ice	☐	☐	☐
* 5. Performs hand hygiene	☐	☐	☐
6. Dons protective equipment before patient contact	☐	☐	☐
7. Explains the procedure and positions the patient	☐	☐	☐
* 8. Assembles and prepares the equipment	☐	☐	☐
* 9. Palpates the puncture site	☐	☐	☐

* **10.** Performs the modified Allen's test or uses an oximeter to assess collateral circulation ☐ ☐ ☐

* **11.** Prepares the site before the puncture ☐ ☐ ☐

   12. Administers an anesthetic, if ordered ☐ ☐ ☐

* **13.** Palpates the puncture site ☐ ☐ ☐

* **14.** Correctly performs the puncture ☐ ☐ ☐

* **15.** Applies firm pressure to the site ☐ ☐ ☐

* **16.** Expels any air from the sample ☐ ☐ ☐

* **17.** Caps and ices the sample ☐ ☐ ☐

* **18.** Checks the circulation distal to the site ☐ ☐ ☐

   19. Ensures patient safety and comfort ☐ ☐ ☐

   20. Cleans up ☐ ☐ ☐

* **21.** Labels and transports the sample ☐ ☐ ☐

* **22.** Checks the site after 20 minutes ☐ ☐ ☐

* **23.** Records the procedure in the chart ☐ ☐ ☐

SCORE: Peer _____ points of possible 62; _____%

                       Lab   _____ points of possible 62; _____%

                       Clinical _____ points of possible 62; _____%

TIME: _____ out of possible 20 minutes

STUDENT SIGNATURES   **INSTRUCTOR SIGNATURES**

PEER: _____   LAB: _____

STUDENT: _____   CLINICAL: _____

PERFORMANCE EVALUATION:
Arterial Line Sampling

Date: Lab _____ Clinical _____ Agency _____

Lab: Pass _____ Fail _____ Clinical: Pass _____ Fail _____

Student name _____ Instructor name _____

No. of times observed in clinical _____

No. of times practiced in clinical _____

PASSING CRITERIA: Obtain 90% or better on the procedure. Tasks indicated by * must receive at least 1 point, or the evaluation is terminated. Procedure must be performed within the designated time, or the performance receives a failing grade.

SCORING: 2 points — Task performed satisfactorily without prompting.
1 point — Task performed satisfactorily with self-initiated correction.
0 points — Task performed incorrectly or with prompting required.
NA — Task not applicable to the patient care situation.

Tasks:	Peer	Lab	Clinical
* 1. Verifies the physician's order	☐	☐	☐
2. Scans the chart	☐	☐	☐
* 3. Verifies the oxygen concentration	☐	☐	☐
4. Gathers the required equipment			
* a. Disposable gloves	☐	☐	☐
* b. Eye protection	☐	☐	☐
* c. 5 mL syringe	☐	☐	☐
* d. Blood gas syringe	☐	☐	☐
* e. Syringe cap or rubber stopper	☐	☐	☐
* f. Ice	☐	☐	☐
* 5. Performs hand hygiene	☐	☐	☐
6. Dons protective equipment before patient contact	☐	☐	☐
7. Explains the procedure and positions the patient	☐	☐	☐
* 8. Assembles and prepares the equipment	☐	☐	☐
9. Turns off the monitor alarms	☐	☐	☐
10. Opens the sampling port			
* a. Removes the cap and sets it on sterile gauze	☐	☐	☐

* **11.** Attaches a disposable syringe   ☐ ☐ ☐

* **12.** Turns the stopcock to fill the syringe and draws 3 mL of blood   ☐ ☐ ☐

* **13.** Turns off the stopcock and removes the syringe   ☐ ☐ ☐

* **14.** Attaches the heparinized blood gas syringe   ☐ ☐ ☐

* **15.** Opens the stopcock and draws a sufficient sample   ☐ ☐ ☐

* **16.** Closes the stopcock and removes the syringe   ☐ ☐ ☐

* **17.** Expels any air from the sample   ☐ ☐ ☐

* **18.** Caps and ices the sample   ☐ ☐ ☐

* **19.** Flushes the sampling port with heparin using the flush control   ☐ ☐ ☐

   20. Ensures the patient's safety and comfort   ☐ ☐ ☐

* **21.** Cleans up the area and disposes of the 3 mL blood sample properly   ☐ ☐ ☐

* **22.** Resets the alarm and observes the monitor for the correct waveform   ☐ ☐ ☐

* **23.** Labels and transports the sample   ☐ ☐ ☐

* **24.** Records the procedure in the chart   ☐ ☐ ☐

SCORE: Peer _____ points of possible 60; _____%

                Lab _____ points of possible 60; _____%

                Clinical _____ points of possible 60; _____%

TIME: _____ out of possible 20 minutes

STUDENT SIGNATURES

PEER: _____

STUDENT: _____

INSTRUCTOR SIGNATURES

LAB: _____

CLINICAL: _____

PERFORMANCE EVALUATION:
Capillary Sampling

Date: Lab _____ Clinical _____ Agency _____

Lab: Pass _____ Fail _____ Clinical: Pass _____ Fail _____

Student name _____ Instructor name _____

No. of times observed in clinical _____

No. of times practiced in clinical _____

PASSING CRITERIA: Obtain 90% or better on the procedure. Tasks indicated by * must receive at least 1 point, or the evaluation is terminated. Procedure must be performed within the designated time, or the performance receives a failing grade.

SCORING: 2 points — Task performed satisfactorily without prompting.
1 point — Task performed satisfactorily with self-initiated correction.
0 points — Task performed incorrectly or with prompting required.
NA — Task not applicable to the patient care situation.

Tasks:	Peer	Lab	Clinical
* **1.** Verifies the physician's order	☐	☐	☐
* **2.** Performs hand hygiene	☐	☐	☐
* **3.** Obtains required supplies			
a. Disposable gloves	☐	☐	☐
b. Eye protection	☐	☐	☐
c. Heparinized capillary collection tubes	☐	☐	☐
d. Clay or rubber stopper	☐	☐	☐
e. Prep pads	☐	☐	☐
f. Hot pack or hot towels	☐	☐	☐
g. Metal rod and magnet	☐	☐	☐
h. 2 × 2-inch gauze pads and adhesive strip	☐	☐	☐
i. Cup filled with ice slush	☐	☐	☐
* **4.** Dons protective equipment before patient contact	☐	☐	☐
5. Positions and interacts with the patient appropriately	☐	☐	☐
* **6.** Applies hot packs for the correct time before sampling	☐	☐	☐
* **7.** Prepares the site before sampling	☐	☐	☐
* **8.** Correctly obtains the blood sample	☐	☐	☐

*   **9.** Correctly cares for the sample

     a. Mixes the heparin   ☐   ☐   ☐

     b. Ices the sample   ☐   ☐   ☐

* **10.** Correctly cares for the puncture site   ☐   ☐   ☐

* **11.** Cleans up after the procedure   ☐   ☐   ☐

* **12.** Labels and transports the sample   ☐   ☐   ☐

* **13.** Records the procedure in the patient's chart   ☐   ☐   ☐

SCORE: Peer   _____ points of possible 48; _____%

                 Lab   _____ points of possible 48; _____%

                 Clinical _____ points of possible 48; _____%

TIME: _____ out of possible 30 minutes

STUDENT SIGNATURES   **INSTRUCTOR SIGNATURES**

PEER: _____   LAB: _____

STUDENT: _____   CLINICAL: _____

CHAPTER 9
Hemodynamic Monitoring

INTRODUCTION

Hemodynamic monitoring provides important clinical information regarding blood pressure, fluid volume, cardiac preload and afterload, cardiac output, and the pulmonary and systemic vascular resistance. Hemodynamic monitoring in its simplest terms is the measurement of pressures within the vascular system, using invasive, indwelling catheters. Besides simply measuring pressures, these catheters provide a convenient route for fluid and drug administration and access for blood sampling (venous and arterial). Not all acutely ill patients will have invasive catheters placed to provide this information; however, the need for such monitoring will be greatest in the most acutely ill patients. It is important for a respiratory practitioner to understand where these catheters are placed anatomically, how the data provided by these catheters relate to cardiac function and fluid balance, how to use these catheters, and the hazards and complications associated with their placement and usage.

KEY TERMS

- Central venous pressure catheter
- Damping
- Distal lumen
- Inflation lumen and balloon
- Pascal's law

- Phlebostatic axis
- Proximal lumen
- Pulmonary artery
- Pulmonary artery catheter
- Pulmonary artery wedge pressure (PAWP)

- Swan-Ganz catheter
- Thermistor
- Thermistor lumen
- Transducer
- Vena cava

THEORY OBJECTIVES

At the end of this chapter, the reader should be able to:

- Describe Pascal's law and how it applies to hemodynamic monitoring.
- Describe what a transducer is and how it is used in hemodynamic monitoring.
- For central venous pressure (CVP) catheters:
  — Describe the preferred routes of vessel access.
  — Describe the correct anatomical placement of the catheter.
  — Identify the parts of a CVP waveform.
  — List the normal values for the CVP.
  — Discuss how a CVP catheter can provide data to help determine:
    — Fluid volume
    — Adequacy of venous return
    — Right ventricular preload
  — Describe what other functions a CVP catheter may serve besides pressure monitoring.
- For pulmonary artery catheters or Swan-Ganz catheters:
  — Identify the parts of a pulmonary artery catheter.
  — Describe the preferred routes of vessel access.

- Describe the correct anatomical placement of the catheter.
- Identify the waveform morphology as the catheter is placed.
- Identify the parts of the pulmonary artery and pulmonary artery wedge pressure tracing.
- List the normal ranges for:
  - Right atrial pressure
  - Right ventricular pressure
  - Pulmonary artery pressure
  - Pulmonary artery wedge pressure
- Discuss how a pulmonary artery catheter can provide data to help determine:
  - Fluid volume
  - Adequacy of venous return
  - Right ventricular preload
  - Right ventricular afterload
  - Left ventricular preload
  - Cardiac output
  - Mixed venous oxygen saturation
  - Pulmonary vascular resistance
  - Systemic vascular resistance

- *Given a set of hemodynamic data, determine which of the following may be occurring:*
  - *Hypovolemia*
  - *Hypervolemia*
  - *Right ventricular failure*
  - *Left ventricular failure*
  - *Effects of positive-pressure ventilation*

- *For an arterial line:*
  - *Describe the preferred routes of vessel access.*
  - *Identify the parts of an arterial pressure waveform.*
  - *List the normal values for the arterial pressure.*
- *Discuss the hazards and complications associated with indwelling vascular catheters, their placement, and usage.*

PASCAL'S LAW

Blaise Pascal was a seventeenth-century investigator. Quite inadvertently, Pascal discovered an important principle in fluid mechanics. He discovered that when the base of a full champagne bottle lying on its side was struck smartly with a mallet, the neck of the bottle would break off and not the base that was struck. Pascal concluded two important concepts from his early experimentation: (1) the pressure of a fluid in a closed container is equal at all points within the container and (2) the pressure acts perpendicularly against the walls of the container (Figure 9-1).

Pascal's law also applies to the vascular system as well as to champagne bottles. For example, for a catheter inserted into the radial artery of a patient, the pressure monitored at the point of insertion is equal to the pressure within the arterial system. We apply Pascal's law to determine arterial, right atrial, and left ventricular end-diastolic pressures using indwelling catheters. Pascal's law holds true as long as the vascular system at the point of interest does not have valves or any other anatomical structures that would alter the reflected pressure being measured.

TRANSDUCERS

A *transducer* is a device that converts one form of energy into another. Hemodynamic monitoring depends heavily on transducers to convert pressures into analog electrical signals, which can then be used to display pressures or graphical waveforms. A typical transducer used in hemodynamic monitoring consists of a diaphragm with a strain gauge embedded into it or attached to it (Figure 9-2). As the pressure applied to the diaphragm increases, the diaphragm distorts, causing the strain gauge to lengthen. The longer the strain gauge becomes, the more resistance it creates to electrical current passed through it. Therefore, a change in electrical current is proportional to a change in pressure (Figure 9-3). These small changes in current are used by the microprocessors in the monitoring systems to provide both the graphical and the digital information used in patient management.

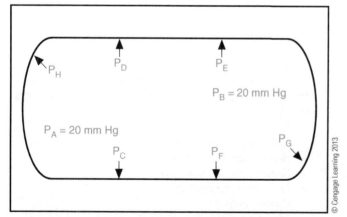

Figure 9-1 A figure illustrating Pascal's law. Note that the pressure at point A is equal to the pressure at point B and that the forces act perpendicular to the walls of the container

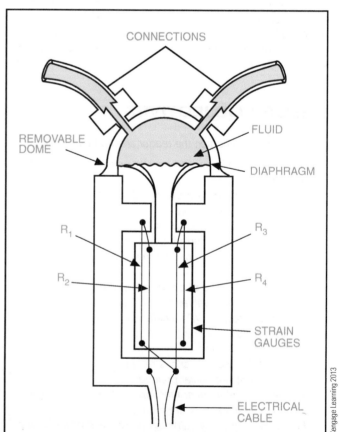

Figure 9-2 A figure illustrating a strain gauge pressure transducer

© Cengage Learning 2013

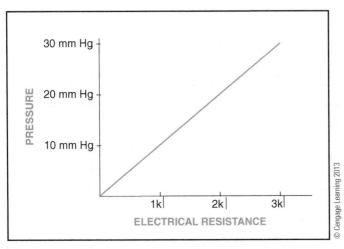

Figure 9-3 A graph illustrating that a change in pressure is proportional to a change in electrical resistance

CENTRAL VENOUS PRESSURE CATHETERS

A *central venous pressure catheter* (CVP catheter) is placed in the venous system so that the distal tip of the catheter rests in the *vena cava* or right atrium (Figure 9-4). The outflow from the vena cava empties into the right atrium. Because there are no heart valves between the vena cava and the right atrium, the pressure in the vena cava is the same as the pressure in the right atrium.

Preferred Routes of Access

Several sites are used for the insertion of CVP catheters. These include the antecubital fossa and the basilic, internal jugular, and subclavian veins. The most commonly used sites are the internal jugular and subclavian sites. A large-bore needle is used percutaneously to puncture the vessel wall and is inserted into the vein. The catheter is advanced while the needle is held steady and then is

threaded through the venous system until the distal tip rests in the vena cava or right atrium.

Central Venous Pressure Waveform and Pressures

Figure 9-5 illustrates a typical CVP tracing, including the *a* wave, *x* wave descent, *c* and *v* waves, and the *y* wave descent. The *a* wave reflects the atrial contraction and follows the P wave on the electrocardiogram (ECG). The height of the *a* wave is dependent on how much pressure is generated by the atrium as it ejects blood into the ventricle at the end of diastole.

The *x* wave descent represents the fall in atrial pressure and CVP as the atrium relaxes. As the muscle fibers relax, fluid pressure diminishes as the muscle fibers elongate to their normal resting potential length. Another factor contributing to the fall in pressure is the downward pull on the atrioventricular (AV) junction during ventricular contraction.

The *c* wave reflects the closure of the tricuspid valve at the beginning of ventricular systole. As the tricuspid valve closes, pressure plateaus as it equalizes against the closed valve.

The *v* wave reflects the filling of the atrium during ventricular systole. As the atrium fills, pressure increases as the muscle fibers become stretched, peaking at a point when the atrium has filled completely with blood prior to contraction.

The *y* wave descent reflects the fall in pressure as the tricuspid valve opens, allowing the right ventricles to fill. As blood is emptied from the atria, CVP falls proportionately as the ventricles fill.

Normal CVP values range from 0 to 7 mm Hg (0 to 10 cm of H_2O). CVP varies with inspiration and expiration. As intrathoracic pressure decreases during a normal inspiratory effort, CVP falls (Figure 9-6). Therefore, CVP is always measured during resting exhalation. Positive intrathoracic pressure—as with mechanical ventilation, positive end expiratory pressure (PEEP), continuous positive

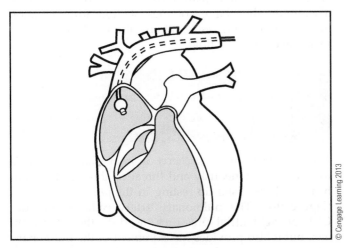

Figure 9-4 The anatomic location of a central venous catheter. Note that the tip rests in the right atrium

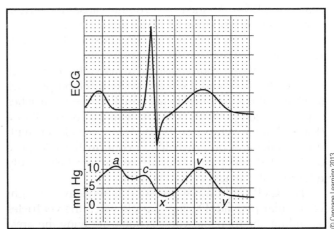

Figure 9-5 The CVP pressure tracing and its component parts—the a, c, x, v, and y waves and the relationship of the waveform to the electrocardiogram

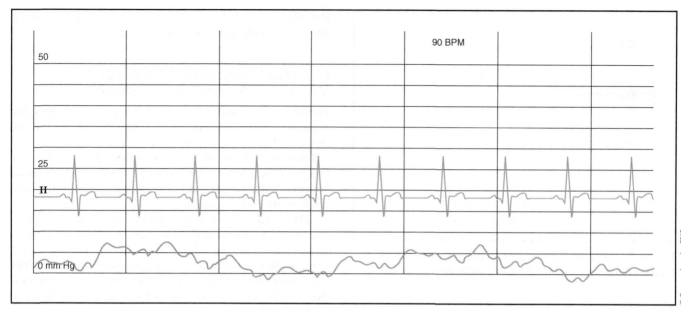

90 BPM

50

25

H

0 mm Hg

© Cengage Learning 2013

Figure 9-6 Note how the CVP pressure varies with the ventilatory cycle, falling during expiration

airway pressure (CPAP), or bilevel positive airway pressure (bi-PAP)—will elevate CVP pressures.

Clinical Applications of the Central Venous Pressure Catheter

The CVP catheter provides useful clinical information that may be applied to determine hypervolemia, hypovolemia, and right ventricular preload, and it is a convenient site for mixed venous blood sampling and for fluid administration. The CVP pressure is a direct reflection of vascular volume and venous return. As vascular volume increases, CVP values will also increase. It is important to correlate increased CVP with fluid intake and output data, daily weights, and blood pressures. An increase in the difference between the CVP and the mean systemic blood pressure (constant blood pressure) reflects an increase in systemic fluid volume (Kiess Daily & Schroeder, 1994). An increased volume causes the atrium to be distended (stretched), increasing the reflected pressure into the vena cava owing to the increased pressures within the chamber.

A decrease in fluid volume causes the difference between the CVP and the mean systemic blood pressure (constant blood pressure) to fall until the pressure reaches zero, at which point the central veins begin to collapse (Kiess Daily & Schroeder, 1994). Again, correlation with fluid intake and output helps to confirm the relevance of the CVP and mean arterial pressure as being truly reflective of changes in fluid volume.

The CVP (right atrial pressure) is reflective of right ventricular preload. During diastole when the ventricles are filling, the tricuspid valve is open, allowing the pressure in the right ventricle to be reflected back to the vena cava (Pascal's law). As CVP values increase, the preload of the right ventricle also increases. Clinically, it

is important to optimize preload to obtain the greatest efficiency from the myocardial contraction. If preload is increased too much, the myocardium loses efficiency (Starling's law); therefore, optimization of preload is clinically important.

The CVP catheter also provides an important route for mixed venous blood sampling. The blood in the right atrium is a mixture of all of the venous blood returning to the heart from all parts of the body. Therefore, a blood sample from the right atrium represents a mixed sample and does not reflect any regional differences in oxygen consumption, as would a sample obtained from a more peripheral vein. Mixed venous samples are important clinically in that they are used to determine oxygen consumption and to determine the clinical shunt fraction.

Fluid administration is also enhanced by the placement of a CVP catheter. The CVP catheter is a large-bore catheter compared with most intravenous catheters. Therefore, when large volumes of fluid administration are required (fluid resuscitation), the CVP catheter can facilitate delivery of fluid.

PULMONARY ARTERY CATHETERS OR SWAN-GANZ CATHETERS

The *pulmonary artery catheter* or *Swan-Ganz catheter* is inserted percutaneously and threaded through the right heart with its distal tip resting in the *pulmonary artery* (Figure 9-7). The pulmonary artery catheter provides CVP or right atrial pressures, as does the CVP catheter, but it also provides measurement of the pulmonary artery pressure and *pulmonary artery wedge pressure (PAWP)*. Today, most Swan-Ganz catheters also have the capability to provide cardiac output data when coupled to an appropriate monitor. In addition to pressure monitoring and cardiac output monitoring, the Swan-Ganz catheter also provides a route for mixed venous sampling and fluid administration, just like the CVP catheter. Clinically, the Swan-Ganz catheter truly represents a leap forward in terms of its capabilities; however, hazards and complications increase proportionately with the length of time the catheter remains indwelling in the right side of the heart.

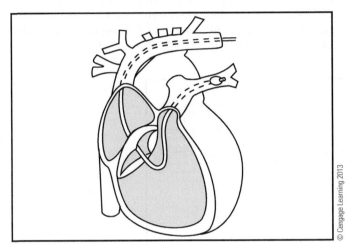

Figure 9-7 Position of a pulmonary artery catheter

Parts of a Pulmonary Artery Catheter

The pulmonary artery catheter is a multilumen catheter with each lumen or port having a specific function. These ports include the proximal lumen, the distal lumen, the thermistor lumen, and the inflation lumen (Figure 9-8). The *proximal lumen*, when the catheter is correctly placed, rests either in the vena cava or in the right atrium. In this position, the pressure information provided by this port or lumen has the same clinical application of the CVP catheter discussed earlier in this chapter.

The *distal lumen* rests in the pulmonary artery when the catheter is correctly placed. The open distal end reflects the pressure in the pulmonary artery (when the balloon is deflated) and is a direct reflection of the right ventricular afterload, or the resistance that the right ventricle must overcome to eject blood.

The *thermistor lumen* is a lumen that contains the electrical conductors emanating from the *thermistor* located near the distal tip of the catheter. The thermistor is a temperature-sensitive resistor (electrical resistance changes proportionally to changes in temperature) that is used to measure cardiac output using the thermal dilution technique, which is discussed later in this chapter.

The *inflation lumen and balloon* are analogous to the pilot line and cuff of an endotracheal or tracheostomy tube. When air (approximately 1 to 2 mL) is injected into the inflation lumen, the balloon inflates. Balloon inflation is used to float the catheter through the right heart.

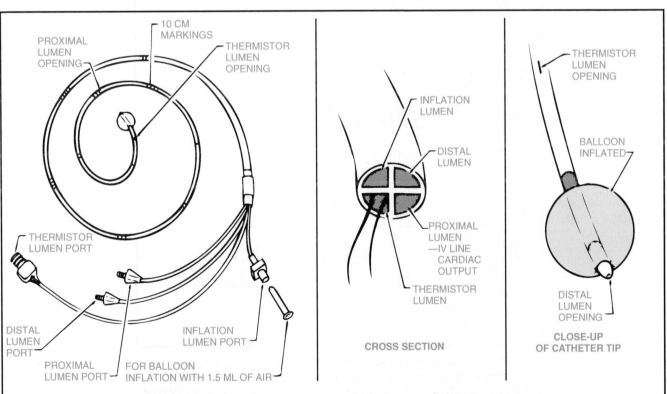

Figure 9-8 A diagram identifying the components of a Swan–Ganz catheter

The pulmonary artery catheter is sometimes called a flow-directed catheter because of the use of the inflated balloon. Blood flow carries the catheter forward into the pulmonary artery until the diameter of the artery diminishes to the point that it becomes stuck, or "wedged." Once the catheter is wedged, the pressure measured at the distal tip (PAWP) reflects the pressure distal to it all the way to the left ventricle (when the mitral valve is opened), in accordance with Pascal's law.

Preferred Routes of Access

Several sites are used for the insertion of pulmonary artery catheters. These include the antecubital fossa and the basilic, internal jugular, and subclavian veins.

The most commonly used sites are the internal jugular and subclavian sites. A large-bore needle is used percutaneously to puncture the vessel wall and is inserted into the vein. The catheter is advanced while the needle is held steady. Once the balloon is inflated, the catheter can be advanced through the venous system until the distal tip rests in the pulmonary artery.

Pulmonary Artery Catheter Waveform Morphology

The morphology of the pressure tracing or waveform obtained from a pulmonary artery catheter varies with its position or location. Waveform characteristics are particularly important to observe and recognize as the catheter is advanced (Figure 9-9). The waveform undergoes

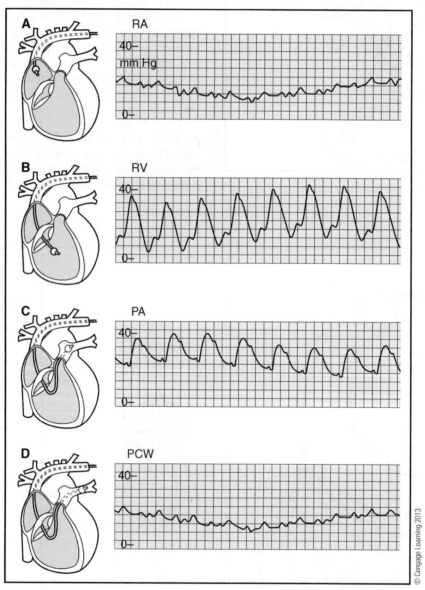

© Cengage Learning 2013

Figure 9-9 Waveform characteristics during advancement of the pulmonary artery catheter: (A) right atrium (RA) and right atrial (central venous) waveform; (B) right ventricle (RV) and right ventricular waveform; (C) pulmonary artery (PA) and pulmonary arterial waveform; and (D) pulmonary capillary wedge (PCW) and pulmonary capillary wedge pressure waveform

distinct morphologic changes as the catheter passes from the right atrium to the right ventricle to the pulmonary artery and finally to its wedged position. The ability to recognize these waveform characteristics is important in the identification of the correct placement of the catheter and in determining whether the catheter has become dislodged from its original placement position. Once the pulmonary artery catheter has been floated into position, the balloon is deflated. The balloon is subsequently inflated only when it is necessary to measure the PAWP.

Pulmonary Artery Pressure and Pulmonary Artery Wedge Pressure Waveform Morphology

It is important to recognize the morphology of the pulmonary artery pressure and PAWP tracings. The morphology of the pressure tracings is a direct result of the underlying physiologic, pathophysiologic, and cardiac cyclic events. Pressure changes are a direct reflection of changes in fluid volume (myocardial preload and afterload), changes in ventricular compliance, or vascular resistance to blood flow.

Pulmonary Artery Pressure Morphology

The pulmonary artery pressure tracing reflects pressure gradients caused by the systolic and diastolic events of the right ventricle. During systole, the ventricle contracts and the pulmonic valve opens, causing a rapid ejection of blood into the pulmonary artery. There is a subsequent rise in pressure as the blood fills the pulmonary artery (Figure 9-10). As the volume of blood decreases, the pressure values also decrease. Once the pressure in the pulmonary artery equals the pressure in the right ventricle, the pulmonic valve closes, causing a small dip in the pressure tracing (dicrotic notch) (see Figure 9-10).

During diastole, the right ventricle is filling. Because no additional blood is ejected into the pulmonary artery (pulmonic valve has closed), the pressure slowly decreases until just before the next systolic event (end-diastole).

The pulmonary artery pressure should be measured at end-diastole.

The respiratory cycle will affect the pulmonary artery pressure tracing. During inspiration (reduced intrathoracic pressure), the pulmonary artery pressure baseline falls. During exhalation (increased intrathoracic pressure), the baseline pressure increases. The pulmonary artery pressure should always be read at end expiration.

Positive-pressure ventilation will also cause changes in the pulmonary artery pressure tracing. Positive intrathoracic pressures reduce venous return to the heart, causing a backup of blood flow in the systemic circulation. The same positive pressure in the lungs causes compression of the pulmonary vasculature, increasing resistance. The net result of these increased pressures is an increase in both CVP and PAWP.

Pulmonary Artery Wedge Pressure Morphology

Once the balloon of the pulmonary artery catheter is inflated, blood flow carries the catheter forward until it wedges or becomes stuck, occluding blood flow as the vessel narrows. Once the catheter is wedged, the distal tip of the catheter reflects pressures distal to the point at which it has become wedged (Figure 9-11). This pressure reflects events occurring in the left atrium and left ventricle (when the mitral valve is opened during diastole). This is so because the pulmonary vasculature lacks the valves present in the systemic vasculature, and Pascal's law applies. The morphology of the PAWP is similar to that of the right atrial or CVP tracing.

The PAWP tracing consists of the *a* wave, the *x* descent, the *v* wave, and the *y* descent (Figure 9-12). These pressure changes are caused by the cardiac cycle of the left atrium and ventricle. The *a* wave is produced as a result of left atrial contraction, the pressure wave building with myocardial fiber contraction. The *x* descent reflects the fall in pressure that occurs following left atrial systole. The *v* wave pressure increase is a result of filling

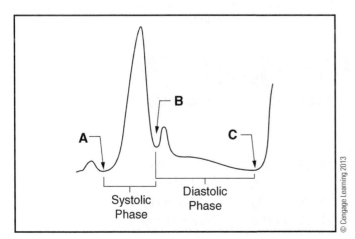

Figure 9-10 Pulmonary arterial pressure (PAP) waveform: (A) beginning systole; (B) dicrotic notch (closure of semilunar valves); and (C) end-diastole

© Cengage Learning 2013

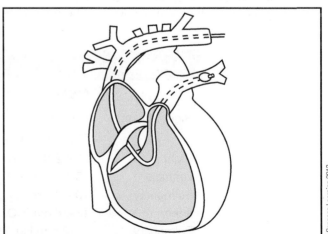

Figure 9-11 The pulmonary artery catheter in the wedge position

© Cengage Learning 2013

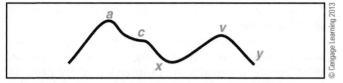

Figure 9-12 Pulmonary capillary wedge pressure (PCWP) waveform: a wave: left atrial contraction; c wave (may be absent): closure of mitral valve; x downslope: decrease of left atrial pressure following atrial contraction; v wave: left ventricular contraction and passive atrial filling; y downslope: decrease of blood volume (pressure) following the opening of mitral valve

of the left atrium during diastole. The *y* descent occurs after the mitral valve opens, when blood passively fills the left ventricle.

Like the pulmonary artery pressure tracing, the PAWP tracing is also affected by spontaneous respiration and positive-pressure ventilation. During inspiration (reduced intrathoracic pressure), the pulmonary artery pressure baseline falls. During exhalation (increased intrathoracic pressure), the baseline pressure increases. The PAWP should always be read at end expiration.

Positive-pressure ventilation will also cause changes in the pulmonary artery pressure tracing. Positive intrathoracic pressures reduce venous return and therefore reduce the preload to the right ventricle, decreasing its output. Therefore, pulmonary artery pressures are typically lower during positive-pressure ventilation because less blood is ejected into the vessels (decreased cardiac output).

NORMAL PRESSURE RANGES

It is important to recognize what the normal pressure ranges are for the right atrial pressure, right ventricular pressure, pulmonary artery pressure, and PAWP. Pressure values reflect right ventricular preload, afterload, and left ventricular preload. Once the normal ranges are committed to memory, abnormal values will become more

readily apparent, enhancing the practitioner's grasp of the clinical applications of the pulmonary artery catheter in patient management. Table 9-1 summarizes the normal ranges for these important pressure values.

CLINICAL APPLICATIONS OF THE PULMONARY ARTERY CATHETER

The pulmonary artery catheter provides very important clinical information regarding fluid volume, right and left heart preloads and function, cardiac output, mixed venous saturation and sampling, and the vascular resistance of the pulmonary and systemic systems. The respiratory practitioner must know the normal values and how abnormal values relate to fluid balance and cardiac function.

Fluid Volume and Venous Return

When the pulmonary artery catheter is positioned correctly, its proximal port rests in the right atrium or vena cava. In the previous discussion of CVP, recall that an increase in CVP or right atrial pressures with a constant systolic blood pressure reflects an increase in fluid volume, and that the converse is also true. As stated previously, it is important to correlate the right atrial pressure or CVP with fluid intake and output, systemic blood pressure, and daily weights because the pressures measured reflect only a small part of the data necessary for correct decision making.

Assessment of Right Ventricular Function

The pulmonary artery catheter provides a means to assess right ventricular function, including preload and after load. As discussed previously, the right atrial pressure (CVP) reflects the preload or stretch of the right ventricle. Increasing right atrial pressures indicate ejection of greater volumes of blood into the right ventricle, and the converse is also true.

TABLE 9-1: Normal Pressure Ranges			
	MEAN	**SYSTOLIC**	**DIASTOLIC**
Right atrium	0–8 mm Hg		
	0–11 cm H₂O		
Right ventricle	10–22 mm Hg	15–28 mm Hg	0–8 mm Hg
	13–30 cm H₂O	20–36 cm H₂O	0–11 cm H₂O
Pulmonary artery	10–22 mm Hg	15–28 mm Hg	5–16 mm Hg
	13–18 cm H₂O	20–36 cm H₂O	7–22 cm H₂O
Pulmonary artery wedge	6–12 mm Hg		
	8–16 cm H₂O		

© Cengage Learning 2013

The pulmonary artery pressure reflects the pressure that the right ventricle must work against to eject blood. Increased pulmonary artery pressure increases the afterload of the right ventricle, increasing the work required to pump blood. Common causes of increased pulmonary artery pressures include increased pulmonary vascular resistance, mitral stenosis, left ventricular failure (decreased compliance), increased fluid volume, and positive-pressure ventilation.

A decrease in pulmonary artery pressure results in a decreased afterload of the right ventricle. A decrease in afterload results in less work that the right ventricle must overcome. Decreased pulmonary artery pressure may be caused by hypovolemia or reduced venous return.

Assessment of Left Ventricular Preload

Measurement of the PAWP (with balloon inflated and wedged) reflects the preload of the left ventricle. The PAWP at end-diastole (while the mitral valve is still open) reflects the filling pressure or preload of the left ventricle. This is so because there is an absence of valves in the pulmonary vascular system, and Pascal's law applies.

It is important to note that the PAWP is independent of pulmonary vascular resistance. This is true because once the catheter is wedged, blood flow distal to the inflated balloon has ceased. *Resistance* by definition is a change in pressure divided by a flow; because blood flow has stopped, resistance must be zero. Therefore, the pressure measured from the distal port of the catheter is the reflected pressure of the left atrium and left ventricle (when the mitral valve is open) during diastole.

A decreased PAWP may be caused by hypovolemia or increased intrathoracic pressures (as with PEEP or CPAP), resulting in reduced venous return. Hypovolemia results in circulation of a lower volume of blood, causing a reduction in left ventricular filling pressure (Starling's law). Positive intrathoracic pressures result in decreased venous return and in reduced right ventricular output and pulmonary artery pressures and, consequently, a lower filling pressure in the left ventricle.

An increased PAWP may be caused by hypervolemia, left ventricular failure, or mitral stenosis. Hypervolemia causes increased left ventricular diastolic pressures because increased blood volume results in the distention of the ventricle (Starling's law). Left ventricular failure may manifest itself as an increased PAWP because a decreased left ventricular compliance causes a concomitant increase in ventricular filling pressure. Mitral stenosis causes an increased resistance as the left ventricle fills, resulting in a higher reflected pressure to the pulmonary artery catheter.

Assessment of Cardiac Output

The pulmonary artery catheter uses a technique called *thermal dilution*, which allows the clinician to assess a patient's cardiac output. Cardiac output is what generates blood pressure and is the "engine" that drives the circulatory system. *Cardiac output* is a product of stroke volume multiplied by heart rate. The thermal dilution technique uses the cardiac output computer monitor and a cold solution to measure cardiac output.

A cold solution, usually 5% dextrose in water (D_5W) or normal (physiologic) saline, is injected through the proximal lumen of the pulmonary artery catheter into the right atrium. The temperature of the solution must be at least 4°C less than the patient's body temperature. If the cardiac output is less than 3 liters per minute or greater than 10 liters per minute, iced (0°C) injectate must be used. Blood flow carries the cold solution downstream to the thermistor lumen, where a temperature drop is detected. The cardiac output computer monitor measures the temperature change using the thermistor located near the distal tip of the catheter. The cardiac output computer monitor factors in the distance (proximal port to thermistor, usually 30 cm), amount of injectate (typically 10 mL), and the temperature change to determine the cardiac output. Thermal dilution cardiac output determination is very technique dependent.

Several factors may alter the results of thermal dilution cardiac output measurements. These include patient position, the time required for injection of cold solution, respiratory phase when injection occurs (inspiration versus expiration), and whether the clinician injects solution unevenly (variance of pressures). Cardiac output should always be determined with the patient in the same position. It is not necessary to position the patient supine. However, the patient should always be in the same position (supine or semi-Fowler's, for example) every time cardiac output is determined. When injecting the cold solution, injection of 10 mL should take no longer than 4 seconds. It will take a strong, quick, and steady push on the syringe to move 10 mL of fluid through the narrow proximal lumen in the required time. Focus on the task at hand and concentrate on maintaining a firm, quick, and even force on the plunger of the syringe. The cold solution should always be injected during the expiratory phase of ventilation. Timing can be tricky, especially at higher ventilatory rates. Because variability exists in the technique, it is important to take several measurements.

When measuring cardiac output using thermal dilution technique, make at least three cardiac output determinations (more will be required if there is a high degree of variability). The respiratory practitioner should strive for all determinations to be within 10% of one another. When three values are plus or minus 10%, calculate the average for those three values.

Determination of Mixed Venous Oxygen Saturation

A pulmonary artery catheter provides a convenient route for mixed venous blood sampling through the proximal port, located in the right atrium. In addition, a specialized catheter is manufactured that incorporates fiberoptic technology into its design, allowing it to continuously monitor mixed venous oxygen saturation. Mixed venous oxygen saturation is normally 68% to 75%. The continuous monitoring of mixed venous saturation allows determination of the patient's oxygen consumption (CaO_2 – CvO_2), and the oxygen supply (10 (CaO_2 × C.O.)) and metabolic demand made by the body.

Determination of Pulmonary Vascular Resistance

As stated earlier, the PAWP (with the balloon inflated) is independent of the pulmonary vascular resistance because blood flow has been halted. Therefore, the difference between the pulmonary artery pressure and the PAWP is reflective of the pulmonary vascular resistance. The pulmonary vascular resistance may be calculated using the following formula:

$$PVR = \frac{PAWP - PA}{\text{cardiac output}} \times 80$$

Pulmonary vascular resistance may be increased by alveolar hypoxemia, acidemia, hypercapnia, positive intrathoracic pressures (as with PEEP or CPAP), vascular blockage, vascular compression, or vascular wall disease. Pulmonary vascular resistance may be decreased owing to pharmacologic agents (oxygen, isoproterenol, aminophylline, or calcium channel blockers) and humoral substances.

Determination of Systemic Vascular Resistance

The pulmonary artery catheter provides a convenient way to determine the systemic vascular resistance, which is the resistance the left ventricle must overcome to pump blood. Systemic vascular resistance may be calculated using the following formula:

$$SVR = \frac{\text{mean arterial pressure} - \text{central venous pressure}}{\text{cardiac output}} \times 80$$

Systemic vascular resistance may be increased owing to hypertension or vasopressor drugs (such as dopamine or norepinephrine). Decreased systemic vascular resistance may be the result of vasodilators (such as nitroglycerin, nitroprusside, or morphine) or hypovolemic or septic shock.

CASE STUDIES ILLUSTRATING THE APPLICATION OF A PULMONARY ARTERY CATHETER

In the previous section, recall how central venous, pulmonary artery, and wedge pressures change in various disease states. It also covers how the pulmonary artery catheter enables the practitioner to measure cardiac output and pulmonary and systemic vascular resistances. In this section, these specific applications of the pulmonary artery catheter are applied to specific case studies or scenarios.

Determination of Hypovolemia

A 23-year-old female patient is admitted to the intensive care unit (ICU) following surgery. She was involved in a motor vehicle accident and suffered a fractured right femur, pelvis, and humerus. Her femoral fracture was a compound fracture requiring open reduction, and she suffered considerable blood loss in the field.

Her admitting blood pressure is 85/60 mm Hg and her heart rate is 125 beats per minute. Because of concerns about her hemodynamic status, a pulmonary artery catheter is inserted. On catheter insertion the following data are obtained:

RA	= 1 mm Hg
PA	= 18/3 mm Hg
PAWP	= 6 mm Hg
C(a–v)O_2	= 8 vol %

where RA is right atrial pressure, PA is pulmonary artery pressure, PAWP is pulmonary artery wedge pressure, and C(a–v)O_2 is the arteriovenous oxygen content difference.

Interpretation of the Data

The data in combination with the patient's history suggest hypovolemia. The right atrial pressure reflects a low blood volume return to the right heart (right ventricular preload). The low pulmonary artery pressure and increased C(a–v)O_2 value suggest a low cardiac output, while the decreased PAWP suggests a low left ventricular preload. The patient was treated by the administration of several units of blood.

Determination of Hypervolemia

The respiratory practitioner is assessing the hemodynamic status of a 43-year-old postoperative patient. Over the course of the past 12 hours, the resident in charge has been treating a low blood pressure with fluid administration. The following hemodynamic data are obtained following the first patient/ventilator system assessment:

BP	= 95/70 mm Hg
RA	= 10 mm Hg
PA	= 48/25 mm Hg
PAWP	= 23 mm Hg
CO	= 7.4 L/min
C(a–v)O_2	= 3 vol %

Interpretation of the Data

The data suggest that the patient is experiencing fluid overload. The right atrial pressure reflects a high preload to the right ventricle from excessive fluid return to the right heart. Elevated pulmonary artery pressure and PAWP also reflect excessive fluid volumes. The elevated cardiac output is a result of the high fluid return and operation of the cardiac muscle at the upper limits of Starling's curve. The patient was treated with vasopressors and aggressive diuresis.

Assessment of Right Ventricular Failure

The respiratory practitioner is caring for an acutely ill 74-year-old patient with chronic obstructive pulmonary disease (COPD) admitted to the ICU. He is currently on 50% oxygen delivered by a Venturi mask. Because of concerns about his hemodynamic status and the possibility of impending respiratory failure, a pulmonary artery catheter is placed. The following set of data is obtained:

RA   = 8 mm Hg
PA   = 42/23 mm Hg
PAWP = 10 mm Hg
CO   = 3.4 L/min

Interpretation of the Data

The elevated right atrial pressure suggests an increased preload on the right ventricle. This could be caused by increased fluid return or by a decreased right ventricular compliance (infarction or failure). The elevated pulmonary artery pressure reflects an increased afterload to the right ventricle. The normal PAWP, however, suggests normal preload to the left ventricle and normal left heart function. The cardiac output is diminished. Upon calculation of the pulmonary vascular resistance, it is substantially elevated. This set of data suggests right heart failure secondary to pulmonary hypertension (history of COPD).

Determination of Left Ventricular Failure

The respiratory practitioner is assessing the hemodynamic status of a patient in the cardiac care unit (CCU). She is 58 years of age and was admitted with an acute myocardial infarction 2 days ago through the emergency department. Her cardiac catheterization last night suggests obstruction in three of her coronary arteries. The practitioner obtains the following set of hemodynamic data before she is transferred for surgery:

RA   = 4 mm Hg
PA   = 32/26 mm Hg
PAWP   = 23 mm Hg
CO   = 3.1 L/min
$C(a–v)O_2$ = 3 vol %

Interpretation of the Data

The normal right atrial pressure reflects a normal return to the right heart and normal preload. The elevated pulmonary artery pressure may be caused by increased pulmonary vascular resistance, mitral stenosis, or decreased left ventricular compliance. The elevated PAWP confirms that left ventricular compliance is decreased. Upon calculation of the pulmonary vascular resistance, it is within normal limits. The decreased cardiac output is also suggestive of ventricular failure.

ASSESSMENT OF THE EFFECTS CAUSED BY POSITIVE-PRESSURE VENTILATION

The respiratory practitioner is assessing the hemodynamic data from a 58-year-old male patient who underwent coronary artery bypass grafting 7 hours earlier. He is on synchronized intermittent mandatory ventilation (SIMV) with a rate of 7 breaths per minute and a PEEP

setting of 10 cm H_2O. The following hemodynamic data are obtained:

RA   = 2 mm Hg
PA   = 23/15 mm Hg
PAWP = 12 mm Hg
BP   = 100/70 mm Hg
CO   = 4.3 L/min

Interpretation of the Data

The right atrial pressure is on the low side of normal, reflecting a decrease in blood volume returning to the heart. Although this could be caused by hypovolemia, in this case it is due to increased intrathoracic pressure. The pulmonary artery pressure and PAWP are normal, reflecting a normal pulmonary vascular resistance and left heart function. The reduction in cardiac output would also match the suggestion of diminished venous return to the heart from elevated intrapleural pressures.

ARTERIAL LINES

An arterial line provides several types of data helpful in the management of critically ill patients. It is a convenient site for arterial blood sampling and real-time measurement of the systemic blood pressure. Besides real-time digital data, an analog graphic display can be used to reflect the systolic and diastolic characteristics of the blood pressure tracing.

Preferred Routes of Vessel Access

The two preferred routes for the insertion of arterial lines are the radial and femoral arteries. Generally, the radial site is preferred owing to presence of collateral circulation (ulnar artery) and ease of vessel access. The femoral site carries with it increased risk of complications, which include loss of the limb with venal injury (because there is no collateral circulation) and the likelihood of arterial plaque that may become dislodged with catheter placement.

When the catheter has been correctly placed, an introducer needle is used to puncture the desired artery. The catheter is advanced while holding the introducer needle steady. After successful placement of the catheter, the introducer needle is removed. The arterial catheter is then secured, resting inside the vessel.

Parts of an Arterial Pressure Waveform

Figure 9-13 illustrates a typical arterial pressure waveform. The rapid upstroke between C and A reflects the rapid change in pressure that occurs as the ventricles contract. As they contract, blood is rapidly ejected into the arterial system, causing a rapid rise in pressure. The downward slope from B to C reflects the fall in pressure that occurs during diastole. During diastole, the

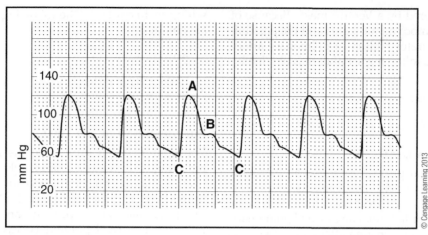

Figure 9-13 Normal arterial pressure waveform. The systolic and diastolic pressures are about 120 mm Hg and 60 mm Hg, respectively: (A) systolic peak; (B) dicrotic notch; (C) end diastole

ventricles are passively filling as the ventricles relax. The dicrotic notch *B* reflects the closure of the semilunar valves. The lowest point on the pressure tracing reflects the end-diastolic pressure, whereas the highest point of the tracing is the systolic pressure. Normal values for arterial pressures are 100 to 140 mm Hg systolic and 60 to 90 mm Hg diastolic.

HAZARDS WITH INDWELLING VASCULAR CATHETERS

Hazards with indwelling vascular catheters include ischemia, infection, and hemorrhage. The pulmonary artery catheter also carries with it the additional risk of cardiac arrhythmias and, in rare instances, pulmonary artery rupture with inflation of the balloon.

Ischemic complications of indwelling vascular catheters are usually secondary to thrombus or embolus formation. The thrombus or embolus then is carried distal to the catheter, where it becomes lodged, result-ing in ischemic injury. The arterial catheter is always maintained with a constant drip of heparin to prevent thrombus formation.

Hemorrhage can occur if the vascular catheter becomes accidentally dislodged or if the sampling port is inadvertently left open. Proper securing of the catheter and care with its use in sampling blood are important in the prevention of this complication.

Infection is always a hazard when any invasive procedure is performed. Therefore, strict use of aseptic techniques is essential; in addition, adherence to standard precautions is required in work with vascular catheters.

The pulmonary artery catheter has its unique hazards and complications. Presence of this catheter may lead to cardiac arrhythmias. Because the catheter passes through the heart, myocardial irritation may result, causing arrhythmias. In rare instances, when the balloon is inflated to measure the PAWP, pulmonary artery rupture may occur (Kiess Daily & Schroeder, 1994). This complication is usually associated with patients of advanced age with hypertension.

PROFICIENCY OBJECTIVES

At the end of this chapter, the reader should be able to:

- *Assemble the equipment required for hemodynamic pressure monitoring.*
- *Demonstrate how to set up the equipment needed for hemodynamic pressure monitoring.*
- *Demonstrate how to zero the pressure-monitoring system.*
- *Demonstrate how to correctly locate the phlebostatic axis and level the transducer to that point.*

- *Recognize and describe four causes of a damped waveform.*
- *Demonstrate how to correctly wedge a pulmonary artery catheter.*
- *Recognize overwedging and describe what may cause it.*
- *Demonstrate how to measure cardiac output using the thermodilution technique.*
- *Demonstrate how to maintain an arterial line.*
- *Demonstrate how to zero an arterial line transducer.*

EQUIPMENT REQUIRED FOR HEMODYNAMIC MONITORING

The equipment required for hemodynamic monitoring is similar for that for CVP, pulmonary artery, and arterial catheters. Table 9-2 lists the equipment required for hemodynamic pressure monitoring.

Infection is one of the hazards of placement and use of indwelling vascular catheters. Therefore, in assembling and preparing the equipment, it is important to maintain aseptic technique.

EQUIPMENT SETUP AND PREPARATION

It is important to prepare the equipment carefully, using aseptic technique as described earlier. Also, embolism is one of the hazards of invasive vascular catheters. Therefore, always remove any air bubbles from the tubing, transducer, and connections. Air bubbles will also cause damping of the waveform (discussed later) because they become compressed and the fluid does not.

Medication Preparation

When preparing equipment to monitor hemodynamic pressures, mix the heparin to the correct concentration. Add 500 units of heparin to the 500 mL normal saline bag. Note the medication and dosage on the medication label and affix it to the solution bag. For heparinizing an arterial solution bag, up to 1000 units may be added to the 500 mL solution bag.

Spiking the Bag and Priming the Tubing

Using the pressurized intravenous (IV) tubing, aseptically spike (pierce) the solution bag. Ensure that the air is removed from the bag. Prime the tubing by allowing solution to flow through it and ensure that all bubbles have been removed; then close the stopcock. Insert the solution bag into the pressure bag. Increase the pressure in the pressure bag to 300 mm Hg by pumping up the hand bulb.

Transducer Preparation

Insert the disposable transducer into its holder. Attach the monitoring cable to its connection on the transducer and the other end to the pressure monitor or patient monitoring system. Attach the infusion IV line to the transducer, locking it into place. Place a three-way stopcock on the other port of the transducer and connect the patient catheter to it.

ZEROING THE TRANSDUCER

All physiologic hemodynamic monitoring is referenced to atmospheric pressure, which by convention is zero. Therefore, it is important to "zero" the transducer before making measurements so that the pressure is always referenced to the same value. The practitioner must zero the transducer on initial setup and preparation and at the beginning of each shift. By doing so, all measurements made will have the same reference point.

When the practitioner zeros the transducer for CVP or pulmonary artery pressure measurements, the transducer should be at the same level as the patient's *phlebostatic axis*. Identification of the phlebostatic axis is described in the next section. Once this reference point has been identified, the transducer should be located at the same height. A carpenter's level is a helpful tool to ensure that the transducer and the phlebostatic axis are on the same plane.

Zero the transducer by first turning off the system to the patient (closing the stopcock) and then opening the reference stopcock to air. This sequence will allow the system to equilibrate to atmospheric pressure. Allow a few seconds for equilibration and then depress the zero button or switch on the monitor.

IDENTIFICATION OF THE PHLEBOSTATIC AXIS

It is assumed that the CVP and pulmonary artery catheters are located in the middle of the chest. When making measurements, ensure that the patient is positioned

TABLE 9-2: Equipment Required for Hemodynamic Monitoring			
	CVP CATHETER	**PA CATHETER**	**ARTERIAL CATHETER**
500 mL bag of 0.9% saline	X	X	X
500 units of heparin	X	X	X
Medication label	X	X	X
Pressure bag	X	X	X
Disposable transducer	X	X	X
Transducer holder	X	X	X
Pressure monitoring cable	X	X	X
IV pressure tubing	X	X	X
Pressure monitor	X	X	X

supine and level. Once the patient has been positioned, identify the phlebostatic axis on the patient's axilla. This reference point is identified by the midaxillary line at the junction of the fourth rib.

Once the axis has been identified as described, position the transducer in the same plane by using a carpenter's level. If the transducer is higher than the phlebostatic axis, pressure readings will be lower. Conversely, if the transducer is located lower than the phlebostatic axis, pressures will be higher. These pressure variations are caused by the gravitational effect on the fluid in the lines.

WAVEFORM DAMPING

A damped (suppressed) waveform is important to recognize. Figures 9-14 and 9-15 illustrate a normal arterial waveform and a damped arterial waveform. Waveform *damping* may occur during monitoring of any hemodynamic data. Damping may be caused by several factors, including air in the system, improper zeroing of the transducer, blood clots in the system, catheter occlusion (clots, balloon, tip touching the vessel wall), leaks in the system, inadequate pressure in the pressure bag, and kinks in the tubing.

OBTAINING A PULMONARY ARTERY WEDGE PRESSURE

As described in previous sections, the PAWP is measured when the balloon on the pulmonary artery catheter is inflated and wedged in the pulmonary artery. Correct wedging is important to obtain accurate data but also for patient safety.

Check to ensure that the transducer is located at the phlebostatic axis and that it is zeroed with the patient in a supine level position. Observe the pressure monitor and verify that the waveform displayed is the pulmonary artery waveform and that pressures correspond as such. Draw air into a tuberculin syringe and attach it to the inflation lumen of the catheter. Run a continuous strip on the monitor. Inject approximately 0.8 cc of air into the inflation lumen while observing the pressure monitor. Inject only enough air to obtain the desired wedged waveform. Observe for the waveform to change from the pulmonary artery pressure morphology to the wedge pressure morphology. Once the catheter is wedged, keep it wedged until pressures stabilize and the patient has breathed for several ventilatory cycles. Evacuate air from the balloon by withdrawing the syringe and observe for the monitor to return to the pulmonary artery waveform characteristics. Last, stop the continuous strip recording.

OVERWEDGING OF THE BALLOON

If too much air is injected, a damped pulmonary artery wedge waveform will result. Do not inject more than 1 to 1.5 cc of air into the inflation lumen of the catheter. If the catheter is believed to be overwedged, withdraw all air from the inflation lumen. Next, verify the correct pulmonary artery waveform morphology is being viewed. Then inject only enough air to obtain the desired pulmonary artery wedge waveform morphology.

CARDIAC OUTPUT DETERMINATION

It is not imperative that the patient always be positioned supine for cardiac output determination; however, the patient should be in the same position

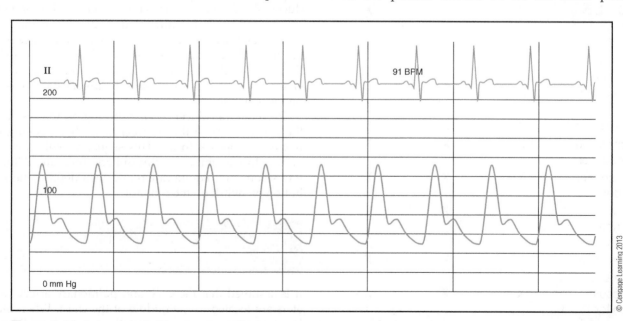

Figure 9-14 A damped arterial pressure waveform

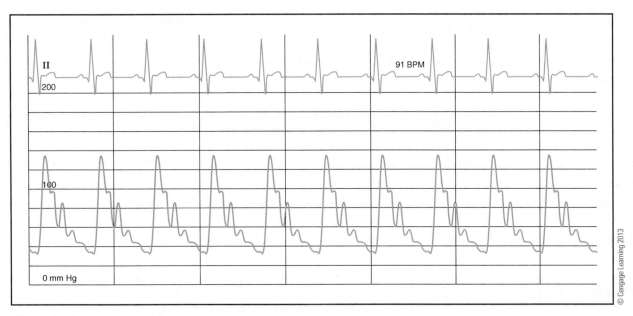

Figure 9-15 A normal arterial pressure waveform

(supine or semi-Fowler's, for example) each time these measurements are performed. Change the monitor's function to cardiac output determination and ensure that there is a supply of cold injectate (D₅W or normal saline). Draw up 10 mL of injectate and attach the syringe to the proximal port. Trigger the monitor to prompt the appropriate time to begin the injection. Once instructed to do so, firmly push the syringe's contents into the proximal port's lumen. The practitioner has approximately 4 seconds to complete the injection. Observe the data and obtain three values within 10% of one another. Take the average of these results for the cardiac output value.

ARTERIAL LINE MAINTENANCE

Maintenance of an arterial line is facilitated by using heparinized solution in the pressure bag. Also, the catheter should be flushed periodically using a syringe and heparinized solution. The catheter should be checked frequently for loose connections because a leak could result in severe hemorrhage. Pulses should also be checked proximal and distal to the catheter to verify that circulation has not been impaired.

ZEROING AN ARTERIAL LINE

The transducer assembly for an arterial line is usually taped to the patient's limb, proximal to the insertion point of the catheter (Figure 9-16). Therefore, the phlebostatic axis or leveling of the transducer is not required. However, the transducer must be zeroed just as for the pulmonary artery and CVP catheters. Turn off the system

to the patient by rotating the stopcock. Open the reference stopcock to atmospheric pressure, allow for equilibration, and zero the monitor.

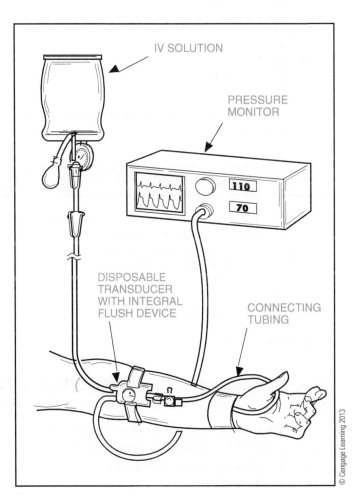

Figure 9-16 The position of a transducer in relation to an arterial catheter

Reference

Kiess Daily, E., & Schroeder, J. S. (1994). *Techniques in bedside hemodynamic monitoring* (5th ed.). St. Louis, MO: Mosby–Year Book.

Additional Resources

Chang, D. W. (2006). *Clinical application of mechanical ventilation* (3rd ed.). Clifton Park, NY: Delmar Cengage Learning.

Des Jardins, T. R. (2008). *Cardiopulmonary anatomy and physiology* (5th ed.). Clifton Park, NY: Delmar Cengage Learning.

Mowreader, M. (1995). *Hemodynamics learning module.* Unpublished manuscript. Sacred Heart Medical Center, Spokane, WA.

Wilkins, R. L. (2005). *Clinical assessment in respiratory care* (5th ed.). St. Louis, MO: Mosby.

Practice Activities: CVP and Pulmonary Artery Catheter Monitoring

1. In the laboratory, assemble all of the equipment required to monitor the CVP and pulmonary artery pressure:
   a. 500 mL normal saline solution bag
   b. 500 units of sodium heparin
   c. Medication label
   d. IV tubing
   e. Disposable transducer and holder
   f. Stopcocks
   g. Pressure bag
   h. Transducer cable
   i. Monitor

2. Using your laboratory setup, prime the tubing and purge it of all air.

3. Close the distal port and practice zeroing the transducer in the laboratory.

4. Using a laboratory partner, correctly position him or her and identify the phlebostatic axis.

5. Level the transducer to the same plane as for the phlebostatic axis, using your laboratory partner.

6. In the laboratory, insert a pulmonary artery catheter into a basin of water. Practice inflating the balloon with air and injecting 10 mL of saline.

Practice Activities: Arterial Line Monitoring

1. In the laboratory, assemble all of the equipment required to monitor arterial pressures:
   a. 500 mL normal saline solution bag
   b. 500 units of sodium heparin
   c. Medication label
   d. IV tubing
   e. Disposable transducer and holder
   f. Stopcocks
   g. Pressure bag
   h. Transducer cable
   i. Monitor

2. Using your laboratory setup, prime the tubing and purge it of all air.

3. Close the distal port and practice zeroing the transducer in the laboratory.

4. Practice flushing an arterial catheter set up in the laboratory using 3 to 5 mL of saline.

Check List: CVP and Pulmonary Artery Catheter Monitoring

1. Assemble and prepare the required equipment:
   _____ a. 500 mL normal saline solution bag
   _____ b. 500 units of sodium heparin
   _____ c. Medication label
   _____ d. IV tubing
   _____ e. Disposable transducer and holder
   _____ f. Stopcocks
   _____ g. Pressure bag
   _____ h. Transducer cable
   _____ i. Monitor

2. Purge all air and prime the system with flush solution.

3. Identify the phlebostatic axis and level the transducer.

4. Zero the transducer.

5. Obtain the pulmonary artery pressure measurement.

6. Wedge the catheter and obtain the pulmonary artery wedge pressure measurement.

7. Measure the cardiac output.

8. Document all findings and affix the strip chart recording to the appropriate location in the patient's chart.

9. Maintain aseptic technique at all times.

Check List: Arterial Line Monitoring

1. Assemble and prepare the required equipment:
_____ a. 500 mL normal saline solution bag
_____ b. 500 units of sodium heparin
_____ c. Medication label
_____ d. IV tubing
_____ e. Disposable transducer and holder
_____ f. Stopcocks
_____ g. Pressure bag
_____ h. Transducer cable
_____ i. Monitor

_____ 2. Purge all air and prime the system with flush solution.
_____ 3. Zero the transducer.
_____ 4. Obtain a tracing and record your values.
_____ 5. Maintain aseptic technique at all times.
_____ 6. Document your results in the patient's chart.

Self-Evaluation Post Test: Hemodynamic Monitoring

1. Which of the following best describes Pascal's law?
   a. Volume changes proportionally with the pressure at the same temperature.
   b. The pressure in a closed system is the same at different points in the system.
   c. Pressure varies inversely with the temperature at the same volume.
   d. Volume varies inversely with temperature at the same pressure.

2. What is the purpose of a transducer in a hemodynamic monitoring system?
   a. It measures pressures.
   b. It converts a physical parameter into an electrical signal.
   c. It separates the blood from the infusion fluid.
   d. It converts cm H_2O to mm Hg.

3. Which of the following can a central venous catheter (CVP) determine?
   I. Right ventricular preload
   II. Right ventricular afterload
   III. Left ventricular preload
   IV. Cardiac output
   a. I   c. I, II, III
   b. I, II   d. I, II, III, IV

4. Which of the following can a pulmonary artery catheter determine?
   I. Right ventricular preload
   II. Right ventricular afterload
   III. Left ventricular preload
   IV. Cardiac output
   a. I   c. I, II, III
   b. I, II   d. I, II, III, IV

5. Which of the following pressures is a measure of right ventricular afterload?
   a. CVP   c. PA
   b. RA   d. PAWP

6. Which of the following pressures is a measure of left ventricular preload?
   a. CVP   c. PA
   b. RA   d. PAWP

7. You are assigned to the ICU and are caring for a patient who experienced traumatic injury. Owing to blood loss, the patient was aggressively fluid resuscitated 24 hours ago. You obtain the following hemodynamic data:
   RA   = 7 mm Hg
   PA   = 48/30 mm Hg
   PAWP = 24 mm Hg
   CO   = 7.3 L/min
   BP   = 110/74 mm Hg
   Which of the following assessments best matches your data?
   a. The patient is hypovolemic.
   b. The patient is experiencing right heart failure.
   c. The patient is experiencing left heart failure.
   d. The patient is experiencing fluid overload.

8. You are assigned to the CCU and are assessing a patient who was admitted yesterday for chest pain. His heart rate is 125 beats per minute. You obtain the following hemodynamic data:
   RA   = 4 mm Hg
   PA   = 40/28 mm Hg
   PAWP = 24 mm Hg
   CO   = 3.2 L/min

Which of the following assessments best matches your data?
a. The patient is hypovolemic.
b. The patient is experiencing right heart failure.
c. The patient is experiencing left heart failure.
d. The patient is experiencing fluid overload.

9. Given the following set of data:

   CO   = 4.3 L/min
   PAWP = 15 mm Hg
   PA   = 45/30 mm Hg
   RA   = 8 mm Hg

calculate the pulmonary vascular resistance:

a. 419 dynes·sec·cm^{-5} c. 279 dynes·sec·cm^{-5}
b. 130 dynes·sec·cm^{-5} d. 539 dynes·sec·cm^{-5}

10. Which of the following is a hazard/are hazards of indwelling vascular catheters?

   I.   Infection
   II. Emboli
   III. Hemorrhage
   IV. Arrhythmias

a. I   c. I, II, III
b. I, II   d. I, II, III, IV

PERFORMANCE EVALUATION:
CVP and Pulmonary Artery Catheter Monitoring

Date: Lab _____ Clinical _____ Agency _____

Lab: Pass _____ Fail _____ Clinical: Pass _____ Fail _____

Student name _____ Instructor name _____

No. of times observed in clinical _____

No. of times practiced in clinical _____

PASSING CRITERIA: Obtain 90% or better on the procedure. Tasks indicated by * must receive at least 1 point, or the evaluation is terminated. Procedure must be performed within the designated time, or the performance receives a failing grade.

SCORING: 2 points — Task performed satisfactorily without prompting.
1 point — Task performed satisfactorily with self-initiated correction.
0 points — Task performed incorrectly or with prompting required.
NA — Task not applicable to the patient care situation.

Tasks:	Peer	Lab	Clinical
* **1.** Practices standard precautions, including hand hygiene	☐	☐	☐
* **2.** Assembles and prepares the required equipment			
a. 500 mL normal saline solution bag	☐	☐	☐
b. 500 units of sodium heparin	☐	☐	☐
c. Medication label	☐	☐	☐
d. IV tubing	☐	☐	☐
e. Disposable transducer and holder	☐	☐	☐
f. Stopcocks	☐	☐	☐
g. Pressure bag	☐	☐	☐
h. Transducer cable	☐	☐	☐
i. Monitor	☐	☐	☐
* **3.** Sets up and primes the tubing, purging it of air	☐	☐	☐
* **4.** Positions the patient, identifying the phlebostatic axis	☐	☐	☐
* **5.** Zeroes the transducer	☐	☐	☐
* **6.** Levels the transducer at the phlebostatic axis	☐	☐	☐
* **7.** Obtains the pulmonary artery pressure measurement	☐	☐	☐
* **8.** Wedges the catheter, obtaining the pulmonary artery wedge pressure	☐	☐	☐
* **9.** Measures the cardiac output	☐	☐	☐

* **10.** Documents all findings and affixes a strip to the chart ☐ ☐ ☐

* **11.** Maintains aseptic technique at all times ☐ ☐ ☐

SCORE: Peer _____ points of possible 38; _____%

Lab _____ points of possible 38; _____%

Clinical _____ points of possible 38; _____%

TIME: _____ out of possible 30 minutes

STUDENT SIGNATURES

PEER: _____

STUDENT: _____

INSTRUCTOR SIGNATURES

LAB: _____

CLINICAL: _____

PERFORMANCE EVALUATION:
Arterial Line Monitoring

Date: Lab _____ Clinical _____ Agency _____

Lab: Pass _____ Fail _____ Clinical: Pass _____ Fail _____

Student name _____ Instructor name _____

No. of times observed in clinical _____

No. of times practiced in clinical _____

PASSING CRITERIA: Obtain 90% or better on the procedure. Tasks indicated by * must receive at least 1 point, or the evaluation is terminated. Procedure must be performed within the designated time, or the performance receives a failing grade.

SCORING: 2 points — Task performed satisfactorily without prompting.
1 point — Task performed satisfactorily with self-initiated correction.
0 points — Task performed incorrectly or with prompting required.
NA — Task not applicable to the patient care situation.

Tasks:	Peer	Lab	Clinical
* 1. Practices standard precautions, including hand hygiene	☐	☐	☐
* 2. Assembles and prepares the required equipment			
a. 500 mL normal saline solution bag	☐	☐	☐
b. 500 units of sodium heparin	☐	☐	☐
c. Medication label	☐	☐	☐
d. IV tubing	☐	☐	☐
e. Disposable transducer and holder	☐	☐	☐
f. Stopcocks	☐	☐	☐
g. Pressure bag	☐	☐	☐
h. Transducer cable	☐	☐	☐
i. Monitor	☐	☐	☐
* 3. Sets up and primes the tubing, purging it of air	☐	☐	☐
* 4. Zeroes the transducer	☐	☐	☐
* 5. Obtains a tracing and records values	☐	☐	☐
* 6. Documents all findings and affixes a strip to the chart	☐	☐	☐
* 7. Maintains aseptic technique at all times	☐	☐	☐

SCORE: Peer   _____ points of possible 30; _____%

                    Lab   _____ points of possible 30; _____%

                    Clinical _____ points of possible 30; _____%

TIME: _____ out of possible 20 minutes

STUDENT SIGNATURES   **INSTRUCTOR SIGNATURES**

PEER: _____   LAB: _____

STUDENT: _____   CLINICAL: _____

CHAPTER 10

Noninvasive Monitoring

INTRODUCTION

Noninvasive patient monitoring has become routine in the acute care setting. Advances in microcomputer and microchip technology with advancements in photospectrometry have allowed the development of small, reliable instruments. Being microprocessor controlled, these instruments display data in real time—as events happen. Clinically, knowing immediately how the patient is responding is a tremendous advantage over having to wait for laboratory results to return.

Noninvasive monitoring, by definition, is ongoing assessment of the patient's condition without entry into the body (through body orifices or via puncture of the skin or vessels). Current noninvasive monitoring allows measurement of transcutaneous (through the skin) oxygen tension ($PtcO_2$), transcutaneous carbon dioxide tension ($PtcCO_2$), arterial oxygen saturation obtained by pulse oximetry (SpO_2), and end-tidal carbon dioxide ($PetCO_2$).

This chapter discusses the purpose and clinical applications of noninvasive monitoring. It also covers how the equipment operates and how to apply it correctly to patients. As with all procedures, there are hazards and limitations associated with noninvasive monitoring techniques. An appreciation of these risks and limitations is important in order to apply these techniques optimally in the acute care setting.

KEY TERMS

- End-tidal CO_2 monitor
- Heating element
- Mainstream monitor
- Noninvasive monitoring
- Pulse oximeter
- Sidestream monitor
- Thermocouple
- Transcutaneous CO_2 monitor
- Transcutaneous PO_2 electrode

THEORY OBJECTIVES

At the end of this chapter, the reader should be able to:

- *Discuss the purpose and clinical applications of noninvasive monitoring.*
- *Describe the principles of operation for the following noninvasive monitors:*
  - *Pulse oximeter*
  - *Transcutaneous CO_2 monitor*
  - *Transcutaneous O_2 monitor*
  - *End-tidal CO_2 monitor*
- *Describe the limitations of noninvasive monitoring.*
- *Discuss the hazards of noninvasive monitoring.*

CLINICAL PRACTICE GUIDELINES

AARC Clinical Practice Guideline Pulse Oximetry

PO 4.0 INDICATIONS:

4.1 The need to monitor the adequacy of arterial oxyhemoglobin saturation.[1,4,6,9]

4.2 The need to quantitate the response of arterial oxyhemoglobin saturation to therapeutic intervention[4,9,10] or to a diagnostic procedure (e.g., bronchoscopy)

4.3 The need to comply with mandated regulations[11,12] or recommendations by authoritative groups[13,14]

PO 5.0 CONTRAINDICATIONS:

The presence of an ongoing need for measurement of pH, $PaCO_2$, total hemoglobin, and abnormal hemoglobins may be a relative contraindication to pulse oximetry.

PO 6.0 HAZARDS/COMPLICATIONS:

Pulse oximetry is considered a safe procedure, but because of device limitations, false-negative results for hypoxemia[4] and/or false-positive results for normoxemia[13,14] or hyperoxemia[17,18] may lead to inappropriate treatment of the patient. In addition, tissue injury may occur at the measuring site as a result of probe misuse (e.g., pressure sores from prolonged application of electrical shock and burns from the substitution of incompatible probes between instruments).[19]

PO 8.0 ASSESSMENT OF NEED:

8.1 When direct measurement of SaO_2 is not available or accessible in a timely fashion, an SpO_2 measurement may temporarily suffice if the limitations of the data are appreciated.[9,10]

8.2 SpO_2 is appropriate for continuous and prolonged monitoring (e.g., during sleep, exercise, bronchoscopy).[1,6,7,9,10,14,31]

8.3 SpO_2 may be adequate when assessment of acid-base status and/or PaO_2 is not required.[1,4,9,10]

PO 9.0 ASSESSMENT OF OUTCOME:

The following should be utilized to evaluate the benefit of pulse oximetry:

9.1 SpO_2 results should reflect the patient's clinical condition (i.e., validate the basis for ordering the test).

9.2 Documentation of results, therapeutic intervention (or lack of), and/or clinical decisions based on the SpO_2 measurement should be noted in the medical record.

Reprinted with permission from *Respiratory Care* 1992; 37; 891–897. The complete AARC Clinical Practice Guidelines are available from the AARC Web site (http://www.aarc.org), from the AARC Executive Office, or from *Respiratory Care* journal.

PO 11.0 MONITORING:

The clinician is referred to Section 7.0 Validation of Results. The monitoring schedule of patient and equipment during continuous oximetry should be tied to bedside assessment and vital signs determinations.

AARC Clinical Practice Guideline Transcutaneous Blood Gas Monitoring for Neonatal & Pediatric Patients

TCM 4.0 INDICATIONS:

4.1 The need to monitor the adequacy of arterial oxygenation and/or ventilation.[11–13]

4.2 The need to quantitate the response to diagnostic and therapeutic interventions as evidenced by $PtcO_2$ and/or $PtcCO_2$ values.[11,12,14,15]

TCM 5.0 CONTRAINDICATIONS:

In patients with poor skin integrity and/or adhesive allergy, transcutaneous monitoring may be relatively contraindicated.[11]

TCM 6.0 HAZARDS/COMPLICATIONS:

$PtcO_2$ and/or $PtcCO_2$ monitoring is considered a safe procedure, but because of device limitations, false-negative and false-positive results may lead to inappropriate treatment of the patient.[12,16–18] In addition, tissue injury may occur at the measuring site (e.g., erythema, blisters, burns, skin tears).[1,9,12,19]

TCM 8.0 ASSESSMENT OF NEED:

8.1 When direct measurement of arterial blood is not available or accessible in a timely fashion, $PtcO_2$ and/or $PtcCO_2$ measurements may temporarily suffice if the limitations of the data are appreciated.[11]

8.2 Transcutaneous blood gas monitoring is appropriate for continuous and prolonged monitoring (e.g., during mechanical ventilation, CPAP, and supplemental oxygen administration).[11,12,24]

8.3 $PtcO_2$ values can be used for diagnostic purposes as in the assessment of functional shunts (e.g., persistent pulmonary hypertension of the newborn, PPHN, or persistent fetal circulation or to determine the response to oxygen challenge in the assessment of congenital heart disease.[30–33]

TCM 9.0 ASSESSMENT OF OUTCOME:

9.1 Results should reflect the patient's clinical condition (i.e., validate the basis for ordering the monitoring).[3,5,7,13,29]

9.2 Documentation of results, therapeutic intervention (or lack of), and/or clinical decisions based on the transcutaneous measurements should be noted in the medical record.

(Continued)

TCM 11.0 MONITORING:

The monitoring schedule of patient and equipment during transcutaneous monitoring should be integrated into patient assessment and vital signs determinations. Results should be documented in the patient's medical record and should detail the conditions under which the readings were obtained:

11.1 The date and time of measurement, transcutaneous reading, patient's position, respiratory rate, and activity level;

11.2 Inspired oxygen concentration or supplemental oxygen flow, specifying the type of oxygen delivery device;

11.3 Mode of ventilatory support, ventilator, or CPAP settings;

11.4 Electrode placement site, electrode temperature, and time of placement;

11.5 Results of simultaneously obtained PaO_2, $PaCO_2$, and pH when available;

11.6 Clinical appearance of patient, subjective assessment of perfusion, pallor, and skin temperature.

Reprinted with permission from *Respiratory Care* 2004; 49: 1070–1072. The complete AARC Clinical Practice Guidelines are available from the AARC Web site (http://www.aarc.org), from the AARC Executive Office, or from *Respiratory Care* journal.

AARC Clinical Practice Guideline Capnography/Capnometry During Mechanical Ventilation
AARC Clinical Practice Guideline Capnography/Capnometry During Mechanical Ventilation: 2011

CO₂ MV 4.0 INDICATIONS

There are 3 broad categories of indications for capnography/capnometry: verification of artificial airway placement; assessment of pulmonary circulation and respiratory status; and optimization of mechanical ventilation.

4.1 Verification of Artificial Airway Placement. Even when the endotracheal tube is seen to pass through the vocal cords and tube position is verified by chest expansion and auscultation during mechanical ventilation, providers should obtain additional confirmation of airway placement with waveform capnography or an exhaled CO_2 or esophageal detector device.[5]

4.1.1 Exhaled CO_2 detectors, including colorimetric and non-waveform, reliably detect intratracheal placement in patients whose cardiac output is not exceedingly low or who have not had prolonged circulatory failure. Their use in prolonged cardiac arrest merits further study.[5,6]

4.1.1.1 When waveform capnography is not available, these methods can be used in addition to clinical assessment as the initial method for confirming correct tube placement in a patient in cardiac arrest.

4.1.2 Capnography may be used as an adjunct to determine that tracheal rather than esophageal intubation has occurred.[4,7,8]

4.1.3 All intubations must be confirmed by some form of $PETCO_2$ measurement.[5,9]

4.1.4 Effective ventilation through a supraglottic airway device such as the laryngeal mask airway (LMA) should result in a capnograph waveform during cardiopulmonary resuscitation (CPR), and after return of spontaneous circulation.[5]

4.1.5 When feasible, monitoring $PETCO_2$ During chest compressions is encouraged.[5]

4.1.5.1 If the $PETCO_2$ is < 10 mm Hg during CPR, the clinician should attempt to improve the quality of compressions.

4.1.5.2 An abrupt and sustained increase in $PETCO_2$ is a sensitive indicator of return of spontaneous circulation.

4.1.6 $PETCO_2$ monitoring is one of the objective standards required for monitoring patients in transport, to ensure integrity of the airway.[6,10,11]

4.1.6.1 Providers should observe a consistent capnographic waveform with ventilation to confirm and monitor endotracheal tube placement in the field, in the transport vehicle, on arrival at the hospital, and after any patient transfer, to reduce the risk of unrecognized tube misplacement or displacement.[5,12]

4.1.7 Capnography can be used to detect inadvertent airway intubation during gastric tube insertion.[13]

4.1.8 Life-threatening airway disasters and ventilator disconnection can be averted with continuous capnography.[14-16]

4.2 Assessment of Pulmonary Circulation and Respiratory Status. Capnography assists in:

4.2.1 Determining changes in pulmonary circulation and respiratory status sooner than pulse oximetry. In patients without lung disease, substantial hypercarbia may present before pulse oximetry notifies the clinician of a change in ventilation.[14,17-20]

4.2.2 Monitoring the adequacy of pulmonary, systemic, and coronary blood flow,[20,21] as well as estimation of the effective (non-shunted) pulmonary capillary blood flow by a partial rebreathing method.[22-24]

4.2.3 Evaluating the partial pressure of exhaled CO_2, especially $PETCO_2$

4.2.4 Screening for pulmonary embolism.[25-28]

(Continued)

4.3 Optimization of Mechanical Ventilation. Capnography during mechanical ventilation allows:

4.3.1 Continuous monitoring of the integrity of the ventilator circuit, including the artificial airway[29] or bag mask ventilation, in addition to potentially detecting mechanical ventilation malfunctions.[30-32]

4.3.2 Decreasing the duration of ventilatory support.[33]

4.3.3 Adjustment of the trigger sensitivity.[34]

4.3.4 Evaluation of the efficiency of mechanical ventilation, by the difference between $PaCO_2$ and the $PETCO_2$.[35]

4.3.5 Monitoring of the severity of pulmonary disease[36,37] and evaluating the response to therapy, especially therapies intended to improve the ratio of dead space to tidal volume (VD/VT) and ventilation-perfusion matching ($\dot{V}/\dot{Q}$).[23,27,38-46]

4.3.6 Monitoring of $\dot{V}/\dot{Q}$ during independent lung ventilation.[47,48]

4.3.7 Monitoring of inspired CO_2 when it is being therapeutically administered.[49]

4.3.8 Graphic evaluation of the ventilator-patient interface. Evaluation of the capnogram may be useful in detecting rebreathing of CO_2, obstructive pulmonary disease, the presence of inspiratory effort during neuromuscular blockade (curare cleft), cardiogenic oscillations, esophageal intubation, and cardiac arrest.[50]

4.3.9 Measurement of the volume of CO_2 elimination to assess metabolic rate and/or alveolar ventilation.[43,51-53]

4.3.10 Monitoring of VD/VT to determine eligibility for extubation in children.[40,54]

4.3.11 There is a relationship between VD/VT and survival in patients with the acute respiratory distress syndrome.[55-57]

CO₂ MV 5.0 CONTRAINDICATIONS

There are no absolute contraindications to capnography in mechanically ventilated patients, provided that the data obtained are evaluated with consideration given to the patient's clinical condition.

O₂ MV 6.0 HAZARDS/COMPLICATIONS

Capnography with a clinically approved device is a safe, noninvasive test, associated with few hazards in most populations. Hazards/complications are different for the 2 types of capnographic device.

6.1 Mainstream

6.1.1 Dead Space. Adapters inserted into the airway between the airway and the ventilator circuit should have a minimal amount of dead space. This effect is inversely proportional to the size of the patient being monitored.[44,58]

6.1.2 The addition of the weight of a mainstream adapter can increase the risk of accidental extubation in neonates and small children.[58]

6.2 Sidestream

6.2.1 The gas sampling rate from some sidestream analyzers may be high enough to cause auto-triggering when flow-triggering of mechanical breaths is used. This effect is also inversely proportional to the size of the patient.[58]

6.2.2 The gas sampling rate can diminish delivered VT in neonates and small patients while using volume targeted or volume controlled ventilation modes.[58]

CO₂ MV 8.0 ASSESSMENT OF NEED

Capnography is considered a standard of care during general anesthesia. The American Society of Anesthesiologists has suggested that capnography be available for patients with acute ventilatory failure on mechanical ventilatory support.[81] The American College of Emergency Physicians recommends capnography as an adjunctive method to ensure proper endotracheal tube position.[75] The 2010 American Heart Association Guidelines for Cardiopulmonary.

Resuscitation and Emergency Cardiovascular Care recommend capnography to verify endotracheal tube placement in all age groups.[6] Assessment of the need to use capnography with a specific patient should be guided by the clinical situation. The patient's primary cause of respiratory failure and the severity of his or her condition should be considered.

CO₂ MV 9.0 ASSESSMENT OF OUTCOME

Results should reflect the patient's condition and should validate the basis for ordering the monitoring. Documentation of results (along with all ventilatory and hemodynamic variables available), therapeutic interventions, and/or clinical decisions made based on the capnogram should be included in the patient's chart.

CO₂ MV 11.0 MONITORING

11.1 During capnography the following should be considered and monitored:

11.1.1 Ventilatory variables: VT, respiratory rate, PEEP, ratio of inspiratory-to-expiratory time, peak airway pressure, and concentrations of respiratory gas mixture.[3,38,44,72,82]

11.1.2 Hemodynamic variables: systemic and pulmonary blood pressure, cardiac output, shunt, and $\dot{V}/\dot{Q}$ imbalances.[23,41,66]

Reprinted with permission from *Respiratory Care* 2011; 56: 503–509. The complete AARC Clinical Practice Guidelines are available from the AARC Web site (http://www.aarc.org), from the AARC Executive Office, or from *Respiratory Care* journal.

RATIONALE FOR NONINVASIVE MONITORING

Noninvasive monitoring allows the respiratory practitioner to monitor in real time (immediately) a patient's oxygen saturation, partial pressure of oxygen, or partial pressure of carbon dioxide. Historically, this information was available only through blood gas analysis. Blood gas analysis is still the standard by which noninvasive monitors are compared, and by which monitoring data are related to the patient's condition. However, noninvasive monitoring has greatly reduced the number of arterial blood gas (ABG) samples drawn in the acute care setting.

By its very nature, noninvasive monitoring is more comfortable for the patient. There is less risk from infection or other complications associated with invasive techniques. Noninvasive monitoring also provides a continuous form of monitoring and tending, which is clinically very useful.

NONINVASIVE MONITORING EQUIPMENT

Pulse Oximeters

Pulse oximeters monitor the oxygen saturation in the arterial blood. Rather than directly measuring the saturation of the blood as a co-oximeter does (SaO_2), the pulse oximeter uses photospectrometry to measure the oxygen saturation of a capillary bed (SpO_2).

Pulse oximeters use two light-emitting diodes (LEDs) and a photodetector (Figure 10-1). One LED emits light that is red at a wavelength of approximately 660 nm, and the other emits infrared light at approximately 900 nm (Craig, 1990). The light passes through the capillary bed, and depending on the amount of saturated hemoglobin, the color of the vascular bed varies (desaturated hemoglobin being darker). Because oxygenated blood is more permeable to red light, the oximeter is able to relate this color change to oxygen saturation.

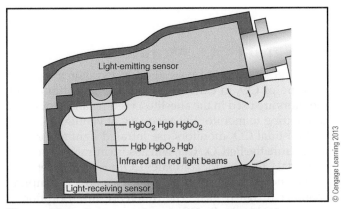

Figure 10-1   A cross section of a pulse oximeter probe.

Common sites of measurement are the fingers, toes, and ears. Different probes are designed for use at specific sites. Newborn and pediatric probes usually wrap around the foot (Figure 10-2).

Masimo Rad-57™ Masimo Corporation, Irvine, California, has introduced the Rad-57™ handheld pulse co-oximeter (Figure 10-3). The Rad-57 uses multiple wavelengths of light, enabling measurement of SpO_2, $SpCO$®, and $SpMet$™. The addition of multiple wavelengths of light allows noninvasive determination of dysfunctional hemoglobin (COHb and METHb). The pulse co-oximeter finger probe is placed on the patient's digit, and once adequate signal strength is obtained, a reading of SpO_2, $SpCO$, and $SpMet$ may be made.

Transcutaneous CO_2 Monitor

The *transcutaneous CO_2 monitor* is a modified PCO_2 electrode (Severinghaus electrode) with a heater incorporated into its design (Figure 10-4). The pH glass membrane is molded into a flat surface that is perpendicular to the surface of the skin. The pH glass membrane separates the measuring and reference electrodes. The *heating element* and *thermocouple* maintain skin temperatures at 44°C. The thermocouple senses the temperature at the skin and regulates the output of the heating element to maintain the desired skin temperature. The increased temperature arterializes the vascular bed under the electrode, increasing circulation to that area.

CO_2 diffuses across the skin and through the membrane (permeable only to CO_2) and is measured by the electrode. An airtight seal around the electrode prevents ambient air from entering the sample site. The transcutaneous electrode should not be placed over bone or on the right chest above the umbilicus. Ideally an area of fatty tissue is best. The probe site will need to be changed periodically to avoid erythema, blisters, burns, and skin tears at the measuring site.

Transcutaneous O_2 Monitor

The *transcutaneous PO_2 electrode* is a modified Clark electrode, incorporating the addition of a heating element and a thermocouple. As in the transcutaneous PCO_2 electrode, the PO_2 electrode's heating element arterializes the sample site by increasing the skin temperature to 44°C. Oxygen diffuses through the skin and is measured by the electrode.

Combination PO_2 and PCO_2 Monitors

Some manufacturers make a combination PO_2 and PCO_2 transcutaneous electrode. In these designs both types of transcutaneous electrodes are incorporated into one sensor assembly. This combination allows the monitoring of the transcutaneous partial pressures of both gases with one instrument.

The principles of operation are identical to those of the individual instruments; only the design differs.

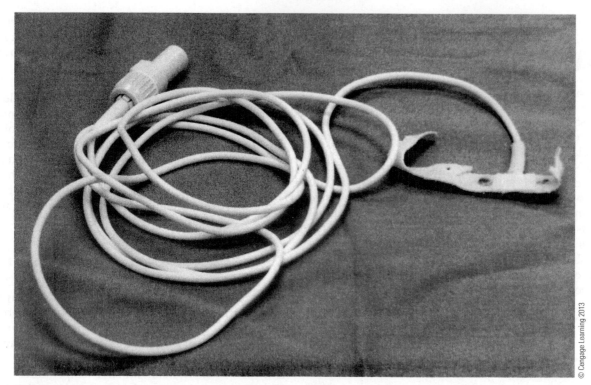

Figure 10-2 A newborn/pediatric pulse oximeter probe

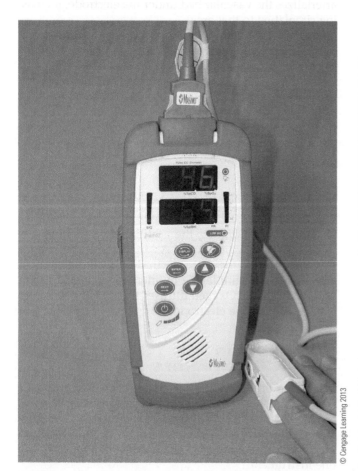

Figure 10-3 A photograph of the Masimo Rad-57 pulse co-oximeter

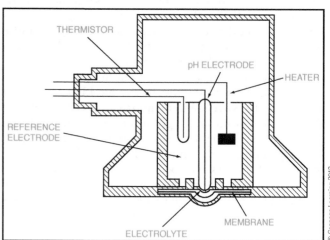

Figure 10-4 A cross section of a transcutaneous CO_2 electrode.

End-Tidal CO_2 Monitors

End-tidal CO_2 monitors are used to monitor the partial pressure of CO_2 in exhaled gas ($PetCO_2$). End-tidal CO_2 monitors are used in the anesthesia setting and the critical care setting to monitor the adequacy of ventilation.

End-tidal CO_2 monitors use infrared light absorption to measure the $PetCO_2$. CO_2 will absorb infrared light. The end-tidal CO_2 monitor compares CO_2 absorption between a reference chamber (no CO_2 present) and a sampling chamber (exhaled gas). The difference in absorption is proportional to the $PetCO_2$.

There are two types of end-tidal CO_2 monitors: mainstream and sidestream. The *mainstream monitors* use a sensor that is attached directly to the airway. The *sidestream monitors* draw the exhaled gas sample from the airway through a capillary tube to an analyzer that is located near the patient.

LIMITATIONS OF NONINVASIVE MONITORING

Although noninvasive monitoring has provided real-time data that facilitate good patient care, the values observed on the monitors do not always reflect the patient's true condition. Noninvasive monitors may provide inaccurate readings owing to the patient's physiologic condition or other environmental influences. Therefore, it is important for the respiratory practitioner to understand the limitations of noninvasive monitors and use each type on patients who will benefit the most from the application of that particular monitor.

Limitations of Pulse Oximetry

Pulse oximetry is widely used in the acute care setting (Allen, 2004). Many respiratory practitioners and other health care workers blindly accept the data obtained with these instruments as correct and accurate, when in fact the results obtained may be inaccurate for a variety of reasons. It is important to understand the limitations of these instruments so that they may be applied and used correctly. The factors that can influence their accuracy are listed in Table 10-1 (Allen, 2004). Accuracy of the reading may be verified by the displayed heart rate by palpation or with ECG monitoring (if available). The pulsatile waveform can also be assessed to verify signal strength.

Upon review of Table 10-1, it is clear that many factors may influence the accuracy of these instruments. Therefore, it is important to correlate the readings from these instruments with ABG values and co-oximetry results. From this comparison the practitioner may recognize discrepancies and trend the data accordingly.

Limitations of Transcutaneous Monitoring

Transcutaneous monitoring, like pulse oximetry and other technologies, has its limitations. Understanding these limitations and knowing when to draw blood for ABG analysis is part of applying these instruments correctly in the acute care setting. The limitations of transcutaneous monitoring are summarized in Table 10-2 (Aloan, 1987; Martin, 1990).

As with pulse oximeters, readings from transcutaneous monitors should be correlated with ABG values and co-oximetry results. Frequent membrane changes, site changes, and calibrations help to minimize some of this technology's limitations.

Limitations of End-Tidal CO_2 Monitoring

End-tidal CO_2 monitoring also has its limitations. These limitations must be recognized, and appropriate tending with blood gas analysis initiated when appropriate. The limitations of end-tidal CO_2 monitoring are summarized in Table 10-3 (Hess, 1990).

HAZARDS OF NONINVASIVE MONITORING

As with most medical procedures and techniques, noninvasive monitoring has its risks as well as its benefits. Understanding the hazards and potential complications is important in the effective clinical application of these techniques. The hazards and complications are summarized in Table 10-4.

TABLE 10-1: Factors Influencing Pulse Oximeter Accuracy

Motion
Sensor misalignment
Dysfunctional hemoglobin
Low perfusion states (patient hemodynamics)
Ambient light interference
Vascular dyes
Skin pigmentation and nail polish

TABLE 10-2: Limitations of Transcutaneous Monitoring

Edema of the skin
Insufficient heat applied to the skin from the electrode
Blistering from skin burns
Use of vasopressive drugs
Poor perfusion to the skin

TABLE 10-3: Limitations of End-Tidal CO_2 Monitoring

Shunt producing pulmonary disease
Pulmonary emboli
Tubing obstructions (sidestream devices)

PROFICIENCY OBJECTIVES

At the end of this chapter, the reader should be able to:

- *Assemble, test for function, and, if required, calibrate the equipment required for noninvasive monitoring:*
  — *Pulse oximeter*
  — *Transcutaneous monitor*
  — *End-tidal CO_2 monitor*
- *Demonstrate how to correctly apply the noninvasive monitor to the patient:*
  — *Pulse oximeter*

— *Transcutaneous monitor*
— *End-tidal CO_2 monitor*

- *Observe the preliminary readings from the instrument and determine if the monitor has been applied correctly and is working normally.*
- *As required, correlate the data from the noninvasive monitor with ABG values.*

TABLE 10-4: Hazards and Complications of Noninvasive Monitoring

PULSE OXIMETRY	TRANSCUTANEOUS MONITORING	END-TIDAL CO_2 MONITORING
Skin burns	Skin burns	Airway occlusion
Pressure necrosis		

TABLE 10-5: Pulse Oximeter Assembly

1. Connect the power cord to a 110 V 60 Hz electrical outlet.
2. Connect the oximeter probe to the monitor:
   a. Finger probe
   b. Ear probe
   c. Pediatric probe
3. Turn on the power switch.
4. Wipe the probe clean using an alcohol prep pad before applying it to the patient.
5. Apply the probe to the patient:
   a. Finger
   b. Toe
   c. Ear
   d. Foot (infant or pediatric patient)
6. Observe for adequate waveforms (pulse signal) and reading.
7. Set alarm limits as required.

ASSEMBLY, TROUBLESHOOTING, AND CALIBRATION

Pulse Oximeter

Assembly

Little assembly is required for most pulse oximeters. Many different pulse oximeters by various manufacturers are used in the acute care setting. A general assembly guide, which should be generic enough for most models, is provided in Table 10-5.

Troubleshooting

Troubleshooting a pulse oximeter is not difficult but may take some sleuthing on your part to correct the problem. Table 10-6 is a summary of the most common problems that may require troubleshooting.

Transcutaneous O_2 and CO_2 Monitors

Assembly

Many different types of transcutaneous monitors are employed in the acute care setting. When assembling the transcutaneous monitor at the clinical site, consult the owner's manual for specific information about that monitor. The information in Table 10-7 is a

summary of assembly instructions that should apply to most monitors.

Troubleshooting

The common problems in transcutaneous monitors that may require troubleshooting are summarized in Table 10-8.

End-Tidal CO_2 Monitors

Assembly

Assembly instructions for end-tidal CO_2 monitors are summarized in Table 10-9.

Troubleshooting

Common sources of problems to look for in troubleshooting are summarized in Table 10-10.

TABLE 10-6: Pulse Oximeter Troubleshooting

1. Patient site may be dirty. Clean the site with an alcohol prep pad.

2. Probe may be dirty. Clean the probe with an alcohol prep pad.

3. Cold extremities or poor perfusion may also affect signal strength and accuracy. Choosing an alternative site may help.

4. Motion artifact can also cause poor readings. Selection of an alternative site where motion is not as prevalent can help.

5. Probe may be misaligned. Check the probe placement and adjust it, or move it to a different site.

6. If the patient is wearing fingernail polish, remove it and reapply the probe.

7. If steps 1 through 4 have been checked and the oximeter is still not functioning, replace the probe.

8. As a final test, place the probe on your own finger to rule out cable/sensor problems.

9. If the room appears unusually bright (strong ambient light), shield the probe from the light using a towel or other covering.

TABLE 10-7: Transcutaneous Monitor Assembly

1. Connect the monitor to a 110 V 60 Hz electrical outlet.

2. Calibrate the monitor to known gas levels of O_2 (using sodium sulfite and room air), CO_2 (usually 5% and 10% CO_2) as recommended by the manufacturer.

3. Adjust the temperature setting to the desired range.

4. Select an appropriate site.

5. Place a drop of contact solution or distilled water onto the electrode and apply the electrode to the skin.

6. Allow the reading to stabilize and correlate the reading to blood gas values.

TABLE 10-8: Transcutaneous Monitor Troubleshooting

1. If readings fluctuate or differ greatly from arterial blood gases:
   a. The membrane may need to be changed.
   b. The site may need to be changed.
   c. The site may be too edematous.
   d. The patient may be receiving vasoactive drugs.
   e. An air leak may be present. Change the site and reapply the electrode to the patient.
   f. If the patient is a premature neonate, persistent or intermittent fetal circulation may compromise perfusion and subsequent transcutaneous CO_2 reading.

TABLE 10-9: End-Tidal CO_2 Monitor Assembly Instructions

1. Connect the monitor to a 110 V 60 Hz electrical outlet.

2. Calibrate the monitor to known CO_2 levels according to the manufacturer's instructions.

3. Connect the monitor to the patient's airway:
   a. Using the special adapter if using a sidestream monitor:
      (1) Adjust the sample flow until a plateau is seen on the capnograph.
   b. Directly to the airway if using a mainstream monitor.

4. Correlate the monitor's readings with ABG values.

TABLE 10-10: Tidal CO_2 Monitor Troubleshooting

1. If the readings vary significantly from blood gas values:
   a. Recalibrate the monitor.
   b. Clear the sampling tubing of moisture or secretions if using a sidestream monitor.
   c. Check the patient's history for indications of chronic obstructive lung disease, pulmonary embolism, left ventricular failure, or low perfusion (shock).

References

Allen, K. (2004). Principles and limitations of pulse oximetry in patient monitoring. *Nursing Times, 100*(41), 34–37.

Aloan, C. A. (1987). *Respiratory care of the newborn*. Philadelphia: Lippincott.

American Association for Respiratory Care. (1991). AARC clinical practice guideline: Pulse oximetry. *Respiratory Care, 36*(12), 1406–1409.

American Association for Respiratory Care. (2011). AARC clinical practice guideline: Capnography/capnometry during mechanical ventilation 2011. *Respiratory Care, 56*(4), 503–509.

American Association for Respiratory Care. (2004). AARC clinical practice guideline: Transcutaneous blood gas monitoring for neonatal & pediatric patients. *Respiratory Care, 49*(9), 1070–1072.

Craig, K. (1990, Summer). *Clinical performance limitations of pulse oximetry* (Progress Notes). Carlsbad, CA: Puritan Bennett Corporation.

Hess, D. (1990). Capnometry and capnography: Technical aspects, physiologic aspects, and clinical applications. *Respiratory Care, 35*(6), 557–576.

Martin, R. J. (1990). Transcutaneous monitoring: Instrumentation and clinical applications. *Respiratory Care, 35*(6), 577–583.

Practice Activities: Noninvasive Monitoring

1. Practice setting up and calibrating (if required) the following noninvasive monitors:
   a. Pulse oximeter
   b. Transcutaneous CO_2 or O_2 monitor
   c. End-tidal CO_2 monitor:
      (1) Mainstream
      (2) Sidestream

2. Practice applying noninvasive monitors to your laboratory partner:
   a. Pulse oximeter
   b. Transcutaneous CO_2 or O_2 monitor
   c. End-tidal CO_2 monitor:
      (1) Mainstream
      (2) Sidestream

3. Troubleshoot the monitors if they fail to function properly.

4. With your laboratory partner, deliberately attempt to make the noninvasive monitor give erroneous readings:

Pulse oximeter:
a. Apply nail polish to your partner.
b. Make the site dirty and apply the probe.
c. Misalign the emitter and detector when applying the probe.
d. Shine a strong light source on the probe when it is applied.

Transcutaneous monitor:
a. Create a small leak around the electrode's membrane.
b. Fail to calibrate the monitor before applying it.
c. Apply the electrode to a poorly perfused site.

End-tidal CO_2 monitor:
a. Fail to calibrate the monitor before applying it.
b. Adjust the sample chamber flow so it is too low.
c. Disconnect the probe to simulate an airway disconnection.

Check List: Pulse Oximeter Monitor

_____ 1. Verify the physician's order for a monitor.
_____ 2. Wash your hands.
3. Obtain the appropriate equipment as required:
_____   a. Pulse oximeter
_____   b. Probe(s)
_____   c. Alcohol prep pads
_____ 4. Explain the procedure to the patient.

_____ 5. Connect the power cord to a 110 V 60 Hz electrical outlet.
6. Connect the oximeter probe to the monitor:
_____   a. Finger probe
_____   b. Ear probe
       c. Pediatric probe

_____ 7. Turn on the power switch.

_____ 8. Wipe the probe clean using an alcohol prep pad before applying it to the patient.

9. Apply the probe to the patient:

_____   a. Finger

_____   b. Toe

_____   c. Ear

_____   d. Foot (infant or pediatric patient)

_____ 10. Observe for adequate waveforms (pulse signal) and reading.

_____ 11. Set alarm limits as required.

_____ 12. Remove any supplies from the patient's room and clean up the area.

_____ 13. Document the procedure and initial readings in the patient's chart.

Check List: Transcutaneous CO_2 and O_2 Monitoring

_____ 1. Verify the physician's order for transcutaneous monitoring.

_____ 2. Wash your hands.

_____ 3. Explain the procedure to the patient or the patient's family (infants).

_____ 4. Connect the monitor to a 110 V 60 Hz electrical outlet.

_____ 5. Calibrate the monitor to known gas levels of O_2 (using sodium sulfite and room air) and of CO_2 (usually 5% and 10% CO_2) as recommended by the manufacturer.

_____ 6. Attach a membrane to the electrode, following the manufacturer's guidelines.

_____ 7. Adjust the temperature setting to the desired range.

_____ 8. Select an appropriate site and prep the site with a clean alcohol prep pad.

_____ 9. Apply a ring of double-sided tape to the electrode.

_____ 10. Place a drop of contact solution or distilled water onto the electrode and apply the electrode to the skin.

_____ 11. Allow the reading to stabilize and correlate the reading with blood gas values.

_____ 12. Clean up the patient's area, removing all disposable supplies.

_____ 13. Document the procedure in the patient's chart, including initial readings.

Check List: End-Tidal CO_2 Monitoring

_____ 1. Verify the physician's order for an end-tidal CO_2 monitor.

_____ 2. Wash your hands.

3. Assemble the appropriate equipment required:

_____   a. End-tidal CO_2 monitor

_____   b. Mainstream or sidestream probe

_____   c. Calibration gases

_____ 4. Explain the procedure to the patient.

_____ 5. Connect the monitor to a 100 V 60 Hz electrical outlet.

_____ 6. Calibrate the monitor to known CO_2 levels according to the manufacturer's instructions.

7. Connect the monitor to the patient's airway:

  a. Use the special adapter if using a sidestream monitor.

_____   (1) Adjust the sample flow until a plateau is seen on the capnograph.

_____   b. Connect directly to the airway if using a mainstream monitor.

_____ 8. Correlate the monitor's readings with ABG values.

_____ 9. Clean up the patient's area, removing all supplies.

_____ 10. Document the procedure in the patient's chart, including the initial readings.

Self-Evaluation Post Test: Noninvasive Monitoring

1. Which of the following instruments is able to measure hemoglobin saturation?
   a. Pulse oximeter
   b. Transcutaneous monitor
   c. Oxygen analyzer
   d. Arterial blood gas analyzer

2. Which of the following instruments measures the partial pressures of oxygen and carbon dioxide noninvasively?
   a. Pulse oximeter
   b. Transcutaneous monitor
   c. Oxygen analyzer
   d. Arterial blood gas analyzer

3. What is the purpose of the heater on the transcutaneous electrode?
   a. It warms the blood before sampling.
   b. It increases perfusion by arterializing the capillary bed.
   c. It improves patient comfort.
   d. It is needed to correct the readings to body temperature.

4. You are setting up an end-tidal CO_2 monitor on a pediatric patient who is intubated and on a ventilator. You are concerned regarding the security of the endotracheal tube and the traction the monitor might place on it. What end-tidal CO_2 monitor might be best in this situation?
   a. Mainstream
   b. Sidestream

5. You are evaluating a patient in the emergency department who was admitted following a motor vehicle accident. The patient's extremities are very cold, and the patient is demonstrating signs and symptoms of shock. The pulse oximeter shows an SpO_2 of 78% and a heart rate of 52 beats per minute, yet the cardiac monitor shows a heart rate of 125 beats per minute. Why is there such a discrepancy between the two heart rates?
   a. The cardiac monitor always reads higher than the pulse oximeter.
   b. They are different because they are measured differently.
   c. The pulse oximeter is not reading accurately because of poor perfusion.
   d. The pulse oximeter is accurate and the cardiac monitor is not.

6. You are called to assess a pediatric patient who is being monitored via pulse oximetry. The nurse is concerned that the patient's saturation is low with activation of the oximeter alarm. When you initially observe the patient, you observe a very active 18-month-old boy who is squirming about his crib with abandon. Which of the following would account for the low reading and alarm condition?
   a. The saturation is low because of the increased patient activity.
   b. The saturation is low because activity increases perfusion.
   c. The saturation is low because the mist tent is powered by room air.
   d. Patient motion is causing artifact.

7. How does an end-tidal CO_2 monitor measure the tension of the exhaled CO_2?
   a. It uses infrared light absorption.
   b. It uses photospectrometry.
   c. It uses a CO_2 electrode similar to that of a blood gas analyzer.
   d. It relies on a chemical change to occur.

8. Which of the following is a hazard/are hazards of pulse oximetry?
   I.   Skin burns
   II. Pressure necrosis
   III. Airway occlusion
   a. I   c. II, III
   b. I, II   d. I, II, III

9. Which of the following is a hazard/are hazards of transcutaneous monitoring?
   I.   Skin burns
   II. Pressure necrosis
   III. Airway occlusion
   a. I   c. II, III
   b. I, II   d. I, II, III

10. Which of the following is a hazard/are hazards of end-tidal CO_2 monitoring?
   I.   Skin burns
   II. Pressure necrosis
   III. Airway occlusion
   a. I   c. III
   b. II   d. II, III

PERFORMANCE EVALUATION:
Pulse Oximeter Monitoring

Date: Lab _____ Clinical _____ Agency _____

Lab: Pass _____ Fail _____ Clinical: Pass _____ Fail _____

Student name _____ Instructor name _____

No. of times observed in clinical _____

No. of times practiced in clinical _____

PASSING CRITERIA: Obtain 90% or better on the procedure. Tasks indicated by * must receive at least 1 point, or the evaluation is terminated. Procedure must be performed within the designated time, or the performance receives a failing grade.

SCORING:
2 points — Task performed satisfactorily without prompting.
1 point — Task performed satisfactorily with self-initiated correction.
0 points — Task performed incorrectly or with prompting required.
NA — Task not applicable to the patient care situation.

Tasks:	Peer	Lab	Clinical
* **1.** Verifies the physician's order for a monitor	☐	☐	☐
* **2.** Performs hand hygiene	☐	☐	☐
* **3.** Obtains the appropriate equipment as required			
a. Pulse oximeter	☐	☐	☐
b. Probe(s)	☐	☐	☐
c. Alcohol prep pads	☐	☐	☐
4. Explains the procedure to the patient	☐	☐	☐
* **5.** Connects the power cord to a 110 V 60 Hz electrical outlet	☐	☐	☐
* **6.** Connects the oximeter probe to the monitor			
a. Finger probe	☐	☐	☐
b. Ear probe	☐	☐	☐
c. Pediatric probe	☐	☐	☐
* **7.** Turns on the power switch	☐	☐	☐
* **8.** Wipes the probe clean using an alcohol prep pad prior to applying it to the patient	☐	☐	☐
* **9.** Applies the probe			
a. Finger	☐	☐	☐
b. Toe	☐	☐	☐

c. Ear

☐ ☐ ☐

d. Foot (infant or pediatric patient)

☐ ☐ ☐

* **10.** Observes for adequate waveforms (pulse signal) and reading

☐ ☐ ☐

* **11.** Sets alarm limits as required

☐ ☐ ☐

12. Removes any supplies from the patient room and cleans up the area

☐ ☐ ☐

* **13.** Documents the procedure and initial readings in the patient's chart

☐ ☐ ☐

SCORE:　　　　Peer　＿＿＿＿＿ points of possible 40; ＿＿＿＿＿%

Lab　＿＿＿＿＿ points of possible 40; ＿＿＿＿＿%

Clinical ＿＿＿＿＿ points of possible 40; ＿＿＿＿＿%

TIME: ＿＿＿＿＿ out of possible 30 minutes

STUDENT SIGNATURES

PEER: ＿＿＿＿＿＿＿＿＿＿＿＿＿＿＿＿＿＿＿＿＿＿＿

STUDENT: ＿＿＿＿＿＿＿＿＿＿＿＿＿＿＿＿＿＿＿＿＿

INSTRUCTOR SIGNATURES

LAB: ＿＿＿＿＿＿＿＿＿＿＿＿＿＿＿＿＿＿＿＿＿＿＿

CLINICAL: ＿＿＿＿＿＿＿＿＿＿＿＿＿＿＿＿＿＿＿＿

PERFORMANCE EVALUATION:
Transcutaneous Monitoring

Date: Lab _____ Clinical _____ Agency _____

Lab: Pass _____ Fail _____ Clinical: Pass _____ Fail _____

Student name _____ Instructor name _____

No. of times observed in clinical _____

No. of times practiced in clinical _____

PASSING CRITERIA: Obtain 90% or better on the procedure. Tasks indicated by * must receive at least 1 point, or the evaluation is terminated. Procedure must be performed within the designated time, or the performance receives a failing grade.

SCORING: 2 points — Task performed satisfactorily without prompting.
1 point — Task performed satisfactorily with self-initiated correction.
0 points — Task performed incorrectly or with prompting required.
NA — Task not applicable to the patient care situation.

Tasks:

		Peer	Lab	Clinical
*	1. Verifies the physician's order	☐	☐	☐
*	2. Performs hand hygiene	☐	☐	☐
	3. Explains the procedure to the patient or family members	☐	☐	☐
*	4. Connects the monitor to a 110 V 60 Hz electrical outlet	☐	☐	☐
*	5. Calibrates the monitor	☐	☐	☐
*	6. Attaches a membrane to the electrode	☐	☐	☐
*	7. Adjusts the temperature setting to the desired range	☐	☐	☐
*	8. Selects an appropriate site and prepares it	☐	☐	☐
*	9. Applies a ring of double-sided tape to the electrode	☐	☐	☐
*	10. Places a drop of contact solution or distilled water onto the electrode and applies it	☐	☐	☐
*	11. Allows the reading to stabilize and correlates it with ABG values	☐	☐	☐
	12. Cleans up the patient's area, removing all supplies	☐	☐	☐
*	13. Documents the procedure in the patient's chart	☐	☐	☐

SCORE: Peer _____ points of possible 26; _____%

                    Lab _____ points of possible 26; _____%

                    Clinical _____ points of possible 26; _____%

TIME: _____ out of possible 30 minutes

STUDENT SIGNATURES   **INSTRUCTOR SIGNATURES**

PEER: _____   LAB: _____

STUDENT: _____   CLINICAL: _____

PERFORMANCE EVALUATION:
End-Tidal Monitoring

Date: Lab _____ Clinical _____ Agency _____

Lab: Pass _____ Fail _____ Clinical: Pass _____ Fail _____

Student name _____ Instructor name _____

No. of times observed in clinical _____

No. of times practiced in clinical _____

PASSING CRITERIA: Obtain 90% or better on the procedure. Tasks indicated by * must receive at least 1 point, or the evaluation is terminated. Procedure must be performed within the designated time, or the performance receives a failing grade.

SCORING:
2 points — Task performed satisfactorily without prompting.
1 point — Task performed satisfactorily with self-initiated correction.
0 points — Task performed incorrectly or with prompting required.
NA — Task not applicable to the patient care situation.

Tasks:	Peer	Lab	Clinical
* 1. Verifies the physician's order for an end-tidal monitor	☐	☐	☐
* 2. Performs hand hygiene	☐	☐	☐
* 3. Obtains the appropriate equipment as required			
a. End-tidal monitor	☐	☐	☐
b. Probes or adapters	☐	☐	☐
c. Calibration gases	☐	☐	☐
4. Introduces self and explains the procedure to the patient	☐	☐	☐
* 5. Connects the monitor to a 100 V 60 Hz electrical outlet	☐	☐	☐
* 6. Calibrates the monitor to known CO_2 levels according to the manufacturer's instructions	☐	☐	☐
* 7. Connects the monitor to the patient's airway			
a. Using the special adapter (sidestream monitor)	☐	☐	☐
(1) Adjusts the sample flow until a plateau is seen on the capnograph	☐	☐	☐
b. Directly to the airway (mainstream monitor)	☐	☐	☐
* 8. Correlates the monitor's readings with ABG values	☐	☐	☐
9. Cleans up the patient's area	☐	☐	☐
* 10. Documents the procedure and the initial readings in the patient's chart	☐	☐	☐

SCORE: Peer _____ points of possible 40; _____%

Lab   _____ points of possible 40; _____%

Clinical _____ points of possible 40; _____%

TIME: _____ out of possible 30 minutes

STUDENT SIGNATURES   **INSTRUCTOR SIGNATURES**

PEER: _____   LAB: _____

STUDENT: _____   CLINICAL: _____

SECTION 2
Therapeutics

CHAPTER 11
Documentation and Goals
Assessment

INTRODUCTION

Documentation is an important part of patient care. Documentation is synonymous with care itself (Castonguay, 2001). Legally, if an event is not documented in the patient's medical record, it was not done. The medical record provides an exact sequential record of the patient's condition, illness, and treatment. The medical record is the common source on a given patient referred to by all health care professionals, including physicians, respiratory practitioners, nurses, physical and occupational therapists, and other allied health practitioners. This record is the one place where nearly all pertinent medical information on a patient is recorded and accessible to all health care professionals caring for that patient.

Assessment(s), treatment(s), procedure(s), and test(s) are all recorded in the patient's medical record. This documentation must be timely, factual, and complete. The medical record serves as legal proof of the nature of care, quality of care, and timeliness of care. The hospital may use the medical record for risk management, reimbursement purposes, continuous quality improvement, case management, or research purposes. Documentation is an important part of patient care. Therefore, the accuracy and completeness of entries are important in the total care of the patient.

Goals assessment is another important part of patient care. Goals are measurable, demonstrated outcomes that can be assessed following patient treatment or intervention. The purpose of the respiratory practitioner's working with a patient is to improve the patient's cardiopulmonary health and quality of life. Specific goals in reference to oxygenation, ventilation, bronchial hygiene, or other interventions may be determined and assessed before and following treatment. The Joint Commission stresses the integration of interdisciplinary teams in the care of the patient (The Joint Commission, 2001). As such, goals assessment and determination are shared among the health care team members collaboratively, mutually benefiting the patient's care. As such, goals and their attainment for each discipline must be documented in the patient's medical record (The Joint Commission, 2001).

KEY TERMS

- **Charting by exception**
- **Clinical goal**
- **Graphic record**

- **HEENT**
- **Objective data**
- **Physician's orders**

- **Progress notes**
- **Subjective data**

THEORY OBJECTIVES

At the end of this chapter, the reader should be able to:

- *Describe the purpose of the medical record.*
- *Describe the components of the medical record.*
- *Discuss the importance of the medical record for legal and reimbursement purposes.*
- *Describe the contents of a complete medical record entry.*
- *Discuss the procedure of charting by exception.*

- *Define a goal or outcome in reference to:*
  - *Oxygenation*
  - *Ventilation*
  - *Bronchial hygiene*
  - *Hyperinflation*
- *Discuss medical record documentation using computer technology.*

THE MEDICAL RECORD

The medical record is a compilation of pertinent facts of a patient's life and health history, illness(es), and treatment(s) written by health care professionals who have contributed to the care of that patient (Huffman, 1994). The purpose of the medical record is to provide a written source of information regarding that patient's health, conditions, and treatments, providing a common source of information for all caregivers. The medical record is the one definitive source referenced by all caregivers about a patient. Because the medical record is such an important source of information, all entries must be clear, concise, and factual.

The medical record is also a legal document. Evidence from the medical record may be entered into a court of law as evidence or as supporting evidence. The entries in a patient's medical record may determine if care was appropriate, timely, and delivered in a competent manner. Therefore, falsification or deletion of information in a patient's medical record can result in legal action against the person or institution altering or destroying the record.

Entries in the patient's medical record are chronologic. Entries begin from the first time the patient is seen or hospitalized and progress from there. Each entry has a date and time, indicating what was assessed, given (medications), or performed (tests or therapies). Because the medical record is chronologic, the practitioner needs to make entries as soon as practicable after working with the patient or giving medications. Timeliness is important because many other health care providers may depend on the entries to provide them with information regarding the patient's status.

Components of the Medical Record

The medical record is organized into several broad content areas. Each area is identified using tabs, color dividers, or other face sheets so that each section may be readily identified and located. Typically, in the acute care (hospital) setting, the medical record is divided into the admission record, physician's orders, progress notes, medical history and physical examination and consultation records, nursing data, graphic record, laboratory reports, imaging reports, operative data, medication administration record, ancillary services, and discharge plan.

Admission Record

The admission record states the date and time the patient was admitted to the acute care facility. The patient's name, birth date, address, Social Security number, telephone number(s), and next of kin are recorded on this form. Insurance information and policy numbers are also recorded on the admission record. The patient's diagnosis must be written out in full without abbreviations. The patient's attending physician is responsible for authenticating the admission diagnosis (Huffman, 1994).

Physician's Orders

Typically, *physician's orders* follow the admission record, proceeding from the front to the back of the medical record. All orders must contain the date and time, the order(s), and the physician's signature. Verbal or telephone orders on hospital admission are typically accepted and countersigned at a later time (The Joint Commission standards specify within 24 hours) when the attending physician first visits the patient in the acute care setting. Each subsequent order follows the initial one in chronologic order. All orders must be signed and dated by the attending or consulting physician(s), including all verbal and telephone orders. New standards may require the time the order was written to also be indicated.

All orders must be clearly printed and not written using cursive. The goal is to achieve legibility, a clear understanding of what is needed with no misunderstandings. Neatness and clarity are the operative points when writing orders. The goal is to prevent mistakes when writing any order on a patient's medical record.

Progress Notes

Every time the patient is visited by a physician, *progress notes* are made in the medical record. Most physicians follow the SOAP (subjective, objective, assessment, plan) format when charting progress notes.

Information provided to the physician by the patient constitutes *subjective data*. When asked specific questions the patient responds, indicating discomfort, dysfunction, pain, and so on. Sometimes patient responses are quite specific and helpful, whereas at other times only vague responses are possible.

Information that is obtained directly constitutes *objective data*. For example, vital signs, breath sounds, jugular venous distention, heart tones, oxygen saturation (SpO_2), bowel sounds, and edema can all be directly assessed and noted.

Assessment is the physician's interpretation of the subjective and objective information. Additional diagnoses or progress may be indicated in this section. For example, "SpO_2 85% on room air," "lung fields remain consolidated," and "temperature within normal limits" all are assessments of the data obtained.

The planning section denotes how the patient will be treated to help resolve some of the continuing problems. Documented plans might include the following: "continue low-flow oxygen for SpO_2 >90%," "continue hyperinflation therapy," and "discontinue IV antibiotics and switch to oral meds."

Physiology and pathophysiology are both dynamic processes. Rarely does a patient go from one moment to the next without a change in some physiologic process. The progress record allows the physician to assess the patient's response to treatment over time and to track the patient's general progress toward wellness.

History and Physical Examination and Consultation Examinations

The patient's history and physical examination are dictated by the attending physician. If the patient is able to communicate, the history may take up to 30 or 40 minutes to obtain. If the patient is unable to communicate, family members or others who are able to relate the facts accurately are solicited for the information.

The initial physical examination is performed by the attending physician. The physical examination includes a head-to-toe assessment of all major organ systems. Included are head, eyes, ears, nose, and throat (*HEENT*) and respiratory, neurologic, musculoskeletal, cardiovascular, gastrointestinal, genitourinary, endocrine, hematologic, and psychosocial assessments. A thorough physical examination may require an additional 20 to 30 minutes to complete.

Any consultations are recorded by the consulting physician (such as a cardiologist or pulmonologist) reporting the patient's history and findings on physical examination. These consultation notes follow chronologically the admission history and physical findings.

Included at the conclusion of each history and physical section is usually a section for assessment—listing diagnosis(es)—and planning. Each potential diagnosis is determined and an initial plan for treatment is specified.

Nursing Data

Nursing data include nursing notes (similar to physician progress notes), nursing assessment records, and nursing teaching records. Usually included in this section are the multidisciplinary plan forms.

The multidisciplinary plan forms are goals or outcomes determined by nursing and other ancillary services (respiratory care, physical therapy, occupational therapy, speech therapy, and so on) for that patient. Each outcome must be measurable, and for each outcome, a treatment or plan to attain it must be specified. Once the outcome or goal is achieved, the date and measured assessment are recorded.

Graphic Record

The *graphic record* contains temperature, pulse, respiration, blood pressure, urine output, oral intake (fluids), and daily weights. The graphic record may be updated as frequently as hourly or as infrequently as every 8 hours in the acute care setting, depending on the patient's acuity level (how ill the patient is).

Laboratory Reports

The laboratory report section includes hematology, chemistry, microbiology, histology, and endocrinology reports. Results of arterial blood gas (ABG) analyses are also typically included in this section.

Imaging Reports

The imaging reports section includes radiographic studies, computed tomography (CT) scans, magnetic resonance imaging (MRI) scans, ultrasound, and other imaging reports. The respiratory practitioner will find that the imaging report (dictated by a radiologist) as well as viewing the actual films (scans) is an important part of patient assessment.

Operative Data

The operative data section includes operative consent(s), operative reports, and anesthesia and postanesthesia records. The operative consent form(s) are signed by the patient or the patient's legal representative and witnessed by a member of the acute care organization's staff (physician or nurse). The operative report is dictated by the surgeon describing the procedure, what was found, and what surgical therapy was performed. The anesthesia/postanesthesia record indicates the anesthetic agent(s) used and the patient's vital signs during and following surgery. In this section some forms are for the physician's use, others for nursing staff, and others may be used by allied health professionals.

Medication Administration Record

The medication administration record provides a chronology of the medications given to the patient, quantity, dosage, route, and date and time of administration. This information is important in the assessment of the patient's response to medical therapy and any adverse reactions that may occur as a result.

Ancillary Services

The ancillary services section is reserved for services such as respiratory care, physical therapy, speech therapy, occupational therapy, and other ancillary services. Various forms (charting by exception), narratives (progress notes), and goal/outcome measure sheets are used by the various ancillary services to denote medical treatments, therapies, or other interventions. Specific respiratory care documentation is discussed in a later section of this chapter.

Discharge Plan

The discharge plan denotes the patient's condition and date and time of discharge. Any prescribed medication(s) and patient teaching for medication administration are documented on this form. The person receiving or accompanying the patient on discharge may also be indicated. If a discharge record is not complete, the patient may have signed out of the facility against medical advice (AMA).

The Medical Record: Legal and Reimbursement Issues

Legal

As stated previously, the medical record is considered a legal document. A patient's medical record may be submitted in court as evidence. Based on the entries in the medical record, the care provided for that patient, including medication, therapies, timeliness of treatment, appropriateness of care, and quality of care, are determined in the court of law. The medical record is the single best source of information regarding the care and treatment of a patient—even though it may have been years since the patient was last admitted or discharged. When making entries in the medical record the respiratory practitioner should imagine trying to reconstruct what was performed based on the documentation.

Because of the legal nature of the medical record, falsification of its contents may result in legal action. Concealment of an incident, attempting to protect oneself or the acute care institution, falsifying data (such as vital signs, ventilator settings, or oxygen concentrations), and intentional deceit (charting something that was not performed) all are forms of falsification. What is documented must be concise, accurate, and truthful. Documentation in any other way is not acceptable and may be punishable in a court of law.

Reimbursement

The medical record is used by third-party payers (such as Medicare, Medicaid, or insurance companies) for purposes of reimbursement. Patients' medical records are periodically audited, verifying that what the acute care institution billed corresponds to what is documented in the medical record. Failure to document activities accurately may result in loss of significant reimbursement. Remember that if it is not documented, it was not performed and, therefore, may not be billable or reimbursed for payment.

The Medical Record Entry

Accuracy, timeliness, and truthfulness all are important when documenting in the patient's medical record. However, for optimal charting, ask the following question: "Of everything performed, what is important to chart?" The medical record entry should include the date and time the event occurred, the practitioner's assessment of the patient, what was done, what technique was employed (including medications administered and dosages when applicable), the length of time spent with the patient, the patient's response (results of what was done), and any special circumstances (unique to the interaction).

The date and time of interaction with the patient and provided respiratory care services should be documented in the entry. The practitioner should never document anything merely in anticipation of doing it; what happens if the practitioner is called away and is unable to return? Document only what *has* been performed, not what is intended to be performed. Time can be important in administering medications. Some medications may not be given too frequently; therefore, the time of administration of the last dosage is important.

The practitioner's assessment of the patient is important. Document vital signs (heart rate, respiratory rate, blood pressure), patient appearance or inspection, breath sounds, oxygen saturation (SpO_2), and specifics of oxygen administration, including the device and flow rate or concentration (if the patient is on supplemental oxygen). Often other health care professionals make determinations based on the respiratory practitioner's assessment (home oxygen, supplemental oxygen for exercise or ambulation, and so on).

Document any therapies performed on the patient (aerosol, oxygen, chest physiotherapy [CPT], and so on) and medications administered, including dosage (in mg or other units as appropriate) and diluents (normal saline, sterile water, etc.). Besides the therapy performed, include what techniques or methods were employed (manual or mechanical percussion, for example). The amount of time spent with the patient should also be documented in the patient's medical record.

The patient's response to therapies may be documented both subjectively and objectively. Subjectively, the patient may state that breathing is easier (less work of breathing), or that his or her chest does not feel as tight. Objectively, the practitioner can assess changes in breath sounds, vital signs (heart rate, respiratory rate, blood pressure), SpO_2 changes, or bedside pulmonary function testing (changes in forced vital capacity [FVC] or in forced expiratory volume in 1 second [FEV_1]). The patient's response is important to document. If the practitioner cannot prove that the desired goal has been accomplished, why be there?

Unique or special circumstances may include adverse reactions, complaints by the patient about the taste of medications, incorrect oxygen settings, and so on. Document how the patient was found (e.g., on oxygen therapy or SpO_2 assessment) and document the patient's state upon leaving.

One important part of the medical record entry is both the practitioner's initials (first and last) and signature followed by the practitioner's professional credentials (such as CRT or RRT). Most medical records have a signature log at the front of the chart (Figure 11-1) or at the bottom of that particular form. Each day when entries are made in the medical record, the person making the entry records his or her initials and signature in full, department or service area, and then printed name and credentials. The signature sheet clearly identifies each person making entries into the medical record.

Charting by Exception

Charting by exception is a method of charting, usually employing fill-in-the-blank forms where only data that change are documented (Figure 11-2). Charting by exception can save considerable time in documentation in the medical record (Short, 1997). Often arrows or other symbols are used to denote that nothing for that data point has changed (see Figure 11-2). Most charting by exception forms allow space for brief narratives, supplied if something significant or unusual occurs. Spaces for the date and time of the occurrence are provided.

GOALS ASSESSMENT AND DOCUMENTATION

Clinical goals are measurable outcomes the patient is expected to achieve following the intervention of a health care practitioner. Every procedure performed should have a desired outcome in which the patient's condition or quality of life can show demonstrated improvement. Clinical goals should be objective measures, rather than subjective as provided by the patient. Documentation of objective

STAFF SIGNATURE SHEET
★PERMANENT CHART FORM. DO NOT DISCARD★

Staff responsible for documentation in this patient's record must record their Initials, Signature, Title, their **PRINTED NAME** and the Date on this form when the first entry is made anywhere in the chart. Entries on individual chart forms may be identified with initials unless form directs otherwise.

DATE	INI	SIGNATURE, TITLE	DEPT.	PRINT NAME

(Addressograph)	**STAFF SIGNATURE SHEET**

Figure 11-1 An example of a signature sheet, documenting all who have made entries into the medical record by date

#	ASSESSMENT/ORDER/ TREATMENT	✓= NORMAL *SIGNIFICANT FINDINGS/COMMENTS						→ = NO CHANGE FROM PREVIOUS*						
1	INHALED MED. PROTOCOL: *Assessment/Reassessment (See Resp. Therapy Assessment Record)													
2	THERAPY MODE: I = IPPB S = SVN M = MDI R = return demonstration from patient with reinforcement/cues Other: _____													
3	MED.:													
4	MED.:													
5	MED.:													
6	HEART RATE PRE:													
	POST:													
7	RESP RATE PRE:													
	POST:													
8	BREATH SOUNDS													
9	VISCOSITY: AMOUNT/COLOR CL = clear; WH = white; GY = grey; B = brown; R = red; Y = yellow; GR = green													
10	O_2 MODE/LITER FLOW*													
11	XIMETRY %													
12	PATIENT EDUCATION: (See purple Multidisciplinary Care Plan—Part 2)													
	DATE													
	TIME													
	INITIALS													

#	DATE	TIME	*SIGNIFICANT FINDINGS/COMMENTS	INI

HM = heat mist;   HF = high flow;   NC = nasal cannula;   T = tent;   USN = ultrasonic nebulizer;   VM = ventimask;   NRB = non rebreather

INI	NAME/TITLE	INI	NAME/TITLE	INI	NAME/TITLE	INI	NAME/TITLE

© Cengage Learning 2013

Figure 11-2 An example of a form used that employs charting by exception. Note that only the data that have changed are documented using this type of form

clinical improvements is one way in which the allied health discipline of respiratory care can demonstrate the clinical benefit by being at the bedside, working with patients.

Oxygenation Goals

Oxygen therapy is indicated for patients with an SpO_2 of less than 90% or a PaO_2 of less than 60 mm Hg (American Association for Respiratory Care [AARC], 1991). Therefore, the clinical goal of oxygen therapy is to increase the SpO_2 to 90% or greater or to increase the partial pressure of oxygen in the arterial blood PaO_2 to 60 mm Hg or greater. The method and delivery device will be dependent on the patient's response to therapy. The desired outcome (ideally) is to reach an end point at which the patient may achieve the clinical goal (SpO_2, PaO_2) without supplemental oxygen (depending on the patient's pathophysiology). In many cases, the desired outcome may not be achieved (long-standing chronic obstructive pulmonary disease [COPD] or pulmonary disease), and the patient may be discharged from the facility on supplemental oxygen.

Ventilation Goals

The best indicator of ventilation is the partial pressure of carbon dioxide in the arterial blood $PaCO_2$ and secondarily the patient's pH. Ventilation goals are often expressed as maintenance of both $PaCO_2$ and pH levels within a specific range. For example, a goal may be to decrease the pressure support but maintain $PaCO_2$ at less than 60 mm Hg and pH at greater than 7.35. The ideal goal or outcome is to achieve the desired $PaCO_2$ and pH without ventilatory assistance (so that the patient is breathing spontaneously). In most patients, this outcome can be successfully met. Those patients in whom this clinical goal cannot be met may be discharged on ventilatory support, using home mechanical ventilators.

Another ventilation goal that is objective and measurable is reversal of atelectasis. Serial chest radiographs may be obtained to evaluate the effectiveness of hyperinflation therapy or chest physiotherapy (CPT). With resolution of atelectasis, ventilation also improves. Patients not receiving ventilatory support (mechanical ventilation) can benefit from adjunctive techniques with the goal of improving ventilation.

Bronchial Hygiene

The goals of bronchial hygiene include production of sputum following coughing, assessment of clinical improvement, improved subjective response, and stabilization of pulmonary hygiene with chronic pulmonary disease and a history of secretion retention (AARC, 1993). Bronchial hygiene techniques may include directed cough, airway aspiration (suctioning), CPT, positive expiratory pressure mask therapy, high-frequency chest wall oscillation (HFCWO), and incentive spirometry. Documentation of sputum production and of the amount, color, consistency, and odor is important. Changes in sputum may indicate the presence of a pulmonary infection, warranting culture and sensitivity testing. The desired clinical goal is for the patient to be able to maintain adequate bronchial hygiene (sputum production and expectoration) without intervention or assistance.

Hyperinflation Goals

Goals of hyperinflation therapy include improvement or reversal of atelectasis, improved vital signs, improved breath sounds, resolution of abnormalities on the chest radiograph, improved PaO_2, and increased vital capacity (VC) and FVC (AARC, 1991). Hyperinflation techniques may include breathing retraining, incentive spirometry, intermittent positive-pressure breathing (IPPB), intrapulmonary percussive ventilation (IPV), and intermittent continuous positive airway pressure (CPAP). Documentation of objective improvement, such as improvement in breath sounds, PaO_2, VC, FVC, and so on, is preferable to subjective assessments. Reversal or lessening of atelectasis may be documented through serial chest x-ray films and also by improvement in breath sounds heard over affected areas. As with other interventions, the ultimate goal is for the patient to maintain spontaneous ventilation without the need for adjunctive medications or intervention.

Computer-Aided Documentation

Computer-aided documentation and medical record keeping are currently in use throughout the world. Eventually, the majority of medical record documentation will be performed using computer technology. Many documentation programs are the fill-in-the-blank

PROFICIENCY OBJECTIVES

At the end of this chapter, the reader should be able to:

- Document a procedure in the medical record using concise, accurate, and descriptive language.
- Demonstrate the ability to use common abbreviations when documenting in the medical record.
- When documenting a procedure, include the following:
  - Date and time
  - Procedures/interventions performed and techniques used
  - The length of time spent with the patient
  - The patient's response
  - Any unusual circumstances or occurrences
  - Initials, signature, and credentials
- Demonstrate the ability to chart by exception.
- Given a therapeutic modality, identify two desirable measurable clinical outcomes.

variety, requiring the user to fill in data into specific fields before the program will allow progression to the next section.

Computer documentation has several advantages (Castonguay, 2001). Computer-aided documentation may improve quality and accuracy, keep the information more up to date, provide prompting for important (required) fields, promote legibility, and improve the availability of information. Once the practitioner becomes accustomed to the computer program, documentation may progress at a much faster pace, conserving time.

DOCUMENTATION GUIDELINES AND ABBREVIATIONS

Documentation of activities in the patient's medical record must be accurate, clear, and concise. The objective is not to write a novel but rather to provide enough information to the reader so that the activities may be accurately reconstructed. Remember that the medical record is a legal document. There always is a potential that at a later time, the practitioner may be on the witness stand, attempting to justify and defend his or her actions based on what was documented in the medical record!

Accuracy in documentation does not mean that it must be lengthy. Accepted abbreviations may be used to conserve space and reduce time. The operative words in documentation are *brevity* and *accuracy*. Common abbreviations are included in Table 11-1. The Joint Commission has adopted a list of abbreviations and symbols that should not be used when documenting in a patient's record (The Joint Commission, 2004). Those abbreviations and symbols are listed in Table 11-2.

Remembering all that occurs at the bedside is often a challenge. The patient, family members, physicians, and other health care professionals may provide distractions at the bedside. Carrying a small spiral notebook (3 × 5 inches) for recording pertinent data will facilitate remembering the patient's vital signs, saturations, breath sounds, and so on. If the practitioner is called away, there is a record of what was done and what was observed that will assist the practitioner in correct documentation later.

Every facility should have in its procedures manual a list of accepted abbreviations that may be used for documentation. What is accepted may vary depending on the facility and the region in which it is located. Therefore, it is important for the respiratory care practitioner to become familiar with all abbreviations used by the facility where the practitioner is employed.

Identification of the Medical Record

Before beginning documentation, the practitioner must correctly identify the patient's medical record. On the front cover or spine of the record are the patient's name

TABLE 11-1: Accepted Abbreviations for Medical Records	
ā	before
bid	twice a day
BS	breath sounds, blood sugar, bowel sounds
c̄	with
cc	cubic centimeters (same as milliliters)
C	Celsius
cm	centimeter
F	Fahrenheit
f̄	frequency
Fr, F	French
gt	drop
HR	heart rate
Hx	history
kg	kilogram
L/min	liters per minute
mg	milligram
mcg,-μg	microgram
p	after
prn	as needed
qh	every hour
q4h	every four hours (also q4 may be used)
qid	four times daily
RR	respiratory rate
Rx	prescription
s̄	without
stat	at once or immediately
tid	three times daily
Tx	treatment

(first and last), room number, and attending physician's name. By checking the cover sheet, the practitioner can verify the patient's full name and medical record number or hospital number, along with the patient's age and gender. Once the correct medical record has been identified, documentation may begin.

Documentation

Documentation in the patient's medical record needs to include date and time; what was performed; the length of time spent; the patient's response; any unusual circumstances; and the practitioner's initials, signature, and credentials. The format this documentation takes will be largely dependent on the type of charting used in the facility (narrative versus tabular versus charting by exception). Clear, concise, and accurate should be descriptors of the documentation.

TABLE 11-2: A "Minimum List" of Dangerous Abbreviations, Acronyms, and Symbols

ABBREVIATION, ACRONYM, OR SYMBOL	PREFERRED DOCUMENTATION
U	Write "unit"
IU	Write "international unit"
Q.D., Q.O.D.	Write "daily" and "every other day"
Trailing zero (i.e., X.0 mg)	Never write a zero by itself after a decimal point
	Always use a zero before a decimal point (i.e., 0.X mg)
MS, MSO$_4$, MgSO$_4$	Write "morphine sulfate" or "magnesium sulfate"
µg	Write "mcg" for microgram
H.S.	Write "half-strength" or "at bedtime"
T.I.W.	Write "3 times weekly" or "three times weekly"
S.C. or S.Q.	Write "Sub-Q", "subQ" or "subcutaneously"
D/C	Write "discharge"
c.c.	Write "ml" for milliliters
A.S., A.D., A.U.	Write "left ear," right ear," or "both ears"; "left eye," "right eye," or "both eyes"

Date and Time

The date and time of the event are important parts of the medical record entry. The date may be abbreviated (01/22/XX or Jan 22, 20XX). Military time (based on a 24-hour clock) is used in most facilities for periods following twelve o'clock noon until midnight. If the practitioner is not familiar with military time, inexpensive watches may be purchased that have both notations on the face of the watch, which may be of help until the practitioner becomes accustomed to it. The time should be documented in hours and minutes. For example, 9:32 PM is documented as 21:32.

What You Performed

This section should accurately describe what was done. This includes assessment of the patient (for heart rate, respiratory rate, breath sounds, SpO$_2$, inspection, and so on); any procedures or tests performed; and any medications given, including dosage (in mg or appropriate units), diluents used, and quantity (in mL). Be brief and concise in the narrative, describing precisely what was done using as few words as possible.

Length of Time

The length of time spent with the patient is also important. This documentation may be used for reimbursement purposes, for determination of patient acuity, or to determine the workload for the facility's respiratory care practitioners. This documentation should be accurate to the nearest minute.

Patient's Response

The patient's response to the procedure should reflect both subjective and objective information. Subjective information provided by the patient may be prefaced by the words "The patient states . . ." or "The patient states she feels . . ." to indicate the subjective nature of the information.

Objective data are measurable information that may provide evidence that clinical objectives are being met. This can include breath sounds, heart and respiratory rates, SpO$_2$, and other data. Documentation of objective criteria is important to validate the benefits of the time and effort spent with the patient. Reimbursement will be closely linked to achievement of objective criteria.

Unusual Circumstances

Documentation of unusual circumstances is also important. These might include adverse reactions or other occurrences that normally may not occur.

Initials and Signature

Each person making the entry in the patient record must be able to be clearly identified. Therefore, the practitioner's initials, full signature, and credentials must be indicated for each entry. Many medical record forms have fill-in-the-blank spaces for initials with spaces at the lower margin for initials followed by the full signature (see Figure 11-2). In addition to the requirement for signing and/or initialing each entry, a signature form may also be included as part of the medical record (see Figure 11-1).

Charting by Exception

Charting by exception is documentation of only items that change from what has been previously documented earlier in time. If the event or item has not changed, arrows, ditto marks, or other shorthand nomenclature may be used to indicate that the data are the same. Only when changes occur is information documented by indicating what changed and what time it changed. See Figure 11-2 for an example of a form using charting by exception.

Clinical Goals

Clinical goals are described in the previous section. It is important to understand the indications and outcomes for each procedure being performed. The AARC has published numerous research-based clinical practice guidelines for the majority of respiratory care modalities. These guidelines are available for purchase or on the AARC's Web site (http://www.aarc.org); many are included in this text. The respiratory care practitioner will find these clinical practice guidelines to be useful resources upon learning the desired clinical outcomes and what it is important to assess to determine if they have been met.

References

American Association for Respiratory Care. (1991). AARC clinical practice guideline: Incentive spirometry. *Respiratory Care*, *36*(12), 1402–1405.

American Association for Respiratory Care. (1993). AARC clinical practice guideline: Directed cough. *Respiratory Care*, *38*(5), 495–499.

Castonguay, D. (2001). Nursing documentation—how important is it? *Nursing News* (New Hampshire), *25*(1).

Huffman, E. K. (1994). *Health information management*. Berwyn, IL: Physicians' Record Company.

Short, M. (1997). Charting by exception on a clinical pathway. *Nurse Manager*, *28*(8), 45–46.

The Joint Commission. (2001). *Hospital accreditation standards*. Oakbrook Terrace, IL: Author.

The Joint Commission. (2004). *A "minimum list" of dangerous abbreviations, acronyms and symbols*. Oakbrook Terrace, IL: Author.

Practice Activities: Documentation

1. Practice the following skills using a laboratory partner:
   a. Auscultation of breath sounds
   b. Physical assessment of the chest
   c. Determination of vital signs
   Once you have completed the skills, document the procedure using a SOAP format.

2. Working together with a laboratory partner, teach the following skills:
   a. Incentive spirometry
   b. Use of a metered dose inhaler (with and without a spacer)
   Upon completion of the instruction, document the procedure.

3. Write three sentences using the following abbreviations:
   a. $\bar{a}$
   b. $\bar{p}$
   c. qid
   Ask a laboratory instructor to check your documentation for correct use of the abbreviations, clarity, and brevity.

4. Using Figure 11-2 as an example, practice charting by exception the information you charted in Practice Activity 1.

5. With a laboratory partner, identify two measurable clinical outcomes for the following modalities and discuss how to assess whether they are met.
   a. Incentive spirometry
   b. Oxygen delivery via nasal cannula
   c. Chest physiotherapy
   d. IPPB therapy

Check List: Documentation and Goals Assessment

_____ 1. Records pertinent information in a small notebook:
_____ a. Vital signs
_____ b. Breath sounds
_____ c. Oxygen saturation
_____ d. Type of therapy/test
_____ e. Medications administered
_____ f. Patient's response
_____ g. Any unusual circumstances

_____ 2. Identifies the patient's medical record:
_____ a. Matches the name
_____ b. Matches the attending physician's name
_____ c. Matches the room number
_____ 3. Identifies the correct section for documentation
_____ 4. Appropriately documents in the medical record:
_____ a. Date/time
_____ b. Patient assessment data

_____ c. Procedures/interventions performed, including technique
_____ d. Medications administered (dose and diluents)
_____ e. The patient's response

_____ f. Any unusual occurrences
_____ g. Signature and credentials
_____ 5. Returns the medical record to its proper location

Self-Evaluation Post Test: Documentation and Goals Assessment

1. Which of the following best describes the patient's medical record?
   a. A document containing subjective information
   b. The one best source of medical information about the patient
   c. A legal document
   d. b and c

2. Which of the following are components of the medical record?
   I. History and physical
   II. Laboratory reports
   III. Discharge summary
   IV. Progress notes
   a. I
   b. I, II
   c. I, II, III
   d. I, II, III, IV

3. Which of the following sections of the medical record are used most by physicians for documentation purposes?
   I. History and physical
   II. Laboratory reports
   III. Medication administration record
   IV. Progress notes
   a. I, II
   b. I, III
   c. II, III
   d. I, IV

4. Which of the following is/are important in documenting in a patient's medical record?
   I. Document only facts.
   II. Be brief.
   III. Use medical terminology.
   IV. Describe precisely what has occurred.
   a. I
   b. I, II
   c. I, II, III
   d. I, II, III, IV

5. The patient's medical record may be:
   a. taken home when the patient is discharged.
   b. used as evidence in a court of law.
   c. falsified to protect the institution caring for the patient.
   d. destroyed on the patient's discharge.

6. Which of the following constitute objective data?
   I. Heart rate
   II. A patient's complaint of dyspnea
   III. Breath sounds
   IV. The patient's statement "I feel crummy"
   a. I, II
   b. I, III
   c. II, III
   d. II, IV

7. Which of the following constitute subjective data?
   I. Heart rate
   II. A patient's complaint of dyspnea
   III. Breath sounds
   IV. The patient's statement "I feel crummy"
   a. I, II
   b. I, III
   c. II, III
   d. II, IV

8. Charting by exception is best described as:
   a. documenting everything that occurs using a narrative style.
   b. documenting only what remains the same.
   c. documenting the data that change.
   d. using computer-aided charting methods.

9. The respiratory practitioner is administering oxygen via nasal cannula at 3 L/min. What are appropriate clinical goals?
   I. Oxygen saturation of >90%
   II. A normal $PaCO_2$
   III. A PaO_2 of >60 mm Hg
   IV. An increased vital capacity
   a. I, II
   b. I, III
   c. I, IV
   d. II, III

10. The physician requests the respiratory practitioner to begin a bronchial hygiene protocol. What are the expected clinical outcomes of this protocol?
    I. Evidence of sputum production
    II. Patient's subjective improvement
    III. Stabilization of pulmonary hygiene in chronic pulmonary disease
    IV. Clinical observation of improvement
    a. I
    b. I, II
    c. I, II, III
    d. I, II, III, IV

PERFORMANCE EVALUATION:
Documentation and Goals Assessment

Date: Lab _____ Clinical _____ Agency _____

Lab: Pass _____ Fail _____ Clinical: Pass _____ Fail _____

Student name _____ Instructor name _____

No. of times observed in clinical _____

No. of times practiced in clinical _____

PASSING CRITERIA: Obtain 90% or better on the procedure. Tasks indicated by * must receive at least 1 point, or the evaluation is terminated. Procedure must be performed within the designated time, or the performance receives a failing grade.

SCORING:
2 points — Task performed satisfactorily without prompting.
1 point — Task performed satisfactorily with self-initiated correction.
0 points — Task performed incorrectly or with prompting required.
NA — Task not applicable to the patient care situation.

Tasks:	Peer	Lab	Clinical
* **1.** Records pertinent information in a small notebook			
a. Vital signs	☐	☐	☐
b. Breath sounds	☐	☐	☐
c. Oxygen saturation	☐	☐	☐
d. Type of therapy/test	☐	☐	☐
e. Medications administered	☐	☐	☐
f. Patient's response	☐	☐	☐
g. Any unusual circumstances	☐	☐	☐
* **2.** Identifies the patient's medical record			
a. Matches the name	☐	☐	☐
b. Matches the attending physician's name	☐	☐	☐
c. Matches the room number	☐	☐	☐
* **3.** Identifies the correct section for documentation	☐	☐	☐
* **4.** Appropriately documents in the medical record			
a. Date/time	☐	☐	☐
b. Patient assessment data	☐	☐	☐
c. Procedures/interventions performed, including technique	☐	☐	☐
d. Medications administered (dose and diluents)	☐	☐	☐

    e. The patient's response ☐ ☐ ☐

    f. Any unusual occurrences ☐ ☐ ☐

    g. Signature and credentials ☐ ☐ ☐

* **5.** Returns the medical record to its proper place ☐ ☐ ☐

SCORE: Peer   _____ points of possible 40; _____%

                 Lab   _____ points of possible 40; _____%

                 Clinical _____ points of possible 40; _____%

TIME: _____ out of possible 15 minutes

STUDENT SIGNATURES   **INSTRUCTOR SIGNATURES**

PEER: _____   LAB: _____

STUDENT: _____   CLINICAL: _____

CHAPTER 12
Oxygen Supply Systems

INTRODUCTION

The respiratory care practitioner will be expected to know how to safely use the various medical gas supply systems available in an institution. These supply systems include medical gas cylinders, medical gas piping systems, liquid systems, and oxygen concentrators.

When used appropriately, these systems are safe and effective. If mishandled, they can be potentially lethal.

In this chapter, the theory of how the systems are constructed, principles of operation, and safety features are discussed. Following this is a section covering the procedure for using the supply systems.

KEY TERMS

- Air/oxygen blender
- American Standard Safety System (ASSS)
- Cracking
- Diameter-indexed safety system (DISS)
- Downstream
- Flowmeter
- Hydrostatic testing
- Oxygen concentrator
- Pin index safety system (PISS)
- Preset reducing valve
- Reducing valve
- Riser
- Spontaneous combustion
- Station outlet
- Tank factor
- Upstream
- Zone valve

THEORY OBJECTIVES

At the end of this chapter, the reader should be able to:

Medical Gas Cylinders

- *Identify the contents of a medical gas cylinder using the United States and International color code system, and the label for the following gases or gas mixtures:*
  - *Air*
  - *Oxygen*
  - *Nitrogen*
  - *Nitrous oxide*
  - *Helium*
  - *Helium/oxygen mixtures*
  - *Carbon dioxide*
  - *Carbon dioxide/oxygen mixtures*
- *Interpret the following data for a full "E" and "H/K" oxygen cylinder:*
  - *Gauge pressure when full*
  - *Contents in liters*
  - *Contents in cubic feet*
- *Describe the two main types of valves found on "E" and "H/K" medical gas cylinders. Identify and describe the function of the following parts:*
  - *Stem*
  - *Outlet*

- *Safety features*
- *Valve plunger*
- *Valve seat*
- *Gas entrance channel*
- *Interpret the markings found on a medical gas cylinder shoulder including:*
  - *Department of Transportation (DOT) specification number*
  - *Cylinder composition code*
  - *Serial number and purchaser/user identification mark*
  - *Inspector's mark and testing date*
  - *Manufacturer's mark*
  - *The mark indicating that a cylinder has successfully passed a hydrostatic test*
  - *The mark indicating that a cylinder may be filled in excess of a service pressure by 10%*
- *List 15 rules for the safe storage and handling of compressed medical gas cylinders.*
- *Given a gauge pressure, cylinder size ("E" or "H/K"), and liter flow rate, calculate the duration of gas flow remaining for an oxygen cylinder.*
- *Describe the appropriate actions to be taken if the contents of a medical gas cylinder are in doubt.*

- *Describe the appropriate actions to be taken when one is requested to transfill a medical gas cylinder.*

Oxygen Piping Systems

- *Describe the safety features associated with an oxygen piping system.*
- *Describe the purpose of a zone valve.*
- *Describe a station outlet and the different types of connections available for the attachment of equipment.*

Liquid Oxygen Systems

- *Describe the physical characteristics of a small liquid oxygen reservoir.*
- *Describe the advantages and disadvantages of a liquid oxygen system for home use.*

Oxygen Concentrators

- *Differentiate between the two types of oxygen concentrators available.*
- *Describe the principles of operation for each type.*
- *Describe how liter flow affects the output of an oxygen concentrator.*

Reducing Valves

- *Differentiate among the three types of reducing valves.*
- *Describe the principle of operation for each type.*
- *Identify the safety features found on a two-stage reducing valve.*

Flowmeters

- *Diagram, label, and trace the flow patterns through the three types of flowmeters.*
- *Describe a Bourdon flowmeter and its principle of operation.*
- *Differentiate between an uncompensated and a compensated Thorpe tube flowmeter.*
- *Discuss the potential hazards associated with using a Bourdon or other uncompensated flowmeter.*

Air/Oxygen Blenders

- *State the purpose of air/oxygen blenders.*
- *Explain how these devices operate.*

MEDICAL GAS CYLINDERS

Cylinders manufactured for the transport of medical gases are constructed in accordance with regulations specifically established by the U.S. Department of Transportation (DOT). The DOT specifies the materials and methods by which medical gas cylinders may be constructed.

In accordance with regulations, medical gas cylinders are generally constructed from seamless steel meeting chemical and physical requirements. Cylinders are formed by either spinning or stamping a flat sheet into the proper shape. Following construction, cylinders are heat treated to retain the steel's tensile strength.

Cylinder Markings

Medical gas cylinders, in compliance with DOT regulations, are required to have specific markings permanently stamped onto the shoulder (Figures 12-1 and 12-2). The first marking stamped on the shoulder of a medical gas cylinder is "DOT 3AA." This indicates that the cylinder meets the DOT standards for 3AA-type compressed gas cylinders. These standards require that the cylinder be of seamless construction and made from high-strength, heat-treated alloy steels with specific chemical compositions. These metals can withstand high stress. Because of the high-tensile-strength alloy construction, this cylinder has a wall thickness less than that of other cylinder types and therefore weighs less than cylinders of comparable size and service pressure.

The next stamp following the cylinder type is the service pressure. This is the pressure, given in *pounds per square inch* (psi), under which the cylinder was designed to operate. The most common service pressure for cylinders in medical use is 2015 psi for oxygen.

The number stamped immediately below the specification number is the serial number for that cylinder. This number is unique and assigned by the manufacturer to that cylinder.

Next, the manufacturer's mark appears below the serial number. The manufacturer's mark may be represented by initials or an abbreviation of the manufacturer's name.

The ownership mark appears on the next line. Like the manufacturer's mark, it may be represented by initials or an abbreviation.

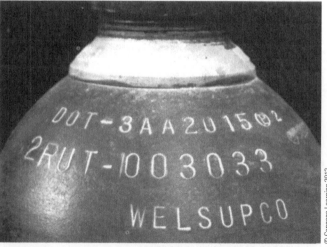

Figure 12-1 Cylinder markings stamped on the cylinder shoulder

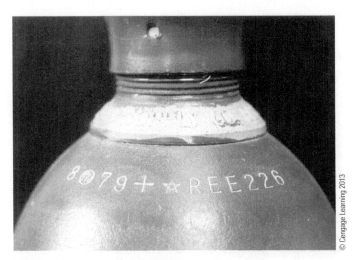

Figure 12-2 Cylinder markings stamped on the cylinder shoulder, indicating month and year of hydrostatic testing and results

© Cengage Learning 2013

If hydrostatic testing has been performed on the cylinder, the date of the hydrostatic test and the inspector's mark will also be stamped on the cylinder shoulder. The inspector's mark may appear between the month and day of the test, or it may appear after the month and day. If a plus sign (+) follows the testing date, this indicates that the cylinder may be charged up to 10% greater than the service pressure. In the case of the cylinder under discussion, the cylinder may be filled to 2200 psi (see Figure 12-2).

Hydrostatic testing every 5 or 10 years is required for all cylinders in service. The test is conducted by placing a cylinder in a vessel filled with water and filling the cylinder to 5/3 the service pressure (for 3A and 3AA cylinders). The expansion of the cylinder is measured while it is under pressure. If the expansion is within acceptable limits, the test date and expansion data are recorded. The cylinder is then stamped with the date of the test and the inspector's mark. If a cylinder fails a hydrostatic test, it is destroyed.

Common Medical Gas Cylinder Sizes

The two most common medical gas cylinder sizes encountered in the clinical setting are "E" and "H/K." Other cylinder sizes are shown in Figure 12-3.

The E cylinder is used for brief intervals owing to its relatively small capacity. Its most common use is for the transport of a patient from one area of the hospital to another, or in ambulance vehicles and short-term therapy where piped gases are not available. The cylinder's small size makes it ideal for use in transport situations. Small mobile cylinder carts make transporting a patient in a wheelchair or gurney much easier.

The H/K cylinder is much larger than the E cylinder and contains a little more than 10 times as much gas. Owing to its size and construction, it is quite heavy, usually weighing approximately 135 pounds. Special cylinder carts have been designed to facilitate the transport of these cylinders from one area to another.

Color Coding

The Compressed Gas Association (CGA) has developed a color code for the different gases and gas mixtures. Each gas or gas mixture has its own unique color code. This code is published by the U.S. Department of Commerce under recommendation from the Bureau of Standards. Table 12-1 illustrates the United States (U.S.) color code system and the International color code system. The only difference between the U.S. and International systems is the color code for oxygen.

Besides the color code, all medical gas cylinders are required to have a label affixed to the cylinder identifying its contents. The label's color code and the cylinder's color code should match.

If in doubt about the contents of a medical gas cylinder (e.g. 3, if a label is missing or if the label and the color code of the cylinder do not match), do not administer gas from that cylinder. Tag the cylinder as being mislabeled and return it to the medical gas supplier.

Only by verifying the color code of the cylinder and matching the label to the color code can the practitioner be certain of the cylinder's contents.

Cylinder Valves and Cylinder Valve Safety Systems

Because of the high pressure contained in a medical gas cylinder, a device is needed to contain the gas and to provide a point of attachment for equipment. These devices are termed *cylinder valves*. The cylinder valves are located at the top of the cylinder and are of two types: direct-acting and diaphragm.

The *direct-acting* cylinder valve is in essence a needle valve. To prevent leakage of the high-pressure gas through the threaded portion of the needle valve, washers and polytetrafluoroethylene (Teflon) gasket material are provided. As the stem of the valve is rotated counterclockwise, the plunger is raised from its seat and gas flows from the cylinder. Figures 12-4A and 12-4B show the component parts of a direct-acting cylinder valve. This type of cylinder valve is able to withstand high pressure and is found on cylinders containing gas at 1500 psi pressure and greater.

The *diaphragm* cylinder valve contains a diaphragm that rests on the seat of the valve. As the valve stem is turned counterclockwise, the pressure in the cylinder displaces the diaphragm and gas flows from the cylinder. In this type of valve, the valve plunger does not act directly on the valve seat. The diaphragm cylinder valve is not prone to leakage but cannot withstand high pressure. It is generally found on cylinders containing less than 1500 psi of pressure. Figures 12-5A and 12-5B depict a typical diaphragm cylinder valve.

There are two safety systems incorporated into cylinder valves: one recommended by the Bureau of Explosives and the other recommended by the CGA. For use in the event that excessive pressure builds up

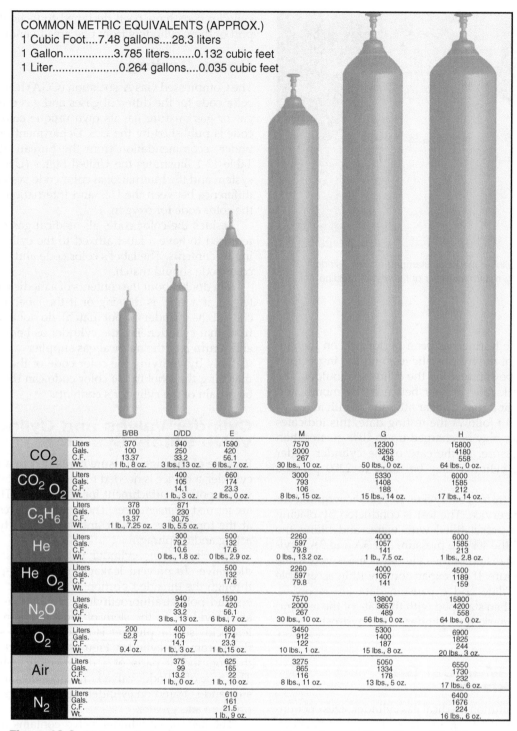

COMMON METRIC EQUIVALENTS (APPROX.)
1 Cubic Foot....7.48 gallons....28.3 liters
1 Gallon................3.785 liters........0.132 cubic feet
1 Liter....................0.264 gallons....0.035 cubic feet

Gas		B/BB	D/DD	E	M	G	H
CO_2	Liters	370	940	1590	7570	12300	15800
	Gals.	100	250	420	2000	3263	4180
	C.F.	13.37	33.2	56.1	267	436	558
	Wt.	1 lb., 8 oz.	3 lbs., 13 oz.	6 lbs., 7 oz.	30 lbs., 10 oz.	50 lbs., 0 oz.	64 lbs., 0 oz.
CO_2 O_2	Liters		400	660	3000	5330	6000
	Gals.		105	174	793	1408	1585
	C.F.		14.1	23.3	106	188	212
	Wt.		1 lb., 3 oz.	2 lbs., 0 oz.	8 lbs., 15 oz.	15 lbs., 14 oz.	17 lbs., 14 oz.
C_3H_6	Liters	378	871				
	Gals.	100	230				
	C.F.	13.37	30.75				
	Wt.	1 lb., 7.25 oz.	3 lb., 5.5 oz.				
He	Liters		300	500	2260	4000	6000
	Gals.		79.2	132	597	1057	1585
	C.F.		10.6	17.6	79.8	141	213
	Wt.		0 lbs., 1.8 oz.	0 lbs., 2.9 oz.	0 lbs., 13.2 oz.	1 lb., 7.5 oz.	1 lbs., 2.8 oz.
He O_2	Liters			500	2260	4000	4500
	Gals.			132	597	1057	1189
	C.F.			17.6	79.8	141	159
	Wt.						
N_2O	Liters		940	1590	7570	13800	15800
	Gals.		249	420	2000	3657	4200
	C.F.		33.2	56.1	267	489	558
	Wt.		3 lbs., 13 oz.	6 lbs., 7 oz.	30 lbs., 10 oz.	56 lbs., 0 oz.	64 lbs., 0 oz.
O_2	Liters	200	400	660	3450	5300	6900
	Gals.	52.8	105	174	912	1400	1825
	C.F.	7	14.1	23.3	122	187	244
	Wt.	9.4 oz.	1 lb., 3 oz.	1 lb.,15 oz.	10 lbs., 1 oz.	15 lbs., 8 oz.	20 lbs., 3 oz.
Air	Liters		375	625	3275	5050	6550
	Gals.		99	165	865	1334	1730
	C.F.		13.2	22	116	178	232
	Wt.		1 lb., 0 oz.	1 lb., 10 oz.	8 lbs., 11 oz.	13 lbs., 5 oz.	17 lbs., 6 oz.
N_2	Liters			610			6400
	Gals.			161			1676
	C.F.			21.5			224
	Wt.			1 lb., 9 oz.			16 lbs., 6 oz.

Figure 12-3   Various cylinder sizes. *(Courtesy of BOC Gases, formerly Airco, Murray Hill, NJ)*

within the cylinder, a safety pressure relief is provided on the cylinder valve. The system recommended by the Bureau of Explosives consists of a frangible disk or a fusible plug. When the frangible disk is exposed to excessive pressure, the disk fragments into small pieces, releasing the pressure in the cylinder. The fusible plug is made from a metal with a low melting point. If the temperature rises beyond the melting point of the metal plug, the plug melts and releases the pressure in the cylinder. A cylinder valve may contain one or both types of safety relief devices (Figure 12-6).

Because medical gas cylinders may contain a variety of gases besides oxygen, a safety system was designed by the CGA to prevent the interchange of cylinders containing dissimilar gases. This system was formally adopted by the American Standards Association and called the American Standard Index system, or the *American Standard Safety System (ASSS)*.

TABLE 12-1: Cylinder Color Coding

| GAS | COLOR CODE | |
	United States	International
Oxygen	Green	White
Carbon dioxide	Gray	Gray
Nitrous oxide	Light blue	Light blue
Cyclopropane	Orange	Orange
Helium	Brown	Brown
Carbon dioxide and oxygen	Gray and green	Gray and white
Helium and oxygen	Brown and green	Brown and white
Air	Yellow	White and black

There are two safety systems designed to prevent the interchange of cylinders containing different gases: one for large cylinders and one for E cylinders and other small cylinder sizes.

The large cylinder safety system consists of different thread sizes and pitches and both internal and external threading. Because of variations in threading, a cylinder containing one gas may not be connected to equipment indexed for a different gas.

In addition to the safety system just described, large medical gas cylinders have a protective cap that covers the cylinder valve. This cap is threaded and matches threads on the cylinder shoulder just below the valve. Whenever the cylinder is transported, safe practice dictates that the protective cylinder valve cap must be kept in place.

Small cylinder (D and E) valves use a yoke connection rather than a threaded connection for equipment attachment. The face of the cylinder valve has two holes drilled in two of six specific positions. The yoke that attaches to the cylinder valve has pins indexed in corresponding positions. If the pin and hole positions do not match, the cylinder and yoke cannot be mated. This indexing is designed to prevent the interchange of equipment or cylinders containing dissimilar gases. This system is commonly known as the *pin index safety system (PISS)*.

Figure 12-7 shows the threaded safety system and the PISS for large and small cylinder sizes.

Safety Precautions with Use of Medical Gas Cylinders

The respiratory care practitioner must use common sense and care when handling compressed gas cylinders. When handled properly and with care, medical gas cylinders are completely safe. However, there are numerous

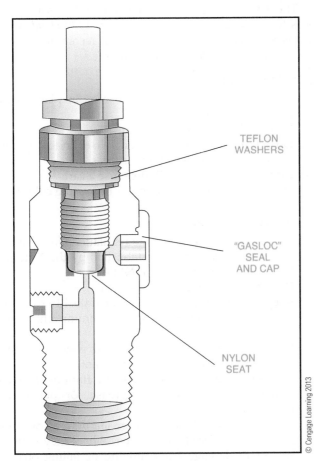

Figure 12-4A A direct-acting cylinder valve

TEFLON WASHERS

"GASLOC" SEAL AND CAP

NYLON SEAT

© Cengage Learning 2013

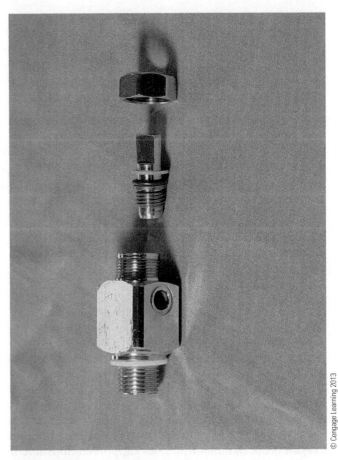

Figure 12-4B A photograph of a direct-acting cylinder valve showing the internal component parts

© Cengage Learning 2013

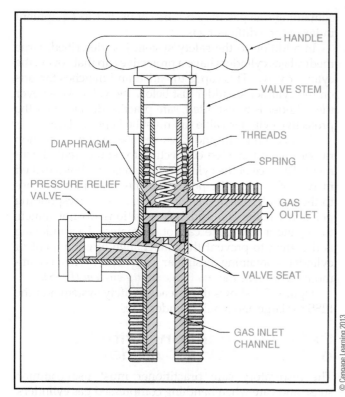

Figure 12-5A A diaphragm cylinder valve

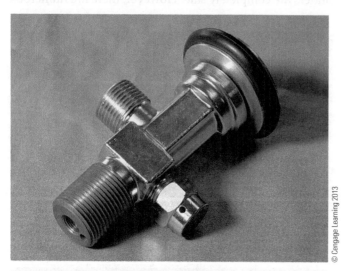

Figure 12-5B A photograph of an indirect-acting cylinder valve showing the internal component parts

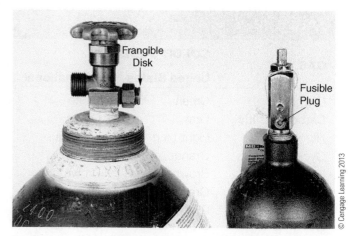

Figure 12-6 The frangible disk and fusible plug safety systems

not to use petroleum products on any cylinder valve fittings or reducing valve fittings.

Certain substances, when exposed to oxygen, may ignite with great force without the addition of heat to initiate the process. This phenomenon is termed *spontaneous combustion*. Such substances that may be encountered in a hospital or transport situation include oil, grease, and petroleum-based products such as Vaseline. Great care must be exercised to prevent the cylinder valves and fittings from making contact with these products.

The CGA has published recommended safe practices for handling medical gases in its 1999 *Handbook of Compressed Gases, Fourth Edition*. These recommendations are summarized in the following lists.

MOVING CYLINDERS

1. Always leave protective valve caps in place when moving a cylinder.
2. Do not lift a cylinder by its cap.
3. Do not drop a cylinder or strike two cylinders against one another, or strike other surfaces.
4. Do not drag or slide cylinders; use a cart.
5. Use a cart whenever loading or unloading cylinders.

STORING CYLINDERS

1. Comply with local and state regulations for cylinder storage as well as those established by the National Fire Protection Association (NFPA).
2. Post the names of the gases stored.
3. Keep full and empty cylinders separate. Place the full cylinders in a convenient spot to minimize handling of cylinders.
4. Keep storage areas dry, cool, and well ventilated. Storage rooms should be fire resistant.
5. Do not store cylinders close to flammable substances such as gasoline, grease, or petroleum products.
6. Protect the cylinders from damage by cuts or abrasion. Do not store them in areas where they may be subject to damage from moving or falling objects. Keep cylinder valve caps on at all times.

documented instances of damage to personnel, buildings, and vehicles resulting from improper handling of cylinders (Compressed Gas Association [CGA], 1999).

The most common gas the practitioner will administer from a medical gas cylinder is oxygen. Knowledge of the physical characteristics of oxygen will help in handling these medical gas cylinders. Oxygen is colorless, odorless, and tasteless. It supports life and is a requirement for combustion of any material. Although oxygen is not flammable, it does support combustion. If anything is burning in close proximity, combustion will occur at a greatly accelerated rate. It is also important

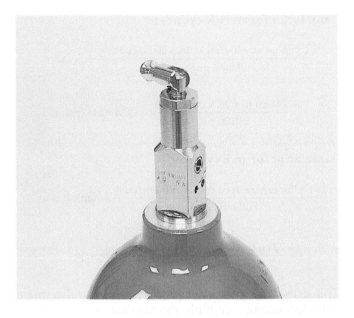

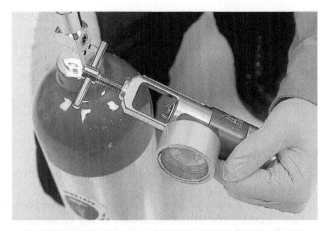

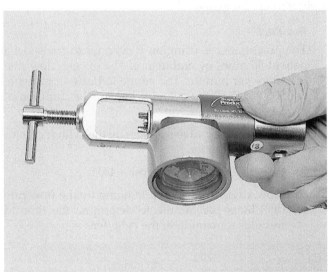

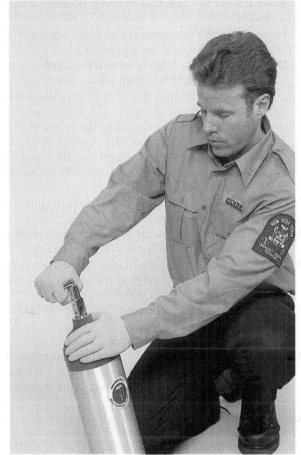

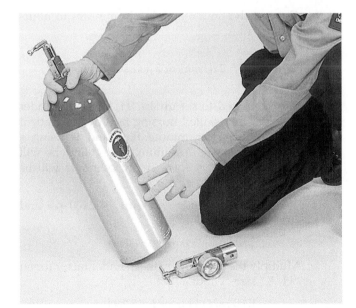

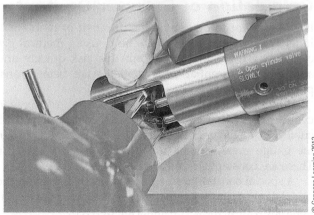

Figure 12-7   The American Standard Safety System (ASSS) and the pin index safety system (PISS)

7. Cylinders may be stored in the open; however, keep them on a platform so that they are above the ground. In some parts of the country, shading may be required because of high temperature extremes. If ice and snow accumulate, thaw at room temperature or use water not exceeding 125°F in temperature.
8. Protect cylinders from potential tampering by untrained, unauthorized persons.

WITHDRAWING CYLINDER CONTENTS

1. Allow cylinders to be handled only by experienced, trained persons.
2. The user of the cylinder is responsible for verifying the cylinder contents before use. If the contents are in doubt, do not use that cylinder. Return it to the supplier.
3. Leave the protective valve cap in place until ready to attach a regulator or other equipment.
4. Use safe practices, making sure the cylinder is well supported and protected from falling over.
5. Use appropriate reducing valves or regulators when attaching equipment designed for lower operating pressures than those contained in the cylinder.
6. Do not force any threaded connections. Verify that the threads in use are designed for the same gas or gas mixture in accordance with the American Standard Index system.
7. Connect a cylinder only to a manifold designed for high-pressure cylinders.
8. Use equipment only with cylinders containing the gases for which the equipment was designed.
9. Open cylinder valves slowly. Never use a wrench or hammer to force a cylinder valve open. Treat cylinders and cylinder valves with care.
10. Do not use compressed gases to dust off body or clothing.
11. Keep all connections tight to prevent leakage.
12. Before removing a regulator, turn off the valve and bleed it to depressurize the connection.
13. Never use a flame to detect leaks with flammable gases.
14. Do not store flammable gases with oxygen. Keep all flammable anesthetic gases stored in a separate area.

Calculation of Cylinder Contents

It is important to determine the duration of time a cylinder will last at a given flow rate in using medical gas cylinders. The ability to perform this task quickly and accurately is essential when patients are being transported.

When full, the most common sizes of oxygen cylinders—H/K and E—contain 244 cubic feet and 22 cubic feet of oxygen, respectively. As discussed earlier, the gauge pressure of a full cylinder is also 2200 psi. These are constants for full cylinders.

A special constant termed a *tank factor* is used in the calculation for each cylinder size. The following calculations show how these constants are derived:

Tank factor for an H/K cylinder:

$$\frac{\text{Cylinder size in cu ft} \times 28.3 \text{ liters/cu ft}}{\text{Full tank pressure}} = \text{tank factor}$$

$$\frac{244 \text{ cu ft} \times 28.3 \text{ liters/cu ft}}{2200 \text{ psi}} = 3.14 \text{ liters/psi}$$

Tank factor for an E cylinder:

$$\frac{\text{Cylinder size in cu ft} \times 28.3 \text{ liters/cu ft}}{\text{Full tank pressure}} = \text{tank factor}$$

$$\frac{22 \text{ cu ft} \times 28.3 \text{ liters/cu ft}}{2200 \text{ psi}} = 0.28 \text{ liters/psi}$$

To use these new tank factors or constants to determine cylinder contents, multiply the constant by the pressure indicated on the gauge.

Problem

The practitioner is using an E cylinder to transport a patient 60 miles by ambulance. The oxygen flow rate is 3 liters per minute. The gauge indicates a pressure of 1500 psi. Will the cylinder last for the duration of the 1-hour 15-minute trip?

a. Multiply the gauge pressure by the cylinder factor for an E cylinder.

$$1500 \text{ psi} \times 0.28 \text{ L/psi} = 420 \text{ L}$$

b. Now, divide the liters remaining by the flow rate of 3 liters per minute to determine the time in minutes remaining in the cylinder.

$$\frac{420 \text{ L}}{3 \text{ L/min}} = 140 \text{ minutes}$$

c. Convert the time remaining in minutes to hours and minutes.

$$\frac{140 \text{ min}}{60 \text{ min/h}} = 2.3 \text{ hours or 2 hours 18 minutes}$$

You are requested to set up an "H/K" size cylinder for a patient in a skilled nursing facility. The patient requires 10 liters per minute flow and is using a nonrebreather mask. Assuming the cylinders will be changed at 500 psi, how many cylinders will be needed to last 7 days?

a. Take the full cylinder pressure of 2200 psi and subtract 500 psi.

$$2200 \text{ psi} - 500 \text{ psi} = 1700 \text{ psi}$$

b. Multiply the pressure by the cylinder factor for an "H/K" size cylinder.

$$1700 \text{ psi } (3.14 \text{ L/psi}) = 5389 \text{ L}$$

c. Divide the liters in the cylinder by the liter flow (10 L/min).

$$5389 \text{ liters}/10 \text{ L/min} = 538.9 \text{ min}$$

d. Divide the answer in minutes by 60 minutes/hour.

$$538.9 \text{ min}/60 \text{ min/hour} = 8.9 \text{ hours or } 9 \text{ hours}$$

e. Divide 24 hours by 9 hours.

$$24 \text{ hr}/9 \text{ hr} = 2.7 \text{ cylinders/day or } 19 \text{ cylinders for } 7 \text{ days}$$

Following this method, it is possible to calculate the amount of time a cylinder of oxygen will last at a given flow rate. However, at the end of the calculated period, the cylinder will be completely empty.

It is common practice to change an oxygen cylinder in use when the gauge pressure reads 500 psi. The pressure at which cylinders are changed may vary with hospital policy. This leaves a slight reserve of oxygen for the patient. Also, by leaving a little pressure in the cylinder, air, water, or other undesirable contaminants cannot enter the cylinder.

Transfilling of Medical Gas Cylinders

The process of transfilling medical gas cylinders involves the connection of an empty cylinder to one that contains gas under pressure. Usually the practice involves the filling of a small portable cylinder from a large H/K cylinder.

Transfilling of medical gas cylinders remains a controversial topic in respiratory care. As with all controversies, there are two schools of thought.

There are definite hazards involved in the transfilling of medical gas cylinders. If transfilling is performed improperly, excessive heat can be generated, posing a potential fire hazard. If the pressure limits of a small cylinder are accidentally exceeded, the result may be a disastrous rupture of the cylinder. There is also the possibility of mixing two dissimilar gases by accident. Serious hazards are associated with the transfilling of gas from one cylinder to another; therefore, it is recommended that the practice be discontinued (CGA, 1999).

Some authors and practitioners maintain that transfilling is a safe, routinely practiced activity. They maintain that if common sense is exercised, cylinders may be transfilled safely.

It is the author's opinion, however, that the benefits of transfilling cylinders are not worth the risk. Requests for transfilling a cylinder should be referred to an appropriate medical gas supply company.

MEDICAL GAS PIPING SYSTEMS

Because of increased convenience, safety, and cost savings, medical gas piping systems have grown in popularity over the years. Like medical gas cylinders, medical gas piping systems are regulated and must conform to specific standards of design and construction. The NFPA is the organization that recommends the standards for construction of medical gas piping systems.

These piping systems may be supplied by a bulk liquid supply of gas or a manifold composed of two or more large medical gas cylinders, or both. Should the bulk supply system run out, a safety system is provided. A piping system is required to have a reserve or backup supply of oxygen. As the pressure in the supply line drops after the main oxygen supply is exhausted, the reserve system is automatically switched on. This reserve system may consist of a liquid bulk supply, a manifold of two or more cylinders, or a combination of the two. The reserve system must be able to meet a facility's oxygen needs for a minimum of 24 hours, according to NFPA regulations.

The bulk gas supply pressure must be reduced to a working pressure of 50 psi by a regulator. From the regulator, oxygen is conducted into the building through a pipe. In a multistoried building, each floor is provided with oxygen by a pipe termed a *riser*. Each riser is required to have a safety shutoff valve in the event of a fire.

Each floor of a building is divided into several zones. Each zone has a safety shutoff valve, termed a *zone valve*. In the event of a fire in one zone or wing of a floor, that zone's oxygen supply can be shut off without affecting other areas on the same floor. If the pressure in either the oxygen or air piping system falls below 45 psi, an alarm will sound alerting personnel to low pressure in the system.

It is important for the respiratory practitioner to know where the riser and zone valves are located in the facility of employment. In the event of a fire, the practitioner may be asked to terminate the oxygen supply to an area to help contain the fire. Figure 12-8 shows a typical zone valve.

The connection for attaching equipment for patient use is termed a *station outlet*. These outlets may have a *diameter-indexed safety system (DISS)* or quick-connect fittings. Both of these fittings have check valves to prevent oxygen loss when they are not in use (Figure 12-9).

The DISS is designed for pressures of 200 psi and lower. It was designed by the CGA. This system prevents the interchange of equipment designed for dissimilar gases or gas mixtures.

Reducing Valves

Medical gas cylinders, as discussed earlier, contain gas under high pressure. This high pressure must be reduced to a working pressure of 50 psi. Respiratory care equipment is designed to function at this lower working pressure. Operating equipment at the lower pressure has obvious safety advantages. A device that reduces the pressure in the medical gas cylinder from 2200 psi to 50 psi is termed a *reducing valve*. There are many types of

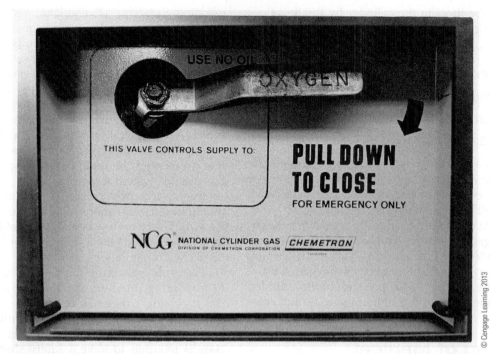

© Cengage Learning 2013

Figure 12-8 A typical zone valve

reducing valves: single-stage, modified single-stage, and multistage valves.

Single-Stage Reducing Valve

A single-stage reducing valve has one chamber for the reduction of cylinder pressure to 50 psi. The single-stage reducing valve operates as a result of two opposing forces (Figure 12-10). The two opposing forces allowing this device to operate are spring tension and gas pressure. The diaphragm allows these two forces to work in opposition. High pressure forces gas into the chamber. As the gas enters the chamber through the nozzle, the valve seat is displaced. If gas flow at the outlet were to remain unobstructed, the valve seat would remain open. Resistance at the outlet causes pressure to build within the chamber. As pressure builds, the diaphragm is forced up against the tension of the spring. When gas pressure in the chamber equals the tension of the spring, the valve seat closes. A pressure drop or decrease in resistance at the outlet allows the cycle to begin again.

Also, note that the portion of the reducing valve housing the spring has openings for atmospheric pressure. This is by design so that movement of the diaphragm does not cause pressure to increase in this portion of the reducing valve. If pressure builds in this section of the reducing valve, there is then an additional force to be overcome as the gas is compressed.

The outlet pressure on some of these reducing valves may be adjusted. By adjusting the tension of the spring using a screw adjustment, pressure may be increased or decreased. If no adjustment is provided, the reducing valve is termed a *preset reducing valve*.

Modified Single-Stage Reducing Valve

A modified single-stage reducing valve is very similar in design to a single-stage reducing valve. The only difference is the addition of a poppet-closing spring (Figure 12-11).

The poppet-closing spring provides a force in addition to gas pressure to oppose the force of the spring tension. The additional force provided by the poppet-closing spring allows the valve to open and close at a faster rate. The faster rate enables this reducing valve to provide higher flow rates than those possible with a standard single-stage reducing valve. Also, because of the faster action of the valve, pressure is more accurately regulated.

The outlet pressure on some of these reducing valves may be adjusted. By adjusting the tension of the spring using a screw adjustment, pressure may be increased or decreased.

Multistage Reducing Valves

A multistage reducing valve consists of two or more single-stage reducing valves working in series. The gas entering the first stage is reduced to an intermediate pressure. This first stage of the reducing valve is usually preset by the factory to a pressure of approximately 200 psi. The gas then enters the second stage and is reduced to the correct working pressure of 50 psi. The second-stage spring tension is less than the spring tension of the first stage—hence the lower pressure (Figure 12-12).

Three or more stages may be connected in series. In clinical practice, two-stage and, on rare occasions, three-stage reducing valves may be encountered.

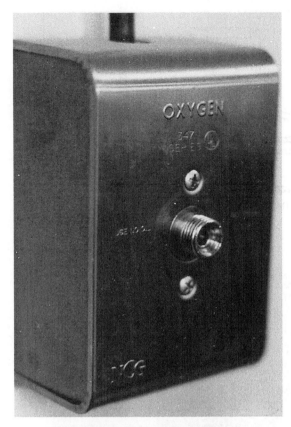

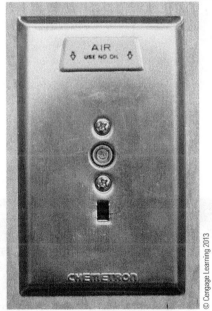

Figure 12-9 DISS (A) and quick-connect (B) fittings

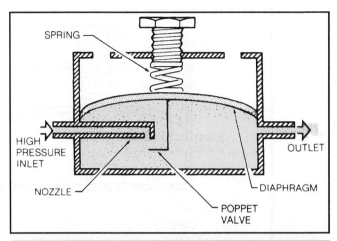

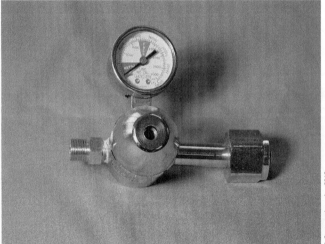

Figure 12-10 A diagram of a single-stage reducing valve

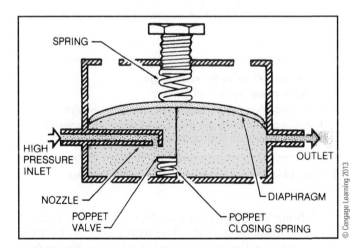

Figure 12-11 A diagram of a modified single-stage reducing valve

The advantages of a multistage reducing valve are more accurate regulation of pressure, smoother operation, and consistently higher flow rates.

Safety Features

In the event of the buildup of excessive pressure within the reducing valve, there are several safety features incorporated into the design. These safety features are listed in Figure 12-13.

Flowmeters

Bourdon Gauge Flowmeters

A Bourdon gauge *flowmeter* may also be referred to as a *fixed orifice flowmeter*. This flowmeter is really not a flowmeter at all but rather a pressure gauge calibrated to measure flow.

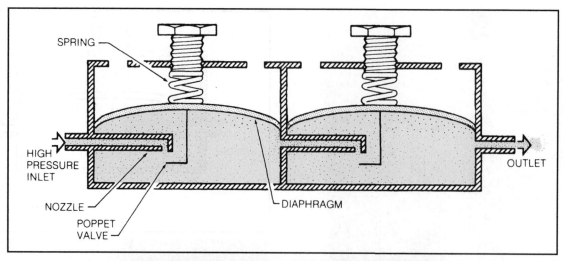

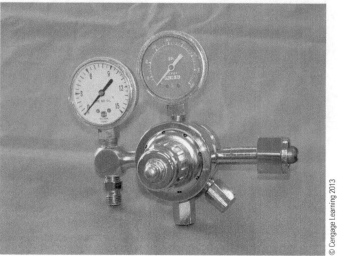

Figure 12-12   A diagram of a two-stage reducing valve

- Safety popoff valve for each stage
- Beveled glass face on all gauges
- Thin, unsealed metal back on the pressure gauge
- American Standard, pin index, and diameter-indexed safety systems as appropriate

Figure 12-13   Oxygen reducing valve safety features

A Bourdon tube flowmeter has a thin tube formed into a portion of a circle. The lower end of the tube is exposed to the pressure released from the reducing valve. The upper end is sealed. Distal to the placement of the Bourdon tube is a restricted orifice (Figure 12-14).

As gas flows past the Bourdon tube and encounters the restricted orifice, pressure builds proximal to the orifice. As the pressure builds, the thin Bourdon tube straightens slightly. As the tube straightens, this motion is translated to rotary motion by a gear mechanism that changes the dial indication on the face of the gauge.

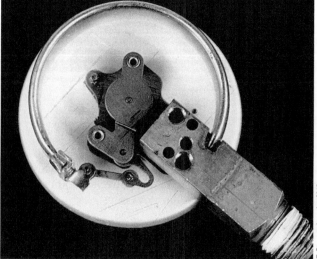

Figure 12-14   A Bourdon gauge flowmeter

These flowmeters are small and quite compact. They have an advantage in that they will operate in any position. This capability has definite advantages in a transport situation.

Certain precautions must be observed with use of this type of flowmeter. The accuracy of the flowmeter is dependent on the size of the orifice of the flowmeter outlet. Therefore, restriction or back pressure at the outlet will render the reading inaccurate. It is possible to occlude the opening of the flowmeter totally so that no flow exists and the gauge will show a flow rate higher than the original setting. Care must be exercised to prevent any restriction to flow with use of this type of flowmeter. When accurate flow rates are required, it is best to use another type of flowmeter.

A fixed orifice flowmeter operates by selecting different-sized orifices that produce specific flow rates. The most common fixed orifice flowmeter is mated to a single-stage reducing valve and a yoke connection for "E" size cylinders (Figure 12-15). It is even more compact than a Bourdon gauge flowmeter (Figure 12-14). This flowmeter is adjustable between off and 15 liters per minute.

Thorpe Tube Flowmeters

Thorpe tube flowmeters employ a Thorpe tube in their design. A Thorpe tube is a tapered tube with a small end at the bottom and a large end at the top. This V-shaped tube provides a variable orifice. The internal diameter of the tube varies from the bottom to the top, increasing in area toward the top.

A float device is suspended in the tube by the flow of gas. In oxygen and air flowmeters, the float is typically a small-diameter steel ball. The ball or float remains suspended as a result of a pressure differential between the top and the bottom of the float. The higher the flow rate, the higher the pressure is below the float, causing the float to be suspended at a higher level. Of course, the higher the float is suspended, the larger the opening around the float. Thus, more gas is allowed to exit

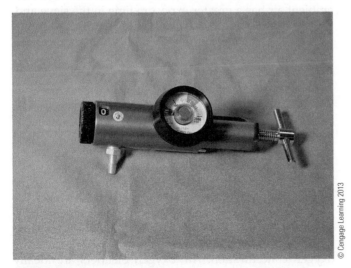

Figure 12-15 A photograph of a fixed orifice (click-type) flowmeter

© Cengage Learning 2013

around the float, allowing the flowmeter to be much shorter. The opposing forces at work are the weight of the ball and the pressure differential that is related to the flow of gas.

Thorpe tube flowmeters can be classified into two general categories: uncompensated and back pressure–compensated. The placement of the needle valve in the flowmeter design determines whether it is uncompensated or back pressure–compensated (Figure 12-16).

Uncompensated Thorpe Tube Flowmeters

The uncompensated Thorpe tube flowmeter has the needle valve placed proximal to the Thorpe tube or *upstream*. With the flowmeter operating normally, the pressure proximal to the needle valve is equal to the line pressure or 50 psi. The pressure distal to the needle valve is equal to the atmospheric pressure.

With partial obstruction of the outlet of the flowmeter, the pressure inside the Thorpe tube would increase owing to the increased resistance. As the pressure within the tube increases, the pressure differential between the top and bottom of the float decreases and the float is suspended at a lower position. This would indicate a lower flow than originally set. In reality, the actual flow rate may not change at all. It is possible, in the face of back pressure distal to the needle valve, to deliver flows higher than indicated by the suspension of the float.

Back Pressure–Compensated Flowmeter

The back pressure–compensated flowmeter has the needle valve placed distal or *downstream* from the Thorpe tube. By placing the needle valve in this position, the pressure within the Thorpe tube proximal to the needle valve remains at the line pressure of 50 psi. The pressure distal to (downstream from) the needle valve is ambient or atmospheric pressure.

If the outlet of a back pressure–compensated flowmeter is partially occluded, the flow rate will still be indicated accurately. As long as there is flow, the pressure distal to the needle valve will not exceed the line pressure of 50 psi. The restriction is simply serving as another needle valve restricting the flow. With total occlusion of the outlet, the pressure distal to the needle valve would be equal to the line pressure of 50 psi and the float would not be suspended, indicating zero flow.

Liquid Oxygen Systems

Liquid oxygen systems have become very popular in home care primarily for economic reasons. A large reservoir is the primary system the patient uses. The reservoir contains as much oxygen as in several H/K cylinders and is less expensive to fill. The large reservoir can power a humidifier, a nebulizer, or positive-pressure breathing devices from its 50 psi outlet. The construction of the liquid reservoir is similar to that of a large thermos bottle. Liquid oxygen is contained in the reservoir at −297°F. When demand causes gas to flow from the reservoir, the liquid moves through condensing coils that vaporize the liquid into a gas.

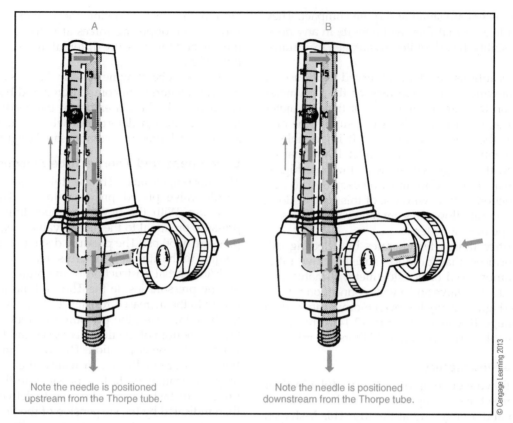

Note the needle is positioned upstream from the Thorpe tube.

Note the needle is positioned downstream from the Thorpe tube.

© Cengage Learning 2013

Figure 12-16 An uncompensated (A) and a compensated (B) Thorpe tube flowmeter

For portable use, a smaller reservoir can be filled from the large one. The smaller reservoir is similar in design and construction to the larger unit. At a low flow rate, the smaller reservoir can last several hours. It is small and compact, weighing approximately 11 pounds when full. Figure 12-17 shows a smaller reservoir mated to the larger one for refilling. It is important to keep these liquid reservoirs in the upright position to prevent loss of liquid oxygen.

Oxygen Concentrators

Within the past 10 years, oxygen concentrators have been developed primarily for low-flow oxygen therapy in the home. An *oxygen concentrator* takes air from the atmosphere and separates the oxygen from the other gases in the air. These units provide an adequate oxygen concentration of between 87% and 94% depending on the type of unit and the flow rate. Some concentrators are capable of flow rates up to 10 liters per minute, but the oxygen percentage delivered falls as flow rate increases.

There are currently two types of oxygen concentrators on the market. The two types are membrane (oxygen enricher) and molecular sieve oxygen concentrators.

The membrane type of oxygen enricher uses a thin membrane made out of a polymer. This membrane is only 1 micrometer thick. A compressor provides a pressure gradient across the membrane. Oxygen and water vapor pass through the membrane at a faster rate than is the case with nitrogen. This type of concentrator can

provide a humidified oxygen concentration of approximately 40%.

The molecular sieve concentrator uses a chemical (sodium–aluminum silicate) to scrub the nitrogen from the air. A compressor forces the ambient air through the sieve. The gas, after passing through the sieve, has a concentration of oxygen between 87% and 94%. At low flow rates (2 L/min or less) the concentration of oxygen is the highest. At a flow rate of 10 liters per minute, the oxygen concentration drops to 87%. At the lower flow rate, the ambient air has a greater exposure time in the sieve and, therefore, more nitrogen is separated. Figure 12-18 shows a typical oxygen concentrator.

Air/Oxygen Blenders

An *air/oxygen blender* is a device that provides a precise oxygen concentration by mixing air and oxygen. The concentration may be adjusted to any value from room air to 100% oxygen. All air/oxygen blenders have a 50 psi outlet, and some have a Thorpe tube flowmeter attached in addition to the outlet.

Air/oxygen blenders have a 50 psi inlet for both air and oxygen. Internally, a proportioning valve mixes the incoming air and oxygen as the oxygen percentage dial is adjusted. Variations in line pressure or in flow or pressure requirements for any attached device will not affect the oxygen concentration. Air/oxygen blenders are ideally suited for use with ventilators or other devices with high flow and pressure demands because oxygen delivery is not affected.

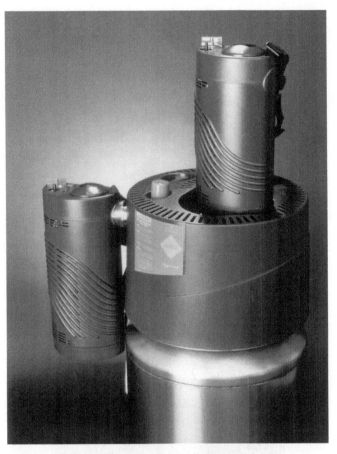

Figure 12-17 A large liquid oxygen reservoir and a portable liquid reservoir for home use. *(Copyright 2011 Chart Industries, Inc. Used with permission, all rights reserved.)*

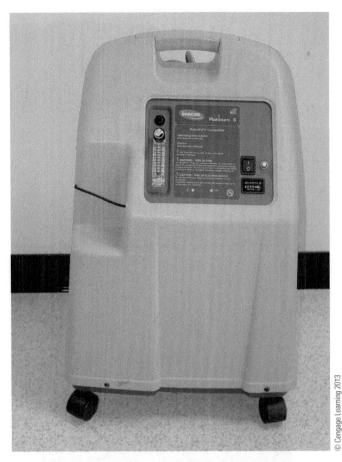

Figure 12-18 An oxygen concentrator

PROFICIENCY OBJECTIVES

At the end of this chapter, the reader should be able to:

- *Correctly select an E or an H/K cylinder for use.*
- *Correctly maneuver a medical gas cylinder onto and off a cylinder cart.*
- *Demonstrate the correct handling of a cylinder and cart on level ground.*

- *Properly prepare a cylinder for attachment of a reducing valve or gas delivery device.*
- *Correctly demonstrate the process of bleeding a reducing valve before removal.*
- *Demonstrate how to prepare an air/oxygen blender for use.*

USING MEDICAL GAS CYLINDERS

Obtaining the Cylinder from Storage

Large medical gas cylinders are stored along a wall where, for optimal safety, chains or straps are provided to secure the cylinders to the wall. The safety chains will prevent the cylinders from accidentally falling from the upright position. A sign will indicate whether cylinders are full or empty.

The first step in obtaining a medical gas cylinder for use is cylinder identification. Color code and the adhesive label affixed to the cylinder should match. If they do not match, do not use that cylinder. Mark the cylinder and return it to the medical gas supplier.

Once the correct cylinder has been identified, the practitioner may maneuver it onto the cart designed to facilitate the safe transport of large cylinders.

Maneuvering Large Medical Gas Cylinders

An oxygen H/K cylinder weighs approximately 135 pounds when full. Care must be exercised when handling this much weight concentrated in a relatively small package. Besides the weight factor, the pressure in a full cylinder, if it is mistreated, could cause serious injury.

To maneuver a cylinder onto the cart, unchain the cylinder or bank of cylinders from the wall. Grasp the cylinder of choice by placing one hand on the protective cap over the cylinder valve and the other hand on

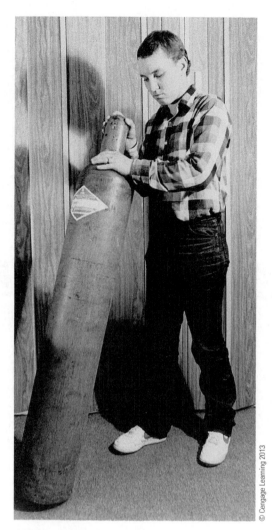

Figure 12-19 Rolling an H cylinder

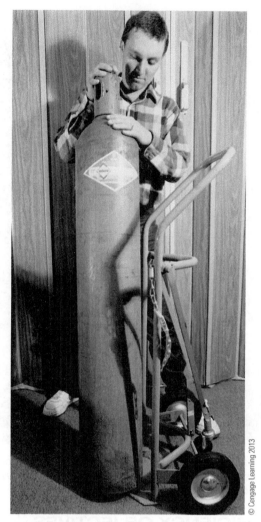

Figure 12-20 A cylinder being rolled onto its cart

the cylinder shoulder. Tilt the cylinder toward the body slightly. With the cylinder in a tilted position, it is easy to roll the cylinder on its base in the desired direction. The hand placed on the safety cap provides stability, while the other hand provides the locomotion (Figure 12-19).

The cylinder cart should be placed in a convenient location close to the bank of cylinders, allowing sufficient room to maneuver. The cart should be in an upright position with the safety wheels in the retracted position.

To maneuver the cylinder onto the cart, block one of the main wheels with a chock or foot to prevent the cart from tipping over when the cylinder is rolled onto it (Figure 12-20). After the cylinder is on the cart, secure it with the chain provided. After the cylinder is secured, lock the safety wheels into position and, by placing a foot on one of the main wheels, rotate the cart onto the extra safety wheels. The cylinder and cart should now be resting on all wheels. Return to the main bank of cylinders and reattach the chain, securing the other cylinders as required.

Transporting the Cylinder and Cart

The practitioner is now ready to transport the cylinder and cart to the desired location. To transport the cylinder and cart, place one hand on the safety cap over the

cylinder valve and the other hand on the handle of the cart. This hand position will provide the best control of the cylinder and cart. Push the cylinder and cart in front of the body while keeping a sharp eye out for other personnel, objects, or hazards. When approaching a corner or busy area, slow down. It is often difficult to see other personnel when approaching these areas.

Cracking the Cylinder

Before attachment of any equipment to a cylinder, the cylinder valve must be cracked. *Cracking* the cylinder removes any dust, or particulate matter, from the outlet of the cylinder valve. This prevents contaminants from entering any equipment. If the materials are flammable, fire hazard is minimized because they are removed before the application of high-pressure oxygen.

To crack a cylinder, place the cart in an upright position and release the third wheel into the retracted position. Remove the safety cap from the cylinder valve. Ideally, this should be done in an area away from patient rooms. Point the outlet of the cylinder valve away from the body and other personnel. Remove the protective cover from the cylinder valve outlet, if one is provided. Announce to any personnel around that you are going to crack the cylinder and that it will make a loud noise. Place a hand around the rim of the cylinder valve handle and quickly rotate the handle one-quarter turn counterclockwise; then quickly rotate it clockwise back to the closed position. When a cylinder is cracked, gas at 2200 psi pressure exiting through the narrow opening of the cylinder valve makes a very loud hissing noise. The sudden noise is enough to startle anyone. The cylinder is now ready for attachment of a reducing valve or other equipment.

Attaching a Reducing Valve

A reducing valve for an H/K cylinder has the American Standard Index thread safety system. The practitioner will need an open-end or crescent wrench to attach the reducing valve to the cylinder.

Place the female end of the American Standard Index fitting of the reducing valve onto the male portion of the cylinder valve. Attach the nut "finger tight" by rotating the nut clockwise. Now, using the wrench, tighten the nut by rotating it farther in the clockwise direction.

After the reducing valve is secure, slowly open the cylinder valve by turning the handle counterclockwise. Keep a hand on the outside of the handle's rim. Never place the palm of the hand so that it covers the entire handle. Listen and feel for leaks at the cylinder valve connection. If in doubt about the presence of a leak, a solution of soapy water may be used to detect it. Open the cylinder valve completely; then rotate it clockwise one-quarter turn. The practitioner is now ready to attach any further equipment requiring a 50 psi oxygen source.

Using an H/K Cylinder in a Patient Area

For use of cylinders at the patient's bedside, there should be safety chains on the wall to secure the cylinder. If chains are not available, a cylinder base may be used to secure the cylinder. For short-term use, the cylinder cart can be tilted in the upright position and the third wheel placed in the retracted position.

It is imperative to place the cylinder in a spot where it will not be disturbed by traffic into or out of the room. Keep it away from heat registers and electrical outlets. Placard the room with signs inside and outside stating "No smoking—oxygen in use." If the patient has a history of smoking and is not coherent, remove any smoking materials.

Do not leave a cylinder standing on its base, unsecured by a chain, cart, or cylinder base.

Maneuvering an E Cylinder

E cylinders are often found in the same storage area as for the larger H/K cylinders. Owing to their smaller size, they are often kept in a divided box, somewhat like an egg crate. This divided box keeps the cylinders upright and separated from one another. Just like H/K cylinders, E cylinders have a special cart to facilitate their transport.

To place an E cylinder onto its cart, lift the cylinder and gently lower it into its cart. Secure the cylinder with one or more wing nuts provided for the purpose (Figure 12-21).

The best way to maneuver an E cylinder cart is to pull it behind. If maneuvering the cart in front of you, the feet can become tangled with the wheels on the cart.

Cracking an E Cylinder

Cracking an E cylinder is quite similar to cracking an H/K cylinder. The same rules apply. Point the cylinder valve outlet in a safe direction and issue a verbal warning before cracking the cylinder. Be sure to use the correct end of the cylinder wrench provided for an E cylinder. Use the small slot that fits the stem of the cylinder valve. The large hexagonal opening fits the upper end of the cylinder valve. If this nut were to be removed, 2200 psi would propel the valve stem with potentially lethal force. Some hospitals cut off the hexagonal end of the wrench to prevent the inadvertent use of the wrong end.

Attaching a Reducing Valve to an E Cylinder

After cracking the cylinder, the practitioner is now ready to attach a reducing valve or other equipment. Unlike an H/K cylinder, an E cylinder uses a doughnut-shaped Teflon

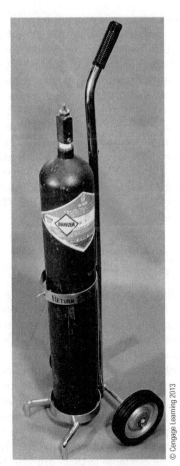

Figure 12-21 An E cylinder secured to its cart

washer between the flat face of the cylinder valve and the yoke. Place the washer onto the male inlet on the yoke, match the PISS safety pins, and tighten the yoke in place using the large wing nut provided. Do not use a wrench. When changing an E cylinder, always change the Teflon washer, putting a new one on with the new cylinder. This precaution will help prevent leaks. After the reducing valve or equipment is secure, slowly turn on the cylinder valve and check any attachments for leaks. Open the cylinder valve completely, and then rotate it clockwise one-quarter of a turn.

Bleeding a Reducing Valve

The process of bleeding a reducing valve relieves the pressure contained in the reducing valve and attachment fittings before removal. The reducing valve should also be bled when the attached device is not in use. To bleed a reducing valve, turn off the cylinder valve. Turn on the flowmeter or the pneumatically powered equipment attached to the reducing valve, allowing the pressure to bleed off. Next, turn off the flowmeter or equipment and remove it from the cylinder.

USE OF PORTABLE LIQUID OXYGEN SYSTEMS

Portable liquid oxygen systems have become popular for home and ambulatory use (see Figure 12-17). The primary liquid systems are relatively small (12 to 15 inches in diameter and 27 to 38 inches tall, weighing between 84 and 160 pounds), whereas the ambulatory systems weigh between 5.3 and 9 pounds and are very compact. These portable systems can contain between 20 and 43 liquid liters of oxygen, whereas the ambulatory systems may contain between 0.6 and 1.2 liquid liters of oxygen. Because each liter of liquid oxygen is equivalent to 861 liters of gaseous oxygen, capacities will vary, ranging between 16,000 and 35,000 liters for the primary systems and 500 and 1025 liters for the ambulatory systems.

Transfilling the Ambulatory System

Before transfilling a portable system from a primary liquid reservoir, it is important to review some important safety considerations. Liquid oxygen is stored at −280°F, and contact with the liquid will result in cryogenic burns. Like gaseous oxygen, liquid oxygen will support and accelerate combustion. Transfilling should never be done in the vicinity of anyone smoking or around any open flames. During the transfilling process and afterward, the couplings are extremely cold and may cause cryogenic burns. Use of protective gloves can prevent injury from cryogenic burns. Always store both the primary liquid reservoir and the portable system upright; tipping them on their side will cause them to vent liquid oxygen.

Attach the ambulatory system to the primary system by coupling them together by connecting the male fill port of the portable system to the female fitting on the primary reservoir. Rotate the portable system until it is locked into place on the primary reservoir. Once the two systems are connected to one another, open the vent port on the portable system to allow liquid to flow from the primary reservoir into the portable system. The vent must be opened for oxygen to flow. Continue filling the portable system until the liquid oxygen being expelled from the vent on the portable system can be observed. Closing the vent valve terminates the flow of oxygen into the portable system. Disconnect the portable system from the primary reservoir by rotating the portable system until it detaches from the primary liquid reservoir.

Primary Liquid Reservoir Use

Connect an oxygen flowmeter to the DISS threaded outlet fitting. Adjust the liter flow to the desired setting and connect an appropriate oxygen delivery device. Some liquid primary reservoirs have a built-in flow control valve: adjust the flow control valve to the desired setting and connect an appropriate oxygen delivery device to the threaded DISS outlet.

Portable System Use

Once the portable system has been transfilled and is full, connect an appropriate oxygen delivery device to the nipple outlet of the portable system. Adjust the flow control valve to the desired setting.

Determining Liquid Oxygen Duration

The duration of liquid oxygen systems is determined by the weight of the reservoir (primary or portable). Each pound of liquid oxygen contains 342.8 liters of gaseous oxygen. To determine the duration of the reservoir, complete the following steps:

1. Weigh the reservoir.
2. Subtract the empty weight of the reservoir from its current weight to determine the weight of the liquid oxygen in the reservoir.
3. Multiply the liquid oxygen weight by 342.8 L/lb and multiply that product by 0.8 (a factor used to allow for variations in spring scales).
4. Divide the result obtained in step 3 by the liter flow rate being used.

Example

Mrs. Jones has filled her portable system. It weighs 9.5 lb following filling and has an empty weight of 6.5 lb. At a liter flow of 3 L/min, how long will her portable system last?

1. 9.5 lb − 6.5 lb = 3 lb liquid oxygen weight
2. (3 lb × 342.8 L/lb)0.8 = 824 L
3. 824 L ÷ 3 L/min = 274 minutes or 4.5 hours

USE OF AN OXYGEN CONCENTRATOR

Oxygen concentrators provide a convenient method for the delivery of oxygen for home or subacute use that is less expensive than use of cylinders or liquid systems. The only expense of these systems, once purchased, is the electricity used to run the unit's compressor because oxygen is separated from atmospheric air.

Place the concentrator in the room in which the patient plans to spend the majority of his or her time. Locate the concentrator away from radiators, heaters, or any hot air registers. Be certain that the back and sides of the unit are at least 6 inches away from any walls, draperies, or surfaces that may interfere with air movement or flow into or out of the concentrator.

When selecting the electrical outlet to power the concentrator, try to select a circuit that has very little additional electrical load on it. Do not choose a circuit that also powers larger, high electrical current–drawing appliances or devices. When plugging the concentrator into the electrical outlet, verify that the power switch is first turned off before connecting the power cord to the outlet.

It is important to check the gross particle filter at the concentrator inlet for cleanliness or obstructions. If the filter is dirty, clean it in a mild solution of water and household dishwashing detergent. Rinse it thoroughly in tap water and use a towel to blot it dry. Reinstall the filter after it has been cleaned. A dirty or obstructed filter will greatly hamper the performance of an oxygen concentrator.

Attach a humidifier or appropriate oxygen delivery device to the outlet of the oxygen concentrator. Additional oxygen extension tubing may be added to facilitate patient mobility and relative freedom for movement about the home. Do not use more than 50 feet of extension tubing. Turn on the power switch and adjust the oxygen flowmeter to the desired setting.

USE OF AIR/ OXYGEN BLENDERS

Preparation of an air/oxygen blender generally consists of the attachment of 50 psi air and oxygen sources to the device. High-pressure hoses are usually the most convenient way to attach the two source gases to the air/oxygen blender. Once the source gases are attached, inlet pressures may be checked on some blenders by checking the attached pressure gauge.

In the event of line pressure failure (<30 psi pressure), an audible alarm will sound. This alarm is strictly a pressure alarm and not an oxygen percentage alarm. This safety feature may be tested by disconnecting either the air or the oxygen source.

Once the inlet gases are attached and the air/oxygen blender is well secured to a stand or wall mount, it is ready for use. Attach the device to be operated to the 50 psi outlet or a flowmeter attached to the outlet. Adjust the desired oxygen concentration and confirm the delivered oxygen concentration with an oxygen analyzer.

Reference

Compressed Gas Association. (1999). *Handbook of compressed gases* (4th ed.). New York: Springer.

Additional Resources

Cairo, J. M., & Pilbeam, S. P. (2010). *Mosby's respiratory care equipment* (8th ed.). St. Louis, MO: Mosby.

Cryogenics Associates Liberator 20, 30, 45, and Stroller, Sprint service manual. (1992). Bloomington, MN: Cryogenics Associates.

DeVilbiss DeVO/MC 44–90 oxygen concentrator service manual. (1987). Somerset, PA: DeVilbiss Health Care.

Nellcor-Puritan Bennett Companion 492a oxygen concentrator service manual. (1990). Lenexa, KS: Nellcor-Puritan Bennett.

Practice Activities: Oxygen Supply Systems

1. Practice maneuvering an H/K cylinder and an E cylinder onto and off a transport cart:
   a. Use good body mechanics.
   b. Use safety chains.
   c. Maintain contact with cylinder at the valve cap and shoulder.

2. Practice maneuvering a cylinder and cart around the laboratory.

3. Practice cracking both cylinder types.
   a. Observe all safety rules.

4. Practice selecting and attaching the appropriate reducing valves:
   a. Identify and describe all safety features.
   b. Determine by inspection whether the reducing valve is single stage or multistage.
   c. Observe all safety rules.

5. Practice bleeding a reducing valve following use.
   a. Observe good safety practices.

6. Practice returning the cylinders to the storage area.
   a. Observe cylinder storage safety rules:
      (1) Empty and full cylinders are separate.
      (2) Flammable anesthetics are not stored with oxygen.
      (3) Cylinders are chained.
      (4) Door is kept closed.

7. Practice preparing an air/oxygen blender for use:
   a. Attach 50 psi air and oxygen sources.
   b. Secure the air/oxygen blender to a stand or wall mount.
   c. Attach a delivery device to the air/oxygen blender.
   d. Adjust the percentage control to the desired concentration.
   e. Confirm the concentration with an oxygen analyzer.

Check List: Oxygen Supply Systems

_____ 1. Obtain an E or H/K cylinder from storage.
2. Release the safety chain.
_____ a. Ensure that other cylinders will not fall or be disturbed.
_____ 3. Maneuver the cylinder onto the cart.
_____ a. Roll or spin the cylinder but do not try to carry it.
_____ b. Observe the principles of good body mechanics.
4. Secure the cylinder to the cart with the safety chain.
_____ a. Secure the safety chain on the cylinders in storage.
5. Tilt the cart upright and release the third wheel.
_____ a. The cart should rest on three wheels for transport.
6. Transport the cylinder to the desired area.
_____ a. Use caution around the other foot or vehicular traffic.

7. Remove the cylinder valve safety cap.
_____ a. Remove the cap outside the patient's room.
8. Crack the cylinder.
_____ a. Use good hand position.
_____ b. Give an audible warning.
9. Select and attach the correct reducing valve for use.
_____ a. Secure it tightly with a wrench.
10. Check and correct for leaks.
_____ a. Look, listen, and feel.
_____ b. Correct for leaks by tightening the connections.
_____ 11. Calculate the time remaining using the gauge pressure and a given flow rate.
_____ 12. After use, push the cart back to storage.
_____ 13. Return all equipment to its proper location.

Check List: Portable Liquid Oxygen Systems

1. Weigh the portable system to determine its need for transfilling or use the electronic indicator gauge to determine the contents of the portable unit if one is provided.

2. Connect the portable system to the stationary reservoir by mating the male fill port fitting to the female fill port on the stationary reservoir, rotating the portable system until it locks into place.

3. Open the vent valve to begin the filling process.

4. Observe all safety rules regarding use of liquid oxygen:
   a. No smoking or open flame is permitted in the area.
   b. Avoid contact with the liquid contents.
   c. Avoid contact with the fill port or filling fittings.
   d. Always store the portable and stationary reservoirs in an upright position.

5. Once liquid oxygen can be observed exiting the vent fitting, close the vent valve to stop the filling process.

6. Disconnect the portable system from the stationary reservoir.

7. Verify by weight or the unit's electronic gauge that the portable system is full.

8. Calculate the duration of time the portable system will last at the desired liter flow rate.

9. Connect the oxygen delivery device to the nipple outlet of the portable system.

10. Set the liter flow to the desired rate using the flowmeter on the portable system.

11. Document the liter flow rate and delivery device in the patient's record.

Check List: Oxygen Concentrator

1. Place the concentrator correctly at the point of use:
   a. Back and sides must be at least 6 inches away from walls, draperies, or potential obstructions to airflow.
   b. Locate the concentrator away from heaters, heat registers, or radiators.
2. Verify that the power switch is in the off position.
3. Connect the power cord to an electrical outlet.
   a. Check to ensure that a minimal load is shared on that particular circuit.
4. Check the gross particle filter at the air inlet for cleanliness or obstructions, and clean it as required.
5. Connect a humidifier to the outlet (if required or prescribed), or connect the oxygen delivery device directly to the outlet of the concentrator.
6. If required for patient mobility, connect up to 50 feet of oxygen extension tubing between the concentrator and the delivery device.
7. Turn on the power switch.
8. Adjust the liter flow to the desired setting.
9. Document the liter flow rate and delivery device in the patient's record.

Self-Evaluation Post Test: Oxygen Supply Systems

1. A molecular sieve oxygen concentrator is delivering oxygen at a flow of 10 L/min. The delivered oxygen percentage is approximately:
   a. 100%.
   b. 80%.
   c. 60%.
   d. 50%.

2. Which of the following safety systems is used for equipment operating at less than 200 psi?
   a. Diameter-indexed safety system
   b. American Standard Safety System
   c. Pin index safety system
   d. Frangible disc and fusible plug combination
   e. American index system

3. With use of a compensated Thorpe tube flowmeter in the face of resistance distal to the flowmeter, the reading on the flowmeter will be:
   a. less than the delivered flow.
   b. greater than the delivered flow.
   c. equal to the delivered flow.
   d. dependent on temperature and pressure.

4. How many liters are there in 1 cubic foot of gaseous oxygen?
   a. 32.8 L
   b. 28.3 L
   c. 3.14 L
   d. 0.28 L

5. If the outlet of a Bourdon gauge became partially obstructed, the indicated flow would:
   a. be higher than you set.
   b. be lower than you set.
   c. indicate no flow (zero).
   d. not change.

6. An H/K cylinder contains how many cubic feet of oxygen when full?
   a. 22 cu ft
   b. 38 cu ft
   c. 220 cu ft
   d. 244 cu ft

7. Stamped on the shoulder of an H/K cylinder are the markings "3AA-2015." These markings indicate the:
   a. DOT code number and filling pressure.
   b. ICC code number.
   c. serial number of the cylinder.
   d. USP purity number.

8. In a compressed gas storage area, oxygen should not be stored with:
   a. carbon dioxide.
   b. helium.
   c. nitrogen.
   d. flammable anesthetics.

9. The difference between a single-stage and a modified single-stage reducing valve is:
   a. an additional pressure relief valve.
   b. a poppet-closing spring.
   c. the presence of two diaphragms.
   d. a second reducing stage.

10. Mr. Brown is a patient with chronic obstructive pulmonary disease (COPD) who is on home oxygen. He wants to go out for dinner. If he takes a full E cylinder and uses 4 L/min, leaving at 6:00 PM, by what time must he return to avoid running out of oxygen?
    a. 6:30 PM
    b. 7:15 PM
    c. 8:20 PM
    d. 9:00 PM

PERFORMANCE EVALUATION:
Oxygen Concentrators

Date: Lab _____ Clinical _____ Agency _____

Lab: Pass _____ Fail _____ Clinical: Pass _____ Fail _____

Student name _____ Instructor name _____

No. of times observed in clinical _____

No. of times practiced in clinical _____

PASSING CRITERIA: Obtain 90% or better on the procedure. Tasks indicated by * must receive at least 1 point, or the evaluation is terminated. Procedure must be performed within the designated time, or the performance receives a failing grade.

SCORING:
2 points — Task performed satisfactorily without prompting.
1 point — Task performed satisfactorily with self-initiated correction.
0 points — Task performed incorrectly or with prompting required.
NA — Task not applicable to the patient care situation.

Tasks:	Peer	Lab	Clinical
1. Places the concentrator correctly at the point of use			
* a. Away from walls or draperies	☐	☐	☐
* b. Away from heaters, heat registers, or radiators	☐	☐	☐
* **2.** Connects the power cord, ensuring that the circuit has minimal electrical load	☐	☐	☐
* **3.** Checks the gross particle filter and cleans as needed	☐	☐	☐
* **4.** Connects a humidifier as required	☐	☐	☐
* **5.** Connects the oxygen delivery device	☐	☐	☐
* **6.** Adds up to 50 feet of extension tubing as needed	☐	☐	☐
* **7.** Turns on the power switch	☐	☐	☐
* **8.** Sets the liter flow rate	☐	☐	☐
* **9.** Documents the procedure in the patient record	☐	☐	☐

SCORE:
Peer _____ points of possible 20; _____%
Lab _____ points of possible 20; _____%
Clinical _____ points of possible 20; _____%

TIME: _____ out of possible 30 minutes

STUDENT SIGNATURES

PEER: _____

STUDENT: _____

INSTRUCTOR SIGNATURES

LAB: _____

CLINICAL: _____

CHAPTER 13

Oxygen Administration

INTRODUCTION

Oxygen therapy, when indicated and when administered by a knowledgeable respiratory practitioner, may have a dramatic effect on the condition of a patient suffering from hypoxemia. However, under certain circumstances, overadministration of oxygen may be harmful and even fatal.

Oxygen is listed in the United States Pharmacopoeia (USP) as a drug. Therefore, it may be administered only upon an order from a physician. Oxygen therapy is frequently abused and misused. It is important that the respiratory practitioner become knowledgeable about the various oxygen delivery devices. Become acquainted with the advantages of each as well as the associated hazards and complications.

Because the initiation of oxygen administration calls for relatively simple skills, it is easy to overlook the hazards and potential complications associated with this modality. The practitioner's knowledge of these factors may prevent injury or even death resulting from the inappropriate administration of oxygen.

KEY TERMS

- **Absorption atelectasis**
- **Air entrainment mask**
- **Anatomic reservoir**
- **FIO$_2$**
- **Head box**
- **High-flow oxygen delivery system**

- **Hypoxemia**
- **Isolette**
- **Low-flow oxygen delivery system**
- **Nasal cannula**
- **Nonrebreathing mask**
- **Oxygen analyzer**

- **Partial rebreathing mask**
- **Retinopathy of prematurity**
- **Simple oxygen mask**
- **Transtracheal catheter**

THEORY OBJECTIVES

At the end of this chapter, the reader should be able to:

- *State the indications for oxygen therapy.*
- *Define high-flow and low-flow oxygen delivery systems, and categorize six administration devices.*
- *Explain the role of the nasopharynx and the oropharynx, and the effect of tidal volume and respiratory rate, on the delivered FIO$_2$ by low-flow oxygen systems.*
- *Explain the principle of operation for the majority of high-flow oxygen delivery systems.*
- *Diagram the flow of oxygen and air through an air entrainment mask.*
- *Given an oxygen flow and entrainment ratio, calculate the total flow.*
- *Differentiate between the indications for the use of a low-flow or high-flow oxygen system.*
- *Explain the rationale for the use of a humidifier with oxygen delivery devices.*

- *List the oxygen delivery devices that can be categorized as enclosures and their advantages and disadvantages and FIO$_2$ ranges.*
- *Describe the oxygen percentages that can be delivered by the different enclosures.*
- *Describe the proper use of an oxygen analyzer.*
- *Describe the two most common types of oxygen analyzers.*
- *Explain the following conditions associated with oxygen administration:*
  - *Absorption atelectasis*
  - *Interruption of hypoxic drive*
  - *Oxygen toxicity*
  - *Retinopathy of prematurity*
- *Discuss the role of arterial blood gas analysis in the administration of oxygen.*

CLINICAL PRACTICE GUIDELINES

AARC Clinical Practice Guideline Oxygen Therapy in the Acute Care Hospital

OT-AC 4.0 INDICATIONS:

4.1 Documented hypoxemia. Defined as a decreased PaO_2 in the blood below normal range.[2] PaO_2 of <60 torr or SaO_2 of <90% in subjects breathing room air or with PaO_2 and/or SaO_2 below desirable range for specific clinical situation.[1]

4.2 An acute care situation in which hypoxemia is suspected[1,3-6] substantiation of hypoxemia is required within an appropriate period of time following initiation of therapy.

4.3 Severe trauma[5,6]

4.4 Acute myocardial infarction[1,7]

4.5 Short-term therapy or surgical intervention (eg, post-anesthesia recovery[5,8], hip surgery[9,10])

OT-AC 5.0 CONTRAINDICATIONS:

No specific contraindications to oxygen therapy exist when indications are judged to be present.

OT-AC 6.0 PRECAUTIONS AND/OR POSSIBLE COMPLICATIONS:

6.1 With PaO_2 > or = 60 torr, ventilatory depression may occur in spontaneously breathing patients with elevated $PaCO_2$.[6,11-14]

6.2 With FIO_2 > or = 0.5, absorption atelectasis, oxygen toxicity, and/or depression of ciliary and/or leukocytic function may occur.[12,15,16]

6.3 Supplemental oxygen should be administered with caution to patients suffering from paraquat poisoning[17] and to patients receiving bleomycin.[18]

6.4 During laser bronchoscopy, minimal levels of supplemental oxygen should be used to avoid intratracheal ignition.[19]

6.5 Fire hazard is increased in the presence of increased oxygen concentrations.

6.6 Bacterial contamination associated with certain nebulization and humidification

OT-AC 7.0 LIMITATIONS OF PROCEDURE:

Oxygen therapy has only limited benefit for the treatment of hypoxia due to anemia, and benefit may be limited with circulatory disturbances.

Oxygen therapy should not be used in lieu of but in addition to mechanical ventilation when ventilatory support is indicated.

OT-AC 8.0 ASSESSMENT OF NEED:

Need is determined by measurement of inadequate oxygen tensions and/or saturations, by invasive or noninvasive methods, and/or the presence of clinical indicators as previously described.

OT-AC 9.0 ASSESSMENT OF OUTCOME:

Outcome is determined by clinical and physiologic assessment to establish adequacy of patient response to therapy.

OT-AC 11.0 MONITORING:

11.1 Patient

11.1.1 Clinical assessment including, but not limited to, cardiac, pulmonary, and neurologic status

11.1.2 Assessment of physiologic parameters: measurement of oxygen tensions or saturation in any patient treated with oxygen

11.1.2.1 In conjunction with the initiation of therapy; or

11.1.2.2 Within 12-hours of initiation with FIO_2 < 0.40

11.1.2.3 Within 8-hours, with FIO_2 > or = 0.40 (including postanesthesia recovery)

11.1.2.4 Within 72 hours in acute myocardial infarction (9)

11.1.2.5 Within 2 hours for any patient with the principal diagnosis of COPD

11.1.2.6 Within 1 hour for the neonate (2)

11.2 Equipment

11.2.1 All oxygen delivery systems should be checked at least once per day.

11.2.2 More frequent checks by calibrated analyzer are necessary in systems.

11.2.2.1 Susceptible to variation in oxygen concentration (e.g., hoods, high-flow blending systems)

11.2.2.2 Applied to patients with artificial airways

11.2.2.3 Delivering a heated gas mixture

11.2.2.4 Applied to patients who are clinically unstable or who require an FIO_2 of 0.50 or higher

11.2.3 The standard of practice for newborns appears to be continuous analysis of F_DO_2 with a system check at least every 4 hours, but data to support this practice may not be available.

Reprinted with permission from *Respiratory Care* 2002; 47(6): 717–720. The complete AARC Clinical Practice Guidelines are available from the AARC Web site (http://www.aarc .org), from the AARC Executive Office, or from *Respiratory Care* journal.

(Continued)

AARC Clinical Practice Guideline Oxygen Therapy in the Home or Extended Care Facility – 2007 Revision & Update

OT-CC 4.0 INDICATIONS:

4.1 Long-term oxygen therapy (LTOT) in the home or alternate site health care facility is normally indicated for the treatment of hypoxemia.[2,3] LTOT has been shown to significantly improve survival in hypoxemic patients with chronic obstructive pulmonary disease (COPD).[4,5] LTOT has been shown to reduce hospitalizations and lengths of stay.[6,7]

4.2 Laboratory indications: Documented hypoxemia in adults, children, and infants older than 28 days as evidenced by [1] $PaO_2 \leq 55$ mm Hg or $SaO_2 \leq 88\%$ in subjects breathing room air or [2] PaO_2 of 56-59 mm Hg or SaO_2 or $SpO_2 \leq 89\%$ in association with specific clinical conditions (eg, cor pulmonale, congestive heart failure, or erythrocythemia with hematocrit > 56).[8,9]

4.3 Some patients may not demonstrate a need for oxygen therapy at rest (normoxic) but will be hypoxemic during ambulation, sleep, or exercise. Oxygen therapy is indicated during these specific activities when the SaO_2 is demonstrated to fall to $\leq 88\%$.[8]

4.4 Oxygen therapy may be prescribed by the attending physician for indications outside of those noted above or in cases where strong evidence may be lacking (eg, cluster headaches) on the order and discretion of the attending physician.

4.5 Patients who are approaching the end of life frequently exhibit dyspnea with or without hypoxemia.[10,11] Dyspnea in the absence of hypoxemia can be treated with techniques and drugs other than oxygen.[12-14] Oxygen may be tried in these patients at 1-3 liters per minute, to obtain subjective relief of dyspnea.[13]

4.6 All oxygen must be prescribed and dispensed in accordance with federal, state, and local laws and regulations.

OT-CC 5.0 CONTRAINDICATIONS:

No absolute contraindications to oxygen therapy exist when indications are present.

OT-CC 6.0 PRECAUTIONS AND/OR POSSIBLE COMPLICATIONS:

6.1 There is a potential in some spontaneously breathing hypoxemic patients with hypercapnia and chronic obstructive pulmonary disease that oxygen administration may lead to an increase in $PaCO_2$.[15-17]

6.2 Undesirable results or events may result from noncompliance with physicians' orders or inadequate instruction in home oxygen therapy.

6.3 Complications may result from use of nasal cannulae[18] or transtracheal catheters.[19]

6.4 Fire hazard is increased in the presence of increased oxygen concentrations.

6.5 Bacterial contamination associated with certain nebulizers and humidification systems is a possible hazard.[20]

6.6 Possible physical hazards can be posed by unsecured cylinders, ungrounded equipment, or mishandling of liquid oxygen. Power or equipment malfunction and/or failure can lead to an interruption in oxygen supply.

OT-CC 7.0 LIMITATIONS OF PROCEDURE:

Oxygen therapy has only limited benefit for the treatment of hypoxia due to anemia and benefit may be limited when circulatory disturbances are present. Oxygen therapy should not be used in lieu of but in addition to mechanical ventilation when ventilatory support is indicated.[21]

OT-CC 8.0 ASSESSMENT OF NEED:

8.1 Initial assessment: Need is determined by the presence of clinical indicators as previously described and the presence of inadequate oxygen tension and/or saturation as demonstrated by the analysis of arterial blood. Concurrent pulse oximetry values must be documented and reconciled with the results of the baseline blood gas analysis if future assessment is to involve pulse oximetry.

8.2 Ongoing evaluation or reassessment: Additional arterial blood gas analysis is indicated whenever there is a major change in clinical status that may be cardiopulmonary-related. Arterial blood gas measurements should be repeated in 1–3 months when oxygen therapy is begun in the hospital in a clinically unstable patient to determine the need for long-term oxygen therapy (LTOT).[14] Once the need for LTOT has been documented, repeat arterial blood gas analysis or oxygen saturation measurements are unnecessary other than to follow the course of the disease, to assess changes in clinical status, or to facilitate changes in the oxygen prescription.[14,15]

OT-CC 9.0 ASSESSMENT OF OUTCOME:

Outcome is determined by clinical and physiologic assessment to establish adequacy of patient response to therapy.

OT-CC 11.0 MONITORING:

11.1 Patient

11.1.1 Clinical assessment should routinely be performed by the patient and/or the caregiver to determine changes in clinical status (e.g., use of dyspnea scales and diary cards). Patients should be visited/monitored at least once a

(Continued)

month by credentialed personnel unless conditions warrant more frequent visits.

11.1.2 Measurement of baseline oxygen tension and saturation is essential before oxygen therapy is begun.[5,15] These measurements should be repeated when clinically indicated or to follow the course of the disease. Measurements of SO_2 also may be made to determine appropriate oxygen flow for ambulation, exercise, or sleep.

11.2 Equipment Maintenance and Supervision: All oxygen delivery equipment should be checked at least once daily by the patient or caregiver. Facets to be assessed include proper function of the equipment, prescribed flow rates, FDO_2, remaining liquid or compressed gas content, and backup supply. A respiratory therapist or equivalent should during monthly visits reinforce appropriate practices and performance by the patient and caregivers and ensure that the oxygen equipment is being maintained in accordance with manufacturers' recommendations. Liquid systems need to be checked to ensure adequate delivery.[25] Oxygen concentrators should be checked regularly to ensure that they are delivering 85% oxygen or greater at 4 L/min.[24]

Reprinted with permission from *Respiratory Care* 2007; 52(1): 1063–1068. The complete AARC Clinical Practice Guidelines are available from the AARC Web site (http://www.aarc .org), from the AARC Executive Office, or from *Respiratory Care* journal.

INDICATIONS FOR OXYGEN THERAPY

The primary indication for oxygen therapy is hypoxemia. *Hypoxemia* is defined as an oxygen tension in arterial blood (PaO_2) that is below normal. The practitioner can estimate PaO_2 for a patient breathing room air by using the following formula: $103.5 - (0.42 \times \text{age}) \pm 4$ (Sabrini, Grassi, Solinas, & Muiesan, 1968). Keep in mind the effects that altitude has on what is considered normal. With increasing altitude, the partial pressure of oxygen decreases because barometric pressure is lower. Therefore, the PaO_2 falls with increasing altitude.

The amount of oxygen required to correct the hypoxemia will vary depending on the patient's clinical condition. The best way to assess the effects of oxygen therapy is by arterial blood gas analysis or monitoring by oximetry. Sampling arterial blood allows the oxygen therapy to be tailored to meet the patient's specific needs.

There are other therapeutic goals for oxygen administration in addition to correction of hypoxemia (American Association for Respiratory Care [AARC], 2002). These goals are listed in Figure 13-1.

Hypoxemia may cause an increase in ventilation and cardiac output as the body compensates (the hypoxic drive). By increasing the oxygen content of the arterial blood, the muscle (energy) requirements of the pulmonary and cardiovascular systems are reduced.

- To correct hypoxemia
- To decrease myocardial work
- To decrease the work of breathing

Figure 13-1 Goals of oxygen therapy

© Cengage Learning 2013

Low-Flow Oxygen Delivery Systems

A *low-flow oxygen delivery system* is defined as a system that supplies oxygen-enriched gas as part of a patient's inspiratory flow needs. The patient must be able to inhale sufficiently to meet ventilatory needs but may require the administration of a limited amount of 100% oxygen, which is then mixed with room air as the patient inhales.

Low-flow devices rely on the nasopharynx and oropharynx to serve as a reservoir, enhancing FIO_2 by temporarily holding a small amount of 100% oxygen. This reservoir is referred to as the *anatomic reservoir*. In an average adult, it is estimated that this reservoir has a volume of about 50 mL (Kacmarek, Dimas, & Mack, 2005).

Because the low-flow devices provide only part of the inspiratory needs, the delivered fraction of inspired oxygen (*FIO_2*, usually expressed as a decimal fraction) may vary depending on several factors. One factor that may alter FIO_2 is the flow of oxygen through the device. Generally, the higher the flow, the higher the FIO_2. The patient's respiratory rate and tidal volume may also affect the FIO_2.

A patient with shallower than normal tidal volumes will receive proportionately more oxygen than that delivered to the patient with a normal tidal volume. The 100% oxygen inhaled from the anatomical reservoir (approximately 50 mL) is proportionately greater in a patient with a 250 mL tidal volume than in a patient with a 500 mL tidal volume. Therefore, the FIO_2 is higher. Keep in mind that the oxygen flow through the device also influences the delivered FIO_2, as noted.

A respiratory rate higher than normal may also dilute the oxygen concentration by not allowing time for the anatomical reservoir to fill sufficiently with oxygen. Under these circumstances, more room air is inspired, diluting the oxygen concentration.

Owing to these variables, the best way to assess the adequacy of oxygen therapy with these devices is by arterial blood gas analysis and careful patient observation.

LOW-FLOW OXYGEN DEVICES

Nasal Cannula

The *nasal cannula* is designed to rest on the upper lip with the two prongs directed into each naris (nostril) of the nose. Oxygen is directed into the nasal passage, where it is warmed and humidified as the gas passes over the turbinates. This device uses the anatomical reservoir to deliver increased FIO_2. In a short time, most patients become quite comfortable with this device and hardly notice its presence.

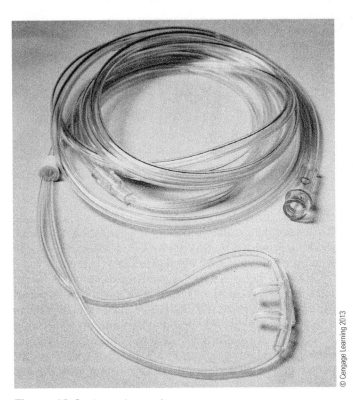

Figure 13-2 A nasal cannula

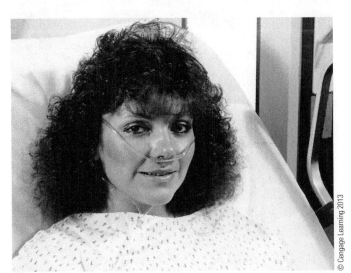

Figure 13-3 A nasal cannula correctly applied on a patient

When the cannula is correctly applied, the cannula tubing is looped over each ear and the slide is adjusted so that it is barely snug under the chin. Application of a cannula in this manner provides for safety. Without the loops, if the patient turns suddenly and stretches the connecting tubing to its limit, the cannula will pull off the face. A cannula applied incorrectly by looping the free tubing around the head may serve as a noose on a confused, combative patient. Figures 13-2 and 13-3 illustrate a nasal cannula and its correct application, respectively. Figure 13-4 is a diagram of the anatomical reservoir.

Oxygen Concentration

The FIO_2 delivered by a nasal cannula will vary with the liter flow and the patient's ventilatory patterns, as discussed earlier. Table 13-1 shows approximate oxygen concentrations at various oxygen flows.

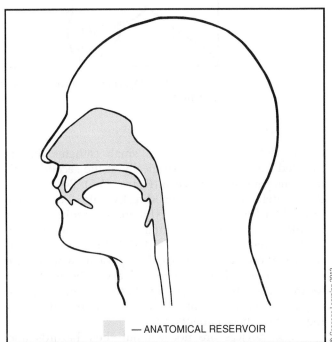

— ANATOMICAL RESERVOIR

Figure 13-4 A cross section of the anatomical reservoir

TABLE 13-1: Nasal Cannula Oxygen Concentrations

OXYGEN 100% O₂ FLOW	APPROXIMATE CONCENTRATION (%)
1 L/min	24
2 L/min	28
3 L/min	32
4 L/min	36
5 L/min	40
6 L/min	44

Reprinted by permission from Shapiro, B. A., Peruzzi, W. T., & Templin, R. (1994). *Clinical Application of Blood Gases* (5th ed.), St. Louis, MO: Mosby

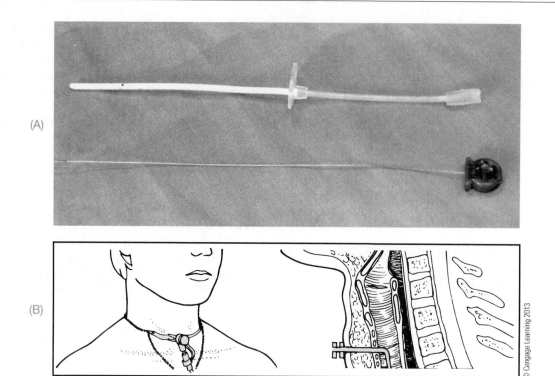

Figure 13-5   (A) A transtracheal catheter; (B) A pictorial representation showing its correct placement

Transtracheal Catheter

A *transtracheal catheter* is a small catheter that is inserted into the trachea surgically at the second cartilaginous ring of the trachea (Figure 13-5). Because this device delivers the oxygen directly into the trachea, lower liter flows may be used than are required with a simple nasal cannula to maintain a desired PaO_2 or SpO_2 (pulse oximeter–determined arterial blood oxygen saturation). These devices are used for patients who require continuous low-flow oxygen delivery. Substantial cost savings may be realized by these patients because often an oxygen flow of 0.25 to 0.50 L/min is all that is required by these patients.

These devices are not without their hazards and complications. Because surgical intervention is required to place them, the risk of infection is always present. Therefore, these catheters must be routinely cleaned and maintained by the patient or the patient's caregiver. Also, the cost advantages must be carefully weighed against the risk of infection and the patient's cosmetic appearance.

Simple Oxygen Mask

The *simple oxygen mask* delivers a low flow of oxygen, meeting only part of a patient's inspiratory flow needs. The underlying principle in use of a mask is to add an oxygen reservoir external to the patient. The volume of the mask serves as this reservoir. Typically, the volume of this reservoir is greater than that of the anatomic reservoir.

The mask is filled with 100% oxygen at the end of inspiration. As the patient inhales, the first portion of the inspired air is the 100% oxygen contained in the mask, followed by a mixture of air and oxygen for the remainder of the inspiratory phase. The room air is allowed to enter the mask through the ports on the side of the mask. Because of the greater volume of oxygen being delivered, the FIO_2 provided by this device is higher than what can be administered using a nasal cannula or catheter.

The FIO_2 delivered by a simple mask ranges between 35% and 55% (Wilkins, 2009). The FIO_2 will vary depending on oxygen flow and the patient's breathing pattern. The oxygen flow should be set at a minimum of 5 L/min to prevent rebreathing of carbon dioxide (CO_2) from exhaled air. Figures 13-6 and 13-7 show a disposable simple oxygen mask and its correct application, respectively.

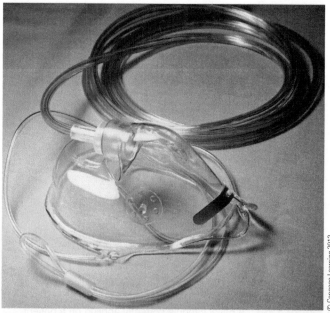

Figure 13-6 A simple oxygen mask

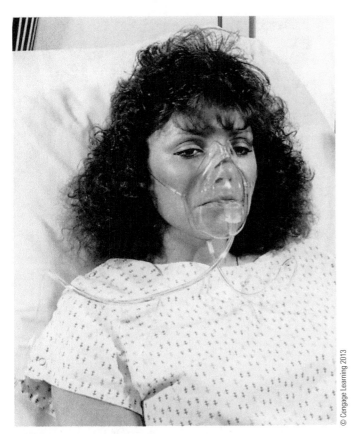

Figure 13-7 A simple oxygen mask correctly applied on a patient

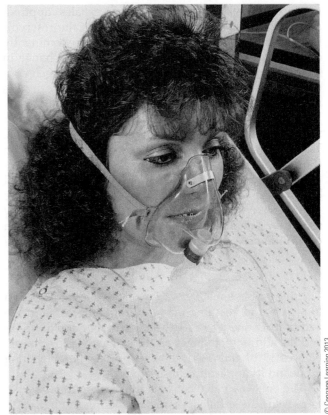

Figure 13-9 A partial rebreathing mask correctly applied on a patient

Partial Rebreathing Mask

A *partial rebreathing mask* takes the reservoir concept of a simple mask one step further by the addition of a reservoir bag. Now, in addition to the mask, a large bag also serves as a reservoir. The oxygen enters the device between the bag and the reservoir. Figures 13-8 and 13-9 show a typical disposable partial rebreathing mask and its application, respectively.

Oxygen enters the mask, filling the reservoir bag. As the patient inhales, part of the breath is inhaled from the bag and mask. The remainder of the breath is air drawn in through the ports on the side of the mask, mixing with

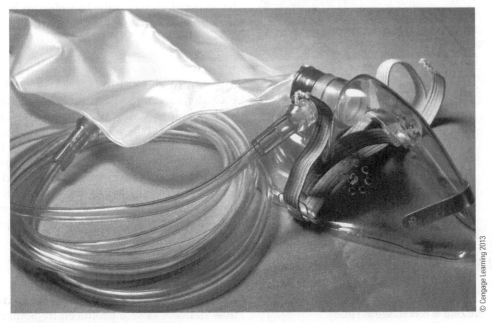

Figure 13-8 A partial rebreathing mask

the incoming oxygen. As the patient exhales, approximately the first third of exhaled gas fills the reservoir bag. This first part of expiratory volume is predominantly dead space and has not participated in gas exchange in the lungs. Therefore, it is relatively high in oxygen concentration. The remainder of the exhaled gas exits the mask through the ports on the side.

Because the partial rebreathing mask has a larger reservoir volume, it is capable of delivering a higher FIO_2. This mask is capable of delivering up to 60% oxygen (Branson, 1993).

When this mask is fitted properly, the flow should be adjusted so that the bag is not allowed to collapse completely on inspiration (Branson, 1993). Oxygen flow should be adjusted such that the bag remains between one-third and one-half full during exhalation.

Nonrebreathing Mask

The disposable *nonrebreathing mask* is similar in design to a partial rebreathing mask. The differences lie in the addition of a one-way valve between the bag and the mask and the addition of valves on the side ports of the mask. Figures 13-10 and 13-11 show a typical nonrebreathing mask and its application, respectively.

The one-way valve between the mask and bag serves to prevent the exhaled gas from entering the bag. This valve may consist of a disk and spring or may be a simple diaphragm valve. Valves over the side ports prevent the entrainment of ambient air on inspiration.

If the fit of the mask is good, both side ports have one-way valves, and if all one-way valves are functional, then it is possible to deliver 60% to 80% oxygen (Branson, 1993). However, with some disposable masks, only one side port is fitted with a one-way valve, and it is rarely possible to obtain a good tight fit. Under these conditions, this type of mask becomes a low-flow device because not

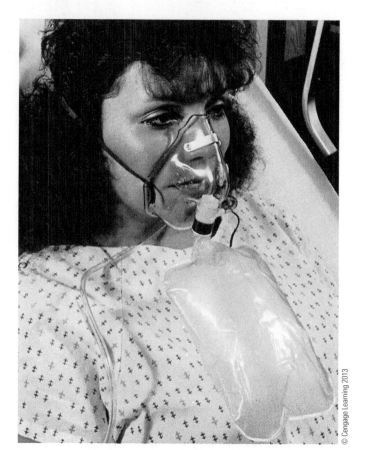

Figure 13-11 A disposable nonrebreathing mask applied on a patient

all of the inspiratory needs of the patient are met. The oxygen delivery would fall considerably below 100% (Branson, 1993).

As with the partial rebreathing mask, it is important to adjust the flow so that the reservoir bag is not allowed to completely collapse on inspiration. Oxygen flow should be adjusted such that the bag remains between one-third and one-half full during exhalation.

Hi-Ox[80]

The Cardinal Health Hi-Ox[80] is a disposable high-FIO_2 delivery mask that incorporates a reservoir bag and multiple one-way valves. The one-way valves are configured in a manifold between the reservoir bag and the mask. Figures 13-12 and 13-13 show the Hi-Ox[80] mask and the flow patterns through the one-way valves. A foam cushion on the bridge of the mask and two straps help the mask to fit tighter and seal better than other disposable reservoir masks. Oxygen concentrations approaching 80% are possible at liter flows of 8 L/min.

OxyMask™

The OxyMask™ (Figure 13-14) is a disposable low-flow delivery device produced by Southmedic, Ontario,

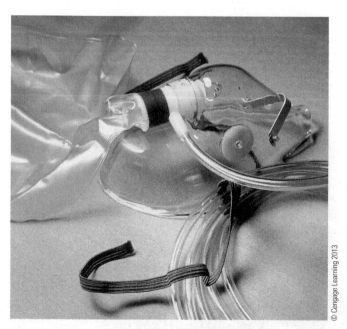

Figure 13-10 A disposable nonrebreathing mask

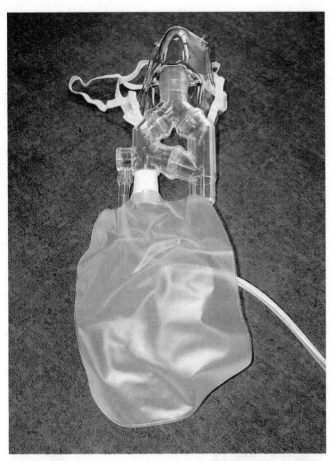

Figure 13-12 A photograph of the HiOx⁸⁰ mask. *(Courtesy of American Association for Respiratory Care, Irving, TX)*

Canada. Depending on the flow rate, the mask delivers between 24% and 90% oxygen (Table 13-2).

The oxygen diffuser (inlet) is proximal to the nose and mouth, delivering 100% oxygen close to the point of entry into the respiratory tract. The larger ports on the sides of the mask improve patient comfort, and they facilitate communication and oral intake of fluids with a straw. The OxyMask™ may be used as a substitute for the majority of disposable oxygen delivery devices (nasal cannula, simple mask, and partial and nonrebreathing masks).

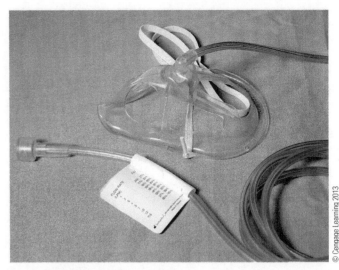

Figure 13-14 The OxyMask™

HIGH-FLOW OXYGEN DELIVERY SYSTEMS

A *high-flow oxygen delivery system* provides all of the total inspiratory flow required by the patient. Any inspired gas is provided solely by the device. Respiratory pattern and rate will not affect the FIO_2 delivered by these devices.

Vapotherm Precision Flow High-Flow Cannula

The Vapotherm precision flow high-flow cannula is a high-flow oxygen therapy system that is capable of delivering oxygen flows from 1 to 40 L/min at humidity contents of 55 mg/L at a temperature of 41°C. Figure 13-15 is a photograph of the Vapotherm precision flow system.

Humidification is achieved using a membrane cartridge, an external water source, and a heater element. The cartridge ensures a large surface area for water/gas interface. Temperature may be selected between 35 and 43°C. A single module controls both flow and temperature.

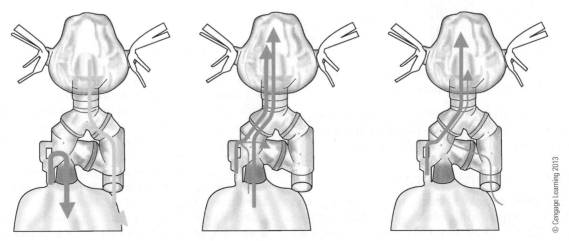

Figure 13-13 Flow path through HiOx⁸⁰ mask's one-way valve system.

TABLE 13-2: OxyMask™ Oxygen Percentage Delivery

OXYGEN FLOW RATE	OXYGEN PERCENTAGE (%)
1 L/min	24–27
2 L/min	27–32
3 L/min	30–60
4 L/min	33–65
5 L/min	36–69
7 L/min	48–80
10 L/min	53–85
12 L/min	57–89
>15 L/min	60–90

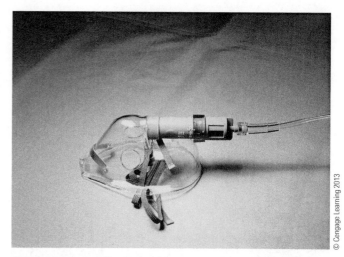

Figure 13-16   A Venturi mask

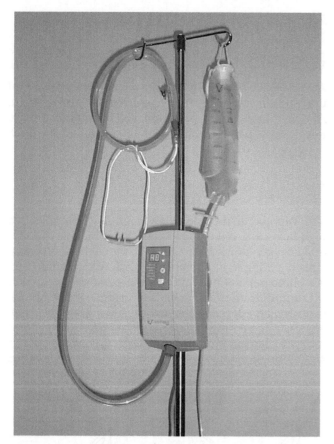

Figure 13-15   The Vapotherm precision high-flow cannula *(Courtesy of Vapotherm, Inc., Annapolis, MD)*

Because the gas delivered to the patient is both warmed and humidified, higher flow may be tolerated when compared with conventional oxygen delivery devices.

Air Entrainment Masks

Other high-flow oxygen systems use jet mixing and precisely mix oxygen and ambient air to deliver a specific FIO₂. Figures 13-16 and 13-17 show a typical *air entrainment mask* and its application, respectively.

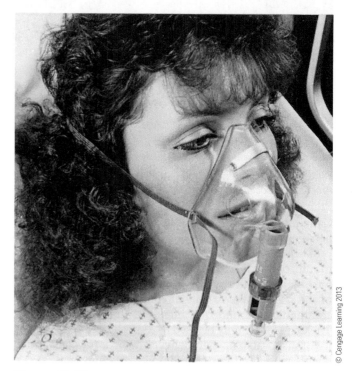

Figure 13-17   A Venturi mask applied on a patient

The way in which these devices function is based on the principles of viscous shearing and vorticity (Scacci, 1979). The high-velocity gas (oxygen) exiting the nozzle (jet) causes shear forces to develop distal to the nozzle orifice and along the axis of the gas flow. These shear forces accelerate the relatively stationary ambient air, forming vortices. The ambient air is entrained by (drawn into) the oxygen flow by these vortices (Figure 13-18). By varying the size of the nozzle (jet) and entrainment ports, air and oxygen may be mixed in precise ratios to achieve known oxygen percentages. These masks are sometimes called Venturi, Venti, or multivent masks. This principle is also employed in many nebulizers to adjust the oxygen concentration.

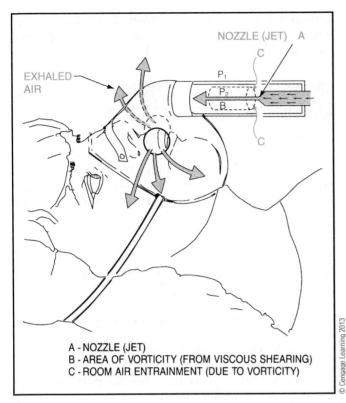

A - NOZZLE (JET)
B - AREA OF VORTICITY (FROM VISCOUS SHEARING)
C - ROOM AIR ENTRAINMENT (DUE TO VORTICITY)

© Cengage Learning 2013

Figure 13-18 Application of viscous shearing and vorticity to entrain room air into a mask to provide a precise concentration of oxygen

TABLE 13-3: Air-to-Oxygen Entrainment Ratios

ROOM AIR-TO-OXYGEN RATIO	OXYGEN CONCENTRATION (%)
25:1	24
10:1	28
8:1	30
5:1	35
3:1	40
1.7:1	50
1:1	60
0:1	100

Entrainment ratios of oxygen to room air used in establishing various FIO_2 concentrations are listed in Table 13-3.

Let us examine the significance of these entrainment ratios and see how the high-flow devices using this principle satisfy total inspiratory needs. Let us assume that the practitioner has set the entrainment device to deliver 35% oxygen with a corresponding entrainment ratio of 5:1. The oxygen flowmeter is set at 6 L/min. According to the entrainment ratio, each liter of oxygen will entrain 5 liters of ambient air. With the oxygen flow at 6 L/min,

the device will entrain 30 liters of ambient air per minute. The entrained ambient air is added to the flow from the oxygen flowmeter for a total flow of 36 L/min. This device, when set at an oxygen flow of 6 L/min, provides a total flow of 36 L/min.

Assuming an average adult has a tidal volume of 500 mL and is breathing at a rate of 14 breaths per minute with an inspiratory-to-expiratory ratio (I:E) of 1:2, the patient would require approximately 22 L/min to meet inspiratory needs. This device floods the patient with oxygen at 35%. It is important to note that the oxygen percentage is changed by adjusting the amount of entrained ambient air, not by adjusting the flowmeter. Increasing the liter flow from 6 L/min to 10 L/min will not affect the delivered FIO_2.

Assume again that the device is adjusted for 35% oxygen at an entrainment ratio of 5:1. Observe in this example that increasing the oxygen flow simply increases ambient air entrainment at the same ratio as before. Although there is an increase in oxygen flow, this does not affect the delivered FIO_2. The total flow to the patient increases, however. In this example, the total flow increases from 36 L/min to 60 L/min, but the ratio remains the same, as does the FIO_2. To prevent dilution of entrained gas by the room air being drawn in around the mask, it is important that the total gas flow exceed the patient minute ventilation (total volume of gas inspired in 1 minute).

Effects of Back Pressure Distal to the Point of Entrainment

Back pressure applied distal to the point of entrainment causes an increase in the delivered FIO_2. This back pressure may occur as a result of a kink in the delivery tubing, water buildup, humidification, secretions in the delivery tubing, or any of a number of other factors.

An obstruction distal to the nozzle (jet) causes pressure to increase upstream to the point of entrainment. If the pressure at the entrainment ports becomes greater than ambient (atmospheric) pressure, ambient air is no longer mixed by vorticity because no air can enter (Scacci, 1979); therefore, the FIO_2 will increase.

CLINICAL APPLICATIONS OF LOW-FLOW AND HIGH-FLOW OXYGEN SYSTEMS

The low-flow oxygen devices are adequate for administering oxygen to the majority of patients. As discussed earlier, the FIO_2 cannot be accurately measured. Therefore, if the patient must receive a precise oxygen concentration, these devices would not be indicated. Also, unusual respiratory rates and depths can significantly alter the FIO_2.

High-flow oxygen systems are indicated for patients who require a constant, precise FIO_2 (Table 13-4).

TABLE 13-4: Effect of Increasing Oxygen Flow through High-Flow Device

ENTRAIN-MENT RATIO	AMBIENT AIR ENTRAIN-MENT	OXYGEN FLOW	OXYGEN CONCEN-TRATION (%)
5:1	30 L/min	6 L/min	35
5:1	50 L/min	10 L/min	35

With use of these devices, FIO_2 will not vary from what has been set. If for physiologic reasons a specific or consistent FIO_2 is desired, the high-flow device would be indicated.

HUMIDIFICATION

Oxygen from a cylinder or piping system is anhydrous. In the manufacture of medical gases, all water and water vapor are removed. The administration of dry gas is very irritating to the mucosa of the upper airway and may lead to thickened secretions, impaired ciliary activity, and retained secretions (Chalon, 1980). These adverse effects can be prevented by proper humidification with administration of oxygen.

All oxygen administration devices should be used with a separate humidifier. If a humidifier or nebulizer is an integral part of the design, it should be used.

With an air entrainment mask, it is more efficient to provide humidification externally by using a collar to attach a nebulizer to the air entrainment port. By the attachment of a nebulizer, the entrained ambient air is humidified before reaching the patient. Figure 13-19 shows the attachment of a large-volume nebulizer to a

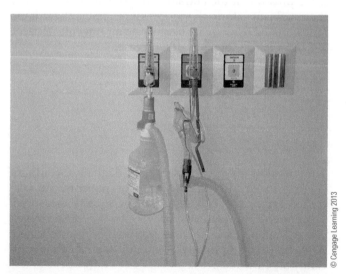

Figure 13-19 Use of a large-volume nebulizer to humidify a Venturi mask

Venturi mask. Note that the external nebulizer, if it is pneumatically driven, should be operated by compressed air so that the FIO_2 is not affected.

ENCLOSURES

Oxygen enclosures are devices designed to contain all or part of the patient's body in an oxygen-enriched atmosphere. The most common applications of these devices are for newborns and infants. The use of adult enclosures is on the decline, owing to the more efficient oxygen administration devices available.

Isolette

An *isolette* is a chamber designed to provide a thermally controlled, oxygen-enriched, humid environment for a newborn. The chamber is constructed of clear Plexiglas with access to the newborn provided by ports on the sides of the isolette.

To maintain a consistent environment, it is important in caring for the newborn to gain access through the ports provided for delivery of care. When the ports are not in use, they should remain closed.

Most isolette models have safety features that prevent administration of high FIO_2 concentrations. Careful monitoring of blood gases (to maintain the PaO_2 between 50 and 80 mm Hg) is important to prevent *retinopathy of prematurity* (ROP). Figure 13-20 shows an isolette.

Head Box or Oxygen Hood

A *head box* is an enclosure designed for use on a newborn infant. It encloses only the head, leaving good access to the rest of the infant's body for nursing care. The head box is typically made from Plexiglas. Some models have removable tops to provide access to the head if needed. Figure 13-21 depicts a typical head box.

Warmed, humidified oxygen is supplied to the box by means of large-bore aerosol tubing. A fitting is provided at the end of the box for the attachment of the tubing. Precautions similar to those taken with the isolette should be employed with head boxes. Careful monitoring of blood gases and FIO_2 is important in the prevention of ROP.

Hazards Associated with Enclosures

Oxygen enclosures having large volumes of oxygen-enriched air can pose a considerable fire hazard if not treated properly.

Children in enclosures should not be allowed to have battery-powered electric toys, radios, or other electrically powered appliances. If possible, limit the child's playthings to stuffed animals or other nonmetallic objects incapable of generating sparks.

All visitors should be prohibited from smoking in the room, and *No smoking* signs should be placed in several conspicuous locations inside and outside the room.

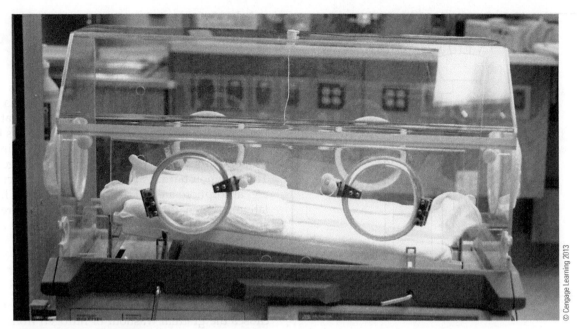

Figure 13-20 An isolette

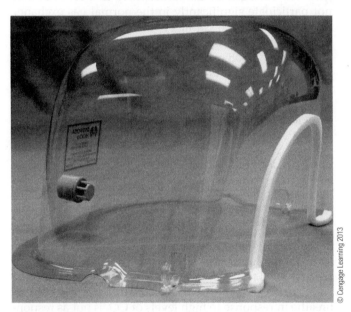

Figure 13-21 An infant head box

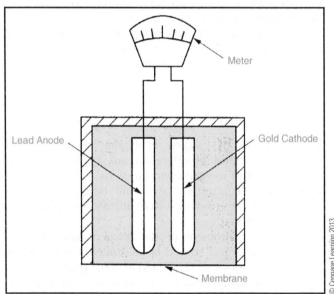

Figure 13-22 A diagram of a galvanic oxygen analyzer

TYPES OF OXYGEN ANALYZERS

Four types of *oxygen analyzer* devices have been produced commercially. These are the physical (based on the principle of paramagnetism), electrical (Wheatstone bridge), and electrochemical, both galvanic and polarographic. Of the four types, the galvanic and polarographic analyzers are the most commonly used types.

Galvanic Oxygen Analyzer

The galvanic oxygen analyzer uses a chemical reaction of oxygen combining with water and electrons to form hydroxyl ions (OH⁻). This reaction is a type of *oxidation-reduction reaction.* The hydroxyl ions migrate to a positive electrode (anode), which reduces the lead, forming more free electrons (Figure 13-22). Formation of these electrons is measured as current flow, and the current is proportional to the oxygen concentration.

Galvanic oxygen analyzers rely strictly on the chemical reaction to produce the electrical current flow that is measured. The response time may be somewhat slower than that with use of a polarographic oxygen analyzer.

Polarographic Oxygen Analyzers

Polarographic oxygen analyzers are similar to galvanic oxygen analyzers with the addition of a battery to polarize the electrodes (Figure 13-23). The polarographic

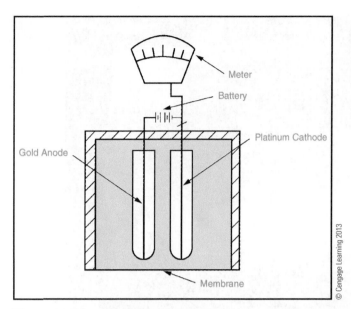

Figure 13-23 A diagram of a polarographic oxygen analyzer

© Cengage Learning 2013

oxygen analyzer uses a similar oxidation-reduction reaction to form free electrons at the anode.

Polarographic analyzers generally have a more rapid response time than galvanic analyzers. The polarization of the electrodes speeds the reaction, reducing the response time.

Use of an Oxygen Analyzer

Various types of oxygen analyzers using different physical principles of operation are available for the measurement of oxygen concentrations. Whenever possible, oxygen concentrations should be measured and documented in the patient's chart at least once each shift, or every 8 hours.

Before measurement of the oxygen concentration, the oxygen analyzer should be calibrated. Calibration is performed at room air (21%) and at 100% (pure oxygen). Calibrate the analyzer at 21% or room air, and then calibrate it at 100% by immersing the probe in a reservoir of 100% oxygen.

To measure the FIO_2, sample the gas as close to the patient as possible. The oxygen concentration may be documented either as a percentage (40% oxygen) or as a fraction of the inspired oxygen (FIO_2 0.40). Do not mix the two methods of documentation.

In some cases, it is very difficult to analyze the oxygen concentration. For example, with a low-flow oxygen delivery system for a patient on a nasal cannula receiving oxygen at 2 L/min, a specific oxygen concentration cannot be measured. In this instance, the oxygen concentration may be documented by the liter flow; for example, the practitioner may chart as follows: "Patient on a nasal cannula at an oxygen flow of 2 L/min." If oxygen concentration cannot be measured, at least document the oxygen flow.

HAZARDS OF OXYGEN THERAPY

There are several hazards and complications associated with oxygen therapy. This section briefly discusses the more common hazards and complications that the practitioner may encounter in clinical practice. It is important to note that the majority may be avoided entirely by the proper administration and monitoring of oxygen therapy. The common hazards and complications discussed here are absorption atelectasis, oxygen-induced hypoventilation, oxygen toxicity, and ROP. For a more in-depth study, consult one of the references listed at the end of this chapter.

Absorption Atelectasis

Prolonged exposure to high concentrations of oxygen causes the gradual washout of nitrogen from the lungs. The atmosphere is composed of approximately 78% nitrogen. The nitrogen in the atmosphere is inert and does not participate significantly in the normal gas exchange across the alveolar-capillary membrane. Because the majority of nitrogen remains in the alveoli, this gas helps to keep the alveoli open at the end of expiration.

As the nitrogen is washed out and replaced by oxygen, the oxygen is absorbed into the blood. As more and more volume is absorbed, the alveolar volume decreases, resulting in a diffuse microatelectasis. In the patient who is compromised and breathing very shallowly, this effect, termed *absorption atelectasis*, can be quite pronounced.

Oxygen-Induced Hypoventilation

Some patients who have a history of chronic obstructive pulmonary disease (COPD) tend to retain higher than normal levels of CO_2 in the blood (hypercapnia). As a result of CO_2 retention, the body's normal stimulus to breathe in response to high levels of CO_2 is not as responsive. The patient with COPD is breathing primarily on an oxygen stimulus rather than a CO_2 stimulus.

When these patients are given moderate to high concentrations of oxygen, the body's chemoreceptors slow respiratory rate and depth as a result of the now adequate levels of PaO_2 (American Association for Respiratory Care, 2002; Robinson, 2000). As a result of the induced hypoventilation, arterial CO_2 levels may rapidly increase, with resulting rapid shifts in pH. Oxygen therapy for these patients should be carefully controlled by observation and by arterial blood gas measurements to ensure that hypercapnia is not made worse by oxygen therapy.

Patients using oxygen at home should be cautioned about the potentially lethal effects of increasing the oxygen flow beyond the level prescribed by their physician.

Oxygen Toxicity

Prolonged exposures to high concentrations of oxygen at ambient pressures have been shown to produce detrimental changes in the pulmonary system. Progressive changes that occur as a result of this exposure may include consolidation, thickening of the capillary beds, formation of hyaline membranes and fibrosis, edema, and atelectasis (American Association for Respiratory Care, 2002).

It is generally accepted that exposure to 100% oxygen for 24 hours is not severely detrimental to the patient. However, the response to oxygen toxicity varies from one person to the next. Exposure to 100% oxygen for longer periods should be viewed with great caution. Serial measurements of the vital capacity have been shown to be helpful in monitoring the effects of oxygen toxicity (Clark, 1974).

If adequate PaO_2 levels cannot be maintained by 100% oxygen administration, continuous mechanical ventilation, bilevel positive airway pressure (bi-PAP®), or continuous positive airway pressure (CPAP) in the spontaneously breathing patient may allow the administration of lower levels of oxygen with subsequent improvement in arterial oxygen tension.

Retinopathy of Prematurity

ROP is a potential complication of oxygen therapy in the newborn. Administration of a high concentration of oxygen causes vasoconstriction in the retina. The vessels become obliterated, and normal growth ceases in the periphery of the retina. Eventually, these changes may lead to partial retinal detachment and blindness. ROP may be prevented by careful monitoring of arterial blood gases. PaO_2 should be maintained between 50 and 80 mm Hg.

It may be difficult to maintain newborns in distress who require high oxygen concentrations. CPAP has helped many newborns by the maintenance of adequate arterial oxygen concentrations on lower FIO_2 levels.

PROFICIENCY OBJECTIVES

At the end of this chapter, the reader should be able to:

* *Correctly assemble, test for function, safely apply, and troubleshoot the following:*
  — *Nasal cannula*
  — *Simple oxygen mask*
  — *Partial rebreathing oxygen mask*
  — *Nonrebreathing oxygen mask*
  — *Venturi oxygen mask*
  — *Oxygen enclosure*
  — *Isolette*
* *Demonstrate how to analyze FIO_2:*
  — *Calibrate the oxygen analyzer.*
  — *Analyze at an appropriate position.*
  — *Adjust the delivery device as appropriate.*
  — *Document the oxygen concentration.*

Review the Patient's Chart

Before proceeding with any prescribed respiratory therapy, take time to review the patient's chart. Check for indications and hazards. In an emergency situation, the practitioner may not have the time to perform this procedure. Obviously, if life is in danger and the order is to proceed, do so.

When reviewing the chart, check for a physician's order. If the order is not written, check with the charge nurse on duty. Ascertain whether the nurse received a verbal or telephone order, verify it, and make sure the order is documented in the patient's chart. It is also important to check the order for completeness (device ordered, liter flow or FIO_2, duration and goal of therapy).

Next, check the laboratory report section of the chart and look for an arterial blood gas analysis report. If an arterial blood gas sample has been drawn, it will indicate the severity of the hypoxemia and the patient's acid-base status. A blood gas analysis report will also help to document the goal of therapy, which is required more frequently as health care providers come under more stringent government regulation.

Gather the Appropriate Equipment

The order for oxygen should specify a delivery device as well as FIO_2. Specified FIO_2 will dictate which equipment is essential or required. Figure 13-24 lists the equipment required for the majority of clinical situations requiring oxygen administration.

Assemble Equipment

After washing the hands, assemble the equipment needed to administer the oxygen therapy ordered by the physician. Most disposable oxygen cannulas and

---

* Oxygen flowmeter
* Humidifier (if required)
* Sterile water (if required)
* Oxygen connecting tubing (if required)
* Oxygen administration device
* *No smoking* sign
* Oxygen analyzer (if appropriate)

Figure 13-24 Equipment required for oxygen administration

© Cengage Learning 2013

masks are packaged with everything needed except the flowmeter, humidifier, *No smoking* sign, and oxygen analyzer. Assembly consists of opening the package, connecting the device to the humidifier or flowmeter, and then applying it to the patient.

Simple oxygen masks, partial rebreathing masks, and nonrebreathing masks generally should not be operated at a flow of less than 5 L/min. This higher flow will ensure that the exhaled CO_2 is adequately flushed from the mask. The head straps should be adjusted to prevent the mask from slipping off the face but should not be so tight as to cause pressure sores to develop.

Enclosures require more assembly. The canopy frame must be set up (if required), nebulizer jar filled (if provided), oxygen connecting tubing attached, ice reservoir filled (if required), and the canopy attached (if required). It is important to practice assembling, testing for function, and troubleshooting the various enclosures commonly used in your geographic region. Only through repeated practice can the practitioner become truly familiar with the equipment required for use.

Explain the Procedure to the Patient

Before actually applying the device to the patient, take a minute to explain who you are, what department you are from, what you will be doing, and why you are doing it. Ask the patient's permission. Patients have the right to know what is being done to their bodies and why.

A little salesmanship on the practitioner's part will help to promote the patient's cooperation and understanding. It takes only a moment. A smile, a polite and concise presentation, and a show of genuine concern for the patient make a great difference to the patient's acceptance of therapy.

Nasal Cannula

Practice applying a nasal cannula with a laboratory partner. Apply the cannula so that the curve of the prongs points down (the airway through the nose progresses posteriorly and then down, not up). Adjust the ear loops or lariat around the back of the ears and then down under the chin. Move the cinch adjustment up so that it is snug enough to keep the prongs in the nose but not so snug as to be uncomfortable.

Turn on the oxygen flow and check it before applying the cannula to the patient. Set the flow between 1 and 6 L/min as ordered by the physician.

Oxygen Masks

Oxygen masks are applied to the bridge of the nose first and then positioned over the chin. The strap should be adjusted snugly around the head to keep the mask in place but not so tight as to cause discomfort or pressure sores.

Liter flows should be adjusted between 6 and 10 L/min. Table 13-5 shows the different liter flows and approximate FIO_2 ranges for the different masks.

TABLE 13-5: Oxygen Mask Application

MASK	FLOW	OXYGEN PERCENTAGE (%)
Simple	6 to 10 L/min	35–55
Partial rebreathing	Enough to keep bag from collapsing	Up to 60
Nonrebreathing	Enough to keep bag from collapsing	Up to 100
OxyMask™	1 - > 15 L/min Adjust based on patient's oxygen saturation (SpO_2)	24–90

Entrainment Masks

The assembly and oxygen flow adjustment will vary depending on the manufacturer of the mask. It is imperative that practitioners familiarize themselves with the various directions supplied by the mask manufacturers because they vary from company to company. Some manufacturers have a separate oxygen dilutor for each desired oxygen percentage (usually color coded). Other manufacturers provide for the oxygen percentage adjustment by adjusting the size of the air entrainment ports. Become familiar with the types of Venturi masks used in your geographic region.

Adjust the liter flow as specified by the manufacturer. Analyze the FIO_2 at the gas entrance port in the mask. Adjust the flow or air entrainment as required to establish the desired FIO_2.

Apply the mask to the bridge of the nose first and then apply it to the chin. Adjust the head strap to keep the mask on the face but not too snugly, as pressure sores may result.

Head Box

It is very difficult to maintain a consistent FIO_2 and humidity for an infant in an isolette because of the constant opening and closing of the enclosure for nursing care. By using a head box to deliver the desired FIO_2 and humidity, adequate access is provided for the rest of the infant's body.

A head box is usually operated from a humidifier capable of delivering 100% body humidity. The FIO_2 adjustments provided on the nebulizer/humidifier may be used, or the humidifier may be operated from an oxygen blender to adjust the FIO_2. Supplemental heat must be provided by use of a heated humidifier with appropriate temperature monitoring.

Using large-bore aerosol tubing, attach the humidifier to the head box. Monitor temperature (35 to 37°C is the desired range) and the FIO_2, using an oxygen analyzer.

Analyze the FIO_2 proximal to the infant's face. Routinely and carefully monitor both the temperature and the FIO_2 as long as the infant requires therapy.

Use of an Oxygen Analyzer

The most common type of oxygen analyzer used in clinical practice is the polarographic oxygen analyzer. It has become popular owing to its small size, its ability to analyze gas in motion, and its rapid response time.

Testing and Calibration

Polarographic analyzers use a battery in their operation. Most manufacturers provide some means to test the battery prior to the use of the analyzer.

Calibrate the oxygen analyzer at 21% or room air. Following this, calibrate the analyzer at 100% by immersing the sensor into a reservoir of 100% oxygen. After calibrating the analyzer at 100%, return the sensor to room air. The reading should stabilize back to 21% within 1 minute.

Analysis

It is important to analyze the oxygen concentration as close to the patient as possible. The practitioner will want to know what the patient is receiving. If the practitioner analyzes distal to the patient, there may be the possibility of room air entrainment between the point of analysis and the patient.

Humidity can shorten the life of some oxygen analyzer sensors. At today's hospital supply prices, one sensor is almost a day's pay for the average respiratory practitioner. If an oxygen analyzer is to be used continuously, make sure that humidity will not adversely affect the sensor.

Dispose of Excess Equipment Properly

After initiating therapy, remove any unneeded equipment. Patient rooms are small and quite cramped for space. Removal of unnecessary equipment will keep the patient area less cluttered and, more important, safer. Extra supplies and plastic are a particular hazard in pediatric units.

Document the Procedure in the Patient Chart

It is helpful to know the liter flow and the FIO_2 on some devices. The oxygen concentration may be documented as a percentage, or as a fraction of inspired oxygen concentration (FIO_2). Use one method or the other, but do not mix the two systems.

Document on the patient's chart the date and time, the equipment used when the practitioner initiated therapy on the patient, and the oxygen concentration or flow—for example: "12/20/2011, 09:00, Mr. J. Smith, room 214, was set up on a simple oxygen mask at a flow of 8 L/min. Respiratory rate is steady at 13 breaths per minute and SpO_2 is 93%."

References

American Association for Respiratory Care. (2002). AARC clinical practice guideline: Oxygen therapy for adults in the acute care facility—2002 revision and update. *Respiratory Care, 47*(6), 717–720.

American Association for Respiratory Care. (2007). AARC clinical practice guideline: Oxygen therapy in the home or alternate site health care facility—2007 revision and update. *Respiratory Care, 52*(1), 1063–1068.

Branson, R. D. (1993). The nuts and bolts of increasing arterial oxygenation: Devices and techniques. *Respiratory Care, 38*(6), 672–686.

Chalon, J. (1980). Low humidity damage to the tracheal mucosa. *Bulletin of the New York Academy of Medicine, 56*, 314–332.

Clark, J. M. (1974). The toxicity of oxygen. *American Review of Respiratory Diseases, 110*(2), 40.

Kacmarek, R. M., Dimas, S., & Mack, C. (2005). *The essentials of respiratory care* (4th ed.). St. Louis, MO: Mosby.

Robinson, T. D. (2000). The role of hypoventilation and ventilation-perfusion redistribution in oxygen-induced hypercapnia during acute exacerbations of chronic obstructive pulmonary disease. *American Journal of Respiratory and Critical Care Medicine, 161*(5), 1524–1529.

Sabrini, C. A., Grassi, V., Solinas, E., & Muiesan, G. (1968). Arterial oxygen tension in relation to age in healthy subjects. *Respiration, 25*(3).

Scacci, R. (1979). Air entrainment masks: Jet mixing is how they work—the Bernoulli and Venturi principles are how they don't. *Respiratory Care, 24*(10), 928–931.

Shapiro, B. A., Peruzzi, W. T., & Templin, R. (1994). *Clinical application of bold gases* (5th ed.). St. Louis, MO: Mosby.

Wilkins, R. L (2009). *Egan's fundamentals of respiratory therapy* (9th ed.). St. Louis, MO: Mosby.

Practice Activities: Oxygen Administration

1. Practice setting up the following equipment using an intubation mannequin or infant resuscitation mannequin as appropriate. Practice with each device until you are familiar with its correct application and operation:
   a. nasal cannula
   b. simple oxygen mask
   c. partial rebreathing mask
   d. nonrebreathing mask
   e. OxyMask™
   f. Venturi mask
   g. head box

2. Practice applying the following devices to a laboratory partner:
   a. nasal cannula at 4 L/min
   b. simple oxygen mask at 8 L/min
   c. partial rebreathing mask at 10 L/min
   d. nonrebreathing mask at 10 L/min
   e. OxyMask™ at 7 L/min
   f. Venturi mask

3. Practice troubleshooting any of the devices by deliberately sabotaging them and then attempting to restore them to normal operation.

4. Practice the calibration of an oxygen analyzer to room air and 100% oxygen settings. Analyze the FIO_2 of a Venturi mask operating at 28%, 35%, and 50%.

Check List: Oxygen Administration

_____ 1. Wash your hands. Help prevent hospital-acquired infections. Protect both your patient and yourself.

2. Obtain the appropriate equipment as required, including:
_____ a. Oxygen flowmeter
_____ b. Humidifier or nebulizer
_____ c. Sterile water (if the humidifier or nebulizer is not prefilled)
_____ d. Oxygen connecting tubing (if required)
_____ e. Oxygen administration device:
_____ (1) nasal cannula
_____ (2) simple oxygen mask
_____ (3) partial rebreathing mask
_____ (4) nonrebreathing mask
_____ (5) OxyMask™
_____ (6) Venturi mask
_____ (7) head box
_____ (8) *No smoking* sign

_____ 3. Assemble the equipment. Assembly will be determined by what oxygen therapy has been ordered.

_____ 4. Identify the patient using the arm band.

_____ 5. Explain the procedure to the patient. Give a brief explanation of the benefits of therapy and do your best to elicit the patient's cooperation.

_____ 6. Apply the device to the patient. As appropriate, adjust the device to an acceptable comfort level for the patient.

_____ 7. Adjust the oxygen concentration or flow as ordered by the physician.

_____ 8. Confirm the delivered oxygen concentration with an oxygen analyzer as appropriate.

_____ 9. Clean up the patient's area. Dispose of any plastic wrappers, excess tubing, or other unused items.

_____ 10. Ensure the patient's comfort and safety.

_____ 11. Wash your hands.

_____ 12. Document in the patient's chart the date, time, oxygen device applied, flow or oxygen concentration, and the patient's condition.

Self-Evaluation Post Test: Oxygen Administration

1. A nasal cannula with a liter flow of 2 L/min applied to a patient with a normal ventilatory pattern delivers an oxygen concentration of approximately:
   a. 24%.
   b. 28%.
   c. 32%.
   d. 36%.

2. Which of these is/are (a) high-flow device(s)?
   a. Partial rebreathing mask
   b. Nasal cannula
   c. Air entrainment mask
   d. Simple oxygen mask

3. Factors that affect the delivered oxygen concentration from a simple mask are:
   I.   patient's tidal volume.
   II. patient's respiratory.
   III. liter flow of oxygen.
   IV. fit of the mask.
   a. I, II
   b. II, III
   c. I, III, IV
   d. I, II, III, IV

4. Which of the following are high-flow delivery systems?
   I.   Nonrebreather mask
   II. Air entrainment mask
   III. High-flow cannula (Vapotherm)
   IV. Partial rebreathing mask
   a. I, III
   b. I, IV
   c. II, III
   d. II, IV

5. If the oxygen cannot be analyzed, it is best to record the concentration delivered in the chart using:
   a. arterial blood gases.
   b. an oxygen analyzer.
   c. liter flows.
   d. duration of therapy.

6. An air entrainment mask set at an air-to-oxygen entrainment ratio of 3:1 delivers:
   a. 30%.   c. 50%.
   b. 40%.   d. 60%.

7. A head box is an example of a(n):
   a. air entrainment device.
   b. tent.
   c. low-flow device.
   d. enclosure.

8. An oxygen analyzer should be calibrated at:
   a. room air.
   c. 100% oxygen.
   b. 50% oxygen.
   d. a and d

9. A low-flow oxygen administration device meets all of a patient's inspiratory needs.
   a. True
   b. False

10. With use of a nonrebreathing mask, the liter flow should be:
    a. at least 2 L/min.
    b. at least 5 L/min.
    c. at least 10 L/min.
    d. high enough to prevent the bag from deflating completely on inspiration.

CHAPTER 14

Introduction to Respiratory Care Pharmacology

The administration of specific drugs that act on the respiratory system is one of many tasks performed by respiratory practitioners. To administer pharmacologic agents safely and effectively, the practitioner must understand the indications and contraindications for these drugs, how they act on the body, their side effects and associated hazards, and common dosages.

This chapter discusses the common drugs administered by respiratory care practitioners as well as how these drugs work, when they are indicated, and their side effects and hazards.

KEY TERMS

- **Alpha receptors**
- **Anticholinergic drugs**
- **Antigen**
- **Antimicrobial agents**
- **Beta-1 receptors**
- **Beta-2 receptors**
- **Cholinergic receptors**
- **Corticosteroids**

- **Degranulation**
- **Dry powder inhaler (DPI)**
- **Histamine**
- **IgE**
- **Leukotrienes**
- **Mast cells**
- **Metered dose inhaler (MDI)**
- **Mucoactive drugs**

- **Muscarinic effect**
- **Nicotinic effect**
- **Phosphodiesterase inhibitors**
- **Prophylactic agent**
- **Prostaglandins**
- **Receptor sites**
- **Spacer**
- **Sympathomimetic drugs**

THEORY OBJECTIVES

At the end of this chapter, the reader should be able to:

- *Discuss the autonomic receptor site theory for the pharmacologic action of the following types of drugs:*
  - *Adrenergic receptors*
  - *Alpha receptors*
  - *Beta-1 receptors*
  - *Beta-2 receptors*
  - *Cholinergic receptors*
- *Describe the mechanisms of bronchospasm:*
  - *Mast cell degranulation*
  - *Leukotrienes*
  - *Histamines*
  - *Prostaglandins*
  - *Release of acetylcholine*
- *Explain how sympathomimetic agents work and state their indications and hazards:*
  - *Salmeterol xinafoate*
  - *Formoterol fumarate*
  - *Pirbuterol acetate*
  - *Albuterol sulfate*
  - *Levalbuterol*
  - *Isoproterenol*

- *Epinephrine*
- *Terbutaline sulfate*
- *Racemic epinephrine*
- *Explain how phosphodiesterase inhibitors work and state their indications and hazards:*
  - *Aminophylline*
  - *Theophylline*
- *Explain how anticholinergic agents work and state their indications and hazards:*
  - *Ipratropium bromide*
  - *Tiotropium bromide*
- *Describe the role of corticosteroids in the management of reactive airways disease:*
  - *Prednisone*
  - *Dexamethasone*
  - *Budesonide*
  - *Triamcinolone*
  - *Beclomethasone*
  - *Flunisolide*
  - *Fluticasone propionate*
  - *Mometasone furoate*

- *Describe the role of combination products in the management of asthma*
  - *Advair (salmeterol and fluticasone propionate)*
  - *Combivent (albuterol and ipratropium bromide)*
  - *Symbicort (formoterol fumarate and budesonide)*
- *Describe the role of cromolyn sodium, nedocromil sodium, montelukast, zafirlukast, and zileuton in the management of reactive airways disease.*
- *Describe the role of mucokinetic agents in respiratory care:*
  - *Acetylcysteine*
  - *Sodium bicarbonate*
  - *Deoxyribonuclease*

- *Describe the role of bland aerosols in humidity therapy.*
- *Describe the role of antimicrobial agents in respiratory care:*
  - *Antibiotics*
  - *Antiviral agents*
  - *Antiprotozoal agents*
- *Explain the advantages and disadvantages of metered dose inhalers (MDIs) in the administration of pharmacologic agents.*
- *Describe a dry powder inhaler (DPI) and its potential advantages over an MDI.*

RECEPTOR SITE THEORY

Throughout the body are *receptor sites*. Receptor sites are specialized cells that will respond predictably to an outside (external to the cell) stimulus. The airways of the lung contain a multitude of receptor sites. Stimulation of some of these sites results in profound bronchospasm, whereas stimulation of others results in bronchodilation. Therefore, it is important that the respiratory practitioner understand these receptor sites and their activity.

Adrenergic Receptor Sites

Alpha Receptors

Alpha receptors are located in the peripheral vasculature, the heart, bronchial muscle, and bronchial blood vessels (Gardenhire, 2008). Stimulation of these receptors causes peripheral vasoconstriction and mild bronchoconstriction in the lungs. Relatively few of these receptor sites are found in the lungs. This accounts for the mild bronchoconstrictive response when these sites are stimulated.

Beta-1 Receptors

Beta-1 receptors are found in the bronchial blood vessels and the heart (Gardenhire, 2008). Stimulation of the beta-1 receptors results in tachycardia, an increased potential for arrhythmias, and an increased cardiac output. In administering drugs to the pulmonary system, stimulation of the beta-1 sites is not desired. However, most respiratory pharmacologic agents have some beta-1 stimulatory effect.

Beta-2 Receptors

Beta-2 receptors are located in the bronchial smooth muscle, the bronchial blood vessels, the systemic blood vessels, and the skeletal muscles. Stimulation of the beta-2 receptors in the lungs causes bronchodilation. A constant goal in the development of new adrenergic drugs for the pulmonary system is to maximize the beta-2 effect while minimizing the beta-1 effect.

Cholinergic Receptors

Cholinergic receptors are cells that respond when stimulated by acetylcholine. Cholinergic receptors cause profound bronchospasm in the lungs when stimulated.

Recall from studying anatomy and physiology that acetylcholine is a chemical unique to the parasympathetic nervous system. Vagal stimulation causes the release of acetylcholine, known as the *muscarinic effect*. The muscarinic system consists of those organs innervated by the 10th cranial nerve (vagus nerve). The other cholinergic effect is the *nicotinic effect*. The nicotinic system consists of the motor nerves of the skeletal muscles.

MECHANISMS OF BRONCHOSPASM

As discussed previously, bronchospasm can result from adrenergic and cholinergic stimulation. Bronchospasm, however, may also result from other mechanisms. The respiratory practitioner needs to understand the mechanisms of bronchospasm so that appropriate drugs can be given to reverse it.

Mast Cell Degranulation

Mast cells are specialized cells in the lungs that are located in the smooth muscle of the bronchi, the intra-alveolar septa, and the submucosal glands (Des Jardins, 2008). The humoral immunity response (allergic response) causes *degranulation* of these cells, releasing chemical mediators such as histamine, heparin, and leukotrienes. The humoral response is caused by an *antigen* (e.g., pollen, animal proteins, feathers) causing the peripheral lymphoid tissue to release immunoglobulin E (*IgE*) antibodies. The IgE (reagin) antibodies sensitize the mast cell. Repeated exposure to the antigen causes the degranulation of the mast cell (Figure 14-1). When the mast cell degranulates, chemical mediators are released, causing bronchospasm and other adverse effects.

Leukotrienes

Leukotrienes are one of many chemical mediators released by the mast cells. Leukotrienes cause a direct, strong bronchoconstriction (Gardenhire, 2008). Leukotrienes also increase vascular permeability, causing edema to occur.

Histamine

Histamine is also a potent bronchoconstrictor. In addition to its bronchoconstrictive activity, histamine increases

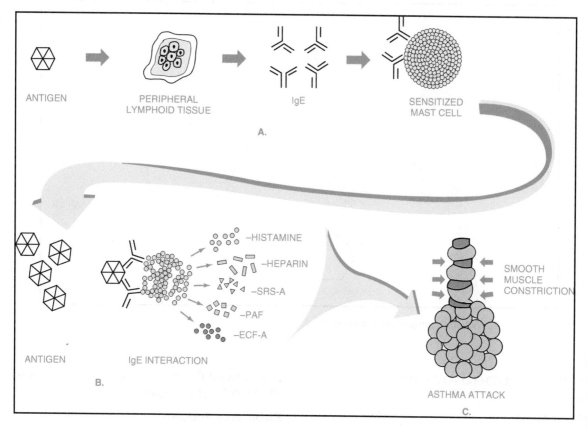

Figure 14-1   Immunologic response causing mast cell degranulation

bronchial gland secretion, causing an increase in the amount of mucus present in the airways (Gardenhire, 2008). Histamine may also have an effect on vascular permeability similar to the effect of SRS-A.

Prostaglandins

Prostaglandins cause a strong bronchospasm, especially in patients with asthma (Gardenhire, 2008). Prostaglandins are produced in the lung and other organs in the body. Prostaglandins have also been implicated in the acute (adult) respiratory distress syndrome (ARDS) (Bulger, 2002).

Acetylcholine

Recall from a previous discussion that release of acetylcholine causes bronchospasm. The muscarinic effect is the one primarily responsible for bronchospasm in the lungs. The bronchospasm from this mechanism is very strong and long lasting.

SYMPATHOMIMETIC DRUGS

Action of Sympathomimetic Drugs

As their name implies, *sympathomimetic drugs* mimic the actions of the sympathetic nervous system. There are

many different drugs that fall under this classification. Sympathomimetic agents are the drugs most commonly used to reverse bronchospasm.

Sympathomimetics stimulate the beta-1 and beta-2 receptor sites. The desired site of stimulation is the beta-2 site, which causes bronchodilation. However, few drugs are purely beta-2 stimulants.

Beta-2 stimulation causes the formation of adenylate cyclase (Figure 14-2). Adenylate cyclase combines with magnesium and ATP (adenosine triphosphate) to form cyclic 3′,5′-AMP (adenosine monophosphate). Cyclic 3′,5′-AMP results in bronchial smooth muscle relaxation and, hence, bronchodilation. Cyclic 3′,5′-AMP is not a long-lived agent. It is readily broken down by another enzyme present in the lungs called phosphodiesterase. Phosphodiesterase breaks 3′,5′-AMP down into 5′-AMP, which no longer causes bronchodilation.

Indications for Sympathomimetic Agents

The primary indication for the administration of sympathomimetic drugs is to reverse bronchospasm. These drugs are very effective and, when given by aerosol route, have few side effects (compared with systemic administration). The different drugs, however, have differing beta-1 and beta-2 effects; therefore, it is important to understand each one so that they can be administered for optimal pharmacologic effect.

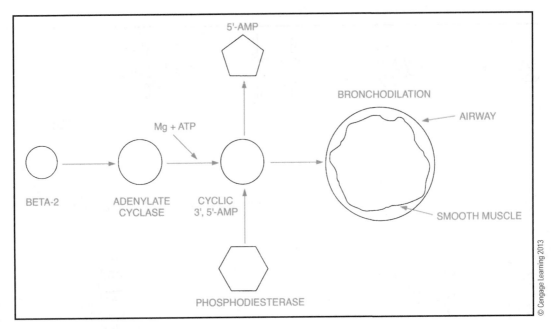

Figure 14-2   Action of sympathomimetic drugs

Specific Sympathomimetic Drugs

Salmeterol Xinafoate

Salmeterol xinafoate (Serevent) is a long-acting beta agonist that has beta-2 effects stronger than its beta-1 effects. It is longer-acting than many other beta agonist drugs, with a 12-hour duration of action and a 60-minute time to onset of action. It is available only as an MDI preparation that delivers 50 micrograms (mcg or µg) per puff. Most patients require two puffs every 12 hours.

Salmeterol is intended for maintenance therapy (typically administered twice per day, morning and night). It is not intended as a rescue drug because its time to onset is at least 60 minutes. Patients using salmeterol usually require a fast-acting beta agonist (such as albuterol) for periods of dyspnea between doses of salmeterol.

Side effects include tachycardia, nausea, palpitations, hypertension, headaches, and tremors. Side effects may be additive if this drug is used in conjunction with other, shorter-acting beta agonists.

Formoterol Fumarate

Formoterol fumarate (Foradil) is a long-acting beta agonist with greater beta-2 effects compared with beta-1 effects. Foradil is administered by an aerolizer in dry powder form (12 mcg twice daily). Like Salmeterol, Foradil is long acting (12 hours) and is administered twice daily.

Formoterol fumarate is intended for maintenance therapy in asthma. It is not intended for use as a rescue agent, in that peak effect is achieved in between 1 and 3 hours. Patients using Foradil may require a short-acting beta agonist such as albuterol for acute periods of dyspnea.

Side effects include tachycardia, nausea, palpitations, hypertension, headaches, and tremors. Side effects may be additive if this drug is used in conjunction with other, shorter-acting beta agonists.

Pirbuterol Acetate

Pirbuterol acetate (Maxair) is another beta agonist available as an MDI preparation (200 mcg/puff). It is also long acting, with a time to onset of action of 5 minutes and a duration of action of 5 hours. Most patients require two puffs every 4 to 6 hours.

Side effects include tachycardia, nausea, palpitations, hypertension, headaches, and tremors. These side effects are related to beta-1 stimulation. However, this drug has more beta-2 effects than beta-1 effects.

Albuterol Sulfate

Albuterol sulfate (Ventolin, Proventil) is a drug with primarily a beta-2 effect. There is some beta-1 effect, but when compared with other sympathomimetics in use in the United States, it has the least beta-1 effect. Albuterol is supplied as a solution for inhalation (0.5% or 5 mg/mL) and as an MDI preparation. It also is available in oral form and in solution for intravenous injection. Recommended dosage is 1.25 to 2.5 mg mixed in normal saline or other diluent given every 4 to 6 hours.

Side effects of albuterol include tachycardia, nausea, palpitations, hypertension, headaches, and tremors. These side effects are related to beta-1 stimulation. Administration via aerosol route can minimize these effects by administration directly to the target organ (the lungs).

Levalbuterol

Levalbuterol (Xopenex) is the R-isomer of the albuterol sulfate (racemic) molecule. It is a short-acting beta-2 agonist for use with asthma and chronic obstructive pulmonary disease (COPD). It is available in both an inhalant solution (0.63, 1.25 mg/mL solution) and as a hydrofluoroalkane (HFA) MDI (45 mcg/puff) every 6 to 8 hours. Side effects of albuterol include tachycardia, nausea, palpitations, hypertension, headaches, and tremors. These side effects are related to beta-1 stimulation. Administration via aerosol route can minimize these effects by administration directly to the target organ (the lungs).

Side effects of levalbuterol may include tachycardia, palpitations, tremors, and other side effects common to other sympathomimetic agents.

Isoproterenol

Isoproterenol (Isuprel) is a powerful bronchodilator. Along with its strong beta-2 effects, it has an almost equally strong beta-1 effect. Isoproterenol is available in solution for aerosol administration (1:200 and 1:100 stock solutions) and is also available for injection. Recommended dosage via aerosol route is 1:1000 final concentration in normal saline or other diluent. The beta-1 side effects are strong enough that Isuprel is rarely used routinely for bronchodilation.

With isoproterenol's strong beta-1 effects, careful monitoring of heart rate, blood pressure, and other symptoms is indicated before, during, and after administration.

Epinephrine

Epinephrine is one of the strongest bronchodilators available. However, it also has the strongest beta-1 side effects and alpha effects. It can be administered by injection or via aerosol. It is most commonly used in the management of acute asthma attacks and is administered intramuscularly. Like Isuprel, epinephrine is not commonly used due to its strong beta-1 side effects.

If epinephrine is given via aerosol, recommended dosage is two deep inhalations spaced about 1 minute apart in a dilution of 1:100 (Wilkins, Stoller, Kackmarek, 2009).

Patients receiving epinephrine should be monitored closely for beta-1 side effects. Be especially alert for adverse effects when it is given to elderly patients. The side effects are similar to those of the other drugs and include tachycardia, nausea, palpitations, hypertension, headaches, and tremors.

Terbutaline Sulfate

Terbutaline sulfate (Brethine) is a sympathomimetic that is available as an oral preparation, in solution for injection or inhalation, and also as an MDI preparation. It has strong beta-2 effects and a lesser beta-1 effect. Recommended aerosol dosage is 0.25 to 0.5 mg diluted in normal saline or other diluent.

Terbutaline has some beta-1 effects although not as strong as those of metaproterenol. The patient should be monitored for the typical symptoms associated with beta-1 stimulation.

Racemic Epinephrine

Racemic epinephrine (Vaponephrine) is a sympathomimetic like the other drugs previously discussed. However, its alpha effects are strong and it is commonly used to relieve croup and epiglottitis symptoms and bronchiolitis

in children. It may also be used for adults following extubation to relieve subglottic edema and its associated airway obstruction. It is supplied in a solution of 2.25% or 22.5 mg/mL. Recommended dosage via aerosol is 7 mg to 14 mg mixed in normal saline or other diluent.

Racemic epinephrine has beta-1 effects as well as beta-2 and alpha effects. Monitoring of the patient for adverse reactions due to beta-1 effects is indicated with use of this drug.

Arformoterol Tartrate (Brovana)

Arformoterol tartrate (Brovana) is a selective beta-2 bronchodilator. Brovana is an R,R enantiomer of formoterol. Brovana is supplied in a 2 mL vial of inhalant solution containing 15 mcg of arformoterol in sterile isotonic saline. It is not necessary to dilute the vial before use. It is recommended that Brovana be used twice daily. Because arformoterol tartrate is a beta-2 adrenergic, the patient should be monitored for adverse reactions such as tachycardia, nervousness, headache, and other common side effects.

PHOSPHODIESTERASE INHIBITORS

Recall that cyclic 3',5'-AMP is broken down into 5'-AMP by the enzyme phosphodiesterase. If the action of phosphodiesterase can be blocked or inhibited, more 3',5'-AMP will remain in the lungs, resulting in better bronchodilation. *Phosphodiesterase inhibitors* act in this way. Common phosphodiesterase drugs are found in the *methylxanthine group*, which are sometimes called just "xanthines." Caffeine and theophylline are two examples of drugs in the xanthine group.

Aminophylline

Aminophylline is a phosphodiesterase inhibitor that is commonly given intravenously for the management of asthma. It is also available for oral administration in tablet form. Aminophylline dosage intravenously is 5 to 10 mg/kg of normal body weight. Serum concentrations should be monitored and dosage adjusted to maintain a therapeutic level (serum theophylline) of 10 to 20 mcg/100 mL. Aminophylline exerts its bronchodilating effect by a pathway other than the sympathomimetic pathway. This difference can be useful clinically.

Aminophylline has several side effects, including nausea, vomiting, nervousness, agitation, and tachycardia. Aminophylline may also cause tachypnea and hyperventilation.

Theophylline

Like aminophylline, theophylline is another methylxanthine. It acts by blocking phosphodiesterase. Theophylline is available in tablet and elixir form. Like aminophylline, it should be titrated until a therapeutic blood level (serum theophylline) of 10 to 20 mcg/100 mL is attained.

Side effects of theophylline and aminophylline are similar and include gastrointestinal discomfort, tachycardia, restlessness, tachypnea, and hyperventilation.

ANTICHOLINERGIC DRUGS

Anticholinergic drugs block the cholinergic receptor sites, preventing that route of bronchospasm. Anticholinergics provide a third pathway for bronchodilation in addition to those described for the sympathomimetics and phosphodiesterase inhibitors.

Ipratropium Bromide

Ipratropium bromide (Atrovent) is another agent that, like atropine, blocks the cholinergic receptor site. It is available as an MDI preparation (18 mcg per puff) and in solution (0.5 mg). Recommended aerosol dosage is two puffs up to 4 times per day or 0.5 mg every 4 hours. The side effects of this drug are similar to atropine's side effects.

Tiotropium Bromide

Tiotropium bromide (Spiriva) is a long-acting anticholinergic agent. It is intended for maintenance therapy for asthma and COPD and is not to be used as a rescue agent. Tiotropium bromide is available as a dry powder and is administered using the HandiHaler administration device. Each capsule contains 18 mcg and is administered once daily.

Side effects may include dry mouth, dysphagia, and dysphonia.

CORTICOSTEROIDS IN RESPIRATORY CARE

Corticosteroids are widely used in the management of the inflammatory process associated with asthma, reactive airways disease, and other pulmonary disorders. Corticosteroids may be administered systemically (orally or via the intravenous route) or via aerosol. Most corticosteroids that are administered via the aerosol route are given using MDIs. It is important for the respiratory practitioner to understand the actions of these drugs and how they are applied in the management of inflammatory disorders.

Prednisone

Prednisone is an oral preparation (tablet) of a glucocorticoid drug. Its action is twofold: (1) inflammation is reduced and (2) the action of sympathomimetic agents is potentiated (enhanced) (Ziment, 1978). Depending on the patient's disease state and need for therapy, prednisone may be given for a 2- to 3-week period followed by a rapid tapering of the dosage, or it may be administered

for a longer term to manage the patient's condition more adequately. A typical dosage would be a loading dose of 4 mg/kg of body weight, and then a maintenance dose of 1 mg/kg is used until a therapeutic level is reached. Therapeutic serum levels are 100 to 150 mcg/100 mL.

Side effects include cushingoid effects, impairment of the immune system, and steroid dependency. The side effects of steroids can be severe, and they are used only when the patient can significantly benefit from their pharmacologic action.

Dexamethasone

Dexamethasone (Decadron) is available as an MDI preparation. The use of this drug in aerosol form allows the physician to target the lungs specifically in its administration. Fewer side effects may be noticed because systemic administration is avoided. Recommended dosage is three puffs 3 or 4 times per day.

The side effects of dexamethasone are similar to those of other steroids and include cushingoid effects, impaired immunity, and steroid dependency. In addition, patients may experience throat irritation or hoarseness from the MDI form of delivery.

Budesonide

Budesonide (Pulmocort) is available as both an inhalant solution (0.25 mg/mL and 0.5 mg/mL once daily) and a dry powder formulation (200 mcg/dose twice daily). In aerosol form, this anti-inflammatory medication targets the lungs specifically with fewer side effects.

Side effects of budesonide are similar to those of other steroids and may include impaired immunity and steroid dependency. In addition, patients may experience throat irritation or hoarseness from the MDI form of delivery.

Beclomethasone Dipropionate

Beclomethasone dipropionate (Beclovent, Vanceril) is two corticosteroids available as an MDI preparation (42 mcg/puff). Most patients require two puffs 3 or 4 times per day. Like other corticosteroids, these drugs act as anti-inflammatory agents. However, because they are inhaled, systemic side effects are fewer than if they were taken orally or intravenously.

Side effects include coughing, oral candidiasis, and dysphonia (difficulty speaking). Side effects may be minimized by thoroughly rinsing the mouth and oropharynx following use of the MDI.

Triamcinolone Acetonide

Triamcinolone acetonide (Azmacort, Pulmicort) is another corticosteroid available as an MDI preparation (100 mcg/puff), given two to four puffs up to 4 times daily. It is also available in a 200 mcg per puff MDI, which is used twice daily. A 0.5 mg/2 mL inhalant solution is available and is used once daily. Azmacort is another anti-inflammatory agent that when given by inhalation has fewer side effects.

Side effects include coughing, oral candidiasis, and dysphonia. Side effects may be minimized by thoroughly rinsing the mouth and oropharynx following use of the MDI.

Flunisolide

Flunisolide (AeroBid) is another MDI corticosteroid preparation (250 mcg/puff). Most patients take two puffs twice each day. Because it is an inhaled corticosteroid, systemic side effects are fewer than with other steroids given parenterally or orally.

Side effects include coughing, oral candidiasis, and dysphonia. Side effects may be minimized by thoroughly rinsing the mouth and oropharynx following use of the MDI.

Fluticasone Propionate

Fluticasone propionate (Flovent) is a synthetic glucocorticoid with good anti-inflammatory properties. It is available in an MDI preparation (44, 110, and 220 mcg/puff) and as a DPI. Most patients use two puffs twice daily for maintenance. As with other inhaled corticosteroids, systemic side effects are fewer than with systemic administration.

Side effects include coughing, oral candidiasis, and dysphonia. Side effects can be minimized by rinsing the mouth following drug administration.

Mometasone Furoate

Mometasone furoate (Asmanex) is an anti-inflammatory agent available in a dry powder formulation administered using a Twisthaler. The formulation is available in both a 220 mcg and 110 mcg per inhalation formulation. Anti-inflammatory medications are intended for maintenance therapy in asthma and are not to be considered rescue agents. When administered via the inhalation route, there are fewer side effects when compared with systemic administration of similar agents.

Side effects include oral candidiasis and dysphonia. Side effects can be minimized by rinsing the mouth following drug administration.

COMBINATION THERAPY DRUGS

Fluticasone Propionate–Salmeterol (Advair)

Fluticasone propionate (Flowvent) and salmeterol (Serevent) have been combined into a DPI preparation (with the trade name of Advair) containing 100 mcg of fluticasone propionate and 50 mcg of salmeterol, 250 mcg of fluticasone and 50 mcg of salmeterol, and 500 mcg of fluticasone and 50 mcg of salmeterol. By taking both drugs together, the long-term effects of both (anti-inflammatory and long-acting bronchodilation) can be achieved. Most patients use two puffs twice each day. Side effects of each have been previously described.

Albuterol Sulfate–Ipratropium Bromide

Albuterol sulfate and ipratropium bromide are available in a combination product with the trade name of Combivent. Combivent contains 3 mg albuterol (equivalent to 2.5 mg albuterol (0.083%) of albuterol base) and 0.5 mg ipratropium bromide (inhalation solution formula) or 103 mcg albuterol and 18 mcg of ipratropium bromide (HFA metered dose formulation), given up to 4 times daily. The two products in combination result in a greater improvement in forced expiratory volume in the first second (FEV_1) in COPD compared with each product when used alone. The action and side effects of these agents have been described previously in this chapter.

Formoterol Fumarate–Budesonide

Formoterol fumarate and budesonide are available together in combination with the trade name of Symbicort. It is available as an MDI preparation with HFA as its propellant. Two doses are available: 80/4.5 mcg of budesonide/foradil and 160/4.5 mcg budesonide/foradil. This combination product is intended for maintenance therapy of asthma and should not be considered a rescue agent. The action and side effects of these drugs have previously been described in this chapter.

CROMOLYN SODIUM AND ASTHMA MANAGEMENT

Cromolyn sodium (Intal) is an agent that inhibits the degranulation of sensitized mast cells. The drug is very useful in the management of extrinsic (allergic) asthma. It is available in a liquid form for nebulization (20 mg/2 mL), and as an MDI preparation (800 mcg/puff). Recommended dosage is 20 to 40 mg per day (of aerosolized solution) or two puffs 4 times per day using the MDI preparation.

Cromolyn sodium is a *prophylactic agent*. That is, it prevents mast cell degranulation. Administration of cromolyn sodium during an acute attack is not indicated. The drug does not have any bronchodilatory action or effect. A patient must use the drug on a regular basis to prevent acute bronchospastic episodes.

Most side effects of the drug are related to the MDI device and include hoarseness and dry mouth. Patients sometimes experience periods of coughing with both the MDI preparation and the aerosolized liquid form of the drug.

Nedocromil Sodium

Nedocromil sodium (Tilade) is a disodium salt of a pyranoquinolone dicarboxylic acid, which is a drug used in asthma management. Nedocromil sodium blocks both the early and late asthmatic responses to a variety of allergic and nonallergic asthma triggers. Like cromolyn sodium, it is most effective when used as a prophylactic agent. Nedocromil sodium is available as an MDI preparation (1.75 mcg/puff) with most patients requiring two puffs between 2 and 4 times per day.

Montelukast (Singulair)

Montelukast (Singulair) is a leukotriene inhibitor used for maintenance therapy in asthma. Leukotrienes are one of many compounds released in an inflammatory response. Leukotrienes can increase vascular permeability, cause bronchospasm, and increase edema. By blocking leukotrienes, this cascade of events can be prevented. Singulair is available in a 4, 5, and 10 mg oral tablet preparation and as a 4 mg packet of oral granules. Dosing is one tablet daily, or for children 6 to 23 months of age, one 4 g packet of oral granules taken once each evening.

Side effects may include headache, gastrointestinal distress (dyspepsia and pain), and cough.

Zarfirlukast

Zarfirlukast (Accolate) is a leukotriene inhibitor used for maintenance therapy in asthma. Accolate is available in both 10 and 20 mg tablets. Dosing is 10 or 20 mg twice daily. Side effects include headache, nausea, and gastrointesntinal pain.

Zileuton

Zileuton (Zyflo) is a leukotriene inhibitor used for maintenance therapy in asthma. Zyflo is available in 600 mg tablets. The typical dosing schedule is two tablets 2 times daily. Side effects include hepatoxicity (elevation of liver enzymes and biliribin levels), sinusitis, nausea, and pharyngeo or laryngeo pain.

MUCOACTIVE AGENTS

Mucoactive drugs are agents that decrease the viscosity of pulmonary secretions, increase mucus production, hydrate retained secretions, or affect the composition of mucus proteins. The goal of all mucoactive therapy is to increase pulmonary clearance through the normal mechanism and to promote coughing.

Acetylcysteine

Acetylcysteine (Mucomyst) is a drug that acts on the disulfide bond of mucus proteins. The action of the drug is to break down the disulfide bonds, weakening the mucus molecule. The net effect is to reduce the viscosity of mucus, thinning it so that it is easier to expectorate. Mucomyst is available in both 10% and 20% solutions. The recommended dosage is 1 to 10 mL of the 20% solution every 2 to 6 hours.

Side effects of acetylcysteine include nausea, bronchospasm in patients with asthma, and rhinorrhea. Usually, acetylcysteine is given with a bronchodilator to prevent the bronchospastic side effect.

Dornase Alfa (Pulmozyme)

Dornase alfa (Pulmozyme) is a purified solution of recombinant human deoxyribonuclease. The action of Pulmozyme is to break the DNA molecules of the mucus, making it less viscous and more easily expectorated. Cystic fibrosis is a disease that is commonly treated with Pulmozyme. Pulmozyme is available as a 2.5 mg inhalant solution. Recommended dosage is once daily.

Side effects of Pulmozyme include voice changes, sore throat, hoarseness, eye irritation, and rash.

USE OF BLAND AEROSOLS IN RESPIRATORY CARE

Bland aerosols are commonly administered in respiratory care. The goals of bland aerosol therapy include humidification of medical gases, mobilization of pulmonary secretions, and sputum induction. Bland aerosols include distilled water, saline solutions, and propylene glycol.

The use of distilled water and saline solutions is discussed in Chapter 15. Propylene glycol is used primarily as a stabilizing agent for other drugs administered via the aerosol route. It stabilizes solutions because of its detergent-like property that reduces surface tension.

AEROSOLIZED ANTIMICROBIAL AGENTS

Antimicrobial agents such as antibiotics have been aerosolized for the treatment of pulmonary infections. The aerosol route targets the lungs specifically while in some cases avoiding systemic side effects (pentamidine administration). It is important to understand these drugs, what they are, and why they are administered.

Antibiotics

The aerosol administration of antibiotics is frequently performed in conjunction with systemic administration of other antibiotics (Wilkins, Stoller, Kackmarek, 2009). Tobramycin and gentamicin are sometimes aerosolized for use in patients with cystic fibrosis and have shown some efficacy in treatment of the recurrent infections these patients experience. One disadvantage of aerosolized antibiotics is the difficulty in controlling dosage.

Tobramycin (Tobi)

Tobramycin (Tobi) is an antibiotic inhalant solution. Each 5 mL ampule contains 300 mg of tobramycin. Tobi is used in the treatment of patients with cystic fibrosis who have *Pseudomonas aeruginosa* pneumonia. Tobi is administered using one ampule nebulized twice daily for 28 days. The patient then does not take Tobi for the following

28 days. Tobi is resumed once again after the alternate 28-day period has passed.

Common side effects of Tobi include increased cough, pharyngitis, rhinitis, headache, and fever.

Antiviral Agents

The primary aerosolized antiviral agent is ribavirin, used in the treatment of respiratory syncytial virus (RSV) infection in pediatric patients. Ribavirin is administered using a special small-particle aerosol generator (SPAG) nebulizer. Ribavirin has been shown to be effective in conjunction with other therapies in the treatment of RSV infection.

Antiprotozoal Agents

Pentamidine is often administered to patients with *Pneumocystis carinii* infections, a secondary complication of human immunodeficiency virus (HIV) infection. Aerosolized pentamidine is more effective and has fewer side effects than are seen with systemic administration of the same drug. When aerosolized, this drug targets the lungs specifically with few systemic effects. Furthermore, a lower aerosolized dosage may be given while achieving higher therapeutic serum levels.

METERED DOSE INHALERS

A *metered dose inhaler (MDI)* is a small, portable aerosol-dispensing device (Figure 14-3). These devices are hand operated and are powered by an HFA propellant, much like an aerosol spray can.

Each activation of the trigger dispenses a known dose of medication. The patient squeezes the MDI trigger during a deep inhalation, depositing the aerosol into the respiratory tract. These devices are convenient to use and with proper technique can be very effective.

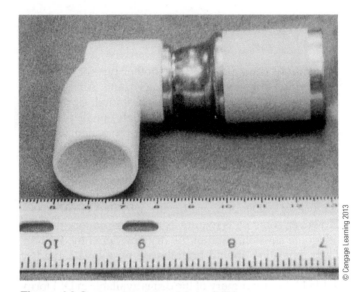

Figure 14-3   A metered dose inhaler (MDI)

The greatest difficulty in MDI application is patient instruction. The patient must understand completely how to use this device. Clear, concise instructions must be given, and a placebo MDI should be used for instructional purposes and demonstration. Ideally, written directions should also be given to the patient for future reference. The medication will be administered as prescribed only when the patient uses the MDI correctly.

MDI Spacer Devices

MDI *spacer* devices are used in conjunction with MDIs and enhance the effectiveness of aerosol deposition and improve medication delivery (Figure 14-4). The spacer helps to increase the evaporation of the MDI propellant, reducing the particle size. The use of a spacer ensures that a smaller particle size is delivered to the patient. Patients who have difficulty coordinating their breathing (inspiration) with hand coordination (squeezing) will achieve better results by using a spacer.

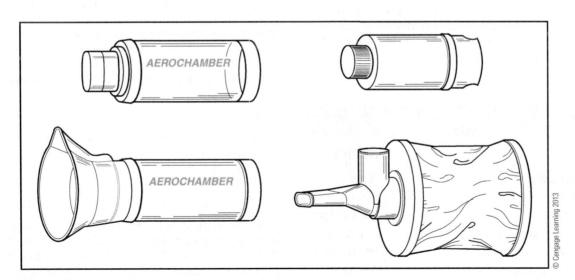

Figure 14-4   A drawing showing different spacer devices

DRY POWDER INHALERS (DPI)

A *dry powder inhaler (DPI)* is another type of device for delivering drugs by the pulmonary route. A DPI creates an aerosol by drawing air through a small dose of dry powder. If the powder is fine enough (small particles), and sufficient airflow is generated by the patient, an aerosol of dry particles will be produced.

Unlike MDIs, DPIs do not require a propellant to expel the medication through the device.

DPIs require less patient coordination than is needed for use of MDIs and are breath activated (Fink, 2000). However, some DPIs require a greater inspiratory flow for adequate aerosolization of the dry powdered medication. Each inhalation should be followed by a breath hold of up to 10 seconds. Figure 14-5 shows an example of a DPI. Table 14-1 is a summary of the drugs available in DPI form.

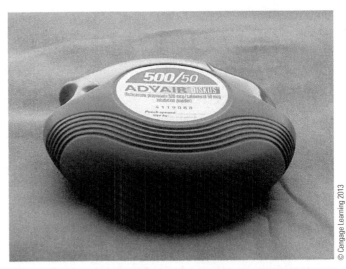

© Cengage Learning 2013

Figure 14-5   A photograph of a dry powder inhaler (DPI)

PROFICIENCY OBJECTIVES

At the end of this chapter, the reader should be able to:

- *Demonstrate how to use a metered dose inhaler (MDI) to deliver a medication.*
- *Demonstrate how to use a spacer device in conjunction with an MDI to deliver a medication.*
- *Demonstrate the use of a dry powder inhaler (DPI).*

METERED DOSE INHALER

It is important to know how to administer a medication using an MDI. The convenience and popularity of this type of aerosol administration have increased in recent years. However, as discussed previously, this method of aerosol administration is very technique dependent; therefore, it is important to understand how to use these devices properly.

Position the Patient

It is important to position the patient properly for optimal administration of medication delivered via MDI. The optimal position is sitting erect or in high Fowler's position. This position allows for good chest expansion.

TABLE 14-1:   Drugs Available in DPI Form

DRUG	DEVICE
Albuterol sulfate	Rotahaler
Salmeterol	Diskus
Budesonide	Turbuhaler
Fluticasone propionate–salmeterol	Diskhaler
Tiotropium bromide (Spiriva)	HandiHaler
Formoterol fumarate (Foradil)	Aerolizer

Ensure that the patient is not wearing any clothing that may interfere with chest wall excursion.

Monitor the Patient

Auscultate the chest and note any abnormal breath sounds or other findings. Measure the heart rate and respiratory rate prior to medication administration. Measure the peak expiratory flow as indicated to measure the effectiveness of bronchodilator therapy.

Instruct the Patient

As discussed previously, it is important to instruct the patient thoroughly to obtain the best results with this type of aerosol administration. Allow the patient opportunity to ask questions about any aspect of the technique he or she does not understand. Ideally, use an MDI containing a placebo and demonstrate the technique yourself.

Assemble the Equipment

Thoroughly shake the MDI prior to use. Attach the mouthpiece to the canister and remove the cap from the mouthpiece.

Administer the Medication

Have the patient hold the MDI a few centimeters from the open mouth. Instruct the patient to inhale slowly and deeply while activating the MDI by squeezing it. Instruct the patient to continue to inhale and to hold the breath at the end of inhalation for 5 to 7 seconds. Have the patient slowly exhale following the medication administration. Repeat the procedure as many times as ordered by the patient's physician, waiting between puffs.

Monitor the Patient following Therapy

Monitor the patient's heart and respiratory rates following medication administration. Auscultate the chest and note any changes in breath sounds. If administering a bronchodilator, measure the peak expiratory flow following aerosol administration.

Clean the Patient's Room and Chart Procedure

Remove any unneeded supplies from the patient's room and ensure that the patient is safe and comfortable. Chart the procedure in the patient's record, noting heart and respiratory rates, breath sounds, peak flows (if measured), and what medication and the number of puffs that were given.

USE OF A SPACER WITH A METERED DOSE INHALER

Spacers are small chambers designed to be used in conjunction with MDI aerosol administration. Spacer devices help to slow the velocity of aerosol particles, enhance the vaporization of the propellant, and reduce the amount of coordination required to obtain optimal results.

Position the Patient

It is important to position the patient properly for optimal administration of medication via MDI. The optimal position is sitting erect or in high Fowler's position. This position allows for good chest expansion. Ensure that the patient is not wearing any clothing that may interfere with chest wall excursion.

Monitor the Patient

Auscultate the chest and note any abnormal breath sounds or other findings. Measure the heart rate and respiratory rate prior to medication administration. Measure the peak expiratory flow as indicated to measure the effectiveness of bronchodilator therapy.

Instruct the Patient

As discussed previously, it is important to instruct the patient thoroughly to obtain the best results with this type of aerosol administration. Allow the patient opportunity to ask questions about any aspect of the technique he or she does not understand. Ideally, use an MDI containing a placebo and demonstrate the technique yourself.

Assemble the Equipment

Thoroughly shake the MDI prior to use. Attach the mouthpiece to the canister and remove the cap from the mouthpiece. Attach the spacer device to the MDI. Ensure that the aerosol can pass through the spacer without obstruction.

Administer the Medication

Have the patient hold the MDI and spacer in the mouth. Instruct the patient to inhale slowly and deeply while activating the MDI by squeezing it. Instruct the patient to continue to inhale and to hold the breath at the end of inhalation for 5 to 7 seconds. Have the patient slowly exhale following the medication administration. Repeat the procedure as many times as ordered by the patient's physician, waiting between puffs.

Monitor the Patient following Therapy

Monitor the patient's heart and respiratory rates following medication administration. Auscultate the chest and note any changes in breath sounds. If administering a bronchodilator, measure the peak expiratory flow following aerosol administration.

Clean the Patient's Room and Chart Procedure

Remove any unneeded supplies from the patient's room and ensure that the patient is safe and comfortable. Chart the procedure in the patient's record, noting heart and respiratory rates, breath sounds, peak flows (if measured), and what medication and the number of puffs that were given. It is also important to note in the record that a spacer was used.

DRY POWDER INHALERS

The correct use of a DPI is dependent on what type of DPI is to be used (Diskhaler, Diskus, Turbuhaler, HandiHaler, Aerolizer, and Twisthaler). Each type requires a slightly different technique, as described in this section. However, it is strongly recommended that the practitioner read the package insert provided by the manufacturer including the directions for use for each DPI prior to teaching the patient how to use the device.

Practice using a DPI containing placebo. Familiarity with the experience of using these devices will enhance the ability to instruct the patient in correct technique.

Diskhaler

Figure 14-6 is a photograph of the Diskhaler. Begin by removing the mouthpiece cover by sliding it off. Pull the tray out from the device (holds the disk), and place the disk on the center wheel of the Diskhaler with the numbers facing up. Rotate the disk by sliding the tray in and out of the Diskhaler. Lift the back of the lid fully upright; this punctures the small blister on the disk, allowing the drug to be released. Keeping the Diskhaler level, insert

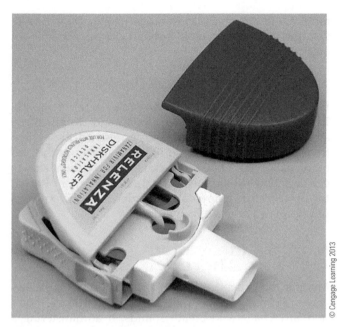

Figure 14-6 A photograph of the Diskhaler

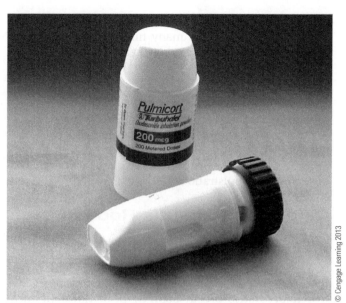

Figure 14-8 A photograph of the Turbuhaler

the open mouthpiece into the mouth. Take a slow deep breath, inhaling the medication. Remove the device from the mouth to exhale.

Diskus

Figure 14-7 is a photograph of the Diskus DPI. Open the device by rotating the inner and outer portions in opposite directions. This exposes the mouthpiece opening. Slide the lever on the side of the device; this advances the foil strip containing medication doses and exposes the contents for inhalation. Keeping the Diskus level, insert the open mouthpiece into the mouth. Take a slow deep breath, inhaling the medication. Remove the device from the mouth to exhale.

Turbuhaler

Like the majority of DPIs, the Turbuhaler contains both the delivery device (DPI) and the medication in one unit

(Figure 14-8). To use the device, remove the cover from the mouthpiece. Holding the Turbuhaler upright (mouthpiece up), rotate the lower grip first right and then left while holding the upper portion (mouthpiece) stationary. When this manuever is performed correctly, a "click" can be heard. Place the mouthpiece into the mouth. Keeping the Turbuhaler level, insert the open mouthpiece into the mouth. Take a slow, deep breath, inhaling the medication. Remove the device from the mouth to exhale. Replace the mouthpiece cover, and store the device in a cool, dry place.

HandiHaler

The HandiHaler must first be loaded with a capsule containing the Spiriva medication. Expose the chamber by opening the hinged dust cap and then opening the hinged mouthpiece (Figure 14-9). Drop the medication capsule into the exposed chamber and close the mouthpiece firmly over it. Press the green piercing button to

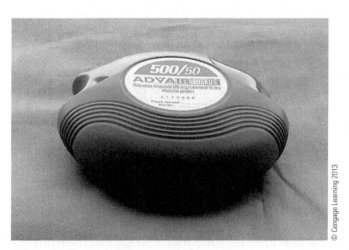

Figure 14-7 A photograph of the Diskus DPI

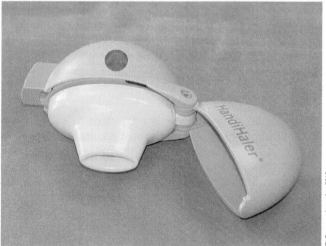

Figure 14-9 A photograph of the HandiHaler

puncture the capsule, releasing the medication. Insert the mouthpiece into the mouth and take a deep breath, aerosolizing the dry powder. Open the chamber again, discarding the spent capsule. Close the mouthpiece and dust cover protecting the chamber from any contamination with foreign material.

Aerolizer

Peel a corner of the blister package back, exposing the medication capsule. Rotate the mouthpiece away from the chamber (Figure 14-10). Drop the capsule into the chamber and rotate the mouthpiece, closing the chamber. Press the side piercing buttons once, piercing the capsule and releasing the dry powder medication. Insert the mouthpiece into the mouth, with the blue buttons positioned horizontally (sideways). Inhale quickly and

deeply to aerosolize the medication. Open the Aerolizer to see if any medication remains. If medication remains, repeat the cycle of inhalation. Open the chamber again and remove the spent capsule. Close the chamber and store the Aerolizer in its box to protect it from contamination by foreign material.

Twisthaler

Hold the Twisthaler upright by grasping the base in one hand. With the other hand, twist the white cap, rotating it counterclockwise (Figure 14-11). When the cap is lifted off the base, the counter at the base of the Twisthaler will count down by one. Exhale fully, insert the white dispenser portion into the mouth and inhale quickly and deeply. Hold your breath for up to 10 seconds, or as long as you can comfortably do so. Replace the cap and turn it clockwise until it "clicks." It is in the proper storage position between uses when the arrow lines up with the dose counter.

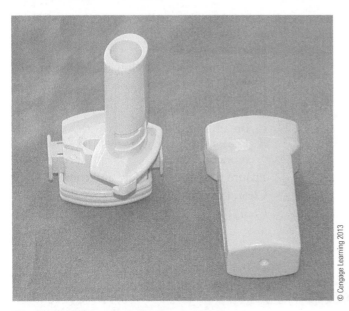

Figure 14-10   A photograph of the Aerolizer

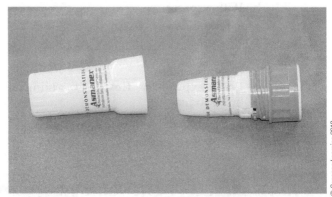

Figure 14-11   A photograph of the Twisthaler

References

Bulger, E. M. (2002). The macrophage response to endotoxin requires platelet activating factor. *Shock, 17*(3), 173–179.

Des Jardins, T. R. (2008). *Cardiopulmonary anatomy & physiology: Essentials for respiratory care* (5th ed.). Clifton Park, NY: Delmar Cengage Learning.

Fink, J. B. (2000). Metered-dose inhalers, dry powder inhalers, and transitions. *Respiratory Care, 45*(6), 623–635.

Gardenhire, D. S. (2008). *Rau's respiratory care pharmacology* (7th ed.). St. Louis, MO: Elsevier.

Scanlan et al., 1995.

Wilkins, R. L., Stoller, J. K., Kacmarek, R. M. (2009). *Egan's fundamentals of respiratory care* (9th ed.). St. Louis, MO: Elsevier.

Ziment, I. (1978), *Respiraotry pharmacology and therapeutics.* Philadelphia: Saunders.

Practice Activities: Introduction to Respiratory Care Pharmacology

1. Using a laboratory partner, practice instructing each other on how to use an MDI. Carefully critique each other's instructions.

2. Using a laboratory partner, practice using an MDI containing a placebo:
   a. With a spacer
   b. Without a spacer

3. Practice charting what you would record in a patient's record following MDI administration.

Check List: Metered Dose Inhaler

_____ 1. Properly identify and position the patient for MDI administration.

_____ 2. Wash your hands.

3. Give complete and thorough instructions on how to use an MDI:
   _____ a. Without a spacer
   _____ b. With a spacer

4. Monitor the patient:
   _____ a. Heart rate
   _____ b. Respiratory rate
   _____ c. Breath sounds
   _____ d. Peak expiratory flows (if giving a bronchodilator)

5. Administer the medication using an MDI:
   _____ a. Without a spacer
   _____ b. With a spacer

6. Monitor the patient following MDI administration.
   _____ a. Heart rate
   _____ b. Respiratory rate
   _____ c. Breath sounds
   _____ d. Peak expiratory flows (if giving a bronchodilator)

_____ 7. Ensure the patient's safety and comfort.

_____ 8. Clean the patient's room.

_____ 9. Chart the procedure in the patient's record.

Self-Evaluation Post Test: Introduction to Respiratory Care Pharmacology

1. Adrenergic receptor sites include which of the following?
   I. Alpha
   II. Beta-1
   III. Beta-2
   IV. Cholinergic
   a. I
   b. I, II
   c. I, II, III
   d. II, III

2. Which of the following mediators is/are released during bronchospasm following mast cell degranulation?
   I. Leukotrienes
   II. Histamine
   III. Prostaglandins
   IV. Acetylcholine
   a. I
   b. I, II
   c. I, II, III
   d. II, III, IV

3. Sympathomimetic agents work by:
   a. releasing acetylcholine.
   b. increasing production of adenylate cyclase.
   c. increasing production of phosphodiesterase.
   d. blocking phosphodiesterase.

4. Examples of sympathomimetic agents are:
   I. albuterol.
   II. atropine.
   III. salmeterol.
   IV. theophylline.
   a. I, II
   b. I, III
   c. II, III
   d. II, IV

5. Albuterol comes in a stock solution of 0.5%. To draw up 1.25 mg of albuterol, you would withdraw how many milliliters from the bottle?
   a. 0.25 mL
   b. 0.50 mL
   c. 0.75 mL
   d. 1 mL

6. Advantages of aerosol administration of respiratory drugs include which of the following?
   I.   The lungs are specifically targeted.
   II. There are fewer systemic side effects.
   III. Dosing is always precise.
   IV. It is less expensive than other routes.
   a. I   c. II, III
   b. I, II   d. II, IV

7. An example of an anticholinergic drug is:
   a. albuterol.
   b. salmeterol.
   c. ipratropium bromide.
   d. prednisone.

8. Advantages of MDIs include:
   I.   ease of use.
   II. portability.
   III. the lungs are specifically targeted.
   IV. fewer systemic side effects.
   a. I   c. I, II, III
   b. I, II   d. I, II, III, IV

9. Which of the following mucoactive agents break chemical bonds in the mucus protein?
   I.   Acetylcysteine
   II. Sodium bicarbonate
   III. Dornase alfa
   IV. Prednisone
   a. I, II   c. II, III
   b. I, III   d. II, IV

10. Which of the following drugs is routinely administered prophylactically to prevent asthma?
    a. Albuterol
    b. Atropine
    c. Cromolyn sodium
    d. Acetylcysteine

PERFORMANCE EVALUATION:
MDI Administration

Date: Lab _____ Clinical _____ Agency _____

Lab: Pass _____ Fail _____ Clinical: Pass _____ Fail _____

Student name _____ Instructor name _____

No. of times observed in clinical _____

No. of times practiced in clinical _____

PASSING CRITERIA: Obtain 90% or better on the procedure. Tasks indicated by * must receive at least 1 point, or the evaluation is terminated. Procedure must be performed within the designated time, or the performance receives a failing grade.

SCORING:
2 points — Task performed satisfactorily without prompting.
1 point — Task performed satisfactorily with self-initiated correction.
0 points — Task performed incorrectly or with prompting required.
NA — Task not applicable to the patient care situation.

Tasks:	Peer	Lab	Clinical
* **1.** Verifies the physician's order	☐	☐	☐
* **2.** Washes hands	☐	☐	☐
* **3.** Identifies the patient and introduces self	☐	☐	☐
* **4.** Obtains the required supplies			
a. MDI	☐	☐	☐
b. Spacer	☐	☐	☐
* **5.** Gives thorough and complete instructions	☐	☐	☐
* **6.** Monitors the patient			
a. Heart rate	☐	☐	☐
b. Respiratory rate	☐	☐	☐
c. Breath sounds	☐	☐	☐
d. Peak expiratory flow	☐	☐	☐
* **7.** Administers aerosol using the MDI			
a. Without a spacer	☐	☐	☐
b. With a spacer	☐	☐	☐
* **8.** Monitors the patient following aerosol administration			
a. Heart rate	☐	☐	☐
b. Respiratory rate	☐	☐	☐

c. Breath sounds

☐ ☐ ☐

d. Peak expiratory flow

☐ ☐ ☐

* **9.** Cleans up after the procedure

☐ ☐ ☐

* **10.** Records the procedure in the patient's chart

☐ ☐ ☐

SCORE:

Peer _____ points of possible 36; _____%

Lab _____ points of possible 36; _____%

Clinical _____ points of possible 36; _____%

TIME: _____ out of possible 30 minutes

STUDENT SIGNATURES

PEER: _____

STUDENT: _____

INSTRUCTOR SIGNATURES

LAB: _____

CLINICAL: _____

PERFORMANCE EVALUATION:
DPI Administration

Date:Lab _____ Clinical _____ Agency _____

Lab: Pass _____ Fail _____ Clinical: Pass _____ Fail _____

Studentname _____ Instructorname _____

No. of times observed in clinical _____

No. of times practiced in clinical _____

PASSING CRITERIA: Obtain 90% or better on the procedure. Tasks indicated by * must receive at least 1 point, or the evaluation is terminated. Procedure must be performed within the designated time, or the performance receives a failing grade.

SCORING:
2 points — Task performed satisfactorily without prompting.
1 point — Task performed satisfactorily with self-initiated correction.
0 points — Task performed incorrectly or with prompting required.
NA — Task not applicable to the patient care situation.

Tasks:	Peer	Lab	Clinical
* **1.** Verifies the physician's order	☐	☐	☐
* **2.** Observes universal precautions, including washing hands	☐	☐	☐
* **3.** Obtains the DPI	☐	☐	☐
* **4.** Identifies the patient and introduces self	☐	☐	☐
* **5.** Gives thorough and complete instructions	☐	☐	☐
* **6.** Monitors the patient			
a. Heart rate	☐	☐	☐
b. Respiratory rate	☐	☐	☐
c. Breath sounds	☐	☐	☐
d. Peak expiratory flow	☐	☐	☐
* **7.** Administers the DPI	☐	☐	☐
* **8.** Monitors the patient following aerosol administration			
a. Heart rate	☐	☐	☐
b. Respiratory rate	☐	☐	☐
c. Breath sounds	☐	☐	☐
d. Peak expiratory flow	☐	☐	☐
9. Cleans up after the procedure	☐	☐	☐
* **10.** Records the procedure in the patient's chart	☐	☐	☐

SCORE: Peer _____ points of possible 32; _____%

                   Lab _____ points of possible 32; _____%

                   Clinical _____ points of possible 32; _____%

TIME: _____ out of possible 30 minutes

STUDENT SIGNATURES   **INSTRUCTOR SIGNATURES**

PEER: _____   LAB: _____

STUDENT: _____   CLINICAL: _____

CHAPTER 15
Humidity and Aerosol Therapy

Humidity and aerosol therapy is a frequently used modality in clinical practice. A great deal of time in respiratory care practice will be spent setting up, monitoring, and troubleshooting humidity and aerosol therapy equipment. It is important for the respiratory practitioner to understand the components and theory of operation of the various types of humidity and aerosol equipment. This knowledge base will allow the practitioner to select and set up appropriate devices to meet clinical goals. The practitioner will also be expected to know how to troubleshoot the equipment, rendering it operational.

This chapter discusses the various types of equipment used to administer humidity and aerosol therapy, their principles of operation, clinical applications, and hazards and complications.

KEY TERMS

- Absolute humidity
- Aerosol
- Amplitude
- Body humidity
- Capacity
- Frequency
- Heat and moisture exchanger (HME)
- Humidifier
- Humidity
- Humidity deficit
- Maximum absolute humidity (capacity)
- Nebulizer
- Relative humidity

THEORY OBJECTIVES

At the end of this chapter, the reader should be able to:

- Define humidity and aerosol.
- Explain the difference between a humidifier and a nebulizer.
- State the three factors that can affect humidity output.
- For the following humidifiers, describe the principles of operation, efficiency, and application in the clinical setting:
  - Bubble humidifier
  - Wick humidifier
- For the following large-volume nebulizers, describe the principles of operation, efficiency, and application in the clinical setting:
  - Large-volume nebulizer
  - MistyOx nebulizers
- Discuss the following features of an ultrasonic nebulizer:
  - Principles of operation
    - Energy generation
    - Function of piezoelectric crystal
    - Significance of amplitude and frequency
  - Clinical application
  - Hazards of use
- Compare and contrast the types of small-volume nebulizers and their clinical applications.

CLINICAL PRACTICE GUIDELINES

AARC Clinical Practice Guideline: Bland Aerosol Administration

BAA 4.0 INDICATIONS:

4.1 The presence of upper airway edema—cool bland aerosol (1,2)

4.1.1 Laryngeotracheobronchitis (LTB) (1,2)

4.1.2 Subglottic edema (1,2)

4.1.3 Postextubation edema (1,2)

4.1.4 Postoperative management of the upper airway

4.2 The presence of a bypassed upper airway (3)

4.3 The need for sputum specimens (3,4)

BAA 5.0 CONTRAINDICATIONS:

5.1 Bronchoconstriction (1,3,5,6)

5.2 History of airway hyperresponsiveness (1,2,5,6)

BAA 6.0 HAZARDS/COMPLICATIONS:

6.1 Wheezing or bronchospasm (1,3,5,6)

6.2 Bronchoconstriction when artificial airway is employed (7–11)

6.3 Infection (12)

6.4 Overhydration (12)

6.5 Patient discomfort

6.6 Caregiver exposure to droplet nuclei of *Mycobacterium tuberculosis* or other airborne contagion produced as a consequence of coughing, particularly during sputum induction.

BAA 8.0 ASSESSMENT OF NEED:

8.1 The presence of one or more of the following may be an indication for administration of a water or isotonic or hypotonic saline aerosol:

8.1.1 Stridor

8.1.2 Brassy, crouplike cough

8.1.3 Hoarseness following extubation

8.1.4 Diagnosis of LTB or croup

8.1.5 Clinical history suggesting upper airway irritation and increased work of breathing (e.g., smoke inhalation)

8.1.6 Patient discomfort associated with airway instrumentation or insult

8.1.7 Bypassed upper airway

8.2 The presence of the need for sputum induction (e.g., for diagnosis of *Pneumocystis carinii* pneumonia [17–19] tuberculosis) is an indication for administration of hypertonic saline aerosol.

BAA 9.0 ASSESSMENT OF OUTCOME:

9.1 With administration of water or hypotonic or isotonic saline, the desired outcome is the presence of one or more of the following:

9.1.1 Decreased work of breathing

9.1.2 Improved vital signs

9.1.3 Decreased stridor

9.1.4 Decreased dyspnea

9.1.5 Improved arterial blood gas values

9.1.6 Improved oxygen saturation as indicated by pulse oximetry (SpO_2)

9.2 With administration of hypertonic saline, the desired outcome is a sputum sample adequate for analysis.

BAA 11.0 MONITORING:

The extent of patient monitoring should be determined on the basis of the stability and severity of the patient's condition:

11.1 Patient subjective response—pain, discomfort, dyspnea, restlessness

11.2 Heart rate and rhythm, blood pressure

11.3 Respiratory rate, pattern, mechanics, accessory muscle use

11.4 Sputum production quantity, color, consistency, odor

11.5 Skin color

11.6 Breath sounds

11.7 Pulse oximetry (if hypoxemia is suspected)

11.8 Spirometry equipment (if concern of adverse reaction)

Reprinted with permission from *Respiratory Care* 2003; 48: 529–533. The complete AARC Clinical Practice Guidelines are available from the AARC Web site (http://www.aarc.org), from the AARC Executive Office, or from *Respiratory Care* journal.

AARC Clinical Practice Guideline: Selection of a Device for Delivery of Aerosol to the Lung Parenchyma

DALP 4.0 INDICATIONS:

The indication for selecting a suitable device is the need to deliver a topical medication (in aerosol form) that has its site of action in the lung parenchyma or is intended for systemic absorption. Such medications may possibly include antibiotics, antivirals, antifungals, surfactants, and enzymes.

DALP 5.0 CONTRAINDICATIONS:

5.1 No contraindications exist for choosing an appropriate device for parenchymal deposition.

5.2 Contraindications related to the substances being delivered may exist. Consult the package insert for product-specific contraindications to medication delivery.

(Continued)

DALP 6.0 HAZARDS/COMPLICATIONS:

6.1 Malfunction of device and/or improper technique may result in underdosing or overdosing.

6.2 In mechanically ventilated patients, the nebulizer design and characteristics of the medication may affect ventilator function (e.g., filter obstruction, altered tidal volume, decreased trigger sensitivity) and medication deposition. (10,11)

6.3 Complications related to specific pharmacologic agents can occur.

6.4 Aerosols may cause bronchospasm or irritation of the airway.

6.5 Exposure to medications (12–23) and patient-generated droplet nuclei may be hazardous to clinicians. (24)

6.5.1 Exposure to medication should be limited to the patient for whom it has been ordered. Nebulized medication that is released into the atmosphere from the nebulizer or exhaled by the patient becomes a form of "secondhand" exposure that may affect health care providers and others in the vicinity of the treatment.

There has been increased awareness of possible health effects of aerosols, such as ribavirin and pentamidine. Anecdotal reports associate symptoms such as conjunctivitis, decreased tolerance to presence of contact lenses, headaches, bronchospasm, shortness of breath, and rashes in health care workers exposed to secondhand aerosols. Similar concerns have been expressed concerning health care workers who are pregnant or are planning to be pregnant within eight weeks of administration. Less often discussed are the potential exposure effects of aerosolized antibiotics (which may contribute to the development of resistant organisms), steroids, and bronchodilators. (25)

Because the data regarding adverse health effects on the health care worker and on those casually exposed are incomplete, the prudent course is to minimize exposure in all situations. (26)

6.5.2 The Centers for Disease Control and Prevention recommends addressing exposure control issues by (1) administrative policy, (2) engineering controls, and (3) personal protective equipment, in that order. (27,28)

6.5.2.1 Administrative controls: Should include warning signs to apprise all who enter a treatment area of potential hazards of exposure. Accidental exposures should be documented and reported according to accepted standards.

Measures to reduce aerosol contamination of room air include:

6.5.2.1.1 Discontinuing nebulization of medication while patient is not breathing the aerosol

6.5.2.1.2 Ensuring that staff who administer medications understand risks inherent with the medication and procedures for safely disposing of hazardous wastes

6.5.2.1.3 Screening of staff for adverse effects of exposure to aerosol medication

6.5.2.1.4 Providing alternative assignments for those staff who are at high risk of adverse effects from exposure (e.g., pregnant women or those with demonstrated sensitivity to the specific agent)

6.5.2.2 Engineering controls:

6.5.2.2.1 Filters or filtered scavenger systems to remove aerosols that cannot be contained

6.5.2.2.2 Frequent air exchanges to dilute concentration of aerosol in room to eliminate 99% of aerosol before the next patient enters and receives treatment in the area

6.5.2.2.3 Booths or stalls for sputum induction and aerosolized medication administration in areas in which multiple patients are treated. Booths or stalls should be designed to provide adequate air flow to draw aerosol and droplet nuclei from the patient and into an appropriate filtration system, with exhaust directed to an appropriate outside vent.

6.5.2.2.4 Handling of filters, nebulizers, and other contaminated components of the aerosol delivery system used with suspect agents (such as pentamidine and ribavirin) as hazardous waste

6.5.2.3 Personal protection devices:

6.5.2.3.1 Personal protection devices should be used to reduce exposure when engineering alternatives are not in place or are not adequate. Use properly fitted respirators with adequate filtration when exhaust flow cannot adequately remove aerosol particles. (28)

6.5.2.3.2 Goggles, gloves, and gowns should be used as splatter shields and to reduce exposure to medication residues and body substances.

DALP 8.0 ASSESSMENT OF NEED (SELECTION CRITERIA FOR DEVICE):

8.1 Availability of prescribed drug in solution or MDI formulation

8.2 Availability of appropriate scavenging or filtration equipment

8.3 Patient preference for a given device that meets therapeutic objectives

(Continued)

8.4 Although specific devices may give known ranges of particle size and output, clear superiority of any one method or device for achieving specific clinical outcomes has not been established. Cost, convenience, effectiveness, and patient tolerance of procedure should be considered. (26,53)

8.5 When spontaneous ventilation is inadequate (e.g., kyphoscoliosis, neuromuscular disorders, or respiratory failure) consider augmentation with mechanical ventilation.

DALP 9.0 ASSESSMENT OF OUTCOME:

Appropriate device selection is reflected by evidence of:

9.1 Use of proper technique in applying device

9.2 Patient compliance with procedure

9.3 A positive clinical outcome (However, appropriate device selection and application does not guarantee a positive outcome.)

DALP 11.0 MONITORING:

11.1 Performance of the device and scavenging system

11.2 Technique of device application

11.3 Assessment of patient response

Reprinted with permission from *Respiratory Care* 1996; 41(7): 647–653. The complete AARC Clinical Practice Guidelines are available from the AARC Web site (http://www.aarc.org), from the AARC Executive Office, or from *Respiratory Care* journal.

AARC Clinical Practice Guideline: Humidification during Mechanical Ventilation

HMV 4.0 INDICATIONS:

Humidification of inspired gas during mechanical ventilation is mandatory when an endotracheal or tracheostomy tube is present. (1–7)

HMV 5.0 CONTRAINDICATIONS:

There are no contraindications [to] providing physiologic conditioning of inspired gas during mechanical ventilation. An HME is contraindicated under some circumstances.

5.1 Use of an HME is contraindicated for patients with thick, copious, or bloody secretions. (8,26–28)

5.2 Use of an HME is contraindicated for patients with an expired tidal volume less than 70% of the delivered tidal volume (e.g., those with large bronchopleurocutaneous fistulas or incompetent or absent endotracheal tube cuffs). (5–25)

5.3 Use of an HME is contraindicated for patients with body temperatures less than 32°C. (8,29)

5.4 Use of an HME may be contraindicated for patients with high spontaneous minute volumes (>10 L/min). (8,26,29)

5.5 An HME must be removed from the patient circuit during aerosol treatments when the nebulizer is placed in the patient circuit. (8–29)

HMV 6.0 HAZARDS/COMPLICATIONS:

Hazards and complications associated with the use of humidification devices include:

6.1 Potential for electrical shock—heated humidifiers (11–14)

6.2 Hypothermia—HME or heated humidifiers; hyperthermia—heated humidifiers (11–14)

6.3 Thermal injury to the airway from heated humidifiers; (30) burns to the patient and tubing meltdown if heated-wire circuits are covered or circuits and humidifiers are incompatible

6.4 Under hydration and impaction of mucus secretions—HME or heated humidifiers (1–7)

6.5 Hypoventilation and/or alveolar gas trapping due to mucous plugging of airways—HME or heated humidifier (1–7)

6.6 Possible increased resistive work of breathing due to mucous plugging of airways—HME or heated humidifiers (1–7)

6.7 Possible increased resistive work of breathing through the humidifier—HME or heated humidifiers (31–34)

6.8 Possible hypoventilation due to increased dead space—HME (8,15–25,26–30)

6.9 Inadvertent overfilling resulting in unintentional tracheal lavage—heated reservoir humidifiers (35)

6.10 The fact that when disconnected from the patient, some ventilators generate a high flow through the patient circuit that may aerosolize contaminated condensate, putting both the patient and clinician at risk for nosocomial infection—heated humidifiers (35)

6.11 Potential for burns to caregivers from hot metal—heated humidifiers

6.12 Inadvertent tracheal lavage from pooled condensate in patient circuit—heated humidifiers (35)

6.13 Elevated airway pressures due to pooled condensation—heated humidifiers

6.14 Patient-ventilator dysynchrony and improper ventilator performance due to pooled condensation in the circuit—heated humidifiers

6.15 Ineffective low-pressure alarm during disconnection due to resistance through HME (36)

HMV 8.0 ASSESSMENT OF NEED:

Humidification is needed by all patients requiring mechanical ventilation via an artificial airway. Conditioning of inspired gases should be instituted using either an HME or a heated humidifier.

(Continued)

8.1 HMEs are better suited for short-term use (< or = 96 hours) and during transport. (8,29)

8.2 Heated humidifiers should be used for patients requiring long-term mechanical ventilation (> 96 hours) or for patients who exhibit contraindications [to] HME use. (8,29)

HMV 9.0 ASSESSMENT OF OUTCOME:

Humidification is assumed to be appropriate if, on regular careful inspection, the patient exhibits none of the hazards or complications listed in HMV 6.0.

HMV 11.0 MONITORING:

The humidification device should be inspected visually during the patient-ventilator system check and condensate should be removed from the patient circuit as necessary. HMEs should be inspected and replaced if secretions have contaminated the insert or filter. The following variables should be recorded during equipment inspection:

11.1 Humidifier setting (temperature setting or numeric dial setting or both). During routine use on an intubated patient, a heated humidifier should be set to deliver an inspired gas temperature of 33 ± 2°C and should provide a minimum of 30 mg/L of water vapor. (8–10)

11.2 Inspired gas temperature. Temperature should be monitored as near the patient's airway opening as possible, if a heated humidifier is used.

11.2.1 Specific temperatures may vary with patient condition, but the inspiratory gas should not exceed 37°C at the airway threshold.

11.2.2 When a heated-wire patient circuit is used (to prevent condensation) on an infant, the temperature probe should be located outside of the incubator or away from the direct heat of the radiant warmer. (12)

11.3 Alarm settings (if applicable). High temperature alarm should be set no higher than 37°C, and the low temperature alarm should be set no lower than 30°C. (8,10)

11.4 Water level and function of automatic feed system (if applicable)

11.5 Quantity and consistency of secretions. Characteristics should be noted and recorded. When using an HME, if secretions become copious or appear increasingly tenacious, a heated humidifier should replace the HME.

Reprinted with permission from *Respiratory Care* 1992; 37: 887–890. The complete AARC Clinical Practice Guidelines are available from the AARC Web site (http://www.aarc.org), from the AARC Executive Office, or from *Respiratory Care* journal.

WHAT IS HUMIDITY AND WHAT IS AEROSOL?

Humidity is water in gaseous form, or vapor. As such, water vapor or humidity cannot be seen. Humidification is used to add water vapor to an anhydrous gas during oxygen administration and to raise the relative humidity of a room to prevent or loosen thick retained secretions. It is also used to provide humidity to the lower airways when the upper airway is bypassed by intubation or tracheostomy.

An *aerosol* is the suspension of particulate water in a gas. Technically, we can generate an aerosol of any matter if there is sufficient energy to suspend it. In the practice of respiratory care, aerosol generation generally serves two purposes: bland aerosol therapy and the aerosolization of medication. A bland aerosol is usually nebulized water or saline and is used to increase the water content of secretions, thereby thinning them. Medications such as bronchodilators may be aerosolized to reverse bronchoconstriction. Mucokinetics may be aerosolized to break down mucus. Decongestants may be aerosolized to shrink swollen mucous membranes by vasoconstriction. Racemic epinephrine is an example and is commonly used to treat croup, epiglottitis, and bronchiolitis.

Humidifiers and Nebulizers

A *humidifier* is a device that produces water in gaseous form (vapor) through the process of evaporation. There are many types of humidifiers that range in efficiency from poor to excellent. An ideal humidifier is capable of completely saturating a gas (100% humidity) at body temperature and pressure (termed *body humidity*: 37°C, 47 mm Hg partial press [H_2O], and 100% saturation).

A *nebulizer* is a device used to aerosolize liquids. Efficiency and particle sizes vary depending on the device and its principle of operation.

Heating a humidifier or nebulizer increases the content of water in the aerosol output, closely matching that of the body. Some people may be sensitive to the nature of the aerosol itself—the water may be irritating as well as the increased temperature. The temperature should be closely regulated to prevent adverse effects on the patient such as fever or burns.

Humidity

The warmer gas is, the more water vapor it can hold. The amount of water vapor contained by a gas at a given temperature is termed *absolute humidity*. If a gas is fully saturated with water vapor (100% saturated), it is said to have *maximum absolute humidity* or at its *capacity*. When the temperature of a gas is increased, its capacity will also increase. A gas heated to body temperature can therefore reach a humidity approaching that of the gas contained in the lungs.

Humidity deficit is the difference between a gas's absolute humidity and body humidity. *Body humidity* is the absolute humidity at body temperature, fully saturated. The conditions of body humidity are 37°C, 100% saturation, and 43.9 mg/L water vapor.

$$Humidity\ Deficit = Body\ Humidity - Absolute\ Humidity$$

Example

A heated humidifier has an output of 35 mg/L at a temperature of 34°C. What is the humidity deficit?

$$\begin{aligned}Humidity\ Deficit &= Body\ Humidity - Absolute\ Humidity\\ &= 43.9\ mg/L - 35\ mg/L\\ &= 8.9\ mg/L\end{aligned}$$

This implies that the patient's airway will need to add 8.9 mg/L water vapor to the inspired gas to fully saturate it with humidity at body temperature.

Relative humidity is the gas's absolute humidity expressed as a percentage of the gas's capacity at any given temperature.

$$Relative\ Humidity = \left(\frac{Absolute\ Humidity}{Capacity}\right)100$$

Example

The temperature is 5°C and the capacity of the gas at 7°C is 4.85 mg/L. What is the relative humidity if the gas's absolute humidity is 3.8 mg/L?

$$Relative\ Humidity = \left(\frac{3.8\,mg/L}{4.85\,mg/L}\right)100 = 78\%$$

Factors Affecting Humidity Output

The three factors that affect humidity output include temperature, surface area, and time for water-gas contact. As described previously, increasing a gas's temperature increases the gas's capacity or ability to hold water vapor.

Surface area and exposure time are other ways to control humidity output. By increasing the surface area for the gas–water interface, more gas is exposed to the water and more water vapor is picked up. Surface areas can be increased to only a limited degree; otherwise, the device would be too large and awkward. The time during which a gas is exposed to the water can also influence humidity output by providing time for evaporation to occur. Time of gas exposure, however, is difficult to influence.

EQUIPMENT FOR HUMIDITY AND AEROSOL THERAPY

Bubble Humidifier

The bubble humidifier is the most commonly used humidifier in clinical practice. These devices are not very efficient in terms of humidity output. Their primary application is in the humidification of oxygen delivered by nasal cannula.

Bubble humidifiers work by conducting gas down a small tube that is submerged in water. The gas passes through a diffuser, which breaks the released gas into small bubbles, increasing the surface area. The bubbles float passively to the surface, absorbing water vapor. The humidified gas then flows through the outlet, out of the unit. Figure 15-1 is a schematic of a typical bubble humidifier.

Bubble humidifiers are disposable units designed for single-patient use. The disposable units are also available prefilled with sterile distilled water.

The outlets of bubble humidifiers have a tapered nipple, designed to fit small-diameter oxygen connecting tubing. The oxygen delivery device used with a bubble humidifier is primarily a low-flow nasal cannula.

This device produces water vapor, or water in gaseous form. The humidity output of this device is not visible. Occasionally, water may be seen in the oxygen connecting tubing if temperature conditions promote condensation.

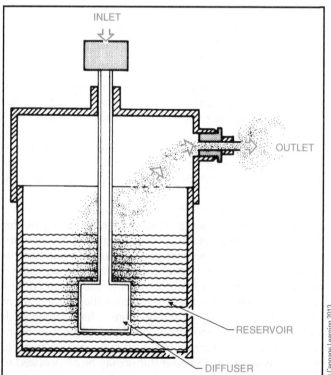

Figure 15-1   A schematic of a typical bubble humidifier

Wick Humidifiers

Wick humidifiers are also very efficient humidifiers. By increasing the temperature and surface area, efficiency is enhanced. The wicks are typically made from a relatively thick blotter-type paper. This paper is very absorbent and quickly conducts water by capillary action.

The Hudson RCI Conchatherm IV wick humidifier has a disposable wick assembly consisting of the wick, aluminum canister to enhance heat transfer, and the gas inlet and outlet. The disposable element is inserted into the servo-controlled heater (Figure 15-2). As the gas passes the wick, water is absorbed by evaporation. The gas can be fully saturated at up to 39°C.

The Hudson RCI Conchaterm IV humidifier is ideal for use with mechanical ventilation, artificial airways, or other applications requiring high flow rates and body humidity. Inlets and outlets on the humidifier are designed for large-bore aerosol tubing, which assists in the conduction of humidified gas at a high volume and flow. Water level is maintained automatically by a continuous feed system and a disposable 1 liter sterile water reservoir (see Figure 15-2).

Heated Pass Over Humidifiers

The Fisher and Paykel MR 850 is another example of a servo-controlled heated pass over humidifier (Figure 15-3). The MR 850 is capable of delivering humidified gas between 30 and 39°C. There is a heated wire option, which, when combined with heated wire ventilator circuits, helps to reduce condensation in the ventilator tubing.

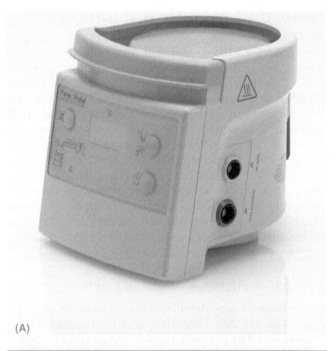

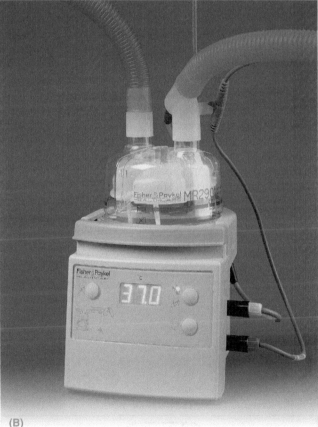

(A)

(B)

Figure 15-3 A photograph of the Fisher and Paykel MR 850 heated humidifier *(Courtesy of Fisher & Paykel Healthcare, Inc.)*

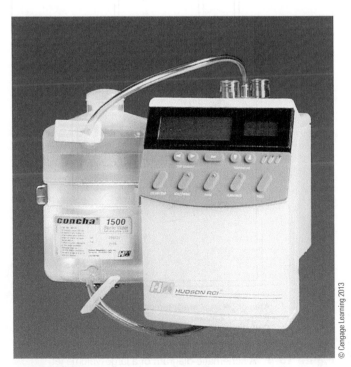

© Cengage Learning 2013

Figure 15-2 A photograph of the RCI Conchatherm IV heated humidifier

Water level is maintained by a float system and disposable containers (similar to intravenous [IV] bags) of sterile water for inhalation. The disposable humidification chamber slides into the servo-controlled heater and is fully self contained.

Heat and Moisture Exchanger

A *heat and moisture exchanger (HME)* is a small hygroscopic device placed proximal to a patient's artificial airway, where it absorbs water vapor and heat from the patient's exhaled gas (Figure 15-4). When the patient breathes or the mechanical ventilator delivers the next breath, the heat and moisture trapped in the HME evaporates, humidifying and heating the airway. The efficiency of these devices varies, ranging from around 70% to 90% at temperatures of 30 to 31°C. These devices are best used for shorter durations (less than 96 hours). The patient should be carefully monitored for increases in airway resistance and increased work of breathing. These devices are not indicated for patients who have excess airway secretions or are having difficulty managing their secretions.

Large-Volume Nebulizers

Use of large-volume nebulizers is very common in respiratory care practice. These devices deliver cool or heated aerosol, and they precisely regulate oxygen concentration using an oxygen diluter.

Jet mixing occurs by viscous shearing and vorticity as described in Chapter 13 to dilute oxygen with room air. These devices provide a range of inspired oxygen levels, operating in a manner similar to that of entrainment masks. Adjustment of the entrainment port size varies the amount of room air added to the oxygen flow. As with other entrainment devices, back pressure distal to the entrainment ports can cause an increase in the fraction of inspired oxygen (FIO_2) delivered. The large-volume nebulizers are especially susceptible to this effect because of their high aerosol output, which may "rain out" and partially obstruct the delivery tubing. Therefore, the tubing should be checked and drained on a routine basis. A drainage bag or 3 liter anesthesia bag may be positioned in line with the delivery tubing to serve as a collection bag for rain-out.

The high-velocity gas exiting from the nozzle (jet) is directed perpendicular to a small capillary tube whose base is immersed in water (Figure 15-5). Shear forces cause water to be removed from the capillary tube into the flow of gas. Because mass has been removed from the capillary tube (water), a void forms because the gas flow across the top of the tube effectively caps it (Scacci, 1979). This void forms a small area of reduced (subambient) pressure within the capillary tube itself. Capillary action draws water up the tube to fill the void (conservation of mass). Once the water level reaches the top, it is removed again by shear forces. This is a continuous process, and the water removed forms a dense aerosol.

Downstream a short distance from the jet is a baffle that serves to stabilize particle size. When the aerosolized particles meet the baffle, larger particles, having greater inertia, are rained out.

The outlet of the nebulizer has a connector for large-bore aerosol tubing. The common applications for the unit are in bland aerosol therapy via aerosol mask or face tent and in humidification of artificial airways via a Briggs adapter (T piece) or tracheostomy mask.

Total gas flow from these nebulizers will vary depending on the FIO_2 setting and entrained room air. Vorticity is used to dilute the source gas with room air entrained by the device. The total flow depends on the entrainment ratio (Table 15-1). It becomes evident that total flow decreases at the higher FIO_2 settings. It is not uncommon to simultaneously use more than one nebulizer to meet the flow needs of the patient.

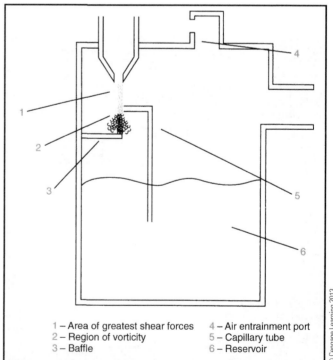

1 – Area of greatest shear forces   4 – Air entrainment port
2 – Region of vorticity   5 – Capillary tube
3 – Baffle   6 – Reservoir

Figure 15-5 A schematic diagram of a large-volume jet nebulizer: 1, Area of greatest shear forces; 2, region of vorticity; 3, baffle to stabilize particle sizes; 4, air entrainment port; 5, capillary tube; 6, liquid reservoir

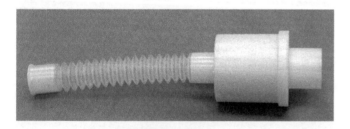

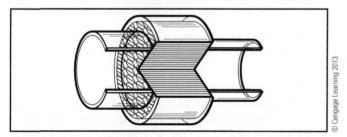

Figure 15-4 A photograph and a cross section of a heat and moisture exchanger (HME)

© Cengage Learning 2013

TABLE 15-1: Air-to-Oxygen Entrainment Ratios	
ROOM AIR-TO-OXYGEN RATIO	**CONCENTRATION (%)**
25:1	24
10:1	28
8:1	30
5:1	35
3:1	40
1.7:1	50
1:1	60
0:1	100

MistyOx Nebulizers

The MistyOx Hi-Fi nebulizer and the MistyOx Gas Injection Nebulizer (GIN), Costa Mesa, CA, are two nebulizers that are designed to provide high-density aerosol delivery at high total flow rates (Figure 15-6). The Hi-Fi nebulizer can provide a flow of 43 L/min at an FIO_2 of 0.96 and of 77 L/min at an FIO_2 of 0.60 from a single oxygen source. The GIN device is capable of providing flows of more than 100 L/min when powered by two gas sources. Tables 15-2 and 15-3 summarize the GIN device oxygen concentrations and flow deliveries.

Both nebulizers have a standard 38 mm threaded fitting that allows connection of the nebulizer to most disposable sterile solution bottles. This capability is advantageous in that significant cost savings can be realized in comparison with other prefilled nebulizer brands. Heated aerosol may be provided by the attachment of the optional TurboHeater.

Ultrasonic Nebulizers

Ultrasonic nebulizers rely on electrical and mechanical energy to generate an aerosol. Because of their greater level of sophistication, they are more expensive and generally more costly to repair than pneumatically powered devices.

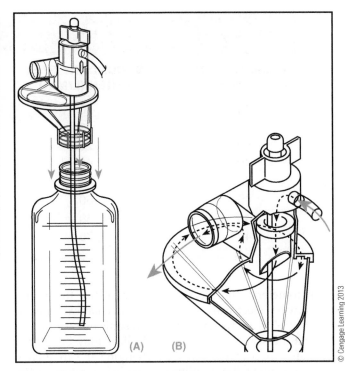

Figure 15-6 (A) An assembly guide and (B) a detailed diagram of the MistyOx Gas Injection Nebulizer (GIN)

© Cengage Learning 2013

The generation of the energy required to produce an aerosol begins with a radio frequency generator (rf generator). An analogy can be drawn by comparing the rf generator with a radio transmitter. However, the frequencies generated are generally higher, in the range of 1.3 to 1.4 megahertz (MHz) (the AM commercial broadcast band is 54 to 160 kilohertz [KHz] and the FM broadcast band is 88 to 108 MHz). The frequencies generated are conducted to a special crystal with a shielded cable.

The special crystal, called a *piezoelectric crystal*, has the ability to change shape in resonance with the rf energy. For each wavelength or impulse of energy, the crystal will oscillate back and forth, creating mechanical energy. These waves are conducted through the water in the reservoir to the surface, breaking the water surface into fine aerosol particles having a mean diameter of 3 to

TABLE 15-2: Concentration of Oxygen as Primary Gas and Total Flow for MistyOx GIN Nebulizer			
PRIMARY GAS: AIR (L/MIN)	**SECONDARY GAS: OXYGEN (L/MIN)**	**TOTAL FLOW**	**CONCENTRATION (%)**
40	0	40	100
40	10	50	84.2
40	20	60	73.6
40	30	70	66.1
40	40	80	60.5
40	50	90	56.1
40	60	100	52.6
40	70	110	49.7

TABLE 15-3: Concentration of Oxygen as Secondary Gas and Total Flow for MistyOx GIN Nebulizer

PRIMARY GAS: AIR (L/MIN)	SECONDARY GAS: OXYGEN (L/MIN)	TOTAL FLOW	CONCENTRATION (%)
40	0	40	20.9
40	10	50	36.8
40	20	60	47.3
40	30	70	54.9
40	40	80	60.5
40	50	90	64.9
40	60	100	68.4
40	70	110	71.3

5 micrometers. The piezoelectric crystal has the ability to convert electrical energy into mechanical energy. Figure 15-7 is a schematic of an ultrasonic nebulizer.

Output from an ultrasonic nebulizer may be altered in one of two ways: either by changing the frequency or by changing the amplitude. *Amplitude* refers to the depth of the waveform from the upper to the lower crest of the wave. Amplitude can vary from a large amplitude to a small amplitude. By increasing the amplitude, the amount of aerosol output increases. *Frequency* refers to the number of waveforms per second. The rf energy in an ultrasonic nebulizer may range from 1.3 million cycles per second to 1.4 million cycles per second. Figure 15-8 shows schematically two different amplitudes and frequencies. By increasing the frequency, more waveforms strike the water surface each second. Because of the greater number of impacts per second, the result is a smaller particle size. The frequency is usually not adjustable on the majority of ultrasonic nebulizers.

Ultrasonic nebulizers are used in the clinical setting to administer bland aerosol therapy. Due to the small particle size, pulmonary deposition is greater than with other nebulizers that have outputs of larger particle size. This therapy is very effective in thinning retained, inspissated secretions.

The hazards of therapy with an ultrasonic nebulizer are related to its output in milliliters of water per minute. An ultrasonic nebulizer is capable of producing 6 mL of aerosol per minute. There is a potential hazard of overhydrating patients if they are exposed to long-term administration. This overhydration may lead to an increased volume of secretions and a narrowing of the airway lumen. These changes will result in increased resistance, wheezing, and dyspnea. Bronchospasm may also be a hazard associated with the use of an ultrasonic nebulizer.

Small-Volume Nebulizers

Small-volume nebulizer therapy has become a very popular means of administering medication in the clinical setting. This is so because of its effectiveness,

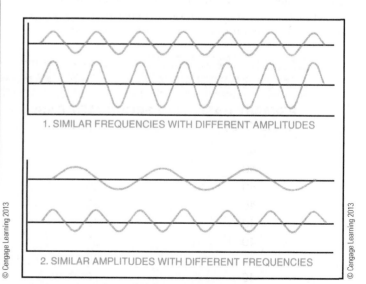

Figure 15-7 A schematic of an ultrasonic nebulizer

Figure 15-8 A comparison of frequency and amplitude

simplicity, and relatively low cost. Small-volume nebulizers provide a convenient, inexpensive way to aerosolize liquid medications.

Mainstream and sidestream devices are the two general types of small-volume nebulizers. The two are differentiated by the placement of the nebulizer in relation to the main flow of gas through the device. The nebulizer in a mainstream device is positioned directly in the path of the gas flow. A sidestream device has the nebulizer positioned adjacent to and connected to the main flow of gas, usually with a Briggs adapter or aerosol T piece. A sidestream nebulizer will generally produce smaller particles owing to the longer pathway the aerosol must travel to reach the main gas flow. Figure 15-9 is a schematic showing both types of nebulizers.

The delivery devices compatible with small-volume nebulizers include a mouthpiece, a Briggs adapter (T piece), an aerosol mask, a tracheostomy mask, and a face tent. The outlet on most nebulizers is designed with an inside diameter that will fit a mouthpiece and an outside diameter to fit larger-bore aerosol tubing.

Commonly Administered Medications

For a more detailed discussion of medications delivered by aerosol, refer to Chapter 14, Introduction to Respiratory Care Pharmacology, or consult any of a number of excellent books on the topic.

Monitoring Therapy for Effectiveness

Small-volume nebulizer therapy may be monitored for effectiveness by measuring the peak flow rate and the forced expired volume in the first second (FEV_1) before and after therapy when administering a bronchodilator. Besides the parameters mentioned previously, breath sounds and sputum should also be monitored. Pretherapy and posttherapy breath sounds should be compared. The patient should be encouraged to cough after therapy, and sputum color, amount, and odor (if present) should be noted.

Heart rate should be monitored before, during, and after therapy. An increase in the heart rate greater than 20 beats per minute over the baseline rate should be the criterion for discontinuing the therapy. The patient should be monitored for other medication side effects, which should be noted on the medical record.

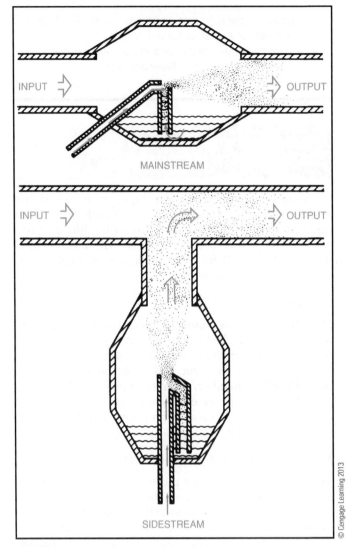

Figure 15-9   Sidestream and mainstream small-volume nebulizers

Hazards and Complications

Hazards and complications of small-volume nebulizer therapy are primarily associated with the side effects from the medications administered. Loosening of secretions may also precipitate obstruction if not cleared by coughing.

PROFICIENCY OBJECTIVES

At the end of this chapter, the reader should be able to:

- *Correctly assemble, test for function, safely apply, and troubleshoot the following humidifiers:*
  - *Bubble humidifier*
  - *Wick humidifier*
  - *Demonstrate use of the humidifiers with appropriate delivery devices.*
  - *Correctly monitor the following as appropriate:*
    - *Oxygen concentration*
    - *Temperature*

- *Correctly assemble, test for function, safely apply, and troubleshoot the following nebulizers:*
  - *Large-volume nebulizer*
  - *MistyOx nebulizers*
  - *Ultrasonic nebulizer*
  - *Demonstrate use of the nebulizers with appropriate delivery devices.*
  - *Correctly monitor the following as appropriate:*
    - *Oxygen concentration*
    - *Temperature*

(Continued)

- *Correctly assemble, test for function, safely apply, and troubleshoot a small-volume nebulizer.*
  - *Demonstrate the use of a small-volume nebulizer with the following delivery devices:*
    - *Aerosol mask*

  - *Briggs adapter/aerosol T piece*
  - *Mouthpiece*
  - *Correctly monitor a patient while delivering a small-volume nebulizer treatment with a bronchodilator.*

HUMIDITY AND AEROSOL THERAPY

Operation of humidification equipment, including assembly, testing, application, and troubleshooting, is quite simple and consists primarily of the filling of reservoirs with sterile, distilled water and the attachment of delivery devices. Refer to the operation manual for the specific device being used.

Wick Humidifier

Mate the disposable humidification chamber or column to the servo-controlled heater assembly. Attach the water reservoir to the chamber or column using the supplied tubing. Connect the inlet and outlet stubbing to the humidification chamber/column. Connect the heater element to an appropriate electrical power source. Connect the temperature probes as appropriate, turn the unit on, and select the desired temperature range.

Heated Pass Over Humidifier

Mate the disposable heater platen/reservoir to the servo-controlled heater base. Attach the temperature probes to the humidifier outlet and locate the proximal probe close to the patient or patient's airway. Connect the water reservoir to the platen/reservoir using the supplied IV tubing. Connect the heater element to an appropriate electrical supply. Set the temperature and monitor the unit to ensure delivery of the desired temperature.

Large-Volume Nebulizers

A large-volume nebulizer is prepared for use by filling the reservoir with sterile, distilled water. It is then attached to a flowmeter with the diameter-indexed safety system (DISS) fitting at the top of the unit. Adjust the oxygen flow rate to between 8 and 12 L/min. Observe the nebulizer for aerosol output. If heat is indicated, a doughnut heater may be used (Figure 15-10). A 115 V AC outlet must be nearby. Adjust the diluter to the desired oxygen percentage and analyze the FIO_2 with an oxygen analyzer. Do not obstruct the outlet when determining the FIO_2 because the back pressure will cause the FIO_2 to increase. Attach a sufficient length of large-bore aerosol tubing to the outlet and position a drainage bag at the lowest point of the tubing. Attach an aerosol mask, tracheostomy mask, Briggs adapter (T piece), or face tent as appropriate.

The majority of problems encountered with this type of nebulizer occur at the diluter jet. The jet often becomes obstructed. Disassembly and cleaning of the jet may be required.

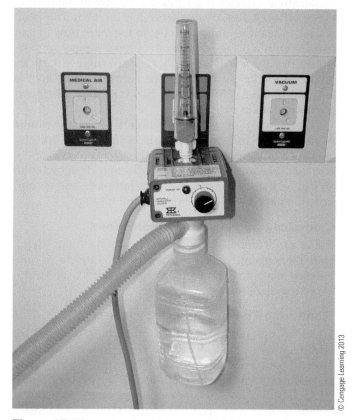

Figure 15-10 A doughnut heater attached to a nebulizer

© Cengage Learning 2013

MistyOx Hi-Fi and GIN Nebulizers

Remove the cap from the sterile solution distilled water bottle, aseptically remove the nebulizer from its packaging, insert the capillary tube into the bottle, and screw the bottle onto the 38 mm fitting on the nebulizer (for both the Hi-Fi and the GIN nebulizers). Make certain that the nebulizer is attached tightly and not cross threaded.

Connect the nebulizer to an oxygen flowmeter or two flowmeters and set the desired oxygen concentration or adjust the flow rates (for the GIN nebulizer; refer to Tables 15-2 and 15-3). If heated aerosol is desired, connect the TurboHeater between the nebulizer and the reservoir bottle and connect it to an electrical outlet. Monitor inspired gas temperature using a thermometer placed close to the patient. Monitor the oxygen concentrations using an oxygen analyzer and adjust the nebulizer to achieve the desired concentration and total flow rate.

Ultrasonic Nebulizers

If the ultrasonic nebulizer in use has a coupling chamber, fill it with tap water; then fill the nebulizer compartment with sterile, distilled water. For an ultrasonic nebulizer without a coupling chamber, simply fill the nebulizer compartment. Attach large-bore aerosol tubing from the fan to the inlet of the nebulizer compartment. Connect the power cord(s) to an appropriate electrical outlet. Turn on the nebulizer and adjust the output control to the desired aerosol output. Attach large-bore aerosol tubing to the outlet and attach an appropriate aerosol delivery device to the distal end of the tubing.

Troubleshooting these devices is often a frustrating experience. Water level in the coupling chamber is critical; too much or too little will decrease the output. Adjust the level for optimal output. The piezoelectric crystal may become contaminated with mineral deposits. Use an ultrasonic nebulizer cleaner and operate the unit for several minutes; then rinse the crystal and chamber with water and try again. Check the electrical connections. Check the tubing for obstruction from rain-out. If all of these efforts fail to restore the nebulizer to an operational condition, send it to the facility's biomedical engineering department for testing and repair or to an authorized service center.

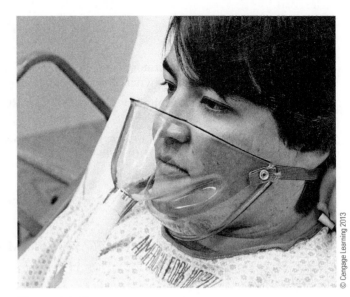

Figure 15-12   Application of a face tent

AEROSOL/OXYGEN DELIVERY DEVICES

There are four commonly used aerosol administration delivery devices. These are the Briggs adapter, aerosol mask, tracheostomy mask, and the face tent. These devices are shown in Figure 15-11. The aerosol mask and tracheostomy mask are used by connecting the large male fitting on the device to the large-bore aerosol tubing.

The Briggs adapter or aerosol T is attached directly to the distal end of the aerosol delivery tubing. In addition, a short, 6-inch piece of aerosol tubing is attached to the opposite end of the Briggs adapter. This serves as a 50 mL oxygen/aerosol reservoir, preventing room air entrainment when the patient first begins inspiration.

The face tent is designed to be positioned under the chin, as shown in Figure 15-12. This device is commonly used in the recovery room following surgery.

Small-Volume Nebulizer Therapy

The assembly of small-volume nebulizers will vary depending on the manufacturer. Some disposable units pull apart into two halves; others have threads that join the two parts. These different designs all provide for the introduction of medication into the reservoir in the proper amount and dilution as ordered by the physician.

Attach an appropriate delivery device to the outlet. An aerosol mask, mouthpiece, Briggs adapter (T piece), tracheostomy mask, or face tent may be appropriate.

Small-diameter oxygen connecting tubing joins the nebulizer to a flowmeter equipped with a nipple adapter or Christmas tree adapter. Oxygen flow is adjusted to between 6 and 8 L/min, depending on the unit. Adjust the flow until a dense aerosol can be observed.

If the nebulizer fails to function properly, check the jet for obstruction and the supply tubing for kinks. If this does not fix the problem, discard the nebulizer and obtain another.

Give the nebulizer to the patient and instruct the patient to take slow, deep breaths with a slight pause before exhaling. This end-inspiratory pause will help the aerosol to deposit in the lungs. If the patient becomes light-headed because of the deep breathing, turn off the flowmeter, and allow the patient to rest for a short period.

Monitor the patient carefully for any side effects caused by the medication you are using. If administering a bronchodilator, measure a pretreatment and posttreatment vital capacity and a peak expiratory flow rate.

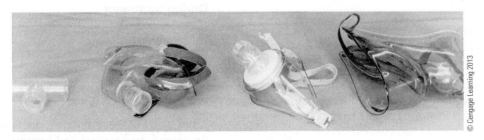

Figure 15-11   Aerosol delivery devices (from left to right: Brigg's adapter, aerosol mask, tracheostomy mask, and face tent)

References

American Association for Respiratory Care. (1996). AARC clinical practice guideline: Selection of a device for delivery of aerosol to the lung parenchyma. *Respiratory Care, 41*(7), 647–653.

American Association for Respiratory Care. (2003). AARC clinical practice guideline: Bland aerosol administration. *Respiratory Care, 48*(5), 529–533.

Scacci, R. (1979). Air entrainment masks: Jet mixing is how they work—the Bernoulli and Venturi principles are how they don't. *Respiratory Care, 24*(10), 928–931.

Additional Resources

Bagwell, T. (1986). U.S. Patent Number: 4,767,576. Costa Mesa, CA: Medical Molding Corporation of America.

Garrett, D., & Donaldson, W. P. (1978). *Physical principles of respiratory therapy equipment.* Madison, WI: Ohio Medical Products.

Practice Activities: Humidity and Aerosol Therapy

1. Practice setting up the following humidifier to the indicated delivery device when appropriate.
   a. Bubble humidifier
   Delivery Device
   (1) Nasal cannula

2. Practice setting up the following humidifiers to the indicated delivery devices. Use large-bore tubing, including a drainage bag and a thermometer, to monitor the inspiratory temperature.
   a. Wick humidifier
   b. Heated pass over humidifier
   Delivery Devices
   (1) Aerosol mask
   (2) Tracheostomy mask
   (3) Face tent
   (4) Briggs adapter

3. Practice setting up the following nebulizers to the indicated delivery devices. Use large-bore tubing, including a drainage bag. When a nebulizer has provisions for a heater, apply a heated aerosol and use a thermometer to monitor the inspiratory temperature.
   a. Large-volume nebulizer
   b. Ultrasonic nebulizer
   Delivery Devices
   (1) Aerosol mask
   (2) Tracheostomy mask
   (3) Face tent
   (4) Briggs adapter (T piece)

4. Practice troubleshooting any of the foregoing humidity or aerosol devices by deliberately sabotaging them and restoring them to an operational condition.

5. Adjust the large-volume nebulizer to 40% oxygen and then to 60% oxygen. Remove the drainage bag and make a large loop in the aerosol tubing below the level of the humidifier and raise the distal end to an appropriate level.
   a. Measure the FIO_2.
   b. Add 100 mL of water into the distal end of the tubing, causing a partial obstruction at the dependent loop.
   c. Measure the FIO_2 with the water partially obstructing the flow.
   (1) How can you explain the difference?

6. Practice applying any of the foregoing humidity or aerosol devices to a laboratory partner. Note how cold and heated humidity/aerosol delivery feels.

7. Practice troubleshooting the small-volume nebulizers by deliberately sabotaging them and restoring them to proper operation.

8. Deliver a small-volume nebulizer treatment to a laboratory partner using normal saline. *Note:* Do not use a bronchodilator without a physician's order. Monitor the following parameters:
   Before treatment
   a. Pulse and respiratory rate
   b. Breath sounds
   c. Peak expiratory flow and FEV_1
   During treatment
   a. Pulse and respiratory rate
   b. Breath sounds
   Following treatment
   a. Pulse and respiratory rate
   b. Breath sounds
   c. Peak expiratory flow and FEV_1

9. Using a blank sheet of paper, document the humidity or aerosol device used and how the "treatment" was administered to your laboratory partner. Have your instructor critique your documentation.

Check List: Humidity and Aerosol Therapy

_____ 1. Verify the physician's order for therapy.

_____ 2. Follow standard precautions, including washing hands.

3. Obtain the appropriate equipment as required:

_____ a. Oxygen flowmeter

_____ b. Sterile water

_____ c. Large-bore aerosol tubing

_____ d. Drainage bag

_____ e. Thermometer (if heated therapy is required)

_____ f. Humidifier or nebulizer

_____ g. _No smoking_ sign

_____ h. Oxygen analyzer, if required

_____ 4. Assemble the equipment.

_____ 5. Identify the patient and introduce yourself.

_____ 6. Confirm operation of equipment and troubleshoot, as required.

_____ 7. Apply the device to the patient.

_____ 8. Reassure the patient.

_____ 9. Monitor temperature and FIO_2, as required.

_____ 10. Clean up any plastic wrappers or unneeded equipment before leaving the room.

_____ 11. Wash your hands.

_____ 12. Document the procedure on the patient's chart.

Check List: Small-Volume Nebulizer Therapy

_____ 1. Verify the order in the chart. Check for medication, amount, dilution, and frequency of therapy.

_____ 2. Follow standard precautions, including handwashing.

3. Obtain and assemble your equipment, which may include:

_____ a. Oxygen flowmeter

_____ b. Small-volume nebulizer

_____ c. Medication

_____ d. Peak expiratory flowmeter

_____ e. Portable spirometer

_____ 4. Prepare the medication as ordered by the physician.

_____ 5. Identify the patient and introduce yourself.

_____ 6. Assemble your equipment.

_____ 7. Explain the procedure, including respiratory pattern.

8. Obtain the following parameters before therapy:

_____ a. Breath sounds

_____ b. Heart and respiratory rate

_____ c. Peak expiratory flow

_____ d. FEV_1

_____ 9. Administer the small-volume nebulizer treatment, encouraging your patient as you progress.

_____ 10. Monitor your patient closely for side effects.

_____ 11. Encourage your patient to cough following therapy. If the cough is productive, note the color, amount, and odor of the sputum.

12. Measure the following parameters after therapy:

_____ a. Breath sounds

_____ b. Heart and respiratory rate

_____ c. Peak expiratory flow rate

_____ d. FEV_1

_____ 13. Clean up the area.

_____ 14. Reassure your patient and check to see if he or she is comfortable.

_____ 15. In the patient's chart, record the date, time, medication (amount and dilution), pretherapy and posttherapy parameters, any sputum production, and the patient's tolerance of the therapy.

Self-Evaluation Post Test: Humidity and Aerosol Therapy

1. Humidity is referred to as:
   a. particulate water.
   b. liquid water.
   c. water vapor.
   d. nebulized water.

2. Why should large-bore tubing used during aerosol therapy have a loop and drainage bag below the patient and the nebulizer?
   a. To prevent condensate from entering the inspiratory site
   b. To prevent back pressure from affecting the Venturi
   c. To prevent condensate from entering the nebulizer
   d. All of the above

3. A patient who received a bronchodilator via a small-volume nebulizer now demonstrates signs of tachycardia and nervousness. The reason is that the:
   a. patient was hyperventilating.
   b. patient received too much bronchodilator.
   c. patient probably received the wrong drug by mistake.
   d. patient received too much oxygen.

4. The piezoelectric crystal of an ultrasonic nebulizer has the ability to:
   a. convert electrical energy to mechanical energy.
   b. convert the couplant fluid to a gas.
   c. cause the particles to form new compounds.
   d. cause variations in the current generated by the rf module.

5. One method to increase the delivered humidity is to:
   a. decrease the temperature.
   b. increase the temperature.
   c. add more tubing between the device and the patient.
   d. increase the line pressure powering the device.

6. A heated wick humidifier:
   I.   is not efficient.
   II. supplies 100% body humidity.
   III. is heated.
   IV. is not heated.
   a. I, II   c. II, III
   b. I, III   d. II, IV

7. An example of a nebulizer that works on the viscous shearing principle and also uses the principle to adjust the oxygen concentration is the:
   a. heated wick nebulizer.
   b. large-volume nebulizer.
   c. bubble humidifier.

8. Body humidity is:
   a. 50% saturated at body temperature and pressure.
   b. 100% saturated at room temperature and pressure.
   c. 50% saturated at room temperature and pressure.
   d. 100% saturated at body temperature and pressure.

9. The use of a baffle in a nebulizer causes:
   a. a mist of larger droplets to be delivered.
   b. no change in the size of the particles.
   c. the mist to be less irritating.
   d. a more uniform-size droplet to be produced.

10. The ideal breathing pattern for maximal aerosol deposition and retention is:
    a. rapid, shallow respirations.
    b. a slow, deep inspiration and a fast, forced exhalation.
    c. a pause of several seconds' duration at the peak of every other breath.
    d. a slow, deep inspiration with an end-inspiratory hold followed by a passive exhalation.

PERFORMANCE EVALUATION:
Small-Volume Nebulizer Therapy

Date: Lab _____ Clinical _____ Agency _____

Lab: Pass _____ Fail _____ Clinical: Pass _____ Fail _____

Student name _____ Instructor name _____

No. of times observed in clinical _____

No. of times practiced in clinical _____

PASSING CRITERIA: Obtain 90% or better on the procedure. Tasks indicated by * must receive at least 1 point, or the evaluation is terminated. Procedure must be performed within the designated time, or the performance receives a failing grade.

SCORING: 2 points — Task performed satisfactorily without prompting.
1 point — Task performed satisfactorily with self-initiated correction.
0 points — Task performed incorrectly or with prompting required.
NA — Task not applicable to the patient care situation.

Tasks:	Peer	Lab	Clinical
* 1. Verifies the physician's order	☐	☐	☐
2. Scans the chart	☐	☐	☐
* 3. Follows standard precautions	☐	☐	☐
4. Obtains the required equipment			
* a. Oxygen flowmeter	☐	☐	☐
* b. Small-volume nebulizer	☐	☐	☐
* c. Peak flowmeter	☐	☐	☐
* d. Respirometer	☐	☐	☐
* 5. Prepares the medication in accordance with the physician's order	☐	☐	☐
* 6. Identifies the patient and introduces self	☐	☐	☐
7. Monitors the patient before therapy			
* a. Pulse and respiratory rate	☐	☐	☐
* b. Peak flow rate	☐	☐	☐
* c. FEV_1	☐	☐	☐
* d. Breath sounds	☐	☐	☐
* 8. Uses the appropriate gas for a propellant	☐	☐	☐
9. Coaches and encourages the patient	☐	☐	☐

10. Monitors the patient

*   a. Pulse   ☐   ☐   ☐

*   b. Respiratory rate   ☐   ☐   ☐

11. Encourages and assists the patient to cough   ☐   ☐   ☐

12. Monitors therapy effectiveness

*   a. Peak expiratory flow rate   ☐   ☐   ☐

*   b. FEV$_1$ ☐   ☐   ☐

* 13. Uses aseptic technique   ☐   ☐   ☐

14. Removes unneeded equipment   ☐   ☐   ☐

15. Leaves the patient area safe and clean   ☐   ☐   ☐

* 16. Charts the therapy appropriately   ☐   ☐   ☐

SCORE: Peer _____ points of possible 48; _____%

                        Lab _____ points of possible 48; _____%

                        Clinical _____ points of possible 48; _____%

TIME: _____ out of possible 20 minutes

STUDENT SIGNATURES   **INSTRUCTOR SIGNATURES**

PEER: _____   LAB: _____

STUDENT: _____   CLINICAL: _____

CHAPTER 16
Bronchial Hygiene Therapy

INTRODUCTION

Bronchial hygiene therapy is an important aspect of respiratory care. Many patients have increased secretion production, impairment of cough, or other pathologic conditions that prevent effective removal of pulmonary secretions. Retained secretions and poor pulmonary hygiene may lead to atelectasis and pulmonary infections. Therefore, it is important for the respiratory practitioner to know the techniques that will assist the patient in the removal of pulmonary secretions.

Postural drainage and chest percussion are indicated for patients who have difficulty mobilizing thick or copious pulmonary secretions. They are simple techniques that can be easily learned and may be performed at home. Like other therapeutic modalities, postural drainage and chest percussion may be performed only when ordered by a physician.

To position a patient safely and properly for postural drainage, an understanding of patient positioning, body mechanics, and the hazards associated with changes in position is required.

Positive expiratory pressure (PEP) mask therapy is the application of positive end-expiratory pressure during active exhalation to functional residual capacity (FRC) following a larger than normal tidal breath. The equipment required is simple and relatively inexpensive. PEP therapy has been shown to be effective in helping to remove secretions in patients with chronic lung diseases such as cystic fibrosis, bronchiectasis, and chronic bronchitis (Giulia, 2006).

Vibratory therapy such as Acapella® or Flutter valve is similar to PEP therapy in that an expiratory resistance device is employed. However, unlike in PEP therapy, the expiratory resistance created by the device varies; as the valve opens and closes, it creates pressure pulses within the chest. Like PEP therapy, vibratory therapy has been successfully employed in the treatment of cystic fibrosis.

Adjunctive breathing techniques include unilateral chest expansion, diaphragmatic breathing, pursed-lip breathing, and controlled cough techniques. All of these techniques are indicated to help the patient improve the ability to clear pulmonary secretions. Through demonstration and patient instruction these techniques are easily learned and may be self-administered by the patient.

This chapter covers the body mechanics and how to correctly position a patient in the common positions used in the hospital setting. Additionally, the respiratory practitioner will learn the 12 positions used to drain the bronchopulmonary segments and how to percuss and vibrate the chest properly to facilitate the removal of secretions from the lungs. Application of PEP and vibratory therapy are also discussed as well as demonstration and teaching of adjunctive breathing techniques to the patient.

KEY TERMS

- Chest percussion
- Diaphragmatic breathing
- Directed cough
- Flutter valve therapy
- High-frequency chest wall oscillation (HFCWO) therapy
- Mechanical percussor
- Patient positions
- Positive expiratory pressure (PEP) therapy
- Postural drainage
- Pursed-lip breathing
- Turning
- Unilateral chest expansion
- Vibration

THEORY OBJECTIVES

At the end of this chapter, the reader should be able to:

- *Describe the role of stance, balance, and body alignment in safe movement by the practitioner.*
- *Explain why body alignment and the use of good body mechanics are important in the positioning of the patient.*
- *Describe the following patient positions:*
  - *Fowler's and semi-Fowler's*
  - *Supine*
  - *Prone*
  - *Side-lying*

- Sims'
- Trendelenburg
- Reverse Trendelenburg
- Explain the use and purpose of these safety devices:
  - Bed rails
  - Restraints
    - Chest
    - Waist
    - Wrist and ankle
  - Nurse call button
  - Code switch
- Explain how chest percussion, postural drainage, and vibration can facilitate the removal of pulmonary secretions.
- Describe the use of adjunct devices to facilitate chest percussion.
- Explain how to use mechanical percussors, noting:
  - Hazards
  - Limitations
- List the components of a complete physician's order for postural drainage and chest percussion.
- Describe the contraindications to and hazards of postural drainage and chest percussion.
- In the absence of a complete physician's order, describe how a patient may be assessed to determine the segments requiring postural drainage and chest percussion.

Pep Therapy

- Define PEP therapy.
- Describe the circuit used for PEP therapy.

- Describe the indications for PEP therapy.
- List the hazards of PEP therapy.

Vibratory Pep Therapy

- Define vibratory PEP therapy.
- Describe the device used for vibratory PEP therapy (Acapella®).
- Describe the indications for vibratory PEP therapy.
- List the hazards of vibratory PEP therapy.

High-Frequency Chest Wall Oscillation (Hfcwo) Therapy

- Define HFCWO therapy and describe the equipment used for HFCWO therapy.
- Describe the indications for HFCWO therapy.
- Discuss the hazards associated with HFCWO therapy.
- Describe how to perform the following adjunctive breathing techniques:
  - Diaphragmatic breathing
  - Unilateral chest expansion
  - Pursed-lip breathing
  - Directed cough
- Discuss the indications for adjunctive breathing techniques and the hazards associated with those techniques.

Respironics Coughassist™ Mi-E Device

- Describe the purpose of the Emerson Coughassist™ MI-E.
- Describe how to use the Emerson Coughassist™ MI-E.
- Discuss potential hazards of using the Emerson Coughassist™ MI-E.

CLINICAL PRACTICE GUIDELINES

AARC Clinical Practice Guideline Postural Drainage Therapy

PDT 4.0 INDICATIONS:

4.1 Turning

4.1.1 Inability or reluctance of patient to change body position (e.g., mechanical ventilation, neuromuscular disease, drug-induced paralysis)

4.1.2 Poor oxygenation associated with position (20,22,48–50) (e.g., unilateral lung disease)

4.1.3 Potential for or presence of atelectasis (24,26,30)

4.1.4 Presence of artificial airway

4.2 Postural drainage

4.2.1 Evidence or suggestion of difficulty with secretion clearance

4.2.1.1 Difficulty clearing secretions with expectorated sputum production greater than 25–30 ml/day (adult) (3,7,9,11,12,27, 38,40,46,51–53)

4.2.1.2 Evidence or suggestion of retained secretions in the presence of an artificial airway

4.2.2 Presence of atelectasis caused by or suspected of being caused by mucous plugging (24,26,29,30,54)

4.2.3 Diagnosis of diseases such ascystic fibrosis, (1,5,6,13–15,18,36,55) bronchiectasis, (4,5,14) or cavitating lung disease

4.2.4 Presence of foreign body in airway (56–58)

4.3 External manipulation of the thorax

4.3.1 Sputum volume or consistency suggesting a need for additional manipulation (e.g., percussion and/or vibration) to assist movement of secretions by gravity in a patient receiving postural drainage

PDT 5.0 CONTRAINDICATIONS:

The decision to use postural drainage therapy requires assessment of potential benefits versus

(Continued)

potential risks. Therapy should be provided for no longer than necessary to obtain the desired therapeutic results. Listed contraindications are relative unless marked as absolute (A).

5.1 Positioning

5.1.1 All positions are contraindicated for:

5.1.1.1 Intracranial pressure (ICP) > 20 mm Hg (59,60)

5.1.1.2 Head and neck injury until stabilized (A)

5.1.1.3 Active hemorrhage with hemodynamic instability (A)

5.1.1.4 Recent spinal surgery (e.g., laminectomy) or acute spinal injury

5.1.1.5 Acute spinal injury or active hemoptysis

5.1.1.6 Empyema

5.1.1.7 Bronchopleural fistula

5.1.1.8 Pulmonary edema associated with congestive heart failure

5.1.1.9 Large pleural effusions

5.1.1.10 Pulmonary embolism

5.1.1.11 Aged, confused, or anxious patients who do not tolerate position changes

5.1.1.12 Rib fracture, with or without flail chest

5.1.1.13 Surgical wound or healing tissue

5.1.2 Trendelenburg position is contraindicated for:

5.1.2.1 Intracranial pressure (ICP) > 20 mm Hg (59,60)

5.1.2.2 Patients in whom increased intracranial pressure is to be avoided (e.g., neurosurgery, aneurysms, eye surgery)

5.1.2.3 Uncontrolled hypertension

5.1.2.4 Distended abdomen

5.1.2.5 Esophageal surgery

5.1.2.6 Recent gross hemoptysis related to recent lung carcinoma treated surgically or with radiation therapy (59)

5.1.2.7 Uncontrolled airway at risk for aspiration (tube feeding or recent meal)

5.1.3 Reverse Trendelenburg is contraindicated in the presence of hypotension or vasoactive medication.

5.2 External manipulation of the thorax

In addition to contraindications previously listed:

5.2.1 Subcutaneous emphysema

5.2.2 Recent epidural spinal infusion or spinal anesthesia

5.2.3 Recent skin grafts, or flaps, on the thorax

5.2.4 Burns, open wounds, and skin infections of the thorax

5.2.5 Recently placed transvenous pacemaker or subcutaneous pacemaker (particularly if mechanical devices are to be used)

5.2.6 Suspected pulmonary tuberculosis

5.2.7 Lung contusion

5.2.8 Bronchospasm

5.2.9 Osteomyelitis of the ribs

5.2.10 Osteoporosis

5.2.11 Coagulopathy

5.2.12 Complaint of chest-wall pain

PDT 6.0 HAZARDS/COMPLICATIONS:

6.1 Hypoxemia

Action to Be Taken/Possible Intervention: Administer higher oxygen concentrations during procedure if potential for or observed hypoxemia exists. If patient becomes hypoxemic during treatment, administer 100% oxygen, stop therapy immediately, return patient to original resting position, and consult physician. Ensure adequate ventilation. Hypoxemia during postural drainage may be avoided in unilateral lung disease by placing the involved lung uppermost with patient on his or her side. (20,22,48–50)

6.2 Increased intracranial pressure

Action to Be Taken/Possible Intervention: Stop therapy, return patient to original resting position, and consult physician.

6.3 Acute hypotension during procedure

Action to Be Taken/Possible Intervention: Stop therapy, return patient to original resting position, and consult physician.

6.4 Pulmonary hemorrhage

Action to Be Taken/Possible Intervention: Stop therapy, return patient to original resting position, call physician immediately. Administer oxygen and maintain an airway until physician responds.

6.5 Pain or injury to muscles, ribs, or spine

Action to Be Taken/Possible Intervention: Stop therapy that appears directly associated with pain or problem, exercise care in moving patient, and consult physician.

6.6 Vomiting and aspiration

Action to Be Taken/Possible Intervention: Stop therapy, clear airway and suction as needed, administer oxygen, maintain airway, return patient to previous resting position, and contact physician immediately.

6.7 Bronchospasm

Action to Be Taken/Possible Intervention: Stop therapy, return patient to original resting position, administer or increase oxygen delivery while contacting physician. Administer physician-ordered bronchodilators.

6.8 Dysrhythmias

Action to Be Taken/Possible Intervention: Stop therapy, return patient to previous resting position, administer or increase oxygen delivery while contacting physician.

(Continued)

PDT 8.0 ASSESSMENT OF NEED:

The following should be assessed together to establish a need for postural drainage therapy:

8.1 Excessive sputum production

8.2 Effectiveness of cough

8.3 History of pulmonary problems treated successfully with PDT (e.g., bronchiectasis, cystic fibrosis, lung abscess)

8.4 Decreased breath sounds or crackles or rhonchi suggesting secretions in the airway

8.5 Change in vital signs

8.6 Abnormal chest x-ray consistent with atelectasis, mucous plugging, or infiltrates

8.7 Deterioration in arterial blood gas values or oxygen saturation

PDT 9.0 ASSESSMENT OF OUTCOME:

These represent individual criteria that indicate a positive response to therapy (and support continuation of therapy). Not all criteria are required to justify continuation of therapy (e.g., a ventilated patient may not have sputum production >30 ml/day, but may have improvement in breath sounds, chest x-ray, or increased compliance or decreased resistance).

9.1 Change in sputum production

If sputum production in an optimally hydrated patient is less than 25 ml/day with PDT, the procedure is not justified. (3,5,7,9,11,12,38,40,46,51–53) Some patients have productive coughs with sputum production from 15 to 30 ml/day (occasionally as high as 70 or 100 ml/day) without postural drainage. If postural drainage does not increase sputum in a patient who produces >30 ml/day of sputum without postural drainage, the continuation of the therapy is not indicated. Because sputum production is affected by systemic hydration, apparently ineffective PDT probably should be continued for at least 24 hours after optimal hydration has been judged to be present.

9.2 Change in breath sounds of lung fields being drained

With effective therapy, breath sounds may "worsen" following the therapy as secretions move into the larger airways and increase rhonchi. An increase in adventitious breath sounds can be a marked improvement over absent or diminished breath sounds. Note any effect that coughing may have on breath sounds. One of the favorable effects of coughing is clearing of adventitious breath sounds.

9.3 Patient subjective response to therapy

The caregiver should ask patient how he or she feels before, during, and after therapy. Feelings of pain, discomfort, shortness of breath, dizziness, and nausea should be considered in decisions to modify or stop therapy. Easier clearance of secretions and increased volume of secretions during and after treatments support continuation.

9.4 Change in vital signs

Moderate changes in respiratory rate and/or pulse rate are expected. Bradycardia, tachycardia, or an increase in irregularity of pulse, or fall or dramatic increase in blood pressure are indications for stopping therapy.

9.5 Change in chest x-ray

Resolution or improvement of atelectasis may be slow or dramatic.

9.6 Change in arterial blood gas values or oxygen saturation

Oxygenation should improve as atelectasis resolves.

9.7 Change in ventilator variables

Resolution of atelectasis and plugging reduces resistance and increases compliance.

PDT 11.0 MONITORING:

The following should be chosen as appropriate for monitoring a patient's response to postural drainage therapy, before, during, and after therapy.

11.1 Subjective response—pain, discomfort, dyspnea, response to therapy

11.2 Pulse rate, dysrhythmia, and ECG if available

11.3 Breathing pattern and rate, symmetrical chest expansion, synchronous thoracico-abdominal movement, flail chest

11.4 Sputum production (quantity, color, consistency, odor) and cough effectiveness

11.5 Mental function

11.6 Skin color

11.7 Breath sounds

11.8 Blood pressure

11.9 Oxygen saturation by pulse oximetry (if hypoxemia is suspected)

11.10 Intracranial pressure (ICP)

Reprinted with permission from *Respiratory Care* 1991; 36: 1418–1426. The complete AARC Clinical Practice Guidelines are available from the AARC Web site (http://www.aarc .org), from the AARC Executive Office, or from *Respiratory Care* journal.

AARC Clinical Practice Guideline: Directed Cough

DC 4.0 INDICATIONS:

4.1 The need to aid in the removal of retained secretions from central airways (3–6)—(the suggestion that FET at lower lung volumes may be effective in preferentially mobilizing secretions in the peripheral airways while larger volumes facilitate movement in the central airways lacks validation).

4.2 The presence of atelectasis (3,7,8)

(Continued)

4.3 As prophylaxis against postoperative pulmonary complications (7)

4.4 As a routine part of bronchial hygiene in patients with cystic fibrosis, (2,4,6,9) bronchiectasis, chronic bronchitis, (3,10,11) narcotizing pulmonary infection, or spinal cord injury (12)

4.5 As an integral part of other bronchial hygiene therapies such as postural drainage therapy (PDT), (2,13) positive expiratory pressure therapy (PEP), and incentive spirometry (IS)

4.6 To obtain sputum specimens for diagnostic analysis

DC 5.0 CONTRAINDICATIONS:

Directed cough is rarely contraindicated. The contraindications listed must be weighed against potential benefit in deciding to eliminate cough from the care of the patient. Listed contraindications are relative.

5.1 Inability to control possible transmission of infection from patients suspected or known to have pathogens transmittable by droplet nuclei (e.g., *M. tuberculosis*)

5.2 Presence of an elevated intracranial pressure or known intracranial aneurysm

5.3 Presence of reduced coronary artery perfusion, such as in acute myocardial infarction (14)

5.4 Acute unstable head, neck, or spine injury
Manually assisted directed cough with pressure to the epigastrium may be contraindicated in presence of:

5.5 increased potential for regurgitation/aspiration (e.g., unconscious patient with unprotected airway)

5.6 acute abdominal pathology, abdominal aortic aneurysm, hiatal hernia, or pregnancy

5.7 a bleeding diathesis

5.8 untreated pneumothorax
Manually assisted directed cough with pressure to the thoracic cage may be contraindicated in presence of:

5.9 osteoporosis, flail chest

DC 6.0 HAZARDS/COMPLICATIONS:

6.1 Reduced coronary artery perfusion (14)

6.2 Reduced cerebral perfusion leading to syncope or alterations in consciousness, such as light-headedness or confusion, (15) vertebral artery dissection

6.3 Incontinence

6.4 Fatigue

6.5 Headaches

6.6 Paresthesia or numbness (15)

6.7 Bronchospasm (11)

6.8 Muscular damage or discomfort

6.9 Spontaneous pneumothorax, pneumomediastinum, subcutaneous emphysema

6.10 Cough paroxysms

6.11 Chest pain

6.12 Rib or costochondral junction fracture

6.13 Incisional pain, evisceration

6.14 Anorexia, vomiting, and retching

6.15 Visual disturbances including retinal hemorrhage (15)

6.16 Central line displacement

6.17 Gastroesophageal reflux (17)

DC 8.0 ASSESSMENT OF NEED

8.1 Spontaneous cough that fails to clear secretions from the airway

8.2 Ineffective spontaneous cough as judged by:

    8.2.1 Clinical observation

    8.2.2 Evidence of atelectasis

    8.2.3 Results of pulmonary function testing

8.3 Postoperative upper abdominal or thoracic surgery patient (7)

8.4 Long-term care of patients with tendency to retain airway secretions

8.5 Presence of endotracheal or tracheostomy tube

DC 9.0 ASSESSMENT OF OUTCOME:

9.1 The presence of sputum specimen following a cough (4)

9.2 Clinical observation of improvement

9.3 Patient's subjective response to therapy

9.4 Stabilization of pulmonary hygiene in patients with chronic pulmonary disease and a history of secretion retention

DC 11.0 MONITORING:

Items from the following list should be chosen as appropriate for monitoring a patient's response to cough technique.

11.1 Patient response: pain, discomfort, dyspnea

11.2 Sputum expectorated following cough to note color, consistency, odor, volume of sputum produced

11.3 Breath sounds

11.4 Presence of any adverse neurologic signs or symptoms following cough (15)

11.5 Presence of any cardiac dysrhythmias or alterations in hemodynamics following coughing

11.6 Measures of pulmonary mechanics, when indicated, may include vital capacity, peak inspiratory pressure, peak expiratory pressure, peak expiratory flow, and airway resistance

---

Reprinted with permission from *Respiratory Care* 1993; 38: 495–499. The complete AARC Clinical Practice Guidelines are available from the AARC Web site (http://www.aarc .org), from the AARC Executive Office, or from *Respiratory Care* journal.

(Continued)

AARC Clinical Practice Guideline: Use of Positive Airway Pressure Adjuncts to Bronchial Hygiene Therapy

PAP 4.0 INDICATIONS:

4.1 To reduce air trapping in asthma and COPD (16,29–31)

4.2 To aid in mobilization of retained secretions (in cystic fibrosis and chronic bronchitis) (14,15,17–24,32,33)

4.3 To prevent or reverse atelectasis (6–13,34–36)

4.4 To optimize delivery of bronchodilators in patients receiving bronchial hygiene therapy (37,38)

PAP 5.0 CONTRAINDICATIONS:

Although no absolute contraindications [to] the use of PEP, CPAP, or EPAP mask therapy have been reported (4,39), the following should be carefully evaluated before a decision is made to initiate PAP mask therapy:

5.1 Patients unable to tolerate the increased work of breathing (acute asthma, COPD)

5.2 Intracranial pressure (ICP) >20 mm Hg

5.3 Hemodynamic instability (4)

5.4 Recent facial, oral, or skull surgery or trauma (4)

5.5 Acute sinusitis (39)

5.6 Epistaxis

5.7 Esophageal surgery

5.8 Active hemoptysis (39)

5.9 Nausea

5.10 Known or suspected tympanic membrane rupture or other middle ear pathology

5.11 Untreated pneumothorax

PAP 6.0 HAZARDS/COMPLICATIONS:

6.1 Increased work of breathing (4) that may lead to hypoventilation and hypercarbia

6.2 Increased intracranial pressure

6.3 Cardiovascular compromise
    6.3.1 Myocardial ischemia
    6.3.2 Decreased venous return (4)

6.4 Air swallowing, (4) with increased likelihood of vomiting and aspiration

6.5 Claustrophobia (4)

6.6 Skin breakdown and discomfort from mask (4)

6.7 Pulmonary barotrauma (4)

PAP 8.0 ASSESSMENT OF NEED:

The following should be assessed together to establish a need for PAP therapy:

8.1 Sputum retention not responsive to spontaneous or directed coughing

8.2 History of pulmonary problems treated successfully with postural drainage therapy

8.3 Decreased breath sounds or adventitious sounds suggesting secretions in the airway

8.4 Change in vital signs—increase in breathing frequency, tachycardia

8.5 Abnormal chest radiograph consistent with atelectasis, mucous plugging, or infiltrates

8.6 Deterioration in arterial blood gas values or oxygen saturation

PAP 9.0 ASSESSMENT OF OUTCOME:

9.1 Change in sputum production—if PEP does not increase sputum production in a patient who produces >30 ml/day of sputum without PEP, the continued use of PEP may not be indicated.

9.2 Change in breath sounds—with effective therapy, breath sounds may clear or the movement of secretions into the larger airways may cause an increase in adventitious breath sounds. The increase in adventitious breath sounds is often a marked improvement over no (or diminished) breath sounds. Note any effect that coughing may have had on the breath sounds.

9.3 Patient subjective response to therapy—the caregiver should ask the patient how he or she feels before, during, and after therapy. Feelings of pain, discomfort, shortness of breath, dizziness, and nausea should be considered in modifying and stopping therapy. Improved ease of clearing secretions and increased volume of secretions during and after treatments support continuation.

9.4 Change in vital signs—moderate changes in respiratory rate and/or pulse rate are expected. Bradycardia, tachycardia, increasingly irregular pulse, or a drop or dramatic increase in blood pressure are indications for stopping therapy.

9.5 Change in chest radiograph—resolution or improvement of atelectasis and localized infiltrates may be slow or dramatic.

9.6 Change in arterial blood gas values or oxygen saturation—normal oxygenation should return as atelectasis resolves.

PAP 11.0 MONITORING:

Items from the following list should be chosen as is appropriate for monitoring a specific patient's response to PAP:

11.1 Patient subjective response—pain, discomfort, dyspnea, response to therapy

11.2 Pulse rate and cardiac rhythm (if ECG is available)

11.3 Breathing pattern and rate, symmetrical lateral costal expansion, synchronous thoracico-abdominal movement

(Continued)

11.4 Sputum production (quantity, color, consistency, and odor)
11.5 Mental function
11.6 Skin color
11.7 Breath sounds
11.8 Blood pressure
11.9 Pulse oximetry (if hypoxemia with procedure has been previously demonstrated or is suspected); blood gas analysis (if indicated)

11.10 Intracranial pressure (ICP) in patients for whom ICP is of critical importance

Reprinted with permission from *Respiratory Care* 1993; 38: 516–521. The complete AARC Clinical Practice Guidelines are available from the AARC Web site (http://www.aarc.org), from the AARC Executive Office, or from *Respiratory Care* journal.

BODY ALIGNMENT AND STANCE

Body alignment and stance are crucial to safe movement in helping patients. A patient who is unable to move is very heavy. When the body is aligned properly, the ability to move is done smoothly. Minimal strain is placed on muscles, tendons, bones, and joints. The muscles assume a state of slight tension or tone.

Injuries are more common when the body is not in alignment. These injuries commonly include muscles of the back, legs, tendons, and joints. Hernias may also result from improper alignment and undue muscle strain. Furthermore, improper alignment adversely affects balance. Balance is critical when assisting a patient to move.

Erect, the body should assume a position as shown in Figure 16-1. The upright body is aligned along an axis with the center of gravity. The feet should be slightly spread to provide a larger base of support. The closer together the feet are, the less stability there is affecting balance.

When lifting heavy objects, always assume a squatting position, as shown in Figure 16-2. Lifting should be performed with the legs, not the back. Keep the object close to the body, minimizing muscle strain. The squatting position should also be assumed for adjusting beds or performing other tasks that are near the floor. This position minimizes the back strain experienced in bending from the waist. In the figure, notice how the feet are spread slightly, facilitating balance.

Patient comfort and prevention of disability from contractures are facilitated with correct body alignment. When the patient's body is properly aligned, the muscles, tendons, and joints are at rest. Pillows aid in providing additional support and removing pressure at contact points in the maintenance of correct alignment.

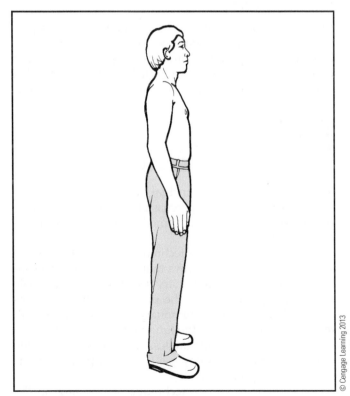

Figure 16-1 Correct body alignment and stance

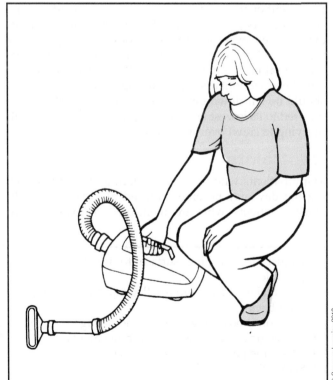

Figure 16-2 Correct lifting stance

© Cengage Learning 2013

GENERAL GUIDELINES FOR MOVING PATIENTS

Common sense is required in moving patients. By following a few simple rules, practitioners will prevent injury to themselves and the task will require less effort. Figure 16-3 is a summary of these rules.

Before attempting to move a patient, check on the patient's general condition and ascertain if a change of position is contraindicated. Some types of surgical procedures limit patient position. A patient who has undergone back surgery may be required to remain supine postoperatively. A patient with a head injury or who has undergone eye surgery may also have limits on positioning. Patients with cardiovascular problems may experience postural hypotension when raised to a sitting or standing position.

Figure 16-4 illustrates the common therapeutic patient positions that are used in the hospital setting. Note the use of pillows for additional comfort and support.

SAFETY DEVICES

Bed Rails

Bed rails are provided on hospital beds for the patient's protection. Under certain circumstances, the patient may become disoriented as to time and place. Bed rails help to minimize the likelihood of a patient's falling out of bed. Bed rails should always be used with confused or elderly patients. Side rails on a crib must always be up unless the practitioner is standing with his or her hands on the child. If the patient emphatically refuses to use bed rails, explain their purpose and try to convince the patient of their benefit. If the patient still refuses to use them, note the refusal on the patient's chart. If a patient is allowed out of bed without assistance during the day, the bed rail should be left down on one side and the bed should be lowered to its lowest level so that the patient does not fall in trying to crawl over the rail.

Restraints

Many patients who are awake, alert, and oriented during the day may become confused at night, especially elderly patients who are medicated. A patient may become confused, combative, or disoriented because of medication, anesthesia, or psychologic conditions. Restraints are used to prevent the patient from removing life support equipment or to prevent self-injury or injury of hospital personnel. Health care facilities have strict rules and regulations regarding the use of restraints, and they must be ordered by a physician or be part of a protocol program that has been preapproved by the medical staff of the facility.

Chest restraints and waist restraints prevent patients from extracting themselves from bed. The restraints should be snug but not tight. Restraints should never impair circulation. It should be easy to insert a finger between the restraint and the patient's skin or gown. The restraint should always be tied to the bed frame, not the side rail.

Wrist and leg restraints reduce the mobility of the limb they are tied to. They are commonly used to prevent the patient from removing endotracheal tubes and intravenous and arterial lines.

Nurse Call Button

The nurse call button is the patient's lifeline. It frequently is the only way a patient can summon help in an emergency situation. Without access to the button, the patient is, in effect, unable to communicate. It is important to leave this device within reach of the patient at all times. If the patient watches television, leave the remote control within reach. Check with the patient before leaving to see if other things need to be within reach. Patients have fallen out of bed trying to reach items placed too far away.

Code Switch

In many intensive care units, a "code" switch is provided to notify appropriate personnel that a life-threatening emergency such as cardiac or respiratory arrest has occurred. The use of the code switch should be limited to appropriate circumstances. False alarms are frowned on.

CHEST PERCUSSION AND POSTURAL DRAINAGE

Manual techniques for bronchial hygiene therapy include postural drainage, chest percussion, and vibration. Chest percussion can also be performed using mechanical percussion devices.

Postural drainage is a technique wherein the patient is positioned in specific ways that allow gravity to facilitate the removal of pulmonary secretions. The rationale for specific positioning is the principle that water runs downhill. The bronchopulmonary tree is complex with the various segments of the lung branching out from the larger airways at unique angles. A thorough knowledge of the pulmonary anatomy is essential for proper performance of this procedure.

Chest percussion is a technique of clapping on the chest wall with cupped hands. The small amount of air

---

- Adjust the working surface to waist level if possible
- Use major muscle groups (legs and arms), not your back
- Use your body weight to your advantage
- Allow gravity to assist in your movements
- Allow the patient to assist if possible
- Seek help if needed

Figure 16-3 Rules for patient positioning

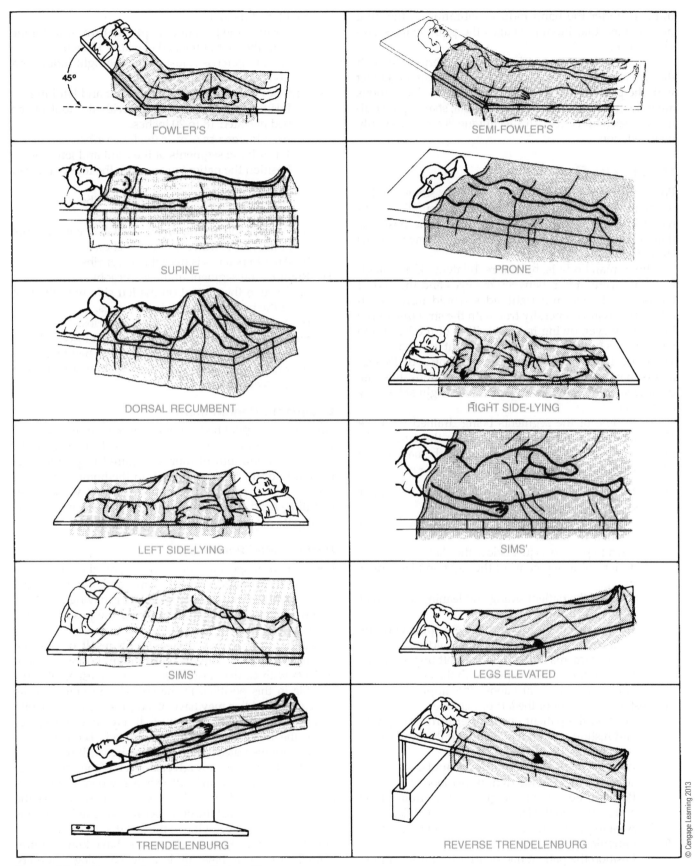

Figure 16-4 Common therapeutic patient positions

trapped under the hand induces vibration in the lung parenchyma that literally shakes the pulmonary secretions loose.

Vibration is an isometric maneuver performed with the arm and hand. The practitioner's hands are in contact with the patient's chest wall, and the induced vibrations are transmitted to the lung parenchyma, shaking the pulmonary secretions free. This technique is employed only on exhalation.

Postural Drainage

Postural drainage may be employed as a single modality or in combination with chest percussion. This technique involves placing the patient in specific positions that ensure that the desired pulmonary segment drains straight down.

The human body is, by nature, bilateral. If an imaginary line were drawn between the eyes and the end of the pelvis, the left and right sides would mirror each other. This is also generally true with the structure of the lungs. However, owing to the position of the heart, the left lung has two lobes, whereas the right lung has three. There are 18 bronchopulmonary segments. All 18 segments may be drained using only 12 positions. In some positions, both segments on the left and right sides may be drained.

An outline of the segments being drained with the 12 positions is listed next and includes the landmarks for percussion. Figure 16-5 is a pictorial schematic of the 12 positions and their segments.

1. Anterior apical segments of the right and left upper lobes
   a. Position the patient sitting and leaning back at about a 45° angle.
   b. Area to percuss is just below the clavicle.
2. Posterior apical segments of the right and left upper lobes
   a. Position the patient sitting and leaning forward at about a 45° angle.
   b. Area to percuss is just above the scapula with the fingers extending up onto the shoulders.
3. Anterior segments of the right and left upper lobes
   a. Position the patient supine with the bed flat.
   b. Area to percuss is just above the nipple.
4. Posterior segment of the left upper lobe
   a. Position the patient one-quarter turn from prone and resting on the right side with the head of the bed elevated 18 inches.
   b. Area to percuss is over the left scapula.
5. Posterior segment of the right upper lobe
   a. Position the patient one-quarter turn from prone and resting on the left side with the bed flat.
   b. Area to percuss is just above the right scapula.
6. Left lingula
   a. Position the patient one-quarter turn from supine and resting on the right side with the foot of the bed elevated 12 inches.
   b. Area to percuss is just above the left nipple and under the armpit.

7. Right middle lobe
   a. Position the patient one-quarter turn from supine with the foot of the bed elevated 12 inches.
   b. Area to percuss is just above the right nipple and under the armpit.
8. Anterior basal segments of the right and left lung
   a. Position the patient supine with the foot of the bed elevated 18 to 20 inches.
   b. Area to percuss is over the lower ribs.
9. Posterior basal segments of the right and left lung
   a. Position the patient prone with the foot of the bed elevated 18 to 20 inches.
   b. Area to percuss is over the lower ribs.
10. Left lateral segment of the lower lobes
    a. Position the patient on the right side with the foot of the bed elevated 18 to 20 inches.
    b. Area to percuss is over the lower ribs.
11. Right lateral segment of the lower lobes
    a. Position the patient on the left side with the foot of the bed elevated 18 to 20 inches.
    b. Area to percuss is over the lower ribs.
12. Superior segments of the right and left lower lobes
    a. Position the patient prone with the bed flat.
    b. Area to percuss is just below the lower margin of the scapula.

Equipment Requirements

An electric hospital bed is not a requirement for postural drainage. Use of several pillows will suffice very nicely. Usually, a minimum of four is required to position the patient to drain the lower lobes. In the home setting, an ironing board propped appropriately will work. Even dangling head down from a coach or sofa has served some patients very well.

Position Modifications

Postural drainage may have effects on the cardiovascular system, intracranial pressure, and arterial partial pressure of oxygen (PaO_2). If a patient is having problems in any of these areas, modification of the positions may be necessary.

Cardiac output may decrease as a result of postural drainage, especially in the head-down position. Those patients with cardiac insufficiency may be especially susceptible in this position. In the critical care unit, patients with an arterial line may have blood pressure conveniently monitored during this procedure. If any adverse changes occur, the therapy may be discontinued. Those patients without sophisticated monitoring devices will need to be carefully observed for any adverse effects of the positioning.

Intracranial pressure will increase when a patient is positioned head down. Blood will tend to pool in the dependent portion of the body because of gravity. Venous return will decrease, owing to the fact that the blood must now flow uphill. Those patients who have known intracranial disease or have undergone neurologic surgery may need to have their positions modified to prevent complications.

PaO_2 may decrease with postural drainage owing to changes in the relationship between ventilation and

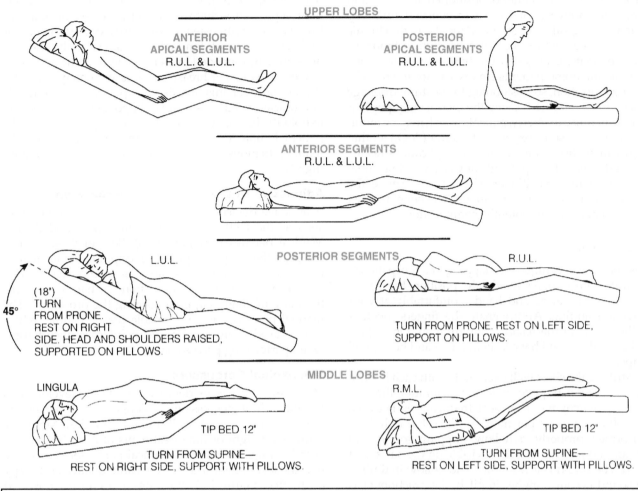

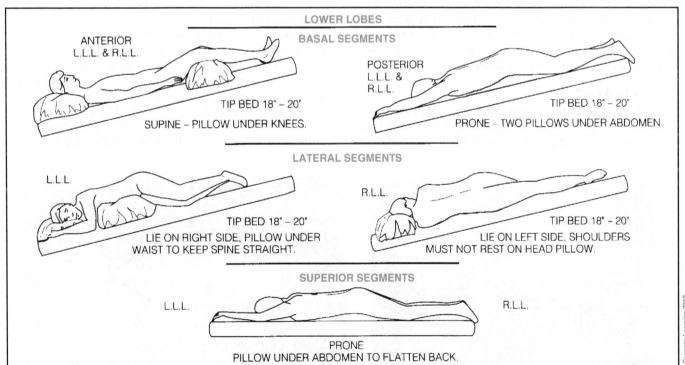

Figure 16-5   The 12 postural drainage positions

perfusion in the lung. Patients positioned so that blood is pooled in an area of atelectasis or consolidation may experience a significant shunt. Patients with chronic obstructive lung disease may also be quite orthopneic. In these patients, changes in position may cause shortness of breath. Some patients simply cannot tolerate the head-down position, so positioning for postural drainage will need to be modified. Using the increasingly popular technique of pulse oximetry, patients at risk may be monitored for a decrease in oxygen saturation (SpO_2) so that therapy can be discontinued before complications result.

The judgment of the patient's physician and personal experience of the practitioner will help determine the modification of the various positions. The benefits must be weighed against any potential complications.

Percussion

Percussion is a technique of clapping on the patient's chest wall with cupped hands. To position the hands properly, rest the arms and hands comfortably at your side while standing. Approximate the fingers together with the hands in the resting configuration. On inspection, the hands should have a slight curve and be cupped in shape.

By striking the chest wall alternately with each hand, a small air pocket is trapped, inducing a vibration through the lung parenchyma. The ideal frequency is between 50 and 60 percussions per minute. When the technique is performed properly, a hollow popping sound will result, and no red marks will be visible on the surface of the skin. The sound is low in pitch and hollow in timbre. If the sound becomes higher in pitch, the practitioner is probably slapping the patient. On inspection of the skin, the practitioner will probably observe some reddening. Percussion is ideally performed over a light covering such as a hospital gown or bedsheet.

Areas to Avoid

Avoid bony structures, the spine, the abdomen, and breast tissue in a female patient. Percussion over bony structures is painful and may result in injury. Percussion over the spine is not indicated because of the severe neurologic injury that may result in the event of a fracture. Patients with osteoporosis are especially susceptible to fractures. The abdominal organs, especially the kidneys, may be damaged by percussing over the abdomen. Finally, a woman's breast tissue is extremely sensitive. Percussion over this area is very painful and definitely not indicated. If access is difficult, politely ask the patient to hold the breast away from the area of percussion. If the patient is unable to cooperate, the practitioner may be required to move the breast while preserving the patient's dignity.

Adjunctive Devices for Chest Percussion

Adjunctive devices for chest percussion include devices such as the DHD Healthcare Palm Cups® and Ballard Medical percussors (Figure 16-6). Both of these devices facilitate the proper cupping or trapping of air against the chest. The Palm Cups® are placed between the first and second digit of the practitioner's hands and take the place of "hand cupping" during the procedure. The manual percussor is on a flexible plastic handle, which can be used in an isolette and helps to reduce fatigue when performing percussion.

Mechanical Percussors

Mechanical percussor devices have been developed to facilitate chest percussion. Prolonged chest percussion requires energy and well-trained muscles. Manually completing eight or nine treatments of 20 to 30 minutes each is tiring. Use of a mechanical percussor can ensure that the last patient receives the same quality of therapy as the first. Figure 16-7 illustrates a electrically powered mechanical precursor.

There are a great variety of mechanical percussors available. Some are well-designed electric and pneumatic devices. Others are not as well designed or effective. Because there are many different percussors available, the one selected determines the mode of application.

There are, however, some general guidelines for the use of mechanical percussors. Use the same anatomical landmarks that are used for manually percussing a

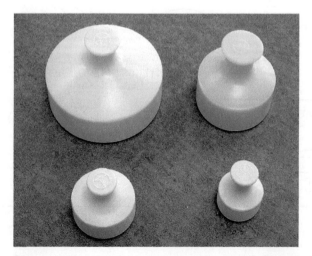
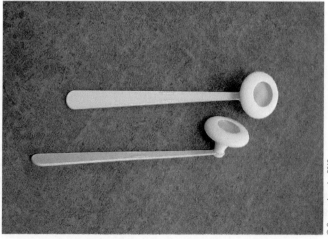

Figure 16-6 A photograph of DHD Palm Cups® and Ballard Medical percussors

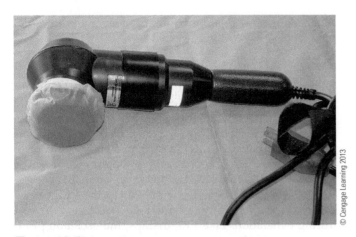

© Cengage Learning 2013

Figure 16-7 A variety of mechanical percussors

patient. Do not apply excessive force, but rather allow the unit to operate at its own speed and frequency. Avoid bony structures, the spine, the abdomen, and breast tissue in female patients. Move the device around in a moderately sized area about 10 to 20 cm in diameter. Constant application of the device to one area may irritate the skin and cause sores to develop.

The practitioner should begin percussion at a lower frequency and gradually increase the frequency to a higher rate as the procedure progresses. This practice helps to alleviate any fear the patient may experience initially.

Do not exert excessive force with the device. Let gravity apply a downward force vector. Use the hands to guide the percussor—not to apply additional force. Some percussors will operate at a lower frequency if pressure is exerted on them.

Hazards Some mechanical devices have a pad or cup attached to a narrow rod about ¼ inch in diameter and 3 to 4 inches long. The cup or pad oscillates back and forth over a range of about 5 cm. Often the pad is held in place by one or two set screws. If the set screws came loose, the pad could easily fall off and the rod could then injure the patient. Always check and tighten the set screws as required before using these percussors.

Limitations The limitations of these devices are primarily dependent on the patient's ability to tolerate their use. Some patients will be able to tolerate them without difficulty and others will not. It is not unusual for a patient to express a fear of mechanical devices, especially in the unfamiliar hospital setting. The therapy of touch as used in manual percussion may be more effective for some patients than the use of mechanical percussors.

Physician's Order

A complete order for postural drainage and chest percussion includes the frequency and duration of therapy and the location or target area. If an order is not complete, it may be up to the respiratory practitioner to determine what is required for optimal treatment of the patient. Check the policy and procedures manual.

In the absence of a complete order, contact the physician in person or by telephone to ascertain the frequency, duration, or location of therapy. If the physician requests that the therapy be performed as indicated, the practitioner will need to rely on his or her diagnostic skills and chest radiograph appearance to determine the areas requiring therapy.

If the practitioner is requested to assess the patient and determine what areas of the chest require therapy, begin with the patient's chart. Check the patient's history for any indications of cardiovascular insufficiency, past surgery on the thorax or spine, or any other abnormalities of the chest or spine that may limit the patient's tolerance to positioning. Look in the chart for any chest radiograph reports. Areas of consolidation or atelectasis constitute areas to drain and percuss. If it is possible, view the chest radiograph to form a mental picture of the areas needing treatment. When the practitioner first sees the patient, auscultate and percuss the chest to help clarify areas of consolidation and hypoaeration. By using these findings, the practitioner is reasonably assured of selecting the correct areas for therapy.

Duration of the therapy should be a minimum of 5 to 10 minutes for a lobe or segment. If all segments are to be drained, the total duration of therapy should not exceed 40 to 45 minutes. Often in this situation, upper lobes are treated in the morning, middle lobes in the afternoon, and lower lobes in the evening.

Contraindications and Hazards

The contraindications to postural drainage and chest percussion are primarily limited to presence of cardiovascular instability and other specific diseases of the pulmonary system. The performance of postural drainage and chest percussion on the patient whose cardiovascular status is unstable may have potentially serious consequences. As discussed previously, decrease in cardiac output and ventilation-perfusion mismatches may be severe enough for the patient to go into shock. Any patient who has a history of cardiovascular instability should be carefully monitored and the drainage positions modified as required.

Pathologic conditions of the lung that may be worsened by postural drainage and chest percussion include an undrained empyema, or lung abscess, and large-volume hemoptysis of unknown cause. In such cases, it is entirely possible for the maneuver of physiotherapy to release suddenly a large amount of loculated fluid or to induce excessive bleeding. Patients may literally drown in their own fluids. The best practice is to have the loculated fluid surgically drained by a physician before proceeding with further therapy.

The safety of patients rests on the judgment of the practitioner. If there are any doubts about a patient's ability to tolerate an ordered procedure, document the reasoning and discuss it with the patient's attending physician. Perhaps with some slight modifications, adequate therapy may be administered without jeopardizing the patient's safety.

OTHER THERAPIES FOR BRONCHIAL HYGIENE

Positive Expiratory Pressure Therapy

Definition and Equipment

Positive expiratory pressure (PEP) therapy is the application of positive pressure (10 to 15 cm H_2O) during active exhalation to increase functional residual capacity (FRC) following a larger than normal tidal breath. The equipment consists of a mouthpiece or mask, T assembly, one-way valve, pressure manometer, threshold resistor or fixed orifice (2.5 to 4 mm diameter), and a nebulizer (optional for aerosol administration) (Figure 16-8). The patient holds the mouthpiece in the mouth and then is instructed to take a deeper than normal breath and to exhale actively, against the resistance, to FRC level. The purpose of PEP therapy is to mechanically (pressure) splint the airways open during exhalation. PEP therapy promotes better distribution of ventilation and improved mucus clearance.

Indications

Indications for PEP therapy include the need to aid in removal of retained secretions, atelectasis, and prophylaxis of pulmonary infections and as routine therapy in the treatment of cystic fibrosis. By splinting the airway open mechanically using positive pressure, PEP therapy allows gas to move distally to obstructed areas. When the patient coughs forcefully, the removal of these secretions is facilitated.

Hazards

The risk of barotrauma and hemodynamic compromise exists with PEP therapy owing to the application of positive intrathoracic pressure. However, with the low pressures involved (10 to 15 cm H_2O), the risk is minimal. As with incentive spirometry, patients may complain of light-headedness or confusion, headaches, fatigue, or other symptoms relating to taking deeper than normal breaths.

Oscillating PEP Therapy

DHD Healthcare's Acapella® oscillating PEP therapy device uses a counterweighted magnet and lever to create a vibratory effect during exhalation (Figure 16-9). As the lever opens and closes, flow is interrupted, causing vibration to the lung parenchyma. Adjustment of the control on the base of the Acapella® moves the magnet closer or farther from the counterweighted lever, adjusting expiratory resistance. The device is similar to the PEP device described earlier, only a vibratory effect is achieved during exhalation. Like PEP therapy, the oscillating PEP device splints the airways open with positive pressure during exhalation.

Indications

Indications for PEP therapy include the need to aid in removal of retained secretions, atelectasis, and prophylaxis of pulmonary infections and as routine therapy in the treatment of cystic fibrosis. By splinting the airway open mechanically using positive pressure, PEP therapy allows gas to move distally to obstructed areas. When the patient coughs forcefully, the removal of these secretions is facilitated.

Hazards

Hazards when using the oscillating PEP device are similar to those for PEP therapy.

Flutter Valve Therapy

Definition and Equipment

Flutter valve therapy is similar to PEP therapy in that an expiratory resistance device is employed during exhalation. The difference, however, is that the Flutter valve has a weighted ball resting on a conical seat (Figure 16-10). The ball rises, then falls, blocking the outlet, and then rises again during exhalation. This happens repeatedly, causing the Flutter device to "chatter"

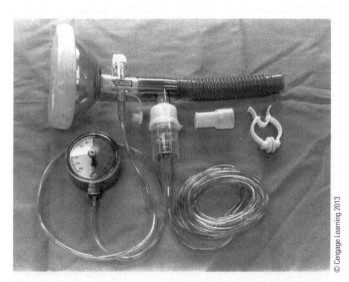

Figure 16-8 A photograph of a PEP mask therapy device with a small volume nebulizer for aerosol delivery attached

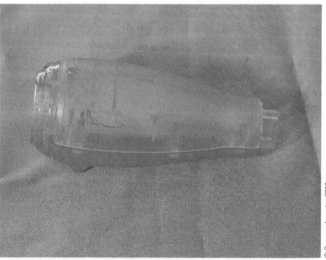

Figure 16-9 A photograph of the DHD Acapella® vibratory PEP device

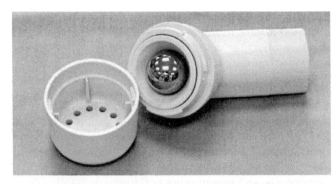

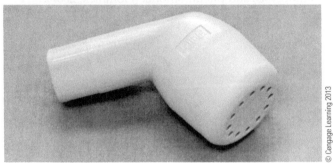

© Cengage Learning 2013

Figure 16-10   An illustration of the Flutter valve. Note the conical seat and the ball that is displaced by exhaling into the seat

during exhalation. The alternating opening and closing of the valve causes pressure pulses to be transmitted throughout the lung parenchyma. The pulsing in conjunction with mechanical splinting of the airways (like PEP therapy) helps to facilitate secretion mobilization. This device is highly position dependent. The conical-shaped valve should be oriented as close to vertical as possible to achieve optimal effect.

Indications

The indications for Flutter valve therapy are similar to those for PEP therapy. Flutter valve therapy is indicated for the need to aid in removal of retained secretions, atelectasis, and prophylaxis of pulmonary infections and as routine therapy in the treatment of cystic fibrosis. When the patient coughs forcefully, the removal of these secretions is facilitated.

Hazards

The hazards of Flutter valve therapy are similar to those of PEP therapy. These hazards are related to the application of positive pressure (barotrauma, cardiovascular compromise) and hyperinflation (light-headedness, headaches).

High-Frequency Chest Wall Oscillation Therapy

High-frequency chest wall oscillation (HFCWO) therapy is the application of pressure pulses to the thoracic cage via a pneumatic inflatable vest (Figure 16-11). The patient applies the vest and connects it to the air-pulse generator, which rapidly inflates and deflates the vest. The alternating inflation and deflation causes oscillatory pressure pulses (5 to 25 times per second) to be transmitted throughout the thorax. This pulsing facilitates the

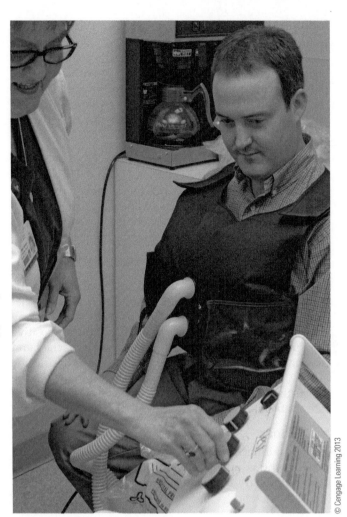

© Cengage Learning 2013

Figure 16-11   A photograph of The Vest® airway clearance system made by Advanced Respiratory, St. Paul, MN

removal of retained secretions and facilitates home self-application of therapy for airway clearance.

Indications

HFCWO therapy is indicated for mucous plugging, retained secretions, and treatment of chronic diseases such as cystic fibrosis. HFCWO facilitates the patient's self-care in the administration of therapy.

Hazards

Patients using HFCWO therapy should follow the physician's and manufacturer's recommendations for the application of the device. Use of HFCWO therapy in patients with fractures of the thoracic cage dictates extreme caution. Disruption of unstable fractures in such cases could result in pneumothorax or other complications.

Adjunctive Breathing Techniques

Adjunctive breathing techniques are breathing exercises that are taught to the patient for self-administration. These exercises include diaphragmatic breathing, unilateral chest expansion, pursed-lip breathing, and directed cough techniques. The goal of these techniques is hyperinflation of the lungs, which will facilitate secretion removal by coughing.

Indications

Indications for adjunctive breathing techniques include removal of retained secretions, atelectasis, and prophylaxis of pulmonary infections and as routine care for patients with cystic fibrosis. These techniques facilitate mobilization of secretions and may be performed independently by the patient in the absence of a caregiver.

Hazards

Hazards of these adjunct breathing techniques are related to the hazards of hyperinflation. Potential symptoms include light-headedness, dizziness, and headaches. Proper patient instruction on awareness of these symptoms and what to do when they occur is important when teaching these adjunctive breathing techniques.

Respironics Coughassist™ MI-E

The Respironics Coughassist™ is an electrically powered pneumatic insufflation-exsufflation device that applies both positive and negative pressure to the airway (Figure 16-12). This ventilator gradually applies a positive pressure to the airway until peak pressure is reached and then rapidly shifts to applying negative pressure to the airway. This rapid shift from positive to negative pressure assists the patient in generating sufficient expiratory flow rates to facilitate coughing.

Indications

The Respironics Coughassist™ may be used on any patient who is unable to generate an effective cough to clear pulmonary secretions because of reduced expiratory flows. Examples may include but are not limited to muscular dystrophy, multiple sclerosis, other neuromuscular diseases affecting ventilator muscle strength or action, and spinal cord injury.

Hazards/Contraindications

Contraindications include a history of bullus emphysema, or pneumothorax. Hazards can include precipitation of cardiac arrhythmias in patients with unstable cardiac status, soreness or chest pain with use, abdominal distention, aggravation of gastroesophageal reflux, hemoptysis, and pneumothorax (Homnick, 2007).

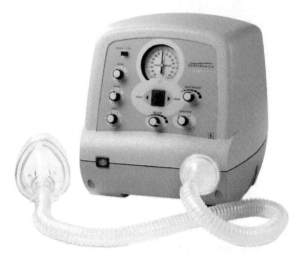

Figure 16-12 A photograph of the Respironics Coughassist™ mechanical insufflator-exsufflator *(Courtesy of Philips Respironics)*

PROFICIENCY OBJECTIVES

At the end of this chapter, the reader should be able to:

* *Demonstrate proper body alignment and stance when performing patient care skills.*
* *Demonstrate the use of good body alignment and body mechanics when positioning or assisting a laboratory partner.*
* *Demonstrate how to properly position a patient in the following positions:*
  — *Fowler's and semi-Fowler's positions*
  — *Supine position*
  — *Prone position*
  — *Side-lying position*
  — *Sims' position*
  — *Trendelenburg position*
* *Demonstrate how to assist a patient from the bed into a chair and back into bed.*
* *Demonstrate how to properly secure the following restraints:*
  — *Chest restraint*
  — *Waist restraint*
  — *Wrist and ankle restraints*
* *Demonstrate the correct use of bed rails and other safety devices while performing patient care.*

* *Using a laboratory partner as a patient substitute, properly perform postural drainage and chest percussion on any specified segment(s) of the lung, including:*
  — *Proper positioning*
  — *Identification of anatomical landmarks*
  — *Proper manual percussion and vibration techniques*
  — *Proper use of a mechanical percussor*
* *Demonstrate use of a PEP mask device:*
  — *Demonstrate how to assemble a PEP mask device with and without a nebulizer.*
  — *Correctly instruct a patient on how to use a PEP device.*
* *Demonstrate use of a Flutter valve:*
  — *Correctly assemble the Flutter valve for use.*
  — *Correctly instruct the patient on how to use the Flutter valve.*
* *Demonstrate use of a vibratory PEP (Acapella®).*
  — *Correctly assemble the Acapella® for use.*
  — *Correctly instruct the patient on how to use the Acapella®.*
* *Demonstrate use of The Vest® airway clearance system.*
  — *Correctly assemble The Vest® airway clearance system.*

— Correctly teach the patient how to use The Vest® airway clearance system.
* Demonstrate the use of the Respironics Coughassist™ Insufflator-Exsufflator, now owned by Phillips.
  — Correctly assemble the Coughassist™.
  — Correctly adjust the controls and settings.
  — Correctly apply the device to the patient.

* Demonstrate the following adjunctive breathing exercises:
  — Diaphragmatic breathing
  — Unilateral chest expansion
  — Pursed-lip breathing
  — Controlled cough, including splinting
  — Acute chest compression coughing

GENERAL GUIDELINES

Bed Rails

Bed rails should always be in the up position except when working on that side of the bed.

Positioning of the Practitioner

The practitioner should always position himself or herself as close to the patient and the side of the bed as possible. It is easier to maintain good body alignment when close to the bed and less strain is placed on the muscles. Additionally, to keep the patient from inadvertently rolling out of bed, the practitioner may use his or her body as a bed rail to prevent a fall.

PATIENT POSITIONING

There are a number of standardized *patient positions*.

Fowler's and Semi-Fowler's Positions

Electric beds have simplified the positioning of patients in the two Fowler's positions. The practitioner may need to pull the patient up in bed so that the bend of the bed is located where the patient bends at the waist. Simply raising or lowering the head of the bed is all that is required. Elevating the knees slightly will help to prevent the patient from sliding to the foot of the bed and relieve pressure on the back and buttocks.

Supine Position

To place the patient in the supine position, lower the bed until it is flat. Position a blanket that has been formed into a roll or small pillow under the knees to slightly flex them and under the small of the back to support the spine. Use of a foot board is helpful to prevent adverse flexing of the feet. Foot drop from the continual pressure of the bedding on the feet can result in permanent disability. Avoid leaving the comatose or helpless patient supine, as there is a danger of vomiting and aspiration.

Prone Position

Positioning a patient in the prone position ideally should be performed by multiple caregivers, especially if the

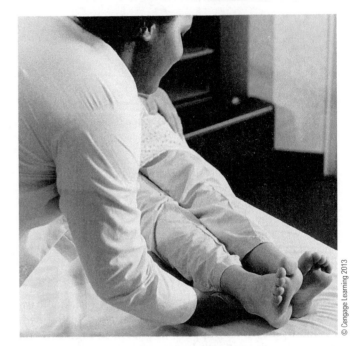

Figure 16-13 Moving a patient by thirds

© Cengage Learning 2013

patient has an artificial airway. Positioning the patient in the prone position requires *turning* the patient. The practitioner must roll the patient first into a side-lying and then into the prone position. Care must be exercised to ensure that enough room is provided to complete the maneuver without rolling the patient out of bed.

Begin by positioning the patient to one side of the bed in the supine position. If the patient is unable to assist, use the following technique: Imagine that the patient is divided into thirds: feet and legs, waist and buttocks, and chest and head. Each third may be easily moved by placing the hands under that portion and then shifting the weight. This is illustrated in Figure 16-13. Slide the patient's feet over first (this is the lightest part). Slide the waist and buttocks over and, finally, the chest and head. Preserve the patient's spinal alignment as much as possible during the procedure.

Once the patient is on one side of the bed, cross the patient's legs and move the patient's arm to the position shown in Figure 16-14. Raise the bed rail and move to the other side of the bed.

Roll the patient into a side-lying position by pulling the patient toward yourself. The practitioner again may accomplish this with a simple weight shift. Continue rolling the patient to the prone position. Realign the patient

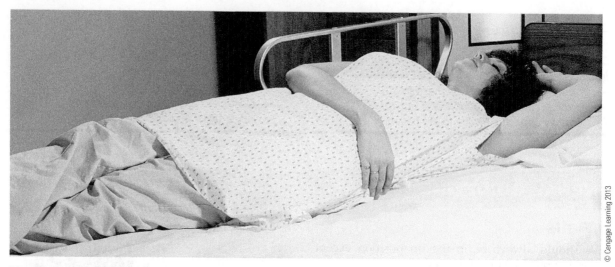

Figure 16-14 Preparing to turn a patient

so that the patient is centered in the bed and the spinal column is in alignment. A small pillow should be placed under the abdomen to maintain proper spinal alignment. Another, larger pillow may be placed under the ankles and lower legs to prevent adverse flexing of the feet, as shown in Figure 16-15.

Side-Lying Position

To position a patient in the side-lying position, turn the patient onto the patient's side, centered in the bed. Position pillows for support, as shown in Figure 16-16. Slightly flex the patient's knees and arms to relieve strain on muscles and tendons.

Sims' Position

Sims' position (Figure 16-17) is similar to the side-lying position, and some patients find it more comfortable. When rolling a patient to the side, care must be taken not to position the lower arm in a location where the patient can roll over onto it.

Trendelenburg Position

Electric beds have simplified the positioning of patients into the Trendelenburg position. Beds vary, so read the printed directions on the bed and follow them to position the patient. If the practitioner does not understand how to work the bed, assistance should be sought.

Once the patient is in Trendelenburg position, monitor the patient closely. Check heart rate, skin color, and respiratory rate for any significant changes. The Trendelenburg position is not a natural position, and complications occasionally arise. Avoid leaving the patient unattended and do not allow the patient to cough spasmodically in this head-down position, as it may increase intracranial pressure to dangerous levels.

Reverse Trendelenburg Position

Using the electric bed, follow the directions and position the patient in the reverse Trendelenburg position. The patient will have a tendency to slide toward the foot of the bed. Use of a foot board will help to prevent this.

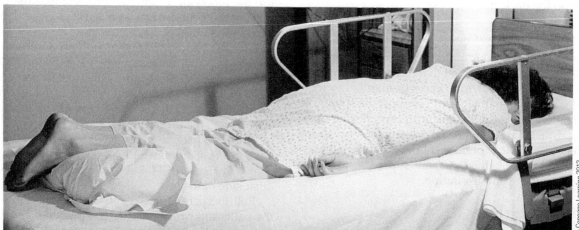

Figure 16-15 Pillow placement for a prone patient

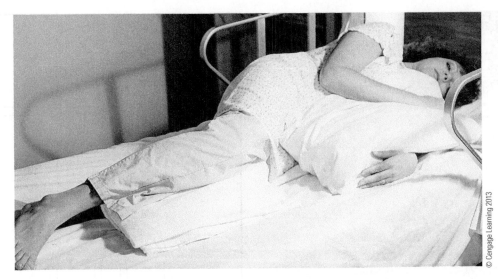

Figure 16-16   A patient in side-lying position

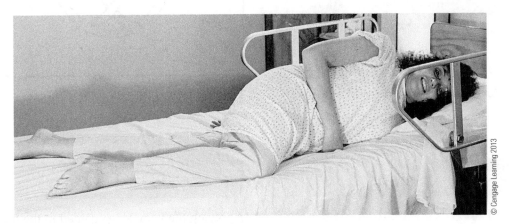

Figure 16-17   A patient in Sims' position

Assisting a Patient into a Chair

Begin by lowering the bed as low as its design permits. Raise the head of the bed to full Fowler's position (as far up as it will go). When raising the bed, be certain that the patient is high enough toward the head of the bed so that the patient will bend at the waist and not the chest. These maneuvers accomplish two things. First, the patient is low enough to make an exit easy. Second, raising the head of the bed reduces the work the practitioner needs to do to assist the patient to a sitting position. The practitioner may wish to allow the patient to sit in this position for a moment to avoid dizziness.

Assist the patient into a dangling position at the side of the bed, as shown in Figure 16-18.

Spread the patient's feet slightly and position your foot closer to the patient between the patient's feet. Grasp the patient under the arms and assist the patient to a standing position, as shown in Figure 16-19. Pivot the patient 90° and lower him or her into the chair.

If this is the patient's first time in a chair after a prolonged period of bed rest, two people should assist. If the patient becomes shaky, two people may be required to prevent a fall.

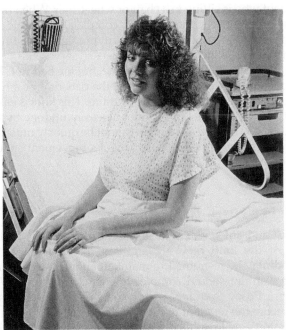

Figure 16-18   A patient in the dangling position, ready to be assisted into a chair

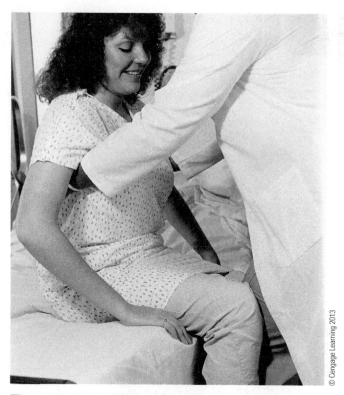

Figure 16-19 Correct foot placement to assist a patient into a chair

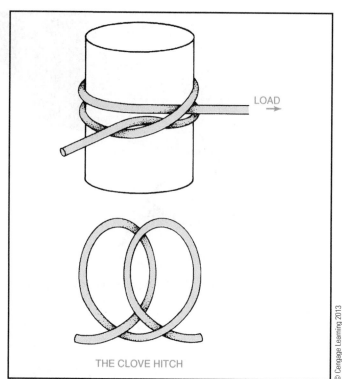

THE CLOVE HITCH

Figure 16-20 How to tie a clove hitch

USE OF RESTRAINTS

Chest and Waist Restraints

Chest restraints are used to prevent the patient from falling or climbing out of bed. They are also used to help a patient who is sitting in a chair or wheelchair. When these devices are used, they should completely encircle the body. Restraints should be snug but not tight, so a finger can be easily slipped underneath.

Tie the restraint to the bed frame, not the bed rail. The knot should be out of the reach of the patient. Use a half-hitch with a loop to secure the restraint. This knot is easily untied by personnel but cannot be easily undone by the patient. Do not use a knot that cannot be quickly untied in an emergency situation. The patient's movement should be only slightly restricted.

Wrist and Ankle Restraints

Wrist and ankle restraints are used to reduce the mobility of the limb they are attached to. Frequently one hand may be restrained to maintain an intravenous line. The restraint should completely encircle the limb. With soft or Posey restraints, a clove hitch is commonly used to secure the restraint to the limb. Figure 16-20 illustrates how to tie a clove hitch. The two free ends are then tied to the bed frame. Like the chest and waist restraints, these should be snug but not tight.

PERCUSSION TECHNIQUE

Applying the knowledge gained in the theory portion of this chapter, practice postural drainage and percussion on a laboratory partner.

Position the hands by letting the arms fall to a resting position at your side while standing. The palmar surface of the hand should face toward the thighs. Keep the fingers together and the hands in the resting configuration. Looking at the shape of the hands, they should be slightly cupped, as shown in Figure 16-21.

Practice chest percussion initially by percussing your own thigh. Try to achieve a hollow, popping sound. Notice the difference in sound and tactile stimulation between a correct and an incorrect technique. Upon mastering the hand positioning, practice percussion on a laboratory partner. Figure 16-22 illustrates correct percussion technique. Using both hands, work

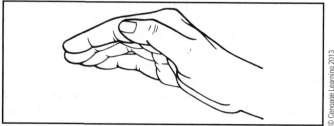

Figure 16-21 Correct hand position for chest percussion

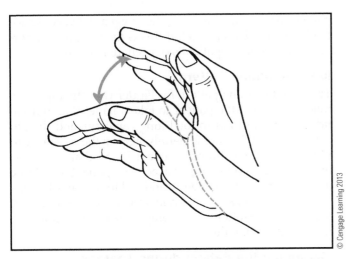

Figure 16-22   Correct percussion technique

toward a frequency of 50 to 60 percussions per minute. The muscle action is predominantly in the wrist and forearm with the wrist acting as a pivot. Observe for red marks on the surface of the skin. Position your laboratory partner into the 12 drainage positions, identify the landmarks for percussion, and properly perform the technique, observing your partner for any adverse effects from the procedure.

POSITIVE EXPIRATORY PRESSURE THERAPY

Verify the Physician's Order

Before initiating PEP therapy, verify the physician's order for PEP therapy. Determine whether or not aerosolized medication delivery is desired along with PEP therapy, the desired pressure level, and the frequency of therapy. If any of these is not clearly stated, contact the patient's physician for clarification.

Scan the Chart

Scan the patient's history documented in the patient's medical record. Verify that the patient does not have acute sinusitis or a history of ear infections or epistaxis. Confirm that facial, oral, or skull surgery has not recently been performed. Also verify that the patient does not have active hemoptysis or an untreated pneumothorax. All of these conditions are contraindications to PEP therapy.

Check the patient's chart, looking for recent blood gas analysis reports, chest radiographs and report, laboratory data, orders for oxygen administration, and any other items that will help to assess the patient's current pulmonary status. Review the physician's progress notes, which may help to determine the goals of PEP therapy. Note the current vital signs, which will provide a frame of reference when the practitioner first sees the patient.

Administration of Therapy

Patient Positioning

The ideal patient position for PEP therapy is sitting comfortably with the elbows resting on a table. This position allows good chest expansion while freeing both hands to provide a good seal around the mouthpiece. If the patient is unable to sit upright, a full Fowler's or high semi-Fowler's position may be adequate. If modifying the patient's position, use good clinical judgment, monitor for any adverse effects, and assess whether the goals and objectives of PEP therapy are being met.

Appropriate Monitoring before Therapy

Prior to beginning PEP therapy, auscultate the patient's chest, measure heart rate and respiratory rate, and observe the patient's ventilatory pattern and symmetry of chest wall motion (by inspection). The goals of PEP therapy are to mobilize secretions, to reverse atelectasis, and to optimize delivery of aerosolized medications. Therefore, quantification of sputum production and determination of pretherapy and posttherapy vital capacity will help to document the effectiveness of therapy. If administering a bronchodilator, measurement of peak expiratory flow or forced expired volume in 1 minute (FEV_1) will be appropriate.

If the patient's oxygen therapy is being interrupted for PEP therapy, monitor the patient's arterial oxygen concentration (SpO_2) with the pulse oximeter before and during therapy. To perform PEP therapy, the patient may need to remove the oxygen delivery device to obtain an adequate seal. If this is the case, it is important to monitor the patient's oxygenation status.

Ideal Breathing Pattern

The ideal breathing pattern for PEP therapy is as follows: Instruct the patient to take a larger than normal tidal breath (but not to total lung capacity), and then to exhale actively, but not forcefully, against the resistance to FRC. The patient should be relaxed, and diaphragmatic breathing should be emphasized. The patient should be instructed to take between 10 and 20 PEP breaths and then to cough. This cycle should be repeated 4 to 6 times. Most PEP therapy sessions take approximately 10 to 20 minutes.

Monitoring the Patient during Therapy

The patient's subjective response (e.g., pain, discomfort, dyspnea) should be monitored and noted. Any dyspnea, tachycardia, or tachypnea should be carefully monitored. If oxygen therapy is being interrupted for PEP therapy, monitor the SpO_2; the practitioner may need to discontinue PEP therapy and place the patient on oxygen therapy if levels drop too low.

Monitor the patient's sputum production. PEP therapy should assist the patient in increasing the quantity of sputum produced. Note the color, consistency, and quantity of the sputum and the presence or absence of odor.

If a bronchodilator is being given, it is important to monitor the heart rate during therapy. Because most sympathomimetic bronchodilators have some cardiac side effects, any significant increase in heart rate warrants stopping therapy and monitoring the patient closely.

FLUTTER VALVE THERAPY

Verify the Physician's Order

Prior to initiating Flutter valve therapy, verify the physician's order for Flutter valve therapy. If the order is not clearly stated, contact the patient's physician for clarification.

Scan the Chart

Scan the patient's history documented in the medical record. Verify that the patient does not have contraindications to Flutter valve therapy. Verify that the patient does not have active hemoptysis or an untreated pneumothorax. Both of these conditions are contraindications to therapy.

Check the patient's chart, looking for recent reports of blood gas analysis, chest radiographs and report, laboratory data, orders for oxygen administration, and any other items that will help assess the patient's current pulmonary status. Review the physician's progress notes, which may help determine the goals of Flutter valve therapy. Note the current vital signs, which will provide a frame of reference when the practitioner first sees the patient.

Administration of Therapy

Patient Positioning

The ideal patient position for Flutter valve therapy is sitting comfortably with his or her elbows resting on a table. This position allows good chest expansion while freeing both hands to provide a good seal around the mouthpiece. If the patient is unable to sit upright, a full Fowler's or high semi-Fowler's position may be adequate. If modifying the patient's position, use good clinical judgment, monitor for any adverse side effects, and assess whether the goals and objectives of Flutter valve therapy are being met. Be aware of the position of the conical valve seat, keeping it as vertical.

Appropriate Monitoring before Therapy

Prior to beginning Flutter valve therapy, auscultate the patient's chest, measure heart rate and respiratory rate, and observe the patient's ventilatory pattern and symmetry of chest wall motion (inspection). The goals of Flutter valve therapy are to mobilize secretions and reverse atelectasis. Therefore, quantification of sputum production and determination of pretherapy and posttherapy vital capacity will help to document the effectiveness of therapy.

If the patient's oxygen therapy is being interrupted for Flutter valve therapy, monitor the patient's SpO_2 before and during therapy. To perform Flutter valve therapy, the patient may need to remove the oxygen delivery device to obtain an adequate seal. If this is the case, it is important to monitor the patient's oxygenation status.

Ideal Breathing Pattern

The ideal breathing pattern for Flutter valve therapy is as follows: Instruct the patient to take a larger than normal tidal breath (but not to total lung capacity), and then to exhale actively, but not forcefully, against the resistance to FRC. The patient should be relaxed, and diaphragmatic breathing should be emphasized. The patient should be instructed to take between 10 and 20 Flutter valve breaths and then to cough. This cycle should be repeated 4 to 6 times. Most Flutter valve therapy sessions take approximately 10 to 20 minutes.

Monitoring the Patient during Therapy

The patient's subjective response (e.g., pain, discomfort, dyspnea) should be monitored and noted. Any dyspnea, tachycardia, or tachypnea should be carefully monitored. If oxygen therapy must be interrupted for Flutter valve therapy, monitor the SpO_2, discontinue therapy, and place the patient on oxygen therapy as required.

Monitor the patient's sputum production. Flutter valve therapy should assist the patient in increasing the quantity of sputum produced. Note the color, consistency, and quantity of sputum and the presence or absence of odor.

VIBRATORY PEP (ACAPELLA®) THERAPY ADMINISTRATION

Verify the Physician's Order

Prior to initiating vibratory PEP therapy, verify the physician's order for therapy. If the order is not clearly stated, contact the patient's physician for clarification.

Scan the Chart

Scan the patient's history documented in the medical record. Verify that the patient does not have contraindications to vibratory PEP therapy. Verify that the patient does not have active hemoptysis or an untreated pneumothorax. Both of these conditions are contraindications to therapy.

Check the patient's chart, looking for recent reports of blood gas analysis, chest radiographs and report, laboratory data, orders for oxygen administration, and any other items that will help assess the patient's current pulmonary status. Review the physician's progress notes, which may help determine the goals of vibratory PEP therapy. Note the current vital signs, which will provide a frame of reference when the practitioner first sees the patient.

Administration of Therapy

Patient Positioning

The ideal patient position for vibratory PEP therapy is sitting comfortably with his or her elbows resting on a table.

This position allows good chest expansion. If the patient is unable to sit upright, a full Fowler's or high semi-Fowler's position may be adequate. If modifying the patient's position, use good clinical judgment, monitor for any adverse side effects, and assess whether the goals and objectives of vibratory PEP therapy are being met.

Appropriate Monitoring before Therapy

Prior to beginning vibratory PEP therapy, auscultate the patient's chest, measure heart rate and respiratory rate, and observe the patient's ventilatory pattern and symmetry of chest wall motion (inspection). The goals of vibratory PEP therapy are to mobilize secretions and reverse atelectasis. Therefore, quantification of sputum production and determination of pretherapy and post-therapy vital capacity will help to document the effectiveness of therapy.

If the patient's oxygen therapy is being interrupted for vibratory PEP therapy, monitor the patient's SpO_2 before and during therapy. To perform vibratory PEP therapy, the patient may need to remove the oxygen delivery device to obtain an adequate seal. If this is the case, it is important to monitor the patient's oxygenation status.

Ideal Breathing Pattern

The ideal breathing pattern for vibratory PEP therapy is as follows: Instruct the patient to take a larger than normal tidal breath (but not to total lung capacity), and then to exhale actively, but not forcefully, against the Acapella® to FRC. The patient should be relaxed, and diaphragmatic breathing should be emphasized. The patient should be instructed to take between 10 and 20 vibratory PEP breaths and then to cough. This cycle should be repeated 4 to 6 times. Most vibratory PEP therapy sessions take approximately 10 to 20 minutes.

Monitoring the Patient during Therapy

The patient's subjective response (e.g., pain, discomfort, dyspnea) should be monitored and noted. Any dyspnea, tachycardia, or tachypnea should be carefully monitored. If oxygen therapy must be interrupted for vibratory PEP therapy, monitor the SpO_2, discontinue therapy, and place the patient on oxygen therapy as required.

Monitor the patient's sputum production. Vibratory PEP therapy should assist the patient in increasing the quantity of sputum produced. Note the color, consistency, and quantity of sputum and the presence or absence of odor.

HIGH-FREQUENCY CHEST WALL OSCILLATION THERAPY ADMINISTRATION

The Vest® Airway Clearance System Assembly

Assist and instruct the patient in applying the vest to the chest. Ensure that the vest is properly secured using the self-fastening straps with the head and arms free to move

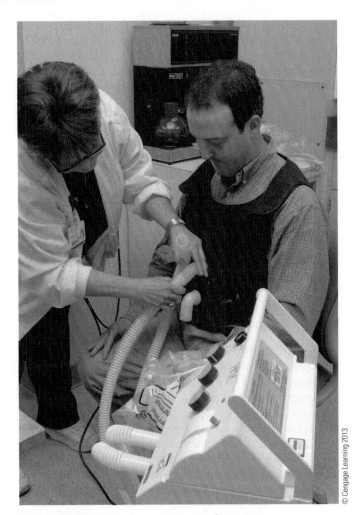

Figure 16-23 Application of The Vest® airway clearance system to the patient's chest

(Figure 16-23). It is important to secure the vest so that it does not ride too high or too low on the chest.

Connect both large-diameter hoses to the air-pulse generator unit, matching left and right sides with the labeled outlets. Connect the power cord to a standard wall electrical outlet, verifying that the voltage is set correctly for the facility. Set the controls (frequency and pressure) to the correct settings.

Verify the Physician's Order

Prior to initiating HFCWO therapy, verify the physician's order for therapy. If the order is not clearly stated, contact the patient's physician for clarification.

Scan the Chart

Scan the patient's history documented in the patient's medical record. Verify that the patient does not have contraindications to HFCWO therapy. Verify that the patient does not have active hemoptysis, an untreated pneumothorax, or unstable chest wall fractures. All of these conditions are contraindications to therapy.

Check the patient's chart, looking for recent results of blood gas analysis, chest radiographs and report, laboratory data, orders for oxygen administration, and any other items that will help assess the patient's current pulmonary status. Review the physician's progress notes, which may help determine the goals of HFCWO therapy. Note the current vital signs, which will provide a frame of reference when the practitioner first sees the patient.

Administration of Therapy

Patient Positioning

The ideal patient position for HFCWO therapy is sitting comfortably erect with the chest in a good position for expansion. If modifying the patient's position, use good clinical judgment, monitor for any adverse effects, and assess whether the goals and objectives of HFCWO therapy are being met.

Technique

Turn the unit on. Have the patient relax and take slow, deep breaths during therapy. If the patient needs to cough, the unit may be turned off if coughing is easier without HFCWO. A typical session takes about 20 minutes.

Monitoring the Patient during Therapy

The patient's subjective response (e.g., pain, discomfort, dyspnea) should be monitored and noted. Any dyspnea, tachycardia, or tachypnea should be carefully monitored. Monitor the patient's SpO_2; place the patient on oxygen therapy as required if oxygen desaturation occurs.

Monitor the patient's sputum production. HFCWO therapy should assist the patient in increasing the quantity of sputum produced. Note the color, consistency, and quantity of sputum and the presence or absence of odor.

COUGHASSIST™ MI-E ADMINISTRATION

The Coughassist™ mechanical in-exsufflator is a device intended to assist a patient in removing pulmonary secretions by providing both positive pressure during inspiration and negative pressure during exhalation. When a patient has insufficient muscle strength or effort to generate high expiratory flow rates, the Coughassist™ device produces a high expiratory flow rate that facilitates secretion removal, mimicking a cough.

Coughassist™ Assembly

Connect the bacteria filter to the patient port on the front panel of the Coughassist™. Attach the 22 mm patient tubing to the bacteria filter. Attach an appropriate patient interface to the distal end of the patient tubing (mask and adapter, mouthpiece or tracheostomy adapter). Connect the unit to a suitable power outlet using the supplied power cord.

Verify Physician's Order

Verify the physician's order for using the Coughassist™. If the order is not clearly stated, contact the physician for clarification.

Scan the Chart

Review the patient's chart, looking for appropriate indications for therapy. These may include but are not limited to neuromuscular disease (muscular dystrophy, multiple sclerosis, etc.), spinal cord injury, reduced peak expiratory flow (<2 to 3 L/sec), or severe fatigue. Review the physician's progress notes, which may help determine the goals of therapy. Note the current vital signs, which will provide a frame of reference when the practitioner first sees the patient.

Administration of Therapy

Patient Positioning

The ideal patient position is sitting or a high Fowler's position. The diaphragm must be free to move, and the lungs should be free to expand. If it becomes necessary to modify the patient's position, exercise good clinical judgment with patient monitoring being paramount. The patient should be monitored during therapy sessions and not be left unattended.

Technique

Turn the Coughassist™ MI-E on by pressing the power toggle switch at the lower left of the front of the unit. Move the manual/auto switch to the manual position and aseptically block the outlet of the patient tubing. Move the pressure rocker switch below the pressure gauge to the exhalation position (left) and adjust the expiratory pressure. An expiratory pressure of 10 to 20 cm H_2O initially allows the patient to become acclimated to the device. Confirm the expiratory pressure using the pressure gauge. Once the patient becomes familiar and accustomed to the unit, pressures may be gradually increased. Expiratory pressures of up to 40 to 45 cm H_2O may be needed to achieve adequate expiratory flow rates.

Now move the pressure rocker switch to the inhalation position (right) and adjust the inspiratory pressure. Set the inspiratory pressure to 10 to 20 cm H_2O and adjust the flow rate control to the right (slowest flow) initially to allow for patient acclimation. Once the patient becomes acclimated to the device, pressures may be gradually increased.

Once exhalation and inhalation pressures are set, manually toggle the pressure rocker switch between the inhalation and exhalation position, verifying the pressure settings on the pressure gauge. Release the rocker switch to the center position, and verify that the pressure returns to zero. The preceding steps should be accomplished while the patient circuit is aseptically blocked.

Adjust the cycle timing using the controls on the left side of the front panel. Using Table 16-1, adjust the cycle timing using the inhale, exhale, and pause controls.

Move the auto/manual control to the manual position. Interface the Coughassist™ to the patient and ensure that there is a tight fit between the interface and the patient (mask, tracheostomy adapter, or mouthpiece). Move the auto/manual control to the auto position to begin the therapy session. Allow the Coughtassist™ to cycle for 4 to 5 inhalation/exhalation/pause cycles. Remove the

TABLE 16-1: Inhalation/Exhalation/Pause Timing

		LOW FLOW SETTING	HIGH FLOW SETTING
Adults	Inhalation	3–4 seconds	1.5–2.5 seconds
	Exhalation	1–2 seconds	1–2 seconds
	Pause	1–2 seconds	1–2 seconds
Children		1–2 seconds	0.5–1.5 seconds
		<1 second	<1 second
		1–2 seconds	1–2 seconds

patient from the interface and allow 20 to 30 seconds rest prior to the next cycle. If secretions are evident, assist the patient with secretion removal or suction as required. Repeat the mechanical insufflation/exsufflation treatment again for 4 to 5 cycles, allowing another rest period of 20 to 30 seconds following the cycle. Four to six repetitions of mechanical insufflation/exsufflation is usually sufficient for a complete treatment. Adjust the pressure and flow rate controls to achieve optimal expiratory flow rates once the patient has become acclimated to the device. The Coughassist™ is not intended for continuous use. The patient must be allowed rest periods between insufflation/exsufflation cycles.

Monitoring the Patient during Therapy

Hyperventilation, chest pain or discomfort, pneumothorax, precipitation of cardiac arrhythmias in unstable cardiac patients, abdominal distention, aggravation of gastroesophageal reflux, and hemoptysis are potential hazards when using the device. Monitor the patient's general condition, response to therapy, and oxygen saturations before and after a therapy session. Monitor the patient's sputum production and assist with secretion removal by suctioning if required.

ADJUNCTIVE BREATHING TECHNIQUES

Adjunctive breathing techniques such as controlled coughing and splinting may be used postoperatively to improve secretion mobilization. Because of pain, a patient may expend considerable energy with weak, ineffective coughs, desperately trying to clear secretions. A low volume combined with a weak effort is insufficient to generate the flow rates necessary to clear any retained secretions.

Diaphragmatic Breathing

Diaphragmatic breathing may be accomplished on both inspiration and expiration. For this technique, the patient is encouraged to distend the abdomen with the inspiratory effort. Use of the abdominal muscles in this way helps to lower the diaphragm, expanding the lungs further. A patient may also be coached to observe the intercostal margin and encouraged to expand it outward. This maneuver takes considerable effort and is the reverse of the breathing pattern most people use (stomach in, chest out).

On expiration, the patient is encouraged to flatten the abdomen, thus pushing the diaphragm up and thereby improving the strength of exhalation. With time, the contractile force of the abdominal muscles will be increased. The patient may feel the effects on the diaphragm by placing the hands over the rib cage at the level of the xiphoid process.

Unilateral Chest Expansion

By placing a hand along the midaxillary line (Figure 16-24), expanding one side of the chest preferentially (unilateral) is facilitated. This position results in a slight kyphosis, compressing the opposite chest. Therefore, when the patient performs deep breathing, the side where the hand is placed preferentially expands. This technique of *unilateral chest expansion* may be helpful in reversing middle or lower lobe atelectasis.

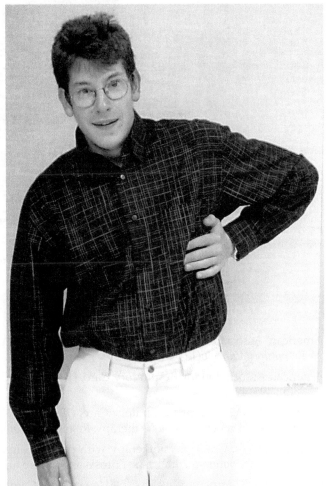

© Cengage Learning 2013

Figure 16-24 An illustration showing unilateral chest expansion

Pursed-Lip Breathing

For *pursed-lip breathing,* the patient is instructed to take a deep breath and exhale through pursed lips. The narrowing of the airway generates a resistance to exhalation, causing pressure to be maintained throughout the bronchial tree. This sustained pressure prevents air trapping and keeps the alveoli inflated for a longer period on exhalation. This is a natural phenomenon that may be observed when a patient is short of breath.

Controlled Coughing

For controlled coughing, or *directed cough,* the patient is instructed to take three breaths as deep as possible. This maneuver will help to reverse atelectasis and to increase the volume available for the cough effort. At the end of the third breath, the patient is encouraged to cough twice very firmly. With the larger volume behind the cough, flow can be improved and the cough becomes more effective.

Splinting is a technique wherein the surgical incision or injured area is supported with the hands, a pillow, or a bath blanket. By applying pressure across the incision and minimizing its movement, pain during coughing is reduced. Splinting may be accomplished by either the practitioner or the patient, if able. Any time pain can be reduced, cooperation is generally better.

Acute Chest Compression

Acute chest compression is effective for those patients with a poor cough effort, which is often due to weak musculature. The patient is instructed to take as deep a breath as possible. Then place the hands on the patient's lateral costal margins. When the patient exhales, apply firm but gentle pressure. This helps to generate the flows and pressures necessary to move secretions into the larger airways from where they may be expelled. Figure 16-25 illustrates the technique of acute chest compression.

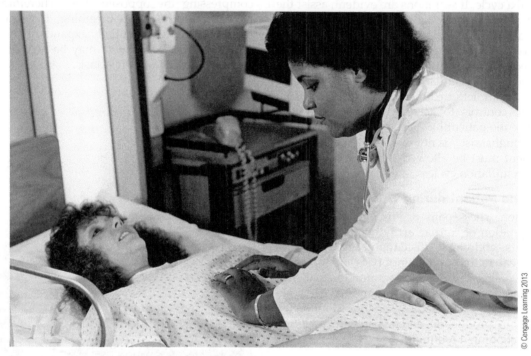

© Cengage Learning 2013

Figure 16-25   A respiratory care practitioner performing acute chest compression

References

American Association for Respiratory Care. (1991). AARC clinical practice guideline: Postural drainage therapy. *Respiratory Care, 36*(12), 1418–1426.

American Association for Respiratory Care. (1993). AARC clinical practice guideline: Directed cough. *Respiratory Care, 38*(5), 495–499.

American Association for Respiratory Care. (1993). AARC clinical practice guideline: Use of positive airway pressure adjuncts to bronchial hygiene therapy. *Respiratory Care, 38*(5), 516–521.

Giulia, P. (2006). Chest physiotherapy with positive airway pressure: A pilot study of short-term effects on sputum clearance in patients with cystic fibrosis and severe airway obstruction. *Respiratory Care, 51*(10), 1145–1153.

J. H. Emerson Company, *Coughassist*[TM] *User's Guide,* Cambridge, MA.

Homnick, D. (2007). Mechanical insufflation-exsufflation for airway mucous clearance. *Respiratory Care, 52*(10), 1296–1305.

Additional Resources

Allsop, K. (1976). *Body mechanics and patient transfer techniques.* Ogden, UT: Weber State College.

DeLaune, S. C., & Ladner, P. K. (2002). *Fundamentals of nursing concepts and procedures* (2nd ed.). Reading, MA: Addison-Wesley.

Fink, J. B. (2007). Forced expiratory technique, directed cough, and autogenic drainage. *Respiratory Care, 52*(9), 1210–1223.

Tyler, M. (1982). Complications of positioning and chest physiotherapy. *Respiratory Care, 27*(4), 458–466.

Van der Schans, C. P. (2007). Conventional chest physical therapy for obstructive lung disease. *Respiratory Care, 52*(9), 1198–1209.

Practice Activities: Patient Positioning and Chest Physiotherapy

1. With a laboratory partner, demonstrate how to position the patient into the following positions:
   a. Fowler's and semi-Fowler's
   b. Dangling
   c. Prone
   d. Side-lying
   e. Sims'
   f. Trendelenburg
   g. Reverse Trendelenburg

2. With a laboratory partner, demonstrate how to use the following restraints:
   a. Chest
   b. Waist
   c. Wrist
   d. Ankle

3. Position a laboratory partner for postural drainage:
   a. Position your partner into the 12 positions, verbally stating what region or structure each position drains.
   b. Ask your partner to test your abilities by specifying a lobe or segment to be drained; then position your partner as appropriate. Observe the following:
      (1) Pulse
      (2) Respiratory rate and depth
      (3) Color

4. With a laboratory partner, practice manual chest percussion. During your practice, observe the following:
   a. Properly identify all anatomical landmarks.
   b. Use correct hand positioning.
   c. Percussion should produce a hollow popping sound.
   d. The skin should not have any evidence of red marks.
   e. Do not percuss bony structures, the spine, the abdomen, or breast tissue in a female patient.

5. With a laboratory partner, practice manual vibration. During your practice, observe the following:
   a. Properly identify all anatomical landmarks.
   b. Use correct hand positioning.
   c. Vibration is performed only on exhalation.

6. With a laboratory partner, practice use of a mechanical percussor. During your practice, observe the following:
   a. Do not use excessive force.
   b. Properly identify all anatomical landmarks.
   c. Do not percuss over bony structures, the spine, the abdomen, or breast tissue in a female patient.
   d. Move the percussor over an area of about 10 to 20 cm.

7. With a laboratory partner, practice setting up and applying the Coughassist™.

8. Using a blank sheet of paper, document the positioning used, the technique (manual or mechanical) of chest percussion, and the lobe and segment treated. Have your laboratory instructor critique your charting.

Practice Activities: PEP Mask Therapy

Circuit Assembly

Connect a mouthpiece to the outlet T assembly with the one-way valves and threshold resistor. Connect a pressure manometer to the opposite side of the T assembly from the threshold resistor for pressure monitoring. If a nebulized medication is desired, connect the nebulizer to the inlet of the T assembly and connect a 6-inch length of aerosol tubing (reservoir) to the opposite end of the nebulizer (Figure 16-26), and connect the nebulizer to a compressed gas source (air or oxygen).

It is important to use nose clips when a mouthpiece is used in that pressure may be lost through the nose without them.

Pressure Adjustment

Adjust the threshold resistor until the desired expiratory pressure is achieved. Most often pressures between 10 and 20 cm H_2O are applied during PEP mask therapy.

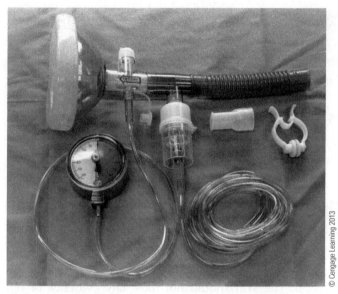

© Cengage Learning 2013

Figure 16-26   The correct assembly of the PEP therapy device

Activities

1. Correctly assemble the circuit for PEP therapy.

2. With a laboratory partner acting as your patient:
   a. Correctly assess your patient prior to therapy.
   b. Correctly instruct your patient on the use of the PEP mask device.
   c. Correctly monitor your patient during therapy.
   d. Correctly monitor your patient following PEP mask therapy.
   e. Using a blank sheet of paper, document the procedure as if you were charting in a medical record and have your laboratory instructor critique your charting.

3. Assemble a PEP device for aerosol delivery.

Practice Activities: Flutter Valve Therapy

1. Correctly assemble the Flutter valve for use.

2. With a laboratory partner acting as your patient:
   a. Correctly assess your patient prior to therapy.
   b. Correctly instruct your patient on the use of the Flutter valve.
   c. Correctly monitor your patient during therapy.
   d. Correctly monitor your patient following Flutter valve therapy.
   e. Using a blank sheet of paper, document the procedure as if you were charting in a medical record and have your laboratory instructor critique your charting.

Practice Activities: Vibratory PEP Therapy (Acapella®)

1. Correctly prepare the Acapella® for use.

2. With a laboratory partner acting as your patient:
   a. Correctly assess your patient prior to therapy.
   b. Correctly instruct your patient on the use of the Acapella®.
   c. Correctly monitor your patient during therapy.
   d. Correctly monitor your patient following vibratory PEP therapy.
   e. Using a blank sheet of paper, document the procedure as if you were charting in a medical record and have your laboratory instructor critique your charting.

Practice Activities: The Vest® Airway Clearance System

1. Assemble the required equipment:
   a. The vest
   b. Two large-bore tubes
   c. The air-pulse generator

2. Using a laboratory partner as your patient, assist in correctly applying the vest.

3. Set the control (frequency) to 15 Hz at a medium pressure.

4. Connect the hoses to the air-pulse generator and plug the unit into an AC electrical outlet.

5. Correctly assess your patient prior to therapy.

6. Instruct the patient on the use of the device.

7. Monitor the patient during therapy:
   a. Shortness of breath
   b. Coughing
   c. Oximetry

8. Using a blank sheet of paper, document the procedure as if you were charting in a medical record and have your laboratory instructor critique your charting.

Practice Activities: Coughassist™ Mechanical In-Exsufflator

1. Assemble the Coughassist™ MI-E:
   a. Coughassist™ MI-E unit
   b. Patient circuit
   c. Patient interface (mask, tracheostomy adapter, or mouthpiece)

2. Using a laboratory partner, correctly assess them prior to therapy.

3. Set the pressure limits (insufflation and exsufflation).

4. Under the direction and observation by your laboratory instructor, practice using the Coughassist™ MI-E using a laboratory partner as your patient. Use a mouthpiece as the patient interface.

5. Following therapy, correctly assess your laboratory partner and assist with secretion clearance as required.

6. Using a blank sheet of paper, document the procedure as if you were charting in a medical record and have your laboratory instructor critique your charting.

Practice Activities: Adjunctive Breathing Techniques

1. With a laboratory partner, practice giving each other directions on how to perform the following techniques:
   a. Diaphragmatic breathing
   b. Unilateral chest expansion
   c. Pursed-lip breathing
   d. Directed cough
   NOTE: When a patient does not seem to do well, it usually may be attributed to poor instruction.

2. Complete the following steps as if you were going to perform these techniques with a patient:
   a. Wash your hands.
   b. Assess the patient:
      (1) Auscultation of breath sounds
      (2) Oximetry
      (3) Determination of heart and respiratory rates
      (4) Assess the work of breathing
   c. Instruct the patient on these techniques:
      (1) Diaphragmatic breathing
      (2) Unilateral chest expansion
      (3) Pursed-lip breathing
      (4) Directed cough
   d. Assist the patient with coughing following the adjunctive exercises.
   e. Wash your hands.
   f. Using a blank sheet of paper, chart the procedure and have your laboratory instructor critique it.

Check List: Patient Positioning

_____   1. Properly identify the patient.
_____   2. Wash your hands.
_____   3. Explain the procedure to the patient.
         4. Use the following guidelines in moving your patient:
_____   a. Stand with correct alignment and balance.
_____   b. Adjust the working surface to waist height.
_____   c. Use the major muscle groups.
_____   d. Use a wide stance for a good base of support.
_____   e. Use your body weight to your advantage.
_____   f. Allow gravity to assist.
_____   5. Operate the electric bed correctly.

         6. Position the patient to the desired position:
_____   a. Allow the patient to assist.
_____   b. Allow the patient to move at his or her own speed.
_____   c. Maintain patient safety at all times.
_____   d. Maintain good body alignment.
         7. Use safety devices properly:
_____   a. Use bed rails correctly.
_____   b. Use restraints properly as required:
_____   (1) Chest and waist
_____   (2) Wrist and ankle
_____   c. Position the nurse call button within reach.
_____   d. Observe the position of the code switch.
_____   8. Check for hazards before leaving the room.

Check List: Postural Drainage and Chest Percussion

_____ 1. Review the patient's chart.
2. Gather the appropriate equipment:
_____ a. Tissues for the patient (if there are none at the bedside)
_____ b. Stethoscope
_____ c. Sputum cup or container
_____ d. Mechanical percussors if required
3. Introduce yourself and explain the procedure.
_____ a. Use simple, easily understood terms.
_____ 4. Follow standard precautions, including hand-washing.
5. Assess your patient as follows:
_____ a. Take the pulse.
_____ b. Inspect skin color.
_____ c. Determine respiratory rate.
_____ d. Auscultate the chest.
_____ e. Percuss the chest.
_____ 6. Position the patient to drain the correct segments or lobes.
7. Following drainage, perform chest percussion or clapping:
_____ a. Identify landmarks.
_____ b. Do not redden the skin.

_____ c. Avoid bony structures, the spine, the abdomen, and breast tissue in a female patient.
8. Perform vibration following percussion.
_____ a. Use proper technique.
_____ b. Vibrate only on exhalation.
_____ 9. Leave the patient in each position for the proper duration.
10. Monitor the following:
_____ a. Pulse
_____ b. Skin color
_____ c. Respiratory rate
_____ d. Redness of the skin
_____ 11. Assist the patient with coughing after treating an area.
12. Leave the patient safe and comfortable.
_____ a. Clean up the area and dispose of materials as appropriate
_____ 13. Reassess breath sounds.
_____ 14. Record the procedure in the patient's chart.

Check List: PEP Therapy

_____ 1. Verify the physician's order.
_____ 2. Scan the chart for relevant information.
_____ 3. Perform hand hygiene.
_____ 4. Obtain and assemble your equipment.
_____ 5. Introduce yourself and explain the procedure.
_____ 6. Position the patient properly.
_____ 7. Assess the patient prior to therapy.
_____ 8. Instruct the patient on PEP therapy.

_____ 9. Assist and coach the patient during therapy.
_____ 10. Periodically have the patient cough.
_____ 11. Monitor the patient during therapy.
_____ 12. Assess the patient following therapy.
_____ 13. Clean up after yourself.
_____ 14. Ensure that the patient is safe and comfortable.
_____ 15. Document the procedure in the patient's chart.

Check List: Flutter Valve Therapy/Vibratory PEP (Acapella®) Therapy

_____ 1. Verify the physician's order.
_____ 2. Scan the chart for relevant information.
_____ 3. Perform hand hygiene.
_____ 4. Obtain and assemble your equipment.
_____ 5. Introduce yourself and explain the procedure.
_____ 6. Position the patient properly.
_____ 7. Assess the patient prior to therapy.
_____ 8. Instruct the patient on Flutter valve therapy.

_____ 9. Assist and coach the patient during therapy.
_____ 10. Periodically, have the patient cough.
_____ 11. Monitor the patient during therapy.
_____ 12. Assess the patient following therapy.
_____ 13. Clean up after yourself.
_____ 14. Ensure that the patient is safe and comfortable.
_____ 15. Document the procedure in the patient's chart.

Check List: HFCWO Therapy—(The Vest® Airway Clearance System)

_____ 1. Verify the physician's order.
_____ 2. Scan the chart for relevant information.
_____ 3. Perform hand hygiene.
4. Obtain and assemble the equipment:
_____   a. The vest
_____   b. Two large-diameter tubes
_____   c. The air-pulse generator
_____ 5. Introduce yourself and explain the procedure.
_____ 6. Position the patient properly.
_____ 7. Assess the patient prior to therapy.

_____ 8. Instruct the patient on applying the vest.
_____ 9. Set the controls correctly.
_____ 10. Assist and coach the patient during therapy.
_____ 11. Periodically, have the patient cough.
_____ 12. Monitor the patient during therapy.
_____ 13. Assess the patient following therapy.
_____ 14. Clean up after yourself.
_____ 15. Ensure that the patient is safe and comfortable.
_____ 16. Document the procedure in the patient's chart.

Check List: Coughassist™ Mechanical In-Exsufflator

_____ 1. Verify the physician's order.
_____ 2. Scan the chart for relevant information.
_____ 3. Perform hand hygiene.
4. Assemble the equipment:
_____   a. Coughassist™ MI-E
_____   b. Patient circuit
_____   c. Patient interface (mask, tracheostomy adapter, or mouthpiece)
_____ 5. Set the insufflation/exsufflation pressures.
_____ 6. Set the time intervals (inhalation, exhalation, pause).
_____ 7. Introduce yourself and explain the procedure.
_____ 8. Position the patient properly.
_____ 9. Assess the patient prior to therapy.
_____ 10. Instruct the patient on how the therapy will proceed.

_____ 11. Assist and coach the patient during therapy.
12. Monitor the patient for adverse events.
_____   a. Hyperventilation
_____   b. Difficulty breathing
_____   c. Cardiac arrhythmias
_____   d. Gastric distention
_____ 13. Allow for rest periods after 4 to 5 cycles.
_____ 14. Assist the patient with secretion removal.
_____ 15. Assess the patient following therapy.
_____ 16. Clean up after yourself following the procedure.
_____ 17. Ensure that the patient is safe and comfortable.
_____ 18. Document the procedure in the patient's chart.

Check List: Adjunctive Breathing Exercises

_____ 1. Verify the physician's order.
_____ 2. Scan the chart for relevant information.
_____ 3. Perform hand hygiene.
_____ 4. Introduce yourself and explain the procedure.
_____ 5. Position the patient properly.
_____ 6. Assess the patient prior to therapy.
7. Instruct the patient on the adjunctive techniques:
_____   a. Diaphragmatic breathing
_____   b. Unilateral chest expansion
_____   c. Pursed-lip breathing
_____   d. Directed cough

_____ 8. Assist and coach the patient during technique performance.
_____ 9. Periodically have the patient cough.
_____ 10. Monitor the patient during therapy.
_____ 11. Assess the patient following therapy.
_____ 12. Clean up after yourself.
_____ 13. Ensure that the patient is safe and comfortable.
_____ 14. Document the procedure in the patient's chart.

Self-Evaluation Post Test: Bronchial Hygiene Therapy

1. The practice of good body mechanics is necessary to:
   a. prevent damage to hospital equipment.
   b. aid in patient rehabilitation.
   c. prevent strain, fatigue, and injuries.
   d. aid in equipment maintenance.

2. To lift a heavy object, you should:
   I. bend at the waist.
   II. use your back.
   III. squat.
   IV. use your legs.
   a. I, IV   c. III, IV
   b. I, II   d. II, III

3. Injuries are more frequent when:
   a. the body is in poor alignment.
   b. the body is balanced.
   c. a wide base of support is used.
   d. large muscle groups are used.

4. The position that facilitates the greatest chest expansion is:
   a. dangling.   c. prone.
   b. Fowler's.   d. supine.

5. The contraindications to PEP therapy may include:
   a. acute sinusitis.   c. pneumonia.
   b. atelectasis.   d. cystic fibrosis.

6. You should never percuss:
   I. the sternum.
   II. breast tissue in an adult female patient.
   III. the spinal column.
   IV. the abdomen.
   a. I   c. I, II, III
   b. I, II   d. I, II, III, IV

7. Which of the following is/are (an) indication(s) for Flutter valve therapy?
   a. Retained secretions
   b. Atelectasis
   c. Routine therapy for cystic fibrosis
   d. All of the above

8. A patient in position for draining the posterior basal segments of both lungs complains of a headache when coughing. The most likely cause is:
   a. increased abdominal pressure.
   b. neck vein engorgement.
   c. increased intrapleural pressure.
   d. increased intracranial pressure.

9. A patient positioned one-quarter turn from prone, resting on the left side and supported against pillows, will experience drainage of the:
   a. superior segment of the right lower lobe.
   b. apical segment of the right upper lobe.
   c. posterior segment of the right upper lobe.
   d. superior segment of the left lower lobe.

10. The Coughassist™ Mechanical In-Exsufflator:
    I. provides positive pressure during inhalation.
    II. provides negative pressure during exhalation.
    III. is intended for intermittent use.
    IV. facilitates secretion removal.
    a. I   c. I, II, III
    b. I, II   d. I, II, III, IV

PERFORMANCE EVALUATION:
Patient Positioning

Date: Lab _____ Clinical _____ Agency _____

Lab: Pass _____ Fail _____ Clinical: Pass _____ Fail _____

Student name _____ Instructor name _____

No. of times observed in clinical _____

No. of times practiced in clinical _____

PASSING CRITERIA: Obtain 90% or better on the procedure. Tasks indicated by * must receive at least 1 point, or the evaluation is terminated. Procedure must be performed within the designated time, or the performance receives a failing grade.

SCORING: 2 points — Task performed satisfactorily without prompting.
1 point — Task performed satisfactorily with self-initiated correction.
0 points — Task performed incorrectly or with prompting required.
NA — Task not applicable to the patient care situation.

Tasks:	Peer	Lab	Clinical
* 1. Properly identifies the patient	☐	☐	☐
2. Explains the procedure to the patient	☐	☐	☐
* 3. Follows standard precautions, including handwashing	☐	☐	☐
4. Uses the following during procedure			
* a. Stands with correct alignment	☐	☐	☐
* b. Adjusts the working surface level	☐	☐	☐
* c. Uses the major muscle groups	☐	☐	☐
* d. Uses a wide base of support	☐	☐	☐
* e. Uses body weight to advantage	☐	☐	☐
* f. Uses gravity when possible	☐	☐	☐
* 5. Operates the electric bed correctly	☐	☐	☐
* 6. Places the patient in the desired position			
* a. Allows the patient to assist	☐	☐	☐
* b. Allows the patient to move at his or her own speed	☐	☐	☐
* c. Maintains patient safety	☐	☐	☐
* d. Maintains good alignment	☐	☐	☐

7. Uses the safety devices properly

*   a. Ensures that restraints are secured correctly

*   b. Places the nurse call button within reach

*   c. Identifies the code switch

   d. Ensures that the bed rails are up

*   **8.** Checks the room for safety hazards

SCORE: Peer _____ points of possible 38; _____%

   Lab _____ points of possible 38; _____%

   Clinical _____ points of possible 38; _____%

TIME: _____ out of possible 20 minutes

STUDENT SIGNATURES

PEER: _____

STUDENT: _____

INSTRUCTOR SIGNATURES

LAB: _____

CLINICAL: _____

PERFORMANCE EVALUATION:
Chest Percussion and Postural Drainage

Date: Lab _____ Clinical _____ Agency _____

Lab: Pass _____ Fail _____ Clinical: Pass _____ Fail _____

Student name _____ Instructor name _____

No. of times observed in clinical _____

No. of times practiced in clinical _____

PASSING CRITERIA: Obtain 90% or better on the procedure. Tasks indicated by * must receive at least 1 point, or the evaluation is terminated. Procedure must be performed within the designated time, or the performance receives a failing grade.

SCORING: 2 points — Task performed satisfactorily without prompting.
1 point — Task performed satisfactorily with self-initiated correction.
0 points — Task performed incorrectly or with prompting required.
NA — Task not applicable to the patient care situation.

Tasks:	Peer	Lab	Clinical
* 1. Verifies the physician's order	☐	☐	☐
* 2. Follows standard precautions, including handwashing	☐	☐	☐
3. Introduces self and explains the procedure	☐	☐	☐
* 4. Places the patient into proper position	☐	☐	☐
5. Percusses the patient's chest			
* a. Does not redden the skin	☐	☐	☐
* b. Makes a loud popping sound	☐	☐	☐
* c. Percusses over segments being drained	☐	☐	☐
* 6. Ensures that vibration does not exert excessive pressure	☐	☐	☐
* 7. Vibrates only on exhalation	☐	☐	☐
8. Percusses and vibrates over a light cover	☐	☐	☐
* 9. Leaves the patient in position for the proper length of time	☐	☐	☐
10. Monitors the patient's condition			
* a. Pulse	☐	☐	☐
* b. Color	☐	☐	☐
* c. Respiratory rate	☐	☐	☐
* 11. Assists the patient to cough	☐	☐	☐
* 12. Has expectoration supplies nearby	☐	☐	☐

13. Leaves the patient safe and comfortable ☐ ☐ ☐

* **14.** Records the procedure on the chart ☐ ☐ ☐

SCORE: Peer _____ points of possible 36; _____%

Lab _____ points of possible 36; _____%

Clinical _____ points of possible 36; _____%

TIME: _____ out of possible 20 minutes

STUDENT SIGNATURES   **INSTRUCTOR SIGNATURES**

PEER: _____   LAB: _____

STUDENT: _____   CLINICAL: _____

PERFORMANCE EVALUATION:
PEP Mask Therapy

Date: Lab _____ Clinical _____ Agency _____

Lab: Pass _____ Fail _____ Clinical: Pass _____ Fail _____

Student name _____ Instructor name _____

No. of times observed in clinical _____

No. of times practiced in clinical _____

PASSING CRITERIA: Obtain 90% or better on the procedure. Tasks indicated by * must receive at least 1 point, or the evaluation is terminated. Procedure must be performed within the designated time, or the performance receives a failing grade.

SCORING: 2 points — Task performed satisfactorily without prompting.
1 point — Task performed satisfactorily with self-initiated correction.
0 points — Task performed incorrectly or with prompting required.
NA — Task not applicable to the patient care situation.

Tasks:	Peer	Lab	Clinical
* **1.** Verifies the physician's order	☐	☐	☐
* **2.** Scans the chart for relevant information	☐	☐	☐
* **3.** Follows standard precautions, including handwashing	☐	☐	☐
4. Obtains and assembles the equipment	☐	☐	☐
5. Introduces self and explains the procedure	☐	☐	☐
6. Positions the patient properly	☐	☐	☐
* **7.** Assesses the patient prior to therapy	☐	☐	☐
* **8.** Instructs the patient on PEP mask therapy	☐	☐	☐
* **9.** Assists and coaches the patient during therapy	☐	☐	☐
10. Periodically has the patient cough	☐	☐	☐
11. Monitors the patient during therapy	☐	☐	☐
12. Assesses the patient following therapy	☐	☐	☐
13. Cleans up	☐	☐	☐
14. Ensures that the patient is safe and comfortable	☐	☐	☐
15. Documents the procedure in the patient's chart	☐	☐	☐

SCORE: Peer   _____ points of possible 30; _____%

                 Lab   _____ points of possible 30; _____%

                 Clinical _____ points of possible 30; _____%

TIME: _____ out of possible 30 minutes

STUDENT SIGNATURES   **INSTRUCTOR SIGNATURES**

PEER: _____   LAB: _____

STUDENT: _____   CLINICAL: _____

PERFORMANCE EVALUATION:

Flutter Valve Therapy/Vibratory PEP (Acapella®) Therapy

Date: Lab _____ Clinical _____ Agency _____

Lab: Pass _____ Fail _____ Clinical: Pass _____ Fail _____

Student name _____ Instructor name _____

No. of times observed in clinical _____

No. of times practiced in clinical _____

PASSING CRITERIA: Obtain 90% or better on the procedure. Tasks indicated by * must receive at least 1 point, or the evaluation is terminated. Procedure must be performed within the designated time, or the performance receives a failing grade.

SCORING: 2 points — Task performed satisfactorily without prompting.
1 point — Task performed satisfactorily with self-initiated correction.
0 points — Task performed incorrectly or with prompting required.
NA — Task not applicable to the patient care situation.

Tasks:	Peer	Lab	Clinical
* 1. Verifies the physician's order	☐	☐	☐
* 2. Scans the chart for relevant information	☐	☐	☐
* 3. Follows standard precautions, including handwashing	☐	☐	☐
4. Obtains and assembles the equipment	☐	☐	☐
5. Introduces self and explains the procedure	☐	☐	☐
6. Positions the patient properly	☐	☐	☐
* 7. Assesses the patient prior to therapy	☐	☐	☐
* 8. Instructs the patient on Flutter valve/Acapella®	☐	☐	☐
* 9. Assists and coaches the patient during therapy	☐	☐	☐
10. Periodically has the patient cough	☐	☐	☐
11. Monitors the patient during therapy	☐	☐	☐
12. Assesses the patient following therapy	☐	☐	☐
13. Cleans up	☐	☐	☐
14. Ensures that the patient is safe and comfortable	☐	☐	☐
15. Documents the procedure in the patient's chart	☐	☐	☐

SCORE: Peer   _____ points of possible 30; _____%

                       Lab   _____ points of possible 30; _____%

                       Clinical _____ points of possible 30; _____%

TIME: _____ out of possible 30 minutes

STUDENT SIGNATURES

PEER: _____

STUDENT: _____

INSTRUCTOR SIGNATURES

LAB: _____

CLINICAL: _____

PERFORMANCE EVALUATION:
HFCWO (The Vest® Airway Clearance System)

Date: Lab _____ Clinical _____ Agency _____

Lab: Pass _____ Fail _____ Clinical: Pass _____ Fail _____

Student name _____ Instructor name _____

No. of times observed in clinical _____

No. of times practiced in clinical _____

PASSING CRITERIA: Obtain 90% or better on the procedure. Tasks indicated by * must receive at least 1 point, or the evaluation is terminated. Procedure must be performed within the designated time, or the performance receives a failing grade.

SCORING: 2 points — Task performed satisfactorily without prompting.
1 point — Task performed satisfactorily with self-initiated correction.
0 points — Task performed incorrectly or with prompting required.
NA — Task not applicable to the patient care situation.

Tasks:	Peer	Lab	Clinical
* 1. Verifies the physician's order	☐	☐	☐
* 2. Scans the chart for relevant information	☐	☐	☐
* 3. Follows standard precautions, including handwashing	☐	☐	☐
4. Obtains and assembles the equipment			
a. The vest	☐	☐	☐
b. Two large-diameter tubes	☐	☐	☐
c. The air-pulse generator	☐	☐	☐
5. Introduces self and explains the procedure	☐	☐	☐
6. Positions the patient properly	☐	☐	☐
* 7. Assesses the patient prior to therapy	☐	☐	☐
* 8. Instructs the patient on applying the vest	☐	☐	☐
* 9. Sets the controls correctly	☐	☐	☐
* 10. Assists and coaches the patient during therapy	☐	☐	☐
11. Periodically has the patient cough	☐	☐	☐
12. Monitors the patient during therapy	☐	☐	☐
13. Assesses the patient following therapy	☐	☐	☐
14. Cleans up	☐	☐	☐

15. Ensures that the patient is safe and comfortable ☐ ☐ ☐

16. Documents the procedure in the patient's chart ☐ ☐ ☐

SCORE: Peer _____ points of possible 36; _____%

Lab _____ points of possible 36; _____%

Clinical _____ points of possible 36; _____%

TIME: _____ out of possible 30 minutes

STUDENT SIGNATURES **INSTRUCTOR SIGNATURES**

PEER: _____ LAB: _____

STUDENT: _____ CLINICAL: _____

PERFORMANCE EVALUATION:
Coughassist™ Mechanical In-Exsufflator

Date: Lab _____ Clinical _____ Agency _____

Lab: Pass _____ Fail _____ Clinical: Pass _____ Fail _____

Student name _____ Instructor name _____

No. of times observed in clinical _____

No. of times practiced in clinical _____

PASSING CRITERIA: Obtain 90% or better on the procedure. Tasks indicated by * must receive at least 1 point, or the evaluation is terminated. Procedure must be performed within the designated time, or the performance receives a failing grade.

SCORING: 2 points — Task performed satisfactorily without prompting.
1 point — Task performed satisfactorily with self-initiated correction.
0 points — Task performed incorrectly or with prompting required.
NA — Task not applicable to the patient care situation.

Tasks:	Peer	Lab	Clinical
* 1. Verify the physician's order	☐	☐	☐
2. Scans the chart for relevant information	☐	☐	☐
* 3. Performs hand hygiene	☐	☐	☐
4. Assembles the equipment			
* a. Coughassist™ MI-E	☐	☐	☐
* b. Patient circuit	☐	☐	☐
* c. Patient interface	☐	☐	☐
* 5. Sets the insufflation/exsufflation pressures	☐	☐	☐
* 6. Sets the time intervals (inhalation, exhalation, pause)	☐	☐	☐
7. Introduces self and explains the procedure	☐	☐	☐
* 8. Positions the patient properly	☐	☐	☐
* 9. Assesses the patient prior to therapy	☐	☐	☐
* 10. Instructs the patient	☐	☐	☐
* 11. Assists and coaches the patient during therapy	☐	☐	☐
12. Monitors the patient for adverse events			
* a. Hyperventilation	☐	☐	☐
* b. Difficulty breathing	☐	☐	☐

*   c. Cardiac arrhythmias   ☐   ☐   ☐

*   d. Gastric distention   ☐   ☐   ☐

* **13.** Allows for rest periods after 4 to 5 cycles   ☐   ☐   ☐

* **14.** Assists the patient with secretion removal   ☐   ☐   ☐

* **15.** Assesses the patient following therapy   ☐   ☐   ☐

16. Cleans up after self following the procedure   ☐   ☐   ☐

* **17.** Ensures that the patient is safe and comfortable   ☐   ☐   ☐

* **18.** Documents the procedure in the patient's chart   ☐   ☐   ☐

SCORE: Peer _____ points of possible 46; _____%

Lab _____ points of possible 46; _____%

Clinical _____ points of possible 46; _____%

TIME: _____ out of possible 30 minutes

STUDENT SIGNATURES   **INSTRUCTOR SIGNATURES**

PEER: _____   LAB: _____

STUDENT: _____   CLINICAL: _____

PERFORMANCE EVALUATION:
Adjunctive Breathing Techniques

Date: Lab _____ Clinical _____ Agency _____

Lab: Pass _____ Fail _____ Clinical: Pass _____ Fail _____

Student name _____ Instructor name _____

No. of times observed in clinical _____

No. of times practiced in clinical _____

PASSING CRITERIA: Obtain 90% or better on the procedure. Tasks indicated by * must receive at least 1 point, or the evaluation is terminated. Procedure must be performed within the designated time, or the performance receives a failing grade.

SCORING: 2 points — Task performed satisfactorily without prompting.
1 point — Task performed satisfactorily with self-initiated correction.
0 points — Task performed incorrectly or with prompting required.
NA — Task not applicable to the patient care situation.

Tasks:	Peer	Lab	Clinical
* 1. Verifies the physician's order	☐	☐	☐
* 2. Scans the chart for relevant information	☐	☐	☐
* 3. Follows standard precautions, including handwashing	☐	☐	☐
4. Introduces self and explains the procedure	☐	☐	☐
* 5. Positions the patient properly	☐	☐	☐
* 6. Assesses the patient prior to therapy	☐	☐	☐
7. Instructs the patient on the adjunctive techniques			
* a. Diaphragmatic breathing	☐	☐	☐
* b. Unilateral chest expansion	☐	☐	☐
* c. Pursed-lip breathing	☐	☐	☐
* d. Directed cough	☐	☐	☐
* 8. Assists and coaches the patient during technique performance	☐	☐	☐
9. Periodically has the patient cough	☐	☐	☐
10. Monitors the patient during therapy	☐	☐	☐
11. Assesses the patient following therapy	☐	☐	☐
12. Cleans up after the procedure	☐	☐	☐
13. Ensures that the patient is safe and comfortable	☐	☐	☐
14. Documents the procedure in the patient's chart	☐	☐	☐

SCORE: Peer _____ points of possible 34; _____%

Lab _____ points of possible 34; _____%

Clinical _____ points of possible 34; _____%

TIME: _____ out of possible 20 minutes

STUDENT SIGNATURES

PEER: _____

STUDENT: _____

INSTRUCTOR SIGNATURES

LAB: _____

CLINICAL: _____

The goal of hyperinflation therapy is to facilitate hyperinflation of the lungs, thereby preventing or reversing atelectasis, facilitating mobilization of secretions, and promoting effective coughing. Incentive spirometry, intermittent positive-pressure breathing (IPPB) therapy, and intrapulmonary percussive ventilation (IPV) therapy all are common modalities used to accomplish these goals.

Incentive spirometry relies on patient effort and muscular strength to accomplish its therapeutic goal. The incentive spirometer is used primarily to monitor and reinforce a patient's effort. It is a relatively inexpensive device that is effective in reducing postoperative complications (Lawrence, 2006).

IPPB therapy uses a mechanical ventilator to deliver positive pressure during inspiration. The extra pressure assists the patient to take deeper breaths.

IPV therapy is a combination of high-frequency phased pulse gas delivery and the administration of a dense aerosol. IPV therapy is administered using a special high-frequency ventilator. The high-frequency pulsed inspiratory gas flow increases mean airway pressure, whereas the percussive effect of the pulses assists in mobilization and clearance of secretions.

The respiratory practitioner must be familiar with the procedures and equipment used. The potential hazards, complications, and the desired therapeutic goals and objectives should be thoroughly understood.

KEY TERMS

- **Incentive spirometer**
- **Incentive spirometry**
- **Intermittent positive-pressure breathing (IPPB)**
- **Intrapulmonary percussive ventilation (IPV)**

THEORY OBJECTIVES

At the end of this chapter, the reader should be able to:

- *Define the following:*
  - *Incentive spirometry*
  - *Intermittent positive-pressure breathing (IPPB) therapy*
  - *Intrapulmonary percussive ventilation (IPV) therapy*
- *Compare and contrast the clinical goals and indications of the following hyperinflation modalities:*
  - *Incentive spirometry*
  - *IPPB therapy*
  - *IPV therapy*
- *State the hazards, contraindications, and complications associated with the following hyperinflation modalities:*
  - *Incentive spirometry*
  - *IPPB therapy*
  - *IPV therapy*
- *Describe how Voldyne or Triflow incentive spirometer measure volume.*

Bird Mark 7A Ventilator

- *Identify the following component parts:*
  - *Ambient chamber*
  - *Pressure chamber*
  - *Center body*
- *Identify and explain the function of the following controls:*
  - *Sensitivity*
  - *Flow rate*
  - *Apneustic time control*
  - *Expiratory timer*
  - *Time/pressure trigger control*
  - *Pressure*
- *Describe the effect each of the controls has on the following:*
  - *Tidal volume*
  - *FIO_2*
  - *I:E ratio*

- *Trace the flow of gas through the Bird Mark 7 breathing circuit.*

IPV Therapy

- *Describe the controls of the IPV-1C ventilator:*
  - *Operational pressure*

  - *Impact control*
  - *Manual inspiration*
- *Identify the components of the Phasitron and how it works.*
- *Describe how to increase tidal delivery and how to increase or decrease the percussive frequency.*

CLINICAL PRACTICE GUIDELINES

AARC Clinical Practice Guideline Incentive Spirometry

IS 5.0 INDICATIONS

5.1 Preoperative screening of patients at risk for postoperative complications to obtain baseline flow or volume.[16,39,40]

5.2 Respiratory therapy that includes daily sessions of incentive spirometry plus deep breathing exercises, directed coughing, early ambulation, and optimal analgesia may lower the incidence of postoperative pulmonary complications.

5.3 Presence of pulmonary atelectasis or conditions predisposing to the development of pulmonary atelectasis when used with:

5.3.1 Upper-abdominal or thoracic surgery[6]

5.3.2 Lower-abdominal surgery[41]

5.3.3 Prolonged bed rest

5.3.4 Surgery in patients with COPD

5.3.5 Lack of pain control[42]

5.3.6 Presence of thoracic or abdominal binders

5.3.7 Restrictive lung defect associated with a dysfunctional diaphragm or involving the respiratory musculature

    5.3.7.1 Patients with inspiratory capacity < 2.5 L[43]

    5.3.7.2 Patients with neuromuscular disease

    5.3.7.3 Patients with spinal cord injury[44]

5.4 Incentive spirometry may prevent atelectasis associated with the acute chest syndrome in patients with sickle cell disease.[42,45]

5.5 In patients undergoing coronary artery bypass graft[46]

    5.5.1 Incentive spirometry and positive airway pressure therapy may improve pulmonary function and 6-minute walk distance and reduce the incidence of postoperative complications.[47,48]

IS 6.0 CONTRAINDICATIONS

6.1 Patients who cannot be instructed or supervised to assure appropriate use of the device

6.2 Patients in whom cooperation is absent or patients unable to understand or demonstrate proper use of the device

6.2.1 Very young patients and others with developmental delays

6.2.2 Patients who are confused or delirious

6.2.3 Patients who are heavily sedated or comatose

6.4 Incentive spirometry is contraindicated in patients unable to deep breathe effectively due to pain, diaphragmatic dysfunction, or opiate analgesia.[5]

6.5 Patients unable to generate adequate inspiration with a vital capacity < 10 mL/kg or an inspiratory capacity < 33% of predicted normal.[5]

IS 7.0 HAZARDS AND COMPLICATIONS

7.1 Ineffective unless performed as instructed

7.2 Hyperventilation/respiratory alkalosis

7.3 Hypoxemia secondary to interruption of prescribed oxygen therapy

7.4 Fatigue

7.5 Pain

IS 8.0 ASSESSMENT OF NEED

8.1 Surgical procedure involving abdomen or thorax

8.2 Conditions predisposing to development of atelectasis, including immobility and abdominal binders

IS 9.0 ASSESSMENT OF OUTCOME

9.1 Resolution or improvement in signs of atelectasis

9.1.1 Decreased respiratory rate

9.1.2 Absence of fever

9.1.3 Normal pulse rate

9.1.4 Improvement in previously absent or diminished breath sounds

9.1.5 Improved radiographic findings

9.1.6 Improved arterial oxygenation (P_{aO_2}, S_{aO_2}, S_{pO_2}), reduced F_{IO_2} requirement

IS 10.0 RESOURCES

10.1 Equipment

10.1.1 Volume-oriented incentive spirometer

    10.1.1.1 volume-oriented incentive spirometers are frequently associated with lower imposed work of breathing and larger

(Continued)

inspiratory lung volume than flow-oriented incentive spirometers.[43,49-52]

10.1.1.2 Incentive spirometers with a low additional imposed work of breathing might be more suitable for postoperative respiratory training.[43]

10.1.2 Flow-oriented incentive spirometer

10.2 Personnel

10.2.1 Clinical personnel should possess:

10.2.1.1 Ability to implement standard/universal precautions

10.2.1.2 Mastery of techniques for proper operation and clinical application of device

10.2.1.3 Ability to instruct patient in proper technique

10.2.1.4 Ability to respond appropriately to adverse effects

10.2.1.5 Ability to identify need for therapy, response to therapy, and need to discontinue ineffective therapy

IS 11.0 MONITORING

Direct supervision of every patient use of incentive spirometry is not necessary once the patient has demonstrated mastery of technique. However, intermittent reassessment is essential to optimal performance.

11.1 Observation of patient performance and utilization

11.1.1 Frequency of sessions

11.1.2 Number of breaths/session

11.1.3 inspiratory volume, flow, and breath-hold goals achieved

11.1.4 Effort/motivation

11.2 Device within reach of patient to encourage performing without supervision

Reprinted with permission from *Respiratory Care* 2011; 56: 1600–1604. The complete AARC Clinical Practice Guidelines are available from the AARC Web site (http://www.aarc.org), from the AARC Executive Office, or from *Respiratory Care* journal.

AARC Clinical Practice Guideline: Intermittent Positive-Pressure Breathing

IPPB 4.0 INDICATIONS:

4.1 The need to improve lung expansion

4.1.1 The presence of clinically significant pulmonary atelectasis when other forms of therapy have been unsuccessful (incentive spirometry, chest physiotherapy, deep breathing exercises, positive airway pressure) or the patient cannot cooperate[13-18]

4.1.2 Inability to clear secretions adequately because of pathology that severely limits the ability to ventilate or cough effectively and failure to respond to other modes of treatment[17]

4.2 The need for short-term ventilatory support for patients who are hypoventilating as an alternative to tracheal intubation and continuous mechanical ventilation.[16-25] Devices specifically designed to deliver noninvasive positive pressure ventilation (NPPV) should be considered.

4.3 The need to deliver aerosol medication.[4] (We are not addressing aerosol delivery for patients on long-term mechanical ventilation.)

4.3.1 Some clinicians oppose the use of IPPB in the treatment of severe bronchospasm (acute asthma or status asthmaticus, and exacerbated COPD);[6,26-28] however, a careful, closely supervised trial of IPPB as a medication delivery device when treatment using other techniques (metered-dose inhaler [MDI] or nebulizer) has been unsuccessful may be warranted.[1,28-36]

4.3.2 IPPB may be used to deliver aerosol medications to patients with fatigue as a result of ventilatory muscle weakness (eg, failure to wean from mechanical ventilation, neuromuscular disease, kyphoscoliosis, spinal injury) or chronic conditions in which intermittent ventilatory support is indicated (eg, ventilatory support for home care patients and the more recent use of nasal IPPV for respiratory insufficiency).[1,19-25,37]

4.3.3 In patients with severe hyperinflation, IPPB may decrease dyspnea and discomfort during nebulized therapy.[38]

IPPB 5.0 CONTRAINDICATIONS:

There are several clinical situations in which IPPB should not be used. With the exception of untreated tension pneumothorax, most of these contraindications are relative:[39]

5.1 Tension pneumothorax (untreated)

5.2 Intracranial pressure (ICP) > 15 mm Hg

5.3 Hemodynamic instability

5.4 Recent facial, oral, or skull surgery

5.5 Tracheoesophageal fistula

5.6 Recent esophageal surgery

5.7 Active hemoptysis

5.8 Nausea

5.9 Air swallowing

5.10 Active untreated tuberculosis

5.11 Radiographic evidence of bleb

5.12 Singulation (hiccups)

IPPB 6.0 HAZARDS/COMPLICATIONS:

6.1 Increased airway resistance and work of breathing[40,41]

6.2 Barotrauma, pneumothorax[40]

6.3 Nosocomial infection[40]

6.4 Hypocarbia[4,42]

6.5 Hemoptysis[4,42]

(Continued)

6.6 Hyperoxia when oxygen is the gas source[40]
6.7 Gastric distention[40]
6.8 Impaction of secretions (associated with inadequately humidified gas mixture)[40]
6.9 Psychological dependence[40]
6.10 Impedance of venous return[40]
6.11 Exacerbation of hypoxemia
6.12 Hypoventilation or hyperventilation
6.13 Increased mismatch of ventilation and perfusion
6.14 Air trapping, auto-PEEP, overdistended alveoli

IPPB 8.0 ASSESSMENT OF NEED:

8.1 Presence of clinically significant atelectasis
8.2 Reduced pulmonary function as evidenced by reductions in timed volumes and vital capacity (eg, FEV1 < 65% predicted, FVC < 70% predicted, MVV < 50% predicted, 68 or VC < 10 mL/kg), precluding an effective cough
8.3 Neuromuscular disorders or kyphoscoliosis with associated decreases in lung volumes and capacities
8.4 Fatigue or muscle weakness with impending respiratory failure
8.5 Presence of acute severe bronchospasm or exacerbated COPD that fails to respond to other therapy
  8.5.1 Based on proven therapeutic efficacy, variety of medications, and cost-effectiveness, the MDI with a spacing device or holding chamber should be the first method to consider for administration of aerosol.[50,63–67,69,70]
  8.5.2 Regardless of the type of delivery device used (MDI with spacer or small volume, large-volume, or ultrasonic nebulizer), it is important to recognize that the dose of the drug needs to be titrated to give the maximum benefit.[45,47]
8.6 With demonstrated effectiveness, the patient's preference for a positive pressure device
8.7 IPPB may be indicated in patients who are at risk for the development of atelectasis and are unable or unwilling to deep breathe without assistance.[71]

IPPB 9.0 ASSESSMENT OF OUTCOME:

9.1 For lung expansion therapy, a minimum delivered tidal volume of at least 1/3 of the predicted IC (1/3 × 50 mL/kg) has been suggested. This corresponds to approximately 1200 mL in a 70 kg adult patient.[71]
9.2 An increase in FEV1 or peak flow
9.3 Cough more effective with treatment
9.4 Secretion clearance enhanced as a consequence of deep breathing and coughing
9.5 Chest radiograph improved
9.6 Breath sounds improved
9.7 Favorable patient subjective response

IPPB 11.0 MONITORING:

Items from the following list should be chosen as appropriate for the specific patient:
11.1 Performance of machine trigger sensitivity, peak pressure, flow setting, FIO_2, inspiratory time, expiratory time, plateau pressure, PEEP
11.2 Respiratory rate
11.3 Delivered tidal volume
11.4 Pulse rate and rhythm from ECG if available
11.5 Patient subjective response to therapy: pain, discomfort, dyspnea
11.6 Sputum production: quantity, color, consistency
11.7 Mental function
11.8 Skin color
11.9 Breath sounds
11.10 Blood pressure
11.11 Arterial hemoglobin saturation by pulse oximetry (if hypoxemia is suspected)
11.12 Intracranial pressure (ICP) in patients for whom ICP is of critical importance
11.13 Chest radiograph

Reprinted with permission from *Respiratory Care* 2003; 48: 540–546. The complete AARC Clinical Practice Guidelines are available from the AARC Web site (http://www.aarc.org), from the AARC Executive Office, or from *Respiratory Care* journal.

HYPERVENTILATION MODALITIES

Incentive Spirometry

Incentive spirometry is a modality that uses the patient's own muscular effort to accomplish hyperinflation of the lungs. A device commonly called an *incentive spirometer* is used to provide biofeedback on the degree of patient inspiratory effort. The patient is then encouraged to perform a voluntary maximal inspiration with a 3- to 5-second inspiratory hold before exhalation is begun.

Intermittent Positive-Pressure Breathing

Intermittent positive-pressure breathing (IPPB) is a therapeutic modality using a ventilator to deliver positive pressure during the inspiratory phase of breathing. The expiratory phase is passive and the patient exhales to ambient pressure. Typically, the breathing circuit includes a nebulizer to deliver a medication during the treatment. IPPB is a short-term therapeutic modality and is not a means of continuous ventilatory support.

Intrapulmonary Percussive Ventilation

Intrapulmonary percussive ventilation (IPV) is applied using a high-frequency ventilator. The delivery of small volumes of gas at a high frequency (100 to 250/min) to the airways via a mouthpiece serves to increase mean airway pressures, while the pulsed gas flow helps to break up secretions and to distribute ventilation more evenly. Coughing following IPV therapy further helps to mobilize and clear secretions. The capability to deliver a dense aerosol during therapy allows administration of bronchodilators or mucokinetic or vasoactive agents to promote bronchial hygiene further.

GOALS OF AND INDICATIONS FOR HYPERINFLATION THERAPY

Although the hyperinflation modalities are different, frequently their clinical goals and indications for therapy are similar.

Reversal of Atelectasis

Postoperative pain and the effects of anesthetics and analgesics reduce the depth of breathing and the frequency of coughing even in relatively normal patients. Often the result is atelectasis and, potentially, pneumonia.

The three hyperinflation modalities provide methods for expanding a patient's lungs. Incentive spirometry relies on a patient's own muscular effort to accomplish the task. To use this modality effectively, the patient must be alert, cooperative, and able to follow directions well. IPPB uses a ventilator to assist the patient. There is no apparent significant difference among hyperinflation methods in preventing postoperative pulmonary complications (Freitas, 2007).

Improvement of the Cough or Cough Mechanism

An increase in tidal volume will enable the patient to generate greater flows and volumes during a cough. The greater the flow, the more effective a cough will be in expelling secretions.

All hyperinflation modalities provide methods for increasing inspiratory volumes. Incentive spirometry can generate large intrapleural pressures. These pressures help to maintain airway patency and to prevent atelectasis. It has also been suggested that hyperinflation stimulates the type II alveolar cells to produce surfactant, a fluid that reduces alveolar surface tension. IPPB may assist some patients by providing augmented volumes to facilitate more effective coughing.

Medication Delivery

IPPB is unique among the three hyperinflation modalities in its ability to deliver medication. Aerosol deposition with volume-oriented IPPB delivery has been found to be equal to that achieved with more simple methods of aerosol therapy (Thomas & McIntosh, 1994). Additionally, some patients who have difficulty coordinating their respiratory pattern may receive more effective bronchodilator therapy with IPPB than with other, simpler methods of aerosol therapy.

HAZARDS AND COMPLICATIONS OF HYPERVENTILATION THERAPY

Hypocapnea Induced by Hyperventilation

Hyperventilation may occur as a result of any hyperinflation modality. Each results in the patient's taking deeper breaths than normal.

Commonly reported signs and symptoms are dizziness, a feeling of light-headedness, a tingling sensation, loss of balance, and headache. These adverse reactions can be prevented to some extent by providing frequent rest periods during therapy sessions. Allow the patient to rest for about 1 minute after five to seven breaths.

Interruption of Hypoxic Drive

Patients with severe chronic obstructive lung disease are stimulated to breathe because with this disease, the body senses a need for oxygen. The normal response to increased CO_2 levels—the hypoxic drive—is absent. If such patients are given too much oxygen, that stimulation to breathe may diminish or cease. Patients with chronic lung disease receiving oxygen therapy must be closely monitored with serial blood gas determinations or oximetry.

IPPB therapy is administered with compressed gas. Departmental policy and the availability of compressed air often determine whether air or oxygen is used. Most hospitals have oxygen piped into almost every room, making its administration convenient. When IPPB is administered with oxygen, the delivered oxygen concentration will range from approximately 64 to 90% if the air-mix mode is used during inspiration (McPherson, 1995). This concentration of oxygen may be very hazardous to the patient with severe chronic obstructive lung disease. If oxygen administration is required, an oxygen blender may be used to regulate precisely the concentration being delivered.

If in doubt, use compressed air as the source gas to power the ventilator. IPPB therapy may be administered safely in this way without the interruption of the hypoxic drive.

Decreased Cardiac Output

The application of IPPB increases the mean intrathoracic pressure during inspiration. The applied pressure is contained within the thoracic cavity, increasing the intrathoracic pressure above normal levels. IPPB therapy, if improperly administered, can compress the mediastinum enough to impede the venous return from the periphery through the vena cava. Impedance of venous return, combined with the squeezing effect on the mediastinum, will result in a markedly decreased cardiac output and a fall in blood pressure. The risk of these abnormalities is especially high if the patient is hypovolemic.

This hazard may be alleviated by maintaining the inspiratory-to-expiratory ratio (I:E ratio) within normal limits or greater. A normal I:E ratio in a spontaneously breathing person is 1:2—if inspiration occurs in 1 second, expiration will take 2 seconds. If IPPB is administered with an I:E ratio of 1:2 or greater, adequate time will be available to allow the great vessels and the heart to fill with blood. The expiratory phase in IPPB therapy is passive with no positive pressure applied. This lack of positive pressure will allow the intrathoracic pressure to return to normal levels.

The I:E ratio may be manipulated during IPPB therapy by the adjustment of the inspiratory flow control (if available) or by proper patient instruction.

Increased Intracranial Pressure

The increased intrathoracic pressure combined with decreased cardiac output may cause an increased intracranial pressure. Impedance of venous return results in backup of blood flow in the cranium. The skull is quite rigid, and expansion due to an increased volume is not possible. If venous return is impeded severely enough, intracranial pressure may go up significantly. Patients with already elevated intracranial pressures, due to head trauma or other causes, are more susceptible to development of increased intracranial pressure from IPPB therapy.

Increased intracranial pressure may be avoided by maintaining the I:E ratio during IPPB therapy at 1:2 or greater. This allows adequate filling of the great vessels and heart between the applications of positive pressure.

Pneumothorax

The incidence of pneumothorax resulting from IPPB therapy is low. If IPPB is administered using excessive volumes, caution should be exercised and the patient should be closely monitored.

Application of pressures exceeding 25 cm H_2O should be approached with caution. Ensure that the I:E ratio is maintained within normal ranges and carefully monitor exhaled volumes. Some patients may be able to tolerate this pressure, but others will not. Carefully monitor the patient when using pressures in this range. Observe the patient for the following signs or symptoms: sudden onset of chest pain and sudden onset of dyspnea. If the patient has either of these symptoms, discontinue therapy and carefully evaluate the patient.

Patients with end-stage emphysema may be especially at risk for this complication. The emphysematous lung's alveolar septa are destroyed in the disease process, leaving large blebs. These blebs trap air on expiration and are not capable of withstanding high pressures.

Untreated Pneumothorax

Administering IPPB therapy to a patient with an untreated pneumothorax is extremely hazardous and therefore contraindicated. A pneumothorax is the presence of free air in the thoracic cavity, predominantly in the pleural space. The usual treatment of the condition involves the placement of a chest tube into the pleural space and evacuation of the free air by the application of vacuum or suction.

Administering IPPB therapy to a patient with an untreated pneumothorax could cause a tension pneumothorax to develop. A tension pneumothorax is the presence of free air in the thoracic cavity at a pressure greater than ambient pressure. The pressure difference will cause lung collapse on the affected side with compression of the heart and great vessels, impeding the ability of the heart to circulate blood. If the pressure continues, eventual circulatory collapse may result.

If the practitioner suspects that a tension pneumothorax has developed during IPPB therapy, auscultate and percuss the chest. With pneumothorax, auscultation on the affected side will indicate absent or diminished breath sounds. Percussion on the affected side will yield a hyperresonant percussion tone. The practitioner may be able to observe deviation of the trachea to the unaffected side as a result of the compression caused by the pressure in the thoracic cavity from the tension pneumothorax. IPPB must be terminated and the pneumothorax must be treated immediately, as it is a life-threatening condition.

If a patient has a patent operating chest tube in place, IPPB therapy may be safely administered.

INCENTIVE SPIROMETERS

Voldyne Volumetric Exerciser

The Voldyne is a single-patient-use, disposable incentive spirometer manufactured by Sherwood Medical, St. Louis, MO. The Voldyne is a relatively simple device consisting of a vertical tube with a piston that indicates the inspired volume and a yellow float to indicate inspiratory flow. Figure 17-1 is a photograph of a Voldyne Volumetric Exerciser. As the patient inhales deeply, a negative pressure is created above the inspiratory float and the piston. The piston rises, indicating the maximum inspired volume. The yellow float will remain suspended as long as inspiratory flow exists. The patient is encouraged to inhale as deeply as possible and to achieve a maximal inspiratory volume. During the maneuver, encourage the patient to keep the yellow float suspended at all times. A movable marker may be raised or lowered, indicating the desired volume for the patient to achieve.

Triflow Incentive Spirometer

The Triflow incentive spirometer is a primary flow measuring incentive spirometer. It indicates inspiratory flow, rather than volume. There are three chambers, each containing a ball (Figure 17-2). When inspiratory flow is greater than 800 mL/second but less than

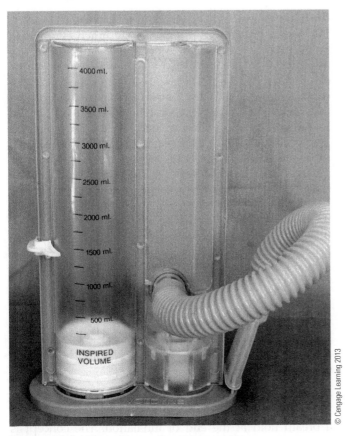

Figure 17-1 The voldyne volumetric exerciser

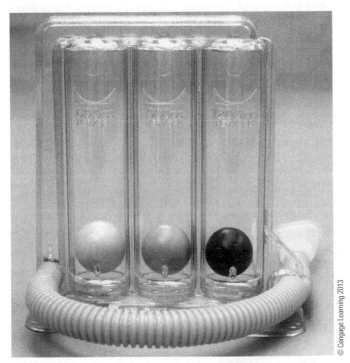

Figure 17-2 The triflow incentive spirometer

1000 mL/second, the first ball is suspended at the top of the chamber. The second ball is suspended when inspiratory flow is greater than 1000 mL/second but less than 1200 mL/second. The third ball is suspended when flow exceeds 1200 mL/second. The goal is to have the patient

suspend the maximum number of balls for a given amount of time (3–5 seconds). Volume is determined by multiplying the indicated flow rate by the number of seconds the ball is suspended at the top of the chamber.

THE BIRD MARK 7A VENTILATOR

The Bird Mark 7A is a pressure-limited patient- or time-cycled ventilator used in IPPB therapy. It is pneumatically powered, requiring a 50 psi compressed gas source for operation. Because of its pneumatic characteristics and delivered tidal volume, flow rate and oxygen concentration tend to change as the patient's respiratory status changes.

The Bird Mark 7A is a small, portable ventilator that may be powered with compressed gas cylinders or hospital piping systems. The Mark 7A is frequently used in the emergency and transport settings. Structurally the device may be divided into three main components: the ambient chamber on the left, made of a transparent green plastic; the center body in the middle, machined from an aluminum alloy; and the pressure chamber on the right, slightly smaller than the ambient chamber and made from a transparent green plastic.

Control Function

There are six controls that control the operation of the Bird Mark 7A ventilator. Figure 17-3 is a photograph of the Bird Mark 7A showing all of the controls. Each control is discussed in sequence in this section. If a Bird Mark 7A ventilator is available, refer to it upon reading the following descriptions.

Pressure

The pressure control regulates the amount of pressure that must build up in the breathing circuit before inspiration is terminated. In this manner it determines the

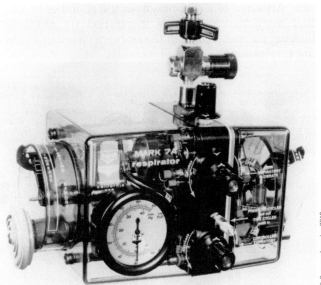

Figure 17-3 A photograph showing the controls on the Bird Mark 7A ventilator

tidal volume being delivered to the patient. The pressure control, in combination with the flow rate control, determines the tidal volume, I:E ratio, and delivered oxygen concentration.

Pressure is controlled by a movable arm on the far right of the ventilator. Figure 17-3 shows the pressure control. The control determines the position of a magnet relative to a metal plate. During inspiration, pressure builds in the pressure chamber and pushes against a diaphragm attached to the center body. Eventually, the force from the pressure exceeds the magnetic pull from the pressure control adjustment and moves the diaphragm to the left. When it does, a switch attached to the diaphragm cycles the ventilator off and inspiration is terminated.

Time/Pressure Trigger Control

The time/pressure trigger control is a pneumatic switch that determines if the ventilator is operating in pressure-triggered mode (IPPB therapy) or a time-triggered mode (patient with apnea). In the pressure-triggered mode, patient effort (subambient pressure) will trigger inspiration. In time-triggered mode, the expiratory timer (timing cartridge) will determine the initiation of inspiration. Time-triggered mode is not used for IPPB therapy.

Expiratory Timer

The expiratory timer is not used for IPPB therapy. It is used to cycle the ventilator on when a patient is apneic. Attempts to use it on a spontaneously breathing patient will cause asynchronous ventilation leading to increased work of breathing as well as frustration for both the practitioner and the patient. It is located at the base of the center body. Figure 17-3 shows the expiratory timer. This control is a pneumatic timer; it controls the ventilatory rate by allowing source gas to leak out of a closed chamber (timing cartridge). The faster the source gas leaks, the more quickly the chamber empties, increasing the ventilatory rate. Conversely, a slow leak will provide a long time interval, decreasing the rate. Attached to a diaphragm in the chamber is a rod that mechanically triggers inspiration by physically moving the metal plate in the ambient chamber, initiating inspiration.

Sensitivity

The sensitivity control regulates how much effort must be exerted by the patient to cycle the ventilator on for inspiration. It is controlled by a movable arm on the extreme left-hand side. Figure 17-3 shows the sensitivity control. Functionally, the sensitivity control determines the position of a magnet relative to a metal disk attached to a diaphragm on the center body. When the magnet is placed closer to the metal plate, more effort is required to initiate inspiration owing to the increased magnetic attraction. To make it easier to initiate inspiration, the sensitivity control arm is rotated toward the rear of the ventilator. This control moves the magnet farther from the metal plate, reducing magnetic attraction, and hence the effort required to initiate a breath.

Flow Rate

Adjustment of the flow rate determines the length of inspiration and, to some extent, the delivered tidal volume. Flow rate is adjusted by a black knob attached to a needle valve located near the top of the center body. Figure 17-3 shows the flow rate control. The flow is determined by the size of the opening created by the position of the needle valve relative to its seat.

Apneustic Time Control

The purpose of the apneustic time control is to provide a breath hold at the end of inhalation. The concept is to provide a period for distribution of gas and aerosol throughout the lungs prior to exhalation. This inspiratory hold is adjustable between 0.3 and 3 seconds. Exhalation is prevented by keeping the exhalation valve located on the patient manifold from depressurizing following breath delivery.

Gas Flow through the Breathing Circuit

Inspiration

During inspiration, gas flows to the patient through both the large-bore tubing and the small-diameter tubing. This flow through both tubes begins simultaneously as inspiration is initiated. Figure 17-4 identifies the components of a disposable circuit.

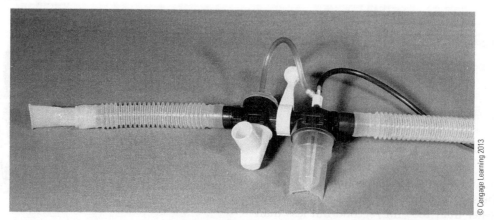

© Cengage Learning 2013

Figure 17-4   Components of a disposable IPPB circuit configured for the Bird ventilator

The large-bore tubing is attached to the outlet of the ventilator. Figure 17-5 shows its attachment. This gas will either be pure source gas or source gas mixed with room air (determined by the air mix control).

The flow through the small-diameter tubing powers the nebulizer and closes the exhalation valve on the breathing circuit. This flow is pure source gas. When the flow closes the exhalation valve, gas flow through the circuit can go only in one direction—toward the patient.

Figure-17-6 is a diagram showing gas flow during inspiration.

Expiration

Whereas inspiration during IPPB occurs with the assistance of positive pressure applied to the airways, expiration is passive. The elastic recoil of the lungs and thorax allows the patient to exhale passively. During expiration, all gas flow through the breathing circuit toward the patient, as well as gas delivered to close the exhalation valve, has stopped. With no flow, the exhalation valve is open. As the patient exhales, the gas flows through the exhalation port out into the room. Figure 17-7 shows gas flow through the breathing circuit on expiration.

PERCUSSIONAIRE IPV-1

The Percussionaire IPV-1C (Figure 17-8) is an acute care ventilator designed for the management of patients with cardiopulmonary disease in whom secretion mobilization is desirable. This ventilator is used to deliver IPV therapy.

Controls

Operational Pressure

The operational pressure control is located on the left front of the ventilator on the control panel. The operational pressure is typically adjusted to between 30 and 40 psi. Operational pressure determines the impact velocity of the percussive pulses. For most patients an initial setting of around 30 psi is recommended.

Percussion Control

The percussion control regulates the frequency of the percussive ventilatory pulses sent to the Phasitron (discussed later). Frequencies are adjustable between 100 and 300 cycles per minute.

Manual Inspiration

By depressing the manual inspiration button, the ventilator can be set to the oscillatory mode. This feature is provided in the event that the ventilator is used for cardiopulmonary resuscitation efforts.

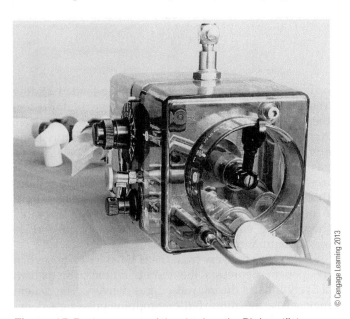

© Cengage Learning 2013

Figure 17-5 Attachment of the circuit to the Bird ventilator

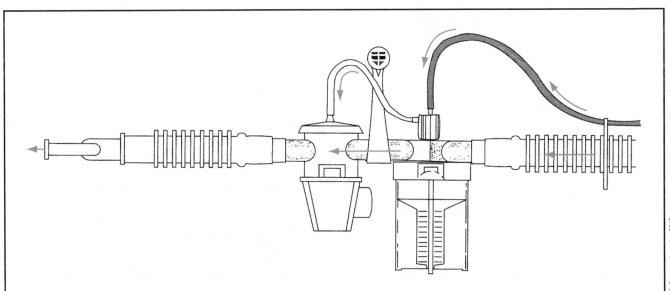

© Cengage Learning 2013

Figure 17-6 Gas flow through the Bird circuit during inspiration

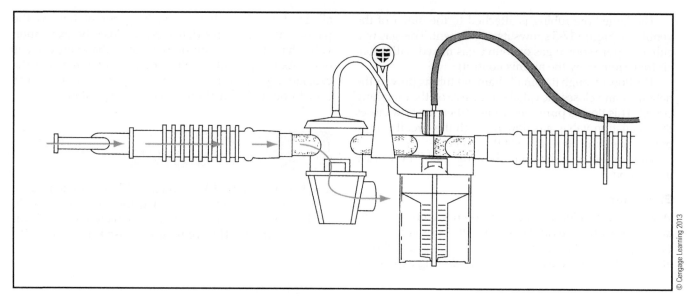

Figure 17-7 Gas flow through the Bird circuit during expiration

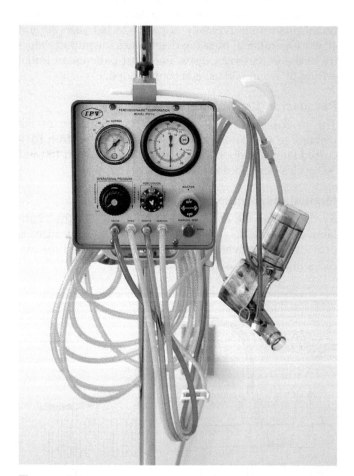

Figure 17-8 A photograph of the Percussionaire IPV®-1C ventilator. *(Courtesy of Percussionaire Corporation, Sandpoint, ID)*

Phasitron

The Phasitron provides a mechanical and pneumatic interface between the IPV ventilator and the patient's airway. The Phasitron (Figure 17-9) consists of a jet, an orifice servo diaphragm, and a spring-loaded sliding Venturi body. Pulsed gas from the IPV ventilator enters the orifice servo diaphragm and jet of the Phasitron. As the diaphragm distorts, the sliding Venturi body advances, closing the expiratory port and delivering gas to the patient. When gas pressure is removed from the orifice diaphragm/jet, spring tension slides the Venturi body back, opening the exhalation port. A dense aerosol is drawn into the Phasitron assembly through the entrainment port adjacent to the orifice servo diaphragm.

Pulsed gas delivery from the IPV device begins when the patient depresses the thumb button. The patient actively inhales during pulsed gas delivery. The patient may release the thumb button, stopping pulsed gas delivery for exhalation, or alternatively may exhale actively against pulsed gas delivered through the Phasitron.

Changing Tidal Volume Delivery and Ventilatory Frequency

Tidal volume delivery is determined by the setting on the operational pressure control. As operational pressure is increased, tidal volume delivery increases. Operational pressure is typically adjusted between 30 and 40 psi. It is suggested to begin therapy at around 30 psi. If chest expansion and percussive effect are inadequate at this setting, increase the operational pressure.

Ventilatory frequency is adjusted using the percussion control. As frequency is increased, the effect of operational pressure is attenuated. At lower frequencies, each pulsed gas delivery is more accentuated than with higher frequencies at the same source pressure. It is suggested that most patients start with the control at mid-position. Rotating the control to the left increases the frequency and decreases the effect of operational pressure (impulse).

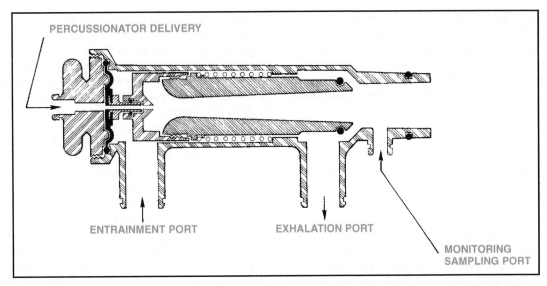

Figure 17-9 A full section showing the Phasitron® *(Courtesy of Percussionaire Corporation, Sandpoint, ID)*

PROFICIENCY OBJECTIVES

At the end of this chapter, the reader should be able to:

- *Demonstrate the use of an incentive spirometer including:*
  - *Patient instruction*
  - *Use of equipment*
  - *Troubleshooting of equipment*
  - *Emphasis of self-motivation on the part of the patient*
- *Demonstrate the correct operation of the Bird Mark 7A*
  - *Establish the ordered pressure.*
  - *Establish the ordered tidal volume.*
  - *Establish the ordered ventilatory rate.*
  - *Maintain an I:E ratio of 1:2 or greater.*
  - *Maintain flow rates and pressures within human physiologic limits.*
  - *Monitor FIO$_2$.*
- *Demonstrate how to administer IPPB therapy with normal saline to a laboratory partner.*
- *Demonstrate the ability to evaluate the signs and symptoms of the adverse effects resulting from IPPB therapy.*
- *State the criteria for terminating IPPB therapy.*

- *Describe the appropriate action that should be taken in the event of terminating IPPB therapy, including:*
  - *Who should be notified*
  - *Correct patient assessment and monitoring*
  - *Correct charting of why the therapy was terminated*
- *Demonstrate appropriate charting following the administration of IPPB therapy.*
- *Demonstrate the correct operation of the Percussionaire IPV®-1C ventilator; given an order for IPV therapy using a test lung:*
  - *Correctly assemble the ventilator for use.*
  - *Establish the correct operational pressure.*
  - *Establish the correct frequency.*
- *With a laboratory partner as your patient, demonstrate how to administer IPV therapy:*
  - *Correctly instruct your patient.*
  - *Correctly adjust the controls for the patient's comfort and efficacy of the therapy.*

INCENTIVE SPIROMETRY

Patient Instruction

The effectiveness of any hyperinflation therapy is dependent on patient cooperation and effort. This can only be accomplished using thorough patient instruction.

Be certain to instruct the patient to inhale through the device. Most patients have a natural tendency to blow through it. A few practice trials and a demonstration by the practitioner using exaggerated technique will help. If incentive spirometry is to be self-administered, be sure the patient can operate the device successfully without prompting.

Incentive Spirometry Equipment

To prepare the Voldyne for use, attach the large-bore tubing to the fitting on the front of the unit. Adjust the yellow pointer to the desired volume.

Instruct the patient to inhale deeply through the mouthpiece. The negative pressure generated will raise the piston from the bottom of the tube.

Troubleshooting amounts to ensuring that all fittings and connections are tight.

To prepare the Triflow incentive spirometer for use, connect the flexible inspiratory tubing to fitting on the lower left side of the device. Attach a mouthpiece to the tubing and ensure that all connections are tight.

Instruct the patient to take a deep breath through the mouthpiece. As inspiratory flow increases, one, two or three balls will be suspended. Encourage the patient to suspend as many balls as he or she can for 3 to 5 seconds.

Troubleshooting amounts to ensuring that all connections between the tubing, spirometer, and mouthpiece are tight.

IPPB THERAPY

Verify the Physician's Order

Prior to administering IPPB therapy, verify the physician's order in the patient's chart. Look for the components of a complete order, including the amount and dilution of medication, frequency, goals of therapy, duration, pressure range, and desired tidal volume. If clarification is needed, contact the physician.

Scan the Chart

Check the patient's chart for the patient's history. A history of chronic obstructive pulmonary disease (COPD) (especially late-stage emphysema), pneumothorax (check for treatment), hypotension, or head injury should alert the practitioner to possible complications resulting from the administration of IPPB therapy.

A quick review of recent results of blood gas analysis will be helpful in assessment of the patient's pulmonary status and of the need for oxygen administration. Also scan the chart for any pulmonary function test reports, laboratory data, physician's progress notes, and radiograph reports. In brief, scan the chart looking for any information that could alert the practitioner to potential complications as a result of IPPB administration.

Administration of Therapy

Patient Positioning

The ideal patient position for IPPB therapy is seated with the legs dangling at the edge of the bed or sitting upright in a chair. This position allows the chest to expand fully without restrictions. An upright position may not be possible with all patients. Full Fowler's or semi-Fowler's position is the next best. Positions may need to be modified depending on the patient's condition. Use good judgment and assess the patient for contraindications.

Appropriate Monitoring before Therapy

Current clinical practice dictates the monitoring of therapy to document its effectiveness. It is difficult to document how effective a therapeutic modality is if the patient is not assessed on what he or she is capable of spontaneously before therapy. Before therapy monitor breath sounds, pulse, respiratory rate, inspiratory capacity, spontaneous tidal volume, peak expiratory flow, and blood pressure.

Ideal Breathing Pattern

The ideal breathing pattern for IPPB therapy is similar to the breathing pattern used for small-volume nebulizer

therapy, discussed in Chapter 15, Humidity and Aerosol Therapy. Instruct the patient to inhale, which will cycle the respirator on. Tell the patient to inhale with the ventilator. By actively assisting the ventilator, the patient will achieve a greater inspiratory capacity. At the end of the inspiratory phase, instruct the patient to pause briefly before exhaling to allow for a more even deposition of the aerosol.

This breathing pattern is unnatural, and success will require both thorough instruction by the practitioner and practice by the patient. It is common for the patient to close the glottis, terminating inspiration, on first experiencing the positive pressure delivered by the ventilator. It is imperative that the patient relax on inspiration to allow the ventilator to fill the lungs.

Exhalation is passive, requiring little effort. Instruct the patient to count to three before beginning the next breath. A short pause will help to decrease the respiratory rate and preserve a more normal I:E ratio.

Monitoring the Patient during IPPB Therapy

During therapy, closely monitor the patient. Measure the pulse and respiratory rate frequently. Constantly assess the patient for any signs or symptoms of the hazards and complications discussed earlier.

Monitor the ventilator tidal volume during therapy using a portable respirometer attached to the exhalation port (Wright, Dragger, or Haloscale). Good IPPB administration will result in a ventilator tidal volume of approximately one third of the predicted inspiratory capacity (50 mL/kg ideal body weight) (AARC, 2003). The practitioner should strive for a ventilator tidal volume approaching the spontaneous inspiratory capacity as long as undue harm is not caused to the patient. With these volumes, monitor delivered pressures closely. Frequent pressure and flow adjustments may be required to achieve a high inspiratory capacity. The physician may indicate a maximum pressure not to be exceeded during therapy.

Monitoring the Patient during Bronchodilator Administration

When administering a bronchodilator, it is important to monitor the patient for any side effects due to the medication. Chapter 15, Humidity and Aerosol Therapy, discusses the most common drugs administered by aerosol and their actions and side effects. Closely monitor the patient's pulse when administering bronchodilators. If it increases by 20/min greater than baseline (depending on the departmental policies), discontinue therapy.

Recognition of Adverse Effects of IPPB Therapy

Hyperventilation

When patients hyperventilate they may complain of light-headedness or dizziness. Some patients complain of a tingling sensation. A headache may often be precipitated. If this effect is severe, the patient may breathe rapidly and deeply without control until a loss of consciousness occurs.

Appropriate Action If any of these signs or symptoms occurs, discontinue therapy. Allow the patient to rest, breathing spontaneously for a few minutes. If hyperventilation continues, contact the patient's attending physician or seek assistance from other personnel.

Interruption of the Hypoxic Drive

With interruption of the hypoxic drive, patients often become very lethargic and drowsy. Spontaneous respiratory rate and depth decrease markedly. If the reaction is severe, the patient may go into respiratory arrest. The administration of IPPB may precipitate an episode of hypoventilation that is not evident for some time. A patient who experiences a significant drop in tidal volume and respiratory rate following therapy, with the foregoing signs and symptoms, should be closely observed.

Appropriate Action At the first indications of these symptoms, discontinue therapy immediately. Stay with the patient and closely monitor the respiratory rate and depth, pulse, and blood pressure. Observe the patient for signs of cyanosis. If possible, call the patient's nurse so that additional appropriate vital signs can be monitored. If respiratory arrest occurs, initiate cardiopulmonary resuscitation (CPR) and get help.

This event may be prevented by reviewing the patient's history first to identify persons at risk (due to COPD) and by administering therapy using compressed air rather than oxygen.

Decreased Cardiac Output

The effects of IPPB on the cardiovascular system may be minimized by maintaining an I:E ratio of 1:2 or greater. Decreased cardiac output is indicated by a fall in blood pressure. If the patient is in the intensive care unit, an arterial line may be present, making blood pressure monitoring easy and convenient. In the absence of these more sophisticated monitoring devices, manual blood pressure measurement is the only means of monitoring for this adverse effect. The practitioner may be able to detect cardiac rhythm changes when monitoring the pulse. Patients at risk (those who have cardiovascular disease) should be monitored closely. A drop in blood pressure may be indicated by complaints of dizziness or faintness, pallor, or diaphoresis or cyanosis.

Appropriate Action At the first sign of cardiac compromise, discontinue therapy and monitor the patient closely. If possible, have a nurse assist in monitoring the patient. If the blood pressure remains low and the cardiovascular system fails to recover after discontinuance of therapy, contact the physician immediately.

Increased Intracranial Pressure

Rising intracranial pressure can impair cerebral circulation and damage brain tissue. Unless the patient is at risk (owing to head trauma or neurologic condition) and the intracranial pressure is already being monitored, an increase in intracranial pressure is very difficult to detect. Some affected patients exhibit bulging and experience increased pressure around the eye orbits. Other symptoms may include changes in sensorium and loss of consciousness. Most patients at risk will have an intracranial pressure monitoring line (ICP line) in place.

Appropriate Action Patients at risk should be closely monitored. If intracranial pressure increases significantly, discontinue therapy. Try to administer therapy with the patient in semi-Fowler's or full Fowler's position, if possible, to help reduce the effects of IPPB on intracranial pressure. Frequently, the physician's order for IPPB will specify a position in these circumstances. If the patient has experienced spinal injury or multiple trauma in addition to the cranial problems, it is wise to request clarification of what position to use during IPPB therapy.

Pneumothorax

Patients with an existing pneumothorax should not receive IPPB therapy unless a chest tube is in place. One hazard of IPPB therapy is a pneumothorax occurring as the result of an air leak in the lung. The result is air in the pleural space, compressing lung tissue.

Patients experiencing a pneumothorax often complain of a sharp chest pain and shortness of breath. With a tension pneumothorax, patients are often gasping.

Appropriate Action Terminate IPPB therapy. Quickly auscultate the chest. Absent or diminished breath sounds may indicate the presence of a pneumothorax. Percuss the chest; if hyperresonance is present and breath sounds are absent or decreased, be very suspicious. If observing a shift in the trachea, contact a physician immediately. If possible, call the patient's nurse to assist in monitoring the patient. Monitor the respiratory rate and depth and pulse frequently.

A STAT chest radiograph is indicated, and if a pneumothorax is present, the physician will place a chest tube.

Do not continue therapy if the patient has a pneumothorax that has not been treated.

Post-IPPB Therapy Monitoring

Following IPPB therapy administration, monitor breath sounds, pulse, respiratory rate, spontaneous tidal volume, peak expiratory flow, and vital capacity.

Charting the Procedure

Appropriate charting includes the following: date and time of administration; medication, amount, and dilution; duration of therapy; pressure; respirator tidal volume; and the patient's parameters before and after therapy.

Also indicate the ability of the patient to cooperate and follow instructions. Indicate whether the patient's coughing was productive and what was expectorated.

In the event of adverse reactions, charting should include why therapy was discontinued (observation of signs and symptoms). The practitioner should indicate how the patient was monitored and what was observed. The people contacted should include the physician, nurse, and a supervisor. Indicate who was contacted, when, and what action was taken.

All charting should conform with the standards and policies of the agency in which the therapy was rendered.

INTRAPULMONARY PERCUSSIVE VENTILATION THERAPY

Verify the Physician's Order

Prior to IPV therapy administration, verify the physician's order in the patient's chart. Look for components of the order, including medication, amount and dilution, and length and frequency of therapy. If clarification is needed, contact the physician.

Scan the Chart

Check the patient's history in the medical record for any indications of untreated pneumothorax, hypotension, or head injuries (elevated intracranial pressure). These problems may be contraindications to IPV therapy because mean intrathoracic pressures will be elevated during therapy. If further clarification is required, contact the patient's physician.

Administration of Therapy

Patient Positioning

The ideal patient position for IPV therapy is seated comfortably in the upright position. If the patient is unable to comply, a high Fowler's or semi-Fowler's position is also acceptable. If modifying the patient's positioning for therapy, be certain that the position chosen does not interfere with achieving the desired clinical goals.

Appropriate Monitoring before Therapy

Prior to beginning therapy, monitor the patient's respiratory rate, heart rate, and breath sounds. Because IPV therapy is effective in mobilization of pulmonary secretions, an increase in sputum production is important to note. If bronchodilators are administered with IPV therapy,

documentation of peak expiratory flow or forced expiratory flow volume in 1 second (FEV_1) pretherapy and posttherapy is appropriate.

Ideal Breathing Pattern

The patient should be instructed to hold the lips tightly around the mouthpiece and to depress the thumb button. Once the button has been depressed, percussive ventilation will begin. The patient should be instructed to inhale and allow the IPV ventilator to fill the lungs and to percuss them for approximately 5 seconds. After the lungs are full, the patient releases the thumb button and exhales completely through the mouthpiece. This process should be repeated until all of the medication in the nebulizer has been delivered.

Monitoring during Therapy

The patient's heart rate, respiratory rate, and breath sounds should be monitored during therapy. If portions of the patient's lungs demonstrated diminished or absent breath sounds prior to therapy, monitor these areas during therapy for improved ventilation. The pressure manometer on the control panel of the IPV ventilator may be monitored to determine peak inspiratory pressures during therapy. When the source pressure is increased, peak pressures during percussion also increase.

The patient's subjective response to therapy such as complaints of dyspnea, pain, or discomfort should be noted. Some patients require time to become accustomed to the high-frequency gas pulsations delivered by the IPV device. Often, increasing the frequency helps the patient to tolerate therapy more easily because the impact of each pulse is lessened.

Monitoring following Therapy

Following IPV therapy, the patient's heart rate, respiratory rate, and breath sounds should be assessed. Quantify sputum production and note its color and consistency and whether any odor is present. If a bronchodilator was used, assess the patient's peak expiratory flow or FEV_1 following therapy.

Charting the Procedure

Document in the patient's chart the date and time of IPV therapy. Note the medications used, including the amount and dilution. Document the source pressure and the patient's subjective response to therapy. Document all vital signs, breath sounds, and sputum production.

References

American Association for Respiratory Care. (1991). AARC clinical practice guideline: Incentive spirometry. *Respiratory Care, 36*(12), 1402–1405.

American Association for Respiratory Care. (2003). AARC clinical practice guideline: Intermittent positive pressure breathing 2003 revision and update. *Respiratory Care, 48*(5), 540–546.

Freitas, E. R. (2007). Incentive spirometry for preventing pulmonary complications after coronary artery bypass graft. *Cochrane Database Systematic Review.*

Lawrence, V. (2006). Strategies to reduce postoperative pulmonary complications after noncardiothoracic surgery: Systematic review for the American College of Physicians. *Annals of Internal Medicine, 144*(8), 596.

McPherson, 1995

Thomas, J. A., & McIntosh, J. M. (1994). Are incentive spirometry, intermittent positive pressure breathing, and deep breathing exercises effective in the prevention of postoperative pulmonary complications after upper abdominal surgery? A systematic overview and meta-analysis. *Physical Therapy, 75*(1), 3–10.

Additional Resources

Bird Corporation. *Instructions for operating the Mark 7 Respirator, Mark 8 Respirator, Mark 10 and Mark 14 ventilators by Bird.* Palm Springs, CA: Author.

Percussionaire Corporation. (1993). *Intrapulmonary percussive ventilation, a twelve year learning curve 1980–1993.* Sandpoint, ID: Author.

Practice Activities: Bird Mark 7A

CIRCUIT ASSEMBLY

Permanent reusable circuits as well as disposables are available for the Bird Mark 7 ventilator. In this activity set you will assemble a disposable universal IPPB circuit and correctly adapt it for the Bird Mark 7 ventilator.

Figure-17-10 shows the contents of a typical disposable universal IPPB circuit. Some of these parts are not required for the Bird Mark 7A circuit.

1. Nebulizer and exhalation valve drive line assembly
   The Bird Mark 7A employs a single small-diameter tube to drive both the nebulizer and the exhalation valve. The small adapter with the short piece of small-diameter tubing is used for this purpose. To assemble:
   a. Insert the tubing adapter onto the nebulizer nipple. Connect the other end of the small-diameter tube to the exhalation valve nipple. Figure 17-11 shows the circuit correctly configured.
   b. Next, take the longer piece of small-diameter tubing and attach it to the adapter. The extra piece of small-diameter tubing with the flared ends may be discarded.

2. Mouthpiece assembly
   a. Attach the short flex tube to the outlet of the manifold assembly. Attach the mouthpiece to the other end of the flex tube. Figure 17-11 shows the circuit correctly assembled.

3. Attachment of the circuit to the ventilator
   a. The large-bore tubing connects the ventilator to the manifold. Attach the large-bore tubing to the outlet on the right side of the ventilator. This attachment may require a 15 mm straight adapter (sometimes called a mask adapter), which may be supplied with the circuit.
   b. Attach the small-diameter tubing that powers the nebulizer and exhalation valve to the small nipple on the right side of the ventilator next to the large-bore outlet.

OPERATION OF THE VENTILATOR

For these activities, remove the mouthpiece on the circuit; replace it with a 15 mm straight adapter (mask adapter) and a rubber test lung. Make sure that the test lung is free of leaks and that the rubber strap is in good condition.

Attach the ventilator to a 50 psi compressed gas source. If the ventilator cycles on prematurely, pull out on the hand-timer rod located in the center of the sensitivity control rod. This control should cycle the ventilator off. If it does not, move the sensitivity control toward the front of the ventilator and rotate the expiratory timer control fully clockwise. Now repeat the procedure of pulling the

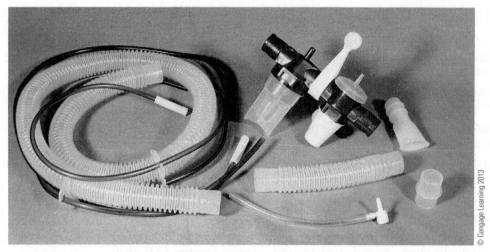

Figure 17-10 A typical disposable IPPB circuit

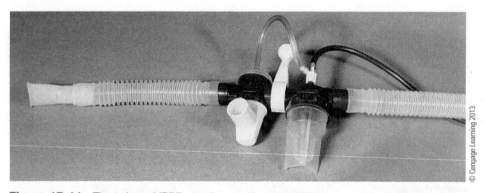

Figure 17-11 The universal IPPB circuit correctly assembled for use with the Bird Mark 7

hand-timer rod. If the ventilator continues to cycle on, ask for assistance from your laboratory instructor.

Activity 1: Pressure Control (1)

Leave the sensitivity control in its current position. Adjust the flow rate control so that is at the 12 o'clock position (pointing straight up). The pressure is controlled by a movable plastic arm or vernier. The manufacturer refers to this control as one of two vernier arms.

1. Adjust the pressure control so the vernier arm is positioned at the 12 o'clock position when facing the control. Push the hand-timer rod in to initiate inspiration. Observe the pressure manometer and note at what pressure the inspiratory phase stops. Adjust the pressure control until the breath stops when the pressure reaches 10 cm H_2O.
   a. Repeat this activity and time the length of the inspiratory phase. Write down your value.

2. Adjust the pressure control so the vernier arm is at the 2 o'clock position when facing the control. Initiate inspiration by pushing the hand-timer rod in. Observe the pressure manometer and note at what pressure the inspiratory phase stops. Adjust the pressure control until the breath stops at 15 cm H_2O.
   a. Repeat this activity and time the length of the inspiratory phase. Write down your value.

3. Adjust the pressure control so the vernier arm is at the 3 o'clock position when facing it.. Push the hand-timer rod in to initiate inspiration. Observe the pressure manometer and note at what pressure the inspiratory phase stops. Adjust the pressure until the breath stops at 25 cm H_2O.
   a. Time the length of the inspiratory phase. Write down your value.

Questions

A. In activity 1, at what pressure did the ventilator terminate inspiration?
B. What effect did moving the pressure control have on the cycling pressure (pressure at which inspiration is terminated)?
C. Compare the inspiratory times for activities 1 through 3. How do you account for the increased inspiratory time when you did not manipulate the flow rate control?
D. Assume that a patient is breathing at a rate of 10 breaths per minute. Calculate the I:E ratios for activities 1 and 3.
E. If you want the pressure delivered in activity 3, but with the I:E ratio in activity 1, what control would you need to manipulate?

Activity 2: Expiratory Timer Control (2)

This control is not normally used with IPPB therapy. It is used only with the patient with apnea. This control is used to set the ventilatory rate.

Activity 3: Sensitivity Control (3)

With the flow rate control set so that it is at the 12 o'clock position, adjust the pressure control on the right of the ventilator to about the 11 o'clock position.

1. Move the sensitivity control toward the back of the ventilator until it automatically cycles on, and then move the control toward the front of the ventilator about ½ inch. The ventilator should be off.
   a. Squeeze the test lung and release it, observing the manometer. How far did the manometer deflect into the negative pressure range?
   b. Move the sensitivity control about ½ inch toward the front of the ventilator. Squeeze the test lung again, observing the manometer. How far did the manometer deflect into the negative pressure range this time?
   c. Move the sensitivity control about 1 inch more toward the front of the ventilator. Squeeze the test lung and observe the manometer. How far did the manometer deflect into the negative pressure range?

Questions

A. Which setting required the least effort (negative pressure) to initiate inspiration?
B. Which setting required the most effort (negative pressure) to initiate inspiration?
C. As a patient working hard to breathe, where do you think you would prefer to have the ventilator set?

Activity 4: Flow Rate Control (4)

Additional Equipment Required:

A watch with a sweep second hand
   Set the sensitivity control to the setting you prefer. Leave the pressure control in the same position.

1. Adjust the flow rate control so that it is at the 12 o'clock position. Initiate inspiration by pushing the hand-timer rod in. Observe how long it takes to complete the inspiratory phase. Write this time down.
2. Adjust the flow rate, rotating it to the right about ¼ turn. Push the hand-timer rod in to initiate inspiration. Observe how long it takes to complete the inspiratory phase. Write this time down.
3. Adjust the flow rate control, rotating it left (past 12 o'clock) about ½ a turn. Push the hand-timer rod in to initiate inspiration. Observe how long it takes to complete the inspiratory phase.

Questions

A. In activity 1, assume that the patient is breathing at a rate of 10 breaths per minute. Using the value you measured for inspiratory time, calculate the I:E ratio.

B. In activity 3, assume that the patient is breathing at a rate of 10 breaths per minute. Using the value you measured for inspiratory time, calculate the I:E ratio.
C. As you progressed from activity 1 to activity 3, what effect did the flow rate control have on inspiratory time?

TIDAL VOLUME DELIVERY WITH IPPB THERAPY

A clinical goal of IPPB therapy is reversal of atelectasis. However, it is difficult to quantify how deeply a patient is breathing strictly by observation. In this activity set, you will monitor delivered tidal volumes and adjust the controls appropriately to increase or decrease the delivered tidal volume while maintaining an I:E ratio of 1:2 or greater.

Additional Equipment Required:

Watch with a sweep second hand
Portable respirometer (Wright or Haloscale)

Activity 1

1. Adjust the sensitivity control so the vernier arm is in the 12 o'clock position. Adjust the flow rate control so that it is at the 12 o'clock position. Adjust the pressure control so that the vernier arm is at the 12 o'clock position.

2. Attach a portable respirometer to the exhalation port of the manifold assembly.

3. Push the hand-timer rod in to initiate inspiration. Measure the tidal volume. Adjust the pressure control until a tidal volume of 300 mL is reached.

4. Rotate the expiratory timer control counterclockwise until a ventilatory rate of 12 breaths per minute is established.

5. Measure the inspiratory time using your watch. Calculate the I:E ratio.

6. Adjust the flow rate control until you have an I:E ratio of 1:2 or greater.
   a. Measure the tidal volume and adjust the pressure to reach 300 mL as required.
   b. Adjust the flow rate control, as required, to maintain an I:E ratio of 1:2.
   c. Repeat the foregoing steps until the desired goal is reached.

Activity 2

1. Adjust the sensitivity control so the vernier arm is in the 12 o'clock position. Adjust the flow rate control so that it is at the 12 o'clock position. Adjust the pressure control so that the vernier is at the 12 o'clock position.

2. Attach a portable respirometer to the exhalation port of the manifold assembly.

3. Push the hand-timer rod in to initiate inspiration. Measure the tidal volume. Adjust the pressure control until a tidal volume of 500 mL is reached.

4. Rotate the expiratory timer control counterclockwise until a ventilatory rate of 10 breaths per minute is established.

5. Measure the inspiratory time using your watch. Calculate the I:E ratio.

6. Adjust the flow rate control until you have an I:E ratio of 1:2 or greater.
   a. Measure the tidal volume and adjust the pressure to reach 500 mL as required.
   b. Adjust the flow rate control, as required, to maintain an I:E ratio of 1:2.
   c. Repeat the foregoing steps until the desired goal is reached.

7. Decrease the tidal volume to 400 mL while maintaining the same I:E ratio and ventilatory rate.

OXYGEN DELIVERY WITH IPPB THERAPY

Oxygen delivery with IPPB therapy is very common. Because the ventilator is pneumatically powered, the use of a 50 psi oxygen source will provide for oxygen delivery. However, the delivered FIO_2 is not consistent throughout the inspiratory phase. If a precise oxygen concentration is desired, it is recommended that you use a blender with a 50 psi outlet to adjust the FIO_2. When using a blender, push the air dilution control in. This will ensure delivery of 100% source gas from the blender.

If the ventilator is powered by a compressed gas cylinder, use a two-stage regulator to ensure that adequate flow rates are provided.

Practice Activities: Percussionaire IPV-1 Ventilator

CIRCUIT ASSEMBLY

In this activity set, you will correctly assemble the circuit for the IPV®-1C intrapulmonary percussive ventilator.

1. Open the nebulizer by rotating the nebulizer bowl counterclockwise. Add medication in the proper dilution and quantity to the nebulizer bowl, and reinstall it to the green tee cap assembly.

2. Connect the Phasitron to the nebulizer assembly by inserting the entrainment port into the nebulizer assembly.

3. Install the four-tube multicolored drive harness to the manifold assembly:
   a. Connect the white tube to the cap on the Phasitron.
   b. Connect the green tube to the socket opposite the thumb switch.
   c. Connect the red tube to the proximal monitoring port near the mouthpiece.
   d. Connect the yellow tube to the base of the nebulizer.

4. Install the four-tube multicolored drive harness to the ventilator by matching the colors of the tube to the sockets located below the pressure manometer.

5. Install the red adapter bushing onto the outlet of the Phasitron and connect the large-bore red tubing to it. This prevents the patient's clothing from becoming spattered with excess aerosolized medication.

6. Connect a 50 psi gas source to the gas inlet on the back of the IPV 1C ventilator.

OPERATION OF THE VENTILATOR

For this activity set, remove the mouthpiece on the circuit and replace it with a 15 mm straight adapter (mask adapter) and a rubber test lung. Make sure that the test lung is free from leaks and that the rubber strap is in good condition.

Adjust the operational pressure control to 30 psi. The operational pressure control is located on the left front of the control panel.

Percussion Control

1. Rotate the percussion control fully clockwise. Activate percussive ventilation by depressing the manual inspiration button or the thumb button on the Phasitron assembly.
   a. Determine the frequency (slow, medium, or fast).
   b. Note approximately how much volume is delivered with each breath.

2. Rotate the percussion control fully counterclockwise. Activate percussive ventilation by depressing the manual inspiration button or the thumb button on the Phasitron assembly.
   a. Determine the frequency (slow, medium, or fast).
   b. Note approximately how much volume is delivered with each breath.

Questions

A. Which setting resulted in the highest ventilatory rate?
B. How did rotating the percussion control affect volume delivery?

Operational Pressure Control

1. Set the percussion control to the 12 o'clock, midrange position. Decrease the operational pressure to 20 psi by rotating the knob counterclockwise. Activate percussive ventilation by depressing the manual inspiration button or the thumb button on the Phasitron assembly.
   a. Determine the frequency (slow, medium, or fast).
   b. Note approximately how much volume is delivered with each breath.

2. Set the percussion control to the 12 o'clock, midrange position. Increase the operational pressure to 40 psi by rotating the knob clockwise. Activate percussive ventilation by depressing the manual inspiration button or the thumb button on the Phasitron assembly.
   a. Determine the frequency (slow, medium, or fast).

b. Note approximately how much volume is delivered with each breath.

Question:

A. What effect did the operational pressure have on volume delivery with each breath?

Practice Activities: Hyperinflation Therapy

1. With a laboratory partner, practice giving each other directions on how to use an incentive spirometer. Include the following information:
   a. Explain what incentive spirometry does physiologically.
   b. Explain how to use the spirometer.
   c. Explain the importance of the patient's cooperation and effort.
   NOTE: When a patient does not seem to do well, it usually can be attributed to poor instruction.

2. Practice incentive spirometry using a laboratory partner. Include in your practice:
   a. Correct assembly
   b. Troubleshooting
   c. Patient instructions

3. Complete the practice activities for the Bird Mark 7 ventilator.

4. Practice administering IPPB with normal saline to a laboratory partner using the IPPB Therapy Check List as a guide.

Safety Precautions

A. IPPB therapy may be hazardous owing to the application of positive pressure in the lungs. Approach high pressures and volumes (greater than 25 cm H_2O and 50% of the inspiratory capacity) with caution.

B. Closely monitor your laboratory partner for signs and symptoms indicating the adverse effects of IPPB therapy. If you observe any of the signs or symptoms described, terminate the therapy and notify your laboratory instructor immediately.

Check List: Incentive Spirometry

_____ 1. Verify the physician's order.

_____ 2. Scan the chart for relevant information.

_____ 3. Observe standard precautions, including handwashing.

_____ 4. Obtain and assemble your equipment.

_____ 5. Identify the patient and introduce yourself, explaining the procedure.

6. Position the patient properly.

_____ a. Semi-Fowler's

_____ b. Full Fowler's

_____ c. Dangling

_____ 7. Assess the patient's spontaneous parameters. Some facilities require a vital capacity determination once each day.

_____ 8. Assist the patient in the performance.

_____ 9. Emphasize self-motivation. With the prevalence of television in patients' rooms, the patient can be encouraged to perform three repetitions on the spirometer during each commercial break.

_____ 10. Leave the spirometer within the patient's reach.

_____ 11. Clean up after yourself.

_____ 12. Ensure that your patient is safe and comfortable.

_____ 13. Record the procedure in the patient's chart. Include date, time, volumes achieved, vital capacity, breath sounds, and, if the cough was productive, the amount, color, and consistency of the sputum.

Check List: IPPB Therapy

_____ 1. Verify the physician's order. In the absence of a complete order, take appropriate action.

2. Scan the patient's chart.
_____ a. History
_____ b. Chest x-ray film and report
_____ c. Blood gas values, if available
_____ 3. Gather the required equipment.
_____ 4. Observe standard precautions, including handwashing.
_____ 5. Identify the patient, introduce yourself, and explain the procedure.

6. During patient monitoring, measure the following:
_____ a. Pulse
_____ b. Respiratory rate
_____ c. Breath sounds
_____ d. Spontaneous inspiratory capacity
_____ e. Peak expiratory flow
_____ f. Blood pressure
_____ 7. Assemble the equipment properly.

8. Instruct the patient on:
_____ a. Proper breathing pattern
_____ b. How to initiate inspiration
_____ c. How to exhale properly
_____ d. Symptoms to be aware of

9. Administer IPPB therapy.
_____ a. Deliver a tidal volume 25% greater than the spontaneous inspiratory capacity.

10. Monitor the patient during therapy:
_____ a. Take the pulse.
_____ b. Determine the respiratory rate.
_____ c. Watch for adverse signs and symptoms.
_____ d. Measure the blood pressure.
_____ 11. Assist your patient with coughing.
_____ 12. Monitor the effectiveness of the therapy by measuring peak flow and vital capacity.
_____ 13. Assess the patient for adverse effects.
_____ 14. Remove all unneeded equipment.
_____ 15. Chart appropriately

Check List: Intrapulmonary Percussive Ventilation Therapy

_____ 1. Verify the physician's order.
_____ 2. Scan the chart for relevant information.
_____ 3. Observe standard precautions, including hand washing.
_____ 4. Obtain and assemble your equipment.
_____ 5. Identify the patient, introduce yourself, and explain the procedure.
_____ 6. Position the patient properly.
_____ 7. Assess the patient prior to therapy.

_____ 8. Instruct the patient on IPV therapy.
_____ 9. Assist and coach the patient during therapy.
_____ 10. Periodically have the patient cough.
_____ 11. Monitor the patient during therapy.
_____ 12. Assess the patient following therapy.
_____ 13. Clean up after yourself.
_____ 14. Ensure that the patient is safe and comfortable.
_____ 15. Document the procedure in the patient's chart.

Self-Evaluation Post Test: Hyperinflation Therapy

1. A goal of incentive spirometry is to:
   a. reduce the practitioner's workload.
   b. provide means of using a patient's muscles to hyperinflate the lungs.
   c. inflict pain and suffering.
   d. place the patient on a fixed schedule of therapy convenient for the practitioner.

2. A sign that your patient may be hyperventilating during incentive spirometry is:
   a. a complaint of feeling light-headed.
   b. a complaint of feeling dizzy.
   c. a tingling sensation.
   d. All of the above

3. Of the following, which is the most important aspect of incentive spirometry?
   a. Duration of therapy
   b. Frequency of therapy
   c. Thorough patient instruction
   d. Practitioner's knowledge of the patient's diagnosis

4. Which of the following is a hazard associated with incentive spirometry?
   a. Oxygen toxicity
   b. Hypercapnia
   c. Hypoxemia
   d. Hypocapnia

5. The contraindications to IPPB therapy may include:
   a. untreated pneumothorax.
   b. atelectasis.
   c. pneumonia.
   d. cystic fibrosis.

6. Which of the following should be included in a complete physician's order for IPPB?
   a. Medication and dilution
   b. Frequency
   c. Duration of therapy
   d. All of the above

7. What is a contraindication to IPPB therapy?
   a. Complaints of pain
   b. Untreated pneumothorax
   c. Productive cough
   d. Shallow tidal volumes

8. To adjust the tidal volume delivery with the Percussionaire IPV-1C ventilator, you must increase the:
   a. operational pressure.
   b. percussion control.
   c. manual control.
   d. nebulizer control.

9. To increase the frequency (respiratory rate) when using the Percussionaire IPV-1C ventilator, you must increase the:
   a. operational pressure.
   b. percussion control.
   c. manual control.
   d. nebulizer control.

10. PEP and Vibratory PEP therapy are:
    I.   performed during inspiration
    II. performed during exhalation
    III. hyperinflation techniques
    IV. intended to help mobilize secrtetions
    a. I
    b. I and II
    c. I, II, and III
    d. I, II, III, and IV

PERFORMANCE EVALUATION:
Incentive Spirometry

Date: Lab _____ Clinical _____ Agency _____

Lab: Pass _____ Fail _____ Clinical: Pass _____ Fail _____

Student name _____ Instructor name _____

No. of times observed in clinical _____

No. of times practiced in clinical _____

PASSING CRITERIA: Obtain 90% or better on the procedure. Tasks indicated by * must receive at least 1 point, or the evaluation is terminated. Procedure must be performed within the designated time, or the performance receives a failing grade.

SCORING:
2 points — Task performed satisfactorily without prompting.
1 point — Task performed satisfactorily with self-initiated correction.
0 points — Task performed incorrectly or with prompting required.
NA — Task not applicable to the patient care situation.

Tasks:	Peer	Lab	Clinical
* 1. Verifies the physician's order	☐	☐	☐
2. Scans the chart	☐	☐	☐
* 3. Obtains and assembles the required equipment	☐	☐	☐
* 4. Observes standard precautions, including handwashing	☐	☐	☐
5. Identifies the patient, introduces self, explains the procedure	☐	☐	☐
* 6. Places the patient into proper position	☐	☐	☐
* 7. Assesses patient parameters	☐	☐	☐
* 8. Assists in the patient's performance	☐	☐	☐
* 9. Emphasizes the importance of self-motivation to the patient	☐	☐	☐
* 10. Leaves the device within the patient's reach	☐	☐	☐
* 11. Uses aseptic technique	☐	☐	☐
12. Removes unneeded equipment	☐	☐	☐
* 13. Records the procedure on the patient's chart	☐	☐	☐

SCORE: Peer _____ points of possible 26; _____%

                     Lab   _____ points of possible 26; _____%

                     Clinical _____ points of possible 26; _____%

TIME: _____ out of possible 20 minutes

STUDENT SIGNATURES   **INSTRUCTOR SIGNATURES**

PEER: _____   LAB: _____

STUDENT: _____   CLINICAL: _____

PERFORMANCE EVALUATION:
IPPB Therapy

Date: Lab _____ Clinical _____ Agency _____

Lab: Pass _____ Fail _____ Clinical: Pass _____ Fail _____

Student name _____ Instructor name _____

No. of times observed in clinical _____

No. of times practiced in clinical _____

PASSING CRITERIA: Obtain 90% or better on the procedure. Tasks indicated by * must receive at least 1 point, or the evaluation is terminated. Procedure must be performed within the designated time, or the performance receives a failing grade.

SCORING: 2 points — Task performed satisfactorily without prompting.
1 point — Task performed satisfactorily with self-initiated correction.
0 points — Task performed incorrectly or with prompting required.
NA — Task not applicable to the patient care situation.

Tasks:	Peer	Lab	Clinical
* 1. Verifies the physician's order	☐	☐	☐
2. Scans the chart	☐	☐	☐
3. Gathers the equipment			
* a. Respirometer	☐	☐	☐
* b. Ventilator	☐	☐	☐
* c. Peak flowmeter	☐	☐	☐
* d. Breathing circuit	☐	☐	☐
* e. Medication	☐	☐	☐
* 4. Assembles and tests the equipment	☐	☐	☐
* 5. Observes standard precautions, including handwashing	☐	☐	☐
* 6. Identifies the patient, introduces self, and explains the procedure	☐	☐	☐
* 7. Positions the patient	☐	☐	☐
8. Monitors the patient			
* a. Pulse and respirations	☐	☐	☐
* b. Breath sounds	☐	☐	☐
* c. Inspiratory capacity	☐	☐	☐
* d. Peak expiratory flow rate	☐	☐	☐
* e. Blood pressure	☐	☐	☐

9. Instructs the patient

  *   a. Explains correct breathing pattern   ☐ ☐ ☐

  *   b. Explains how to initiate a breath   ☐ ☐ ☐

  *   c. Explains how expiration occurs   ☐ ☐ ☐

  *   d. Explains the warning signs and symptoms   ☐ ☐ ☐

10. Administers therapy

  *   a. Adjusts the ventilator as required   ☐ ☐ ☐

  *   b. Monitors the tidal volume   ☐ ☐ ☐

  *   c. Monitors the respiratory and heart rates   ☐ ☐ ☐

  *   d. Monitors the blood pressure   ☐ ☐ ☐

11. Assists and encourages the patient to cough   ☐ ☐ ☐

12. Monitors therapy effectiveness

  *   a. Inspiratory capacity   ☐ ☐ ☐

  *   b. Peak expiratory flow rate   ☐ ☐ ☐

13. Removes unneeded equipment   ☐ ☐ ☐

* 14. Practices aseptic techniques   ☐ ☐ ☐

* 15. Records the procedure on the patient's chart   ☐ ☐ ☐

SCORE: Peer   _____ points of possible 58; _____%

                    Lab   _____ points of possible 58; _____%

                    Clinical _____ points of possible 58; _____%

TIME: _____ out of possible 15 minutes

STUDENT SIGNATURES

PEER: _____

STUDENT: _____

INSTRUCTOR SIGNATURES

LAB: _____

CLINICAL: _____

PERFORMANCE EVALUATION:

Intrapulmonary Percussive Ventilation (IPV)

Date: Lab _____ Clinical _____ Agency _____

Lab: Pass _____ Fail _____ Clinical: Pass _____ Fail _____

Student name _____ Instructor name _____

No. of times observed in clinical _____

No. of times practiced in clinical _____

PASSING CRITERIA: Obtain 90% or better on the procedure. Tasks indicated by * must receive at least 1 point, or the evaluation is terminated. Procedure must be performed within the designated time, or the performance receives a failing grade.

SCORING: 2 points — Task performed satisfactorily without prompting.
1 point — Task performed satisfactorily with self-initiated correction.
0 points — Task performed incorrectly or with prompting required.
NA — Task not applicable to the patient care situation.

Tasks:

		Peer	Lab	Clinical
*	1. Verifies the physician's order	☐	☐	☐
*	2. Scans the chart for relevant information	☐	☐	☐
*	3. Observes standard precautions, including handwashing	☐	☐	☐
	4. Obtains and assembles the equipment	☐	☐	☐
	5. Identifies the patient, introduces self, and explains the procedure	☐	☐	☐
	6. Positions the patient properly	☐	☐	☐
*	7. Assesses the patient prior to therapy	☐	☐	☐
*	8. Instructs the patient on IPV therapy	☐	☐	☐
*	9. Assists and coaches the patient during therapy	☐	☐	☐
	10. Periodically has the patient cough	☐	☐	☐
	11. Monitors the patient during therapy	☐	☐	☐
	12. Assesses the patient following therapy	☐	☐	☐
	13. Cleans up	☐	☐	☐
	14. Ensures that the patient is safe and comfortable	☐	☐	☐
	15. Documents the procedure in the patient's chart	☐	☐	☐

SCORE: Peer _____ points of possible 30; _____%

                    Lab _____ points of possible 30; _____%

                    Clinical _____ points of possible 30; _____%

TIME: _____ out of possible 30 minutes

STUDENT SIGNATURES   **INSTRUCTOR SIGNATURES**

PEER: _____   LAB: _____

STUDENT: _____   CLINICAL: _____

CHAPTER 18
Bronchoscopy Assisting

INTRODUCTION

Bronchoscopy is visual examination of the tracheobronchial tree. This procedure may be performed using a rigid or a flexible fiberoptic bronchoscope. Bronchoscopy is frequently employed in the management of patients in the acute care setting and in physicians' clinics. The respiratory practitioner will be expected to understand how to assist the physician in this very important diagnostic and therapeutic procedure.

This chapter addresses the indications and contraindications, hazards and complications, and technique and equipment required for the procedure, and how to correctly monitor the patient. In respiratory care practice in the acute care setting, this procedure will be most commonly performed in the short-stay outpatient area and in the intensive care unit in both adult and pediatric patients.

KEY TERMS

- **Bronchoalveolar lavage (BAL)**
- **Bronchoscopy**
- **Cytology brush**
- **Diagnostic bronchoscopy**
- **Fiberoptic bronchoscope**
- **Forceps**
- **Rigid bronchoscope**
- **Therapeutic bronchoscopy**
- **Wang needle**

THEORY OBJECTIVES

At the end of this chapter, the reader should be able to:

- *Differentiate between therapeutic and diagnostic bronchoscopy.*
- *Describe the indications for therapeutic and diagnostic bronchoscopy.*
- *Differentiate between a flexible and rigid bronchoscope and state when the use of a rigid bronchoscope is indicated.*
- *Describe the construction of a flexible fiberoptic bronchoscope.*
- *Describe the specialized instruments used during bronchoscopy.*
- *List the types of laboratory tests performed on samples obtained via bronchoscopy.*
- *List the different solutions used for cytologic, histologic, and microbiologic analysis of bronchoscopy samples.*

- *Describe the appropriate personal protective equipment that should be worn during a bronchoscopy procedure.*
- *Describe the components of a designated bronchoscopy room or suite for outpatient bronchoscopy procedures.*
- *Describe the structure and function of both rigid and flexible bronchoscopes.*
- *Describe the medications used to provide anesthesia and analgesia for a patient prior to bronchoscopy and the potential hazards and adverse effects of these medications.*
- *Describe how to appropriately monitor the patient during the bronchoscopy procedure.*
- *Describe how bronchoscopy may be performed on a patient receiving mechanical ventilation via an endotracheal tube or tracheostomy tube.*
- *Describe the hazards and complications of bronchoscopy.*

CLINICAL PRACTICE GUIDELINES

AARC Clinical Practice Guideline
Fiberoptic Bronchoscopy Assisting

BA 4.0 INDICATIONS

Indications include but are not limited to

4.1 The presence of lesions of unknown etiology on the chest radiograph film or the need to evaluate recurrent pneumonia, persistent atelectasis or pulmonary infiltrates 1,2,4–9

4.2 The need to assess patency or mechanical properties of the upper airway 1,2,4,6,8

4.3 The need to investigate hemoptysis, persistent unexplained cough, dyspnea, localized wheeze, or stridor 1,2,4–8,10

4.4 Suspicious or positive sputum cytology results 1,2,4–6

4.5 The need to obtain lower respiratory tract secretions, cell washings, and biopsies for cytologic, histologic, and microbiologic evaluation 1,2,4,7,9,11,12

4.6 The need to determine the location and extent of injury from toxic inhalation or aspiration 1,2,4,6

4.7 The need to evaluate problems associated with endotracheal or tracheostomy tubes (tracheal damage, airway obstruction, or tube placement) 1,2,4–7

4.8 The need for aid in performing difficult intubations or percutaneous tracheostomies 1,2,4,6,7

4.9 The suspicion that secretions or mucus plugs are responsible for lobar or segmental atelectasis 1,2,4–6

4.10 The need to remove abnormal endobronchial tissue or foreign material by forceps, basket, or laser 1,2

4.11 The need to retrieve a foreign body (although under most circumstances, rigid bronchoscopy is preferred) 6,7,13

4.12 Therapeutic management of endobronchial toilet in ventilator associated pneumonia 14

4.13 Achieving selective intubation of a main stem bronchus 14

4.14 The need to place and/or assess airway stent function 14

4.15 The need for airway balloon dilatation in treatment of tracheobronchial stenosis 15,16

BA 5.0 CONTRAINDICATIONS

Flexible bronchoscopy should be performed only when the relative benefits outweigh the risks.

5.1 Absolute contraindications include

5.1.1 Absence of consent from the patient or his/her representative unless a medical emergency exists and patient is not competent to give permission 1,2

5.1.2 Absence of an experienced bronchoscopist to perform or closely and directly supervise the procedure 1,2,4

5.1.3 Lack of adequate facilities and personnel to care for such emergencies such as cardiopulmonary arrest, pneumothorax, or bleeding 1,2,4

5.1.4 Inability to adequately oxygenate the patient during the procedure 1,2

5.2 The danger of a serious complication from bronchoscopy is especially high in patients with the disorders listed, and these conditions are usually considered absolute contraindications unless the risk-benefit assessment warrants the procedure 1,2,4

5.2.1 Coagulopathy or bleeding diathesis that cannot be corrected 1,2,4

5.2.2 Severe refractory hypoxemia 1,2,4

5.2.3 Unstable hemodynamic status including dysrhythmias 1,2,4

5.3 Relative contraindications (or conditions involving increased risk), according to the American Thoracic Society Guidelines for Fiberoptic Bronchoscopy in adults, 1,2 include

5.3.1 Lack of patient cooperation

5.3.2 Recent (within 6 weeks) myocardial infarction or unstable angina 17

5.3.3 Partial tracheal obstruction

5.3.4 Moderate-to-severe hypoxemia or any degree of hypercarbia

5.3.5 Uremia and pulmonary hypertension (possible serious hemorrhage after biopsy)

5.3.6 Lung abscess (danger of flooding the airway with purulent material)

5.3.7 Obstruction of the superior vena cava (possibility of bleeding and laryngeal edema)

5.3.8 Debility and malnutrition

5.3.9 Disorders requiring laser therapy, biopsy of lesions obstructing large airways, or multiple transbronchial lung biopsies

5.3.10 Known or suspected pregnancy (safety concern of possible radiation exposure)

5.4 The safety of bronchoscopic procedures in asthmatic patients is a concern, but the presence of asthma does not preclude the use of these procedures 11,18

5.5 Recent head injury patients susceptible to increased intracranial pressures 19

5.6 Inability to sedate (including time constraints of oral ingestion of solids or liquids 17

BA 6.0 HAZARDS/COMPLICATIONS

6.1 Adverse effects of medication used before and during the bronchoscopic procedure 4,7,20,21

6.2 Hypoxemia 4,22

6.3 Hypercarbia

6.4 Bronchospasm 23

6.5 Hypotension 24

(Continued)

6.6 Laryngospasm, bradycardia, or other vagally mediated phenomena 4,7,20

6.7 Mechanical complications such as epistaxis, pneumothorax, and hemoptysis 7,20,23,25

6.8 Increased airway resistance 4,26

6.9 Death 27

6.10 Infection hazard for health-care workers or other patients 28–31 (see also Section 13)

6.11 Cross-contamination of specimens or bronchoscopes 28–31

6.12 Nausea, vomiting 23

6.13 Fever and chills 23

6.14 Cardiac dysrhythmias 32

BA 8.0 ASSESSMENT OF NEED:

Need is determined by bronchoscopist assessment of the patient and treatment plan in addition to the presence of clinical indicators as described in Section 4.0, and by the absence of contraindications as described in Section 5.0.1,2,4

BA 9.0 ASSESSMENT OF OUTCOME:

Patient outcome is determined by clinical, physiologic, and pathologic assessment. Procedural outcome is determined by the accomplishment of the procedural goals as indicated in Section 4.0, and by quality assessment indicators listed in Section 11.0.

BA 11.0 MONITORING

Patient monitoring should be done before, at regular intervals during, and after bronchoscopy until the patient meets appropriate discharge criteria. For no or minimal sedation, less monitoring is necessary. For moderate and deep sedation, more monitoring should be done. 47 The following should be monitored before, during, and/or after bronchoscopy, continuously, until the patient returns to his pre-sedation level of consciousness.

11.1 Patient

11.1.1 Level of consciousness 46

11.1.2 Medications administered, dosage, route, and time of delivery 46

11.1.3 Subjective response to procedure (eg, pain, discomfort, dyspnea) 46

11.1.4 Blood pressure, breath sounds, heart rate, rhythm, and changes in cardiac status

11.1.5 SpO_2, FIO_2 and $ETCO_2$ 17,46,48

11.1.6 Tidal volume, peak inspiratory pressure, adequacy of inspiratory flow, and other ventilation parameters if subject is being mechanically ventilated

11.1.7 Lavage volumes (delivered and retrieved)

11.1.8 Monitor and document site of biopsies and washings. Record which lab tests were requested on each sample

11.1.9 Periodic post-procedure follow-up monitoring of patient condition is advisable for 24–48 hours for inpatients. Outpatients should be instructed to contact the bronchoscopist regarding fever, chest pain or discomfort, dyspnea, wheezing, hemoptysis, or any new findings presenting after the procedure has been completed. Oral instructions should be reinforced by written instructions that include names and phone numbers of persons to be contacted in emergency.

11.1.10 Chest radiograph one hour after transbronchial biopsy to exclude pneumothorax 43

11.2 Technical Devices

11.2.1 Bronchoscope integrity (fiberoptic or channel damage, passage of leak test) 36

11.2.2 Strict adherence to the manufacturer's and institutional recommended procedures for cleaning, disinfection, and sterilization of the devices, and the integrity of disinfection or sterilization packaging 35,36

11.2.3 Smooth, unhampered operation of biopsy devices (forceps, needles, brushes)

11.3 Recordkeeping

11.3.1 Quality assessment indicators as determined appropriate by the institution's quality assessment committee

11.3.2 Documentation of monitors indicated in Sections 11.1 and 11.2.

11.3.3 Identification of bronchoscope used for each patient

11.3.4 Annual assessment of the institutional or departmental bronchoscopy procedure, including an evaluation of quality assurance issues

> **11.3.4.1** Adequacy of bronchoscopic specimens (size or volume for accurate analysis, sample integrity)
>
> **11.3.4.2** Review of infection control procedures and compliance with the current guidelines for semicritical patient-care objects 34,35
>
> **11.3.4.3** Synopsis of complications
>
> **11.3.4.4** Control washings to assure that infection control and disinfection/sterilization procedures are adequate, and that cross-contamination of specimens does not occur
>
> **11.3.4.5** Annual review of the bronchoscopy service and all of the above listed record

Reprinted with permission from *Respiratory Care* 2007; 52: 74–80. The complete AARC Clinical Practice Guidelines are available from the AARC Web site (http://www.aarc.org), from the AARC Executive Office, or from *Respiratory Care* journal.

THERAPEUTIC AND DIAGNOSTIC BRONCHOSCOPY

Bronchoscopy is commonly performed for two reasons: therapeutic and diagnostic. Therapeutic indications usually involve secretion removal, foreign body removal, or airway management problems. Diagnostic bronchoscopy is performed to identify or rule out pathologic conditions.

Therapeutic Bronchoscopy

Therapeutic bronchoscopy is performed to remove excessive pulmonary secretions or foreign material suspected of causing lobar or segmental atelectasis. By performing bronchoscopy, the material (secretions or foreign bodies) may be removed and the lobe or segment reinflated (Ernst, 2003).

Therapeutic bronchoscopy may also be performed to evaluate placement of an endotracheal tube or to perform difficult intubation. Occasionally, an endotracheal tube can become dislodged or obstructed. The flexible bronchoscope provides a convenient way to assess endotracheal tube placement and to check the tube for obstruction. In some cases, difficult intubation may be performed by passing a flexible bronchoscope through the endotracheal tube and advancing it during direct visualization. The ability to direct the flexible tip of the bronchoscope facilitates the placement of the endotracheal tube (Ernst, 2003).

Diagnostic Bronchoscopy

Diagnostic bronchoscopy is performed to obtain lower respiratory tract secretions or tissue samples for cytological, histologic, or microbiologic study (Ernst, 2003). Cytologic testing is frequently performed on tissue samples obtained from lesions of unknown etiology as observed on the chest radiograph.

INDICATIONS FOR BRONCHOSCOPY

The indications for both therapeutic and diagnostic bronchoscopy are briefly discussed in the previous section. Table 18-1 lists the indications for both therapeutic and diagnostic bronchoscopy, as adapted from the American Association for Respiratory Care, *Clinical Practice Guideline: Fiberoptic Bronchoscopy Assisting* (AARC, 2007).

RIGID AND FLEXIBLE BRONCHOSCOPES

The *rigid bronchoscope* (Figure 18-1) has some unique advantages and disadvantages. The rigid bronchoscope is frequently used for the removal of foreign bodies.

TABLE 18-1: Bronchoscopy Indications

Therapeutic Indications

- Removal of secretions or mucous plugs causing lobar or segmental atelectasis

- Removal of abnormal endobronchial tissue or foreign bodies

- Evaluation of endotracheal tube placement or performance of difficult intubation

Diagnostic Indications

- Evaluation of lesions of unknown etiology as observed on chest x-ray

- Assessment of patency or mechanical properties of the upper airway

- Investigation of hemoptysis, persistent cough, localized wheezing, or stridor

- Sampling of lower respiratory tract secretions for cytologic, histologic, or microbiologic analysis

- Investigation of suspicious or positive cytologic findings

- The need to determine the location and extent of injury from toxic inhalation or aspiration

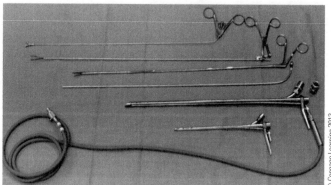

© Cengage Learning 2013

Figure 18-1 A photograph of a rigid bronchoscope

It has a much larger channel that allows the bronchoscopist to pass larger instruments, which are more effective in grasping and removing foreign objects. The larger channel also facilitates removal of large quantities of liquid or more purulent material because a greater amount of subambient pressure may be applied to the larger channel.

The disadvantages of the rigid bronchoscope are that it must be used with the patient under general anesthesia and that it provides a limited view of the tracheobronchial tree, as it cannot pass beyond the main bronchi.

The flexible *fiberoptic bronchoscope* (Figure 18-2) may be used to assess areas located more distally than the rigid bronchoscope can reach. The flexible fiberoptic bronchoscope has a control operated by the bronchoscopist's thumb that enables maneuvering of the bronchoscope tip in a desired direction. This capability allows the bronchoscope to make the sharp bends and turns required to assess the upper lobes. Most recently, video bronchoscopy has gained popularity (Figure 18-3). The video bronchoscope incorporates a miniaturized television camera that allows the bronchoscopist to observe the procedure on a large-screen color monitor. Videotaping of the procedure can also be performed, which provides a real-time permanent record of the bronchoscopy.

Construction of a Flexible Fiberoptic Bronchoscope

The fiberoptic bronchoscope consists of several parts (Figure 18-4). The light channel conducts light from the portable light source to the bronchoscope via fiberoptic bundles. The tip of the bronchoscope is marked in centimeters to assist the bronchoscopist in determining the placement of the scope. The fiberoptic bronchoscope has one or two light channels, an objective lens, and a suction channel (see Figure 18-4). The light channels conduct light from the light source to the distal tip of the bronchoscope. The objective lens focuses the image onto a fiberoptic bundle that conducts the image to the lens set at the proximal end of the bronchoscope, where the bronchoscopist can focus the image. The suction channel is used to aspirate secretions or blood and is also used to pass specialized instruments such as the cytology brush, forceps, and basket.

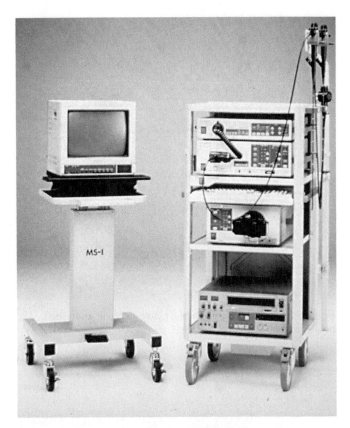

Figure 18-3 A photograph of a videobronchoscope. *(Courtesy of Olympus Medical Corporation)*

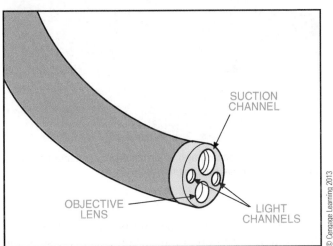

Figure 18-4 A cross section showing the light channels, suction channel, and objective lens of a fiberoptic bronchoscope

TYPES OF INSTRUMENTS

The instruments used during flexible bronchoscopy include the cytology brush, Wang needle, forceps, and basket. The *cytology brush* is a small brush (Figure 18-5) that is designed to be passed through the suction channel and brushed against the location of interest in the tracheobronchial tree. Cytology brushes may be sheathed or unsheathed. A sheathed brush (Figure 18-6) is used

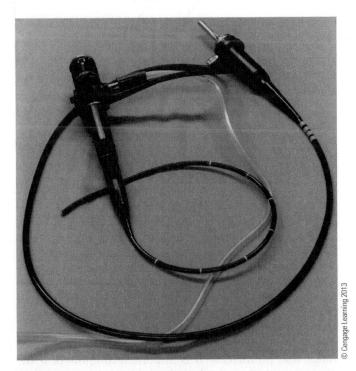

Figure 18-2 A photograph of a flexible fiberoptic bronchoscope

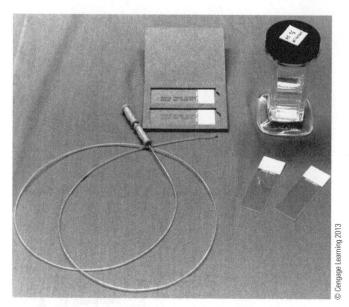

Figure 18-5   A photograph of a cytology brush, dry slide holder, and 95% alcohol fixative

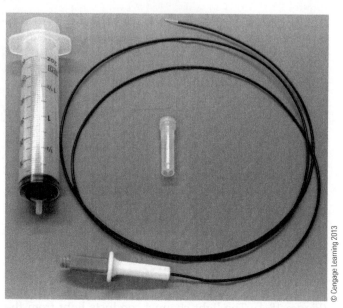

Figure 18-7   A photograph of a Wang needle used for needle biopsy, a 20 mL syringe, and fixative solution

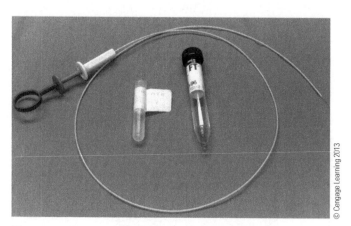

Figure 18-6   A photograph of a sheathed or protected cytology brush and Saccomanno's solution

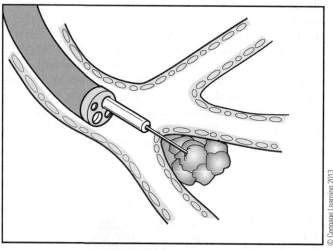

Figure 18-8   An illustration showing the applications of the Wang needle

to obtain a sample that does not become contaminated during retrieval through the suction channel. Use of the sheathed brush is described later in the chapter.

The *Wang needle* is used to sample an area of interest that lies on the opposite side of the bronchial wall from where the bronchoscope is located (Figure 18-7). The Wang needle passes through the bronchial wall and material is then aspirated for analysis (Figure 18-8). Use of the Wang needle is discussed later in this chapter.

The *forceps* are used to sample areas of interest by "biting" off small chunks of tissue (Figure 18-9). Forceps may also be used to retrieve small foreign objects that may be easily grasped. However, once the object has been grasped, the entire bronchoscope must be withdrawn because few foreign objects will pass through the small suction channel.

TYPES OF SAMPLE TESTING AND ANALYSIS

Types of testing and analysis performed on samples obtained by bronchoscopy include cytologic, histologic, and microbiologic testing. Cytologic testing is performed to study a cell's structure, function, or origin. Tissue samples obtained by bronchoscopy are frequently suspected of being cancerous. Histologic testing primarily focuses on the structure of cells, their composition, and how they are organized. Microbiologic testing is used to identify the cause of various pulmonary infections, including those due to bacteria, viruses, fungi, and protozoans. It is important to know how the physician wishes to analyze the samples obtained during

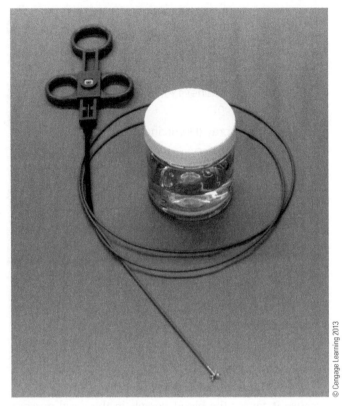

Figure 18-9 A photograph of a pair of biopsy forceps and fixative solution

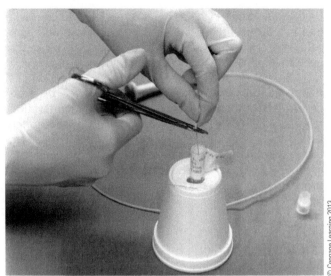

Figure 18-10 A photograph showing the biopsy brush being clipped into a test tube of Saccomanno's solution

bronchoscopy because the fixative agent or treatment of the sample for the laboratory will vary depending on the tests that will be performed.

SOLUTIONS USED TO FIX OR PREPARE SAMPLES FOR TESTING

Depending on the type of tests to be performed on the samples obtained during bronchoscopy, the respiratory practitioner will be expected to know how to prepare the samples properly for the pathologist. Cytologic, histologic, or microbiologic testing determines what solutions are used to prepare the samples.

If cytologic studies will be performed, the samples are usually obtained via brushing or washings. Gently streak or smear the slide with the sample brush using an S-shaped motion. Fix the slide in 95% alcohol. Alternatively, Saccomanno's solution may be used, in which case the brush may be clipped off with scissors and dropped into a test tube containing the solution (Figure 18-10).

Histologic testing requires that the sample be fixed in a formalin solution. Usually, test tubes or small sample collection containers that contain formalin solution are prepared in advance. The samples are then introduced into the solution, capped or sealed, and sent to the laboratory for analysis.

Samples for microbiologic testing may not be fixed at all. The 95% alcohol, Saccomanno's, and formalin solutions could potentially kill or seriously hamper the growth of microorganisms. Physiologic saline (0.9%) or Ringer's lactate is frequently used for preparation of microbiology samples to quantify organisms per milliliter.

PERSONAL PROTECTIVE EQUIPMENT

Bronchoscopy is an invasive procedure in which the bronchoscopist and the bronchoscopy assistant are at risk for body substance contact via splashing or direct contact; therefore, the standard precautions as recommended by the Centers for Disease Control and Prevention (CDC) should be strictly adhered to (Siegel & the Health Care Infection Control Practices Committee, 2007). Personal protective equipment includes a waterproof gown, gloves, mask and goggles or full face shield or mask-shield combination, and a radiation dosimeter badge.

A waterproof gown is required because body fluids may come in contact with the bronchoscopist or the bronchoscopy assistant. Without the use of a waterproof gown, it is likely that clothing could become soiled with the patient's secretions or body fluids during the procedure.

The use of gloves is mandatory. The practitioner will be handling instruments (brushes, forceps, or baskets) and syringes (used in sampling of bronchoalveolar lavage fluid) that have come in contact with the patient's body fluids. Therefore, a protective barrier is required to prevent these fluids from coming in contact with the skin.

A mask over the mouth and nose is worn as protection from inhaling or aspirating aerosolized droplets that can be produced by the patient's coughing during the procedure. If the presence of acid-fast bacilli (AFB) is suspected, both the bronchoscopist and the bronchoscopy assistant should wear high-efficiency particulate air (HEPA) masks in accordance with CDC and Occupational Safety and Health Administration (OSHA) guidelines.

Goggles, a full face shield, or a mask-shield combination is worn to protect the eyes from splashes and aerosolized droplets. The specific type of personal protective eyewear is a matter of personal preference; however, it should be worn at all times.

A radiation dosimeter badge should also be worn because often bronchoscopy is performed under fluoroscopy so that the bronchoscopist may more accurately assess the placement of the bronchoscope. The dosimeter badge should be analyzed for radiation exposure according to both OSHA and institutional policies and procedures.

BRONCHOSCOPY ROOM OR SUITE

Frequently, outpatient bronchoscopy is performed in a specialized room or suite specifically designed for the procedure. The bronchoscopy suite has multiple banks of fluorescent lighting that provide a high degree of illumination while not producing excessive heat. Irradiation by ultraviolet (UV) lights placed high in the room is used to destroy AFB bacteria that may be aerosolized during coughing. The room also has special filtration and air-changing requirements, in which the air is circulated at a faster rate than in other areas. The bronchoscopy suite is also equipped with piped oxygen, air, and vacuum services that may be required to run equipment and provide supplemental oxygen for the patient during the procedure.

MEDICATIONS EMPLOYED FOR ANESTHESIA AND ANALGESIA

The respiratory practitioner is expected to know how to prepare the patient properly for the bronchoscopy procedure, which includes both anesthesia and analgesia. The medications frequently used for bronchoscopy are listed in Table 18-2.

For initial preparation of the patient, 4 mL of 4% lidocaine is aerosolized using a small-volume nebulizer. A bronchodilator such as albuterol may be mixed with and aerosolized along with the lidocaine solution. Then the patient inhales the mixture and should be encouraged to exhale through the nose to help anesthetize the nasal passages more completely. The nebulizer treatment may be followed by use of Hurricane or Cetacaine spray. Upper airway reflexes and the effectiveness of topical anesthesia may be tested by using a long cotton-tipped swab to manipulate the uvula while the patient holds the mouth open widely.

The absence of the gag reflex is an encouraging sign of the effectiveness of the efforts to provide topical anesthesia.

Long cotton-tipped swabs may be used to anesthetize the nasal passages further. The swabs are dipped into lidocaine jelly (4%) and then passed into the nasal passages. Some physicians prefer to use cocaine topically

TABLE 18-2: Medications Used in Bronchoscopy

Medications for Anesthesia

- Lidocaine (Xylocaine) 1%, 2%, 4%; 0.5% for pediatric patients
- Benzocaine spray (Hurricane spray)
- Benzocaine-tetracaine-butamben (Cetacaine) spray

Medications for Secretion or Bleeding Management

- Atropine
- Epinephrine (1:20,000 concentration)

Medications for Sedation

- Diazepam (Valium)
- Midazolam (Versed)
- Lorazepam (Ativan)

because it causes the blood vessels in the nasal mucosa to constrict, opening the passage further and helping to control any bleeding.

A venous catheter (an intravenous [IV] line) may be placed to facilitate the administration of analgesics such as diazepam, midazolam, or lorazepam. Use of these medications achieves the desired analgesic effect, reducing the patient's anxiety regarding the procedure; however, these drugs may produce unwanted hazards and complications.

Hazards and Complications of the Medications Used for Bronchoscopy

The lidocaine (2% distal to the vocal cords) that is aerosolized prior to the procedure, and which may also be administered during the procedure through the suction channel, has potential unwanted effects. In some patients it is possible to achieve low but measurable plasma concentrations of lidocaine from the doses given before and during bronchoscopy. Adverse effects with low plasma concentrations may include vertigo, restlessness, tinnitus, and difficulty in focusing the eyes. Further increases in plasma concentration can lead to skeletal muscle twitching and seizures (Langmack, Martin, Pak et al. 2000). Therefore, with administration of this drug, the patient should be monitored for these signs and symptoms.

The use of analgesic agents such as diazepam, midazolam, and lorazepam may cause depression of the respiratory drive in some patients. This effect may be observed primarily as a decrease in respiratory rate and tidal volume. Patients should be closely monitored for signs and symptoms of respiratory depression when these drugs are given.

PATIENT MONITORING

Patient variables that should be monitored during bronchoscopy include blood pressure, heart rate and rhythm, oxygen saturation (SpO$_2$), and fraction of inspired oxygen (FIO$_2$). The patient's blood pressure should be measured and recorded prior to anesthetic administration. In the event of an adverse drug effect, baseline blood pressure is very helpful in patient management.

Heart rate and rhythm are easily monitored in real time by the use of electrocardiographic (ECG) monitoring equipment. Usually cardiac leads are placed and lead II is monitored. Changes in rate and rhythm may be easily assessed at any point during the procedure. Alarm limits may also be set to alert the bronchoscopist and the assistant of potential problems.

SpO$_2$ may be monitored using a pulse oximeter with alarm limits set to signal impending problems. FIO$_2$ may also need to be monitored if the patient is receiving high-flow oxygen or is being mechanically ventilated during the procedure.

HAZARDS AND COMPLICATIONS OF BRONCHOSCOPY

Hazards and complications of bronchoscopy include hypoxemia (AARC, 2007), wheezing, hypotension, bradycardia, hemoptysis, bleeding, and infection.

Hypoxemia is a common complication of bronchoscopy. Many patients undergoing the procedure have underlying lung disease. The insertion of the bronchoscope and the application of subambient pressure result in the removal of oxygen from the airways, causing hypoxemia, in much the same manner as described in Chapter 20.

Wheezing may be precipitated by the irritation of the patient's airway by the bronchoscope. This stimulation can result in bronchospasm, causing wheezing. Frequently, a bronchodilator such as albuterol is mixed with the lidocaine and given prior to bronchoscopy to help to prevent this effect.

Hypotension, bradycardia, and other vagal reflex effects may be caused by the physical stimulation of the bronchoscope in the airway via the vagus nerve. The patient should be monitored for these effects; early detection is facilitated by the electrocardiographic monitor and automatic blood pressure monitoring if available.

Localized bleeding during bronchoscopy is usually controlled by the administration of 1:20,000 epinephrine through the suction channel of the bronchoscope and application of direct pressure with the tip of the bronchoscope. The patient may experience hemoptysis following the procedure as these localized areas of bleeding gradually resolve.

Because bronchoscopy is an invasive procedure, infection is always a concern. The likelihood of infection and cross-contamination may be minimized through the proper care and cleaning of the bronchoscope between patients.

PROFICIENCY OBJECTIVES

At the end of this chapter, the reader should be able to:

- *Demonstrate how to prepare the equipment required for bronchoscopy.*
- *Demonstrate how to prepare the paperwork and charting forms needed for this procedure.*
- *Demonstrate how to prepare the medications used for the procedure.*
- *Demonstrate how to connect the proper monitoring equipment to the patient and set the alarms appropriately.*
- *Demonstrate how to start an IV line or insert a heparin lock.*
- *Demonstrate how to administer preoperative medications, including those for analgesia and anesthesia.*
- *Demonstrate how to provide supplemental oxygen during the procedure.*
- *Demonstrate how to assist the bronchoscopist during the procedure, including administration of medications and collection of specimens for analysis.*

- *Demonstrate how to properly prepare specimens for analysis by the laboratory, including those for cytological, histological, and microbiological study.*
- *Demonstrate how to assist the physician during a bronchioalveolar lavage (BAL).*
- *Correctly monitor the patient during the procedure for adverse effects.*
- *Demonstrate how to perform bronchoscopy on a patient who is being mechanically ventilated.*
- *Demonstrate how to monitor the patient after the procedure and prepare the bronchoscope for cleaning.*
- *Demonstrate correct documentation of the procedure, including medications administered and patient monitoring data.*
- *Correctly clean the bronchoscope following the procedure.*
- *Demonstrate how to correctly deliver the specimens obtained during the procedure to the laboratory for analysis.*

EQUIPMENT PREPARATION

Bronchoscopy can progress smoothly and almost effortlessly, or it may be conducted in a tense environment in which nothing seems to go correctly. The ease of the procedure is largely dependent on how well the bronchoscopy assistant has set up and prepared for the procedure. Therefore, it is very important to prepare everything and have all required equipment ready at hand and organized in such a way that it can easily be retrieved when it is required.

Bronchoscope Preparation

Attach the bronchoscope to the light source and connect the light source to a suitable electrical outlet (120 V 60 Hz or 220 V 60 Hz). Turn on the light source and check to ensure that light is conducted to the distal end of the bronchoscope and that the light source is functioning properly.

If required, attach the suction valve to the bronchoscope and connect the bronchoscope to a suction source. Adjust the vacuum level to the maximum setting. It is also advisable to have a second vacuum source ready with a Yankauer suction tool attached to it. Place the bronchoscope onto the bronchoscopy cart or tray and cover it with a sterile towel.

Have a bite block at hand so that if the physician wishes to pass the bronchoscope orally the bronchoscope may be protected. The preferred route is to pass the bronchoscope nasally rather than orally. Even with the use of a bite block, an orally placed instrument can occasionally slip out of position so that the patient bites down reflexively, ruining the fiberoptics.

Medication Preparation

First, draw up 50 mL of 2% lidocaine and transfer it into a sterile container such as a urology analysis container. Label the container "2% lidocaine" and locate it on the bronchoscopy cart or tray where it can be easily reached. Have two 10 mL syringes with "slip tips" nearby for drawing up the solution as required.

Then draw up 50 mL of normal saline (0.9%) and transfer it into a sterile container such as a urology analysis container. Label the container "normal saline" and locate it on the bronchoscopy cart or tray where it can be easily reached. Have two 10 mL syringes with "slip tips" nearby for drawing up the solution as required.

Finally, draw up 20 mL of 1:20,000 epinephrine and transfer it into a sterile container such as a urology analysis container. Label the container "1:20,000 epinephrine" and locate it on the bronchoscopy cart or tray where it can be easily reached. Have two 10 mL syringes with "slip tips" nearby for drawing up the solution as required.

Also have available several unit dose containers (4 mL) of 20% acetylcysteine (Mucomyst) should the physician wish to instill it through the bronchoscope. Have available a 10 mL syringe for injecting the solution through the bronchoscope.

Sample Solution Preparation

Have slide containers with 95% alcohol, formalin, and normal saline (0.9%) available. Additionally, test tubes containing those solutions and Saccomanno's solution should be at hand. Attach blank labels to the specimen containers and have a pen readily available to label the container as to where the sample was obtained during the procedure. Clean sterile slides should be available to make smears for cytologic study. Often a slide dispenser is used to prepare specimens. Dry slides are frequently used for AFB and mycologic culturing. Organize the containers into groupings (cytology, histology, and microbiology) so that during the procedure it is not necessary to hunt to find what is needed.

Emergency Equipment

Ensure that a "code cart" is in the procedure room. Check the cart for appropriate Advanced Cardiac Life Support (ACLS) emergency medications; a manual resuscitator; a defibrillator; and intubation supplies, including a suction catheter.

Personal Protective Equipment

Check to be sure that personal protective equipment is available for all personnel participating in the procedure. This equipment includes waterproof gowns, masks (HEPA if required), gloves, and eye protection.

Equipment for the Patient

It is desirable to have certain pieces of equipment available for the patient. These items include tissues, an emesis basin, a denture cup (if required), a washcloth, and a small hand towel.

DOCUMENTATION PREPARATION

This procedure requires an informed consent form that must be signed by the patient and a witness. The form explains the procedure and the hazards and complications associated with it. It may be necessary to explain to the patient in nontechnical language what the form means; therefore, the practitioner should be familiar with it and what it says. If the bronchoscopy procedure is to be performed in the intensive care unit setting and the patient is unable to sign the form, a member of the patient's immediate family may give consent if such a person is available.

Have any charting forms required by the institution at hand with the patient's name and identification number imprinted or written in ink on the forms. Also have any laboratory testing request forms available and marked with the patient's name and identification number.

PATIENT PREPARATION

Prior to performing the bronchoscopy procedure, it is important to prepare the patient for the procedure. This includes establishing appropriate monitoring and administration of anesthesia and analgesia and having the patient sign the appropriate consent forms.

Monitoring

Attach cardiac leads so that lead II may be monitored. Connect the patient to an ECG monitor and verify that heart rate and rhythm are appropriately displayed.

Measure the patient's blood pressure, and if a blood pressure cuff is available, apply it and attach it to an automatic sphygmomanometer. Set the time interval to the desired frequency of blood pressure measurement.

Initiate continuous pulse oximetry monitoring. The use of a finger or ear probe is usually best for this procedure. An ear probe is less likely to experience artifact due to patient motion during the procedure. Check the oximeter against the ECG monitor to verify that the signal is appropriate.

Anesthesia and Analgesia

Start an IV line or insert a heparin lock so that IV access is available for the administration of analgesic agents.

Nebulize 4 to 5 mL of 4% lidocaine and, depending on institutional policy, add 2.5 mg albuterol to the solution to achieve bronchodilation. Have the patient inhale deeply and slowly. Request that the patient exhale through the nose to help anesthetize the upper airway more fully. Following the administration of the lidocaine, Hurricane or Cetacaine spray may be used to anesthetize the upper airway further. Evaluate the numbness of the upper airway by manipulating the uvula with a long cotton-tipped swab. If the patient does not gag, the airway has been well anesthetized.

Using long cotton-tipped swabs, apply 4% lidocaine jelly to the nasal passages and into the region of the turbinates. This will help to lubricate the airway and also to anesthetize it further.

When the physician arrives, determine whether or not analgesic medication is desired and what dose is to be administered intravenously. Draw up the medication according to the physician's instructions and administer the drug through the IV line or heparin lock.

SUPPLEMENTAL OXYGEN

Supplemental oxygen may be provided by using a nasal cannula with one prong "clipped off" or plugged, or by using a simple mask in which one side has had an opening cut into it so that the bronchoscope may be passed through it. Monitor the patient's SpO_2 and adjust the oxygen delivery to maintain saturations greater than 90% during the procedure.

BRONCHOSCOPY ASSISTING

Bronchoscopy assisting involves many skills, including medication administration, assistance with tissue sampling, and specimen preparation.

Medication Administration

The physician will advance the bronchoscope through either naris and advance it through the upper airway. If the patient begins to cough or fight the procedure, be prepared to instill 2% lidocaine upon the physician's request.

Once the bronchoscope enters the larynx, the coughing reflex is commonly encountered. Again, be prepared to administer 2% lidocaine on the physician's request. Depending on how the procedure progresses, the physician will request that you instill 2% lidocaine, normal saline, or if secretions are very thick, 20% acetylcysteine.

Tissue Sampling

Tissue sampling is frequently performed to obtain small samples for laboratory analysis. The most common instruments used are the biopsy forceps and the brush (either protected or unprotected).

Forceps

If tissue samples are required for diagnostic purposes, the physician will perform biopsy using the forceps, brush, or the Wang needle. If biopsy is to be performed, the practitioner will be requested to pass the forceps through the suction channel. Be certain that the forceps are closed upon passing them through the suction channel. Open forceps will damage the fiberoptics of the bronchoscope. The physician will then direct the tip of the scope, guiding the forceps to the desired location, and will advance the forceps near the tissue site. The physician will request "open," which means the practitioner must open the forceps by pushing the thumb control. The physician will then push the open forceps into the tissue to be sampled and request "closed," which means the practitioner must then retract the thumb control to close the forceps. Before the procedure, manipulate the forceps to determine which position is open and which is closed.

Brushes

Brushing is usually performed for cytologic or histologic analysis. The brushes used may be protected or unprotected. If protected brushing is performed, a protected brush is passed through the suction channel much like the forceps. The physician will request "out," which means the practitioner must advance the inner brush through the wax seal, exposing it past the outer sheath, by manipulating the thumb control; then the brush is advanced. The physician will brush the desired site multiple times and request "retract" or "in," which means the practitioner must then retract the brush once again into the protective sheath. The brush is then withdrawn, and slides are made or the brush is clipped off and dropped into the proper solution for the test.

Wang Needle

The Wang needle is used to sample areas that are on the opposite side of the bronchial wall from the bronchoscope (extrabronchial). As for the forceps, the practitioner must pass the Wang needle with the needle retracted. Failure to do so will ruin the bronchoscope's fiberoptics. The Wang needle is passed through the bronchoscope in a similar way to the forceps and brush. The physician will request "out," which means the practitioner must advance the needle, exposing it past the sheath, by manipulating the thumb control. The physician will then "dart" the desired site multiple times and request "retract" or "in," which means the practitioner must then retract the brush once again into the protective sheath. Often the Wang needle is used under a fluoroscope to determine its location more precisely. Suction is applied to the end of the Wang needle with a syringe to aspirate a sample for analysis. Very small samples are secured by this method, so look closely to ensure that an adequate specimen was obtained. Prepare the sample as required for cytological or histological analysis.

Bleeding Control

Often during sampling, bleeding may occur. The physician may control bleeding by direct pressure, instillation of 1:20,000 epinephrine, or a combination of both. It is important to have good suction through the bronchoscope to protect the airway in the event of profound bleeding. If bleeding is profound, a pulmonary tamponade balloon may be inserted, inflated, and left in place to control bleeding.

SPECIMEN PREPARATION

As described earlier, it is important to have ready the different solutions that may be needed to prepare samples for analysis. Properly prepared and labeled samples make it easier for the pathologist to achieve an accurate diagnosis. If the practitioner can make it easier for the pathologist and the pulmonologist performing the procedure through preparation and proficiency, the practitioner is in effect marketing his or her services.

Label all samples with the patient's name and the anatomical location from which the samples were taken. Ask the physician to name all lobes and segments sampled to ensure that specimens from different areas are not inadvertently mislabeled.

If in doubt, ask the pulmonologist whether the sample is for cytologic, histologic, or microbiologic analysis and prepare the sample accordingly by using the correct solution.

BRONCHOALVEOLAR LAVAGE

Bronchoalveolar lavage (BAL) is performed when the area to be sampled is distal to the segmental or subsegmental bronchi in which the bronchoscope is resting. The bronchoscopist advances the bronchoscope until it is "wedged," totally occluding the airway. The bronchoscopist will then request the practitioner to instill 30 to 50 mL of normal saline (0.9%) rapidly through the suction channel and then withdraw the syringe plunger firmly, attempting to aspirate as much of the instilled saline as possible through the bronchoscope. The concept is to lavage the area distal to the bronchoscope with saline and then to recover as much of the saline as possible. The recovered solution will contain the cells that the physician wishes to analyze. When performing BAL, be sure to turn off the suction to the bronchoscope, or install a trap, so that if the physician occludes the suction port, the sample will not be lost to the wall suction unit! BAL may be performed several times until the physician is satisfied that the area has been adequately sampled. BAL is often performed to obtain specimens for microbiologic analysis. Visually inspect the sample, observing for a foamy head, almost like that on beer, indicating that surfactant is present and a good sample has been obtained.

PATIENT MONITORING

As described earlier, the patient must be monitored for signs of hypoxemia, wheezing, hypotension, bradycardia, hemoptysis, and bleeding. Through the use of appropriate monitoring devices and paying attention to the patient, early signs may be detected. Remember that the physician is more focused on the bronchoscope and its location and may not necessarily be closely watching the patient. Therefore, it is the practitioner's responsibility as the assistant to report adverse signs or symptoms. This may easily be performed using the ECG monitor, blood pressure monitor, and pulse oximeter. The practitioner's knowledge and assessment skills are what make the respiratory practitioner uniquely qualified to assist in this procedure.

Following the procedure, closely monitor the patient's level of consciousness and evaluate the patient for the return of the protective reflexes of the upper airway as the local anesthetic wears off. Evidence of the return of reflexes includes coughing and appropriate swallowing. The medications used for analgesia may be reversed using agents such as naloxone or flumazenil. Before the patient is allowed to leave the area, be certain that he or she is alert enough to walk and behave appropriately. It is frequently recommended that another person drive the patient home following the procedure. It is also important to instruct the patient not to eat or drink anything for at least 2 hours following the procedure because aspiration may be likely owing to the local anesthesia.

BRONCHOSCOPY DURING MECHANICAL VENTILATION

Bronchoscopy may be performed on patients who are receiving mechanical ventilation. This is accomplished by inserting the instrument through a swivel adapter that has a soft Silastic seal, which helps to prevent volume loss in passing the bronchoscope (Figure 18-11). The bronchoscope is advanced through the endotracheal or tracheostomy tube. If the patient is orally intubated, a bite block should be inserted to protect the bronchoscope.

Ventilator settings will need to be modified during the procedure. Usually the tidal volume is reduced, the flow rate reduced, the FIO_2 increased, and the respiratory rate increased. Experience is required to determine the optimal settings that still achieve adequate ventilation and oxygenation without the occurrence of ventilator pressure cycling (high-pressure alarm) with each breath.

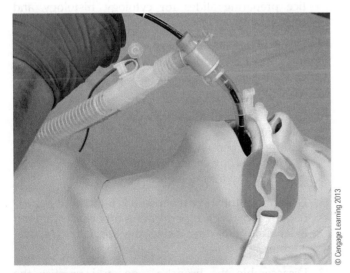

© Cengage Learning 2013

Figure 18-11 A photograph showing how a swivel adapter is used to perform bronchoscopy on a patient on ventilatory support through an endotracheal tube

DOCUMENTATION

Bronchoscopy assisting requires appropriate documentation of the procedure just as for other respiratory care procedures. Documentation should include the patient's baseline blood pressure, ECG strip, and SpO_2. The preparation of the patient, including medications used, IV access, and routes of delivery, should also be documented. Appropriate notations during the procedure of blood pressure, respiratory rate, ECG, and SpO_2 should also be provided.

The amount and type of medications given during the procedure should also be documented. If you know you started with 50 mL each of lidocaine and normal saline and 20 mL of 1:20,000 epinephrine, measuring what you have left and subtracting it from what you started with will tell you the amount you used. Any use of other medications such as acetylcysteine and analgesia-reversal agents should also be documented.

The location of samples obtained and the types of tests (cytologic, histologic, or microbiologic) the samples were prepared for should also be noted. If BAL was performed, note how much aspirate was recovered and the number of attempts that were made.

The patient's recovery data, including respiratory rate, ECG, and blood pressure, should be documented. It is also important to document the return of reflexes by noting coughing, swallowing, and so forth.

CLEANING THE BRONCHOSCOPE

The bronchoscope is initially prepared for cleaning by aspirating about 100 to 200 mL of normal saline through the suction channel. A cleaning brush may be passed through the bronchoscope a few times and more saline aspirated before transporting the bronchoscope to the decontamination area.

At the decontamination area, the bronchoscope is disassembled and those parts that can be decontaminated using surgical instrument soap are washed and rinsed. The outer surface of the bronchoscope is cleaned with a disinfection solution and a soft cloth.

The bronchoscope's suction channel is cleaned by aspirating a cold disinfection agent such as Cidex or Control III through the suction channel and brushing it with the cleaning brush. Following cleaning, the bronchoscope should then be tested for leaks. The bronchoscope may then be placed into an automatic endoscope washer, in which alternately a cold disinfection solution and sterile water are passed through the bronchoscope, cleaning it. Alternatively, the bronchoscope may be immersed in a cold disinfection solution and allowed to stand for the required period.

Following disinfection, the bronchoscope is rinsed with sterile water and then 95% alcohol is injected through the suction channel, which promotes drying. The bronchoscope is then aseptically covered until it will be used again.

SAMPLE DELIVERY

Once the samples are labeled and properly prepared, they should be delivered to the laboratory for analysis. Any institutional slips required for testing should be filled out completely and submitted with the samples. Most laboratories require time and date stamping of when samples are received; therefore, comply with the requirements and use the stamping machine to accomplish this on the laboratory slips. Prompt delivery and handling of the specimens will help to ensure that an accurate diagnosis may be made. Remember the practitioner is marketing services not only to the patient and the pulmonologist but also to the pathologist!

References

American Association for Respiratory Care. (2007). AARC clinical practice guideline: Fiberoptic bronchoscopy assisting. *Respiratory Care, 52*, 74–80.

Ernst, A. (2003). Interventional pulmonary procedures: Guidelines from the American College of Chest Physicians. *Chest, 123*(2), 1693–1717.

Langmack EL, Martin RJ, Pak J, et al. (2000). Serum lidocaine concentrations in asthmatics undergoing research bronchoscopy. *Chest, 117*(4), 1055–1060.

Siegel, J. D., & the Health Care Infection Control Practices Committee. (2007, December). 2007 Guideline for isolation precautions: Preventing transmission of infectious agents in healthcare settings. *American Journal of Infection Control, 35*([10] Suppl. 2), S65–164.

Practice Activities: Bronchoscopy Assisting

1. Organize and set up a bronchoscopy tray or cart, including:
   a. Fixative solutions
   b. Microscope slides
   c. Instruments: biopsy forceps, brushes, and Wang needle
   d. Saline
   e. Topical anesthetics
   f. Analgesics
   g. Intravenous supplies
   h. 10 mL syringes

2. Once the cart or tray has been organized, practice bronchoscopy assisting with a laboratory partner with one partner calling for a particular item and the other retrieving it.

3. Using water-soluble lubricant, practice making S-shaped smears on microscope slides with the brush. Practice evenly distributing the material throughout your smear.

4. Make a list of all of the emergency supplies that you might want when performing bronchoscopy, should an emergency situation occur.

5. Assemble the bronchoscope and test it for function:
   a. Light source   b. Suction source

6. Practice using the biopsy forceps, protected brush, and Wang needle until you can change from the open to the closed position without having to concentrate or think about it.

7. Using an intubation mannequin for practice, practice performing the bronchoscopy procedure with a laboratory partner, alternating roles as the bronchoscopist and the bronchoscopy assistant.

8. Using a water-soluble lubricant as a "sample," practice preparing slides for cytology, histology, and microbiology analysis.

9. Using a laboratory partner as a patient, properly instrument the patient for monitoring during bronchoscopy, including blood pressure, ECG, and pulse oximetry.

10. Using your institution's charting forms, prepare the following:
    a. Informed consent
    b. Bronchoscopy charting form
    c. Laboratory testing requests

11. Using an intubation mannequin, intubate the mannequin and practice performing bronchoscopy with a laboratory partner using the specialized swivel adapter.

12. Disassemble the bronchoscope, and practice the cleaning procedure according to your institutional policy.

Check List: Bronchoscopy Assisting

_____ 1. Follow standard precautions, including hand washing.

2. Gather the appropriate equipment and supplies:
_____ a. Bronchoscope and light source
_____ b. Fixative solutions
_____ c. Microscope slides
_____ d. Instruments: biopsy forceps, brushes, and Wang needle
_____ e. Saline
_____ f. Topical anesthetics
_____ g. Analgesics
_____ h. Intravenous supplies
_____ i. 10 mL syringes
_____ j. Personal protective equipment

3. Prepare the documentation for the procedure:
_____ a. Informed consent form
_____ b. Charting forms
_____ c. Laboratory request forms

_____ 4. Organize the bronchoscopy tray or cart.

_____ 5. Assemble and test the bronchoscope.

_____ 6. Identify the patient and introduce yourself.

_____ 7. Correctly instrument the patient for monitoring.

_____ 8. Gown and glove for the procedure.

_____ 9. Initiate an IV line or insert a heparin lock.

10. Administer anesthesia topically:
_____ a. Small-volume nebulizer
_____ b. Cotton-tipped swabs

_____ 11. Evaluate adequacy of anesthesia.

_____ 12. Administer analgesia per physician's request.

_____ 13. Assist the physician with the procedure.

14. As required, obtain tissue samples for analysis:
_____ a. Brushing
_____ b. Biopsy specimens
_____ c. BAL

_____ 15. Assist the physician with bleeding control as required.

_____ 16. Monitor the patient during the procedure.

_____ 17. Correctly document the procedure.

_____ 18. Evaluate the patient following the procedure.

_____ 19. Properly clean and care for the bronchoscope.

Self-Evaluation Post Test: Bronchoscopy Assisting

1. Which of the following rationales is/are indicated for a therapeutic bronchoscopy?
   I. Removal of secretions or mucous plugs
   II. Assessment of the patency or mechanical properties of the upper airway
   III. Removal of abnormal endobronchial tissue or foreign bodies
   IV. Investigation of hemoptysis, persistent cough, localized wheezing, or stridor
   a. I, II   c. II, III
   b. I, III   d. II, IV

2. Which of the following rationales is/are indicated for a diagnostic bronchoscopy?
   I. Removal of secretions or mucous plugs
   II. Assessment of the patency or mechanical properties of the upper airway
   III. Removal of abnormal endobronchial tissue or foreign bodies
   IV. Investigation of hemoptysis, persistent cough, localized wheezing, or stridor
   a. I, II   c. II, III
   b. I, III   d. II, IV

3. For which of the following indications might a rigid bronchoscope be preferred over a fiberoptic bronchoscope?
   a. Removal of foreign bodies
   b. Diagnosis of peripheral lung disease
   c. Bronchoalveolar lavage
   d. Brushing for cytology

4. Which of the following may be performed on samples obtained from bronchoscopy?
   I. Cytology testing
   II. Histology testing
   III. Microbiology testing
   a. I   c. II, III
   b. I, II   d. I, II, III

5. Which of the following is/are considered appropriate personal protective equipment for bronchoscopy?
   I. Waterproof gown
   II. Gloves
   III. Eye shields or goggles
   IV. Mask or HEPA mask
   a. I   c. I, II, III
   b. I, II   d. I, II, III, IV

6. Which of the following make(s) a bronchoscopy suite or room different from the typical outpatient examination room?
   I. Air filtration rate
   II. Ultraviolet lights
   III. Increased lighting
   IV. Presence of piped gases
   a. I   c. I, II, III
   b. I, II   d. I, II, III, IV

7. Which of the following are medications employed for anesthesia?
   I. Lidocaine (Xylocaine)
   II. Lorazepam (Ativan)
   III. Benzocaine (Hurricane spray)
   IV. Midazolam (Versed)
   a. I, II   c. II, III
   b. I, III   d. II, IV

8. Which of the following are medications employed for analgesia?
   I. Lidocaine (Xylocaine)
   II. Lorazepam (Ativan)
   III. Benzocaine spray (Hurricane spray)
   IV. Midazolam (Versed)
   a. I, II   c. II, III
   b. I, III   d. II, IV

9. Which of the following is/are appropriate for monitoring the patient during bronchoscopy?
   I. Heart rate and rhythm
   II. Blood pressure
   III. Pulse oximetry
   IV. Respiratory rate and rhythm
   a. I   c. I, II, III
   b. I, II   d. I, II, III, IV

10. Which of the following may be (a) hazard(s) of bronchoscopy?
    I. Bleeding
    II. Hemoptysis
    III. Wheezing
    IV. Hypotension
    a. I   c. I, II, III
    b. I, II   d. I, II, III, IV

PERFORMANCE EVALUATION:
Bronchoscopy Assisting

Date: Lab _____ Clinical _____ Agency _____

Lab: Pass _____ Fail _____ Clinical: Pass _____ Fail _____

Student name _____ Instructor name _____

No. of times observed in clinical _____

No. of times practiced in clinical _____

PASSING CRITERIA: Obtain 90% or better on the procedure. Tasks indicated by * must receive at least 1 point, or the evaluation is terminated. Procedure must be performed within the designated time, or the performance receives a failing grade.

SCORING:
2 points — Task performed satisfactorily without prompting.
1 point — Task performed satisfactorily with self-initiated correction.
0 points — Task performed incorrectly or with prompting required.
NA — Task not applicable to the patient care situation.

Tasks:	Peer	Lab	Clinical
* **1.** Observes standard precautions, including hand washing	☐	☐	☐
* **2.** Prepares all documentation forms			
a. Informed consent	☐	☐	☐
b. Charting forms	☐	☐	☐
c. Laboratory request slips	☐	☐	☐
* **3.** Organizes and sets up a bronchoscopy tray or cart, including:			
a. Fixative solutions	☐	☐	☐
b. Microscope slides	☐	☐	☐
c. Biopsy forceps, brushes, and Wang needle	☐	☐	☐
d. Saline	☐	☐	☐
e. Topical anesthetics	☐	☐	☐
f. Analgesics	☐	☐	☐
g. Intravenous supplies	☐	☐	☐
h. 10 mL syringes	☐	☐	☐
* **4.** Ensures that emergency supplies are available	☐	☐	☐
* **5.** Assembles the bronchoscope and tests its function	☐	☐	☐
* **6.** Identifies the patient and introduces self	☐	☐	☐

* **7.** Prepares the patient for monitoring

    a. ECG   ☐ ☐ ☐

    b. Blood pressure   ☐ ☐ ☐

    c. Oximetry   ☐ ☐ ☐

* **8.** Applies personal protective equipment   ☐ ☐ ☐

* **9.** Starts an IV line or inserts a heparin lock   ☐ ☐ ☐

* **10.** Administers local anesthesia

    a. Nebulizes 4% lidocaine   ☐ ☐ ☐

    b. Administers lidocaine jelly on swabs   ☐ ☐ ☐

* **11.** Administers analgesia per physician's request   ☐ ☐ ☐

* **12.** Assists the physician with the procedure   ☐ ☐ ☐

* **13.** Prepares the samples for laboratory analysis   ☐ ☐ ☐

* **14.** Monitors the patient   ☐ ☐ ☐

* **15.** Correctly documents the procedure   ☐ ☐ ☐

* **16.** Correctly disassembles and cleans the bronchoscope   ☐ ☐ ☐

* **17.** Delivers the specimens to the laboratory for analysis   ☐ ☐ ☐

SCORE: Peer _____ points of possible 58; _____%

               Lab _____ points of possible 58; _____%

               Clinical _____ points of possible 58; _____%

TIME: _____ out of possible 30 minutes

STUDENT SIGNATURES

PEER: _____

STUDENT: _____

INSTRUCTOR SIGNATURES

LAB: _____

CLINICAL: _____

CHAPTER 19
Equipment Processing and Surveillance

INTRODUCTION

A variety of methods are used for the decontamination of respiratory therapy equipment. Because of the presence of water, saline, and body secretions in warm reservoirs, respiratory therapy equipment may serve as an excellent vector for the growth and transmission of disease. Knowledge of the organisms, the general principles of microbiology, and the effects the processing methods have on microorganisms is essential to process equipment correctly. An understanding of how the different methods affect rubber and plastics is also required to prevent costly errors.

This chapter reviews basic microbiology. The respiratory practitioner will learn how the various processing methods affect microorganisms and the equipment being processed. Bacteriologic surveillance and how it is an integral part of equipment processing is also covered.

KEY TERMS

- Antisepsis
- Bacilli
- Bacteriologic surveillance
- Capsule
- Cocci
- Disinfection
- Endotoxins
- Ethylene oxide
- Eukaryotic bacteria
- Gamma irradiation
- Glutaraldehyde
- Gram stain
- Pasteurization
- Prokaryotic bacteria
- Quaternary ammonium compounds
- Spirilla
- Steam autoclaving
- Sterilization

THEORY OBJECTIVES

At the end of this chapter, the reader should be able to:

- *Differentiate between eukaryotic and prokaryotic organisms.*
- *Differentiate among the following bacterial shapes:*
  - *Cocci*
  - *Bacilli*
  - *Spirilla*
- *Differentiate between capsules and endospores and their significance for equipment processing.*
- *Differentiate between the cell wall structure of gram-positive and gram-negative bacteria.*
- *Describe the structural characteristics of viruses.*
- *Define the following terms:*
  - *Sterilization*
  - *Disinfection*
  - *Antisepsis*
- *Differentiate among the following processing methods and how they kill microorganisms:*
  - *Steam autoclaving*
  - *Pasteurization*
  - *Ethylene oxide processing*
  - *Glutaraldehyde processing*
  - *Exposure to quaternary ammonium compounds*
  - *Gamma irradiation*
- *Diagram and explain the rationale for the design of an equipment processing facility.*
- *Explain the purpose of a bacteriologic surveillance program.*
- *Differentiate among the following sampling methods and state the most appropriate application for each:*
  - *Aliquot*
  - *Output*
  - *Rinse*
  - *Rodac plate*
  - *Swab*
- *Explain how the data from a bacteriologic surveillance program are used.*

RELATED MICROBIOLOGY

Eukaryotic and Prokaryotic Cell Types

Eukaryotic bacteria have a true nucleus containing genetic material (chromosomes). The nucleus is a membrane-enclosed structure separate from other structures within the cell. The cell reproduces by *mitosis*, wherein the genetic material is duplicated and the cell divides in two. Eukaryotic organisms are more complex than prokaryotes.

Prokaryotic bacteria have a single naked DNA molecule within the cell. Internal structures are fewer and far less complex than those of eukaryotes. Replication is accomplished by cell division, not mitosis as in eukaryotic organisms. There are significant differences in the cell wall structure, as discussed later when the Gram stain is explained.

Bacterial Shapes

Bacterial shapes further help to classify prokaryotic bacteria. The most common shapes are cocci, bacilli, and spirilla. These shapes are illustrated in Figure 19-1. The shapes are relatively constant and more or less independent of environmental influences.

Cocci are spherical in shape. A rounded shape enables this bacterial type to resist desiccation because of its smaller surface area.

Bacilli are rod-shaped. They are greater in length than in diameter. The greater surface area makes them more susceptible to desiccation but also allows these bacteria to absorb nutrients more easily from the environment.

Spirilla are spiral in configuration. A spiral shape aids in motility through fluids.

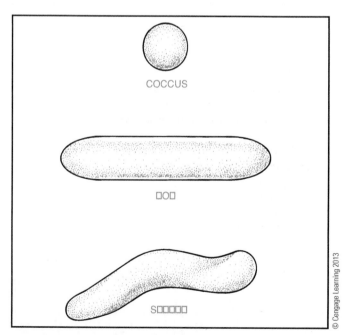

© Cengage Learning 2013

Figure 19-1   Common bacterial shapes

Gram Stain

The *Gram stain* is used to differentiate further among the prokaryotic bacteria. The Gram stain demonstrates differences in composition of the cell walls of bacteria. The prokaryotes are divided into *gram-positive* and *gram-negative* organisms according to their response to the Gram stain.

Gram-positive bacteria have cell walls that are composed of a single layer and are thicker than cell walls of gram-negative bacteria. The wall is composed of peptidoglycan (a material composed of two sugars and a small group of amino acids). Figure 19-2 compares the cell wall structures of gram-positive and gram-negative organisms. During the Gram stain process, the thickness of the cell wall causes the alcohol or acetone to seal it by dehydration, thereby preventing the release of the crystal violet solution. The captured stain makes the organism appear purple in color.

Gram-negative bacteria have a more complex, multilayered cell wall. These bacteria have a peptidoglycan layer and also a lipopolysaccharide and protein layer in their cell walls. Frequently this outer layer containing lipopolysaccharides is toxic to humans. This occurs primarily when the cell lyses and harmful substances called *endotoxins* are released from the cell wall. During the Gram stain process, the alcohol or acetone dissolves the crystal violet compound in the cell wall so that the color is washed away. As a result, gram-negative bacteria appear colorless.

Capsules and Endospores

Some bacteria secrete a slimy or gummy material on the surface of the cell wall. When this material forms a closely compacted structure, it is termed a *capsule*. These capsules are usually composed of polysaccharides, polypeptides, or polysaccharide-protein complexes (Madigan, Dunlap, & Clark, 2009). Presence of a capsule brings a survival or protective advantage to the bacteria. The capsule makes it difficult for the body's phagocytes to ingest the bacteria. The presence of capsules may also cause the formation of antibodies. Generally speaking, encapsulated bacteria are more difficult to destroy.

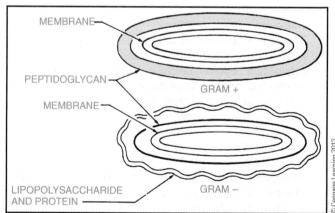

© Cengage Learning 2013

Figure 19-2   A comparison of gram-positive and gram-negative cell wall structures

Some prokaryotic bacteria reproduce by means of endospores. *Bacillus* and *Clostridium* are common bacteria that reproduce in this way. Genetic material within the endospore is encapsulated within the cell by a very resistant wall. Eventually, the cell lyses, releasing the endospore. The spore can lie dormant for years, surviving very unfavorable conditions. The spore is very resistant to heat, ionizing radiation, and chemicals. When conditions are right, the spore germinates, forming a new vegetative organism. Because of the resistance spores possess, special techniques for equipment processing must be employed to destroy them.

Common Causative Organisms

Table 19-1 summarizes the common organisms that are responsible for many hospital-acquired infections. As shown in the table, many of these organisms are present in sinks, water reservoirs, and the body's secretions. Aseptic techniques and proper decontamination and equipment processing will help to reduce the incidence of hospital-acquired infections.

EQUIPMENT PROCESSING TERMS

Before the different methods of equipment processing are discussed, it is important to understand some of the terms used in the process. The different methods accomplish different results depending on the techniques employed and the effects the methods have on microorganisms.

Sterilization

Sterilization is the complete destruction of all forms of microorganisms, including spores. The equipment or surface is completely free of any living microorganisms. This does not imply that the equipment or surface does not have dead "carcasses" of microorganisms. They are there; however, further life is not possible, and replication does not occur when they are cultured.

Disinfection

Disinfection is the complete destruction of vegetative forms of pathogenic microorganisms. Note that spores are not included in this definition. Only vegetative, or living, forms are destroyed.

Antisepsis

Antisepsis is the application of chemical agents to a surface to inhibit microbial growth and reproduction. It does not kill organisms; it just slows them down. Typically, chemical agents may be applied to the skin or the surface of equipment to accomplish this end. For example, wiping a mouthpiece with alcohol before its use is one application of antisepsis.

EQUIPMENT PROCESSING METHODS

There are several methods employed in equipment processing. It is important to understand whether the method sterilizes or disinfects and what effect it has

TABLE 19-1: Organisms Commonly Implicated in Hospital-Acquired Infections

ORGANISM	DISEASE	SOURCE	FORM	PROCESSING
Haemophilus influenzae	Meningitis Pneumonia Epiglottitis	Upper respiratory tract	Gram–bacillus	Pasteurize
Klebsiella pneumoniae	Klebsiella pneumonia	Solutions, reservoirs	Gram–bacillus	Pasteurize
Legionella pneumophila	Legionnaires' disease	Sinks, showers, air ducts	Gram–bacillus	Pasteurize
Mycobacterium tuberculosis	Tuberculosis	Secretions, vectors	Spore	Sterilize
Neisseria	Meningitis Sexually transmitted disease (STD)	Secretions	Gram–diplococci	Pasteurize
Pseudomonas aeruginosa	*Pseudomonas* pneumonia	Secretions, reservoirs, soap, sinks	Gram–bacillus	Pasteurize
Serratia	Pneumonia	Solutions, reservoirs	Gram–bacillus	Pasteurize
Staphylococcus aureus	Staphylococcal infections	Secretions, nasal passage, vectors, wounds	Gram+cocci	Pasteurize
Streptococcus pneumoniae	Pneumonia	Secretions	Gram+cocci	Pasteurize

on equipment that has plastic or rubber parts. Each method has its own specific equipment and procedural requirements that, if not met, will render the processing ineffective. It is important to understand each method and its requirements to ensure the destruction of harmful microorganisms. No matter what manner is used, the handling, packaging, and storage after processing have a direct effect on the cleanliness of equipment used at the patient's bedside. Also, equipment does not remain decontaminated forever. Each method of sterilization has an expiration date. This length of time will vary with the method and packaging used. Therefore, rotation of supplies is important. All processed equipment should be dated at the time processing is complete. Stock should be checked to ensure that supplies are not out of date.

Steam Autoclaving

Steam autoclaving is one of the more common methods employed in the processing of medical equipment. This method will sterilize any equipment that is properly prepared and processed.

The steam autoclave works by combining high heat, moisture, and pressure. Moist heat is more penetrating than dry heat. This may easily be understood by comparing two climates: A warm day with a temperature of 90°F is more comfortable in Salt Lake City than in Washington, DC because of the differences in moisture content of the air. A similar principle is employed in the steam autoclave. Steam (water vapor) is combined with high heat (121 to 126°C) and increased pressure (1 to 2 atm) to penetrate cellular structures effectively, thereby destroying microorganisms.

Correct preparation of equipment for this processing method is important. Equipment should be disassembled and washed in a detergent solution to remove gross particles and body secretions. The equipment is then rinsed and packaged in a porous material such as muslin, linen, kraft or brown paper, crepe paper, or Mylar (a polyester film).

The equipment must be loosely packed so that the steam can penetrate all surfaces. Any liquid containers must be loosely capped to allow penetration of the steam.

Exposure time, temperature, and pressure are critical to ensure this method's effectiveness. Before exposure, all air must first be evacuated from the autoclave and replaced by steam. A typical setting is 121°C at 15 psi for 15 minutes or 121°C at 30 psi for 3 minutes. Masking tape indicators are used to verify that exposure has been sufficient for sterilization. If the conditions and time are correct, the indicator will change color. Similar indicators are available for use with the ethylene oxide processing method.

Autoclaving may be detrimental to some equipment. It tends to dull surgical instruments and to speed deterioration of rubber and some plastics, and it cannot be used on electrical/electronic devices. If in doubt about the ability of equipment to withstand autoclaving, contact the equipment manufacturer before use.

Pasteurization

Pasteurization of respiratory therapy equipment is popular. Its advantages include a temperature that is not high enough to destroy many plastics (unlike the temperature in autoclaving). It uses only water so that employee exposure to chemicals does not occur and no residue is left on the equipment. Water is also less expensive than chemicals or other methods.

Pasteurization is a process that involves heating a liquid to temperatures sufficient to destroy vegetative organisms (living organisms capable of reproduction). This process is employed commercially in the processing of milk and beer. In respiratory care, equipment is immersed in a hot water bath at 77°C for 30 minutes. This is a disinfection method and does not sterilize equipment. The moist heat coagulates the cellular protein of microorganisms. Spores are not destroyed by this method, as their resistance to heat is much greater.

Correct preparation of equipment is important for this method to succeed. Equipment must be disassembled and washed in a detergent solution to remove any gross particles and body secretions, as they may protect and insulate the organism from the heat. The equipment should then be rinsed before pasteurizing. Small items are usually contained in a nylon net or mesh to prevent them from sinking to the bottom of the pasteurizer and making retrieval difficult. The pasteurizer temperature should be checked and the equipment immersed for the proper time.

Following pasteurization, the equipment should be aseptically removed and allowed to dry in a special drying cabinet that filters bacteria and particles from the air. Following this, items should be assembled, packaged, and dated.

Ethylene Oxide Processing

Ethylene oxide is a toxic gas that is combined with moisture and heat to sterilize equipment. Its effectiveness depends on equipment preparation, gas concentration, humidity, and temperature.

Ethylene oxide works by affecting the enzymes, reproduction, and metabolism of microorganisms. It will kill spores if the method is correctly applied for the correct time.

Equipment must be properly prepared for this processing method by disassembling and washing in detergent to remove mucus and body secretions. Because this method employs a gas, any microorganisms protected within mucus may not be affected by the gas. After washing, the equipment should be rinsed and allowed to dry. Water combines with the ethylene oxide to form ethylene glycol. This toxic chemical is potentially dangerous if inhaled or ingested through contact with medical equipment. After drying, the equipment should be packaged in porous packages such as wrapping paper, muslin or other cloth, or Mylar. A sterilization indicator is used for each package. It changes color if conditions and exposure time are correct and sterilization occurs. This indicator may be a special tape used to close the package or a device that is placed inside the package.

Gas concentration, temperature, and humidity all must be closely regulated for this method to be successful. Ethylene oxide concentration should be between 800 and 1000 mg/L. The ethylene oxide gas should be mixed with carbon dioxide or Freon to reduce the hazard of gas explosion. The temperature should range between 49 and 57°C. If the temperature becomes higher than 60°C, ethylene oxide will polymerize and become ineffective. The humidity should be maintained between 30% and 60%. Time exposure is typically 3 to 4 hours.

Following ethylene oxide exposure, the equipment should be aerated in a special cabinet to remove the gas. Aeration time may be as long as 24 hours or several days, depending on the material composition of the equipment.

This method may be harmful to some plastics because they retain and hold the gas. Polyvinyl chloride (PVC) and neoprene rubber require extended aeration times (Lucas, 2003). Because of the detrimental effects on some materials and the longer time involved for processing, a larger stock of supplies is required.

Glutaraldehyde Processing

Glutaraldehyde is a chemical that is used to cold-sterilize or disinfect equipment by immersion. Cidex is an example of a glutaraldehyde preparation. Heat is not used in glutaraldehyde processing.

Glutaraldehyde is manufactured in an alkaline (requires activation) and Cidex OPA® (*ortho*-Phthalaldehyde) forms.

Equipment is processed by immersion in the activated chemical. The acid or alkaline environment glutaraldehyde provides destroys microorganisms. Organisms are destroyed by alkylation of enzymes.

To process equipment for the method, begin by disassembling it and washing it in detergent. Following the detergent wash, rinse the equipment and shake it dry before immersing it in the solution.

Equipment should be immersed for 10 to 20 minutes to disinfect and for 6 to 10 hours to sterilize it. After immersion, the equipment should be aseptically rinsed of any glutaraldehyde residue (it is toxic) with a sodium bisulfite solution (1 ounce to 1 gallon of water) and allowed to dry in a drying cabinet with filter elements to remove particles and microorganisms from the air. Because of glutaraldehyde's toxicity, some persons using this processing technique may show signs of dermal sensitivity or allergy to the fumes. This sensitivity may be a potential drawback.

Because this method involves the use of a liquid, it is not compatible with most electronic equipment. Rubber and plastic products seem to tolerate it without adverse effects. The life of the product ranges from 14 to 30 days, depending on the product. At the end of this time interval, it must be discarded and new solution prepared.

Processing with Quaternary Ammonium Compounds

Quaternary ammonium compounds ("quats") are special cationic detergents that destroy microorganisms by disrupting or lysing the cell membrane. Most quats are specific for one or a few types of organisms. Therefore, quats are frequently combined to broaden their destruction of microorganisms.

These liquids are used in a way similar to that for the glutaraldehyde method. Clean equipment is immersed for 10 to 20 minutes. Equipment preparation is essentially the same as for the former method. The exposure time varies with the product being used. It is typically 10 to 20 minutes. This method accomplishes disinfection but not sterilization—spores and some viruses will survive exposure.

Most respiratory care equipment will tolerate this processing method. The exception is electronic equipment because a solution is used. Another disadvantage to this method is that the life of the solution is very short, on the order of 1 to 2 weeks. However, the cost is usually less than that for glutaraldehyde.

Gamma Irradiation

Gamma radiation is a form of ionizing radiation that destroys microorganisms by affecting the cells' enzymes and DNA. *Gamma irradiation* is a method of sterilization.

The equipment required for this method is expensive and the protective shielding is cumbersome. Its use is usually limited to manufacturers of medical equipment.

Owing to the nature of the radiation, the physical structure and composition of some materials may be altered by exposure. If the facility uses this method, consult the equipment manufacturer before subjecting equipment to this method.

FACILITY DESIGN FOR EQUIPMENT PROCESSING

The facility design for equipment processing is important in the maintenance of asepsis and the prevention of cross-contamination. Figure 19-3 shows a sample design of an equipment processing area. Note that the equipment "flows" through the facility in only one direction and that equipment in storage is physically separated from equipment being processed. The facility is divided into three main areas: decontamination, processing, and storage. The flow of equipment begins at decontamination, where it is disassembled, washed, and rinsed. Ideally, a pass-through is provided between the decontamination area and processing. The processing area is the area in which the equipment is disinfected or sterilized, reassembled, tested, and packaged for storage. As noted, the storage area should be physically separate from the other two. The design should prevent contact between clean and dirty equipment and traffic flow through the clean equipment, assembly, and storage areas.

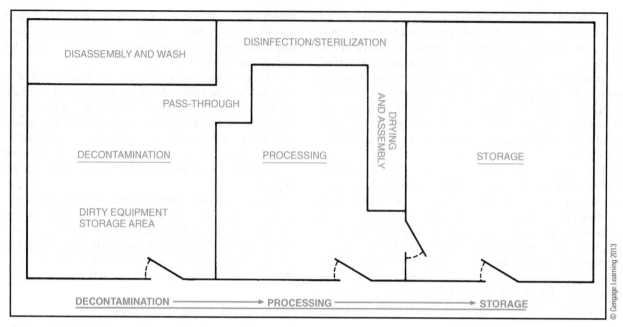

Figure 19-3 Equipment flow pattern in an equipment processing facility

BACTERIOLOGIC SURVEILLANCE PROGRAMS

Bacteriologic surveillance provides data on the effectiveness of disinfection and sterilization methods, equipment handling, storage procedures, and how frequently in-use equipment should be changed. Various methods are used to culture clean and in-use equipment. Each method has its advantages, disadvantages, and most suitable application.

Aliquot Culturing

Aliquot culturing is a method of culturing solutions.

A sterile sample is drawn. Then serial dilutions are made from the sample and cultured. Colony counts are made and the colonizing organisms are identified. This method is qualitative—the data obtained indicate what, but not how much, is there. Aliquot culturing is used to detect contamination in fluids.

Rinse Sampling

The rinse sampling technique involves sloshing sterile broth aseptically in respiratory therapy equipment tubing, recovering it, and allowing the broth to incubate. Colonies are then counted and colonizing organisms identified. This method is quantitative and very sensitive. Procedures must be carefully followed so as not to introduce sampling errors. This method is used primarily to culture processed equipment for assessing the effectiveness of the processing method.

Rodac Plate Sampling

Rodac plate sampling involves the use of a special raised-bed culture plate. The plate is pressed against the equipment being cultured and then incubated. This method samples a very small area and therefore may not detect contamination in other parts of the equipment. It is qualitative, providing only data on what, but not how much, is there. This method is used primarily to sample clean equipment for contamination. Because the plate is flat, its use is somewhat limited.

Swab Sampling

Swab sampling is one of the most common methods used in bacteriologic surveillance. A special swab containing culture medium is aseptically withdrawn from its container and rubbed onto the surface being cultured. The swab is then aseptically rubbed onto a culture plate.

The plate is then incubated. Colonies are identified and counted. This method is very convenient in that small cotton-tipped applicators are used as swabs. The method is qualitative and samples only a small area.

DATA UTILIZATION

Culturing of clean equipment should be performed monthly. The data obtained will help to identify the effectiveness of processing, storage procedures, and equipment assembly practices. If positive results (indicating the presence of pathogens) are obtained, equipment handling and processing procedures must be reviewed and scrutinized to find the source of contamination. Samples at each step of the process should be cultured in an attempt to identify the point at which contamination is occurring. Once the source is identified, the procedures should be modified to eliminate the contamination problem.

In-use equipment is exposed to an environment teeming with microorganisms. Positive culture results, indicating contamination by pathogenic organisms, necessitate further investigation. If specimens from the patient using the equipment yield similar culture results, the source is the patient. If the patient's sputum culture is negative for the organism, other sources such as cross-contamination, personnel, airborne transmission, solutions, and compressed gases must be considered and investigated. The source must be identified and the contamination problem corrected.

If *Staphylococcus epidermidis* or other nonpathogenic members of the normal flora are cultured on clean or in-use equipment, the most likely contamination source is the person conducting the culturing. This is one source of sampling error. Contamination may be introduced during collection, sample handling, or culturing. Maintenance of aseptic technique during all phases is important.

Not all schools or facilities will have the equipment required to perform the procedures outlined in this section. The hospital laboratory, microbiology school, or microbiology department may be willing to provide the supplies necessary to complete these activities if they are not available. Not all personnel in respiratory care will be responsible for the performance of these procedures. However, by completing these activities, the practitioner will gain a better understanding of the surveillance process.

PROFICIENCY OBJECTIVES

At the end of this chapter, the reader should be able to:

- *Demonstrate the correct technique for swab sampling.*
- *Demonstrate how to fill out a bacteriologic surveillance record.*
- *Demonstrate how to decontaminate and process respiratory care equipment:*
  - *Wash the equipment in detergent and water, removing all gross contamination.*
  - *Rinse all equipment, removing residual detergent.*
  - *If steam autoclaving or gas sterilizing, wrap equipment in approved wrapping material, enclosing appropriate indicators.*
  - *Correctly sterilize or disinfect the equipment.*
  - *Correctly assemble and package equipment following disinfection.*
  - *Label and store the processed equipment, rotating the stock.*

SWAB SAMPLING

Obtain the Required Supplies

Obtain the supplies required for this method of sampling. In addition to the culturing device, obtain the required paperwork for the procedure that will be filled out on collection of the sample.

Hand Hygiene

Handwashing is important during this procedure to prevent inadvertent introduction of microorganisms. Aseptic technique is very important to prevent sampling errors.

Aseptically Withdraw the Swab and Sample the Area

Aseptically remove the swab from its container and rub it onto the surface being cultured. Return the swab to its container and rub it onto the culture medium. Label the swab as to what was cultured—for example, "baffle in [a particular] Ohio Deluxe nebulizer."

SURVEILLANCE RECORDS

A surveillance record should contain the information listed in Figure 19-4. It is very important that the records be correctly maintained and that all parts be completely filled out.

- Date
- Personnel who did the sample
- For in-use equipment
  - Patient's name
  - Hospital number
  - Diagnosis
  - Nursing unit or location (room number)
- Type of equipment
- Equipment number or serial number if available
- Equipment status
  - Clean
  - In-use (number of hours in service)

Figure 19-4 Elements of the bacteriologic surveillance record

Transport the Plate to the Laboratory Facility

Fill out the paperwork associated with the surveillance program and deliver the labeled plate to the laboratory facility for culturing.

PROCESSING RESPIRATORY CARE EQUIPMENT

Washing

All equipment must be washed prior to processing. Washing removes sputum, blood or blood products, and other organic contamination. The removal of contamination is important because some processing methods (e.g., gas sterilization) may not penetrate to the surface of the equipment. Soiled parts also frequently do not function properly in an assembly, binding or not conducting gas or fluids as they should.

Equipment should be washed in water using a surgical detergent. The detergent reduces the surface tension of the water, facilitating the removal of contamination (Howie, 2008). Some detergents also have a bacteriostatic action. Use plenty of friction and water to remove stubborn contamination. Friction combined with detergent and water will remove most contamination.

Rinsing

Immediately after washing the equipment, it is important to rinse it, removing all detergent residues. The chemicals used in some processing methods (e.g., quaternary ammonium compounds and glutaraldehyde) are diluted by detergents, reducing their effectiveness.

For gas sterilization, it is important to dry the equipment before packaging and processing. Water combines with ethylene oxide to form ethylene glycol, a very toxic compound.

Packaging

Two sterilization methods—steam autoclaving and gas sterilization—require that the equipment be packaged in permeable wrapping prior to processing. The permeable wrapping allows the steam or gas to penetrate to the equipment and helps to prevent the contamination of sterile articles following processing. A device made up of several components should be packaged loosely to allow the steam or gas to reach all exposed surfaces.

An indicator is placed in the wrap with each piece of equipment, or special indicator tape is used to seal the wrap. The indicator will change color if sterilization conditions have been met. The color change of the indicator assures the processing technician that the processing method has met the minimum conditions for sterilization.

Processing the Equipment

Equipment processing will result in either sterilization or disinfection, depending on what method is being used. Processing in the acute care setting usually involves one of the following: (1) steam autoclaving, (2) gas sterilization, (3) use of glutaraldehydes, or (4) use of quaternary ammonium compounds. For each method, it is important to use correct temperatures, pressures, or concentrations to ensure desired results.

Package Equipment Following Disinfection

Equipment should be rinsed, dried, and packaged following processing. Aseptic procedures should be followed including a 5-minute scrub and use of a gown, shoe covers, and a hair net. Following assembly, the equipment should be checked for function and tested prior to packaging if possible. The respiratory practitioner's diligence and close attention to details may avert a crisis in the emergency department, operating suite, or intensive care unit.

Label and Store the Equipment

All equipment should be labeled showing the date of processing and initialed by the processing technician. The equipment should be stored with other clean equipment. All reusable equipment that has been processed should be rotated such that the most recently processed equipment is to the rear of the shelf or bin and older stock is moved forward for use.

References

Howie, R. (2008). Survival of enveloped and non-enveloped viruses on surfaces compared with other micro-organisms and impact of suboptimal disinfectant exposure. *Journal of Hospital Infection, 69*(4), 368–376.

Lucas, A. D. (2003). Residual ethylene oxide in medical devices and device material. *Journal of Biomedical Materials Research Part B: Applied Biomaterials, 66*(2), 548–552.

Madigan, M. T., Dunlap, P. V., & Clark, D. P. J. (2009). *Brock biology of microorganisms* (12th ed.). Upper Saddle River, NJ: Benjamin Cummings.

Additional Resource

Association of Perioperative Registered Nurses. (2005). Recommended practices for high-level disinfection, *AORN Journal, 81*(2), 402–412.

Practice Activities: Equipment Processing and Surveillance

1. Practice swab sampling on the following equipment:
   a. Tubing dryer
   b. Oxygen humidifier
   c.

IN YOUR PRACTICE

(1) Obtain the required supplies.
(2) Wash your hands.
(3) Practice aseptic technique.
(4) Correctly prepare the equipment for sampling.
(5) Sample for the appropriate length of time.
(6) Label and transport the sample.
(7) Complete all paperwork.

2. Obtain specimens for culture from your hands, nasal passages, and the sink in the laboratory and identify what organisms grow.

3. Practice processing respiratory care equipment, including:
   a. Washing
   b. Rinsing
      (1) Drying if required (gas sterilizing and steam autoclaving)
   c. Packaging for processing (gas sterilizing and steam autoclaving)
   d. Processing:
      (1) Steam autoclaving
      (2) Gas sterilizing
      (3) Glutaraldehyde processing
      (4) Processing with quaternary ammonium compounds
   e. Rinsing and drying if required
   f. Assembling and testing the equipment following processing
   g. Packaging the equipment aseptically:
      (1) Labeling all equipment
   h. Stocking the equipment in the clean equipment room

Check List: Bacteriologic Surveillance

_____ 1. Gather the appropriate supplies:
_____   a. Sampling swabs
_____   b. Required paperwork
_____ 2. Wash your hands before obtaining a sample.
_____ 3. Prepare a sampling device for use.
_____ 4. Aseptically obtain the sample.

_____ 5. Correctly handle the sampling device after sample collection.
_____ 6. Label and transport the sample to the laboratory.
_____ 7. Complete all paperwork.

Check List: Equipment Processing

_____ 1. Perform a 5 minute scrub.
_____ 2. Cover your clothing:
_____   a. Use a gown.
_____   b. Put on shoe covers.
_____   c. Put on gloves.
_____   d. Put on a hair net.
_____ 3. Disassemble and wash the equipment.
_____ 4. Rinse the equipment and dry it if gas sterilization is used.
_____ 5. Package the equipment before processing by gas sterilization or steam autoclaving:

_____   a. Use the correct wrapping material.
_____   b. Use an indicator.
_____ 6. Process the equipment correctly:
_____   a. Use the correct time exposure.
_____   b. Use the correct temperature.
_____   c. Use the correct concentration.
_____ 7. Assemble the equipment following processing.
_____ 8. Test the equipment.
_____ 9. Package the equipment.
_____ 10. Label and store the equipment.

Self-Evaluation Post Test: Equipment Processing and Surveillance

1. Prokaryotic bacteria are differentiated by:
   I. shape.
   II. Gram stain.
   III. color.
   IV. size.
   V. cell wall structure
   a. I, III
   b. I, II
   c. II, IV
   d. III, V

2. Of eukaryotes and prokaryotes, the more complex organisms are the:
   a. prokaryotes.
   b. eukaryotes.

3. The complete destruction of all microorganisms is:
   a. termed sterilization.
   b. accomplished by pasteurization.
   c. termed asepsis.
   d. termed disinfection.

4. A method of disinfection is:
   a. ethylene oxide processing.
   b. steam autoclaving.
   c. gamma irradiation.
   d. exposure to quaternary ammonium compounds.

5. Which of the following principles are incorporated into the design of an equipment processing facility?
   I. Equipment flows in one direction.
   II. Stored and processed equipment are separated.
   III. Reassembly takes place in the decontamination area.
   IV. Disinfection/sterilization takes place in the processing area.
   a. I, III, IV
   b. I, II, IV
   c. II, III, IV
   d. I, II

6. An indicator is used to:
   a. establish when equipment is out of date.
   b. tell when equipment has been cleaned.
   c. identify when sterilization has occurred.
   d. tell when equipment has been contaminated.

7. Gram-negative bacteria appear:
   a. red.
   b. violet.
   c. blue.
   d. colorless.

8. Gram-positive bacteria appear:
   a. red.
   b. violet.
   c. blue.
   d. colorless.

9. The most common types of sampling methods are:
   I. aliquot.
   II. rinse.
   III. Rodac plate.
   IV. swab.
   a. I, III
   b. II, IV
   c. I, IV
   d. I, V

10. Prior to using any disinfection method on any respiratory care equipment:
    a. equipment should be disassembled, washed in surgical soap, and rinsed.
    b. you should check for a physician's order.
    c. equipment should be properly packaged.
    d. equipment should be sterilized first.

PERFORMANCE EVALUATION:
Bacteriologic Surveillance

Date: Lab _____ Clinical _____ Agency _____

Lab: Pass _____ Fail _____ Clinical: Pass _____ Fail _____

Student name _____ Instructor name _____

No. of times observed in clinical _____

No. of times practiced in clinical _____

PASSING CRITERIA: Obtain 90% or better on the procedure. Tasks indicated by * must receive at least 1 point, or the evaluation is terminated. Procedure must be performed within the designated time, or the performance receives a failing grade.

SCORING: 2 points — Task performed satisfactorily without prompting.
1 point — Task performed satisfactorily with self-initiated correction.
0 points — Task performed incorrectly or with prompting required.
NA — Task not applicable to the patient care situation.

Tasks:	Peer	Lab	Clinical
* 1. Gathers the appropriate equipment	☐	☐	☐
* 2. Observes standard precautions, including hand washing	☐	☐	☐
* 3. Aseptically prepares the sampling device	☐	☐	☐
* 4. Correctly samples the equipment	☐	☐	☐
* 5. Correctly handles the culturing device following sampling	☐	☐	☐
* 6. Labels and transports the sample to the laboratory for culture	☐	☐	☐
* 7. Completes all required paperwork	☐	☐	☐

SCORE: Peer _____ points of possible 14; _____%

Lab _____ points of possible 14; _____%

Clinical _____ points of possible 14; _____%

TIME: _____ out of possible 20 minutes

STUDENT SIGNATURES

PEER: _____

STUDENT: _____

INSTRUCTOR SIGNATURES

LAB: _____

CLINICAL: _____

PERFORMANCE EVALUATION

Date: Lab _____ Clinical _____ Agency _____

Lab: Pass _____ Fail _____ Clinical: Pass _____ Fail _____

Student name _____ Instructor name _____

No. of times observed in clinical _____

No. of times practiced in clinical _____

PASSING CRITERIA: Obtain 90% or better on the procedure. Tasks indicated by "*" must receive at least 1 point or the evaluation is terminated. Procedure must be performed within the designated time or the performance receives a failing grade.

SCORING:

2 points — Task performed satisfactorily without prompting.
1 point — Task performed satisfactorily with self-initiated correction.
0 points — Task performed improperly or with prompting required.
NA — Task not applicable to the patient care situation.

Tasks:	Peer	Lab	Clinical
1. Gathers the appropriate equipment	☐	☐	☐
2. Observes standard precautions, including hand washing	☐	☐	☐
3. Aseptically prepares the sampling device	☐	☐	☐
4. Correctly samples the equipment	☐	☐	☐
5. Correctly handles the culturing device following sampling	☐	☐	☐
6. Labels and transports the sample to the laboratory for culture	☐	☐	☐
7. Completes all required paperwork	☐	☐	☐

SCORE:

Peer _____ points of possible 14

Lab _____ points of possible 14

Clinical _____ points of possible 14

STUDENT SIGNATURES	INSTRUCTOR SIGNATURES
PEER	LAB
STUDENT	CLINICAL

PERFORMANCE EVALUATION:
Equipment Processing

Date: Lab _____ Clinical _____ Agency _____

Lab: Pass _____ Fail _____ Clinical: Pass _____ Fail _____

Student name _____ Instructor name _____

No. of times observed in clinical _____

No. of times practiced in clinical _____

PASSING CRITERIA: Obtain 90% or better on the procedure. Tasks indicated by * must receive at least 1 point, or the evaluation is terminated. Procedure must be performed within the designated time, or the performance receives a failing grade.

SCORING: 2 points — Task performed satisfactorily without prompting.
1 point — Task performed satisfactorily with self-initiated correction.
0 points — Task performed incorrectly or with prompting required.
NA — Task not applicable to the patient care situation.

Tasks:	Peer	Lab	Clinical
* **1.** Performs a 5 minute scrub	☐	☐	☐
* **2.** Wears gloves during disassembly and decontamination	☐	☐	☐
* **3.** Disassembles and washes the equipment	☐	☐	☐
* **4.** Rinses the equipment and dries it if gas sterilization is used	☐	☐	☐
* **5.** Packages the equipment before processing if required			
a. Uses the correct packaging	☐	☐	☐
b. Uses an indicator	☐	☐	☐
* **6.** Processes the equipment correctly			
a. Uses the correct time exposure	☐	☐	☐
b. Uses the correct temperature	☐	☐	☐
c. Uses the correct concentration	☐	☐	☐
* **7.** Assembles the equipment following disinfection	☐	☐	☐
* **8.** Tests the equipment before packaging	☐	☐	☐
* **9.** Labels and stores the equipment	☐	☐	☐

SCORE: Peer   _____ points of possible 22; _____%

                    Lab   _____ points of possible 22; _____%

                    Clinical _____ points of possible 22; _____%

TIME: _____ out of possible 90 minutes

STUDENT SIGNATURES   **INSTRUCTOR SIGNATURES**

PEER: _____   LAB: _____

STUDENT: _____   CLINICAL: _____

SECTION 3
Emergency Management

CHAPTER 20
Emergency Airway Management

INTRODUCTION

Emergency airway management is an important role of the respiratory practitioner. Respiratory failure may result from many underlying disorders. When it occurs, a patent airway must quickly be established and ventilation resumed.

A simple method of airway management is patient positioning to relieve obstruction so that the patient's own respiratory efforts may resume. Alternatively, airway management may involve placement of an artificial airway and manual ventilation of the patient using a manual resuscitator.

It is important to understand the rationale, techniques, and equipment for emergency airway management and the associated hazards and complications. This chapter teaches patient positioning to open the airway, how to use a manual resuscitator, and intubation techniques.

KEY TERMS

- Anterior mandibular displacement
- Combitube airway
- Endotracheal pilot tube and balloon
- Endotracheal tube
- Endotracheal tube cuff
- Extubation
- Head tilt
- Intubation
- Laryngeal mask airway (LMA)
- Laryngeal obstruction
- Laryngoscope
- Macintosh blade
- Miller blade
- Nasopharyngeal airway
- Oropharyngeal airway
- Soft tissue obstruction

THEORY OBJECTIVES

At the end of this chapter, the reader should be able to:

- Identify the anatomical structures of the upper airway.
- Identify the reflexes encountered in descending order from the mouth to the carina, and state the significance of these reflexes in relation to the level of consciousness.
- Explain the etiology of upper airway obstruction.
- Explain the mechanisms of the manual maneuvers used to open the airway:
  — Head tilt and chin lift
  — Anterior mandibular displacement
- Differentiate between a self-inflating and a flow-inflating manual resuscitator.
- Describe the types of valves commonly used in manual resuscitators. Explain the advantages and disadvantages of each type.
- Describe the following for the commonly used self-inflating manual resuscitators:
  — FIO_2 delivery with and without reservoir attachment
  — Identify those that deliver oxygen-enriched gas during spontaneous ventilation
  — Ease of cleaning aspirate

- State the importance of maintaining an I:E ratio of at least 1:2 or greater while ventilating a patient with a manual resuscitator.
- Describe the hazards and complications associated with the use of a manual resuscitator on the nonintubated patient.
- Explain the mechanism of airway maintenance with the following devices, and state their indications, advantages, disadvantages, and associated hazards:
  — Nasopharyngeal airway
  — Oropharyngeal airway
  — Combitube airway
- Describe the laryngeal mask airway (LMA) and its insertion.
- Describe the routes of intubation and their advantages and disadvantages:
  — Oral route
  — Nasal route
- Describe the two types of laryngoscopes and blades used for intubation, including:
  Laryngoscopes
  — Conventional
  — Fiberoptic

Laryngoscope blades
— *Macintosh*
— *Miller*

- *Describe the construction and design of a modern endotracheal tube, and state the significance of the following components in relation to their function:*
  — *Murphy eye*
  — *Cuff*

— *Bivona foam cuff*
— *Standard cuff*
  — *Pilot tube*
  — *Markings*
— *Pilot balloon*

- *Describe the early and late complications of intubation.*
- *List the indications for intubation and the criteria for extubation.*

CLINICAL PRACTICE GUIDELINES

AARC Clinical Practice Guideline: Resuscitation and Defibrillation in the Health Care Setting 2004 Revision & Update

RAD 4.0 INDICATIONS:

Cardiac arrest, respiratory arrest, or the presence of conditions that may lead to cardiopulmonary arrest as indicated by rapid deterioration in vital signs, level of consciousness, and blood gas values—included in those conditions are

4.1 Airway obstruction—partial or complete
4.2 Acute myocardial infarction with cardiodynamic instability
4.3 Life-threatening dysrhythmias
4.4 Hypovolemic shock
4.5 Severe infections
4.6 Spinal cord or head injury
4.7 Drug overdose
4.8 Pulmonary edema
4.9 Anaphylaxis
4.10 Pulmonary embolus
4.11 Smoke inhalation
4.12 Defibrillation is indicated when cardiac arrest results in or is due to ventricular fibrillation.[1-5]
4.13 Pulseless ventricular tachycardia

RAD 5.0 CONTRAINDICATIONS:

Resuscitation is contraindicated when
5.1 The patient's desire not to be resuscitated has been clearly expressed and documented in the patient's medical record[6-9]
5.2 Resuscitation has been determined to be futile because of the patient's underlying condition or disease[9-18]
5.3 Defibrillation is also contraindicated when immediate danger to the rescuers is present due to the environment, patient's location, or patient's condition.

RAD 6.0 PRECAUTIONS/HAZARDS AND/OR COMPLICATIONS:

The following represent possible hazards or complications related to the major facets of resuscitation:

6.1 Airway management[10,11]
   6.1.1 Failure to establish a patent airway[19-21]
   6.1.2 Failure to intubate the trachea[19,20]
   6.1.3 Failure to recognize intubation of the esophagus[19,22,23]
   6.1.4 Upper airway trauma, laryngeal, and esophageal damage[24-29]
      6.1.4.1 Vocal cord paralysis[28]
   6.1.5 Aspiration[21,23,24,30]
   6.1.6 Cervical spine trauma[24,31,32]
   6.1.7 Unrecognized bronchial intubation[19,30,33]
   6.1.8 Eye injury[21]
   6.1.9 Facial trauma[30]
   6.1.10 Problems with ETT cuff[21,34-36]
   6.1.11 Bronchospasm[19,21,23]
   6.1.12 Laryngospasm[37]
   6.1.13 Dental accidents[24,30]
   6.1.14 Dysrhythmias[37,38]
   6.1.15 Hypotension and bradycardia due to vagal stimulation[37]
   6.1.16 Hypertension and tachycardia[37,39]
   6.1.17 Inappropriate tube size[30,34,40]
   6.1.18 Bleeding
   6.1.19 Pneumonia[41]
6.2 Ventilation
   6.2.1 Inadequate oxygen delivery (FDO$_2$)[42-45]
   6.2.2 Hypo- and/or hyperventilation[43-47]
   6.2.3 Gastric insufflation and/or rupture[45,48,49]
   6.2.4 Barotrauma[50,51]
   6.2.5 Hypotension due to reduced venous return secondary to high mean intrathoracic pressure[52,53]
   6.2.6 Vomiting and aspiration[21,54]
   6.2.7 Prolonged interruption of ventilation for intubation[55]
6.3 Circulation/Compressions
   6.3.1 Ineffective chest compression[56,57]
   6.3.2 Fractured ribs and/or sternum[24,54,58,59]
   6.3.3 Laceration of spleen or liver[24,54,58,60-62]
   6.3.4 Failure to restore circulation despite functional rhythm
      6.3.4.1 Severe hypovolemia[63,64]
      6.3.4.2 Cardiac tamponade[58,64]

(Continued)

6.3.4.3 Hemo- or pneumothorax[63,64]

6.3.4.4 Hypoxia

6.3.4.5 Acidosis

6.3.4.6 Hyperkalemia

6.3.4.7 Massive acute myocardial infarction[63]

6.3.4.8 Aortic dissection[63]

6.3.4.9 Cardiac rupture[59,65]

6.3.4.10 Air embolus, pulmonary embolism[58,66]

6.3.5 Central nervous system impairment[58]

6.4 Electrical therapy

6.4.1 AEDs may be hazardous in patients weighing <25 kg[67]

6.4.2 Failure of defibrillator[68]

6.4.3 Shock to team members[69]

6.4.4 Pulse checking between sequential shocks of AEDs delays rapid identification of persistent ventricular fibrillation, interferes with assessment capabilities of the devices, and increases the possibility of operator error.[67]

6.4.5 The initial 3 shocks should be delivered in sequence, without delay, interruption for CPR, medication administration, or pulse checks for ventricular fibrillation and pulseless ventricular tachycardia.[2,4,70-72]

6.4.6 Induction of malignant dysrhythmias[73,74]

6.4.7 Interference with implanted pacemaker function[75-77]

6.4.8 Fire hazard

6.4.8.1 AEDs may be hazardous in an oxygen-enriched environment.[78]

6.4.8.2 Alcohol should never be used as conducting material for paddles because serious burns can result.[79]

6.4.8.3 Superficial arcing of the current along the chest wall can occur as a consequence of the presence of conductive paste or gel between the paddles.[80]

6.4.8.4 The aluminized backing on some transdermal systems can cause electric arcing during defibrillation, with explosive noises, smoke, visible arcing, patient burns, and impaired transmission of current;[81-84] therefore, patches should be removed before defibrillation.

6.4.9 Muscle burn[81,85]

6.4.10 Muscle injury resulting in acute renal failure[86,87]

6.4.11 If transthoracic impedance is high, a low energy shock (<100 J) may fail to generate enough current to achieve successful defibrillation.[88-91]

6.4.12 Attention must be paid to factors influencing total and transthoracic impedance.[67,79,88,90,91]

6.4.12.1 Paddle electrode pressure

6.4.12.2 The use of an appropriate conductive medium that can withstand high current flow

6.4.12.3 Electrode/paddle size—should be 8.5 to 12 cm for adults

6.4.12.4 Electrode placement

6.4.12.5 Time interval between shocks

6.4.12.6 Distance between electrodes (size of the chest)

6.4.12.7 Energy selected

6.4.12.8 Paddle-skin electrode material

6.4.12.9 Number of previous shocks

6.4.12.10 Phase of ventilation

6.4.12.11 Diaphoretic patients should be dried to prevent contact problems with adhesive defibrillation pads and/or electrodes.

6.5 Drug administration

6.5.1 Inappropriate drug or dose

6.5.2 Idiosyncratic or allergic response to drug

6.5.3 Endotracheal-tube drug-delivery failure[91-94]—The endotracheal tube dose should be 2 to 2.5 times the normal I.V. dose, diluted in 10 mL of normal saline (or distilled water).

RAD 8.0 ASSESSMENT OF NEED:

8.1 Assessment of patient condition

8.1.1 Pre-arrest—Identification of patients in danger of imminent arrest and in whom consequent early intervention may prevent arrest and improve outcome. These are patients with conditions that may lead to cardiopulmonary arrest as indicated by rapid deterioration in vital signs, level of consciousness, and blood gas values (see Section 4.00).

8.1.2 Arrest—absence of spontaneous breathing and/or circulation

8.1.3 Post-arrest—Once a patient has sustained an arrest, the likelihood of additional life-threatening problems is high, and continued vigilance and aggressive action using this Guideline are indicated. Control of the airway and cardiac monitoring must be continued and optimal oxygenation and ventilation assured.

8.1.3.1 After arrival of defibrillator: The patient should be evaluated immediately for the presence of ventricular fibrillation or ventricular tachycardia by the operator (conventional) or the defibrillator (automated or semi-automated). Inappropriate defibrillation can cause harm.

RAD 9.0 ASSESSMENT OF PROCESS AND OUTCOME:

9.1 Timely, high-quality resuscitation improves patient outcome in terms of survival and level of function. Despite optimal resuscitation performance,

(Continued)

outcomes are affected by patient-specific factors. Patient condition post-arrest should be evaluated from this perspective.

9.2 Documentation and evaluation of the resuscitation process (eg, system activation, team member performance, functioning of equipment, and adherence to guidelines and algorithms) should occur continuously and improvements be made[91,95-99]

9.3 Equipment management issues. Use of standard checklists can improve defibrillator dependability.[100]

9.4 Defibrillation process issues

9.4.1 System access[101]

9.4.2 Response time[91,102,103]

9.4.3 First-responder actions[91,102-104]

9.4.4 Adherence to established algorithms[105]

9.4.5 Patient selection and outcome

9.4.6 First responder authorization to defibrillate[91,103,106]

RAD 11.0 MONITORING:

11.1 Patient

11.1.1 Clinical assessment—continuous observation of the patient and repeated clinical assessment by a trained observer provide optimal monitoring of the resuscitation process. Special consideration should be given to the following:

11.1.1.1 Level of consciousness

11.1.1.2 Adequacy of airway

11.1.1.3 Adequacy of ventilation

11.1.1.4 Peripheral/apical pulse and character

11.1.1.5 Evidence of chest and head trauma

11.1.1.6 Pulmonary compliance and airway resistance

11.1.1.7 Presence of seizure activity

11.1.2 Assessment of physiologic parameters— Repeat assessment of physiologic data by trained professionals supplements clinical assessment in managing patients throughout the resuscitation process. Monitoring devices should be available, accessible, functional, and periodically evaluated for function. These data include but are not limited to[95]

11.1.2.1 Arterial blood gas studies (although investigators have suggested that such values may have a limited role in decision-making during CPR[158]

11.1.2.2 Hemodynamic data[152,158-160]

11.1.2.3 Cardiac rhythm[153,154]

11.1.2.4 Ventilatory frequency, tidal volume, and airway pressure[95,96]

11.1.2.5 Exhaled CO_2[146-150]

11.1.2.6 Neurologic status

11.2 Resuscitation process—properly performed resuscitation should improve patient outcome. Continuous monitoring of the process will identify areas needing improvement. Among these areas are response time, equipment function, equipment availability, team member performance, team performance, complication rate, and patient survival and functional status.

11.3 Equipment—All maintenance should be documented and records preserved. Included in documentation should be routine checks of energy output, condition of batteries, proper functioning of monitor and recorder, and presence of disposables needed for function of defibrillator, including electrodes and defibrillation pads. Defibrillators should be checked and documented each shift for presence, condition, and function of cables and paddles; presence of defibrillating and monitoring electrodes, paper, and spare batteries (as applicable); and charging, message/ light indicators, monitors, and ECG recorder (as applicable).[91] AEDs should be checked and documented each day for function and appropriate maintenance.[67]

11.4 Training—Records should be kept of initial training and continuing education of all personnel who perform defibrillation as part of their professional activities.

Reprinted with permission from *Respiratory Care* 2004; 49: 1085–1099. The complete AARC Clinical Practice Guidelines are available from the AARC Web site (http://www.aarc.org), from the AARC Executive Office, or from *Respiratory Care* journal.

AARC Clinical Practice Guideline Management of Airway Emergencies

MAE 4.0 INDICATIONS:

4.1 Conditions requiring management of the airway, in general, are impending or actual (1) airway compromise, (2) respiratory failure, and (3) need to protect the airway. Specific conditions include but are not limited to:

4.1.1 Airway emergency prior to endotracheal intubation

4.1.2 Obstruction of the artificial airway

4.1.3 Apnea

4.1.4 Acute traumatic coma (1)

4.1.5 Penetrating neck trauma (2)

4.1.6 Cardiopulmonary arrest and unstable dysrhythmias (3)

(Continued)

4.1.7 Severe bronchospasm (4–8)

4.1.8 Severe allergic reactions with cardiopulmonary compromise (9,10)

4.1.9 Pulmonary edema (11,12)

4.1.10 Sedative or narcotic drug effect (13)

4.1.11 Foreign body airway obstruction (3)

4.1.12 Choanal atresia in neonates (14)

4.1.13 Aspiration

4.1.14 Risk of aspiration

4.1.15 Severe laryngospasm (15)

4.1.16 Self-extubation (16,17)

4.2 Conditions requiring emergency tracheal intubation include, but are not limited to:

4.2.1 Persistent apnea

4.2.2 Traumatic upper airway obstruction (partial or complete) (18–20)

4.2.3 Accidental extubation of the patient unable to maintain adequate spontaneous ventilation (16,17)

4.2.4 Obstructive angioedema (edema involving the deeper layers of the skin, subcutaneous tissue, and mucosa) (21–23)

4.2.5 Massive uncontrolled upper airway bleeding (2,24)

4.2.6 Coma with potential for increased intracranial pressure (25)

4.2.7 Infection-related upper airway obstruction (partial or complete):

4.2.7.1 Epiglottitis in children or adults (26,27)

4.2.7.2 Acute uvular edema (28)

4.2.7.3 Tonsillopharyngitis or retropharyngeal abscess (29)

4.2.7.4 Suppurative parotitis (30)

4.2.8 Laryngeal and upper airway edema (31)

4.2.9 Neonatal- or pediatric-specific:

4.2.9.1 Perinatal asphyxia (32,33)

4.2.9.2 Severe adenotonsillar hypertrophy (34,35)

4.2.9.3 Severe laryngomalacia (36,37)

4.2.9.4 Bacterial tracheitis (38–40)

4.2.9.5 Neonatal epignathus (41,42)

4.2.9.6 Obstruction from abnormal laryngeal closure due to arytenoid masses (43)

4.2.9.7 Mediastinal tumors (44)

4.2.9.8 Congenital diaphragmatic hernia (45)

4.2.9.9 Presence of thick and/or particulate meconium in amniotic fluid (46–48)

4.2.10 Absence of airway protective reflexes

4.2.11 Cardiopulmonary arrest

4.2.12 Massive hemoptysis (49)

4.3 The patient in whom airway control is not possible by other methods may require surgical placement of an airway (needle or surgical cricothyrotomy). (20,50,51)

4.4 Conditions in which endotracheal intubation may not be possible and in which alternative techniques may be used include but are not limited to:

4.4.1 Restriction of endotracheal intubation by policy or statute

4.4.2 Difficult or failed intubation in the presence of risk factors associated with difficult tracheal intubations (52) such as:

4.4.2.1 Short neck, (53) or bull neck (54)

4.4.2.2 Protruding maxillary incisors (53)

4.4.2.3 Receding mandible (53)

4.4.2.4 Reduced mobility of the atlanto-occipital joint (55)

4.4.2.5 Temporomandibular ankylosis (55)

4.4.2.6 Congenital oropharyngeal wall stenosis (56)

4.4.2.7 Anterior osteophytes of the cervical vertebrae, associated with diffuse idiopathic skeletal hyperostosis (57)

4.4.2.8 Large substernal and/or cancerous goiters (58)

4.4.2.9 Treacher Collins syndrome (59)

4.4.2.10 Morquio-Brailsford syndrome (60)

4.4.2.11 Endolaryngeal tumors (61)

4.4.3 When endotracheal intubation is not immediately possible

MAE 5.0 CONTRAINDICATIONS:

Aggressive airway management (intubation or establishment of a surgical airway) may be contraindicated when the patient's desire not to be resuscitated has been clearly expressed and documented in the patient's medical record or other valid legal document. (62–64)

MAE 6.0 PRECAUTIONS/HAZARDS AND/OR COMPLICATIONS:

The following represent possible hazards or complications related to the major facets of management of airway emergencies:

6.1 Translaryngeal intubation or cricothyrotomy is usually the route of choice. It may be necessary occasionally to use a surgical airway. Controversy exists as to whether intubation is hazardous in the presence of an unstable injury to the cervical spine. In one series the incidence of serious cervical spine injury in a severely injured population of blunt trauma patients was relatively low, and commonly used methods of precautionary airway management rarely led to neurologic deterioration. (65–67)

6.1.1 Failure to establish a patent airway (68–70)

6.1.2 Failure to intubate the trachea (68,69)

6.1.3 Failure to recognize intubation of esophagus (25,68,71–81)

(Continued)

6.1.4 Upper airway trauma, laryngeal, and esophageal damage (82)

6.1.5 Aspiration (70,74,82,83)

6.1.6 Cervical spine trauma (67,84,85)

6.1.7 Unrecognized bronchial intubation (25,68,72,82,86,87)

6.1.8 Eye injury (70)

6.1.9 Vocal cord paralysis (88)

6.1.10 Problems with ETT tubes:

6.1.10.1 Cuff perforation (89)

6.1.10.2 Cuff herniation (89)

6.1.10.3 Pilot-tube-valve incompetence (90)

6.1.10.4 Tube kinking during biting (70,89)

6.1.10.5 Inadvertent extubation (17,25, 68,72,86,91–93)

6.1.10.6 Tube occlusion (17,72,82,89,93,94)

6.1.11 Bronchospasm (68,70,74)

6.1.12 Laryngospasm (72)

6.1.13 Dental accidents (70)

6.1.14 Dysrhythmias (94)

6.1.15 Hypotension and bradycardia due to vagal stimulation (94)

6.1.16 Hypertension and tachycardia (94,95)

6.1.17 Inappropriate tube size (89,96–99)

6.1.18 Bleeding

6.1.19 Mouth ulceration (82)

6.1.20 Nasal-intubation specific:

6.1.20.1 Nasal damage including epistaxis

6.1.20.2 Tube kinking in pharynx

6.1.20.3 Sinusitis (100–102) and otitis media

6.1.21 Tongue ulceration

6.1.22 Tracheal damage including tracheoesophageal fistula, tracheal innominate fistula, tracheal stenosis, and tracheomalacia (103–107)

6.1.23 Pneumonia (108)

6.1.24 Laryngeal damage with consequent laryngeal stenosis, (82,101,107,109,110) laryngeal ulcer, granuloma, polyps, synechia

6.1.25 Surgical cricothyrotomy or tracheostomy-specific (111,112)

6.1.25.1 Stomal stenosis (82,113)

6.1.25.2 Innominate erosion (113)

6.1.26 Needle cricothyrotomy–specific (114–118)

6.1.26.1 Bleeding at insertion site with hematoma formation

6.1.26.2 Subcutaneous and mediastinal emphysema (117)

6.1.26.3 Esophageal perforation

6.2 Emergency ventilation

6.2.1 Inadequate oxygen delivery (119–121)

6.2.2 Hypo- or hyperventilation (122–124)

6.2.3 Gastric insufflation and/or rupture (125,126)

6.2.4 Barotrauma (127–129)

6.2.5 Hypotension due to reduced venous return secondary to high mean intrathoracic pressure (130–132)

6.2.6 Vomiting and aspiration (125)

6.2.7 Prolonged interruption of ventilation for intubation (3,126)

6.2.8 Failure to establish adequate functional residual capacity in the newborn (133–135)

6.2.9 Movement of unstable cervical spine (more than by any commonly used method of endotracheal intubation) (136)

6.2.10 Failure to exhale due to upper airway obstruction during percutaneous transtracheal ventilation (118,136)

MAE 8.0 ASSESSMENT OF NEED:

The need for management of airway emergencies is dictated by the patient's clinical condition. Careful observation, the implementation of basic airway management techniques, and laboratory and clinical data should help determine the need for more aggressive measures. Specific conditions requiring intervention include:

8.1 Inability to adequately protect airway (e.g., coma, lack of gag reflex, inability to cough) with or without other signs of respiratory distress

8.2 Partially obstructed airway. Signs of a partially obstructed upper airway include ineffective patient efforts to ventilate, paradoxical respiration, stridor, use of accessory muscles, patient's pointing to neck, choking motions, cyanosis, and distress. Signs of lower airway obstruction may include the above and wheezing.

8.3 Complete airway obstruction. Respiratory efforts with no breath sounds or suggestion of air movement are indicative of complete obstruction.

8.4 Apnea. No respiratory efforts are seen. May be associated with cardiac arrest.

8.5 Hypoxemia, hypercarbia, and/or acidemia seen on arterial blood gas analysis, oximetry, or exhaled gas analysis.

8.6 Respiratory distress. Elevated respiratory rate, high or low ventilatory volumes, and signs of sympathetic nervous system hyperactivity may be associated with respiratory distress.

(Continued)

MAE 9.0 ASSESSMENT OF PROCESS AND OUTCOME:

Timely intervention to maintain the patient's airway can improve outcome in terms of survival and level of function. Under rare circumstances, maintenance of an airway by nonsurgical means may not be possible. Despite optimal maintenance of the airway, patient outcomes are affected by patient-specific factors. Lack of availability of appropriate equipment and personnel may adversely affect patient outcome. Monitoring and recording are important to the improvement of the process of emergency airway management. Some aspects (e.g., frequency of complications of tracheal intubation or time for establishment of a definitive airway) are easy to quantitate and can lead to improvement in hospitalwide systems. Patient condition following the emergency should be evaluated from this perspective.

MAE 11.0 MONITORING:

11.1 Patient

11.1.1 Clinical signs—Continuous observation of the patient and repeated clinical assessment by a trained observer provide optimal monitoring of the airway. Special consideration should be given to the following: (174)

11.1.1.1 Level of consciousness

11.1.1.2 Presence and character of breath sounds

11.1.1.3 Ease of ventilation

11.1.1.4 Symmetry and amount of chest movement

11.1.1.5 Skin color and character (temperature and presence or absence of diaphoresis)

11.1.1.6 Presence of upper airway sounds (crowing, snoring, stridor)

11.1.1.7 Presence of excessive secretions, blood, vomitus, or foreign objects in the airway

11.1.1.8 Presence of epigastric sounds

11.1.1.9 Presence of retractions

11.1.1.10 Presence of nasal flaring

11.1.2 Physiologic variables—Repeated assessment of physiologic data by trained professionals supplements clinical assessment in managing patients with airway difficulties. Monitoring devices should be available, accessible, functional, and periodically evaluated for function. These data include but are not limited to: (142,175)

11.1.2.1 Ventilatory frequency, tidal volume, and airway pressure

11.1.2.2 Presence of CO_2 in exhaled gas

11.1.2.3 Heart rate and rhythm

11.1.2.4 Pulse oximetry

11.1.2.5 Arterial blood gas values

11.1.2.6 Chest radiograph

11.2 Endotracheal tube position—Regardless of the method of ventilation used, the most important consideration is detection of esophageal intubation.

11.2.1 Tracheal intubation is suggested but may not be confirmed by:

11.2.1.1 Bilateral breath sounds over the chest, symmetrical chest movement, and absence of ventilation sounds over the epigastrium (174,175,177)

11.2.1.2 Presence of condensate inside the tube, corresponding with exhalation (174,176,177)

11.2.1.3 Visualization of the tip of the tube passing through the vocal cords

11.2.1.4 Esophageal detector devices may be useful in differentiating esophageal from tracheal intubation (178,179)

11.2.2 Tracheal intubation is confirmed by detection of CO_2 in the exhaled gas, (180–182) although cases of transient CO_2 excretion from the stomach have been reported. (183)

11.2.3 Tracheal intubation is confirmed by endoscopic visualization of the carina or tracheal rings through the tube.

11.2.4 The position of the endotracheal tube (i.e., depth of insertion) should be appropriate on chest radiograph.

11.3 Airway management process—A properly managed airway may improve patient outcome. Continuous evaluation of the process will identify components needing improvement. These include response time, equipment function, equipment availability, therapist performance, complication rate, and patient survival and functional status.

Reprinted with permission from *Respiratory Care* 1995; 40(7): 749–760. The complete AARC Clinical Practice Guidelines are available from the AARC Web site (http://www.aarc .org), from the AARC Executive Office, or from *Respiratory Care* journal.

ANATOMY OF THE UPPER AIRWAY

Tongue

The tongue is the first structure visible in the patient's mouth when looking down the airway. The tongue falling back against the posterior pharynx is a common cause of upper airway obstruction. In the unconscious patient, it is amazing how flaccid the tongue is.

Figure 20-1 illustrates what is seen when looking down the airway. Refer to this illustration upon reading the description of the structures.

Vallecula

The vallecula is a notch between the base of the tongue and the epiglottis. When a Macintosh laryngoscope blade is used, the distal tip is placed in the vallecula. The vallecula may be found by advancing the blade along the tongue until advancement terminates.

Epiglottis

The epiglottis is a lidlike cartilaginous structure that serves as a cover over the trachea. When closed, it protects the trachea from food or other foreign material. The structure is located superiorly looking down the airway. When the Miller (straight) laryngoscope blade is used, the epiglottis is lifted. This is the farthest a laryngoscope blade is ever advanced down the airway.

Arytenoid Cartilages

The arytenoid cartilages are fairly large structures having right and left sides just beyond the epiglottis. These are oval-shaped structures in the lower portion of the field of view.

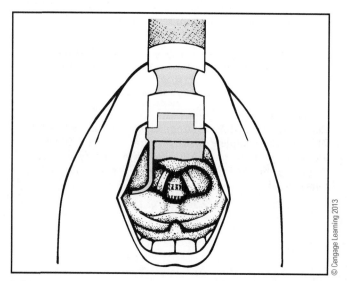

Figure 20-1   Anatomy of the upper airway as viewed through a laryngoscope

© Cengage Learning 2013

Vocal Cords

The vocal cords are the target when orally intubating a patient. The paired cords appear as a white inverted *V* near the top of the field of view. Upon advancing the endotracheal tube, aim for these. The practitioner should be able to visualize the tube passing through the vocal cords.

The vocal cords will move with inspiration and expiration. It may be necessary to wait until the vocal cords open before passing the endotracheal tube through them.

REFLEXES OF THE UPPER AIRWAY

The upper airway is protected by a variety of reflexes. The presence of foreign substances or irritation stimulates various reflexes at different levels. These protective reflexes help to maintain airway patency and protect it from obstruction. They also serve to protect the lower airways from foreign objects and noxious gases or fumes.

Swallow

The first reflex encountered in the upper airway, in progressing from the mouth toward the lower airway, is the swallow reflex. Toward the posterior portion of the oropharynx are nerve receptors termed *swallowing receptors*. Stimulation of this area by food or a foreign object will cause an involuntary reflex, resulting in pharyngeal muscle contractions that propel the food or object posteriorly toward the esophagus. Lack of the swallow reflex may allow oral secretions to pool in the posterior oral pharynx. The integrity of the remaining reflexes is essential to prevent aspiration of these secretions.

A patient without the swallow reflex needs oral suctioning frequently. Positioning the patient lying on the side with the head turned toward the lower shoulder will allow the secretions to drain out of the mouth.

Gag

Toward the posterior oropharynx are vagal receptors that will cause gagging with sufficient stimulation. The gag reflex may induce vomiting, further compromising the patency of the airway. The gag reflex is a strong reflex with some patients being more susceptible to gagging than others. The reflex may be depressed with central nervous system (CNS) depression, anesthesia, or drug overdose, or it may be intentionally depressed using lidocaine topically. Topical lidocaine is frequently used prior to bronchoscopy to depress the protective reflexes. A patient awakening from anesthesia may gag on an oropharyngeal airway as the patient returns to consciousness. While the patient is under anesthesia, the airway may be used without reflex stimulation. However, few patients can tolerate these airways when conscious.

Laryngeal

Stimulation of the larynx will cause the epiglottis to slam shut and the vocal cords to approximate (come together). The approximation of the vocal cords causes *laryngospasm*. All of us have experienced this reflex when food "goes down the wrong pipe." Other causes for laryngospasm are anaphylaxis and epiglottitis. Under these circumstances, the laryngospasm may be severe enough to totally occlude the airway.

Tracheal

Stimulation of the trachea will induce a cough. The trachea is very sensitive to stimulation by foreign material. The presence of secretions mobilized by airflow is sufficient to stimulate a cough. The placement of an artificial airway into the trachea may also stimulate a cough by irritation.

Carinal

The carina, which is where the trachea branches into the right and left mainstem bronchi, is extremely sensitive to stimulation. Stimulation of this area causes a cough reflex.

Reflexes and Loss of Consciousness

As a person loses consciousness, the reflexes protecting the airway are lost, in descending order, from the swallow reflex to the carinal reflex. The level of consciousness is reflected in the presence or absence of the reflexes. Upon intubating a patient, observe for the presence of reflexes. The presence of reflexes at one or more levels will indicate the patient's level of consciousness. Conversely, reflexes are regained in ascending order from the carinal reflex to the swallow reflex. This information is also useful in evaluating coma and in assessing the need for intubation in neurologically depressed patients, such as those suffering from drug intoxication.

UPPER AIRWAY OBSTRUCTION

Causes

Upper airway obstruction may result from soft tissue or laryngeal obstruction. Contributing factors include CNS depression as the result of drug overdose or anesthesia; cardiac arrest; loss of consciousness; space-occupying lesions such as tumors; edema; and the presence of foreign material, aspirate, vomitus, or blood in the airway. The most common cause is soft tissue obstruction from the loss of muscle tone resulting in the tongue slipping back against the soft palate. *Laryngeal obstruction* is more commonly the result of muscle spasm (laryngospasm), edema from croup, epiglottitis, or the presence of foreign material. Laryngeal obstruction resulting from laryngeal spasm may occur as a result of anaphylactic reaction, postintubation, or foreign body aspiration or in the near-drowning victim.

Clinical Findings

Upper airway obstruction is often accompanied by very noisy inspiratory efforts. The noise may vary from a mild snoring sound to a roar. Silence may indicate total obstruction. Generally speaking, the louder the noise is, the worse the obstruction. Frequently in severe obstruction, the practitioner may observe retraction of the intercostal muscles accompanied by sternal and clavicular retraction. Retractions are more easily observed in the infant or child. If prolonged, upper airway obstruction can lead to hypoxemia and hypercapnia. Total airway obstruction may lead to death in 5 to 10 minutes.

Positional Maneuvers to Open the Airway

The goal of airway management is the prompt restoration of airway patency. The majority of upper airway obstructions can be relieved using simple positional maneuvers. Once an airway is established, evaluate the adequacy of ventilation. Often, relief of the airway obstruction will allow spontaneous respirations to resume.

In the clinical setting, patients at risk for airway obstruction should be positioned to prevent its occurrence. Patients who have CNS depression, or who are under anesthesia or are comatose, should be placed on their side with the head tilted toward the lower shoulder to prevent aspiration. The placement of an artificial airway (as tolerated), such as a nasopharyngeal or an oropharyngeal airway, will also help to prevent airway obstruction.

Head Tilt

The *head tilt* maneuver involves tilting the head back to relieve *soft tissue obstruction* from the tongue and soft palate. It may be accomplished in one of two ways. The head tilt-chin lift maneuver is performed by tilting the head back and lifting the chin to open the airway. The other maneuver is most easily performed while standing behind the patient. Using both hands, place one hand on the forehead and push back; with the other hand, lift the mandible. Performance of this maneuver is effective and rapid. Figure 20-2 shows the proper hand placement and patient position. In the event of obvious trauma, as from a motor vehicle accident, use of this maneuver may be contraindicated. If the vertebral column has been involved in the trauma, permanent nerve damage may be caused by this maneuver. In such cases, a better choice of technique is anterior mandibular displacement.

Anterior Mandibular Displacement

Anterior mandibular displacement is performed by grasping the jaw at the ramus on each side and lifting the jaw forward. This maneuver can be accomplished without tilting or moving the head, making it the treatment of choice in suspected vertebral column trauma. Figure 20-3 shows the maneuver to open the airway.

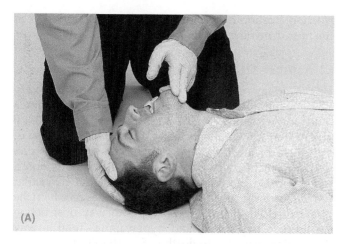

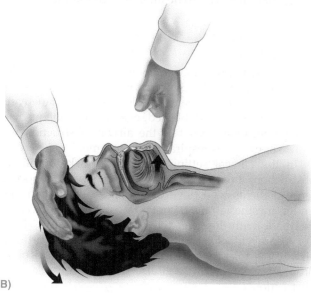

© Cengage Learning 2013

Figure 20-2   The head tilt maneuver to relieve upper airway obstruction

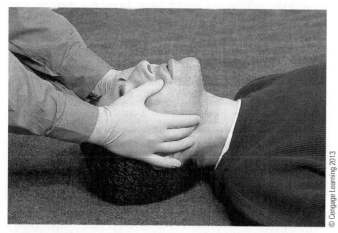

© Cengage Learning 2013

Figure 20-3   Anterior mandibular displacement to relieve airway obstruction

Triple Airway Maneuver

The triple airway maneuver is a combination of the head tilt, anterior mandibular displacement, and the separation of the teeth to open the mouth.

RESUSCITATORS

Once a patent airway has been restored, the adequacy of spontaneous respirations must be evaluated. Ventilatory assistance may be administered with a manual resuscitator.

There are two main types of manual resuscitators: self-inflating and flow-inflating. Each has advantages and disadvantages. Owing to the differences in operation, the technique for using each is also different. The respiratory practitioner will be expected to be thoroughly familiar with each type.

A self-inflating resuscitator, as the name implies, will automatically inflate after the bag is squeezed for inspiration. These resuscitators are constructed so that the walls have a stiffness or rigidity to them that causes the bag to return to its original shape after compression. Because of the stiffer wall design, it may be difficult to feel the compliance of a patient's lungs and thorax. Because of the structure of the bag, it is easily operated with one hand as the mask is held to the patient's face with the other hand. These resuscitators are useful in the emergency setting because they do not require a compressed gas source for operation. Compressed oxygen may be added to them to deliver an oxygen-enriched atmosphere.

A flow-inflating resuscitator, as the name implies, depends on the flow of source gas to inflate. This resuscitator will not operate without a compressed gas source. The construction of this resuscitator is such that the bag is very floppy and compliant. This makes it easy to assess the compliance of a patient's lungs and thorax. It is possible to deliver 100% oxygen with this resuscitator. Use of this device with a resuscitation mask is more difficult and requires considerable practice.

Gas-Powered Resuscitators

Gas-powered resuscitators are available that operate using a 50 psi oxygen source. A gas-powered resuscitator works as either a pressure-limited resuscitator, delivering a preset pressure (usually no more than 50 cm H₂O), or as a demand valve, so that the patient is able to initiate the inspiration. These resuscitators have a standardized patient connection (15 mm inner diameter and 22 mm outer diameter) that enables them to be used with a resuscitation mask or an artificial airway. An advantage of these devices is that 100% oxygen is delivered and some fatigue from prolonged manual ventilation is relieved. Before using this type of device, verify that it has a safety popoff valve to prevent delivery of excessive pressures. Verify that it works.

Valve Types Used in Self-Inflating Manual Resuscitators

The purpose of all valves used in manual resuscitators is to deliver gas to the patient during inspiration and to allow the patient to exhale to the ambient atmosphere on exhalation. Additional criteria used in the design of these valves include sensitivity to the patient's inspiratory efforts, ease of cleaning should they become fouled with vomitus, compact size, and ease of disassembly for cleaning and parts replacement.

Several types of valves and different valve combinations are used to accomplish the stated objectives. Figure 20-4 shows the different types of valves used for manual resuscitators. Table 20-1 compares the characteristics of these valve types with one another.

Besides having a working knowledge of the valves used in the self-inflating manual resuscitators, the practitioner should also be aware of the different capabilities of each device (fraction of inspired oxygen [FIO_2] delivery, spontaneous ventilation from the reservoir). Table 20-2 compares the different manual resuscitators.

IMPORTANCE OF INSPIRATORY-EXPIRATORY RATIO DURING RESUSCITATION

The use of a manual resuscitator involves applying pressure or squeezing the bag and forcing gas into the airway to ventilate the patient's lungs. This method of ventilation is similar in principle to intermittent positive-pressure breathing (IPPB), and, therefore, the hazards and complications are similar. The reader may want to review the effects of positive intrathoracic pressure found in Chapter 17, Hyperinflation Therapy.

Increased intrathoracic pressure can decrease venous return to the heart through the vena cava. Decreased

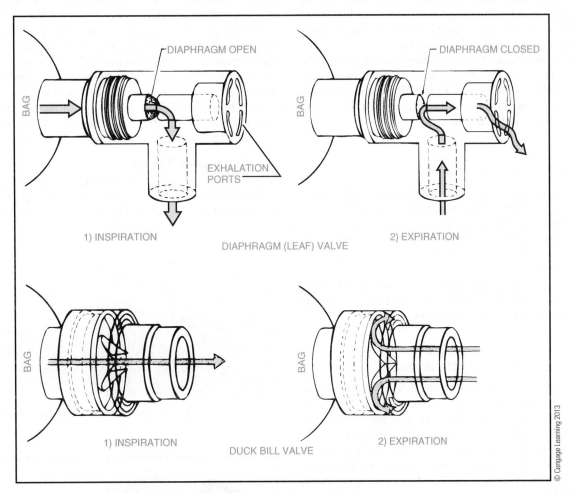

Figure 20-4   Valve types found in self-inflating manual resuscitators

TABLE 20-1: Types of Self-Inflating Manual Resuscitation Valves			
TYPE	**EASE OF CLEANING**	**EASE OF DISASSEMBLY**	**SENSITIVITY**
Diaphragm (leaf)	Good	Good	Good
Duck bill	Good	Good	Good

TABLE 20-2: Comparison of Self-Inflating Manual Resuscitators

RESUSCITATOR	VALVE TYPE	SPONTANEOUS VENTILATION FROM BAG	FIO₂ WITH RESERVOIR
Ambu SPUR II	Leaf diaphragm	Yes	84–96%
Allegiance Resuscitation Bag with 40-inch Tubing Reservoir	Duck bill	Yes	78–86%
Hudson RCI Lifesaver	Diaphragm	Yes	98–100%
Mercury Medical Adult CPR Bag	Duck bill	Yes	88–91%

venous return, combined with the compression of the mediastinum, can lead to a significant decrease in cardiac output. In an emergency situation, one of the primary goals is the improvement of circulation.

The adverse effects may be avoided by ventilating the patient using an inspiratory-expiratory (I:E) ratio of 1:2 or greater. An I:E ratio of 1:2 will allow sufficient time for the heart to fill during the expiratory phase when there is no positive pressure in the thoracic cavity.

Hazards of Manual Resuscitation

The major hazards associated with manual resuscitation include gastric distention, aspiration, and diminished cardiac output. Gastric distention can result when inflation pressures open the esophagus, admitting air into the stomach. The etiology of decreased cardiac output has been previously discussed.

Another hazard is inadequate ventilation due to poor technique or an ill-fitting mask. Equipment malfunctions may also reduce effective ventilation.

Pharyngeal Airways in Manual Resuscitation

Pharyngeal airways are specialized devices employed to maintain a patent airway. This is accomplished through bypassing the site of the obstruction or preventing the tongue from slipping back against the soft palate. The most common airways used in ventilating a nonintubated patient with a manual resuscitator are the nasopharyngeal and oropharyngeal airways, laryngeal mask airways (LMAs), and Combitube airways.

Pharyngeal airways are not tolerated well once the patient is awake or alert. They do not provide a direct passage to the lower airway, and they do not protect the patient from aspiration in the case of diminished protective reflexes as intubation would. These airways are intended for short-term management.

Nasopharyngeal Airway

The *nasopharyngeal airway* is often referred to as a nasal horn or trumpet, names acquired due to its shape.

Figure 20-5 shows a nasal trumpet. The nasopharyngeal airway is inserted through one of the nares of the nose and past the turbinates, with the tip separating the tongue from the posterior soft palate. Figure 20-6 shows the airway in proper position. This airway is far from stable, but it is usually well tolerated. Its position at the opening of the naris should be checked frequently to ensure it has not slipped anteriorly, or worse, posteriorly. Some styles have a means to secure the airway to the patient's face, using tape or a tie of some type.

Oropharyngeal Airway

The *oropharyngeal airway* is larger than the nasopharyngeal airway. It is designed to be inserted into the mouth and then rotated with the tip resting against the

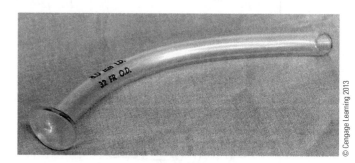

Figure 20-5 A photograph of a nasopharyngeal airway

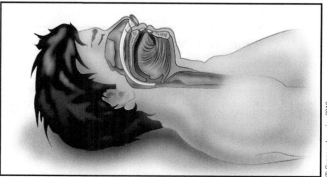

Figure 20-6 Correct placement of a nasopharyngeal airway

© Cengage Learning 2013

base of the tongue. It is designed to separate the tongue from the posterior palate. It does not provide a tube for the patient to breathe through, so its fit is essential to accomplish the job. This airway is not tolerated well by the conscious patient. It may cause a severe gag reflex and vomiting. Figure 20-7 shows the airway and its proper insertion.

Like the nasopharyngeal airway, this airway is unstable. Patients with this airway in place should not be left alone. Gagging and vomiting as well as displacement of the airway are common complications. It is easy for the patient to manipulate the airway with the tongue, often spitting it out.

Several types of these airways are available. Figure 20-8 shows some of the varieties that are manufactured.

Laryngeal Mask Airway (LMA)

The *laryngeal mask airway (LMA)* is illustrated in Figure 20-9. It is a small triangular-shaped inflatable mask that is secured to a tube, similar in size to an endotracheal tube. The LMA is designed to be inserted such that once the mask is inflated, the tip rests against the upper esophageal sphincter and the sides face into the pyriform fossae, lying just under the base of the tongue. This device is designed to seal the esophagus, preventing gastric aspiration while providing a patent airway for positive-pressure ventilation to the trachea.

Combitube Airway

The *Combitube airway* is a double-lumen airway that is inserted blindly (without visualization using a laryngoscope) into the oropharnyx and advanced into the esophagus or trachea. It has features similar to the esophageal gastric airway (no longer manufactured) and the endotracheal tube. Once inserted, the proximal and distal cuffs are inflated. The resuscitator attempts ventilation through the shorter tube and observes for adequate chest expansion, condensate in the airway, and confirmation by end-tidal CO_2 monitoring. If adequate ventilation is not observed, ventilation is then attempted through the longer tube and similar signs of adequate ventilation are

confirmed as described before. The tube may be inserted into the esophagus or trachea and ventilation can be established (Figure 20-10). The Combitube airway is more effective than a bag-mask device and an oropharyngeal airway.

Upon removal of a Combitube airway, it is important to have adequate suctions supplies (Yankauer suction catheter and 14 Fr suction catheter kit) available. If the Combitube airway has been inserted into the esophagus, the subsequent gastric distention and gastric contents can be easily aspirated upon removal of the airway. Therefore, it is important to protect the airway when extubation is performed.

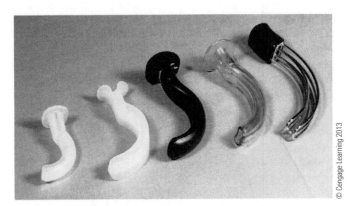

Figure 20-8 A variety of oropharyngeal airways

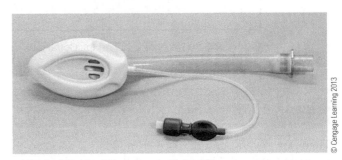

Figure 20-9 A photograph of a laryngeal mask airway (LMA)

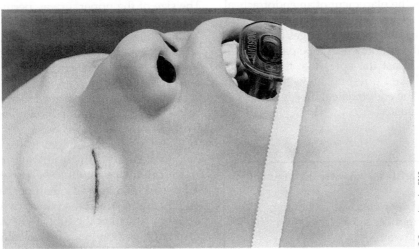

Figure 20-7 Correct use of an oropharyngeal airway

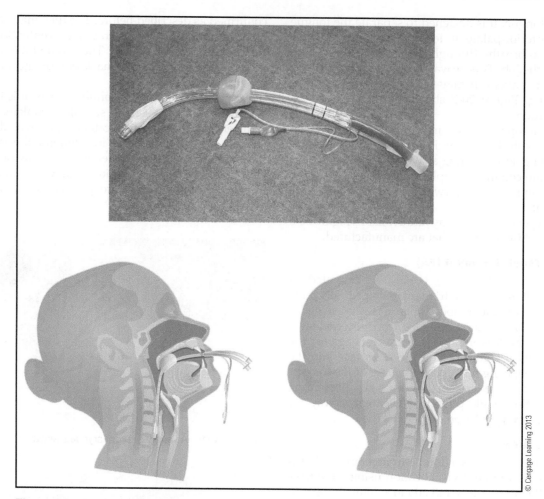

Figure 20-10 A photograph of the Combitube airway

© Cengage Learning 2013

INTUBATION: WHAT IS IT?

There are several criteria used in making a decision to intubate a patient. One or more of these criteria is justification for the intubation of a patient. Figure 20-11 lists these criteria.

Intubation involves the placement of an endotracheal tube into the trachea. There are two routes: oral and nasal. Each route has its inherent advantages and disadvantages. Ultimately, the endotracheal tube passes down the posterior pharynx, past the epiglottis, through the vocal cords with the distal tip resting 1.5 inches or 5 cm above the carina. With the endotracheal tube in place, the patient is said to be intubated.

- Failure of other artificial airways to maintain a patent airway
- Need for repeated deep tracheal suctioning
- Need for long-term mechanical ventilation
- Protection of the airway

© Cengage Learning 2013

Figure 20-11 Criteria for intubation

Oral Route

The oral route of intubation is the fastest and most direct. It is usually the first route learned by most respiratory practitioners. During the procedure, the vocal cords are directly visualized by the use of a laryngoscope while the endotracheal tube is inserted. If the cords are visualized, the chances of esophageal intubation are minimized. The size of the upper airway permits the use of a larger endotracheal tube, minimizing the resistance through the artificial airway (Poiseuille's law). When the procedure is properly performed, trauma to the oral and laryngeal structures is minimal. If the first attempt does not meet with success, a repeat attempt may be made after allowing sufficient time for reventilation and oxygenation before the repeat attempt. Intubation attempts should not last for more than 15 seconds.

There are disadvantages to the oral route of intubation. Oral care is difficult owing to the presence of the large endotracheal tube. The presence of tape or other supportive materials also hampers access to the oral cavity for care. A conscious patient will often gag or cough from movement of the tube in the airway. Because of the size of the oral cavity in relationship to the endotracheal tube and the presence of copious oral secretions, it is difficult to stabilize the endotracheal tube securely.

Nasal Route

Some facilities do not allow respiratory practitioners to perform nasal intubation of the patient. This description is provided so that the respiratory practitioner may better assist the physician performing this procedure.

- Failure of other artificial airways to maintain a patent airway
- Need for repeated deep tracheal suctioning
- Need for long-term mechanical ventilation
- Protection of the airway

Patients may be intubated nasally if they have experienced oral or facial trauma, making the oral intubation route impossible or impractical. An anesthesiologist will often nasally intubate patients during the administration of general anesthesia. Nasal intubation is common enough that the respiratory practitioner should be familiar with the technique and know how to secure the endotracheal tube properly after the procedure has been performed.

There are several advantages to this route of intubation. As mentioned, if a patient has suffered trauma to the mouth or face, making the oral route impractical, the patient may still be intubated nasally. Generally speaking, conscious patients tolerate nasal intubation better than oral intubation because the gag reflex is not as strongly stimulated. The absence of the endotracheal tube in the mouth makes oral care much easier, allowing sufficient access. The naris of the nose provides a natural anatomical structure to stabilize the endotracheal tube. Just a small amount of tape to prevent the tube from moving in or out is all that is required.

There are several disadvantages to the nasal route. Owing to the size of the nasal passage, a smaller tube, which increases resistance, must be used. This can be significant during mechanical ventilation and in weaning the patient because of the increased work of breathing. Smaller tubes may also make suctioning the airway more difficult. During nasal intubation, the vocal cords are not directly visualized, making this procedure "blind." The length of time taken for the procedure is longer. The tube must be first inserted through the nasal passages and then advanced down through the lower airway. Sometimes, this procedure is performed using a laryngoscope and Magill forceps to visualize the distal end of the tube and guide the tube through the vocal cords. The long-term placement of an endotracheal tube through the nasal passages may result in necrosis of the nasal tissue caused by the pressure of the tube decreasing the blood flow through the capillaries.

Equipment for Endotracheal Intubation

Laryngoscopes

There are two main types of laryngoscopes in use. One is termed conventional and the other fiberoptic.

The conventional *laryngoscope* is the most common type in use today. It consists of a handle containing batteries, a switch, and a socket into which different blades can be snapped in place. It works much like a flashlight. To turn it on, position the blade at a right angle to the handle by snapping it up. A blade is inserted by holding the handle vertically and aligning the socket on the blade with the handle socket. Pull each part together as if trying to pull each past the other. Figure 20-12 shows a laryngoscope with a Miller blade and its assembly.

The fiberoptic laryngoscope uses fiberoptics to transmit light to its distal tip. It has a self-contained battery pack and a flexible fiberoptic bundle that takes the place of a conventional blade. Owing to its small diameter and flexibility, it may be inserted into the endotracheal tube, and together the two can be advanced into position. An advantage of this laryngoscope is the ability to visualize the carina once the tube is in place. Exercise caution in the use of this equipment. Fiberoptics are fragile. Biting down on the laryngoscope by the patient could cause permanent damage to it.

Blades

There are two types of laryngoscope blades commonly used: the Miller and the Macintosh. The *Miller blade* is the straight blade. Figure 20-13 shows several sizes of Miller blades. When using this blade, the epiglottis is physically lifted. The *Macintosh blade* is a curved blade. It is inserted into the vallecula. As the laryngoscope is lifted, the epiglottis will follow, exposing the vocal cords and laryngeal structures. Many practitioners find it easier to visualize the cords with this blade.

Characteristics of Endotracheal Tubes

Modern endotracheal tubes are made of polyvinyl chloride (PVC), which is inert and nontoxic to tissue. The polymer is semirigid and is molded into a gentle curve that matches the curve of the airway. Upon looking closely at an *endotracheal tube*, the practitioner will see

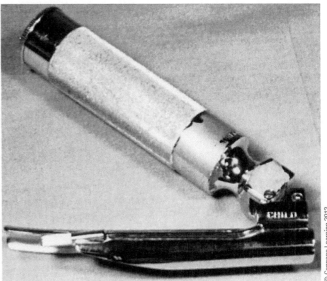

Figure 20-12 A conventional laryngoscope with a Miller blade attached

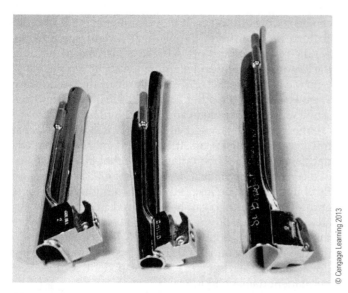

Figure 20-13   Different sizes of Miller laryngoscope blades

a stripe that runs almost the full length of the tube. This stripe is radiopaque and will show as a white band on the radiograph, helping to locate the exact position of the tip. Figure 20-14 shows an endotracheal tube. These tubes come in different diameters and are cut to an approximate length.

Murphy Eye Endotracheal Tube

A Murphy endotracheal tube has an eye or opening opposite the bevel on the distal end of the tube. Figure 20-15 shows this eye. In the event the distal tip becomes occluded, airflow may still pass through this eye (although resistance will be significantly greater).

Endotracheal Tube Cuff

The *endotracheal tube cuff* is an inflatable balloon near the tip of the tube. It creates a seal against the tracheal wall.

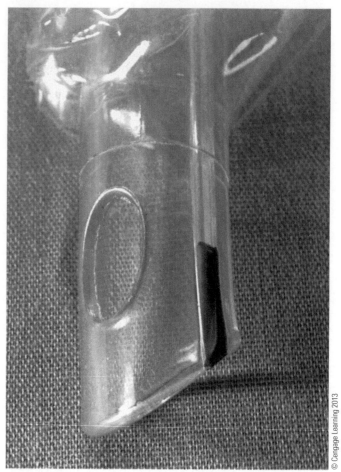

Figure 20-15   The Murphy eye on an endotracheal tube

An inflated cuff permits the application of positive pressure to the lungs and protects the airway from aspiration. It is best to use a high-volume, low-pressure cuff. This will distribute the pressure over a greater area, minimizing damage to the mucosa.

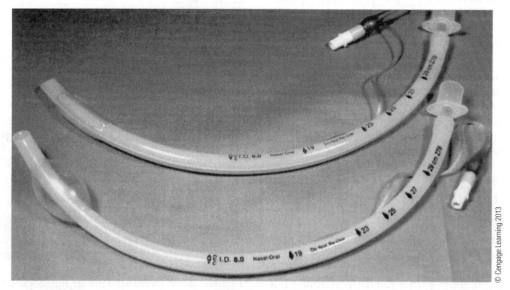

Figure 20-14   A contemporary endotracheal tube

One type of cuff is designed not to be inflated. It is the Bivona foam cuff. To use this cuff, first evacuate all of the air and seal it with the stopper provided. Once the tube is in place, open the pilot tube to atmospheric pressure. The foam in the cuff will reexpand, exerting minimal pressure to the tracheal wall. Figure 20-16 shows two Bivona cuffs, one evacuated and one expanded.

Pilot Tube and Balloon

The *endotracheal pilot tube* conducts air to the cuff of the tube. Be careful not to inadvertently cut the pilot tube. If this occurs, the patient will need to be reintubated.

If the pilot tube on a Bivona endotracheal tube is cut, the practitioner will be unable to deflate the cuff to extubate the patient. Repair kits using blunt needles can be used to restore cuff inflation/deflation following loss of integrity to the pilot line or pilot balloon.

The endotracheal pilot balloon is located on the proximal end of the pilot tube. It will indicate whether air is present in the endotracheal tube cuff. The larger the balloon is, the more air (volume) is in the cuff. It is advisable to measure cuff volume and cuff pressure twice each shift.

Markings

The proximal end of an endotracheal tube is conveniently marked in centimeter increments. This can provide a rough guide as to how far a tube has been advanced. However, it is best to rely on a chest radiograph to determine tube placement in relation to the carina. The patient's head should be in a neutral position (not hyperextended or flexed) when the radiograph is taken. After a chest radiograph has verified the position, the markings may be used to establish whether it has slipped in or out from the original location.

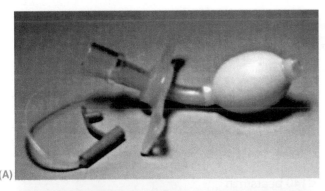

(A)

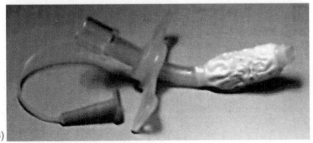

(B)

© Cengage Learning 2013

Figure 20-16   The Bivona foam cuff

COMPLICATIONS OF INTUBATION

The complications of intubation may be divided into early and late complications. Early complications generally occur during the procedure itself, whereas late complications occur hours or days after intubation.

Early Complications

One of the most common early complications is esophageal intubation. This may be assessed by auscultating the chest and by a chest radiograph. On auscultation, breath sounds will be diminished or absent. End-tidal CO_2 may also be used to confirm esophageal intubation. If the esophagus is intubated, the exhaled CO_2 will quickly fall to zero. Observe the abdomen while ventilating the patient. If the esophagus is intubated, the abdomen will rise and fall. Auscultate the abdomen: if sounds are present on inspiration, esophageal intubation is likely. A chest radiograph will ultimately confirm that the tube is improperly placed. However, often the practitioner cannot afford the time required for a radiograph in an emergency situation.

Trauma to the dentition or the oral cavity may result from a difficult intubation. If the patient is conscious, administration of a fast-acting paralytic agent (such as succinylcholine) by a physician or a nurse anesthetist will facilitate intubation and minimize trauma. At the very least, a conscious patient should receive intravenous midazolam and/or etomidate to decrease anxiety and to facilitate the procedure.

If the endotracheal tube is advanced too far, the right or left mainstem bronchus will be intubated. Advance the endotracheal tube only a short distance past the vocal cords. After placement, obtain a chest radiograph to verify that its position is 1.5 inches above the carina.

On intubation, there is a possibility of kinking the tube, making the resistance to airflow very high. If the practitioner suspects that the tube has kinked, try to pull it out slightly and then try to ventilate the patient again. If required, extubate the patient and insert another endotracheal tube.

Vomiting and aspiration may occur during the procedure. Have both a Yankauer (tonsil tip) and a suction catheter readily available to clear vomitus. Clear the oropharynx with the Yankauer suction first, and then intubate.

Late Complications

Vocal cord damage may occur as a result of the cord being approximated by the endotracheal tube and the friction resulting from it. It is not uncommon for a patient to sound hoarse for several hours after extubation.

Tracheal stenosis—narrowing of the trachea by scar tissue—may be a long-term complication of intubation. The decrease of capillary circulation combined with the irritation of the tube itself may cause tracheal damage. The best way to manage this condition is to prevent it.

If cuff pressure is maintained at a level greater than 25 cm H_2O for extended periods, capillary circulation will be impeded, resulting in tissue necrosis. It is best to keep cuff pressures at 20 cm H_2O or lower. Another method to determine cuff inflation is to establish a *minimal occlusion volume* (MOV). To perform this technique, inflate the lungs with positive pressure while simultaneously inflating the cuff. Stop cuff inflation just when the airway is occluded and escaping air is no longer heard. If cuff pressure is measured, it will generally be 25 cm H_2O or lower. If pressures are much greater, it is likely that too small an endotracheal tube was inserted. With the *minimal leak technique*, a slight leak is allowed during inspiration. To perform this technique, inflate the cuff under positive pressure. Stop cuff inflation when a small leak is heard at the mouth during inspiration.

Infection is a common complication from intubation. The introduction of bacteria into the lower airway is probably due to the bypassing of the upper airway defense mechanisms.

Extubation

Once the patient is able to manage secretions or the underlying cause for intubation has been resolved, *extubation* may be performed. Prior to extubation, patients should undergo a spontaneous breathing trial of between 30 and 120 minutes to determine readiness for removal from mechanical ventilation and extubation (refer to Chapter 28, Weaning and Discontinuance of Mechanical Ventilation). Objective measures in addition to a spontaneous breathing trial are listed in Table 20-3 (MacIntyre, 2007). Failure of ventilator discontinuance and reintubation can be attributed to several factors including advanced age, severity of illness, anemia, mental status, and excessive airway secretions (Mokhlesi, 2007).

The complications of extubation are associated primarily with edema, laryngospasm, and aspiration.

The artificial airway is irritating to the tracheal and laryngeal structures. Following its removal, the tissue frequently swells in response to the irritation, narrowing the lumen of the airway. Laryngospasm may occur in some patients as the endotracheal tube is withdrawn through the larynx. Aspiration may occur when the cuff is deflated and secretions that have pooled above the cuff drain inferiorly down the trachea. The epiglottis may not function normally for a few hours, also increasing the risk of aspiration.

Knowledge of these potential complications can help to avoid them. Edema may be relieved by the application of cool aerosol following extubation. Aspiration complications may be avoided by complete suctioning prior to extubation and keeping the head elevated by placing the patient in a semi-Fowler's position. Epiglottitis and edema may be treated by the administration of racemic epinephrine via small-volume nebulizer following extubation to reduce mucosal edema by stimulating the alpha receptors in the mucosal circulatory system.

TABLE 20-3: Objective Criteria for Ventilator Discontinuance and Extubation

OXYGENATION	CRITERIA
PaO_2	≥60 mm Hg on FIO_2 ≤ 0.4; PEEP ≤ 5–10 cm H_2O
PO_2/FIO_2	≥150–300
SpO_2	≥85–90%
Cardiovascular	
Heart Rate	≤140 beats/min
Blood Pressure	Stable with no or minimal vasopressor use
Ventilation	
pH	≥7.25
Minute Volume (V_E)	≤10–15 L/min
Negative Inspiratory Force (NIF)	≥−20 to −30 cm H_2O
Respiratory Rate	≤30–38 breaths/min
Tidal Volume (V_T)	325–408 mL
Rapid Shallow Breathing Index (f/V_T)	60–105/L

PROFICIENCY OBJECTIVES

At the end of this chapter, the reader should be able to:

* *Demonstrate the manual maneuvers to open the airway.*
* *Using an intubation mannequin, demonstrate the correct use of an oropharyngeal and a nasopharyngeal airway.*
* *Demonstrate how to assemble and prepare for use, including testing for function prior to use, a self-inflating manual resuscitator.*
* *Using a self-inflating manual resuscitator and a mask, maintain a patent airway and ventilate a resuscitation mannequin for 3 minutes, according to the following criteria:*
  * *Maintain an I:E ratio of 1:2 or greater.*
  * *Maintain a rate of 12 breaths per minute.*
  * *Observe the patient for the following:*
    * *Vomiting*
    * *Skin color*
    * *Chest expansion*
    * *Gastric distention*

* *Using an intubated resuscitation mannequin, demonstrate the use of a flow-inflating resuscitator, ventilating the mannequin according to the following criteria:*
  * *Maintain an I:E ratio of 1:2 or greater.*
  * *Maintain a rate of 12 breaths per minute.*
  * *Observe the "patient" for the following:*
    * *Skin color*
    * *Chest expansion*
* *Demonstrate oral intubation of a resuscitation mannequin using first a Miller and then a Macintosh laryngoscope blade.*
* *Discuss the rationale for hyperinflation and oxygenation prior to intubation.*
* *Describe the procedure used for nasal intubation, and demonstrate how to secure a nasal endotracheal tube.*
* *Using an orally intubated mannequin, demonstrate how to extubate the mannequin.*

PATIENT POSITIONING TO RELIEVE UPPER AIRWAY OBSTRUCTION

The positional maneuvers employed to relieve upper airway obstruction are discussed earlier in this chapter. The procedures and techniques are not covered here. It is suggested the reader review this portion of the chapter before proceeding.

AIRWAY INSERTION

Insertion of the Nasopharyngeal Airway

Nasopharyngeal airways come in different diameters and lengths. They are made from a soft rubber or plastic. Some manufacturers shape and mark them for use in the right or left naris.

Use of a nasopharyngeal airway is contraindicated in patients receiving anticoagulant therapy or those who have bleeding disorders. The insertion of this airway may cause trauma to the nasopharynx with associated bleeding.

For proper sizing of a nasopharyngeal airway, place the distal end of the airway at the tragus of the ear. The length of the airway should span from the tragus of the ear to the tip of the nose. As a general rule, use the largest diameter tube that can easily be inserted without undue force or trauma.

The technique of nasopharyngeal airway insertion begins with lubrication of the entire length of the airway with a water-soluble lubricant. Insert the airway gently through the nostril, parallel to the floor of the nasal cavity, matching the curve of the airway with the patient's airway.

If the airway has a beveled distal tip, the bevel should face medially. The nasal passage progresses posteriorly along the floor of the nasal cavity, then inferiorly. Do not attempt to insert the airway up the nose toward the eyes. Gently advance the airway. If resistance is encountered, redirect or rotate the airway slightly. Do not force the insertion of the airway. If unable to successfully insert an airway in one naris, try the other rather than attempting insertion by force. The tip of the airway should be just past the level of the posterior tongue, separating it from the posterior oropharynx. Once the airway is in place, the flared end will help to prevent further advancement of the airway down the nasal passage. However, check its placement frequently. Figure 20-6 shows the airway's placement.

The practitioner may not be able to insert this airway into a patient with a deviated septum. The use of this airway under this circumstance is not indicated.

Potential complications of using this type of airway include hearing problems caused by irritation of the eustachian tubes and mucosal irritation and trauma. The airway should be changed every 8 hours, and the new airway should be inserted into the alternate nare.

Insertion of the Oropharyngeal Airway

The airway is inserted by rotating the tip so that it is directed toward the hard palate. The airway is advanced toward the rear of the oropharynx and then rotated 180° so the tip now points down toward the throat. The rotation of the airway displaces the tongue forward and opens the passage between the tongue and the posterior pharynx. Figure 20-7 shows the airway's placement.

This airway should not be used if its placement stimulates gagging and vomiting. The patient should be positioned to minimize aspiration and should be closely watched.

PREPARATION OF MANUAL RESUSCITATORS

This section describes the preparation of manual resuscitators for use with a resuscitation mask. Any of the manual resuscitators may be used directly on an endotracheal tube or tracheostomy tube by removing the resuscitation mask. The patient connection on all of these devices is standardized, having an inside diameter of 15 mm and an outside diameter of 22 mm. It provides a direct connection with endotracheal tubes, tracheostomy tubes, masks, and manual resuscitators.

Check the valves for correct assembly and operation. Visually inspect the valve to ensure that it is assembled correctly and squeeze the bag several times to verify valve operation.

Attach the reservoir assembly to the manual resuscitator. Attach the oxygen connecting tubing to an oxygen flowmeter and set the flow to at least 15 L/min. Reassess the operation of the valves by squeezing the bag several times. Occlude the patient outlet, and squeeze the bag. Pressure should be maintained within the bag, indicating that the valve(s) are functioning properly.

To assemble a flow-inflating manual resuscitator, the following components are necessary: an anesthesia elbow with an oxygen inlet, a 3- or 5-liter anesthesia bag (cut off the very tip of the distal end), a length of oxygen connecting tubing, and an oxygen flowmeter. Attach the anesthesia bag to the anesthesia elbow. This may require the use of a mask adapter (22 mm outside diameter, 15 mm inside diameter). Attach the oxygen connecting tubing between the anesthesia elbow and the flowmeter. Figure 20-17 shows the completed assembly.

VENTILATION WITH A MANUAL RESUSCITATOR

Patient Positioning

Place the patient in a supine position and open the airway using one of the manual maneuvers. It is easiest to ventilate a patient in this position. It also allows for the observation of chest expansion and gastric distention. This position also permits cardiac compression, if it is required.

Mask Placement

Place the mask on the patient's face, applying the mask to the bridge of the nose first and then securing a tight seal below the lower lip. With a little practice, the mask's position can be maintained with the thumb and index finger of one hand, freeing the third, fourth, and fifth fingers on that hand to hook under the mandible, displacing it anteriorly to maintain a patent airway. Figure 20-18 shows the mask placement and finger positions. The other hand is free to compress the bag, inflating the lungs. The maintenance of an absolutely tight seal between the mask and face is required at all times for a flow-inflating manual resuscitator.

Ventilation

If the patient is apneic, ventilation may begin immediately. Ventilate the patient at a rate of 8 to 12 breaths per minute during administration of CPR or 10 to 12 breaths per minute with a perfusing heart rhythm (American Heart Association, 2005). Tidal volumes should range between 6 and 7 mL/kg normal body weight or 500 to 600 mL/breath. Watch for chest expansion to ensure that adequate volumes are delivered. Ventilate the patient with an I:E ratio of at least 1:2 or better to minimize the effects of positive intrathoracic pressure on the cardiovascular system.

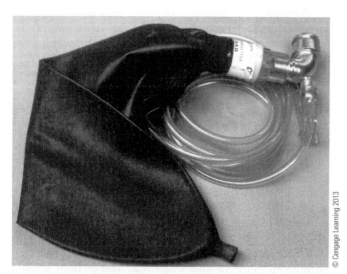

© Cengage Learning 2013

Figure 20-17   Assembly of a flow-inflating manual resuscitator

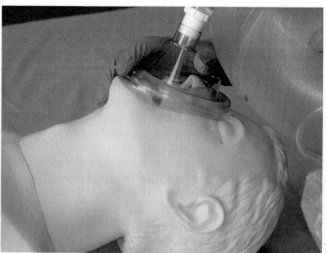

© Cengage Learning 2013

Figure 20-18   Correct use of a mask to manually ventilate a patient

It is important not to hyperventilate the patient. Often the rush of the emergency setting may cause health care personnel to become overly zealous. Hyperventilation will cause a rapid change in partial pressures of carbon dioxide in the arterial blood ($PaCO_2$) in patients who have been hypoventilating for long periods. Hyperventilation of these patients may potentially result in seizures.

If the patient has spontaneous respiratory efforts, match the ventilation efforts with the patient's efforts. When the patient begins inspiration, deliver a breath with the manual resuscitator. Knowledge of which resuscitators allow spontaneous ventilation is helpful under these circumstances.

Ventilation with a flow-inflating manual resuscitator requires the distal end of the bag to be pinched during compression. With exhalation, the practitioner must release the distal end to allow the exhaled gas to exit the bag. Oxygen flow will flush the exhaled CO_2 from the bag. A person unfamiliar with the operation of a flow-inflating bag will frequently have the flow set too high. A high oxygen flow will cause the bag to balloon, making it very difficult to manage with one hand. Either turn down the flow rate or compress the bag from the middle portion, decreasing the volume of the bag (as long as minute ventilation and tidal volume are adequate).

Patient Assessment during the Procedure

As mentioned previously, observe the patient for chest expansion, which indicates adequate volume delivery. Note the amount of resistance encountered upon ventilating the patient. This resistance is a direct reflection of the compliance of the lungs and thorax. If resistance is increased, it may indicate decreased compliance or a partial obstruction of the airway. Reassess the airway patency and continue ventilation. This is easier to assess with use of a flow-inflating manual resuscitator. Another person, if available, should auscultate the chest to assess ventilation.

Observe the patient frequently for signs of cyanosis. Watch for any signs of gastric distention. Gastric insufflation is a dangerous potential complication of bag and mask ventilation, as it may result in vomiting and aspiration. Decompression may be accomplished by the insertion of a nasogastric tube. If long-term resuscitation is expected, the early insertion of a nasogastric tube is recommended. Do not attempt to decompress the stomach by pushing on it until the patient is intubated. This maneuver may result in the patient's vomiting with the aspirate being driven into the tracheobronchial tree by the positive-pressure ventilation.

Assess the patient's pulse frequently. Another advantage of using the third, fourth, and fifth fingers to displace the mandible is that the last two fingers may assess the pulse, using the facial artery just anterior to the angle of the mandible. Other health care personnel available should assess carotid and femoral pulses to ensure adequate circulation. Cardiopulmonary complications may be minimized by using an I:E ratio of 1:2 or greater.

EQUIPMENT PREPARATION AND ASSEMBLY FOR INTUBATION

The equipment required for endotracheal intubation may be conveniently stored on a small tray or in a small fishing tackle box. The supplies needed are listed in Figure 20-19.

Preparation of the Laryngoscope

The laryngoscope should be assembled and a blade attached. Check the light for operation. If the light fails to illuminate, change the batteries and the bulb. If this fails to render it operational, change handles and repair the first unit later when time permits.

Oropharyngeal Airways

Lay out the airways in a convenient way that allows grabbing one quickly as the need arises. For female adult patients, small to medium sizes should be used. A male patient usually requires a medium to large airway size. The airway is sized properly when the flange rests on the patient's lips and the distal tip keeps the posterior tongue separated from the soft palate.

Yankauer Suction

Connect the Yankauer suction (tonsil tip) to a vacuum gauge and suction trap. Adjust the vacuum level to 120 mm Hg. Have the suction ready at hand where it may instantly be picked up. Have a 14 Fr sterile suction catheter or suction kit handy for use after the patient is intubated.

10 mL (or Larger) Syringe

Fill the syringe with 6 to 9 mL of air. Have it ready for attachment to the pilot balloon after the patient is intubated.

- Gloves, goggles, or face shield
- Laryngoscope
- Laryngoscope blades
- Spare batteries
- Spare bulbs
- Oropharyngeal airways (several sizes)
- Yankauer suctions (tonsil tip)
- Endotracheal tubes sized from 6.5-mm to 10-mm inner diameter
- 10-mL (or larger) syringe
- Cloth first-aid tape
- Water-soluble lubricant
- Magill forceps
- Stylet

Figure 20-19 Equipment needed for intubation

Commercial Endotracheal Tube Holder

Several manufacturers produce commercial endotracheal tube securing devices. Many of these devices incorporate a bite block as well as a means of securing the endotracheal tube. In lieu of a commercial device, tape may be used to temporarily secure an endotracheal tube.

Tear several strips about 15 inches long from a roll of 1-inch cloth first-aid tape. You will need this later to secure the tube. Stick the tape on a nearby wall or other surface where it will be handy and will not tangle.

Water-Soluble Lubricant

Squeeze out some lubricant onto a sterile 4 × 4-inch gauze pad for lubricating the endotracheal tube prior to insertion.

Magill Forceps

Keep these handy in case the patient needs to be nasally intubated.

Endotracheal Tubes

Check the cuff on the endotracheal tube prior to insertion by inflating it with about 10 mL of air (depending on cuff size, use more or less). Make sure the cuff is not torn and is capable of withstanding the pressure. Endotracheal tube sizes for female adult patients range from 7.5 to 8.5 mm inner diameter, whereas male patients' sizes range from 8.5 to 9.5 mm inner diameter. Nasal intubation requires a longer length tube than that needed for oral intubation.

Stylet

The stylet is a flexible metal wire used to stiffen the endotracheal tube. This will help during insertion of the tube to keep the tip anterior and guide it into the trachea. The stylet should never extend beyond the tip of the endotracheal tube.

General Notes

If the patient has been hypoxic for an extended period, or if it is an emergency situation, the person with the most intubation experience should make the attempt. It is best for a new respiratory practitioner to gain experience under more controlled circumstances. Ideally, this occurs in the operating room under the supervision of an anesthesiologist or a nurse anesthetist.

No more than 30 seconds should elapse from the time the laryngoscope enters the mouth until the endotracheal tube has been inserted. If the tube has not been inserted in this time frame, withdraw the laryngoscope and ventilate the patient with a manual resuscitator for 1 or 2 minutes and reattempt the intubation. For intubation of a patient in the clinical setting, no more than three attempts should be made. If unable to insert the tube, ventilate the patient and get someone who can.

Patient Positioning

The patient should be positioned supine with a small roll under the shoulders and the head slightly hyperextended. Imagine walking up to a rosebush to sniff the roses, and visualize the head position as the neck extends to get the nose closer to the blossom. That is the position the patient should be in. Figure 20-20 shows a patient in the "sniffing" position. Figure 20-21 shows what happens to the anatomy of the upper airway in this position versus having the head at a right angle to the body.

Hyperinflation and Oxygenation

Intubation is an emergency procedure often performed on patients with apnea and hypoxia. The procedure may stimulate the vagus nerve, causing bradycardia and the cough reflex if present. Two or three minutes of vigorous resuscitation with 100% oxygen will enable patients to tolerate the procedure better with fewer complications.

INTUBATION TECHNIQUES

Oral Intubation

First, prepare all of the equipment as described previously in the section on preparation.

Position the patient in the "sniffing" position, slightly hyperextending the head. Insert an airway and manually ventilate the patient on 100% oxygen for 2 to 3 minutes. After ventilation, remove the airway.

Miller Blade (Straight Blade)

The Miller blade is inserted into the mouth at a slight angle. Upon facing the patient, standing at the top of the head, insert the tip of the blade in the right corner of the mouth. Advance the tip of the blade at an angle toward

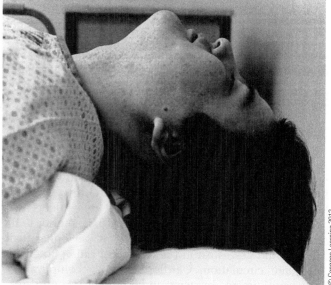

Figure 20-20 A patient in the "sniffing" position

© Cengage Learning 2013

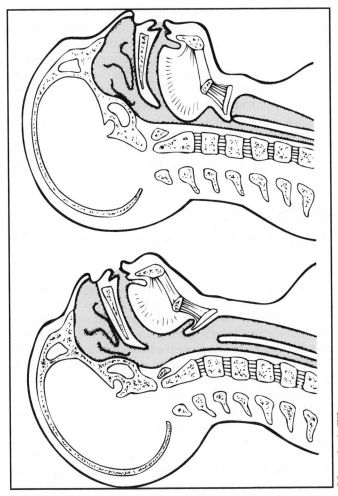

Figure 20-21 A comparison of the airway of a patient in two supine positions

the lower left of the tongue; then slide the handle and blade to the left. This will lift and displace the tongue to the left side of the mouth, allowing visualization of the airway. Continue to advance the blade until the epiglottis is visualized. Pick up the epiglottis with the tip of the blade by lifting straight up. The vocal cords should now be visualized.

Macintosh Blade (Curved Blade)

The Macintosh blade is inserted into the mouth in the same way as the Miller blade. The difference lies in the advancement of the blade. The blade is advanced until the epiglottis is visualized. At this point, the tip of the blade should be in the vallecula. Lift straight up. Upon lifting, the epiglottis will also be lifted, allowing visualization of the vocal cords.

Evaluation

Once the tube is in place, remove the blade and attach the resuscitator to the patient connection. Inflate the cuff and ventilate the patient with several breaths. Watch for chest expansion and auscultate the chest for bilateral breath sounds. It is important to realize that at this point the endotracheal tube is highly unstable. The

practitioner should hold on to it at all times until it is permanently secured.

Once bilateral breath sounds are confirmed, tape the tube in place. The use of tincture of benzoin will help the adhesive tape adhere to the skin better. Figure 20-22 shows one technique of taping a tube. Obtain a chest radiograph to verify tube placement. Adjust the tube placement as required, and secure it more thoroughly using tape or a commercial harness as shown in Figure 20-23.

Use of End-Tidal CO_2 Detectors or Esophageal Detectors

End-tidal CO_2 monitoring (capnographic or colormetric) may be used to determine endotracheal tube placement. If the endotracheal tube is in the airway, end-tidal CO_2 detection can be useful in determining correct endotracheal tube placement (American Heart Association, 2005).

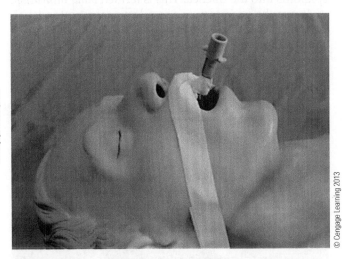

Figure 20-22 One method of securing an oral endotracheal tube with adhesive tape

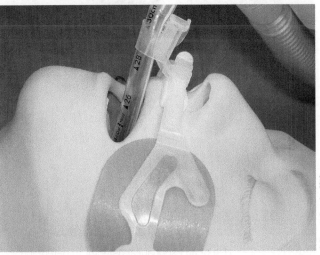

Figure 20-23 Use of a commercially made harness to secure an oral endotracheal tube

An esophageal detector consists of a bulb that, once squeezed, is placed on the endotracheal tube once the cuff is inflated (Figure 20-24). If the endotracheal tube is in the esophagus, it will not reexpand. If the endotracheal tube is in the lungs, the bulb will reexpand when released.

Nasal Intubation

Nasal intubation is a more difficult procedure than oral intubation. Usually it is performed by a physician with the respiratory practitioner assisting.

Begin by assembling and testing all of the equipment as described in the section on equipment preparation.

Position the patient in a "sniffing" position. Manually ventilate the patient for 2 or 3 minutes using 100% oxygen. Anesthetize the nasal passage with lidocaine or cocaine, or both.

Lubricate the endotracheal tube well with water-soluble lubricant. Advance the tube down the nasal passage. If the patient is breathing spontaneously, wait for the inspiratory phase and try to advance the tube past the epiglottis into the trachea. This is termed *blind intubation*.

It may be necessary to use a laryngoscope to visualize the airway. Either a Miller or a Macintosh blade may be used. Forceps may be required to direct the tube into the trachea.

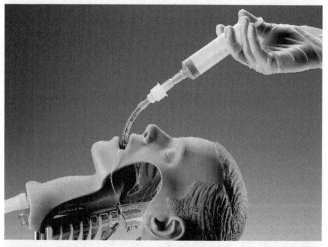

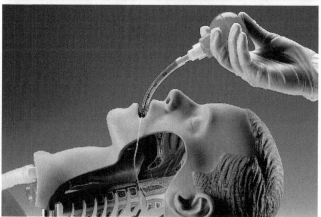

Figure 20-24 Use of an esophageal detector to determine esophageal intubation. Note that the bulb has not reinflated upon release. *(Courtesy of Ambu, Inc., Linthicum, Maryland)*

Note the position of the tube by the markings on it. Inflate the cuff and ventilate the patient with a manual resuscitator. Auscultate the chest for bilateral breath sounds. Obtain a chest radiograph to verify correct tube placement.

Secure the tube using a commercial device or a 1-inch-wide cloth first-aid tape. If using tape, tear off two lengths approximately 9 inches long. Tear the tape in half lengthwise for about 4 inches. Secure the wide end next to the nose above the upper lip. Wrap one small tail around the tube and secure the other tail to the upper lip. Repeat the process on the other side. Figure 20-25 shows the tube secured this way.

EXTUBATION

Extubation Technique

Extubation is one of the highlights of being a respiratory practitioner. The patient has finally become well enough that the artificial airway is no longer needed. Removal of the endotracheal tube is easier than insertion, but care must be taken not to contaminate the lower airway. Whenever a patient is extubated, always have the supplies needed to intubate the patient again if required.

Position the patient in full Fowler's position.

Hyperinflate and oxygenate the patient with a manual resuscitator. Suction the airway prior to removing the endotracheal tube.

Attach the syringe to the pilot balloon. Wrap the catheter around the fourth and fifth fingers of the dominant hand (the one wearing the sterile glove for suctioning), allowing the distal 4 inches of the catheter to rest in the oropharynyx. Hold the syringe between the third finger and the first segment of the fourth finger. Position the endotracheal tube between the second and third fingers. Figure 20-26 shows this seemingly complex hand position.

Inflate the lungs using the manual resuscitator. Apply an end-inspiratory hold while simultaneously withdrawing air from the endotracheal tube cuff by extending the thumb to pull out the plunger on the syringe and remove air from the cuff. This positive pressure jets out around the tube, propelling secretions into the mouth where the cath-

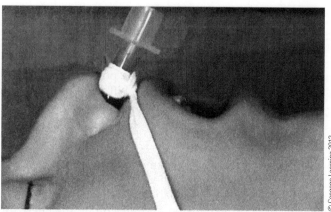

Figure 20-25 One method of securing the tube of a nasally intubated patient

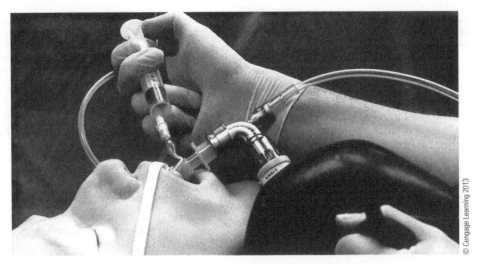

Figure 20-26   Use of a flow-inflating manual resuscitator, suction catheter, and a syringe during extubation

eter evacuates them, preventing them from sliding back down the airway. Now extubate the patient by removing the endotracheal tube. After the tube is removed, instruct the patient to cough vigorously. Administer supplemental oxygen as ordered by the physician.

Monitoring after Extubation

Following extubation, careful monitoring is important to ensure that the patient is able to maintain adequate ventilation and to control secretions effectively. Auscultate the chest to ensure that the lungs are clear. Assess the patient's breathing for stridor, which may indicate laryngospasm or edema. Ensure that the patient's swallow reflex is intact. Inform the patient that although speaking is now permissible, the patient will be hoarse for a while and should minimize speech for about 8 hours. Also, do not administer liquids by mouth for 8 hours or until the swallow reflex is fully regained.

References

American Association for Respiratory Care. (1995). AARC clinical practice guideline: Management of airway emergencies. *Respiratory Care, 40*(7), 749–760.

American Association for Respiratory Care. (2004). AARC clinical practice guideline: Resuscitation and defibrillation in the health care setting. *Respiratory Care, 49*, 1085–1099.

American Heart Association. (2005). Adjuncts for airway control and ventilation. *Circulation, 112*(11), IV-51–IV-57.

MacIntyre, N. (2007). Discontinuing mechanical ventilatory support. *Chest, 132*(3), 1049–1056.

Mokhlesi, B. (2007). Predicting extubation failure after successful completion of a spontaneous breathing trial. *Respiratory Care, 52*(12), 1710–1717.

Additional Resource

Mazzolini, D. (2004). Evaluation of 16 adult disposable manual resuscitators. *Respiratory Care, 49*(12), 1509–1514.

Practice Activities: Manual Resuscitation

1. Using a laboratory partner as your patient, place the patient in a supine position and open the airway using the following positional maneuvers:
   a. Head tilt-chin lift
   b. Anterior mandibular displacement

2. Using an intubation mannequin, practice the insertion of the following airways:
   a. Nasopharyngeal
   b. Oropharyngeal

3. Practice assembling, testing for function, and troubleshooting the following self-inflating manual resuscitators:
   a. AmbuSPUR II
   b. Allegiance Resuscitation Bag
   c. Hudson RCI Lifesaver
   d. Mercury Medical Adult CPR Bag

4. Attach a portable respirometer (Wright, Dragger, Haloscale) to a manual resuscitator and measure the tidal volume you can deliver using one hand and then using both hands.

5. Practice ventilating a resuscitation mannequin using the following self-inflating manual resuscitators:
   a. AmbuSPUR II
   b. Allegiance Resuscitation Bag
   c. Hudson RCI Lifesaver
   d. Mercury Medical Adult CPR Bag
   Include the following:
   (1) Ventilate the mannequin with a I:E ratio of 1:2 or greater.
   (2) Maintain a rate of 12 breaths per minute.
   (3) Observe for chest expansion, gastric distention, and skin color.

6. Using the following manual resuscitators and a respirometer, measure the tidal volume delivered using one hand and then using both hands to compress the bag:
   a. Ambu SPUR II
   b. Allegiance Resuscitation Bag
   c. Hudson RCI Lifesaver
   d. Mercury Medical Adult CPR Bag
   Calculate the following:
   (1) Using the stroke volume measured, calculate the minute volume you would deliver if you were ventilating a patient at a rate of 12 breaths per minute.
   (2) Using the stroke volume measured, calculate the minute volume you would deliver if you were ventilating a patient at a rate of 20 breaths per minute.

7. Assemble, test for function, and troubleshoot a flow-inflating manual resuscitator.

8. Using an intubated resuscitation mannequin, practice ventilating the mannequin with a flow-inflating manual resuscitator, including the following:
   a. Maintain an I:E ratio of 1:2 or greater.
   b. Maintain a rate of 12 breaths per minute.
   c. Observe the following:
   (1) Chest expansion
   (2) Gastric distention
   (3) Skin color

9. Using a laboratory partner as a patient, practice assisting the patient's ventilation with a self-inflating manual resuscitator.

INTUBATION PRACTICE ACTIVITIES

1. Assemble all of the equipment required for intubation.

2. Assemble the laryngoscope and test it for proper operation.

3. Check the self-inflating manual resuscitator for proper operation.

4. Place an intubation mannequin or a laboratory partner in proper position for intubation.
   a. Supine
   b. "Sniffing" position

5. Using an intubation mannequin, practice using both the Miller (straight) blade and the Macintosh (curved) blade.
   a. Miller blade:
   (1) Hold the laryngoscope in your left hand.
   (2) Insert it at an angle and slide it left into position.
   (3) Slowly advance the blade.
   (4) Pick up the epiglottis with the tip of the blade.
   b. Macintosh blade:
   (1) Hold the laryngoscope in your left hand.
   (2) Insert the blade at an angle and slide it left into position.
   (3) Slowly advance the blade.
   (4) When the epiglottis is visualized, lift straight up, exposing the vocal cords.

6. Using an intubation mannequin, practice oral intubation, including the following steps:
   a. Equipment assembly and testing
   b. Patient positioning
   c. Hyperinflation and oxygenation with 100% oxygen
   d. Correct laryngoscope use
   e. Insertion of the endotracheal tube within 15 seconds
   f. Stabilization of the endotracheal tube until secured with tape
   g. Ventilation of the patient with adequate volumes and I:E ratio

h. Auscultation of the chest for tube placement

i. Evaluation of placement using end-tidal CO_2 monitoring or an esophageal detector

j. Securing the endotracheal tube with a commercial holder or first-aid tape

7. Using an intubation mannequin, insert an endotracheal tube nasally and secure it properly with first-aid tape.

8. Orally intubate an intubation mannequin and practice the extubation procedure, including the following:

a. Positioning the patient

b. Hyperinflation and oxygenation

c. Aspirating the airway prior to removal

d. Deflation of the cuff under positive pressure

e. Aspirating expelled secretions

f. Removal of the endotracheal tube

g. Monitoring the patient

Check List: Manual Resuscitation

_____ 1. Wash your hands.

2. Gather the appropriate equipment:

_____ a. Manual resuscitator

_____ b. Oxygen flowmeter

_____ c. Resuscitation mask

_____ d. Oxygen connecting tubing

_____ e. Artificial airway

_____ f. Personal protective equipment (gloves, goggles, or face shield)

3. Assemble and check equipment function.

_____ a. Check the valve assembly.

_____ b. Assemble the resuscitator.

_____ c. Attach:

(1) Mask

(2) Connecting tubing

(3) Flowmeter set at 10 to 15 L/min

4. Apply the mask to the patient:

_____ a. Apply to the bridge of the nose first.

_____ b. Obtain a good seal.

_____ c. Anteriorly displace the mandible with free fingers.

5. Ventilate the patient.

_____ a. Deliver an adequate volume.

_____ b. Ventilate with an I:E ratio of 1:2 or greater.

6. Assess the patient during the procedure for:

_____ a. Cyanosis

_____ b. Vomiting/gagging

_____ c. Gastric distention

_____ d. Airway placement

_____ 7. Following procedure, clean up the area.

Check List: Intubation

1. Assemble all needed equipment:

_____ a. Laryngoscope

_____ b. Laryngoscope blades

_____ c. Spare batteries

_____ d. Oropharyngeal airways

_____ e. Yankauer suction and supplies

_____ f. 10 mL (or larger) syringe

_____ g. Stylet

_____ h. Cloth first-aid tape

_____ i. Water-soluble lubricant

_____ j. Magill forceps

_____ k. Self-inflating manual resuscitator

_____ l. Oxygen flowmeter

_____ m. Endotracheal tubes sized 6.5 mm to 10 mm

_____ n. End-tidal CO_2 monitor or esophageal detector

_____ o. Personal protective equipment (gloves, goggles, or face shield)

_____ 2. Test all equipment to ensure proper function.

_____ 3. Hyperinflate and oxygenate the patient using a manual resuscitator prior to attempting intubation.

4. Position the patient properly.

_____ a. Supine

_____ b. "Sniffing" position

_____ 5. Use the laryngoscope properly.

_____ 6. Insert the endotracheal tube within 30 seconds.

7. Ventilate the patient with a manual resuscitator, using:

_____ a. Adequate volume delivery

_____ b. I:E ratio of at least 1:2

_____ 8. Stabilize the tube at all times until it is taped securely.

_____ 9. Auscultate the chest for tube placement.

_____ 10. Evaluate tube placement using end-tidal CO_2 or an esophageal detector

_____ 11. Obtain a chest x-ray film.

_____ 12. Tape the tube securely.

Check List: Extubation

_____ 1. Verify the physician's order.

_____ 2. Scan the chart to ensure that the patient is ready for extubation.

_____ 3. Measure spontaneous parameters and blood gases.

4. Gather the required equipment:

_____ a. Intubation tray

_____ b. 20 mL syringe

_____ c. Suction supplies

_____ d. Oxygen/aerosol equipment

_____ e. Personal protective equipment (gloves, goggles, or face shield)

_____ 5. Wash your hands.

_____ 6. Introduce yourself and explain the procedure.

_____ 7. Position the patient in full Fowler's position.

_____ 8. Suction the patient thoroughly.

_____ 9. Oxygenate the patient with 100% oxygen using a flow-inflating manual resuscitator.

_____ 10. Deflate the cuff while the patient is exhaling forcefully and withdraw the tube.

_____ 11. Have the patient cough several times and speak to allow you to assess for hoarseness and to clear the airway.

_____ 12. Administer cool aerosol as ordered.

_____ 13. Evaluate the patient following extubation.

_____ 14. Clean up the area.

_____ 15. Chart the procedure.

Self-Evaluation Post Test: Emergency Airway Management

1. When using a flow-inflating bag, you should:
   a. connect it to a 50 psi oxygen source.
   b. pinch the tail of the bag when delivering a breath.
   c. release the tail during the expiratory phase.
   d. Both b and c

2. The most commonly used airway for ventilating a patient with a manual resuscitator is the:
   a. nasopharyngeal airway.
   b. oropharyngeal airway.
   c. nasal trumpet.
   d. tracheostomy tube.

3. Patient observation during manual resuscitation should include:
   I.   skin color.
   II. chest expansion.
   III. gastric distention.
   IV. the presence of vomiting.
   a. I, II   c. II, III, IV
   b. I, II, III   d. I, II, III, IV

4. Two advantages of a flow-inflating manual resuscitator are:
   I.   size.
   II. its self-inflation characteristics.
   III. oxygen delivery.
   IV. ease of assessing patient compliance.
   V.   ease of using it with a resuscitation mask.
   a. I, II   c. III, IV
   b. II, IV   d. IV, V

5. A common complication of manual resuscitation is:
   a. vagal stimulation.   c. gastric distention.
   b. bradycardia.   d. pneumothorax.

6. When using a Miller (straight) laryngoscope blade, you should:
   a. insert the tip of the blade into the vallecula.
   b. insert the tip of the blade through the vocal cords.
   c. lift the epiglottis with the tip of the blade.
   d. insert the tip of the blade into the larynx.

7. Attempts to insert the endotracheal tube should be limited to:
   a. 10 seconds.   c. 20 seconds.
   b. 15 seconds.   d. 30 seconds.

8. The first thing you should do to assess the placement of an endotracheal tube is to:
   a. auscultate the chest.
   b. order a chest x-ray film.
   c. check for cyanosis.
   d. observe the stomach expanding on inspiration.

9. The best way to prevent equipment malfunction is to:
   a. use new equipment.
   b. carefully check equipment before use.
   c. have all supplies ready.
   d. Both b and c

10. The last reflex a patient loses when progressing into unconsciousness is the:
    a. gag reflex.
    b. laryngeal reflex.
    c. tracheal reflex.
    d. carinal reflex.

PERFORMANCE EVALUATION:
Manual Resuscitation

Date: Lab _____ Clinical _____ Agency _____

Lab: Pass _____ Fail _____ Clinical: Pass _____ Fail _____

Student name _____ Instructor name _____

No. of times observed in clinical _____

No. of times practiced in clinical _____

PASSING CRITERIA: Obtain 90% or better on the procedure. Tasks indicated by * must receive at least 1 point, or the evaluation is terminated. Procedure must be performed within the designated time, or the performance receives a failing grade.

SCORING: 2 points — Task performed satisfactorily without prompting.
1 point — Task performed satisfactorily with self-initiated correction.
0 points — Task performed incorrectly or with prompting required.
NA — Task not applicable to the patient care situation.

Tasks:	Peer	Lab	Clinical
* 1. Observes standard precautions, including handwashing	☐	☐	☐
2. Applies personal protective equipment	☐	☐	☐
3. Obtains the required equipment			
* a. Oxygen flowmeter	☐	☐	☐
* b. Manual resuscitator	☐	☐	☐
* c. Resuscitation mask	☐	☐	☐
* d. Oxygen connecting tubing	☐	☐	☐
* e. Artificial airway	☐	☐	☐
* f. Gloves, goggles, or face shield	☐	☐	☐
* 4. Assembles and checks the equipment	☐	☐	☐
5. Applies the mask			
* a. Seats the mask on the bridge of the nose first	☐	☐	☐
* b. Obtains a good seal	☐	☐	☐
* c. Lifts the mandible with the fingers	☐	☐	☐
6. Ventilates the patient appropriately			
* a. Maintains an I:E ratio of 1:2 or greater	☐	☐	☐
* b. Delivers adequate volumes	☐	☐	☐

7. Reassesses the patient for

*   a. Cyanosis   ☐   ☐   ☐

*   b. Vomiting   ☐   ☐   ☐

*   c. Gastric distention   ☐   ☐   ☐

*   **8.** Ventilates for an appropriate time   ☐   ☐   ☐

*   **9.** Removes the equipment after the procedure   ☐   ☐   ☐

SCORE: Peer   _____ points of possible 38; _____%

                     Lab   _____ points of possible 38; _____%

                     Clinical _____ points of possible 38; _____%

TIME: _____ out of possible 5 minutes

STUDENT SIGNATURES   **INSTRUCTOR SIGNATURES**

PEER: _____   LAB: _____

STUDENT: _____   CLINICAL: _____

PERFORMANCE EVALUATION:
Intubation

Date: Lab _____ Clinical _____ Agency _____

Lab: Pass _____ Fail _____ Clinical: Pass _____ Fail _____

Student name _____ Instructor name _____

No. of times observed in clinical _____

No. of times practiced in clinical _____

PASSING CRITERIA: Obtain 90% or better on the procedure. Tasks indicated by * must receive at least 1 point, or the evaluation is terminated. Procedure must be performed within the designated time, or the performance receives a failing grade.

SCORING: 2 points — Task performed satisfactorily without prompting.
1 point — Task performed satisfactorily with self-initiated correction.
0 points — Task performed incorrectly or with prompting required.
NA — Task not applicable to the patient care situation.

Tasks:	Peer	Lab	Clinical
* 1. Observes standard precautions, including handwashing	☐	☐	☐
2. Obtains the required equipment			
* a. Oxygen flowmeter	☐	☐	☐
* b. Manual resuscitator	☐	☐	☐
* c. Resuscitation mask	☐	☐	☐
* d. Laryngoscope and blades	☐	☐	☐
* e. Artificial airways	☐	☐	☐
* f. 10 mL (or larger) syringe	☐	☐	☐
* g. End-tidal CO_2 monitor or esophageal detector	☐	☐	☐
* h. Endotracheal tubes	☐	☐	☐
* i. Stylet	☐	☐	☐
* j. Lubricant	☐	☐	☐
* k. Tape	☐	☐	☐
* l. Suctioning supplies	☐	☐	☐
* m. Gloves, goggles, or face shield	☐	☐	☐
* 3. Assembles and checks the equipment	☐	☐	☐
* 4. Positions the patient	☐	☐	☐
* 5. Hyperinflates and oxygenates the patient	☐	☐	☐

*   **6.** Correctly uses the laryngoscope ☐ ☐ ☐

*   **7.** Inserts the tube within 15 seconds ☐ ☐ ☐

*   **8.** Ventilates following intubation

*   a. Gives adequate volumes ☐ ☐ ☐

*   b. Maintains an I:E ratio greater than 1:2 ☐ ☐ ☐

*   **9.** Stabilizes the tube until taped ☐ ☐ ☐

* **10.** Auscultates for tube position ☐ ☐ ☐

* **11.** Tapes the tube ☐ ☐ ☐

* **12.** Assesses tube placement using end-tidal CO_2 or An esophageal detector ☐ ☐ ☐

* **13.** Orders a chest x-ray film ☐ ☐ ☐

* **14.** Cleans up the patient area afterward ☐ ☐ ☐

* **15.** Uses aseptic technique ☐ ☐ ☐

SCORE: Peer _____ points of possible 56; _____%

                   Lab _____ points of possible 56; _____%

                   Clinical _____ points of possible 56; _____%

TIME: _____ out of possible 10 minutes

STUDENT SIGNATURES   **INSTRUCTOR SIGNATURES**

PEER: _____   LAB: _____

STUDENT: _____   CLINICAL: _____

PERFORMANCE EVALUATION:
Extubation

Date: Lab _____ Clinical _____ Agency _____

Lab: Pass _____ Fail _____ Clinical: Pass _____ Fail _____

Student name _____ Instructor name _____

No. of times observed in clinical _____

No. of times practiced in clinical _____

PASSING CRITERIA: Obtain 90% or better on the procedure. Tasks indicated by * must receive at least 1 point, or the evaluation is terminated. Procedure must be performed within the designated time, or the performance receives a failing grade.

SCORING:
2 points — Task performed satisfactorily without prompting.
1 point — Task performed satisfactorily with self-initiated correction.
0 points — Task performed incorrectly or with prompting required.
NA — Task not applicable to the patient care situation.

Tasks:	Peer	Lab	Clinical
* 1. Verifies the physician's order	☐	☐	☐
* 2. Scans the chart to ensure that the patient is ready for extubation	☐	☐	☐
* 3. Performs spontaneous breathing trial, measures spontaneous parameters and blood gases	☐	☐	☐
* 4. Gathers the required equipment	☐	☐	☐
a. Intubation tray	☐	☐	☐
b. 20 mL syringe	☐	☐	☐
c. Suction supplies	☐	☐	☐
d. Oxygen/aerosol equipment	☐	☐	☐
e. Gloves, goggles, or face shield	☐	☐	☐
* 5. Observes standard precautions, including handwashing	☐	☐	☐
6. Introduces self and explains the procedure	☐	☐	☐
* 7. Positions the patient in full Fowler's position	☐	☐	☐
* 8. Suctions the patient thoroughly	☐	☐	☐
* 9. Oxygenates the patient with 100% oxygen using a flow-inflating manual resuscitator	☐	☐	☐
* 10. Deflates the cuff under positive pressure and withdraws the tube	☐	☐	☐
* 11. Has the patient cough several times and speak to assess hoarseness and clear the airway	☐	☐	☐

* **12.** Administers cool aerosol ☐ ☐ ☐

* **13.** Evaluates the patient ☐ ☐ ☐

* **14.** Cleans up the area ☐ ☐ ☐

* **15.** Charts the procedure ☐ ☐ ☐

SCORE: Peer _____ points of possible 38; _____%

Lab _____ points of possible 38; _____%

Clinical _____ points of possible 38; _____%

TIME: _____ out of possible 20 minutes

STUDENT SIGNATURES

PEER: _____

STUDENT: _____

INSTRUCTOR SIGNATURES

LAB: _____

CLINICAL: _____

CHAPTER 21
Artificial Airway Care

INTRODUCTION

As a respiratory practitioner, you will be responsible for the routine care of the artificial airway. Artificial airway care includes humidification (see Chapter 15); suctioning; cuff care; and for tracheostomy tubes, stoma care. This routine care is necessary to ensure a patent airway and to protect the lower airway from aspirated secretions and infection. Stoma care is needed to prevent the accumulation of secretions or exudate at the stoma site. You will be expected to perform these procedures correctly and safely.

KEY TERMS

- Closed suction system
- Decannulation
- Fenestrated tracheostomy tube
- Minimal leak technique
- Minimal occlusion volume (MOV) technique
- Passy-Muir valve
- Suction catheters
- Suctioning
- Tracheostomy
- Tracheostomy button
- Washout volume

THEORY OBJECTIVES

At the end of this chapter, the reader should be able to:

- State the rationale for nasotracheal and artificial airway aspiration (suctioning).
- Compare and contrast the functional characteristics of the following suction catheters and the advantages of each:
  - Whistle tip
  - Coudé tip
  - Closed suction systems
- State the complications of airway aspiration and describe how to minimize them.
- State the rationale for the use of hyperinflation and oxygenation before and after suctioning.
- Describe the use of a mechanical ventilator (volume ventilator) to oxygenate and hyperinflate the patient for suctioning.
- Explain the importance of maintaining proper cuff pressures.
- List the importance of the following in prevention of ventilator-associated pneumonia (VAP):
  - Head of bed elevation between 30 and 45°
  - Use of subglottic secretion drainage
  - Maintenance of cuff pressure
  - Maintenance of appropriate humidity
- List the indications for a tracheostomy.
- Explain the purpose of tracheostomy and stoma care, and state the associated hazards and complications.
- Identify the following types of tracheostomy cannulas, and describe their clinical application:
  - Single cannula tracheostomy tube
  - Single cannula tracheostomy tube with a disposable inner cannula
  - Single cannula fenestrated tracheostomy tube
  - Silver Hollinger or Jackson tracheostomy tube
  - Bivona foam cuff
- Identify the following specialized tracheostomy tubes and tracheostomy appliances, and describe their clinical application:
  - Pitt Speaking Tube/Communi-Trach
  - Trach button
  - Kistner button
  - Passy-Muir valve
  - Olympic Trach-Talk

CLINICAL PRACTICE GUIDELINES

AARC Clinical Practice Guideline: Nasotracheal Suctioning – 2004 Revision and Update

NTS (NASOTRACHEAL SUCTIONING) 4.0 INDICATIONS:

The need to maintain a patent airway and remove saliva, pulmonary secretions, blood, vomitus, or foreign material from the trachea in the presence of:

4.1 Inability to clear secretions when audible or visible evidence of secretions in the large/central airways that persist in spite of patient's best cough effort. [1,5,6,25–27] This is evidenced by one or more of the following

   4.1.1 Visible secretions in the airway [1,27]

   4.1.2 Chest auscultation of coarse, gurgling breath sounds, rhonchi[1, 14,21,27,28] or diminished sounds [21]

   4.1.3 Feeling of secretions in the chest (increased tactile fremitus) [21]

   4.1.4 Suspected aspiration of gastric or upper airway secretions[1]

   4.1.5 Clinically apparent increased work of breathing [1]

   4.1.6 Deterioration of arterial blood gas values suggesting hypoxemia or hypercarbia [1,21]

   4.1.7 Chest radiographic evidence of retained secretions resulting in atelectasis or consolidation [1,27]

   4.1.8 Restlessness [21,28]

4.2 To stimulate cough [1,2,27,29] or for unrelieved coughing [21]

4.3 To obtain a sputum sample for microbiological or cytological analysis [1,2,27]

NTS 5.0 CONTRAINDICATIONS

Listed contraindications are relative unless marked as absolute.

5.1 Occluded nasal passages [1,6]

5.2 Nasal bleeding [1]

5.3 Epiglottitis or croup (absolute) [1,6]

5.4 Acute head, facial, or neck injury [1,2,6]

5.5 Coagulopathy or bleeding disorder [1,3,6]

5.6 Laryngospasm [1,3,6]

5.7 Irritable airway [1]

5.8 Upper respiratory tract infection [1]

5.9 Tracheal surgery [6]

5.10 Gastric surgery with high anastomosis [6]

5.11 Myocardial infarction [6]

5.12 Bronchospasm [2]

NTS 6.0 HAZARDS/COMPLICATIONS:

6.1 Mechanical trauma (mucosal hemorrhage, tracheitis, epitaxis from laceration of nasal turbinates, and perforation of the pharynx) [1,6,14,17,26,27, 30–34]

   6.1.1 Laceration of nasal turbinates [8,35]

   6.1.2 Perforation of the pharynx [36]

   6.1.3 Nasal irritation/bleeding [7]

   6.1.4 Tracheitis [1,17]

   6.1.5 Mucosal hemorrhage [2,32]

   6.1.6 Uvular edema [37]

6.2 Hypoxia/hypoxemia [1,2,6,17,27,33,38–41]

6.3 Cardiac dysrhythmias/arrest [2,4,6,14,33–35]

6.4 Bradycardia [1,2,6,27,38,41–44]

6.5 Increase in blood pressure [1,2,6,38,40,45]

6.6 Hypotension [1,38]

6.7 Respiratory arrest [35]

6.8 Uncontrolled coughing [1,2,7,34]

6.9 Gagging/vomiting [1,6,7,46]

6.10 Laryngospasm [1,3,35]

6.11 Bronchoconstriction/bronchospasm [1,14,33,34]

6.12 Discomfort [7,41] and pain [1,2,7,41]

6.13 Nosocomial infection [1,2,27,34,44]

6.14 Atelectasis [2,8,14,17,27,33]

6.15 Misdirection of catheter [6,7,34]

6.16 Increased intracranial pressure (ICP) [6,28,40, 41,45,47–49]

   6.16.1 Intraventricular hemorrhage [14,40,50]

   6.16.2 Exacerbation of cerebral edema

6.17 Pneumothorax [17]

NTS 8.0 ASSESSMENT OF NEED:

8.1 Personnel should perform a baseline assessment for indications of respiratory distress and the need for NTS as recognized by presenting indications as listed above. This should include but not be limited to

   8.1.1 Auscultation of chest [1,3,9,12,14,27,53,54]

   8.1.2 Monitor patient's heart rate [3,12,14]

   8.1.3 Respiratory rate [12]

   8.1.4 Cardiac rhythm [12,14]

   8.1.5 Oxygen saturation [12,14]

   8.1.6 Skin color and perfusion [12]

   8.1.7 Personnel should assess effectiveness of cough [1]

8.2 Prepare the patient for the procedure by providing an appropriate explanation along with adequate sedation and pain relief as needed. [2,9,12]

NTS 9.0 ASSESSMENT OF OUTCOME:

Effectiveness of NTS should be reflected by assessing patient post suction for

9.1 Improved breath sounds [1,36]

9.2 Removal of secretions [1,36]

9.3 Improved blood gas data or pulse oximetry [1]

9.4 Decreased work of breathing (decreased respiratory rate or dyspnea) [1]

(Continued)

NTS 11.0 MONITORING:

The following should be monitored before, during and following the procedure.

11.1 Breath sounds 1,3,12,27,59

11.2 Skin color 1,6,12,61

11.3 Breathing pattern and rate 1,6,12

11.4 Pulse rate, dysrhythmia, electrocardiogram if available 1,6,12,14,27,41

11.5 Color, consistency, and volume of secretions 1,6

11.6 Presence of bleeding or evidence of physical trauma 1,6

11.7 Subjective response including pain 1,2,7,41,46

11.8 Cough 1

11.9 Oxygenation (pulse oximeter) 1,2,3,6,12,14

11.10 Intracranial pressure (ICP), if equipment is available 1

11.11 Arterial blood pressure if available 6

11.12 Laryngospasm 6

Reprinted with permission from *Respiratory Care* 2004; 49: 1080–1084. The complete AARC Clinical Practice Guidelines are available from the AARC Web site (http://www.aarc .org), from the AARC Executive Office, or from *Respiratory Care* journal.

AARC Clinical Practice Guideline: Endotracheal Suctioning of Mechanically Ventilated Patients with Artificial Airways 2010

ETS 1.0 DESCRIPTION

Endotracheal suctioning (ETS) is one of the most common procedures performed in patients with artificial airways. It is a component of bronchial hygiene therapy and mechanical ventilation that involves the mechanical aspiration of pulmonary secretions from a patient's artificial airway to prevent its obstruction. 1 The procedure includes patient preparation, the suctioning event, and follow-up care. There are 2 methods of endotracheal suctioning based on the selection of catheter: open and closed. The *open* suctioning technique requires disconnecting the patient from the ventilator, while the *closed* suctioning technique involves attachment of a sterile, closed, in-line suction catheter to the ventilator circuit, which allows passage of a suction catheter through the artificial airway without disconnecting the patient from the ventilator. There are also 2 methods of suctioning based on the catheter suction depth selected during the procedure: deep and shallow. *Deep suctioning* is defined as the insertion of a suction catheter until resistance is met, followed by withdrawal of the catheter by 1 cm before application of negative pressure, and *shallow suctioning* as the insertion of a suction catheter to a predetermined depth, usually the length of the artificial airway plus the adapter. 2

ETS 2.0 PATIENT PREPARATION

It is recommended to use smaller catheters whenever possible, since suction pressure seems to have less influence on lung volume loss than catheter size. 3 For a given diameter of the endotracheal tube (ETT), the level of negative pressure transmitted to the airway is determined by the combination of the catheter size and the suction pressure. The larger the diameter of the catheter size, the less attenuation of the suction pressure through the airways. 4

2.1 Diameter of the suction catheter should not exceed one half the inner diameter of the artificial airway in adults, providing an internal-to-external diameter ratio of 0.5 in adults, 5,6 and 0.5–0.66 in infants and small children. 7

2.2 In preparation for the suctioning event, delivery of 100% oxygen in pediatric 8 and adult patients 9 and 10% increase of baseline in neonates 10–12 for 30–60 seconds prior to the suctioning event is suggested, especially in patients who are hypoxemic before suctioning. 13,14 This may be accomplished either:

2.2.1 by adjusting the FIO_2 setting on the mechanical ventilator, or

2.2.2 by use of a temporary oxygen-enrichment program available on many microprocessor ventilators. 15

2.2.3 Manual ventilation of the patient is not recommended, as it has been shown to be ineffective for providing delivered FIO_2 of 1.0.16,17 Practitioners should ensure that PEEP is maintained if no other alternative is available to hyper-oxygenate.

2.3 The negative pressure of the unit must be checked by occluding the end of the suction tubing before attaching it to the suction catheter, and prior to each suctioning event. Suction pressure should be set as slow as possible and yet effectively clear secretions. Experimental data to support an appropriate maximum suction level are lacking. Negative pressure of 80–100 mmHg in neonates 18 and less than 150 mmHg in adults have been recommended. 19

2.4 The *closed suctioning technique* facilitates continuous mechanical ventilation and oxygenation during the suctioning event. 20,21

2.4.1 It may prevent lung derecruitment associated with the use of open-suction system in patients at higher risk of desaturation (eg, premature newborns). 22–29

2.4.2 It should be considered in patients requiring high FIO2 and PEEP (eg, acute lung injury). 30–36

2.4.3 It neither increases nor decreases the risk of ventilator-associated pneumonia. 37–39

2.4.4 Daily changes of in-line suction catheters do not decrease the risk of ventilator-associated pneumonia and is not cost-effective. 40,41

(Continued)

2.5 A patient should be placed on a pulse oximeter to assess oxygenation during and following the procedure.

ETS 3.0 PROCEDURE

The suctioning event consists of the placement of a suction catheter through the artificial airway into the trachea and the application of negative pressure as the catheter is being withdrawn. Each pass of the suction catheter into the artificial airway is considered a suctioning event. 42

3.1 Shallow suctioning is recommended to prevent trauma to the tracheal mucosa.

3.2 Deep suctioning has not shown superior benefit over shallow suction 43 and may be associated with more adverse events. 44–46

3.3 The duration of each suctioning event should be no more than 15 seconds. 8,47,48

3.4 Sterile technique is encouraged during open suctioning technique. 2

3.5 **Normal saline instillation**. Instillation refers to the administration of aliquots of saline directly into the trachea via an artificial airway. It is hypothesized that normal saline instillation may loosen secretions, increase the amount of secretions removed, and aid in the removal of tenacious secretions. However, there is insufficient evidence to support this hypothesis. Normal saline instillation appears to enhance secretion clearance through cough stimulation in adults, 49 and a recent report suggests that normal saline instillation prior to suctioning is associated with decreased incidence of ventilator-associated pneumonia in ventilated adult patients. 50 The great majority of the references used to update this guideline indicate that normal saline instillation is unlikely to be beneficial, and may in fact be harmful. 17,48,51–53 Therefore, it should not be routinely performed prior to performing endotracheal suctioning.

ETS 4.0 FOLLOW-UP CARE

Following the suctioning event:

4.1 Hyper-oxygenation for at least 1 min by following the same technique(s) used to pre-oxygenate the patient may be used, especially in patients who are hypoxemic before and/or during suctioning. 10

4.2 Hyperventilation should not be routinely used.

    4.2.1 Lung-recruitment maneuvers may be attempted in patients with clear evidence of derecruitment. 30,54,55

4.3 The patient *should be* monitored for adverse reactions.

ETS 5.0 SETTING

Endotracheal suctioning may be performed by properly trained persons in a wide variety of settings that include (but are not limited to):

5.1 Hospital

5.2 Extended care facility

5.3 Home

5.4 Out-patient clinic

5.5 Physician's office

5.6 Transport vehicle

ETS 6.0 INDICATIONS

6.1 The need to maintain the patency and integrity of the artificial airway

6.2 The need to remove accumulated pulmonary secretions as evidenced by one of:

    6.2.1 sawtooth pattern on the flow-volume loop on the monitor screen of the ventilator and/or the presence of coarse crackles over the trachea are strong indicators of retained pulmonary secretions. 56,57

    6.2.2 increased peak inspiratory pressure during volume-controlled mechanical ventilation or decreased tidal volume during pressure-controlled ventilation 58

    6.2.3 deterioration of oxygen saturation and/or arterial blood gas values 58

    6.2.4 visible secretions in the airway 58

    6.2.5 patient's inability to generate an effective spontaneous cough

    6.2.6 acute respiratory distress 58

    6.2.7 suspected aspiration of gastric or upper-airway secretions

6.3 The need to obtain a sputum specimen to rule out or identify pneumonia or other pulmonary infection or for sputum cytology

ETS 7.0 CONTRAINDICATIONS

Endotracheal suctioning is a necessary procedure for patients with artificial airways. Most contraindications are relative to the patient's risk of developing adverse reactions or worsening clinical condition as result of the procedure. When indicated, there is no absolute contraindication to endotracheal suctioning, because the decision to withhold suctioning in order to avoid a possible adverse reaction may, in fact, be lethal.

ETS 8.0 HAZARDS/COMPLICATIONS

8.1 Decrease in dynamic lung compliance 59 and functional residual capacity 60

8.2 Atelectasis 32,37

8.3 Hypoxia/hypoxemia 61,62

8.4 Tissue trauma to the tracheal and/or bronchial mucosa 63

8.5 Bronchoconstriction/bronchospasm 1,60

8.6 Increased microbial colonization of lower airway 5,64

8.7 Changes in cerebral blood flow 65,66 and increased intracranial pressure 67–69

8.8 Hypertension 70

8.9 Hypotension 17

8.10 Cardiac dysrhythmias 17

(Continued)

8.11 Routine use of normal saline instillation may be associated with the following adverse events:

8.11.1 excessive coughing 49

8.11.2 decreased oxygen saturation 53,71–75

8.11.3 bronchospasm

8.11.4 dislodgement of the bacterial biofilm that colonizes the ETT into the lower airway 50,76–78

8.11.5 pain, anxiety, dyspnea 79,80

8.11.6 tachycardia 53

8.11.7 increased intracranial pressure 70,81

ETS 9.0 LIMITATIONS OF METHOD

Endotracheal suctioning is not a benign procedure, and operators should remain sensitive to possible hazards and complications and take all necessary precautions to ensure patient safety. Secretions in peripheral airways are not and should not be directly removed by endotracheal suctioning.

ETS 10.0 ASSESSMENT OF NEED

Qualified personnel should assess the need for endotracheal suctioning as a routine part of the patient/ventilator system assessment as detailed in section 6.0 Indications.

ETS 11.0 ASSESSMENT OF OUTCOME

11.1 Improvement in appearance of ventilator graphics and breath sounds 57,58

11.2 Decreased peak inspiratory pressure with narrowing of peak inspiratory pressure-plateau pressure; decreased airway resistance or increased dynamic compliance; increased tidal volume delivery during pressure-limited ventilation

11.3 Improvement in arterial blood gas values or saturation, as reflected by pulse oximetry (SpO_2)

11.4 Removal of pulmonary secretions

ETS 12.0 RESOURCES

12.1 Necessary Equipment

12.1.1 Vacuum source

12.1.2 Calibrated, adjustable regulator

12.1.3 Collection bottle and connecting tubing

12.1.4 Disposable gloves

12.1.4.1 Sterile (open suction)

12.1.4.2 Clean (closed suction)

12.1.5 Sterile suction catheter

12.1.5.1 For selective main-bronchus suctioning, a curved-tip catheter may be helpful. 82 The information related to the effectiveness of head turning for selective suctioning is inconclusive.

12.1.6 Sterile water and cup (open suction)

12.1.7 Goggles, mask, and other appropriate equipment for standard precautions 83

12.1.8 Oxygen source with a calibrated metering device

12.1.9 Pulse oximeter

12.1.10 Manual resuscitation bag equipped with an oxygen-enrichment device for emergency backup use

12.1.11 Stethoscope

12.2 Optional Equipment

12.2.1 Electrocardiograph

12.2.2 Sterile sputum trap for culture specimen

12.3 Personnel. Licensed or credentialed respiratory therapists or individuals with similar credentials (eg, MD, RN) who have the necessary training and demonstrated skills to correctly assess need for suctioning, perform the procedure, and adequately evaluate the patient after the procedure.

ETS 13.0 MONITORING

The following should be monitored prior to, during, and after the procedure:

13.1 Breath sounds

13.2 Oxygen saturation

13.2.1 Skin color

13.2.2 Pulse oximeter

13.3 Respiratory rate and pattern

13.4 Hemodynamic parameters

13.4.1 Pulse rate

13.4.2 Blood pressure, if indicated and available

13.4.3 Electrocardiogram, if indicated and available

13.5 Sputum characteristics

13.5.1 Color

13.5.2 Volume

13.5.3 Consistency

13.5.4 Odor

13.6 Cough characteristics

13.7 Intracranial pressure, if indicated and available

13.8 Ventilator parameters

13.8.1 Peak inspiratory pressure and plateau pressure

13.8.2 Tidal volume

13.8.3 Pressure, flow, and volume graphics, if available

13.8.4 FIO_2

ETS 14.0 FREQUENCY

Although the internal lumen of an ETT decreases substantially after a few days of intubation, due to formation of biofilm, 84 suctioning should be performed *only* when clinically indicated in order to maintain the patency of the artificial airway used. 85–87 Special consideration should be given to the potential complications associated with the procedure.

ETS 15.0 INFECTION CONTROL

15.1 Centers for Disease Control guidelines for standard precautions should be followed. 83

(Continued)

15.1.1 If manual ventilation is used, care must be taken not to contaminate the airway.
15.1.2 Sterile technique is encouraged during the entire suctioning event.
15.2 All equipment and supplies should be appropriately disposed of or disinfected.

ETS 16.0 RECOMMENDATIONS

The following recommendations are made following the Grading of Recommendations Assessment, Development, and Evaluation (GRADE) 88,89 criteria:

16.1 It is recommended that endotracheal suctioning should be performed only when secretions are present, and not routinely. (1C)
16.2 It is suggested that pre-oxygenation be considered if the patient has a clinically important reduction in oxygen saturation with suctioning. (2B)
16.3 Performing suctioning without disconnecting the patient from the ventilator is suggested. (2B)
16.4 Use of shallow suction is suggested instead of deep suction, based on evidence from infant and pediatric studies. (2B)
16.5 It is suggested that routine use of normal saline instillation prior to endotracheal suction should *not* be performed. (2C)
16.6 The use of closed suction is suggested for adults with high FIO_2, or PEEP, or at risk for lung derecruitment (2B), and for neonates (2C).
16.7 Endotracheal suctioning without disconnection (closed system) is suggested in neonates. (2B)
16.8 Avoidance of disconnection and use of lung recruitment maneuvers are suggested if suctioning induced lung derecruitment occurs in patients with *acute lung injury*. (2B)

16.9 It is suggested that a suction catheter is used that occludes less than 50% of the lumen of the ETT in children and adults, and less than 70% in infants. (2C)
16.10 It is suggested that the duration of the suctioning event be limited to less than 15 seconds. (2C)

17.0 ETS CPG IDENTIFYING INFORMATION AND AVAILABILITY

17.1 Adaptation Original Publication: Respir Care 1993; 38(5):500–504.
17.2 Guideline Developers American Association for Respiratory Care Clinical Practice Guidelines Steering Committee Ruben D Restrepo MD RRT FAARC, Chair Joel M Brown II RRT John M Hughes MEd RRT AEC
17.3 Source(s) of funding None
17.4 Financial disclosures/conflicts of interest No conflicts of interest.
17.5 Availability Interested persons may photocopy these clinical practice guidelines (CPGs) for noncommercial purposes of scientific or educational advancement. Please credit the American Association for Respiratory Care (AARC) and RESPIRATORY CARE. All of the AARC CPGs can be downloaded at no charge at http://www. rcjournal .com/cpgs.

SUCTIONING

Rationale for Suctioning

The cough is one of the normal defense mechanisms that protects the airway. It rids the airway of foreign matter and expels excess secretions. An effective cough is dependent on the ability to close the glottis to generate high intrathoracic pressure. The sudden opening of the glottis results in forceful expulsion of gas, which is the cough. Patients with respiratory disabilities or disease may have excessive secretions that they are unable to manage. Because excessive secretions provide an excellent medium for bacterial growth, pneumonia may result, with subsequent atelectasis, hypoxemia, and increased work of breathing.

A patient's cough can be augmented or assisted through directed spontaneous coughing or by use of the forced expiratory technique (huff cough). The directed cough begins by encouraging the patient to take several slow deep inspirations followed by passive quiet exhalation. After two to three breaths, the patient is instructed to close the glottis, to contract the abdominal muscles, and to forcefully cough.

The forced expiratory technique, or huff cough, is performed with an open glottis. The patient is instructed to take a deeper than normal breath (mid to low lung volumes); during exhalation the patient is instructed to forcefully exhale with an open glottis (huff). The forced exhalation can be assisted by the patient briskly adducting the arms from shoulder level to the chest wall during the exhalation effort.

The cough reflex may be depressed, bypassed, or even absent for a variety of reasons. These may include central nervous system (CNS) depression (such as with drug overdose), brainstem injury, cerebrovascular accident (CVA), pain, and muscle weakness. The presence of an artificial airway precludes effective utilization of the cough mechanism. In these instances and others, it may be necessary to intervene by suctioning the secretions from the airway. This intervention is known as airway aspiration or suctioning.

What Is Suctioning?

Suctioning is an invasive procedure that involves the insertion of a small catheter into the airway and the application of a vacuum (subambient pressure) to aspirate secretions or foreign material. Once in place, a vacuum is applied, and the catheter is withdrawn, evacuating secretions.

Because this is an invasive procedure, scrupulous aseptic technique should be observed at all times to prevent the inadvertent introduction of bacteria into the tracheobronchial tree. Sterile technique is encouraged throughout the performance of this procedure (AARC, 2010).

Suction Catheter Designs

With advances in pulmonary medicine and in the practice of respiratory care, an evolution has occurred in the design of *suction catheters.* Generally, advancements have improved efficiency, reduced mucosal trauma, and improved cost containment.

Whistle Tip

The whistle tip catheter design incorporates an eye or side port on the side of the catheter proximal to the distal opening. Figure 21-1 shows a typical suction catheter design. The advantage of this design is that if the tip comes in contact with the mucosa, the side port provides a relief for the applied vacuum. In this manner, inadvertent "biopsy" of mucosal tissue is prevented.

Coudé Tip

The Coudé tip is an angled tip design. This design permits the selective entry into the right or left mainstem bronchus. Figure 21-2 shows an example of the Coudé tip design. To maximize the usefulness of this catheter design, you must pay close attention to the tip position on entering the patient's airway or an artificial airway. By advancing the catheter and selectively rotating the

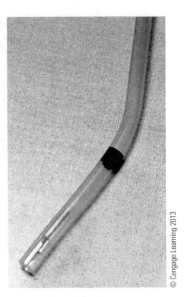

Figure 21-2 A Coudé tip suction catheter

tip right or left, the chance of entering the desired bronchus is increased. Guaranteed 100% entry is not possible; however, the likelihood of accurate entry is greater with this design than with a straight-tipped catheter.

Closed Suction Systems

The closed suction catheter is a sterile suction catheter contained in a protective sheath that is attached in-line to the ventilator circuit or artificial airway by means of the T piece, which is part of the system. Figure 21-3 shows the Trach Care catheter, manufactured by Kimberly Clark, which is one example of many *closed suction systems.* The catheter is encased in a sealed plastic protective sheath. The distal end is attached to a modified aerosol T and the proximal end is attached to a control valve. The suction system is a replaceable item; the closed suction system should be changed as recommended by the manufacturer or as indicated by institutional policy.

The system is unique in that disconnection from mechanical ventilation or the patient's oxygen source is not required for suctioning (owing to the design of the modified aerosol T).

Whenever the patient requires suctioning, the same catheter is used. A question was raised regarding infection control and the possible introduction of bacteria resulting from the use of this system. Investigators found no significant difference in colony counts between the multiple-use catheter system and a conventional design (Topeli, 2004). This design improves convenience, prevents physiologic problems associated with ventilator disconnection, and reduces costs to the patient.

Complications and Hazards of Suctioning

Various investigators have studied the complications of suctioning. The complications identified include tissue trauma, hypoxemia, microatelectasis, cardiac arrhythmias,

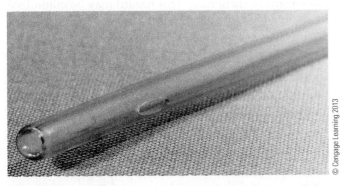

Figure 21-1 A photograph of a single-use disposable suction catheter

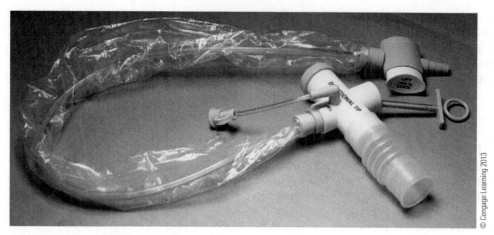

© Cengage Learning 2013

Figure 21-3   The Trach Care closed suction system

and hospital-acquired infection (mainly associated with nasotracheal aspiration) (AARC, 2010).

Tissue Trauma

Tissue trauma caused by suctioning usually involves the invagination (infolding) of airway mucosal tissue into the catheter tip or side port (Fiorentini, 1992). The applied vacuum may be strong enough to draw the mucosal tissue into the openings. Minimal trauma may result in a slight reddening of the tissue, representing an area of irritation. More severe trauma results in petechiae, or in actual inadvertent "biopsy" of tissue.

Trauma may be minimized in three ways. First, set the vacuum levels as described in Table 21-1. Suction pressures should be set as low as possible while still permitting effective removal of secretions (AARC, 1993). Last, limit the suction attempt to no more than 15 seconds (AARC, 2004, 2010).

Hypoxemia

It has been shown that tracheobronchial suction will induce hypoxemia (AARC, 1993; Lasocki, 2006). Hypoxemia is the result of the evacuation of oxygen from the tracheobronchial tree. One study demonstrated an 18% decrease in arterial partial pressure of oxygen (PaO_2), which persisted for up to 15 minutes following suctioning (Lasocki, 2006). In current clinical practice, similar effects may be easily observed with oximetry.

Hypoxemia may be prevented by preoxygenation and postoxygenation and hyperinflation of the lungs with 100% oxygen (AARC, 1993, 2004). It is very important to perform these procedures before and after suctioning to prevent hypoxemia and to reverse atelectasis.

The selection of the proper catheter size is important in suctioning the artificial airway so that the inadvertent application of excessive vacuum is prevented. A good general rule to follow is that the outside diameter of the catheter should not exceed one half of the inside diameter of the artificial airway (AARC, 2010). Using a catheter that is too large could cause the application of excessive vacuum, resulting in atelectasis or, worse, the collapse of a total segment of the lung (Table 21-2).

Cardiac Arrhythmias

Cardiac arrhythmias are common during suctioning of the unstable patient in the intensive care unit (ICU). They may be induced by vagal stimulation or hypoxemia. The vagus nerve innervates the trachea and the carinal areas. Stimulation may result in bradycardia and premature ventricular contractions (PVCs). These and other arrhythmias are also associated with hypoxemia. Those patients who have a predisposing condition of hypoxemia or cardiac irritability should be carefully monitored while being suctioned. Careful attention should be paid to preoxygenation and postoxygenation. If nasotracheal suction is performed, excessive manipulation of the catheter should be avoided.

Pneumonia

Pneumonia as a complication of bronchoscopy as well as suctioning has been documented (Combes, 2000; Demers, 1982). The introduction of bacteria into the lower airway is a hazard of suctioning. This hazard may be minimized by maintenance of sterile technique (AARC, 2010).

TABLE 21-1: Vacuum Pressures for Suctioning

Infant	80–100 mm Hg
Pediatric	80–100 mm Hg
Adult	80–120 mm Hg (never exceed 150 mm Hg)

TABLE 21-2: Suction Catheter Sizing

AIRWAY INNER DIAMETER (ID)	SUCTION CATHETER SIZE (Fr)
8.0 mm–9.5 mm	14 Fr
5.0 mm–7.0 mm	10 Fr
4.0 mm–4.5 mm	8 Fr
2.5 mm–3.5 mm	6 Fr

Oxygenation and Hyperinflation Using Mechanical Ventilation

It is a common practice in the critical care setting to use the ventilator for hyperinflation and oxygenation in patients who are receiving ventilatory support. This involves increasing the delivered oxygen level to 100% and allowing sufficient time for at least 30 to 60 seconds. This regimen is then followed by suctioning the patient. It is easy to overlook the effects of *washout volume* of the ventilator circuit prior to suctioning. Washout volume is the volume internal to the ventilator (internal reservoir used by some ventilators) and the ventilator circuit. It takes time for this volume to be replaced by fresh gas when a change in fraction of inspired oxygen (FIO_2) is made. Failure to keep this concept in mind may result in inadequate preoxygenation prior to suctioning.

Positive End-Expiratory Pressure

Patients receiving positive end-expiratory pressure (PEEP) are more susceptible to hypoxemia when they are disconnected from mechanical ventilation for suctioning. The sudden removal of PEEP will often result in a dramatic fall in PaO_2. Also, once PEEP is removed and then resumed again, it may take some time to regain the level of oxygen saturation the patient had before disconnection of PEEP. Other investigators studied a closed suction system, suctioning without preoxygenation or disconnection from PEEP or mechanical ventilation, and found that there was no significant drop in oxygen saturation (Lasocki, 2006).

These studies indicate that the best way to suction patients on PEEP is not to disconnect them from mechanical ventilation, if at all possible. The closed suction systems provide a convenient and cost-effective means to provide artificial airway care for these patients without disconnecting them from PEEP.

Prevention of Ventilator-Associated Pneumonia (VAP)

Ventilator-associated pneumonia (VAP) is one of the most common hospital-acquired infections in the United States (Kollef, 2005). VAP accounts for countless deaths and increased length of stay. Evidence supports that when several techniques are employed together, VAP may be reduced or prevented (Muscedere, 2008).

Elevation of the Head of the Bed

Elevation of the head of the bed to 30 to 45° reduces the risk of silent aspiration (Hess, 2005; Muscedere, 2008). Evidence supports a reduction in gastric content aspiration in patients in the semirecumbent position. The Centers for Disease Control and Prevention (CDC) state, "In the absence of medical contraindication(s), elevate at an angle of 30–45 degrees of the head of the bed of a patient at high risk for aspiration (e.g., a person receiving mechanically assisted ventilation and/or who has an enteral tube in place)" (CDC, 2004). This is a simple intervention that may easily be monitored by all health care providers at the bedside of each patient who is intubated.

Subglottic Secretion Drainage

Secretions pool above the endotracheal tube's cuff when the cuff is inflated. These secretions may consist of oropharyngeal drainage as well as gastric secretions. There is a risk of these secretions leaking past the cuff and contaminating or inoculating the lower airway (Emili, 2005). The use of specialized endotracheal tubes, such as the Hi-Lo Evac (Figure 21-4), can help to remove these secretions, preventing aspiration. The Hi-Lo Evac endotracheal tube has a second lumen molded into the tube that terminates proximal to the tube's cuff. When this lumen is connected to continuous suction, pooled secretions are removed from the area above the tube's cuff, reducing the likelihood of aspiration (Emili, 2005).

Maintenance of Cuff Pressures

Maintenance of cuff pressures is an important factor in preventing aspiration. A discussion follows in this chapter regarding cuff pressure monitoring.

Humidification of Inspired Gases

Heating and humidifying inspired gas is standard of care for patients on a ventilator. Heat and humidity can be provided by a heat and moisture exchanger (HME) or a heated humidifier. If the patient is expected to be ventilated for less than 96 hours, an HME can provide adequate humidification (AARC, 1993). If the patient has thick and/or copious pulmonary secretions, or is expected to be on the ventilator longer than 96 hours, a heated humidifier is preferable (Branson, 2007).

Studies indicate that the use of an HME can reduce the risk of VAP (Hess, 2003; Kranabetter, 2004). These studies and others conclude that the rate of VAP when using an HME is less than when a heated humidifier is used. However, the mechanism of action as to why is not understood (Branson, 2005).

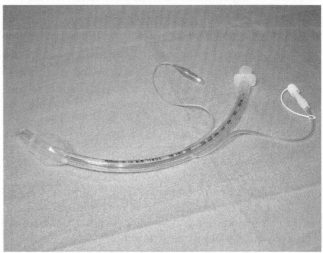

Figure 21-4 Hi-Lo Evac endotracheal tube.

© Cengage Learning 2013

CUFF PRESSURE MONITORING

Maintenance of appropriate cuff pressure is important in the prevention of silent aspiration and VAP. Cuff pressures should be maintained as low as possible but not more than 25 to 30 cm H_2O (Emili, 2005). Cuff pressures should be monitored regularly to prevent tracheal mucosal damage and VAP. The use of minimal occlusive volume (MOV) by inflating the cuff enough to provide a seal (no leak auscultated at the larynx) is recommended. Once the cuff seals against the trachea, it is important to measure and monitor the cuff pressure.

Cuff pressures are determined by three commonly used techniques; minimal occlusion volume, minimal occlusion pressure, and minimal leak. MOV is accomplished by inflating the cuff with a syringe until all air leakage under positive pressure stops. Auscultation at the larynx with a stethoscope is an easy way to detect any leak past the cuff.

Minimal occlusion pressure is similar to MOV, except a pressure manometer is used in lieu of a syringe. The cuff is inflated until any leak under positive pressure stops. As with MOV, auscultation at the larynx is an easy method to detect leakage past the cuff.

Minimal leak technique is one in which the cuff is inflated until a slight leak is heard past the cuff during inspiration. The cuff is inflated until no leak is detected, then a small amount of air is removed from the cuff until a slight leak occurs. This technique is the least common in that there is an increased risk of silent aspiration past the airway's cuff.

Indications for a Tracheostomy

There are several indications for a tracheostomy. These indications are summarized in Figure 21-5.

TRACHEOSTOMY AND STOMA CARE

Purpose of Tracheostomy and Stoma Care

Tracheostomy and stoma care is essential to prevent infection and to preserve the patency of the airway. A *tracheostomy* is created by a surgical procedure requiring, like other surgical procedures, that the incision be

kept clean and dry to promote healing and to reduce the likelihood of infection. A tracheostomy is a particularly dirty area owing to the expectoration of secretions through the tracheostomy tube and seepage around it. Secretions, if not removed from the tube and airway by suctioning and periodic cleaning, may become encrusted, reducing or compromising the lumen of the airway. Administration of adequate humidification aids liquefaction of secretions. Accumulated secretions may also become colonized by bacteria, infecting the lower airway.

Hazards and Complications of Tracheostomy Care

Displacement and Decannulation of the Tracheostomy Tube

In performing tracheostomy care, it is essential that the tracheostomy tube be stabilized at all times. This is especially true if the surgical procedure to create the tracheostomy was performed in the previous 24 hours (a "fresh trach"). Displacement of the tracheostomy tube from the trachea may result in its lodging in the subcutaneous tissue, thus compromising the airway. Loss of ventilation and subcutaneous emphysema may result from this complication.

If the tracheostomy is fresh, a surgeon should be immediately consulted to replace the tracheostomy tube. It is very difficult to locate the incision in the trachea early after a tracheostomy is performed. Later on, the stoma becomes more established and it is easier to reinsert the tracheostomy tube.

Decannulation is the removal of the tracheostomy tube. This may occur accidentally during tracheostomy care or as a result of a strong cough or other movements by the patient if the tube is not well secured.

Like tracheostomy tube displacement, decannulation of a fresh trach requires the immediate services of a surgeon. If the stoma is well established, a practitioner may easily reinsert the tracheostomy tube.

Infection

A tracheostomy is created by a surgical procedure. Because of the nature of the surgical site, infection is a potential complication. Infection may be minimized by adequate maintenance of the airway (suctioning) and proper tracheostomy care. Initially, tracheostomy care may be required every 4 hours. As the tracheostomy begins to heal, tracheostomy care may be reduced to once every shift and may eventually be performed on a daily basis, depending on the patient's condition.

Types of Tubes

Single Cannula Tracheostomy Tube

The single cannula disposable single patient use tracheostomy tube is the most common type of tube used. Figure 21-6 shows this type of tube. It is generally made of PVC 9, which is a nontoxic type of plastic. These tubes do not have a removable inner cannula; therefore, if occlusion occurs, they may need to be changed.

- To provide a patent airway following intubation or when intubation is contraindicated
- To protect the lower airway from aspiration
- To permit frequent aspiration of secretions
- To allow long-term mechanical ventilation
- To reduce anatomical dead space

© Cengage Learning 2013

Figure 21-5 Indications for a tracheostomy

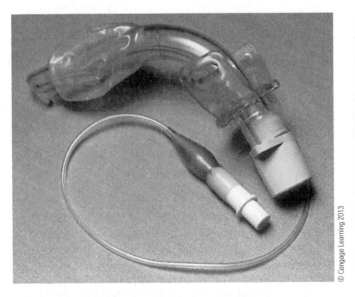

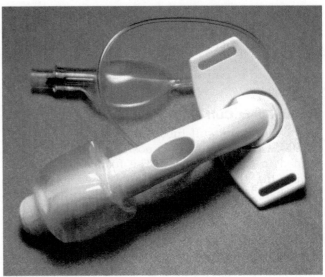

Figure 21-8 A fenestrated tracheostomy tube

Figure 21-6 A single cuff disposable tracheostomy tube

Single Cannula Tracheostomy Tube with a Disposable or Removable Inner Cannula

This type of tube is similar to the single cannula tracheostomy tube with the exception of the removable inner cannula. Figure 21-7 shows a double lumen tube with a removable inner cannula. By removing the inner cannula, cleaning is facilitated and it becomes easier to maintain the patency of the airway. Some of these tubes have disposable inner cannulas, whereas others are cleaned and then reinserted. This cleaning eliminates the need to change the tracheostomy tube periodically.

Single Cannula Fenestrated Tracheostomy Tube

The *fenestrated tracheostomy tube* has a fenestration or window in the outer cannula. Figure 21-8 shows a single cannula fenestrated tracheostomy tube. By removing

the inner cannula and deflating the cuff, the patient can breathe through the upper airway. This will facilitate weaning the patient from the tracheostomy appliance. Cleaning is facilitated by the removal of the inner cannula. If the patient's upper airway becomes obstructed or if mechanical ventilation is needed, the inner cannula may be inserted and the cuff reinflated. The fenestrated tube then is functionally similar to a single cannula tube with a removable inner cannula.

Silver Holinger Tracheostomy Tube

The silver Holinger or Jackson tube is a nondisposable, reusable tracheostomy tube with a removable inner cannula. Figure 21-9 shows this tracheostomy tube. This tube is cuffless and has a removable inner cannula. These tubes are made of sterling silver. This

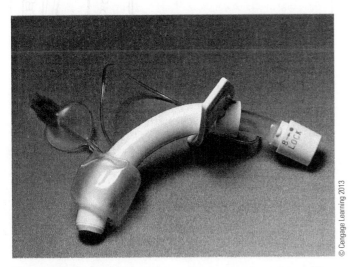

Figure 21-7 A single cuff disposable tracheostomy tube with a removable inner cannula

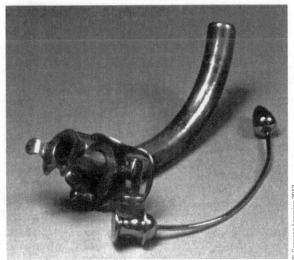

Figure 21-9 A Jackson tracheostomy tube

type of tube is commonly used in patients with long-term tracheostomy because of its superior durability and ease of cleaning. A tube of like construction, but shorter, is called a *laryngectomy tube* and may be encountered in patients who have had a laryngectomy performed.

Bivona Foam Cuff

The Bivona foam cuff tube has a foam cuff that self-inflates. Once the tube is in position, the pilot tube is opened to the atmosphere. The foam then expands, sealing the airway. The cuff is designed to exert no more than 25 mm Hg of pressure against the tracheal wall. Prior to insertion of this airway, all air must be first evacuated from the cuff. Once the airway is in position, the pilot line is opened to the atmosphere, allowing the cuff to self-inflate. It is important never to inflate this type of cuff, as this makes it a high-pressure cuff.

Specialized Tracheostomy Tubes and Appliances

Communi-Trach

This tracheostomy tube is similar to the Pitt Speaking Tube. A fitting is provided that directs a flow of oxygen above the cuff of the tube. When the patient occludes a thumb port, gas flows up and through the vocal cords, allowing the patient to speak. Figure 21-10 shows this device. Speech is accomplished without deflating the cuff. The phonation is rather hoarse, but the patient may be understood. It takes some coordination to attempt speech independent of diaphragmatic motion.

Tracheostomy Button

A *tracheostomy button* is a useful device that facilitates weaning the patient from a tracheostomy. Figure 21-11 shows an Olympic Trach button. Spacer rings are provided to adjust the length of the button to

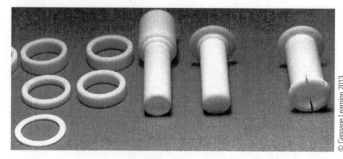

Figure 21-11 An Olympic Trach button

accommodate various neck sizes. An intermittent positive-pressure breathing (IPPB) adapter may be inserted into the button to facilitate attachment of devices for ventilation, or a plug may be inserted to allow the patient to breathe through the upper airway.

The tracheostomy button is inserted into the stoma with the distal tip resting just inside the trachea. Figure 21-12 shows a cross section of the airway and the tracheostomy button's placement. With the plug or IPPB adapter removed, the airway may be suctioned, facilitating airway management.

Kistner Button

The Kistner tracheostomy tube is a plastic tube that is somewhat similar to the Olympic Trach button in its use and placement. Figure 21-13 shows this appliance. This device is inserted into the stoma with the distal end resting just inside the trachea. A plastic

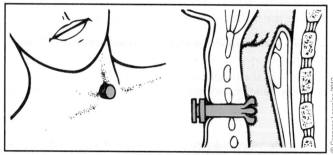

Figure 21-12 Anatomical placement of a trach button

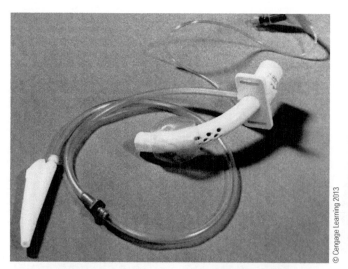

Figure 21-10 The Communi-Trach tracheostomy tube

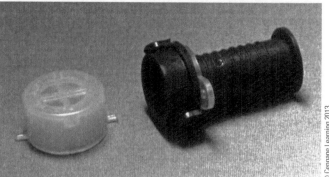

Figure 21-13 A Kistner button

cap containing a one-way valve is then inserted over the tube. With the cap in place, the patient may inhale through the tube; on exhalation the one-way valve closes, forcing air up through the upper airway. With this device, the patient may speak and develop sufficient intrathoracic pressures to cough effectively.

Olympic Trach-Talk

Olympic Trach-Talk is a modified aerosol T with a one-way valve. Figure 21-14 is a photograph of this device. When the device is used, the cuff of the tracheostomy tube is deflated and the Trach-Talk is then placed on the tube. When the patient inhales, the one-way valve opens, allowing gas to flow into the lower airway. On exhalation, the valve closes, forcing air up through the upper airway. Like the Kistner trach tube, this device facilitates speech and effective coughing. The Olympic Trach-Talk should be used only in alert patients who are capable of managing their own secretions.

Passy-Muir Valve

The *Passy-Muir valve* is a tracheostomy valve manufactured by Passy-Muir, Inc., Irvine, CA (Figure 21-15). This device consists of a leaf or diaphragm valve, which during inspiration allows the patient to inhale through the tracheostomy tube and which during exhalation closes and forces air through the upper airway. When this device is used, *it is important to deflate the cuff of the tracheostomy tube prior to installing the Passy-Muir valve onto the airway.* Failure to deflate the cuff prior to installing the Passy-Muir valve results in the patient not having the ability to exhale!

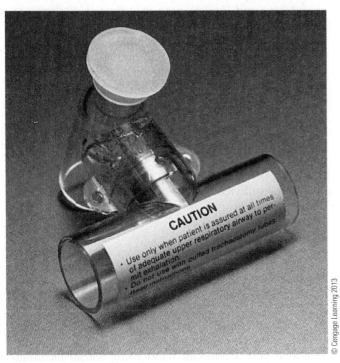

Figure 21-14 The Olympic Trach-Talk

© Cengage Learning 2013

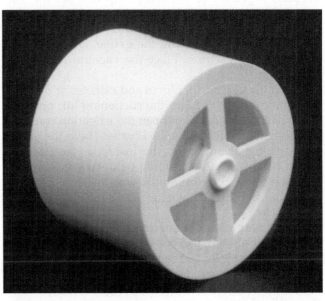

Figure 21-15 A photograph of the Passy-Muir valve. *(Courtesy of Passy-Muir, Inc., Irvine, CA)*

PROFICIENCY OBJECTIVES

At the end of this chapter, the reader should be able to:

- *Assemble the equipment required for airway aspiration and test it for proper operation before use.*
- *Using an intubation mannequin, demonstrate nasotracheal suctioning.*
- *Using an intubated mannequin, demonstrate artificial airway aspiration.*
- *Using an intubated intubation mannequin or a tracheostomy mannequin, demonstrate cuff deflation and inflation and how to check cuff pressure.*
- *Demonstrate the proper procedure for cleaning a double cannula tracheostomy tube.*
- *Using a tracheostomy mannequin, demonstrate how to perform stoma care.*
- *Verbally describe the action to be taken in the event of accidental decannulation or tube displacement.*

SUCTIONING PROCEDURE

Equipment Needed for Suctioning

The equipment needed for suctioning may be assembled individually, or a suction kit may be used. The kit is very convenient and contains the majority of the supplies required. Figure 21-16 lists the equipment required for suctioning. The first three items—suction catheter, gloves, and goggles—are normally contained in most suction kits. The packaging wrapper serves as a convenient sterile field for preparing the equipment.

Equipment Preparation

Assemble and test the manual resuscitator for proper operation and set the oxygen flowmeter between 10 and 15 L/min.

After assembling your equipment, connect the vacuum regulator or suction pump and set the vacuum level between −60 and −180 mm Hg according to the size of the patient. Do this by occluding the suction line and observing the gauge. Do not exceed −120 mm Hg vacuum. Place the vacuum line within easy reach.

Open the package of gloves and catheter or open the suctioning kit. To prepare the suctioning kit, open the package so it lies flat. Pop open the irrigation container and fill it with sterile distilled water. Have the gloves and catheter arranged on the inside of the package, which has become your sterile field, so you may easily reach them. Squeeze a little water-soluble lubricant onto the sterile field where you can later lubricate the catheter.

Unit dose packages of normal saline usually used in aerosol therapy are also convenient for irrigation. The packages are sterile, and each contains between 2.5 and 5 mL of fluid. If these are not available, draw up 10 mL of sterile normal saline into a syringe for irrigation of the artificial airway.

Open the sterile distilled water container and pour some into the sterile basin to irrigate the suction line following suctioning. Arrange all of your irrigation fluids so they are convenient and easily accessible.

- Sterile suction catheter
- Sterile gloves
- Goggles or face shield
- Sterile basin or container
- Sterile normal saline for irrigation
- Sterile distilled water to clean the catheter
- Vacuum regulator or pump with suction trap
- Flow-inflating or self-inflating manual resuscitator
- Water-soluble lubricant

© Cengage Learning 2013

Figure 21-16 Equipment needed for suctioning

Positioning for Artificial Airway Aspiration

The preferred patient position for artificial airway aspiration is semi-Fowler's. The artificial airway ensures that the catheter will enter the airway, so positioning is less critical. The semi-Fowler's position affords better chest expansion for hyperinflation, and if the patient gags and vomits, the airway is somewhat more protected.

Preaspiration Patient Assessment

Auscultate the chest, paying close attention near the large airways. The presence of crackles is a good indication for suctioning. In some patients the use of a stethoscope will not be required. When these patients breathe, they will have very noisy, gurgling respirations.

Suctioning should be performed only if secretions are present and if suctioning is indicated. If suctioning is needed, perform the procedure, but do not suction the patient's airway without careful assessment as to the need for the procedure. Suctioning has many complications, and the routine practice of suctioning without an indicated need should be avoided (Branson, 2007).

Oxygenation of the Patient

When using a mechanical ventilator for this task, and the patient has an artificial airway in place, turn the oxygen percentage control to 100%, or press the 100% suction soft key. Allow sufficient time to compensate for the ventilator washout volume.

Nasotracheal Suctioning Procedure

Two common patient positions are used in nasotracheal suctioning: semi-Fowler's and supine with a roll under the shoulders. The latter position is often referred to as the "sniffing" position. Both of these positions facilitate entry into the airway.

Glove your dominant hand using sterile technique. Pick up the catheter with your gloved hand, wrapping it around your fingers to maintain its cleanliness and keep it under control at all times. Figure 21-17 shows the catheter coiled in this way. Expose approximately 8 to 10 inches of the distal end of the catheter and lubricate it with water-soluble lubricant.

Connect the distal end of the suction catheter to the vacuum line, which should already be set to the correct level of vacuum.

Gently insert the catheter into one of the nares with your gloved hand, matching the droop of the catheter with the natural curve of the airway. Slowly advance the catheter. If resistance is encountered, withdraw and gently redirect the catheter. Do not use force.

After inserting approximately 8 to 10 inches of the catheter, watch the patient inhale. The objective is to slip the catheter past the epiglottis into the trachea. During

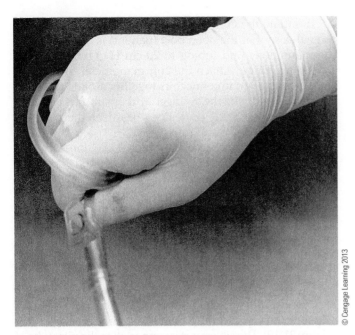

© Cengage Learning 2013

Figure 21-17 The suction catheter wrapped around the gloved hand

inspiration, the epiglottis is open. If this does not work, instruct your patient to cough and slip the catheter into the larynx. Sometimes having the patient say "E" during expiration will help, or request the patient to take a deep breath.

You will be able to tell when the catheter is inserted into the trachea because the patient will be coughing violently. The patient's color will often turn red and then almost ashen. As soon as the catheter has entered the trachea, begin application of vacuum. As you withdraw the catheter, if you feel resistance or pulling, release vacuum by lifting your thumb off the control port. Withdraw the catheter 1 or 2 cm and reapply vacuum. Limit the application of vacuum to no more than 15 seconds.

Following the procedure, oxygenate the patient for 1 or 2 minutes. If the patient is alert, you may use a nonrebreathing mask and instruct the patient to take slow, deep breaths. Otherwise, a manual resuscitator may be used. After each suctioning attempt and after the procedure is completed, it is important to oxygenate the patient to prevent a fall in PaO_2.

Return the patient to any previous oxygen therapy. Using your stethoscope, assess the patient to ensure that the airway has been cleared.

Following the procedure, dispose of your equipment and clean up the area. Clear the vacuum line by aspirating sterile distilled water. Reassure the patient and ensure that the patient is safe and comfortable.

Use of a Nasopharyngeal Airway

Patients needing frequent nasotracheal suctioning may benefit from placement of a nasopharyngeal airway. The airway will facilitate repeated suctioning while minimizing trauma to the nose and nasopharynx.

Artificial Airway Aspiration

The artificial airway provides a direct passage to the airway below the larynx. Normal physiologic protective mechanisms are bypassed. Introduction of pathogenic bacteria into the airway could possibly result in pneumonia, an extended hospital stay, or death.

Apply gloves to both hands. Using your dominant hand pick up the catheter, wrapping it around your fingers to control it and to preserve its cleanliness. Connect the proximal end to the vacuum line.

It is common practice to instill normal saline prior to suctioning to thin secretions. Installation of saline will induce coughing with an intact cough reflex. Concerns regarding this practice have suggested the possibility of inoculation of the lower respiratory tract with secretions from the biofilm on the endotracheal tube. Current evidence does not support the routine installation of normal saline to thin secretions (Branson, 2007).

Gently insert the catheter down the airway until resistance is felt. Withdraw the catheter 1 to 2 cm and apply intermittent suction. If you feel resistance or pulling on the catheter, release vacuum by lifting your thumb off the control port. Withdraw the catheter 1 to 2 cm, and reapply vacuum. Limit your suctioning to a total of 15 seconds. As you withdraw the catheter, wrap it around your gloved hand or roll it up and hold it between your fingers.

Oxygenate the patient for 1 or 2 minutes, using a manual resuscitator or a mechanical ventilator.

Repeat the suctioning procedure as required to clear the airway. Clear the catheter and the suction line by aspirating sterile distilled water before repeating your suction attempt.

Following the procedure, oxygenate and hyperinflate the patient's lungs for 1 or 2 minutes. These measures are important to prevent drastic changes in PaO_2 following suctioning.

Assess the patient by auscultating the chest to ensure that the airways are clear.

Clean up the area and dispose of your equipment appropriately. Ensure that the patient is safe and comfortable and return the patient to oxygen therapy.

Use of a Closed Suction System

The closed suction system is much easier to use than a conventional catheter in that aseptic technique is facilitated by the design of the system.

Connect the control valve to a vacuum source set between −80 and −120 mm Hg.

Perform oxygenation and hyperinflation of the lungs for 1 or 2 minutes prior to suctioning the patient's airway. If the patient is receiving ventilatory support, the ventilator may be used for oxygenation. Investigators have found that oxygenation is not required if the patient is not disconnected from mechanical ventilation for suctioning (Lasocki, 2006). Desaturation was less using the closed suction system.

Advance the catheter into the airway, compressing the protective sheath as the catheter is advanced. Apply vacuum when withdrawing the catheter. If resistance or pulling is felt, withdraw the catheter 1 to 2 cm and apply vacuum. Limit total suctioning time to 15 seconds or less.

Oxygenate the patient with 100% oxygen between suction attempts.

Attach a syringe (without a needle) or unit dose normal saline to clear the catheter and vacuum line following suctioning.

Repeat the suctioning procedure as required to clear the airway.

Following the procedure, oxygenate the patient for 1 or 2 minutes.

Assess the patient by auscultating the chest to ensure that you have cleared the airway of secretions.

Turn off the control valve on the closed suction system to prevent the inadvertent application of vacuum.

Return the patient to previous oxygen therapy regimen.

CUFF PRESSURE MEASUREMENT

Measurement of cuff pressures and the inflation of the cuff may be performed using one of three methods: the *minimal occlusion volume (MOV) technique* the *minimal leak technique,* and the minimal occlusion pressure (MOP) technique.

Pressure Manometer and Three-Way Stopcock

Cuff pressures are measured using a pressure manometer calibrated in cm H_2O. A small-diameter tube, a three-way stopcock, and a syringe are attached as shown in Figure 21-18. By rotating the valve of the stopcock, you choose which ports are open to one another. By pointing the valve toward the patient's pilot tube, the syringe and pressure manometer are open to one another and the pilot tube is off. When the valve is rotated opposite to the syringe, all three ports (patient, pressure manometer, and syringe) are open to one another.

To inflate the cuff to obtain MOV pressure, first turn the valve so that the open port (patient) is off. Pressurize the manometer and tubing to 20 cm H_2O by adding air from the syringe. Attach the cuff manometer to the pilot tube by pushing the connectors together. Rotate the valve so that it is opposite the syringe. Add or subtract air using the syringe just until no leak is heard at the patient's mouth. Measure the cuff pressure.

To inflate the cuff to obtain minimal leak pressure, first turn the valve so that the open port (patient) is off. Pressurize the manometer and tubing to 20 cm H_2O by adding air from the syringe. Attach the cuff manometer to the pilot tube by pushing the connectors together. Rotate the valve so it is opposite the syringe. Add or subtract air using the syringe just until a small leak is heard at the patient's mouth during a positive-pressure breath. Measure the cuff pressure.

Posey Cufflator

The Posey Cufflator combines the functions of a syringe, stopcock, and pressure manometer into one single unit (Figure 21-19). The silver port is connected to the pilot tube of the artificial airway. Once they are connected, cuff pressure is recorded on the manometer. If there is insufficient air in the cuff, you may squeeze the bulb, adding air into the cuff. If too much pressure is present, the red toggle valve on the side of the device may be depressed, venting excess pressure to the atmosphere. Both addition and subtraction of pressure may be accomplished using one hand. The MOV, MOP, or minimal leak technique may be employed with this device.

TRACHEOSTOMY CARE PROCEDURE

Equipment Required for Tracheostomy Care

The equipment requirements for tracheostomy and stoma care are minimal. Often, most of the required equipment is contained in a disposable single-use tracheostomy care kit. Figure 21-20 is a listing of the required supplies.

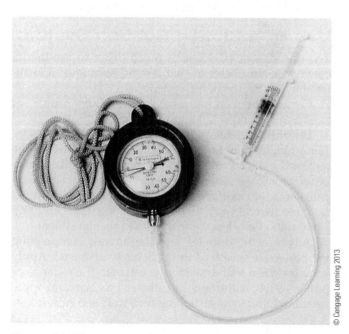

Figure 21-18 A photograph of a cuff pressure manometer

© Cengage Learning 2013

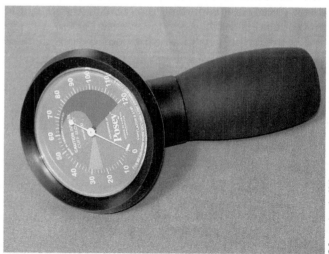

Figure 21-19 A photograph of the Posey Cufflator

© Cengage Learning 2013

*• Sterile cotton applicators
*• Sterile 4 × 4-inch gauze pads
*• Fabric tracheostomy ties
*• Sterile brush or cotton pipe cleaners
*• Sterile gloves
• Sterile water
• Hydrogen peroxide (3%)
• Scissors
• Supplemental oxygen source
• Spare sterile tracheostomy tube
• Self-inflating or flow-inflating resuscitator
• Syringe
• Cuff pressure manometer

*The first five items are usually contained in a disposable tracheostomy care kit.

© Cengage Learning 2013

Figure 21-20   Equipment needed for tracheostomy care

Cuff Deflation and Inflation

The deflation and inflation of a tracheostomy cuff constitute a routine part of caring for a tracheostomy.

Before deflating the cuff, suction the airway to ensure it is clear and free from secretions. Following airway aspiration, suction the oropharynx. Leave the suction catheter positioned at the posterior portion of the oropharynx and deflate the cuff while simultaneously applying positive pressure to the airway with a manual resuscitator. This will expel any secretions pooled above the cuff into the mouth, where they may be suctioned.

Inflate the cuff to MOV. Using a pressure manometer, measure the cuff pressure. Ensure that the cuff pressure is less than 25 to 30 cm H_2O.

Components of Tracheostomy Care Procedure

Physician's Order for Care

Often, a physician's order will not include tracheostomy care. Tracheostomy care is a routine procedure performed on any patient following a tracheostomy. It is always prudent, however, to check the respiratory care department's policy and procedure manual to ensure that this clinical procedure is covered by departmental policies.

Auscultate the Chest

It is necessary to auscultate the chest prior to performing tracheostomy care for two reasons: (1) to determine if the patient's lungs are clear of secretions, and (2) if secretions are present, to determine whether suctioning is required prior to performing tracheostomy care. You will feel very frustrated if you neglect this part of the procedure if, after performing tracheostomy care, the patient coughs a large amount of secretions over your work, necessitating that you repeat it. Listen for equal bilateral breath sounds. This will provide a rough indicator as to the placement of the tracheostomy tube. If

the tube is accidentally displaced during the procedure, breath sounds after completion of tracheostomy care will be diminished, absent, or unequal.

Prepare a Sterile Field and Apply Sterile Gloves

Tracheostomy care is treated as a sterile procedure. It is essential that you perform this procedure as aseptically as possible. Begin the procedure by unfolding the sterile towel supplied in the tracheostomy care kit to prepare a sterile field. All of the sterile supplies should be placed on this sterile field, arranged so they are convenient and accessible. Pour the sterile water and hydrogen peroxide into the two basins. You are now ready to put on the sterile gloves. (When using a tracheostomy kit, uncap the sterile water and hydrogen peroxide, don gloves, and assemble the equipment in order of use.)

Gloves are worn for this procedure to protect both you and the patient. Treat the stoma site as an incision or a surgical site. It should be considered the *clean* area. All cleansing motions should originate at the stoma site and then progress outward, in a radiating pattern.

Remove and Clean the Inner Cannula

Using one hand, stabilize the tracheostomy tube by holding the flange. With the other hand, remove the inner cannula by twisting the lock or rotating it to the unlocked position and removing it. If the patient requires mechanical ventilation, insert a tracheostomy adapter and reconnect the patient to the ventilator. If supplemental oxygen is required, a tracheostomy mask may be used to provide oxygen while the inner cannula is being cleaned.

Soak the inner cannula in the hydrogen peroxide and scrub it with a brush or cotton applicator. Remove any dried or inspissated secretions both inside and outside of the cannula. Ensure that the lumen is unobstructed. Thoroughly clean the area that mates with the flange and ensure that the locking mechanism is free of secretions. Use clean cotton swabs soaked in hydrogen peroxide.

Rinse the inner cannula in sterile water and shake it dry. If you attempt to reinsert the inner cannula without removing the excess water, any water dripping down the trachea may stimulate a cough reflex.

Reinsert the Inner Cannula

Using a similar two-handed technique, replace the inner cannula. Following the replacement of the cannula, return the patient to the previous mode of therapy (mechanical ventilation or supplemental oxygen as required).

STOMA CARE PROCEDURE

Tracheostomy care and stoma care are usually performed together as one procedure. In this text, each is identified as a separate procedure for the sake of clarity. Both procedures are sterile procedures and should be performed as aseptically as possible. Stoma care involves the cleaning of the stoma site and the application of clean tracheostomy ties and a dressing.

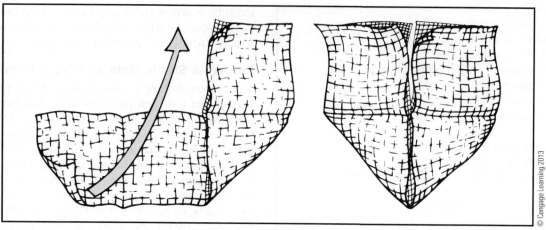

Figure 21-21   Folding a 4 × 4-inch gauze pad to make a tracheostomy dressing

Assess the Tracheostomy Tube Position

If this procedure is performed separately, auscultate the chest to assess the breath sounds before performing the procedure. Determine whether the patient requires suctioning, and listen for bilateral breath sounds.

Remove the Old Dressing and Ties

After determining that all supplies are at hand and prepared, stabilize the tracheostomy tube with one hand and remove the old dressing. Then cut and remove the old ties. It is essential, once the ties are cut, that the tube be stabilized at all times. It is very easy for accidental decannulation to occur once the ties are removed. A sudden movement or cough may be all that is required for displacement of the tube or decannulation. A spare tube should be available for immediate use if decannulation occurs.

Clean the Stoma Site

Initially, it may be necessary to clean the stoma area with 4 × 4-inch gauze pads dipped in hydrogen peroxide if a large amount of secretions are present. Begin cleaning at the stoma and move out from the site. Use each pad for a single pass only, and discard used pads by placing them in your dirty area. Carefully observe the stoma for unusual redness, swelling, tissue breakdown, or pulsation of the tracheostomy tube.

Following the removal of the majority of the secretions, use cotton-tipped applicators dipped in hydrogen peroxide for the detail cleaning. Clean very carefully around the stoma and the flanges of the tracheostomy tube.

After completing the cleaning using hydrogen peroxide, rinse the site using gauze pads dipped in sterile water. Pat the area dry with sterile gauze pads.

In some facilities, a small amount of povidone-iodine ointment is applied to help retard the growth of any microorganisms. This is not a universal practice and may require a physician's order. Check your hospital procedure manual to verify whether the ointment is used. Care should be exercised not to apply any non–water-soluble ointments around the stoma site.

Apply a Clean Dressing and New Ties

Never cut a gauze pad to make a dressing. Small cotton filaments separate from the gauze and may be absorbed into the healing stoma and later cause an abscess. A clean dressing may be constructed using a sterile 4 × 4-inch gauze pad if a dressing is not supplied in the tracheostomy care kit. Figure 21-21 shows how to fold the dressing for use. A variety of feltlike materials are used for commercial stoma dressings.

Apply new ties. The ties should be cut prior to performing the procedure so that the tube may be stabilized at all times. Tie a square knot to secure the tracheostomy tube. Never use a bow knot, as it is too easy to untie. A square knot is secure and easy to untie if necessary. A square knot may be tied by passing the right tie over the left, forming a half-hitch and then passing the left tie over the right, forming another half-hitch. Figure 21-22

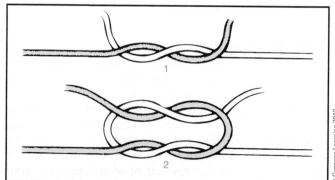

Figure 21-22   How to tie a square knot

shows how to tie this knot. Many hospitals are using manufactured trach ties that secure with Velcro. Be sure to understand how to apply the specific type of device used.

Alternatively, the new ties may be threaded through the flange and tied prior to removing the old ties. Using this technique, the chance of decannulation is minimized because the old ties help to secure the tracheostomy tube while the new ties are being placed. The disadvantage of this technique is that the old ties and secretions may soil the new ties with the patient's secretions.

Reassess the Tracheostomy Tube Position

Auscultate the chest following the procedure to assess the tube position. If the placement of the tube is in doubt, assess the adequacy of the patient's ventilation. If the patient is not in distress, summon help and attempt to reinsert the tube (unless the trach is less than 24 hours old). If the patient is in distress, cover the stoma site with a sterile 4×4-inch gauze pad and ventilate the patient by mouth until a physician arrives to assist in reinserting the tube.

References

American Association for Respiratory Care. (1993). AARC clinical practice guideline: Humidification during mechanical ventilation. *Respiratory Care, 37*(8), 887–890.

American Association for Respiratory Care. (2004). AARC clinical practice guideline: Nasotracheal suctioning–2004 revision and update. *Respiratory Care, 49*(9), 1080–1084.

American Association for Respiratory Care. (2010). AARC clinical practice guideline: Endotracheal suctioning of mechanically ventilated patients with artificial airways 2010. *Respiratory Care, 55*(6), 758–764.

Branson, R. (2007). Secretion management in the mechanically ventilated patient. *Respiratory Care, 52*(10), 1328–1347.

Centers for Disease Control and Prevention (CDC). (2004, March). *Guidelines for preventing healthcare-associated pneumonia.* Atlanta, GA: Author.

Combes, P. (2000). Nosocomial pneumonia in mechanically ventilated patients: A prospective randomized evaluation of the Stericath closed suctioning system. *Intensive Care Medicine, 26*(7), 878–882.

Demers, R. R. (1982). Complications of endotracheal suctioning procedures. *Respiratory Care, 27*(4), 453–457.

Emili, D. (2005). Ventilator-associated pneumonia: Issues related to the artificial airway. *Respiratory Care, 50*(7), 900–909.

Fiorentini, A. (1992). Potential hazards of tracheobronchial suctioning. *Intensive and Critical Care Nursing, 8*(4), 217–226.

Hess, D. R. (2003). AARC Evidence-based clinical practice guidelines: 9 Care of the ventilator circuit and its relation to ventilator-associated pneumonia, *Respiratory Care, 48*(9), 869–879.

Hess, D. R. (2005). Patient positioning and ventilator-associated pneumonia. *Respiratory Care, 50*(7), 892–899.

Kollef, M. (2005). Ventilator-associated pneumonia and why is it important? *Respiratory Care, 50*(6), 714–724.

Kranabetter, R. (2004). The effects of active and passive humidification on ventilation-associated pneumonia. *Anesthesist, 53*(1), 29–35.

Lasocki, L. (2006). Open and closed-circuit endotracheal suctioning in acute lung injury: Efficiency and effects on gas exchange. *Anesthesiology, 104*(1), 39–47.

Muscedere, J. (2008). Comprehensive evidence-based clinical practice guidelines for ventilator-associated pneumonia: Prevention. *Journal of Critical Care, 23*(1), 26–37.

Topeli, A. (2004). Comparison of the effect of closed versus open endotracheal suction systems on the development of ventilator-associated pneumonia. *Journal of Hospital Infection, 58*(1), 14–19.

Additional Resource

Lyons, R. J. (1979). *Tracheostomy care.* Pleasanton, CA: Shiley.

Practice Activities: Suctioning

1. Assemble the equipment required for airway aspiration, including the following:
   a. Sterile catheter
   b. Sterile gloves
   c. Goggles or face shield
   d. Sterile basin or container
   e. Sterile distilled water
   f. Sterile normal saline
   g. Flow-inflating or self-inflating manual resuscitator
   h. Vacuum gauge or pump and suction trap
   i. Water-soluble lubricant

2. Verify the operation of the vacuum gauge or pump and set the vacuum level between −80 and −120 mm Hg.

3. Assemble and test the manual resuscitator for proper operation.

4. With a laboratory partner as your patient, position the patient for:
   a. Nasotracheal suctioning
      (1) Semi-Fowler's
      (2) Supine in "sniffing" position
   b. Artificial airway aspiration
      (1) Semi-Fowler's
      (2) Supine in "sniffing" position

5. Using an intubation mannequin or a laboratory partner, practice oxygenation and hyperinflation:
   a. Without an artificial airway
   b. With an artificial airway

6. Using an intubation mannequin, practice nasotracheal and artificial airway aspiration using the following criteria:
   a. Equipment assembly and testing
   b. Patient assessment
   c. Preoxygenation and hyperinflation using a self-inflating or flow-inflating manual resuscitator
   d. Suctioning
      (1) Vacuum range between −80 and −120 mm Hg
      (2) Application of vacuum limited to 15 seconds
      (3) Vacuum is applied intermittently
      (4) Sterile technique is maintained
   e. Oxygenation following airway aspiration
   f. Airway aspiration repeated as required
   g. Oxygenation and hyperinflation following the procedure
   h. Patient assessment following the procedure

7. Using an intubated intubation mannequin, practice using the Trach Care suctioning system, including the following:
   a. Patient assessment
   b. Preoxygenation and hyperinflation
   c. Suctioning
      (1) Vacuum range between −80 and −120 mm Hg
      (2) Application of vacuum limited to 15 seconds
      (3) Vacuum applied intermittently
   d. Oxygenation and hyperinflation following aspiration
   e. Aspiration repeated as required
   f. Oxygenation and hyperinflation following the procedure
   g. Patient assessment following the procedure
   h. Control valve is turned off

8. Using an intubated intubation mannequin, practice measuring cuff pressures with the following techniques:
   a. MOV technique
   b. Minimal leak technique

Practice Activities: Tracheostomy and Stoma Care

1. Practice preparing a sterile field:
   a. Glove using sterile technique.
   b. Arrange supplies without contamination.

2. Using a tracheostomy mannequin, practice tracheostomy care:
   a. Auscultate the chest.
   b. Prepare a sterile field and supplies.
   c. Remove and clean the inner cannula.
      (1) Use hydrogen peroxide.
      (2) Clean the inner cannula thoroughly.
      (3) Rinse the inner cannula in sterile water.
      (4) Provide supplemental oxygen or ventilation as required.

3. Check for tube placement by auscultating the chest.

4. Using a tracheostomy mannequin, practice stoma care:
   a. Auscultate the chest.
   b. Perform the procedure aseptically.
   c. While stabilizing the tube at all times:
      (1) Remove the old dressing and ties.
      (2) Clean the stoma site.
         (a) Use 4 × 4-inch gauze pad and hydrogen peroxide to clean large amounts of secretions.
         (b) Use cotton-tipped applicators for detail cleaning.
         (c) Rinse the area with sterile water using 4 × 4-inch gauze pads.
         (d) Apply povidone-iodine ointment as required.
         (e) Replace the tracheostomy ties.
         (f) Replace the dressing.
   d. Evaluate the breath sounds to determine tracheostomy tube placement.

Check List: Nasotracheal Suctioning

_____ 1. Assemble the equipment.

_____ 2. Prepare and test the equipment.

_____   a. Arrange a sterile field.

_____   b. Check the vacuum level.

_____   c. Pour the solutions.

_____ 3. Properly position the patient.

_____ 4. Assess the patient.

_____   a. Auscultate the trachea.

_____   b. Auscultate around the large airways.

_____ 5. Oxygenate and hyperinflate the patient for 1 or 2 minutes on 100% oxygen.

    6. Suction the patient.

_____   a. Vacuum range between −80 and −120 mm Hg

_____   b. Application of vacuum limited to 15 seconds

_____   c. Vacuum applied intermittently

_____   d. Sterile technique maintained

_____ 7. Oxygenate following aspiration.

_____ 8. Repeat suctioning until the airway is clear.

_____ 9. Oxygenate and hyperinflate the patient for 1 or 2 minutes on 100% oxygen following the procedure.

_____ 10. Reassess the patient.

_____ 11. Return the patient to previous oxygen therapy.

_____ 12. Clean up the area.

_____ 13. Record the procedure in the chart.

Check List: Artificial Airway Aspiration

_____ 1. Assemble the required equipment.

_____ 2. Prepare and test the equipment.

_____   a. Check the vacuum level.

_____   b. Arrange a sterile field.

_____   c. Pour the solutions.

_____ 3. Position the patient.

_____ 4. Assess the patient by auscultation.

_____ 5. Oxygenate and hyperinflate the patient:

_____   a. Using a manual resuscitator

_____   b. Using the mechanical ventilator, allowing for washout volume

    6. Suction the patient.

_____   a. Vacuum range between −80 and −120 mm Hg

_____   b. Application of vacuum limited to 15 seconds

_____   c. Vacuum applied intermittently

_____   d. Sterile technique maintained

_____ 7. Oxygenate following aspiration.

_____ 8. Repeat aspiration until the airway is clear.

_____ 9. Oxygenate following the procedure with 100% oxygen for 1 or 2 minutes.

_____ 10. Assess the patient following the procedure.

_____ 11. Return the patient to previous oxygen therapy.

_____ 12. Clean up the area.

_____ 13. Record the procedure in the chart.

Check List: Cuff Pressure Monitoring

_____ 1. Assemble and test the equipment needed prior to measurement of cuff pressures.

_____ 2. Follow standard precautions, including handwashing.

_____ 3. Pressurize the manometer and tubing to 18 cm H_2O.

_____ 4. Attach the manometer to the pilot tube by pushing the connectors together.

    5. Measure the cuff pressure:

_____   a. MOV technique

_____   b. Minimal leak technique

_____ 6. Turn off the stopcock to the pilot tube.

_____ 7. Disconnect the cuff manometer from the pilot tube.

_____ 8. Remove any unneeded equipment.

_____ 9. Assess the patient's breath sounds.

_____ 10. Record your findings in the chart.

Check List: Tracheostomy and Stoma Care

_____ 1. Verify the order or policy and review the chart for pertinent information.

_____ 2. Explain the procedure.

_____ 3. Assemble the required equipment.

4. Auscultate the chest.

_____   a. Determine tube placement.

_____   b. Determine the need for suctioning and suction as required.

_____ 5. Prepare a sterile field and arrange all supplies aseptically.

_____ 6. Using sterile technique, glove for the procedure.

7. Remove and clean the inner cannula.

_____   a. Use hydrogen peroxide.

_____   b. Rinse in sterile water.

_____   c. Provide supplemental oxygen or ventilation as required.

_____   d. Stabilize the tube at all times.

_____ 8. Replace the inner cannula.

9. While stabilizing the tube at all times:

_____   a. Remove the old ties and dressing.

    b. Clean the stoma area.

_____   (1) Use 4 × 4-inch gauze pad.

_____   (2) Use cotton applicators for fine detail.

_____   (3) Rinse the stoma site with sterile water.

_____   c. Replace the ties.

_____   d. Replace the dressing.

_____ 10. Evaluate th ebreath sounds following the procedure.

_____ 11. Remove the supplies and clean up the area.

_____ 12. Reposition the patient as required.

_____ 13. Record the procedure in the patient's chart.

Self-Evaluation Post Test: Artificial Airway Care

1. When suctioning a patient, you should limit the suctioning time to:
   a. no more than 10 seconds.
   b. no more than 15 seconds.
   c. no more than 20 seconds.
   d. no more than 30 seconds.

2. The level of vacuum on the vacuum gauge should be set at:
   a. −80 to −120 mm Hg.
   b. 120 to 150 mm Hg.
   c. less than 80 mm Hg.
   d. 70 to 80 cm H_2O.

3. During nasotracheal suctioning, mucosal irritation can be reduced by:
   a. using a larger catheter.
   b. leaving the catheter in place.
   c. leaving the catheter in place and disconnecting it from the vacuum source.
   d. ensuring that the vacuum is greater than 150 mm Hg.

4. The advantages of the closed suction system include:
   I. cost effectiveness.
   II. the ability to suction without disconnection.
   III. decreased mucosal trauma.
   IV. selective entry into the right or left bronchi.
   a. I, II   c. I, IV
   b. I, III   d. I, II, IV

5. Which of the following are complications of suctioning?
   I. Tissue trauma
   II. Decreased cardiac output
   III. Hypoxemia
   IV. Cardiac arrhythmias
   V. Infection
   a. I, II, V   c. I, III, IV
   b. II, III, V   d. I, III, IV, V

6. A potential complication of stoma care is:
   a. obturator occlusion.
   b. inner cannula obstruction.
   c. decannulation.
   d. hypoventilation.

7. Tracheostomy tube displacement is most rapidly assessed by:
   a. chest x-ray.
   b. fluoroscopy.
   c. auscultation.
   d. arterial blood gas analysis.

8. The purpose of tracheostomy and stoma care is:
   a. to keep the stoma site clean and dry.
   b. to keep the airway patent.
   c. to remove secretions from the stoma site.
   d. All of the above.

9. When using a gauze pad to make a dressing, you should:
   a. cut the dressing to fit.
   b. never use gauze for a dressing.
   c. fold the dressing to fit.
   d. use a lot of tape to hold the dressing.

10. Before performing tracheostomy and stoma care you should:

I. auscultate the chest.
II. take the respiratory rate.
III. draw specimens for arterial blood gas (ABG) analysis.
IV. suction the patient if needed.

a. I, II
b. I, III
c. I, IV
d. II, IV

PERFORMANCE EVALUATION:
Nasotracheal Suctioning

Date: Lab _____ Clinical _____ Agency _____

Lab: Pass _____ Fail _____ Clinical: Pass _____ Fail _____

Student name _____ Instructor name _____

No. of times observed in clinical _____

No. of times practiced in clinical _____

PASSING CRITERIA: Obtain 90% or better on the procedure. Tasks indicated by * must receive at least 1 point, or the evaluation is terminated. Procedure must be performed within the designated time, or the performance receives a failing grade.

SCORING:
2 points — Task performed satisfactorily without prompting.
1 point — Task performed satisfactorily with self-initiated correction.
0 points — Task performed incorrectly or with prompting required.
NA — Task not applicable to the patient care situation.

Tasks:	Peer	Lab	Clinical
* 1. Follows standard precautions, including hand washing	☐	☐	☐
2. Obtains the required equipment			
* a. Suction kit or	☐	☐	☐
(1) Sterile catheter	☐	☐	☐
(2) Sterile gloves	☐	☐	☐
(3) Sterile basin	☐	☐	☐
(4) Eye protection (goggles or face shield)	☐	☐	☐
* b. Manual resuscitator	☐	☐	☐
* c. Sterile water	☐	☐	☐
* d. Water-soluble lubricant	☐	☐	☐
* e. Vacuum gauge or pump and trap	☐	☐	☐
* 3. Assembles and checks the equipment	☐	☐	☐
* 4. Positions the patient	☐	☐	☐
* 5. Assesses the need for suctioning	☐	☐	☐
* 6. Hyperinflates and oxygenates the patient	☐	☐	☐
* 7. Inserts the catheter	☐	☐	☐

   8. Suctions the airway

*   a. Vacuum level of −80 to −120 mm Hg   ☐   ☐   ☐

*   b. Application of vacuum limited to no more than 15 seconds   ☐   ☐   ☐

*   c. Sterile technique maintained   ☐   ☐   ☐

* **9.** Oxygenates following suctioning   ☐   ☐   ☐

* **10.** Repeats aspiration as required   ☐   ☐   ☐

* **11.** Repositions the patient   ☐   ☐   ☐

* **12.** Returns the patient to previous oxygen therapy   ☐   ☐   ☐

* **13.** Cleans up the area after the procedure   ☐   ☐   ☐

* **14.** Records the procedure in the patient's chart   ☐   ☐   ☐

SCORE: Peer _____ points of possible 42; _____%

                   Lab   _____ points of possible 42; _____%

                   Clinical _____ points of possible 42; _____%

TIME: _____ out of possible 20 minutes

STUDENT SIGNATURES

PEER: _____

STUDENT: _____

INSTRUCTOR SIGNATURES

LAB: _____

CLINICAL: _____

PERFORMANCE EVALUATION:
Endotracheal Suctioning

Date: Lab _____ Clinical _____ Agency _____

Lab: Pass _____ Fail _____ Clinical: Pass _____ Fail _____

Student name _____ Instructor name _____

No. of times observed in clinical _____

No. of times practiced in clinical _____

PASSING CRITERIA: Obtain 90% or better on the procedure. Tasks indicated by * must receive at least 1 point, or the evaluation is terminated. Procedure must be performed within the designated time, or the performance receives a failing grade.

SCORING:
2 points — Task performed satisfactorily without prompting.
1 point — Task performed satisfactorily with self-initiated correction.
0 points — Task performed incorrectly or with prompting required.
NA — Task not applicable to the patient care situation.

Tasks:	Peer	Lab	Clinical
* 1. Follows standard precautions, including hand washing	☐	☐	☐
2. Obtains the required equipment			
* a. Suction kit or	☐	☐	☐
(1) Sterile catheter	☐	☐	☐
(2) Sterile gloves	☐	☐	☐
(3) Sterile basin	☐	☐	☐
(4) Eye protection (goggles or face shield)	☐	☐	☐
* b. Manual resuscitator	☐	☐	☐
* c. Sterile water	☐	☐	☐
* d. Water-soluble lubricant	☐	☐	☐
* e. Vacuum gauge or pump and trap	☐	☐	☐
* 3. Assembles and checks the equipment	☐	☐	☐
* 4. Positions the patient	☐	☐	☐
* 5. Assesses the need for suctioning	☐	☐	☐
6. Hyperinflates and oxygenates the patient			
* a. Uses a manual resuscitator, or	☐	☐	☐
* b. Uses a ventilator, allowing for washout volume	☐	☐	☐

* **7.** Inserts the catheter ☐ ☐ ☐

   8. Suctions the airway

*   a. Vacuum level of −80 to −120 mm Hg ☐ ☐ ☐

*   b. Application of vacuum limited to no more than 15 seconds ☐ ☐ ☐

*   c. Sterile technique maintained ☐ ☐ ☐

   9. Oxygenates following suctioning

*   a. Uses a manual resuscitator, or ☐ ☐ ☐

*   b. Uses a ventilator, allowing for washout volume ☐ ☐ ☐

* **10.** Repeats aspiration as required ☐ ☐ ☐

* **11.** Oxygenates and hyperinflates for 1 or 2 minutes following the procedure ☐ ☐ ☐

* **12.** Repositions the patient ☐ ☐ ☐

* **13.** Returns the patient to previous oxygen therapy ☐ ☐ ☐

* **14.** Cleans up the area after the procedure ☐ ☐ ☐

* **15.** Records the procedure in the patient's chart ☐ ☐ ☐

SCORE: Peer _____ points of possible 48; _____%

            Lab _____ points of possible 48; _____%

            Clinical _____ points of possible 48; _____%

TIME: _____ out of possible 20 minutes

STUDENT SIGNATURES

PEER: _____

STUDENT: _____

INSTRUCTOR SIGNATURES

LAB: _____

CLINICAL: _____

PERFORMANCE EVALUATION:
Monitoring Cuff Pressures

Date: Lab _____ Clinical _____ Agency _____

Lab: Pass _____ Fail _____ Clinical: Pass _____ Fail _____

Student name _____ Instructor name _____

No. of times observed in clinical _____

No. of times practiced in clinical _____

PASSING CRITERIA: Obtain 90% or better on the procedure. Tasks indicated by * must receive at least 1 point, or the evaluation is terminated. Procedure must be performed within the designated time, or the performance receives a failing grade.

SCORING:
2 points — Task performed satisfactorily without prompting.
1 point — Task performed satisfactorily with self-initiated correction.
0 points — Task performed incorrectly or with prompting required.
NA — Task not applicable to the patient care situation.

Tasks:	Peer	Lab	Clinical
* **1.** Assembles and tests the equipment	☐	☐	☐
* **2.** Follows standard precautions, including hand washing	☐	☐	☐
* **3.** Pressurizes the manometer and tubing to 18 cm H_2O	☐	☐	☐
* **4.** Attaches the manometer to the pilot tube	☐	☐	☐
* **5.** Measures the cuff pressure			
a. MOV technique	☐	☐	☐
b. Minimal leak technique	☐	☐	☐
* **6.** Turns off the stopcock to the pilot tube	☐	☐	☐
* **7.** Disconnects the cuff manometer	☐	☐	☐
8. Removes any unneeded equipment	☐	☐	☐
* **9.** Auscultates the chest	☐	☐	☐
* **10.** Charts the procedure	☐	☐	☐

SCORE:
Peer _____ points of possible 22; _____%
Lab _____ points of possible 22; _____%
Clinical _____ points of possible 22; _____%

TIME: _____ out of possible 15 minutes

STUDENT SIGNATURES

PEER: _____

STUDENT: _____

INSTRUCTOR SIGNATURES

LAB: _____

CLINICAL: _____

Date: Lab _____ Clinical _____ Agency _____

Lab: Pass _____ Fail _____ Clinical: Pass _____ Fail _____

Student name _____ Instructor name _____

No. of times observed in clinical _____

No. of times practiced in clinical _____

PASSING CRITERIA: Obtain 90% or better on the procedure. Tasks indicated by * must receive at least 1 point, or the evaluation is terminated. Procedure must be performed within the designated time, or the performance receives a failing grade.

SCORING: 2 points — Task performed satisfactorily without prompting.
1 point — Task performed satisfactorily with self-initiated correction.
0 points — Task performed incorrectly or with prompting required.
NA — Task not applicable to the patient care situation.

Tasks:	Peer	Lab	Clinical
* 1. Verifies the order or policy	☐	☐	☐
* 2. Scans the chart for pertinent information	☐	☐	☐
* 3. Introduces self and identifies the patient	☐	☐	☐
4. Explains the procedure	☐	☐	☐
* 5. Gathers the appropriate equipment	☐	☐	☐
* 6. Follows standard precautions, including hand washing	☐	☐	☐
* 7. Auscultates the chest	☐	☐	☐
* 8. Suctions the patient as required	☐	☐	☐
* 9. Prepares a sterile field	☐	☐	☐
* 10. Gloves aseptically	☐	☐	☐
11. Removes the inner cannula			
* a. Stabilizes the tube	☐	☐	☐
* b. Provides supplemental oxygen or ventilation as required	☐	☐	☐
12. Cleans the inner cannula			
* a. Uses hydrogen peroxide	☐	☐	☐
* b. Cleans inside and outside	☐	☐	☐
* c. Rinses with sterile water and shakes dry	☐	☐	☐

* **13.** Reinserts the inner cannula   ☐   ☐   ☐

* **14.** Removes the old dressing and ties   ☐   ☐   ☐

15. Performs stoma care

*   a. Stabilizes the tube at all times   ☐   ☐   ☐

*   b. Cleans from the stoma out   ☐   ☐   ☐

*   c. Uses hydrogen peroxide   ☐   ☐   ☐

*   d. Rinses with sterile water   ☐   ☐   ☐

* **16.** Applies the new ties and dressing   ☐   ☐   ☐

* **17.** Auscultates the chest   ☐   ☐   ☐

* **18.** Cleans up the area and removes the supplies   ☐   ☐   ☐

* **19.** Returns the patient to previous therapy   ☐   ☐   ☐

* **20.** Records the procedure in the patient's chart   ☐   ☐   ☐

SCORE: Peer   _____ points of possible 52; _____ %

                Lab   _____ points of possible 52; _____ %

                Clinical _____ points of possible 52; _____ %

TIME: _____ out of possible 20 minutes

STUDENT SIGNATURES

PEER: _____

STUDENT: _____

INSTRUCTOR SIGNATURES

LAB: _____

CLINICAL: _____

CHAPTER 22
Chest Tubes

INTRODUCTION

Caring for the acutely ill patient will require that you understand how to manage and troubleshoot chest tubes. As a respiratory practitioner, you may be required to assist the physician in the placement of chest drains or chest tubes and then to maintain them once they are placed. In this chapter, you will learn about what chest tubes are and what they do, how to assist the physician in placing these tubes, and how to maintain and troubleshoot them once they are placed.

KEY TERMS

- Chest drain
- Chest tube
- Collection chamber
- Suction control chamber
- Trocar
- Water seal chamber

THEORY OBJECTIVES

At the end of this chapter, the reader should be able to:

- State the indications for placement and the purpose of chest tubes.
- Differentiate between a chest drain and a chest tube.
- Describe why a chest tube might be placed anteriorly or posteriorly in the thoracic cavity.
- Describe the function of the three components of a disposable chest drainage system:
  — Collection chamber
  — Water seal chamber
  — Suction control chamber
- Describe the consequences of the presence of too much or too little water in the water seal chamber.
- Describe the consequences of the presence of too much or too little water in the suction control chamber.
- Describe how to assess whether the vacuum source is correctly regulated.
- Describe how to assess the chest drainage system for leaks and how to correct them.
- Describe the actions to take should an emergency occur with the chest tube drainage system.
- Describe the Heimlich valve.

CHEST TUBES: BASIC PRINCIPLES

Indications for Chest Tube Placement

Chest tubes are indicated to remove blood, pus, pleural fluid, or air from the thoracic cavity (McMahon-Parkes, 1997). Chest drains may be placed in the mediastinal space or the pleural space.

Mediastinal drain placement may be indicated postoperatively (as after coronary artery bypass grafting or open heart surgery) to remove blood or to remove air (pneumopericardium). Mediastinal drains are important in the prevention of postoperative cardiac tamponade, which may cause the cardiac output to fall to dangerous levels. Once the postoperative bleeding has resolved, the drains are then removed.

Pleural drains may be placed to remove blood, pleural fluid, pus, or air from the pleural space. Air or fluid in the pleural space will cause a loss of lung volume on the affected side. Often the patient will present with dyspnea, a fall in oxygen saturation, and dullness or hyperresonance to percussion (depending on whether the problem is air or fluid). Often when a drain is placed to remove air from the pleural space (pneumothorax), it is called a chest tube. Chest tubes may be indicated following trauma or postoperatively (thoracic surgery) or to manage barotrauma from mechanical ventilation.

Chest Drains versus Chest Tubes

Frequently the terms *chest tube* and *chest drain* are used interchangeably. A drain is a device that has the purpose of removing fluid. In this textbook, the term *chest tube* is used to describe drains (placed for fluid removal) as well as tubes placed to remove air. In the case of thoracic applications, fluids may include blood, pleural fluid, or pus. A chest tube is placed in the pleural space to remove air (pneumothorax). Figure 22-1 is a photograph of a chest tube. Note the trocar in the photograph (lower solid piece). The *trocar* is a rigid metal rod that is inserted into the chest tube for insertion. The trocar provides stiffness to the otherwise flexible polyvinyl chloride (PVC) tube

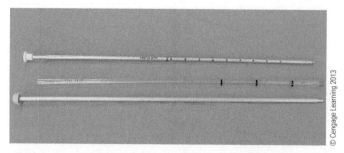

Figure 22-1 A photograph of a chest tube with the trocar. Note how the trocar is inserted into the chest tube, providing rigidity for insertion

© Cengage Learning 2013

(made of the same material as for endotracheal tubes), allowing it to be advanced into place by separating tissue. Once the tube is properly positioned, the trocar is removed, leaving the hollow chest tube to perform its function.

Rationale for Placement

Chest tubes or pleural drains are placed either anteriorly high in the thoracic cavity or posteriorly in the thoracic cavity. The rationale for placement depends on whether the tube is to function as a chest drain or as a chest tube. Note that gravity will cause the fluid to collect in the lowest part of the thorax, owing to its greater density. Therefore, to act as a drain, a drain is placed posteriorly along the base of the lung to remove fluid as it is collected (Figure 22-2).

Air will migrate preferentially to the least gravity-dependent (highest) area owing to its decreased density. Therefore, chest tubes are placed anteriorly near the apex of the lung to remove the free pleural air (see Figure 22-2).

CHEST DRAINAGE SYSTEM

Components of a Chest Drainage System

There are currently seven different brands of disposable chest drainage systems on the market (Carroll, 2000; Schiff, 2000). Even though brands vary, all of the disposable systems have common components. The collection system is divided into three parts: the collection chamber, the water seal chamber, and the suction control chamber (Figure 22-3).

The *collection chamber* is the part of the drainage system that collects fluids from the patient. It is calibrated in milliliters (mL) and is commonly subdivided into columns of 600 to 1000 mL per column. By observing the collection chamber, you can assess the amount of drainage, and its color and consistency, over time. You can mark the collection chamber using a piece of tape or marking pen, noting the amount and date and time of measurement, to detect trends in fluid drainage (McMahon-Parkes, 1997).

The *water seal chamber* is the center portion of the collection system (see Figure 22-3). The water seal chamber acts as a one-way valve, allowing air to escape from the pleural or mediastinal space but not allowing it to enter those spaces from the atmosphere. To appreciate the principle of operation, immerse one end of a drinking straw in a glass of water. You can blow air through the straw into the glass, but you cannot draw air in through the straw if it is below the level of the liquid. Typically, the water seal chamber is filled only to a depth of 2 cm. This allows air to freely escape the pleural or mediastinal space while protecting the patient from drawing ambient air into those areas (Smith, Fallentine, & Kessel, 1995).

The *suction control chamber* is the chamber most distal from the patient's chest tube (see Figure 22-3). The purpose of this chamber is to regulate the amount of vacuum

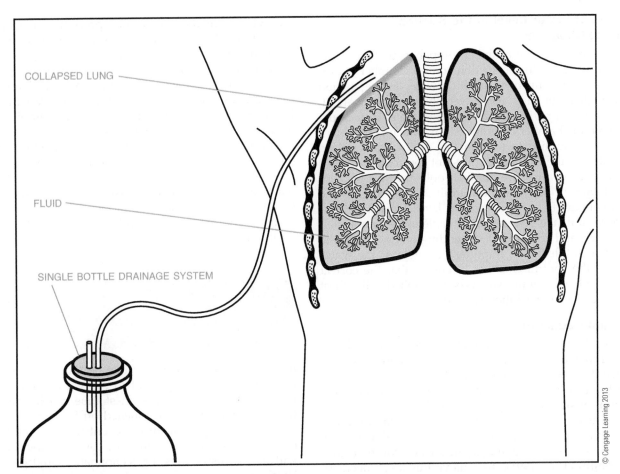

Figure 22-2 An illustration showing placement of a pleural drain and a chest tube. (A) The pleural drain is low in the thoracic cavity and posterior to remove fluid as gravity pulls it to the most dependent area. (B) The chest tube is placed anteriorly near the apex of the lung to capture air as it migrates away from the gravity-dependent areas

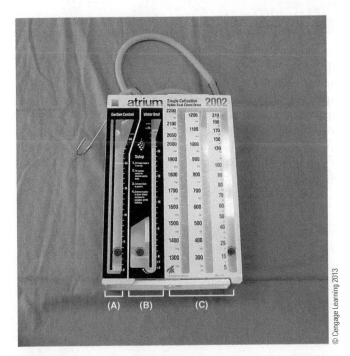

Figure 22-3 An illustration of the three parts of a chest drainage system. (A) The collection chamber. (B) The water seal chamber. (C) The suction control chamber

applied to the chest tube and thus to the patient's thoracic cavity. For most adult patients, the suction control chamber is filled to a depth of 20 cm. This depth provides application of continuous vacuum at a pressure of 20 cm H_2O below ambient pressure. If the depth is increased (to, say, 25 cm), a pressure of 25 cm H_2O below ambient pressure would be applied. The level of vacuum that is applied is directly proportional to the depth in the suction control chamber. If it is low, less vacuum is applied and, conversely, if it is high, more vacuum is applied.

Important Principles of Operation

Effects of Water Level in the Water Seal Chamber

Maintenance of the correct water level in the water seal chamber is important. If too little water is in the chamber (less than 2 cm), there is increased risk that with a deep breath (increased subambient pressure in the thorax), air could be drawn into the thoracic cavity. Conversely, too much water in the water seal chamber (greater than 2 cm) will inhibit air from leaving the thoracic cavity because it must overcome a greater pressure (depth in the chamber) to escape (Smith et al., 1995).

Effects of Water Level in the Suction Control Chamber

As for the water seal chamber, proper regulation of the amount of water in the suction control chamber is also important. Too much or too little water in the suction control chamber may also adversely affect the patient. As described previously, the depth of water in the suction control chamber determines how much subambient pressure is applied to the thoracic cavity. The vacuum regulator on the wall outlet does not control the amount of subambient pressure applied; only the suction control chamber does. For most adults, 20 cm H_2O is the most commonly applied vacuum level. However, most modern drainage systems are capable of being adjusted between 5 and 25 cm H_2O, depending on how deep the chamber is filled. It is important to monitor the water level in the control chamber to ensure that the correct level of subambient pressure is being applied to the chest tube and the patient's thoracic cavity.

Vacuum Regulation

Besides the depth of water in the suction control chamber, proper adjustment of the vacuum regulator connected to the wall vacuum outlet is also important. The level in the suction control chamber regulates the amount of subambient pressure applied to the thoracic cavity, as described before. However, it is important to adjust the vacuum regulator correctly as well to achieve continuous gentle bubbling in the suction control chamber (Smith et al., 1995). To achieve this level, decrease the vacuum level by turning down the suction regulator control until bubbling ceases. Then increase the vacuum level applied from the regulator until bubbling is continuous but gentle. If the bubbling is too vigorous, evaporation can occur in the suction control chamber, decreasing the level of subambient pressure applied to the thoracic cavity.

Assessment for Leaks

Leaks are identified by observing continuous bubbling in the water seal chamber. Normally, the water seal chamber will occasionally bubble as air is evacuated from the pleural or mediastinal space. If continuous bubbling occurs, there is an air leak either within the thorax or externally in the tubing and connections.

First, assess the patient. Determine if the patient is in distress. Auscultate and percuss the chest to determine if the pneumothorax has increased in size or if a tension pneumothorax may be present. If a tension pneumothorax has occurred, contact the patient's physician immediately.

If the patient is not in distress and appears out of any danger, assess the system for leaks. First, check all tubing connections. Connections should be tight and taped with pink surgical tape (airtight and watertight) to prevent leaks. If the leak persists, using a toothless clamp (one that will not puncture the surgical tubing), briefly clamp the tubing where it attaches to the patient's chest tube. If the bubbling stops, the leak is in the patient's chest (Carroll, 1995). Air leaks are common

following many thoracic surgical procedures (e.g., pneumonectomy, lobectomy). The surgeon may wish to be notified when leaks persist following surgery; note it in the patient's chart and notify the physician as appropriate. If the leak persists when the tubing is clamped at the patient's chest tube, the leak is in the system itself. Move the clamp in short intervals, briefly clamping each time while moving closer to the collection chamber. If the bubbling stops, the leak is in the connecting tubing (between the chest tube and the collection chamber). The tubing has a hole and must be replaced. If you reach the collection chamber itself and clamp the tubing where it enters the chamber and the leak stops, the leak is in the drainage system and the whole unit must be replaced (Carroll, 1995).

EMERGENCY MANAGEMENT OF THE CHEST DRAINAGE SYSTEM

If the chest tube drainage system becomes disconnected from suction, it is important to prevent air from entering the pleural space. The chest tube can be clamped (using a Kelly clamp) or pinched off by folding it over and securely taping it. In the event that the chest tube becomes inadvertently removed, cover the incision site with an occlusive dressing (cellophane, vinyl glove, or Vaseline-impregnated gauze dressing), taping it securely to the chest wall to prevent air entry.

HEIMLICH VALVE

The Heimlich valve is a one-way valve that is attached to the chest tube that prevents air from entering the pleural space. Air can escape through the valve to the atmosphere (e.g., during a cough), but air cannot go through the valve back into the pleural space (Figure 22-4). The valve may make a "fluttering" or "honking" sound as air passes through it from the chest, which is normal. The valve must remain connected to the chest tube at all times.

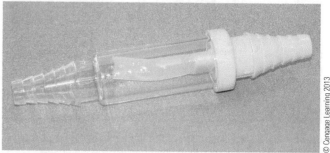

Figure 22-4 A photograph of the Heimlich valve

PROFICIENCY OBJECTIVES

At the end of this chapter, the reader should be able to:

- Collect and assemble the equipment required to assist the physician with the placement of a chest tube.
- Demonstrate how to assist the physician with the placement of a chest tube.
- Demonstrate how to assess the placement of a chest tube radiographically.

- Demonstrate how to set up a three-chamber disposable water seal chest drainage system.
- Demonstrate how to monitor and troubleshoot a chest drainage system.
- Demonstrate how to identify and correct leaks in the system.

ASSISTING WITH CHEST TUBE PLACEMENT

Equipment Required for Chest Tube Placement

As a respiratory care practitioner, you may be required to assist the physician with the placement of a chest tube. The most common settings in which this occurs are the emergency department, the intensive care unit (ICU), and the surgical floor in the acute care hospital. Common equipment required includes a chest tube insertion tray, sterile gloves, chest tubes, local anesthetic, antiseptic, the chest drainage system, and a vacuum regulator for the wall suction.

The chest tube tray typically includes sterile drapes, a scalpel, suture material, cotton-tipped or sponge swabs, antiseptic (usually povidone-iodine), and a sterile dressing. The chest tube insertion tray contains most of the supplies required to insert a chest tube. You will additionally need to obtain the chest tubes, local anesthetic, syringes, and the chest drainage system.

Draw up 4% lidocaine into a syringe in preparation for the procedure. The physician will use local anesthetic at the point of insertion. The physician may also order an analgesic, such as midazolam, prior to the procedure to help relax the patient. It is helpful to draw up and prepare medications in advance in case you are required to maintain sterile technique during the procedure.

Open the chest drainage system. Fill the suction control chamber to 20 cm H_2O and fill the water seal chamber to 2 cm H_2O. Connect the vacuum regulator to the wall outlet. Connect the drainage system to the wall outlet with surgical tubing. Do not apply vacuum to the system at this time. Set everything up in preparation for the procedure.

Assisting the Physician with the Procedure

Using a bedside tray or counter space, open the sterile chest tube insertion tray. Use the packaging wrap to form a sterile field. Assist the physician with applying sterile gloves if requested to do so.

Place the patient in a high Fowler's or semi-Fowler's position for anterior tube placement if the patient's condition permits it. You may be requested to pour or squeeze povidone-iodine solution into a sterile cup molded into the tray. The physician will apply the antiseptic to the site of the chest tube insertion. Following application of antiseptic, the physician may use disposable sterile drapes to form a sterile field. Many disposable drapes have adhesive strips to help them stay in place and are usually applied directly to the skin. Once the site is prepped and draped, the physician will inject the site with local anesthetic.

Most chest tubes that are to drain air are inserted on the anterior chest in the second or third intercostal space along the midclavicular line. An incision is made right over the rib and will dissect up and over the rib in an angular fashion. This will aid in closing the opening when the tube is withdrawn.

Chest tubes placed to drain fluid will be placed lower in the chest, in the fourth or lower intercostal space along the midaxillary line. The patient is placed lying on the side with the affected side superior. Once the incision is made, the chest tube will be advanced posteriorly, toward the base of the lung, where gravity will draw the fluid.

Assist the physician by opening the chest tube package such that he or she can obtain it, maintaining sterile technique. The physician will insert the chest tube with the trocar in place, directing it superiorly toward the apex of the lung (air moves away from the gravity-dependent areas). The patient may experience discomfort during the procedure. Considerable pressure is required to insert the tube through the muscle layers and into the pleural space.

Once the chest tube is placed, the physician will suture it into place to minimize the chance of its becoming displaced. Suturing the skin will also pull it up tight around the chest tube, helping to prevent leaks. Once it is sutured, assist the physician by opening the sterile petrolatum gauze dressing, which may be applied around the chest tube. A sterile airtight dressing is then applied over the gauze dressing to prevent dissection of air into the pleural space around the tube through the incision site.

Assessment of Chest Tube Placement

Chest tube placement is assessed by obtaining a chest x-ray film. Most patients in the ICU setting will have portable anteroposterior films taken. Like endotracheal tubes, chest tubes have a radiopaque line that promotes their visibility on an x-ray film. Verify that the chest tube is located properly and directed properly (superiorly for air, inferiorly for fluid).

SETUP AND MAINTENANCE OF THE CHEST DRAINAGE SYSTEM

Setting up the Drainage System

If you followed the steps outlined previously for equipment assembly, you have the drainage system's suction control and water seal chambers filled with water and the unit connected to the vacuum regulator. Using latex surgical tubing, connect the patient's chest tube to the latex tubing using a barbed connector as shown in Figure 22-5. If you anticipate a large amount of drainage, you may wish to trim the opening of the barbed connector, enlarging it so that fluids may flow more freely (Figure 22-6) (Smith et al., 1995). Once the connections are made at the chest tube, tape the connection using pink watertight/airtight surgical tape. Taping the connection will help to minimize the possibility of a leak at the connection.

Connect the surgical tubing to the drainage system and tape that joint as well. Make certain that there are no dependent loops in the tubing between the patient

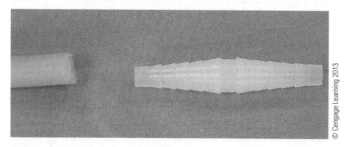

Figure 22-5 Connecting the chest tube to the latex surgical tubing using a barbed connector

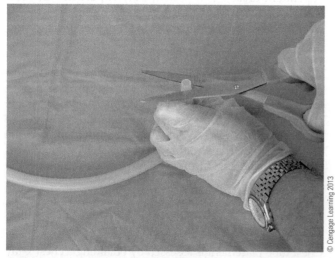

Figure 22-6 Trimming the barbed connector, enlarging the opening

and the drainage system. Any dependent loops can collect fluid, stopping flow. You want an uninterrupted downward pathway from the chest tube to the drainage system.

Adjust the vacuum regulator until gentle continuous bubbling is observed in the suction control chamber. Gentle continuous bubbling ensures that enough vacuum is being applied (greater than the water depth in the suction control chamber). However, the depth of water in the suction control chamber is what regulates the amount of subambient pressure applied to the patient's chest tube. Gentle, not vigorous, bubbling is important. Vigorous bubbling increases water evaporation in the suction control chamber, ultimately decreasing the level of subambient pressure applied to the patient's chest tube.

Monitoring and Troubleshooting the Drainage System

Monitoring a chest drainage system involves measuring and documenting fluid collection and monitoring and maintaining water levels in the water seal chamber and suction control chamber. Fluid drainage should be monitored initially every 30 to 60 minutes (Smith et al., 1995). If the patient's drainage exceeds 100 mL per hour and appears to be increasing, notify the physician. Once the drainage slows, monitoring may be performed every 2 hours. Marking on the collection chamber with a permanent marker or using tape is helpful in detecting trends in the patient's drainage. Mark the amount, date, and time of the measurement using the marking pen or affix a piece of tape with the same information. The amount, color, and consistency of drainage should be documented.

At least every 4 hours, monitor the water levels in the suction control chamber and the water seal chamber. With time, water will evaporate from the suction control chamber, and addition of water will be required to maintain the subambient pressure level. If the chamber becomes overfilled, most drainage systems have a diaphragm or port where fluid may be removed from the suction control chamber (Pettinicchi, 1998).

Proper water level (2 cm H_2O) is very important in the water seal chamber. Too much water in the chamber makes it more difficult for air or fluid to drain, whereas too little water increases the risk of entry of atmospheric air into the patient's thoracic cavity. If the water level in the water seal chamber increases (without addition of water by yourself), too much vacuum is being applied to the system. Press and hold the negative-pressure relief valve (usually located on the top of most drainage systems) to relieve the excess pressure (Pettinicchi, 1998). Once the pressure is relieved, the water level will return to normal.

Identifying and Correcting Leaks

Leaks in the chest drainage system are potentially dangerous because ambient air may enter through leaks in the system into the patient's thoracic cavity. Therefore, it is important for you to be able to identify and correct leaks.

During normal operation, the water seal chamber will periodically bubble. As air is drawn from the pleural space, it passes through the collection chamber and then bubbles through the water seal chamber. You can even notice the water level in the water seal chamber rise and fall with ventilation. The level rises during spontaneous exhalation and falls during inspiration. This slight change in fluid level is due to changes in pressure within the thoracic cavity with ventilation. If the patient is on mechanical ventilation, during inspiration the level rises (positive intrapleural pressure) and during exhalation it will fall. This normal rise and fall of the fluid level is termed *tidaling* (Carroll, 1995).

Continuous bubbling in the water seal chamber is a sign of a leak. It is important to distinguish whether the leak is the patient's chest (intrathoracic) or in the system, external to the patient. External leaks can be corrected. To differentiate the location of the leak, momentarily clamp the chest tube where it exits the patient's chest. Only clamp the chest tube briefly, using a toothless clamp or one protected with tape or rubber guards. If the bubbling stops, the leak is within the patient's chest. Sometimes air leaks are common with some thoracic surgical procedures (e.g., bullectomies, lobectomies). If bubbling persists, now you must check the drainage system.

Move the clamp to just below the joint between the patient's chest tube and the surgical tubing. Briefly clamp this location and observe the water seal chamber. If the bubbling stops, your leak is at that joint. Remove the tape, make sure the connector is tightly inserted into both the chest tube and the surgical tubing, and retape the joint. Repeat the clamp test to ensure that the leak has stopped. If bubbling persists when this location is clamped, the leak is distal to the point it was clamped.

Move distal from the patient, clamping the surgical tubing briefly in about 10 cm increments. If the bubbling stops, you have identified a leak in the tubing. Have the patient exhale and hold the breath. Clamp the chest tube about 4 to 6 cm from the point where the tube exits the patient's chest, using a protected clamp. Place a second clamp 2.5 cm distal to the first. Now you may aseptically change the tubing. Once the tubing is changed, remove the clamps and have the patient resume normal ventilation. If you progressively move along the entire length of the tubing and bubbling persists, the leak is in the drainage system.

To change the drainage system, set up a new system by initially filling the suction control and water seal chambers with water to their proper levels. Instruct the patient to exhale and then hold the breath. Clamp the chest tube with a protected or toothless clamp. Place a second padded clamp 2.5 cm distal to the first and clamp the chest tube again. Aseptically change the drainage system. Remove the clamps and instruct the patient to resume normal ventilation. Record the initial drainage and ensure that the new unit is functioning properly.

References

Carroll, P. (1995). Chest tubes made easy. *RN, 58*(12), 46–55.

Carroll, P. (2000). Exploring chest drain options. *RN, 63*(10), 50–52.

McMahon-Parkes, K. (1997). Management of pleural drains. *Nursing Times, 24*(52).

Pettinicchi, T. A. (1998, March). Troubleshooting chest tubes. *Nursing 1998*, 58–59.

Schiff, L. (2000). Market choices. Chest drainage systems. *RN, 63*(10), 57–58.

Smith, R. N., Fallentine, J., & Kessel, S. (1995). Underwater chest drainage bringing the facts to the surface. *Nursing '95, 25*(2), 60–63.

Practice Activities: Chest Tubes

1. Have your laboratory partner critique your aseptic technique while you prepare a chest tube insertion tray for use.

2. Properly prepare a chest drainage system for use:
   a. Fill the suction control chamber with water.
   b. Fill the water seal chamber with water.
   c. Connect the unit to a vacuum regulator.

3. Use a resuscitation mannequin as a "patient." With your laboratory partner, role-play the parts of a physician inserting a chest tube and a respiratory care practitioner assisting in the procedure.
   a. Prepare the chest tube insertion tray for use.
   b. Draw up local anesthetic (4% lidocaine).
   c. Assist the physician with surgical prep and draping.
   d. Assist the physician by passing instruments.
   e. Assist the physician with placement of the sterile airtight dressings.
   f. Assist the physician by connecting the newly placed chest tube with the drainage system.

4. With your laboratory instructor, view several chest x-ray films of patients who have chest tubes placed. Determine if the tube is for a pneumothorax, pleural drainage, or mediastinal drainage.

5. Monitor a chest drainage system:
   a. Drainage
   b. Suction control chamber water level
   c. Water seal chamber water level

6. Using a resuscitation mannequin as a patient, practice troubleshooting a chest drainage system:
   a. Determine if the leak is within the patient's thorax or the drainage system.
   b. Troubleshoot the system for leaks.

7. Using a blank sheet of paper, practice what you would chart when monitoring a chest drainage system. When you have finished, have your laboratory instructor critique your charting.

Check List: Chest Tubes

_____ 1. Wash your hands.
2. Assemble the required equipment:
_____ a. Chest tube insertion tray
_____ b. Local anesthetic and syringes
_____ c. Chest tubes
_____ d. Chest drainage system
_____ e. Vacuum regulator
3. Prepare the chest drainage system for use:
_____ a. Fill the suction control chamber.
_____ b. Fill the water seal chamber.
_____ c. Connect the vacuum regulator to a wall source.
_____ d. Connect the chest drainage system to the vacuum regulator and check the system for operation.
4. Prepare the chest tube insertion tray for use:
_____ a. Aseptically open the tray, creating a sterile field.
_____ b. Draw up topical anesthetics.
_____ c. Organize supplies for easy retrieval and access.

5. Assist the physician with the procedure:
_____ a. Assist with surgical prep and draping.
_____ b. Assist by passing instruments.
_____ c. Assist with placement of the sterile airtight dressings.
_____ d. Assist by connecting the newly placed chest tube with the drainage system.
6. Monitor the drainage system:
_____ a. Drainage output
_____ b. Water level in the suction control chamber
_____ c. Water level in the water seal chamber
7. Assess the chest drainage system for leaks:
_____ a. Determine if the leak is intrathoracic (patient) or in the chest drainage system.
_____ b. If the leak is in the drainage system, systematically identify it.
_____ 8. Following the procedure, clean up the area by disposing of unused and opened supplies.
_____ 9. Wash your hands.
_____ 10. Document the procedure in the patient's chart.

Self-Evaluation Post Test: Chest Tubes

1. Indications for placement of a chest drainage system for fluid drainage include:
   I.   coronary artery bypass graft surgery.
   II. pleural effusion.
   III. pneumothorax.
   IV. blunt chest trauma.
   a. I   c. III
   b. I, II   d. III, IV

2. Indications for placement of a chest tube for removal of air include:
   I.   coronary artery bypass graft surgery.
   II. pleural effusion.
   III. pneumothorax.
   IV. blunt chest trauma.
   a. I   c. III
   b. I, II   d. III, IV

3. A chest tube placed for evacuation of air would be:
   I.   placed at the second or third intercostal space.
   II. placed at the fourth or lower sixth intercostal space.
   III. directed superiorly toward the apex.
   IV. directed inferiorly toward the base.
   a. I, III   c. II, III
   b. I, IV   d. II, IV

4. A chest tube placed for fluid evacuation would be:
   I.   placed at the second or third intercostal space.
   II. placed at the fourth or lower sixth intercostal space.
   III. directed superiorly toward the apex.
   IV. directed inferiorly toward the base.
   a. I, III   c. II, III
   b. I, IV   d. II, IV

5. Which of the following chambers regulates the amount of subambient pressure applied to the patient's chest?
   a. Collection chamber
   b. Water seal chamber
   c. Suction control chamber
   d. Vacuum regulator

6. Which of the following chambers prevents ambient air from entering the patient's thoracic cavity?
   a. Collection chamber
   b. Water seal chamber
   c. Suction control chamber
   d. Vacuum regulator

7. When monitoring the chest drainage system for a postoperative thoracotomy patient, you find that the water seal chamber is filled to 8 cm H_2O. As a respiratory care practitioner, you should:
   a. ignore it because the levels should range between 5 and 20 cm H_2O.
   b. press and hold the negative-pressure relief valve.
   c. ensure that the chamber is filled to 2 cm H_2O.
   d. Both b and c.

8. Too much water in the water seal chamber:
   I. inhibits air/fluid from being evacuated from the chest.
   II. facilitates evacuation of air/fluid from the chest.

   III. causes more pressure having to be generated for air/fluid to be removed.
   IV. causes less pressure having to be generated for air/fluid to be removed.
   a. I, III   c. II, III
   b. I, IV   d. II, IV

9. Vigorous bubbling in the suction control chamber:
   a. is required to maintain adequate subambient pressure.
   b. may result in excess subambient pressure being applied to the chest.
   c. may cause increased evaporation of water.
   d. None of the above.

10. Constant bubbling in the water seal chamber:
    a. is normal and should be ignored.
    b. is a sign of a leak.
    c. indicates that too much pressure is being applied at the vacuum regulator.
    d. indicates that the suction control chamber is filled too much.

PERFORMANCE EVALUATION:

Chest Tubes

Date: Lab _____ Clinical _____ Agency _____

Lab: Pass _____ Fail _____ Clinical: Pass _____ Fail _____

Student name _____ Instructor name _____

No. of times observed in clinical _____

No. of times practiced in clinical _____

PASSING CRITERIA: Obtain 90% or better on the procedure. Tasks indicated by * must receive at least 1 point, or the evaluation is terminated. Procedure must be performed within the designated time, or the performance receives a failing grade.

SCORING: 2 points — Task performed satisfactorily without prompting.
1 point — Task performed satisfactorily with self-initiated correction.
0 points — Task performed incorrectly or with prompting required.
NA — Task not applicable to the patient care situation.

Tasks:	Peer	Lab	Clinical
1. Washes hands	☐	☐	☐
2. Assembles the required equipment			
a. Chest tube insertion tray	☐	☐	☐
b. Local anesthetic and syringes	☐	☐	☐
c. Chest tubes	☐	☐	☐
d. Chest drainage system	☐	☐	☐
e. Vacuum regulator	☐	☐	☐
* **3.** Prepares the chest drainage system for use			
a. Fills the suction control chamber	☐	☐	☐
b. Fills the water seal chamber	☐	☐	☐
c. Connects the regulator to a wall source	☐	☐	☐
d. Connects the chest drainage system to the vacuum regulator and checks the system for operation	☐	☐	☐
4. Prepares the chest tube insertion tray for use			
a. Opens the tray, creating a sterile field	☐	☐	☐
b. Draws up the topical anesthetics	☐	☐	☐
c. Organizes the supplies for easy retrieval	☐	☐	☐

5. Assists the physician with the procedure

   a. Assists with surgical prep and draping ☐ ☐ ☐

   b. Assists by passing the instruments/supplies ☐ ☐ ☐

   c. Assists with placing the dressings ☐ ☐ ☐

   d. Connects the chest tube to the drainage system ☐ ☐ ☐

6. Monitors the drainage system

   a. Drainage output ☐ ☐ ☐

   b. Water level in the suction control chamber ☐ ☐ ☐

   c. Water level in the water seal chamber ☐ ☐ ☐

7. Assesses the chest drainage system for leaks

   a. Determines if the leak is intrathoracic or in the chest drainage system ☐ ☐ ☐

   b. Identifies the leak's location in the system ☐ ☐ ☐

8. Cleans up the area ☐ ☐ ☐

9. Washes hands ☐ ☐ ☐

10. Documents the procedure in the patient's chart ☐ ☐ ☐

SCORE:

Peer _____ points of possible 50; _____%

Lab _____ points of possible 50; _____%

Clinical _____ points of possible 50; _____%

TIME: _____ out of possible 45 minutes

STUDENT SIGNATURES

PEER: _____

STUDENT: _____

INSTRUCTOR SIGNATURES

LAB: _____

CLINICAL: _____

CHAPTER 23

Insertion and Maintenance of Intravenous Lines

Stephen S. Pitts

David A. Field

INTRODUCTION

The insertion and maintenance of peripheral intravenous (IV) catheters constitute an advanced skill practiced by many respiratory practitioners today. For safe and effective technique in clinical practice, both an understanding of the theory of IV administration and a comprehensive training program are necessary.

In this chapter you will learn the theory behind IV therapy as well as the specifics of IV insertion and maintenance and associated complications.

KEY TERMS

- Air embolism
- Butterfly catheter
- Catheter fragment embolism
- Catheter shear
- Cellulitis
- Chevron
- gtt

- Hypertonic solution
- Hypotonic solution
- Infiltration
- Infusion pumps
- Isotonic solution
- KVO
- Over-the-needle catheter

- Patency
- Phlebitis
- prn
- Thrombus
- TKO
- Wheal

THEORY OBJECTIVES

At the end of this chapter, the reader should be able to:

- *Explain the rationale(s) for the insertion of intravenous (IV) needles, to include:*
  - *The administration of medications on a continuous or prn (as needed) basis*
  - *The administration of fluids to maintain normal hydration of the patient*
  - *The administration of fluids in the presence of shock*
  - *The administration of blood and blood products*
- *Differentiate among isotonic, hypertonic, and hypotonic solutions, and explain their effects on the vascular system and the cells of the body.*

- *Describe the procedure for locating an acceptable anatomical site for the insertion of an IV needle.*
- *Describe the complications associated with the insertion and maintenance of an IV line.*
- *Explain the steps associated with the maintenance of an existing IV line and how to correct problems with the line.*
- *Perform calculations necessary to run a solution at the prescribed rate.*

This section deals with the reasoning and indications for IV catheter placement and the maintenance of the solutions that can be infused through them.

THE PRINCIPLES OF INTRAVENOUS THERAPY

IV access is established in a patient for a variety of reasons. These include the administration of medications over a long-term period as an infusion, or as a single dose given as needed (*prn*). Both methods of medication administration are made easier and more comfortable for the patient if an indwelling IV catheter is in place. The existence of this catheter eliminates the necessity of repeated injections that can be both painful and frightening to the patient.

Another reason for the establishment of an IV line is to help maintain the normal fluid status of the patient. It is not uncommon for a patient who is unable to eat or drink normally to become dehydrated and need the assistance of IV "feedings." Patients who are under long-term care and continue to be unable to maintain normal caloric intake can be given IV infusions that include all of the necessary electrolytes, fatty acids, and carbohydrates as well as fluid to maintain a homeostatic state.

In the presence of shock, whether it be from hypovolemia, sepsis, anaphylaxis, or any other cause, normal tissue perfusion can be drastically altered and in severe cases ceased completely. With the aid of the IV line, fluids, blood, and blood products can be infused to assist in returning the body to its normal state.

Blood and blood products, such as plasma, packed red blood cells, and platelets, can also be administered through an established IV line. In the case of a patient who may require many such transfusions, the presence of a patent catheter makes such procedures very easy and expedient.

INTRAVENOUS FLUID PROPERTIES

There are numerous types of IV fluids that are available for both direct undiluted infusion and as the diluent in medication administration. Examples of these include D$_5$W (5% dextrose in water), lactated Ringer's solution (which contains electrolytes and lactate as a buffer), normal (physiologic) saline (0.9% sodium chloride [NaCl] in water), and many combinations of these, such as D$_5$–0.45% NaCl and D$_5$–LR.

Many medications will become inactivated or their action decreased if they are mixed in the incorrect solution. Proper use of these medications requires that they be mixed only in a specific solution. For example, the anticoagulant heparin is mixed with D$_5$W for administration to the patient.

Most of the IV solutions that are used for mixing medications and for fluid replacement are isotonic with

extracellular fluid (i.e., they have the same tonicity as measured by solute concentration). With the administration of an *isotonic solution*, there is very little, if any, net movement of fluid into or out of the cells. This is most desirable for maintaining a normal environment for cellular function. A *hypertonic solution* will cause water to be drawn from inside the cell and into the vascular space. This effect may be desirable in cases of cerebral edema or fluid retention due to renal failure or overhydration. An example of a hypertonic solution is mannitol, which is used in some head injury cases. A *hypotonic solution*, which has a solute concentration lower than that of the fluid inside the cells, will result in a net movement of water from the vascular space to inside the cell. This effect may be helpful in cases of severe dehydration where the function of cells is hampered owing to the absence of necessary intracellular fluid. A 0.225% NaCl solution is considered a hypotonic solution.

LOCATING ACCEPTABLE SITES FOR INTRAVENOUS NEEDLE PLACEMENT

In assessing a possible site for IV needle insertion, several factors must be taken into consideration. Many times, the IV line will remain for an extended period. This may be dictated by the length of stay of the patient, hospital policy regulating the length of time that an IV may remain in place, the failure of an IV to remain patent, or any combination of these. When the IV site is chosen, it should be assumed that the site will remain for an extended time and the location chosen accordingly.

A basic knowledge of the location of the major superficial veins that are generally used for IV cannulation is very helpful. Figure 23-1 shows the location of many of these vessels and where they are located on the lower portion of the arm. Although IV catheters can be placed in the leg or foot in adults, and in a scalp vein in newborns and infants, these sites carry their own special considerations and are not addressed here.

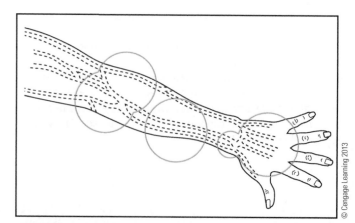

© Cengage Learning 2013

Figure 23-1 The major veins of the forearm are good sites for insertion of IV catheters. The areas within the circles are common sites that are used

In choosing a site, it is preferable to select the non-dominant hand or arm of the patient (i.e., the left arm of a right-handed patient). This will allow the patient to be less restricted in performing normal daily functions. It is also suggested that the catheter be placed in a location that does not "stick out" or extend away from the extremity in such a manner that it will be constantly bumped or jarred and consequently disrupt the *patency* of the IV.

Areas directly over joints and bony prominences are less desirable sites, as it is possible to make contact with the bone during insertion of the IV needle. This can lead to infection and is also quite painful. Catheter positions on the inside of a joint, or in the area that forms the "crease" in a joint, are also not the first sites of consideration owing to problems created when the joint is moved. This could lead to "kinking" of the catheter, which could restrict or stop the flow of fluids. These sites also limit the range of motion for the patient.

Another consideration is the amount of pain experienced by the patient during the procedure of inserting the catheter into the vein. Generally, the underside of the lower arm and the inside of the wrist are more sensitive than the back of the hand, the anterior and inferior portions of the lower arm, and the inside of the elbow. Although some institutions require the use of a local anesthetic, this is not always the case, so consideration for the comfort of the patient is of importance.

With some medical conditions, a tourniquet cannot be applied to the patient's arm. These include the placement of a shunt for renal dialysis and a previous mastectomy. The extremity opposite the side affected by these conditions should be selected.

A tourniquet is applied above or proximal to the site that is selected for the insertion of the catheter. This restrictive band is usually made of rubber and can be either a flat band or a tubular piece of latex, such as a Penrose drain. Generally, a wider band of 1 inch to 1½ inches is more comfortable than a narrower ¼ inch or ½ inch band. A blood pressure cuff can also be used to occlude venous flow. The cuff is inflated so that it reads 20 to 30 mm Hg below the systolic number of the patient's blood pressure. After the placement of the tourniquet, you should be able to palpate the radial pulse distal to the tourniquet placement site.

To hold the tourniquet in place temporarily, make a loop around the patient's arm with one free end of the band. This end is then folded over itself and tucked under the other end of the tourniquet. It is important to leave the free end of the folded-over section exposed so that it may be grasped and pulled free to loosen the tourniquet when you desire to do so (Figure 23-2).

Once the tourniquet has been properly applied, the restriction of venous flow will cause the veins of the arm to distend and become engorged with blood. Visualization and palpation of the vessels will make the selection of a proper site possible. Select a site that is relatively straight and free of palpable "knots" or "Ys." These "knots" are valves in the vein that help to maintain the flow of blood in the correct direction; they will not allow the passage of

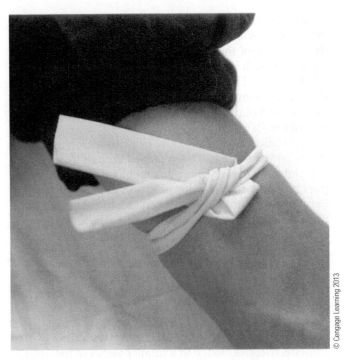

Figure 23-2 This method of tying the tourniquet allows easy removal by grasping the end of the folded-over section and pulling quickly

the IV catheter. The bifurcations or "Ys" are junctions of two vessels and should be avoided.

The vessel should be large enough to accept the catheter that has been chosen. In situations in which the IV line is being established strictly for the administration of medications, a smaller catheter may be acceptable. When large amounts of fluids or blood products will be given, a larger catheter may be desired, and a larger vessel is chosen. Again, the comfort of the patient should be taken into consideration, and a catheter no larger than necessary should be chosen for performing the procedure.

COMPLICATIONS OF INTRAVENOUS THERAPY

With the practice of good aseptic technique and attention to detail in proper IV needle insertion, most "starts" will be accomplished without a great deal of difficulty. However, there are certain problems inherent to this procedure that may be unavoidable, and recognition of their existence is important to both the comfort and the safety of the patient.

Infiltration

Infiltration occurs when the fluid or medication that is being infused leaks out of the blood vessel that was cannulated. This results in a swelling at the site, which can be quite painful. This problem may be caused by a small laceration or puncture to the vessel incurred during the process of inserting the needle or may be due simply to the vessel's inability to maintain its integrity owing to previous medications (e.g., cortico steroids) or the structure of the vessel itself. In some circumstances, the IV line will continue to function, but this is not usually the case. The infusion should be discontinued, the IV catheter removed, direct pressure applied to the site for at least 5 minutes, and a new site selected for reinsertion of the IV.

Infiltration may also occur prior to attaching the IV fluids if the needle has been passed entirely through the vessel during the insertion, so that blood flows out of the puncture site. Many times, this will appear as a hematoma or bruise that is visible beneath the skin. Again, in this case, the catheter should be removed, direct pressure and a bandage applied, and another site chosen.

Thrombosis

After the successful introduction of an IV catheter, it is possible for a blood clot to form at the site of insertion, at the end of the catheter, or in the cannulated vessel. This *thrombus* could break free and potentially become an embolus that may lodge in a smaller vessel of the lung or brain, creating the symptoms of pulmonary embolism or cerebrovascular accident (CVA or stroke).

Any complaint of pain, tenderness, or swelling at the IV site should be investigated thoroughly and evaluated for the possibility of thrombus formation. Gentle palpation at the site may reveal a mass or lump around or near the end of the catheter. Under many circumstances, the IV infusion will have slowed dramatically or stopped altogether. Under no circumstances should the clot be "flushed" or cleared by application of pressure to the IV bag or by use of a fluid-filled syringe to force the clot out of the catheter. A syringe can be attached to the IV tubing and negative pressure applied by drawing back on the plunger of the syringe to attempt to draw the clot out of the catheter and into the syringe. This technique should be attempted gently; if it is unsuccessful, discontinue the infusion, remove the catheter, dress the site appropriately, and obtain IV access elsewhere.

Phlebitis and Cellulitis

Phlebitis, or inflammation of the vein, may occur simply owing to the presence of a foreign body such as the IV catheter. *Cellulitis,* or an inflammation of the surrounding tissues, may also occur. These problems are not necessarily an indication of poor technique or infection. Both can be present with symptoms of tenderness, swelling, and possibly heat at the site. In these cases, the IV infusion may continue to run at its normal rate. However, if either is suspected, it is much better to discontinue the infusion, decannulate the vessel, dress the site, and attempt to locate another site for the infusion to be started.

Air Embolism

The infusion of approximately 50 mL of air into an IV line may be fatal to the normal adult. Care must be taken when assembling the tubing to the bag, and the subsequent flushing of the line, to ensure that all air is removed before the tubing is connected to the catheter. Maintaining the IV bag in an upright (vertical orientation) position at all times will also reduce the possibility of air entering the tubing, causing an *air embolism*. Most modern infusion pumps are equipped to detect the presence of air in the tubing and will alarm if the condition exists.

It is also possible for air to enter the tubing at any of the connections in the circuit, such as at the connection between the catheter and the tubing or at the connection between an extension set and the primary IV tubing. If these connections are loose, air can be drawn into the circuit by the Venturi effect. Proper technique in assembling the IV tubing and any of its components, as well as ensuring that the tubing is attached tightly to the IV catheter, will help to prevent the aspiration of air into the circuit.

Catheter Shear or Catheter Fragment Embolism

During the placement of an IV needle, it is possible for the flexible catheter to become slightly bent or distorted after the metal stylet is removed. For this reason, the metal needle should never be reinserted or advanced back into the catheter. This may cut off or "shear" the end of the catheter, which may subsequently enter the vascular system, leading to problems discussed earlier. This complication is termed *catheter shear* or *catheter fragment embolism.*

MAINTENANCE OF INTRAVENOUS INFUSIONS

Once an IV infusion has been established, it is important that the site, the fluid level in the bag, and the rate of infusion be monitored. This will ensure that the site remains patent and that the IV infusion is running at the prescribed rate. With the widespread use of *infusion pumps*, the rate and the desired amounts to be given to the patient are easily programmed and then monitored by the pump. The indwelling catheter, however, must be visually inspected by the technician.

Each institution specifies predetermined lengths of time for which IV catheters may remain in place. This period varies but is typically between 24 and 72 hours. You should become familiar with the policies in your facility that dictate this period. At the site of insertion, the date and time of the start and your name or initials should be recorded on a piece of tape. This allows for easy identification of how long the IV line has been in place.

Inspection of the site should include looking to ensure that the infusion has not infiltrated and that there are no signs of phlebitis or cellulitis. This visualization should include looking for any swelling, redness, or tenderness around the catheter. The infusion should be running at the correct rate, and the IV bag should contain the correct fluid and any additives that have been prescribed. If any problems are discovered, you should report them immediately to the person in charge of the patient's care.

DRIP RATE CALCULATIONS

In some instances, it may be necessary or desirable to run an IV infusion without the assistance of an infusion pump. It is therefore necessary that you be able to perform the appropriate calculations and run the infusion at the prescribed rate.

The terms *TKO* (to keep open) and *KVO* (keep vein open) can be used interchangeably and refer to a rate that is just fast enough to keep the infusion running and to prevent a clot from forming in the catheter. The type of infusion set that is being used will determine the correct rate. You should become familiar with the type and brand of sets in use at your institution and with the number of drops (*gtt*) in the drip chamber that equal 1 mL for each type. Common drip sets and their drops per milliliter (gtt/mL) rates are minidrips, which produce 60 gtt/mL, and macrodrips, which produce 10, 12, or 15 gtt/mL. The sterile packages that contain the sets should have information printed on them to indicate the drops per milliliter rate. Some sets have the number printed on the tabs next to the drip chamber. Rates of 10 to 15 drops per minute (gtt/min) with a 60 gtt/mL set will ensure that the vein will remain open and that the infusion will continue to run. Five to eight drops per minute are appropriate with the other administration sets. Understanding drip rate calculations can be useful with some continuous nebulizer setups as well.

There are two ways in which IV infusions are commonly ordered. The first is to infuse a set amount over a given time (e.g., 1 liter over 4 hours). The second is to run the infusion at a set rate per hour (e.g., 100 mL per hour). The formulas for calculating the infusion rate are very similar in both cases.

In the first instance, the *drops per minute* will equal the volume to be infused multiplied by the drops per milliliter of the infusion set. The product is then divided by the total time the infusion is to run in minutes.

Example

1 liter of 0.9% NaCl over 3 hours
The administration set delivers 15 gtt/mL.

$$\text{gtt/minute} = 1000 \text{ mL} \times 15 \text{ gtt/mL}/180 \text{ minutes}$$
$$= \text{approximately } 84 \text{ gtt/mL}$$

To figure a rate in *milliliters per hour*, the drops per minute equals the volume to be infused multiplied by the drops per milliliter of the infusion set; the product is then divided by 60 minutes.

Example

Lactated Ringer's to run at 100 mL per hour
The administration set delivers 15 gtt/mL.

$$\text{gtt/minute} = 100 \text{ mL} \times 15 \text{ gtt/mL}/60 \text{ minutes}$$
$$= 25 \text{ gtt/mL}$$

These simple formulas will work for all rates of infusion and administration sets, and the respiratory practitioner should be familiar with them and be able to perform the calculations quickly.

PROFICIENCY OBJECTIVES

At the end of this chapter, the reader should be able to:

- *Collect and assemble all of the equipment necessary for starting an IV infusion.*
- *Using a laboratory partner or a mannequin arm for simulation, demonstrate proper technique for the application of a tourniquet and selection of an appropriate IV insertion site.*
- *Demonstrate, using aseptic technique and standard precautions, the insertion of an IV needle and establishment of a patent IV.*
- *Demonstrate proper technique for securing the IV needle and the administration set to the patient.*
- *Demonstrate the proper disposal of all used and unused supplies.*
- *Demonstrate the calculations necessary to run the IV infusion at the prescribed rate, and adjust the flow of the IV accordingly.*
- *Demonstrate the steps for maintenance of an ongoing IV infusion.*
- *Demonstrate the steps for discontinuing an IV infusion.*

A physician's order is required for this procedure to be performed. This order may be in the form of a protocol or given as the result of a consultation or examination. You should be familiar with the type of system in place in your facility.

SUPPLIES NEEDED FOR INTRAVENOUS CANNULATION

Prior to beginning the venipuncture technique, it is necessary to select and gather all of the necessary equipment to perform the procedure.

Needle Selection

An understanding of the numbering system for the size of IV catheters is necessary to help you select a range of catheters of appropriate size when planning to establish an IV line. The gauge of the portion of the catheter that remains in the vein is used. Catheters can range from as small as a tiny 27-gauge butterfly to a much larger 14-gauge polytetrafluoroethylene (Teflon) or plastic over-the-needle catheter. An easy rule to remember is the larger the number, the smaller the catheter.

There are several types of IV needles available. Each type has its advantages and disadvantages, and many have very specific uses in the clinical setting. This chapter deals only with the hollow butterfly needle and the over-the-needle types of catheters.

The *butterfly needle*, so named because of the plastic tabs that extend away from the needle much like a butterfly's wings, has a fairly limited use. Because the needle that remains in the vein is metal, it is possible for the vein to become lacerated or punctured with any movement or contact. These needles are also typically very small, for example, 25 gauge or 27 gauge. Their primary use is in infants and the elderly, who have very small veins and in whom the desired infusion rate of the IV is typically very slow. The needle must be secured in a very stable manner; an arm board can also be used to ensure that minimal movement of the extremity around the needle is allowed. These needles can also be used in the tiny scalp veins of infants.

The *over-the-needle catheter* is a plastic or Teflon sleeve that has a hollow metal needle running through its length. This allows for the use of the metal needle to initiate the insertion and obtain access to the lumen of the vein, but after the removal of this metal stylet, the only remaining portion is the flexible, relatively blunt catheter. These needles typically range in size from the very small 24 gauge up to a large-bore 14 gauge. The needle is usually two gauges smaller than the plastic catheter (e.g., an 18-gauge IV catheter uses a 20-gauge needle/stylet). Figure 23-3 shows a typical butterfly and an over-the-needle catheter.

When selecting the catheter to be used for the insertion, remember that the needle must be small enough to fit into the vein but large enough to allow the infusion to run at the prescribed rate. Experience, institution policy, and the advice of experienced coworkers will help in these decisions.

Other Supplies

Preparation of all necessary equipment prior to the actual performance of the venipuncture will aid in making the process go smoothly. Knowledge of your institution's policies and procedures will help you to assemble correctly the administration set, including any extension tubing or T-connectors, and to perform the preferred method for anchoring the IV catheter to the patient.

If at all possible, the IV fluid and administration set should be prepared outside of the patient's room. This will help to avoid creating anxiety in the patient.

The prescribed fluid bag should be obtained. Prior to opening, confirm that the correct fluid is being selected, such as 0.9% NaCl (physiologic saline). The expiration date of the fluid should be visible through the opaque or transparent covering. Open the protective covering by tearing at the precut tab.

Inspect the integrity of the bag by squeezing it firmly to look for any small leaks (Figure 23-4). The fluid inside should be clear and free from particulate matter. At this time if there are any medications that need to be added, they can be injected into the port with the yellow rubber stopper, located either on the bottom of the bag or in the lower front portion.

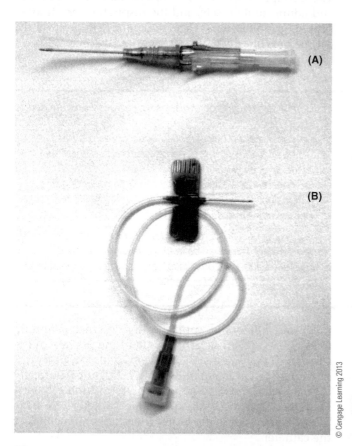

(A)

(B)

© Cengage Learning 2013

Figure 23-3 Two common types of catheters are the butterfly, on the right with the small tubing attached, and the over-the-needle type of catheter

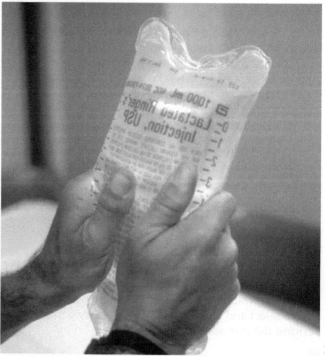

© Cengage Learning 2013

Figure 23-4 Firmly squeezing the intravenous solution bag allows for the detection of any small holes in the container

Select the proper administration set. If an infusion pump will be used, make sure that the set is compatible with the pump to be used. Occlude the tubing by either closing the roller clamp or using one of the small slide clamps.

Remove the protective cap from the end with the drip chamber attached. Remove the protective cap from the IV bag. Insert the "spike" from the administration set into the port on the IV bag (Figure 23-5). Care must be used because the plastic spike is very sharp and it is possible to push the spike through the side of the port, where it may injure your hand or fingers.

Fill the drip chamber halfway by squeezing the chamber once or twice. Allow the flow to stop before unclasping the tubing to help reduce the number of small air bubbles that enter the tubing. In the event that the chamber becomes overfilled, simply invert the chamber and the bag and then squeeze some of the fluid back into the bag.

Flush the administration tubing by releasing the roller or slide clamp. It may be necessary to remove the protective cap from the end of the set to allow the fluid to flow more freely. Care must be taken to not touch the end of the tubing, however, as it is sterile. Hold the end of the tubing lower than the bag to allow the fluid to flow. If a cassette for an infusion pump is in line, this portion of the tubing may have to be held inverted to clear all air and allow for proper function.

Once the entire tubing has been flushed, replace the protective cap on the male end if it has been removed.

Another type of administration set that may be used is a heparin or saline lock. This allows for the administration of prn medications without having a solution bag and administration tubing attached. The set consists of a male adapter plug that can be directly attached to the IV catheter or a short T-connector. The plug and any tubing attached to it must be flushed using a syringe filled with either normal saline solution or a very dilute heparin solution used specifically for heparin locks. Again, check with institution policy to see which is preferred.

There are commercial IV start kits that may be available. These kits include all of the necessary supplies except for gloves and the catheter itself.

If you need to assemble the necessary supplies yourself, here is a list of what you will need:

1. Protective gloves
2. Mask
3. Protective eyewear (in case of inadvertent splashing of blood)
4. A selection of IV catheters
5. Tape
6. Tourniquet
7. 2 × 2-inch gauze
8. Alcohol swabs
9. Povidone-iodine swabs
10. Sterile, transparent dressing for covering the insertion site
11. Local anesthetic, if required
12. Approved sharps container

Take all supplies to the patient's bedside. Organize the supplies in such a manner that all can be reached easily.

VENIPUNCTURE PROCEDURE

With practice, venipuncture can be accomplished quickly and professionally. Developing a plan or system that suits your preferences will help ensure success.

Standard Precautions

Blood and blood products are body fluids that require adherence to Standard Precautions. It is important to wear protective gloves, a mask, and eyewear to minimize the risk of acquiring an illness owing to inadvertent exposure to these fluids.

General Considerations

A physician's order is required before the performance of IV cannulation. The patient's chart should be reviewed for such an order. If your institution has established

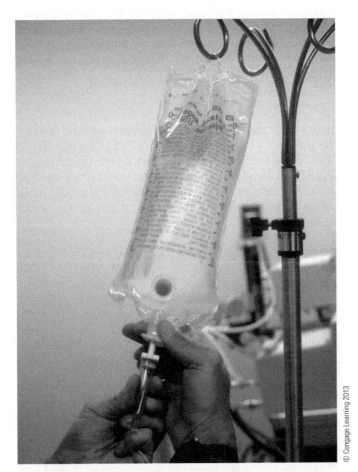

© Cengage Learning 2013

Figure 23-5 Insertion of the spike of the administration set into the fluid bag allows fluid to flow into the tubing. Care must be taken because the spike is sharp and can cause injury

protocols covering IV insertion, you should be familiar with them.

The patient should be educated about the procedure and any questions answered prior to beginning. Many people have a fear of needles; therefore, a professional, knowledgeable manner will help to alleviate some of this anxiety.

The patient should be asked about any allergies relating to iodine products and tape. There are many different types of tape that can be used to lessen reactions due to sensitivity or allergy. Alcohol only can be used if the patient has had previous reactions to iodine products.

It may be necessary to shave the arm of the patient with a safety razor to remove hair that would interfere with securing the IV. An area approximately 2 inches square should be shaved around the planned insertion site.

Local Anesthetic Use

Many institutions require that a local anesthetic be used prior to the insertion of an IV needle. The puncture site should be prepared in the same manner as for IV insertion described later in the chapter. Draw up 0.1 to 0.2 mL of 2% lidocaine, without epinephrine, into a tuberculin syringe with a 25-gauge needle. Puncture the skin at the site chosen for IV placement. The needle should be in the dermal layer. Draw back on the plunger. If blood appears, the needle has entered a vessel and should be removed and moved to another location.

Slowly inject the anesthetic into the skin to produce a *wheal* at the site. The wheal should be approximately 1 cm in diameter. Withdraw the needle and dab any blood that may appear with a 2 × 2-inch gauze sponge. Allow 1 or 2 minutes before performing the venipuncture.

Do not recap the syringe. Place the used syringe in an approved sharps container.

Site Preparation

Once the equipment has been assembled and the procedure explained to the patient, a site for insertion of the catheter can be chosen. Wash your hands and don protective gloves.

Apply the tourniquet above the location on the arm where you will be looking for an acceptable vein. In most cases the tourniquet can be placed above the elbow (Figure 23-6). This allows evaluation of the entire lower arm for suitable vessels. However, the tourniquet can be placed above the wrist or in the middle of the forearm.

After the application of the tourniquet, palpate for a radial pulse to ensure that arterial blood flow has not been occluded. Have the patient place the arm in a dependent position. The patient can also be asked to clench the fist several times to aid in distending the veins.

Visually locate a vein that appears suitable. Gently palpate the vein with your finger for any valves or bifurcations. The distended vein should rebound quickly when palpated. If local anesthetic will be used, release the tourniquet, cleanse the area appropriately, and inject the anesthetic. After 1 or 2 minutes, reapply the tourniquet.

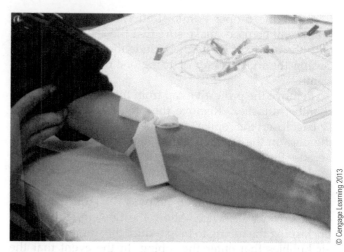

Figure 23-6 The tourniquet is used to occlude venous flow and distend the veins with blood. This allows for visualization and palpation of the vein to determine its usefulness for venipuncture

Cleanse the area chosen for insertion with the povidone-iodine solution. This should be done in a circular motion (Figure 23-7), beginning at the center and moving outward.

The povidone-iodine is removed using an alcohol swab (Figure 23-8). Begin at the top center of the area and wipe toward the hand. Move to the side of the area just cleansed, and again wipe the swab from top to bottom. Continue this process until the entire area has been cleansed. The site chosen for insertion should be roughly in the center of this clean area.

Technique

Select an IV catheter of the appropriate size and remove the protective sleeve (Figure 23-9). Grasp the catheter in your dominant hand (Figure 23-10) with your fingers located on the plastic of the stylet. Do not grasp the hub of the catheter, as it will simply slide off the needle when insertion is attempted. The bevel of the metal needle

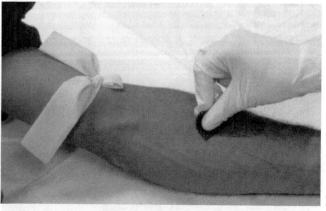

Figure 23-7 The site chosen for venipuncture is cleansed with a povidone-iodine solution. This should be performed beginning at the center and proceeding outwards in ever-widening circles

should be facing directly upward. In a well-lit room, the light will reflect off the bevel (Figure 23-11).

Using your other hand, apply gentle traction to the skin by pulling it toward the patient's hand. This will help to stabilize the vein and will prevent the skin from bunching up as the needle is inserted.

With the needle held at an angle of approximately 10° to 30° up from the skin (Figure 23-12), enter the skin with a quick, firm motion (Figure 23-13). Remember that you are attempting not to enter the vein at this point but simply to get through the dermal layers.

While maintaining the same or slightly shallower angle from the skin, advance the needle toward the vein. A "flash" of blood in the clear chamber of the catheter (Figure 23-14) indicates that the vessel has been entered. It is also common to feel a slight "pop" as the needle enters the vein. Advance the entire needle approximately 5 to 10 mm to ensure that the catheter has also entered the

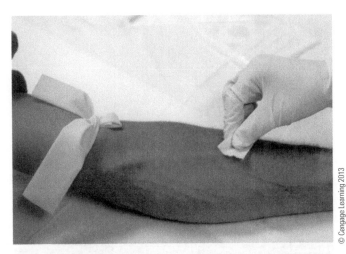

Figure 23-8 The povidone-iodine is removed using an alcohol swab. When the site cleansing is complete, an area approximately 2 inches square will be prepped

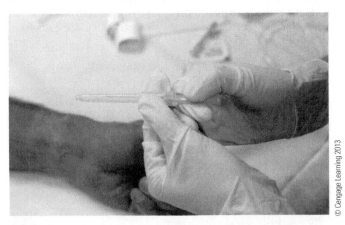

Figure 23-9 Grasping the plastic portion of the catheter in one hand and the protective cover in the other, remove the cover by pulling in opposite directions

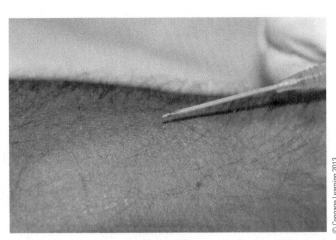

Figure 23-11 With proper lighting, the bevel of the needle can be easily located and should be kept facing directly up from the patient's skin

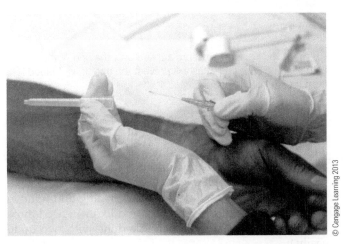

Figure 23-10 After removal of the protective cover, maintain your fingers on the plastic portion of the stylet. Begin looking for the bevel of the needle

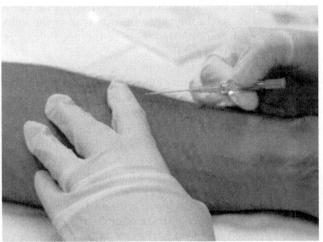

Figure 23-12 The correct angle of insertion between the patient's skin and the needle is between 10° and 30°

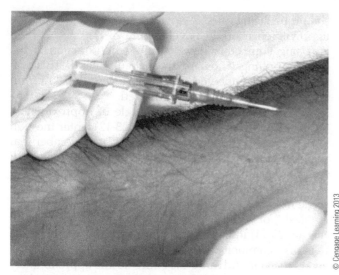

Figure 23-13 The initial step of insertion is to get the needle through the dermal layers of the skin, not directly into the vein

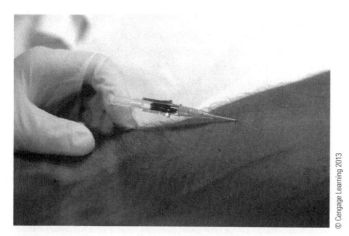

Figure 23-14 As the needle enters the vein, blood will appear in the flash chamber of the needle. The entire unit should then be advanced about 1 cm

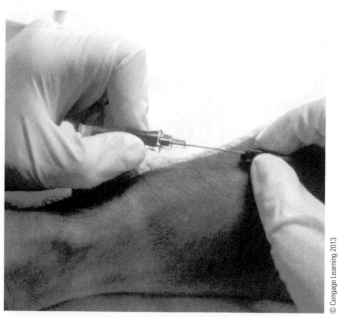

Figure 23-15 After the hub of the catheter has been advanced so that it is touching the skin, remove the stylet with one hand while applying pressure on the skin over the end of the catheter with the other hand

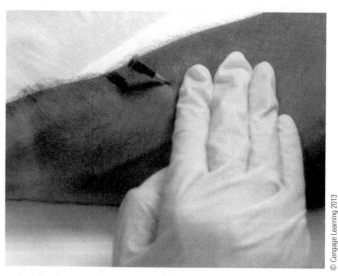

Figure 23-16 Firm pressure applied over the end of the catheter with your fingertips will prevent the free flow of blood from the end of the catheter

vein. Care must be taken at this point so that the needle is not allowed to go through the opposite wall of the vein, resulting in infiltration. The angle of the needle can be lowered to help prevent this.

The nondominant hand can now release traction on the skin and grasp the hub of the catheter. Gently slide the catheter off the needle/stylet and advance it until the front part of the hub is in contact with the skin. Do not withdraw the needle as you are doing this (Figure 23-15), as it provides direction and stabilization for the flexible catheter.

With the nondominant hand, reach up and grasp the folded-over end of the tourniquet, and with a quick pull, remove the tourniquet.

After the catheter is in place, with the hub against the skin, one or two fingers of the nondominant hand should be firmly placed on the skin (Figure 23-16) over the area where the end of the plastic catheter is lying. This will help to prevent a rush of blood out of the catheter when the needle is removed.

Remove the needle/stylet with the dominant hand and place it in the sharps container (Figure 23-17). Place a 2 × 2-inch gauze sponge under the hub of the catheter to catch any blood that may leak out. Grasp the end of the administration set or male adapter plug and remove the protective cover. (This may sound like you need three hands, but with practice, it can be done with two quite easily.)

Insert the end of the tubing or plug into the hub of the catheter and, with a slight twisting motion, push the two together (Figure 23-18).

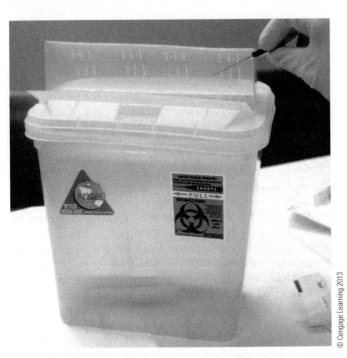

Figure 23-17   All needles should be disposed of in an approved sharps disposal container

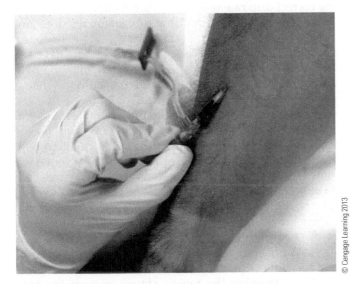

Figure 23-18   Attach the end of the administration set tubing into the hub of the catheter. This can be done with a slight twisting motion to ensure a patent, leak-free connection

While holding the catheter in place, open the roller clamp slowly. Watch the drip chamber for evidence of flow. If it appears that the IV infusion is not running, the catheter tip may be against the vessel wall, impeding the flow. Slowly withdraw the catheter, up to 1 cm, while watching the drip chamber. When good flow is obtained, discontinue withdrawing the catheter and hold it in position.

Cover the site with the sterile, transparent dressing. The dressing should cover only the hub of the catheter and the actual puncture site (Figure 23-19). Do not cover

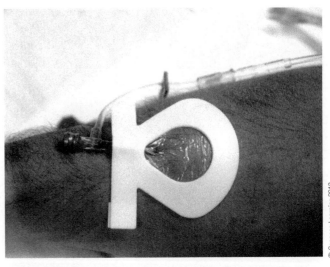

Figure 23-19   A sterile transparent dressing should cover the site of insertion. This allows for continuing visualization of the site for any signs or symptoms of redness or swelling

the end of the administration tubing. This allows for easy change of the tubing if necessary without the risk of disengaging the catheter from the vessel.

During the next steps, care must be taken that the patient does not move the extremity. Explain to the patient that you are going to tape the IV catheter in place. Gross movement may dislodge the IV, as it is being kept in place only by the transparent dressing.

Slide a 1/2-inch-wide piece of tape, approximately 3 inches long, under the end of the tubing where it connects to the catheter, sticky side facing up, centering the tubing and hub in the piece of tape. Cross one end of the tape over the tubing and stick the tape to the patient's skin. Cross the remaining end over and stick it to the skin. This taping pattern, called a *chevron,* helps to secure the end of the tubing and the hub of the catheter in place (Figure 23-20). Place a 2-inch piece of tape over the chevron, securing it to the patient. Approximately 1 to 2 inches from the first piece of tape, place another 2-inch piece of tape across the tubing.

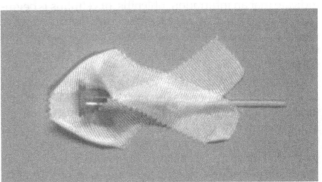

Figure 23-20   A chevron results when the tape is placed under the catheter hub sticky side up, and the ends of the tape are then criss-crossed over the catheter hub

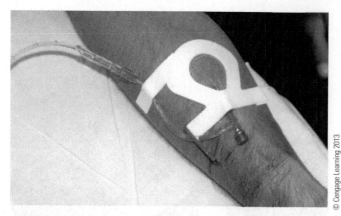

© Cengage Learning 2013

Figure 23-21 A loop of tubing and adequate securing with tape will help to prevent the inadvertent dislodging of the catheter

Make either a half loop or a full loop out of the administration tubing (Figure 23-21), and secure it with tape. This excess tubing serves as a safety device in case the tubing is inadvertently pulled. The loop changes the direction of pull so that the catheter is not pulled in the opposite direction in which it was inserted.

At this time, either place the cassette in the pump and begin administering the fluids or adjust the roller clamp so that the fluid flows at the prescribed rate. The calculations necessary should have been performed prior to the beginning of the insertion procedure.

If it is necessary to place an arm board to prevent the catheter from being occluded secondary to patient movement, do so at this time. The board should be padded for patient comfort and should be long enough to extend both above and below the insertion site far enough to prevent movement. When taping the board in place, do so in a manner that does not restrict the flow of blood or the fluid infusing from the IV.

An important element to remember in securing the tubing and catheter in place is that tape should not cover any of the Y injection ports located in the tubing. These sites are for administration of medications into the tubing and should be left uncovered.

Explain to the patient that the procedure is complete. Educate the patient about signs and symptoms that may indicate that an infiltration, phlebitis, or cellulitis is beginning. Have the patient alert the care provider of any pain, swelling, or redness that may occur. Also give the patient time to address any questions or concerns that he or she may have.

Make sure that all used needles have been placed in an approved container. Collect all used supplies and their wrappers, protective covers, and so on, and place them in the appropriate waste containers. Clean up any spilled blood with the approved antiseptic cleaner. Remember that any items contaminated with blood or body fluids should be placed in a biohazard waste container. Remove your gloves, wash your hands, and record the procedure in the patient's chart. Local policy will dictate the manner in which this is done.

MAINTENANCE OF INTRAVENOUS INFUSIONS

The IV infusion line should be checked on a regular basis to ensure that the infusion is running properly, that the fluid level in the bag is appropriate, and that there are no signs of impending problems with the site. These checks also allow for the changing of tubing as it is required.

When performing the maintenance of IV infusions, attempt to develop a routine that will allow you to perform these checks in a timely and efficient manner. In this routine, the fluid level of the IV solution should be checked. If it is necessary to change the fluid, obtain a new bag of solution and confirm that it is clear, not outdated, and the correct type of fluid. Open the protective bag and remove the solution. Clamp the administration set tubing with either the roller clamp or a slide clamp. Remove the protective plug or cap from the new bag. Holding the drip chamber in an upright position, tip the solution bag upside down, and pull the drip chamber "spike" from the bag. Inverting the solution bag will prevent any remaining fluid from running out when the drip chamber is removed. Reinsert the drip chamber spike into the new solution bag. Hang the bag and reset the correct drip rate using the roller clamp.

Ensure that the administration set tubing does not need to be changed. Many institutions use color-coded labels or dated labels to track how long a tubing has been in use. If the tubing needs to be changed, obtain a new administration set that matches the one currently being used. Prepare a small syringe, 1 mL or 3 mL, by filling it with the same fluid that is being infused into the patient. This can be done by withdrawing the fluid from one of the ports on the side or bottom of the IV solution bag. Remove the needle, dispose of it in the sharps container, and set the syringe aside where it can be easily reached. Take care not to contaminate the syringe hub. A male adapter plug can be used in place of the syringe if this adheres to hospital policy. Remember that the plug must be flushed with solution to remove any air before it is used. Wash your hands and put on protective gloves, a mask, and eye protection.

After clamping the tubing closed, remove the tape from the tubing beginning at the end nearer the solution bag. As you get closer to the hub of the catheter and the end of the tubing, take care that you do not inadvertently pull the catheter from the vein. Once all of the tape has been removed from the tubing, gently pull the end of the tubing from the hub of the catheter. While you are doing this, use one or two fingers to apply pressure to the skin over the end of the catheter to prevent the flow of blood from the catheter hub. Place the syringe or male adapter plug into the hub of the catheter.

Invert the solution bag, remove the old administration set, and dispose of it in a biohazard waste container. Remove the protective cover from the "spike" of the new set and insert it into the solution bag. Squeeze the drip chamber until it is half full and flush the air from the tubing by opening the clamp and allowing the solution to flow. Reattach the tubing to the catheter hub after removing the syringe or plug, and retape the tubing to secure it to the patient. Clean up any spilled fluid or blood; remove your gloves, mask, and eyewear; and wash your hands again.

DISCONTINUING INTRAVENOUS THERAPY

IV therapy can be discontinued for any number of reasons. You should be familiar with how to remove the catheter and dress the site to minimize patient discomfort, prevent unnecessary hematoma formation, and help prevent infection.

Once the decision has been made to remove the catheter, the procedure is quite simple. Aseptic technique and standard precautions should be observed.

After washing your hands and putting on protective gloves, a mask, and eyewear, clamp the IV tubing to discontinue the flow of the solution. Open one or two packages of sterile 2 × 2-inch gauze sponges and have them easily accessible. Begin untaping the tubing from the patient's arm. When the tape is removed, carefully peel the edges of the transparent dressing away from the patient's skin. It is not necessary to remove the dressing from the hub of the catheter, as attempting to do so may inadvertently pull the catheter out.

Once the tubing and catheter are no longer secured to the patient, place a folded 2 × 2-inch sponge over the insertion site and press gently. Grasp the hub of the catheter and quickly pull it from the skin. Continue to press firmly over the insertion site to help minimize bleeding both at the skin and at the vessel. You should continue to hold pressure over the site for at least 5 minutes.

Inspect the catheter that has been removed to ensure that it is intact. If you suspect that a portion of the catheter was not removed, immediately notify the person in charge of the patient's care.

After ensuring that the site is not actively bleeding, place a different folded 2 × 2-inch sponge over the site and secure it with a piece of tape. In some institutions it is acceptable to use an adhesive strip-type bandage in place of the 2 × 2-inch sponge. Use of antibiotic ointment may be desirable prior to placing the 2 × 2-inch sponge dressing.

Clean up the area that has been used and dispose of all supplies, including the IV bag, tubing, and catheter, in a biohazard waste container. Remove your gloves and wash your hands.

References

American Heart Association. (2006). *Advanced cardiac life support provider manual*. Dallas, TX: Author.

Caroline, N. L. (1993). *Emergency care in the streets* (3rd ed.). Boston: Little, Brown.

Grant, H. D., O'Keefe, M., Limmer, D., Murry, R., & Bergeron, J. (1990). *Brady emergency care*. Englewood Cliffs, NJ: Prentice-Hall.

Additional Resources

Bruner, P. M., Sineltzer, S., & Bare, B. (1984). *Textbook of medical-surgical nursing*. Philadelphia: Lippincott.

Potter, P. (1987). *Basic nursing theory and practice*. St. Louis, MO: Mosby.

Saxton, D. F., Pelikan, P. K., Nugent, P. M., & Hyland, P. A. (1983). *Addison-Wesley manual of nursing practice*. Menlo Park, CA: Addison-Wesley.

Practice Activities: Intravenous Line Insertion and Maintenance

1. Prepare the IV solution to be used:
   a. Identify the proper solution per physician order.
   b. Open the package (save the package/bag).
   c. Recheck the proper solution and expiration date.
   d. Gently squeeze the bag to ensure that there are no leaks.
   e. Remove the protective covering from the outlet port of the fluid bag.
   f. Hang the fluid bag on an IV pole or hook (use anything applicable).
   g. Remove the protective covering from the spike/sharp end of the infusion tubing.
   h. Insert the sharp end of the infusion tubing into the uncovered port of the fluid bag (make sure that it is snug).
   i. Fill the infusion tubing drip chamber by squeezing it several times until the drip chamber is half filled.
   j. Remove the protective covering from the patient end of the infusion tubing, being careful not to touch this end and keeping it sterile.

k. Making use of gravity and using the package/bag that the solution came in to catch the drips, allow the IV solution to flow freely out the patient end until all bubbles are cleared from the infusion tubing. (NOTE: Watch for bubbles that collect in the injection ports upstream.)

2. Prepare and gather the IV supplies:
   a. Lay all the supplies needed close to where you will be performing the procedure:
      (1) IV pole with solution and tubing
      (2) Tourniquet
      (3) Razor
      (4) Povidone-iodine swab
      (5) Alcohol-based swab
      (6) IV catheter
      (7) Securing tape/holder

3. Prepare your patient:
   a. Set the patient at ease.
   b. Explain what you are going to do.
   c. Explain why you are doing it.
   d. Position yourself and the patient comfortably.

4. Using a laboratory partner as your patient, perform the following for the listed venous puncture sites:
   a. Properly position the patient.
   b. Locate the probable insertion site.
   c. Palpate the site.

   Puncture sites:
      (1) Medial vein of the forearm
      (2) Radial vein in the wrist
      (3) Cephalic vein on the back of the hand

5. Apply a tourniquet to the arm to cause venous distention.
   a. Place a tourniquet 10 cm or 5 inches above the insertion site.
   b. Have your partner clench and unclench the fist several times.

c. Palpate the insertion site.
d. Practice tying and releasing the tourniquet several times.

6. Prepare the insertion site:
   a. Wash your hands.
   b. Don disposable gloves.
   c. Scrub the area directly over the vein using a povidone-iodine swab. Move the swab in ever-widening circles away from the center of the puncture site, out approximately 4 cm.
   d. Scrub the area directly over the vein using an alcohol-based swab. Move the swab in ever-widening circles away from the center of the puncture site, out approximately 4 cm.

7. Prepare the IV catheter:
   a. Open the catheter in a manner that preserves its sterility. (Follow the manufacturer's directions.)
   b. Remove the catheter from the package using the two to three fingers that you will use to insert the catheter (take care not to touch the needle end of the catheter with your fingers).

8. Using a venous arm simulator:
   a. Practice preparing the IV solution to include when flushing the infusion tubing.
   b. Practice accumulating the supplies you will need.
   c. Observe Standard Precautions and aseptic technique.
   d. Practice placement of the tourniquet.
   e. Practice holding the catheter with your fingers.
   f. Practice the angle of catheter insertion.
   g. Practice your insertion skill.
   h. Practice removing the tourniquet.
   i. Practice hooking up the infusion tubing.
   j. Practice the proper disposal of sharps and waste.
   k. Practice the proper securing of the catheter.

Check List: Peripheral IV Insertion

_____ 1. Verify the physician's order.
_____ 2. Check the patient's chart for contraindications and pertinent information.
   3. Gather the supplies:
_____   a. Disposable gloves
_____   b. Razor
_____   c. Povidone-iodine swab
_____   d. Alcohol-based swab
_____   e. Tourniquet
_____   f. IV fluid
_____   g. IV solution
_____   h. IV catheter of appropriate size
_____   i. Tape or securing system
_____   j. Sharps container
_____   k. Waste container

_____ 4. Wash your hands.
_____ 5. Don disposable gloves.
_____ 6. Explain the procedure to the patient.
_____ 7. Position the patient.
_____ 8. Position yourself.
   9. Palpate the arm for an appropriate site:
_____   a. Medial vein of the forearm
_____   b. Radial vein of the wrist
_____   c. Cephalic vein on the back of the hand
_____ 10. Apply the tourniquet.
_____ 11. Repalpate the arm and choose a specific site.
   12. Prep the site:
_____   a. Use a razor if hair will interfere.
_____   b. Use povidone-iodine swab.
_____   c. Use alcohol-based swab.

_____ 13. Open the package using sterile technique and position the catheter for insertion.

14. Perform the IV puncture:

_____ a. Use the correct angle (10° to 30° and aligned with the vein).

_____ b. Ensure that the bevel is up.

_____ c. Penetrate the skin.

_____ d. Advance the needle to flashback.

_____ e. Advance the catheter only into the vein.

_____ f. Remove the needle and place it in the sharps container.

_____ g. With the free hand, apply firm pressure with the fingers directly to the cannulated vein at least 2 cm above the hub.

_____ 15. Insert the infusion tubing into the hub of the catheter snugly.

_____ 16. Release the tourniquet.

_____ 17. Release the finger pressure of the free hand.

_____ 18. Secure the catheter hub using a sterile transparent dressing.

_____ 19. Secure the infusion tubing to the arm.

_____ 20. Run the solution per the physician's order.

21. Observe for complications:

_____ a. Infiltration

_____ b. Impaired flow of the solution

22. Document the procedure:

_____ a. Time

_____ b. Date

_____ c. Catheter size

_____ d. Site

_____ e. Number of attempts

_____ f. Solution used

_____ g. Rate of infusion

Self-Evaluation Post Test: Intravenous Line Insertion and Maintenance

1. Complications of a peripheral IV insertion include:
   a. hematoma.   c. infection.
   b. air embolus.   d. All of the above

2. It is acceptable to have a few air bubbles left in your infusion tubing before hooking it up to the patient/catheter.
   a. True
   b. False

3. All of the following supplies will be required to insert an IV catheter *except*:
   a. scalpel.
   b. povidone-iodine swab
   c. IV catheter.
   d. tape.

4. A tourniquet should be placed:
   a. between the puncture site and the shoulder.
   b. 6 to 12 cm above the puncture site.
   c. below the site.
   d. 5 to 10 cm above the puncture site.

5. Upon insertion, the bevel of the needle should be:
   a. up.
   b. down.
   c. pointed to the left side.
   d. pointed to the right side.

6. The proper angle of the IV insertion is:
   a. 30° to 60° and aligned with the vein.
   b. 10° to 30° degrees and aligned with the vein.
   c. 60° and aligned with the vein.
   d. 45° and aligned with the vein.

7. Which of the following is an indicator confirming that you are in the vein and that it is patent?
   a. Good flashback
   b. Little resistance to the advancing catheter
   c. Free-running IV solution
   d. All of the above

8. It is considered acceptable to take off one of your gloves to get a better feel for the vein.
   a. True   b. False

9. After catheter insertion, but before tourniquet removal, finger pressure on the cannulated vein allows:
   a. for pain control.
   b. time for the infusion tubing to be attached before blood flow begins to back up.
   c. time to flush the infusion tubing to get it ready.
   d. time for the disposal of sharps.

10. When documenting an IV insertion, you should include:
    a. date/time.   c. number of attempts.
    b. catheter/size.   d. site.

PERFORMANCE EVALUATION:
Intravenous Line Insertion and Maintenance

Date: Lab _____ Clinical _____ Agency _____

Lab: Pass _____ Fail _____ Clinical: Pass _____ Fail _____

Student name _____ Instructor name _____

No. of times observed in clinical _____

No. of times practiced in clinical _____

PASSING CRITERIA: Obtain 90% or better on the procedure. Tasks indicated by * must receive at least 1 point, or the evaluation is terminated. Procedure must be performed within the designated time, or the performance receives a failing grade.

SCORING:
2 points — Task performed satisfactorily without prompting.
1 point — Task performed satisfactorily with self-initiated correction.
0 points — Task performed incorrectly or with prompting required.
NA — Task not applicable to the patient care situation.

Tasks:	Peer	Lab	Clinical
* **1.** Verifies the physician's order	☐	☐	☐
2. Scans the chart	☐	☐	☐
* **3.** Gathers the necessary supplies			
a. Disposable gloves	☐	☐	☐
b. Razor	☐	☐	☐
c. Iodine-based swab	☐	☐	☐
d. Alcohol-based swab	☐	☐	☐
e. Tourniquet	☐	☐	☐
f. IV catheter	☐	☐	☐
g. Securing tape/transparent sterile dressing	☐	☐	☐
h. IV solution	☐	☐	☐
i. Infusion tubing	☐	☐	☐
* **4.** Follows standard precautions, including handwashing	☐	☐	☐
* **5.** Dons gloves, a mask, and protective eyewear	☐	☐	☐
* **6.** Prepares the IV solution	☐	☐	☐
* **7.** Prepares the infusion tubing without bubbles	☐	☐	☐
8. Positions self and the patient	☐	☐	☐
9. Explains the procedure to the patient	☐	☐	☐

* **10.** Palpates the probable sites ☐ ☐ ☐

* **11.** Applies the tourniquet ☐ ☐ ☐

* **12.** Repalpates and chooses a specific site ☐ ☐ ☐

* **13.** Prepares the insertion site

     a. Preps the area with iodine-based swab ☐ ☐ ☐

     b. Cleans the area with alcohol-based swab ☐ ☐ ☐

* **14.** Prepares the IV catheter

     a. Opens the package, maintaining a sterile catheter ☐ ☐ ☐

     b. Holds the catheter in the fingers ☐ ☐ ☐

* **15.** Inserts the IV catheter

     a. Bevel is up ☐ ☐ ☐

     b. Correct angle is at 10° to 30° ☐ ☐ ☐

     c. Advances to flashback ☐ ☐ ☐

     d. Advances the catheter into the vein ☐ ☐ ☐

     e. Removes the needle to the sharps container ☐ ☐ ☐

     f. Applies finger pressure to the vein proximal to the site ☐ ☐ ☐

* **16.** Inserts the infusion tubing ☐ ☐ ☐

* **17.** Removes the tourniquet ☐ ☐ ☐

* **18.** Secures the catheter hub with tape ☐ ☐ ☐

* **19.** Secures the infusion tubing with tape ☐ ☐ ☐

* **20.** Runs the solution per physician's order ☐ ☐ ☐

* **21.** Watches for complications ☐ ☐ ☐

   22. Cleans up the area and removes unused supplies ☐ ☐ ☐

* **23.** Documents the procedure ☐ ☐ ☐

SCORE:　　　　Peer _____ points of possible 70; _____%

　　　　　　　　　Lab _____ points of possible 70; _____%

　　　　　　　　　Clinical _____ points of possible 70; _____%

TIME: _____ out of possible 20 minutes

STUDENT SIGNATURES

PEER: _____

STUDENT: _____

INSTRUCTOR SIGNATURES

LAB: _____

CLINICAL: _____

SECTION IV
Ventilation

CHAPTER 24

Noninvasive Positive-Pressure Ventilation

INTRODUCTION

Noninvasive positive-pressure ventilation (NPPV) is the application of positive pressure via the upper respiratory tract to augment alveolar ventilation (American Respiratory Care Foundation [ARCF], 1997). For the purposes of this chapter, NPPV is further defined as the application of positive-pressure ventilation to the upper respiratory tract using either a nasal or a full-face mask as the ventilator-patient interface. NPPV is not new but has been used for many years (Pierson, 1997). Application of NPPV is becoming more common. NPPV may eliminate the need for intubation or placement of a tracheostomy.

Ventilators used for NPPV include any of the acute care ventilators employed in the intensive care setting. However, the ventilators most commonly applied for this purpose are the portable pressure-targeted ventilators (PTVs) such as *continuous positive airway pressure (CPAP)* and *bilevel positive airway pressure (Bi-PAP®)* ventilators (Kacmarek, 1997). Recent advances in technology have improved the monitoring capabilities of these ventilators. These advances, combined with concurrent advances in electrocardiography (ECG), oximetry, and blood pressure monitoring, have reduced some of the risks associated with managing patients using NPPV. In addition to dedicated CPAP or Bi-PAP® ventilators, many critical care ventilators have the capability of NPPV. These ventilators have an advantage of comprehensive monitoring capability and alarms.

KEY TERMS

- **Bilevel positive airway pressure (Bi-PAP®)**
- **Continuous positive airway pressure (CPAP)**
- **Expiratory positive airway pressure**
- **Full-face mask**
- **Inspiratory positive airway pressure**
- **Nasal mask**

- **Nasal pillows**
- **Nasogastric tube**
- **Pressure-targeted ventilation (PTV)**
- **Rapid-shallow-breathing index**

- **Spacers**
- **Spontaneous breath**
- **Timed mode**
- **Total™ Mask**

THEORY OBJECTIVES

At the end of this chapter, the reader should be able to:

- *Define noninvasive positive-pressure ventilation (NPPV).*
- *List the indications for NPPV.*
- *Describe the assessment of a patient for NPPV.*
- *Compare and contrast the advantages and disadvantages of nasal and full-face masks as the patient-ventilator interface.*
- *State the hazards and complications associated with NPPV.*

- *Describe the effects of changes in resistance and compliance on volume delivery with pressure-targeted ventilation (PTV).*
- *Describe the modes of NPPV.*
- *Explain how to provide supplemental oxygen.*
- *State what monitoring devices should be used when a patient is receiving NPPV.*

DEFINITION OF NONINVASIVE POSITIVE-PRESSURE VENTILATION

Noninvasive positive-pressure ventilation (NPPV) is the application of positive pressure via the upper respiratory tract to augment alveolar ventilation (ARCF, 1997). NPPV is increasingly used to provide improved alveolar ventilation to those patients in acute respiratory failure, especially when intubation is not desirable (Brochard et al., 1995; Wunderink & Hill, 1997). By using a nasal or full-face mask as the interface between the patient and the ventilator, the associated complications of intubation may be avoided. Advantages of avoiding intubation include better ability of the patient to communicate and the ability to take fluids and medications orally.

INDICATIONS FOR NONINVASIVE POSITIVE-PRESSURE VENTILATION

The indications for NPPV are summarized in Table 24-1.

Many authors have investigated the efficacy of NPPV in acute respiratory failure (Brochard et al., 1995; Kramer, Meyer, Meharg, Cece, & Hill, 1995; Martin et al., 2000). The greatest number of patients in which this modality has been used is acute exacerbation of chronic obstructive pulmonary disease (COPD). NPPV can be effective in augmenting alveolar ventilation with the goals of reducing partial pressure of carbon dioxide in the arterial blood ($PaCO_2$), increasing partial pressure of oxygen in the arterial blood (PaO_2), increasing oxygen saturation (SpO_2), and normalizing arterial pH. Intubation and mechanical ventilation may accomplish many of these same goals; however, NPPV avoids the hazards and complications of intubation as described in Chapter 20.

TABLE 24-1: Indications for NPPV in Acute Respiratory Failure

Acute exacerbation of chronic obstructive pulmonary disease

Acute hypoxemic respiratory failure

Acute cardiogenic pulmonary edema

Weaning from ventilatory support

Community-acquired pneumonia

Postoperative respiratory failure

Severe acute asthma

Do not resuscitate/do not intubate orders

Patients with COPD benefit from NPPV by avoiding intubation (Brochard et al., 1995; Wunderink & Hill, 1997). Often, once intubated, these patients tend to have an extended ventilator course and may be difficult to wean and extubate. NPPV may help the patient through the period of acute respiratory failure, allowing time for antibiotics, diuretics, and other medications to work, so that intubation is avoided.

Hypoxic respiratory failure may also be an indication for NPPV. This is especially true in cases in which the patient or the patient's family has requested not to intubate or resuscitate. In these cases, NPPV may assist the patient through the acute respiratory failure phase, giving other medications time to work. NPPV can temporarily reverse the hypoxemia and hypercarbia associated with acute respiratory failure.

NPPV may also play a role in acute cardiogenic pulmonary edema (Mehta et al., 1997). NPPV can again provide augmented alveolar ventilation until other medications have time to work (diuretics and cardiac medications). NPPV helps the patient through the period of acute respiratory failure, and once the pulmonary edema resolves, the patient may resume spontaneous respiration.

In some cases, the patient fails initial weaning and extubation from mechanical ventilation. NPPV can provide a means of augmenting alveolar ventilation without reintubation and initiation of conventional ventilation. NPPV can again provide time, permitting the patient to gain ventilatory strength and to complete the weaning process successfully.

Community-acquired pneumonia can lead to ventilatory failure and corresponding hypercapnia and hypoxemia. In these cases, NPPV may provide the muscle unloading and ventilatory assistance required, overcoming the patient's short-term ventilatory failure. The potential benefits of short-term NPPV include avoidance of intubation and providing time (ventilatory support) for the antibiotics and other medications to work.

NPPV may also be helpful in postoperative respiratory failure. Postoperative respiratory failure is characterized by hypoxemia and hypercarbia. NPPV can provide ventilatory assistance without intubation, supporting these patients until the underlying cause of respiratory failure has resolved.

NPPV has been successfully used in asthma and status asthmaticus (Meduri et al., 1991; Pollack, Torres, & Alexander, 1996). In asthma, the patient may present with hypercarbia and hypoxemia. NPPV can support the patient's ventilation without intubation and, therefore, has been shown to have benefit.

Many patients with chronic disease have made the determination, with or without family consensus, to not be intubated and mechanically ventilated when they become terminally ill. NPPV has been used to provide ventilatory support in these patients, potentially allowing time to overcome the cause of ventilatory failure.

ASSESSMENT OF THE PATIENT FOR NONINVASIVE POSITIVE-PRESSURE VENTILATION

Patient assessment for NPPV is similar to assessment of patients for intubation and continuous mechanical ventilation. Assessment should include determination of ventilatory parameters, arterial blood gases, oxygen saturation, and work of breathing and detection of changes in the patient's vital signs.

Ventilatory parameters include tidal volume, minute volume, frequency, and the rapid-shallow-breathing index. Tidal volumes of less than 3 to 5 mL/kg are indicative of impending ventilatory failure. A patient cannot move sufficient volume (greater than dead space volume) to sustain ventilatory needs when the tidal volume falls to this level. A minute volume in excess of 10 L/min is also indicative of impending failure. Excessive muscle work is required to sustain this level of ventilation, and, therefore, it cannot be maintained for long periods. A respiratory rate of greater than 35 per minute is also indicative of impending failure. Like increased minute ventilation, increased ventilatory rates require more muscle effort to sustain and, therefore, cannot be maintained for long periods. The *rapid-shallow-breathing index (RSBI)* is often used as a weaning criterion (Krieger, Isber, Breitenbucher, Throop, & Ershowsky, 1997). The rapid-shallow-breathing index is the frequency divided by the tidal volume (in liters).

$$RSBI = \frac{frequency}{tidal\ volume\ (L)}$$

An index of 130 or greater is an indication of impending failure. The RSBI quantifies the relationship between the ventilatory rate (frequency) and the tidal volume.

Arterial blood gas analysis is also used to identify impending ventilatory failure. The pH, $PaCO_2$, and PaO_2 are measured and compared with the patient's baseline values to determine impending ventilatory failure. A pH of less than 7.25, a $PaCO_2$ greater than 55 mm Hg (except in chronic hypercapnia), and a PaO_2 of less than 50 mm Hg on an FIO_2 (fraction of inspired oxygen) greater than 0.5 are indicative of impending failure. It is important to trend results of arterial blood gas analysis against the patient's normal values. Taking these values and using them as absolute guidelines in the chronically ill patient may often lead to the wrong conclusion about the patient's condition. Refer to Table 24-2.

A declining oxygen saturation or a saturation of less than 90% is also not a good sign. Oxygen saturation as measured by pulse oximetry (SpO_2) is widely used to determine oxygenation. In using pulse oximetry, it is important to ensure that the signal strength is adequate and to compare the pulse rate with the heart monitor. If both are adequate, the reading will probably be valid as well.

TABLE 24-2: Criteria for Noninvasive Positive-Pressure Ventilation (NPPV)

Tidal Volume	<3–5 mL/kg
Rapid-Shallow-Breathing Index (RSBI)	>130
Minute Volume	>10 L/min
Respiratory Rate	>35/min
pH	<7.35
$PaCO_2$	>55 mm Hg
PaO_2	<50 mm Hg on FIO_2 >0.5

Work of breathing is best assessed by inspection (refer to Chapter 3). Use of accessory muscles, retractions, and pursed-lip breathing all are signs of increased ventilatory work. Careful inspection combined with the patient's subjective comments regarding the perceived work of breathing combined with the ventilatory parameters will complete the picture of the patient's actual work of breathing.

Impending ventilatory failure will also result in changes in the patient's vital signs. Hypoxemia, hypercapnia, and increased ventilatory work all have an impact on the vital signs. Typically tachycardia, arrhythmias, and hypertension will present concomitantly with the changes in ventilatory status.

PATIENT-VENTILATOR INTERFACE IN NONINVASIVE POSITIVE-PRESSURE VENTILATION

The interface of the ventilator with the patient—the mask and headgear—is critical to the success of NPPV (Turner, 1997). Patient comfort is important in tolerance of NPPV. Therefore, the type of mask (nasal versus full-face), type of harness, and the fit of the mask are imperative to the success of NPPV. A patient who is uncomfortable wearing the mask will pull it off the face if he or she is able to do so. As a clinician you must decide what type, size, and fit are best for the patient.

Patients who are claustrophobic often tolerate a *nasal mask* better. The nasal mask fits over the nose and upper lip, leaving the mouth relatively free (Figure 24-1). Advantages of the nasal mask include decreased risk of aspiration and improved verbal communication. The cushion that seals the mask should be of very soft, nonallergenic material. When the mask is fitted properly, little force should be required by the harness to maintain a good seal.

Nasal pillows are a soft, conical-shaped interface designed to be inserted into the nares (Figure 24-2). Nasal pillows are typically supported with fewer straps when compared with the nasal mask. The use of fewer straps on

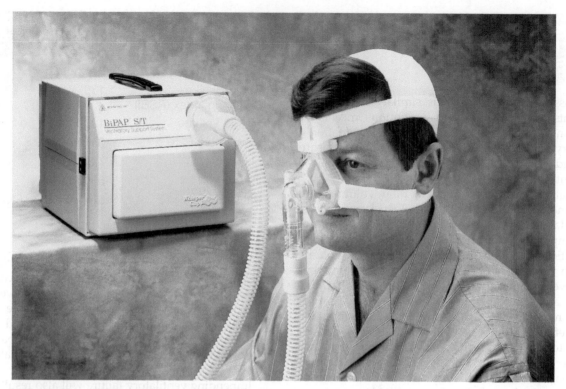

Figure 24-1 The nasal mask used for NPPV. Note how it fits over the nose and upper lip, leaving the mouth relatively free. *(Courtesy of Respironics, Inc., Pittsburgh, PA)*

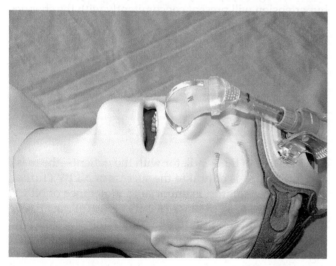

Figure 24-2 A photograph of nasal pillows as the patient interface. *(Courtesy of Philips Respironics, Inc., Pittsburgh, PA.)*

the headgear and the pillows not completely covering the nose may make this interface seem less confining to some patients and therefore more comfortable. This interface is common for patients who wear nocturnal CPAP for the treatment of obstructive sleep apnea.

The *full-face mask* fits over the entire mouth and nose (Figure 24-3). The face mask has the advantage of lower resistance to flow than with the nasal mask (Turner, 1997). However, the full-face mask carries the risk of increased aspiration. Therefore, a *nasogastric tube* is often placed to decompress the stomach and reduce the risk of aspiration.

Other disadvantages of the full-face mask include the inability of the patient to take any food or liquids by mouth and decreased ability to communicate verbally without removing the mask.

The *Total™ Mask* is a variation of a full-face mask (Figure 24-4). The Total™ Mask covers the entire face. The perimeter of this mask is sealed with a soft silicone seal. This mask may be helpful when obtaining a good seal is difficult when using a nasal mask or full-face mask. Some patients experience skin breakdown on the bridge of the nose or on the forehead due to contact by the mask itself or the headgear. The Total™ Mask may help alleviate this since these pressure points are avoided, and positive pressure from the ventilator helps to seal the perimeter of the mask, reducing pressure applied to the skin.

HAZARDS AND COMPLICATIONS OF NONINVASIVE POSITIVE-PRESSURE VENTILATION

Hazards and complications of NPPV include leaks, nasal or sinus pain or discomfort, gastric insufflation, eye irritation, barotrauma, aspiration pneumonia, mucous plugging, and hypoxemia (Hill, 1997).

Leaks in the circuitry used in NPPV are common. Most ventilators used for NPPV are able to tolerate and compensate for some amount of leak. However, too much of a leak will result in decreased ventilation (lower pressure),

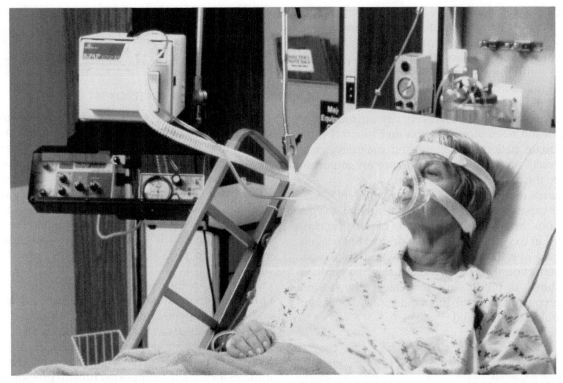

Figure 24-3 The full-face mask. Note how it fits, covering both the mouth and nose. *(Courtesy of Respironics, Inc., Pittsburgh, PA.)*

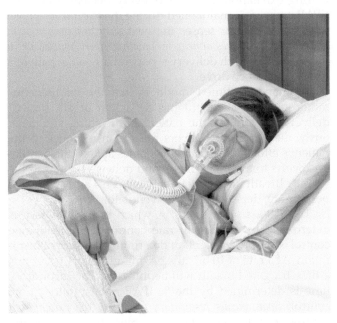

Figure 24-4 The Total™ Mask interface applied to a patient *(Courtesy of Philips Respironics, Inc., Pittsburgh, PA.)*

leading to hypoxemia and hypercarbia. The fit of the mask and harness is important to minimize leaks. Your skill as a clinician in fitting the mask and adjusting the harness is important to the success of NPPV. Therefore, it is important for you to become proficient at fitting and selecting the best mask and to have a variety of masks available for use.

Nasal or sinus pain is a frequent complaint of patients being ventilated by mask. The increased flow and pressure through the sinuses from the ventilator cause this

discomfort. If possible, initiate NPPV at lower pressures and gradually work toward the desired target pressure to achieve the desired tidal volume and minute ventilation. Humidification may be helpful in reducing some of the effects of the elevated pressure and increased inspiratory flow rates.

Pressure sores and ulcerations may also occur owing to excessive pressure of the mask against the face. The bridge of the nose is the most common site for these pressure sores. Again, proper mask fit is imperative to the success of NPPV. This is a common problem when a wrong-size mask is used and excessive strap pressure is used to compensate.

Gastric insufflation is often reported as a consequence of NPPV. Gastric insufflation occurs because the pressure and flow from the ventilator may be transmitted to the esophagus as well as the trachea. Like intermittent positive-pressure ventilation (IPPB), discussed in Chapter 17, NPPV can result in gastric insufflation. Sometimes a nasogastric tube is used in conjunction with NPPV to decompress the stomach, preventing gastric insufflation.

Eye irritation occurs because of flow around the mask up into the eyes. This flow is caused by leaks. If the mask fits properly, eye irritation can be minimized. Check by holding your hand near the bridge of the mask. Use of *spacers*, proper mask fit, and correct adjustment of the headgear or harness can minimize leaks, correcting this problem.

Barotrauma may result from the application of too much pressure in ventilating a patient with NPPV. NPPV has the potential to cause a pneumothorax by rupturing a bleb in a patient with bullous lung disease.

Aspiration pneumonia is a potential complication of NPPV. Because the airway is not as secure as with an endotracheal or a tracheostomy tube, aspiration into the lower airway is possible. If the patient's protective reflexes are compromised or absent, intubation and conventional ventilation should be considered.

NPPV ventilators often are used without humidification. The increased flow of relatively dry air may result in drying of the respiratory mucosa and mucous plugging. Adequate patient hydration and maintenance of adequate cough and pulmonary clearance are important to minimize this potential complication.

Hypoxemia can occur with NPPV. Not all NPPV ventilators are capable of providing supplemental oxygen concentrations. Many NPPV ventilators require the clinician to bleed in oxygen to achieve the desired SpO_2 levels. A tee inserted into the circuit is used to add the oxygen (O_2), by connecting it to a flowmeter using oxygen connecting tubing. If NPPV fails to achieve the desired oxygenation outcomes, intubation and conventional ventilation should be considered.

HOW RESISTANCE AND COMPLIANCE AFFECT NONINVASIVE POSITIVE-PRESSURE VENTILATION

NPPV is really *pressure-targeted ventilation (PTV)* (Kacmarek, 1997). In PTV, a set pressure is applied to achieve a desired tidal volume. NPPV ventilators do not have tidal volume controls or adjustment capability as in most acute care ventilators. Rather, the clinician selects an inspiratory pressure that is then delivered by the ventilator to achieve the desired tidal volume. Volume and flow both vary during inspiration and are not adjustable or set by the clinician. Therefore, volume delivery varies, just as volume delivery varies with IPPB.

Changes in resistance affect inspiratory time. Increases in airway resistance (R_{AW}) result in increased inspiratory times, in that pressure rises more slowly to the target level (Strumpf, Carlisle, Millman, Smith, & Hill, 1990). With increased R_{AW}, volumes may also concomitantly decrease during the typical 1- to 2-second inspiratory times during ventilation.

Changes in compliance have a profound effect on volume delivery at a set pressure. Decreased compliance (from a stiffer lung or thorax) causes decreased volume delivery for a given pressure. Increased compliance results in greater volume delivery for a given set pressure.

Because both R_{AW} and compliance affect volume delivery, it is important to monitor delivered tidal volumes, SpO_2, and blood gases to ensure that the patient is being adequately ventilated. Volume delivery will vary breath by breath depending on how the patient's condition changes. This requires the practitioner to be aware of potential hypoventilation. Many NPPV ventilators have provisions for monitoring tidal volumes and have alarms that may be set to alert the practitioner to unsafe conditions and events.

MODES OF NONINVASIVE POSITIVE-PRESSURE VENTILATION

Bilevel Ventilators

The modes of NPPV ventilation include pressure adjustment, spontaneous, spontaneous/timed, and timed ventilation. Pressure adjustment entails adjusting both inspiratory and expiratory pressures. Inspiratory pressure is often named *inspiratory positive airway pressure* (IPAP) in bilevel pressure ventilation. On some ventilators this may be labeled as pressure support. IPAP is the peak inspiratory pressure that is achieved when the ventilator delivers a breath. IPAP is typically adjustable between 4 and 40 cm H_2O depending on the unit. *Expiratory positive airway pressure* (EPAP) is the pressure level maintained in the circuit during the expiratory phase. On some ventilators this may be labeled as positive end-expiratory pressure (PEEP). EPAP may be adjusted between 4 and 20 cm H_2O, depending on the ventilator.

Spontaneous mode is what the name implies. The ventilator senses the patient's inspiratory effort (flow) and initiates a ventilator-supported breath (pressure delivery). Inspiratory flow rapidly increases, and the desired pressure is maintained for the set inspiratory time (% IPAP). During exhalation, pressure delivery decreases and the EPAP pressure is maintained during the expiratory phase until the ventilator senses the next *spontaneous breath. If the patient becomes apneic, no breath delivery will occur in this mode.* All breath delivery is dependent on the patient's intact respiratory drive.

Spontaneous/timed mode is like the spontaneous mode just described but has a backup breath (timed) delivery. As long as the patient is breathing spontaneously, the ventilator delivers breaths in response to the patient's effort. If the patient becomes apneic, the ventilator reverts to the timed mode and delivers breaths at the set rate. Breath rates may be set between 4 and 40 breaths per minute, depending on the ventilator.

Timed mode is a mode in which breath delivery is determined by the breath rate control. The breath rate control is simply a timer that determines the start of inspiration. At a rate of 10 breaths per minute, every 6 seconds a time-triggered breath will be initiated. The inspiratory time is determined by the % IPAP or inspiratory time control. *Spontaneous respiratory efforts by the patient will not trigger inspiration in this mode.* Since this is a pressure mode, it does not mean the patient is being sufficiently ventilated.

SUPPLEMENTAL OXYGEN DELIVERY

The PTV ventilators used in NPPV were originally employed in the home setting for treatment of sleep apnea. As such, they were designed initially to run on household electrical power and be independent of any gas source. As the application of these ventilators was expanded into the acute care setting, the need for supplemental oxygen delivery became required. Some ventilators now provide for the adjustment of oxygen concentrations (% oxygen) just as with other acute care ventilators. However, if this adjustment is not available, oxygen must be bled into the circuit.

Often, supplemental oxygen is provided by bleeding in oxygen through an adapter at the outlet of the ventilator (Figure 24-5). Alternatively, oxygen may be

provided by bleeding it into a port on the nasal mask. SpO_2 and arterial blood gases should be monitored to ensure that the patient's oxygenation needs are being met. Additionally, tidal volumes should be monitored to ensure that they are also adequate to meet the patient's needs and have not changed owing to the addition of supplemental oxygen.

Acute Care Ventilators

Several acute care ventilators have the ability to deliver noninvasive ventilation. Noninvasive ventilation delivered by these ventilators has the advantage of built-in oxygen delivery and sophisticated monitoring capability that many bilevel ventilators do not have. In order to use this mode on acute care ventilators, the patient interface should be a snug-fitting mask without any bleed holes and a compliant seal for a good fit.

Mode

The choice of acute care ventilator will determine which mode is selected for noninvasive ventilation. Table 24-3 compares several acute care ventilators capable of providing noninvasive ventilation and the settings needed for spontaneous noninvasive ventilation.

Ventilator Circuit

The ventilator circuit employed by acute care ventilators is the traditional "wye"-type circuit. A circuit with an exhalation swivel is not required as it is for most bilevel ventilators.

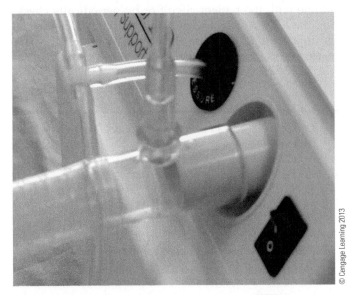

Figure 24-5 Supplemental oxygen being bled into the circuit at the ventilator outlet

© Cengage Learning 2013

TABLE 24-3: Noninvasive Ventilation Using Acute Care Ventilators			
VENTILATOR	**MODE**	**BREATH DELIVERY**	**SPONTANEOUS SETTINGS**
Viasys AVEA	Pressure support	Spontaneous	1. Pressure support 2. Continuous positive airway pressure (CPAP) 3. Leak compensation 4. FIO$_2$ 5. Flow trigger sensitivity
Puritan Bennett 840	Noninvasive ventilation (NIV)	A/C, synchronized intermittent mandatory ventilation (SIMV), spontaneous	1. Pressure support 2. CPAP 3. Leak compensation 4. FIO$_2$ 5. Flow trigger sensitivity
Maquet Servo^i	NIV	Pressure support, pressure control	1. Pressure support 2. CPAP 3. Leak compensation 4. FIO$_2$ 5. Flow trigger sensitivity

PATIENT MONITORING

Patients on NPPV require careful monitoring and considerable one-on-one care during initiation of NPPV. Monitors used should include oxygen saturation, cardiac, blood pressure, and oxygen analysis monitors.

Oximetry is important in determining whether NPPV is meeting the patient's oxygenation requirements. Oximeters with alarms (set off by low SpO_2) are helpful in signaling a decrease in the patient's oxygen saturation. When you use an oximeter, the measured heart rate should be compared with the patient's heart rate (as monitored or palpated), and the signal strength should also be verified when you are taking readings.

Heart monitors are important in detecting arrythmias and changes in heart rate. Critically ill patients should be monitored closely for cardiac complications. Continuous ECG monitoring is the standard of care for these patients.

Blood pressure may be monitored by the use of noninvasive blood pressure monitors. At set intervals, the automated blood pressure cuff inflates and the readings are obtained. Hypotension from NPPV is a rare complication (Hill, 1997). Appropriate blood pressure monitoring will alert you to changes in the patient's status.

Oxygen analyzers are used to monitor the FIO_2 delivered when supplemental oxygen is used. Monitoring may be performed continuously by placing the sensor in-line with the patient circuit or by periodically checking the FIO_2. As always, in using an oxygen analyzer, it is important to calibrate the device periodically (once each shift).

PROFICIENCY OBJECTIVES

At the end of this chapter, the reader should be able to:

* *Demonstrate the assessment of a patient for the need for NPPV:*
  — *Respiratory frequency*
  — *Tidal volume*
  — *Minute ventilation*
  — *Rapid-shallow-breathing index*
  — *Vital capacity*
  — *SpO₂*
  — *Arterial blood gases*
* *Demonstrate how to assemble and test an NPPV ventilator prior to use.*
* *Demonstrate how to select a mask for NPPV:*
  — *Demonstrate the use of both nasal and full-face masks.*
  — *Demonstrate how to use the harness/headgear correctly.*
  — *Demonstrate how to size the mask correctly for the patient's face.*

* *Demonstrate how to establish appropriate ventilator settings:*
  — *IPAP*
  — *EPAP*
  — *% IPAP*
  — *Mode*
  — *FIO₂*
  — *Alarms*
* *Demonstrate how to establish appropriate monitoring for the patient on NPPV:*
  — *ECG monitoring*
  — *Oximetry*
  — *Noninvasive blood pressure monitoring*
  — *Oxygen analysis*
* *Demonstrate how to chart NPPV in the patient's flow sheet or chart.*

PATIENT ASSESSMENT FOR NPPV

Prior to initiation of NPPV, the patient must be closely assessed to determine the need for ventilation. This assessment may include physical assessment, oximetry, arterial blood gas analysis, and determination of ventilatory parameters.

Physical assessment and spontaneous parameters are described in Chapters 4 and 5. The acutely ill patient may be hypoxemic and hypercapneic; therefore, caution and common sense are required when the mechanics of ventilation are assessed. The patient may require supplemental oxygen to maintain adequate oxygen saturation even without any undue stress. Arterial blood gas analysis is important in establishing the patient's baseline

pH, $PaCO_2$, and PaO_2 prior to NPPV. Periodically, repeat arterial blood gases may be obtained following commitment to NPPV to determine whether the patient is being adequately ventilated.

ASSEMBLY AND TESTING OF THE VENTILATOR

The ventilator circuit required for NPPV is relatively simple (Figure 24-6). Connection and assembly of the circuit are described for the NPPV ventilators in the practice activities section of this chapter.

Testing of the circuit's integrity can be accomplished by blocking the mask interface and placing the ventilator into the timed mode with a set rate. Observe for the

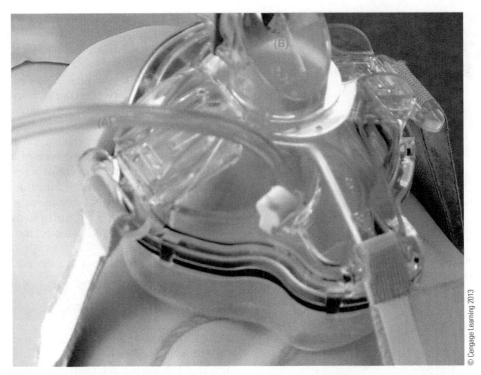

Figure 24-6 A photo of the NPPV ventilator circuit connected to a full-face mask. Note the main circuit tubing (A), proximal pressure line (B), and mask interface

pressure to rise to the set IPAP level for the appropriate percentage of the inspiratory time. If the pressure fails to rise to the IPAP level, you have a leak. Check all connections for leaks and make sure all connections are tight.

MASK SELECTION

Mask selection and fitting constitute one of the most important determinants of success with NPPV. Selection and fitting of the mask require both knowledge and skill. As a new respiratory practitioner, you will need time and practice under the supervision of a seasoned practitioner to master this skill.

Fitting of nasal masks can be facilitated using the size guide rings (Figure 24-7). Once the patient's nose is matched to the size, a mask can then be selected. Besides size, the type of cushion is also important to the correct mask fit. If a mask is correctly selected, minimal pressure will be required to make it seal. Figure 24-8 shows a nasal mask correctly fitted to the patient's face.

Full-face masks must cover both the nose and the mouth. Sizes vary from small to large. The cushion is important as well as the size to obtain the proper seal. Once the correct mask size is selected, the four-point harness is used to hold the mask in position. As with the nasal mask, if it is fitted correctly, minimal pressure will be required to secure the full-face mask. Figure 24-9 shows the full-face mask correctly fitted to the patient.

The head gear or straps are important in securing the mask and keeping it in place. A common mistake made

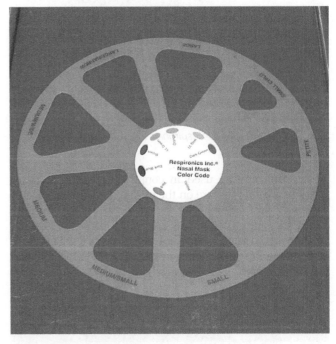

Figure 24-7 A sizing ring being used to determine the correct manufacturer's mask size for a patient *(Courtesy of Philips Respironics Inc., Pittsburgh, PA.)*

by inexperienced respiratory practitioners is to tighten the straps too much. Too much tension can cause pressure sores to develop quickly, making the mask very uncomfortable for the patient. Remember that if the mask is correctly fitted, little pressure will be required to seal it.

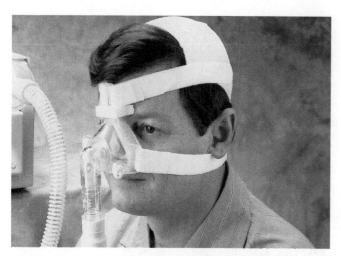

Figure 24-8 A photograph of a nasal mask correctly fitted and secured to a patient's face. *(Courtesy of Philips Respironics Inc., Pittsburgh, PA)*

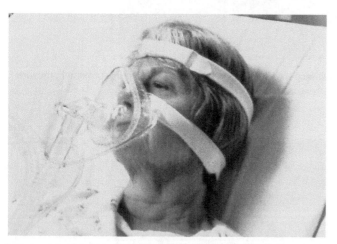

Figure 24-9 The full-face mask correctly fitted to the patient's face. *(Courtesy of Philips Respironics Inc., Pittsburgh, PA)*

Spacers may be used in conjunction with the nasal mask to relieve pressure on the bridge of the nose. Spacers generally rest against the forehead, reducing pressure along the apex of the mask. Spacers come in varying thickness and materials. Choose the spacer that fits the patient the best and helps to improve the mask fit and patient comfort.

VENTILATOR SETTINGS

The physician may order specific pressures (IPAP and EPAP), rate, and FIO_2 for NPPV. Alternatively, the physician may order a desired tidal volume range; in this case, as a clinician you must adjust the IPAP and EPAP to achieve it. In either case, you must be able to adjust both IPAP and EPAP controls as well as the inspiratory time (% IPAP) to achieve the desired ventilation.

Most often, spontaneous/timed mode is used for NPPV. This allows the ventilator to detect the patient's spontaneous efforts, triggering ventilator-supported breaths. In this mode, if the patient fails to initiate a breath, the ventilator's backup rate will ensure ventilation.

FIO_2 levels may be adjusted by "bleeding in" oxygen or by setting the % oxygen control. In either case, monitoring the FIO_2 using an oxygen analyzer must be done to confirm the correct settings.

Alarms will vary depending on the NPPV ventilator that is used. The simplest type of alarm is a pressure disconnect alarm. In the event of a severe leak or tubing disconnect, pressure will fall and the alarm will sound. Other NPPV ventilators have more sophisticated alarm and monitoring systems. Alarm systems specific to NPPV ventilators are discussed later in the practice activities portion of this chapter.

PATIENT MONITORING

The ECG leads should be placed and connected to the patient monitor. Verify that the ECG waveform is correct and that the leads have been correctly placed.

Connect the patient to a continuous oximeter monitor. Verify that the heart rate display matches the ECG heart rate. Also ensure that the signal strength is adequate for a good reading. Patient motion, bright ambient light, fingernail polish, and other factors can influence the accuracy of pulse oximeters.

If noninvasive blood pressure monitoring is desired, connect the blood pressure cuff to the patient's arm and program the unit for the desired blood pressure measurement interval. Press the manual pressure measurement button to verify that it is connected correctly and working properly.

If continuous oxygen (FIO_2) monitoring is desired, connect the oxygen analyzer in-line at the ventilator outlet. If oxygen is bled into the circuit, where you bleed in the oxygen and where you place the monitor is important. Do not place the monitor upstream from the point of oxygen addition and expect to have an accurate reading. If oxygen is bled into the system, you may wish to consider spot checks of FIO_2 rather than continuous monitoring.

PATIENT CHARTING

At a minimum, patient charting should include breath sounds, heart rate, SpO_2, work of breathing, IPAP, EPAP, mode, ventilatory rate, tidal volume, estimated leak, ventilator rate (backup), and FIO_2. Often a flow sheet is used to record the data in a checklist format. Monitoring may be performed as frequently as every hour or more often, depending on the patient's status. At initiation of NPPV, it takes considerable time to fit the mask, make the ventilator adjustments, and work with the patient to relieve anxiety and to faciliatate getting used to the NPPV system.

References

American Respiratory Care Foundation (ARCF). (1997). Consensus conference: Noninvasive positive pressure ventilation. *Respiratory Care, 42*(4), 364–369.

Brochard, L., Mancebo, J., Wysocki, M., Lofaso, F., Conti, G., Rauss, A., et al. (1995). Noninvasive ventilation for acute exacerbations of chronic obstructive pulmonary disease. *New England Journal of Medicine, 333*, 817–822.

Hill, N. (1997). Complications of noninvasive positive pressure ventilation. *Respiratory Care, 42*(4), 432–442.

Kacmarek, R. M. (1997). Characteristics of pressure-targeted ventilators used for noninvasive positive pressure ventilation. *Respiratory Care, 42*(4), 380–388.

Kramer, N., Meyer, T. J., Meharg, J., Cece, R. D., & Hill, N. S. (1995). Randomized, prospective trial of noninvasive positive pressure ventilation in acute respiratory failure. *American Journal of Respiratory and Critical Care Medicine, 151*, 1799–1806.

Krieger, B. P., Isber, J., Breitenbucher, A., Throop, G., & Ershowsky, P. (1997). Serial measurements of the rapid-shallow-breathing index as a predictor of weaning outcome in elderly medical patients. *Chest, 112*(4), 1029–1034.

Martin, T. J., Hovis, J. D., Costantino, J. P., Bieman, M. I., Donahoe, M. P., Rogers, R. M., et al. (2000). A randomized, prospective evaluation of noninvasive ventilation for acute respiratory failure. *American Journal of Respiratory and Critical Care Medicine, 161*, 807–813.

Meduri, G. U., Abou-Shala, N., Fox, R. C., Jones, C. B., Leeper, K. V., & Wunderink, R. G. (1991). Noninvasive positive pressure ventilation via face mask: First-line intervention in patients with acute hypercapnia and hypoxemic respiratory failure. *Chest, 100*(2), 445–454.

Mehta, S., Jay, G. D., Woolard, R. H., Hipona, R. A., Connolly, E. M., Cimini, D. M., et al. (1997). Randomized, prospective trial of bilevel versus continuous positive airway pressure in acute pulmonary edema. *Critical Care Medicine, 25*, 620–628.

Pierson, D. J. (1997). Noninvasive positive pressure ventilation: History and terminology. *Respiratory Care, 42*(4), 370–379.

Pollack, C., Jr., Torres, M. T., & Alexander, L. (1996). Feasibility study of the use of bi-level positive airway pressure for respiratory support in the emergency department. *Annals of Emergency Medicine, 27*(2), 189–192.

Strumpf, D. A., Carlisle, C. C., Millman, R. P., Smith, K. W., & Hill, N. S. (1990). An evaluation of the Respironics BiPAP® bi-level CPAP device for delivery of assisted ventilation. *Respiratory Care, 35*(5), 415–422.

Turner, R. (1997). NPPV: Face versus interface. *Respiratory Care, 42*(4), 389–393.

Wunderink, R. G., & Hill, N. S. (1997). Continuous and periodic applications of noninvasive positive pressure ventilation in respiratory failure. *Respiratory Care, 42*(4), 394–402.

Practice Activities: Respironics BiPAP® Vision

CIRCUIT ASSEMBLY

Assembly of the BiPAP® Vision circuit is illustrated in Figure 24-10 where it is ready to attach to the ventilator. Note that the circuit consists of two pieces of tubing: the patient tubing (22 mm diameter) and the proximal pressure line. The tubing must terminate at the patient end with a Whisper Swivel. The Whisper Swivel is equivalent to an exhalation valve, allowing the patient to exhale to the ambient air, and acts as a one-way valve during inspiration. The mask (nasal or full-face) attaches to the Whisper Swivel.

VENTILATOR PREPARATION

1. Connect a main flow bacteria filter to the ventilator outlet. A standard bacteria filter commonly employed with acute care ventilators will work for this application.

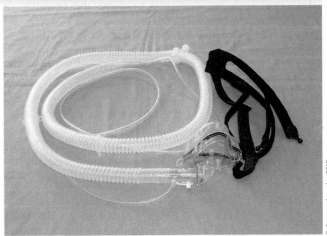

Figure 24-10 The Vision and V60 patient circuit

2. Connect the large-diameter (22 mm) tubing to the ventilator's outlet and connect the proximal pressure line to the proximal pressure port above it.

3. Connect the ventilator to a 50 psi oxygen source using a high-pressure hose and the diameter-indexed safety system (DISS) adapter located on the rear of the ventilator.

4. Verify that the voltage is set correctly for your facility by checking the voltage setting window above the alternating current (AC) power connection on the rear of the ventilator.

5. Verify that the Start/Stop switch is in the Stop position. Connect the power cord to your facility's AC electrical outlet.

6. Move the Start/Stop switch to the Start position. The BiPAP® Vision will conduct a 15-second self-test on initial start-up.

7. Press the "Test Exh Port" soft key on the upper left part of the display screen. This will begin the exhalation port test. It is important to perform this test before each use and following each circuit change. This test will calculate the leak in the circuit, allowing monitoring for patient leaks and of tidal volume delivery.
   a. Occlude the mask port on the patient circuit.
   b. Press the "Start Test" soft key at the upper right of the screen.
   c. The test will take about 15 seconds to complete.
   d. In the event that the ventilator detects a problem, follow the prompts on the screen, checking the circuit or proximal line, and repeat the test by pressing the "Start Test" soft key.

8. Press the "Monitoring" key on the lower left corner of the control panel. The ventilator is now ready for use.

VENTILATOR OPERATION VERIFICATION

Prior to using the ventilator, as a clinician you should verify that it is functioning properly. The self- and exhalation port tests are designed to check the majority of the ventilator's systems. By checking the modes and pressure settings, you can be assured of the ventilator's operation.

1. Complete steps 1 through 8 in the Ventilator Preparation section.

2. Occlude the patient circuit and press the "Options" soft key at the lower right corner of the monitoring screen. If an alarm is active, press the "Reset" hard key (one with the two diagonal slashes at the upper right part of the control panel).

3. Press the "Test Alarms" soft key located in the middle of the left-hand side of the display screen. This test will verify the function of the audible and visual alarms. The "Vent Inop" and "Check Vent" icons will illuminate below the "Reset" hard key.

4. Press the "Mode" key (center hard key to the right of the "Monitoring" key), and select "S/T" (Spontaneous/ Timed) mode key. Set the ventilator to the following settings:
   IPAP: 15 cm H_2O
   EPAP: 5 cm H_2O
   Rate: 16/min
   Timed Inspiration: 1 second
   Rise Time: 0.1 second

5. Press the "Alarms" hard key and make the following alarm settings:
   High Pressure: 20 cm H_2O
   Low Pressure: 10 cm H_2O
   Low Pressure Delay: 20 seconds
   Apnea: Disabled
   Low Minute Ventilation: 0 L/min
   High Rate: 40/minute
   Low Rate: 10/minute

6. Press the "Monitoring" key and return to the monitoring screen. Occlude the circuit outlet port and verify IPAP, EPAP, rate, and inspiratory time.

7. Create a small leak at the circuit outlet. Verify that the ventilator cycles into inspiration. Once the breath is triggered, occlude the port again.

8. Press the "Alarms" hard key to obtain the current alarm settings. Change the high pressure alarm to 10 cm H_2O. Verify that the high pressure alarm activates on the next breath cycle (with the outlet port occluded). Reset the alarm to 20 cm H_2O.

9. Open the circuit outlet simulating a patient disconnect. Wait about 30 seconds to verify that the low pressure alarm activates. Occlude the circuit outlet and press the "Alarm Reset" key.

10. Press the "Apnea" soft key on the lower left portion of the display screen. Adjust the apnea parameter to 20 seconds. Keep the circuit outlet occluded and verify that the alarm activates. Readjust the "Apnea" parameter to "Disabled" and press the "Alarm Reset" key.

ACTIVITIES

To complete these practice exercises, it is recommended that you use a lung analog/simulator such as a Medishield or Manley test lung. With these units, you may easily adjust resistance (R_{AW}) and compliance for the following exercises to simulate changes in the patient's condition.

Exercise 1: Continuous Positive Airway Pressure (CPAP) Mode

CPAP mode is a spontaneous mode; there is no backup ventilatory support. If the patient fails to take a breath, the ventilator will not respond by providing one. When performing this exercise, you must provide the test lung with a spontaneous effort by expanding the bellows, simulating inspiration.

The active controls are CPAP (pressure) and % O_2.

1. Assemble the ventilator's circuit and prepare the ventilator for operation as described earlier.

2. Press the "Mode" key (lower left part of the control panel), and select CPAP mode by pressing its soft key.

3. Adjust the CPAP level to 10 cm H_2O by pressing the "CPAP" soft key and rotating the adjustment knob adjacent to the ventilator outlet.

4. Select the "Activate New Mode" soft key at the lower right corner of the display screen. CPAP mode and a pressure of 10 cm H_2O have now been selected and activated.

5. Simulate spontaneous breathing by moving the test lung's bellows. Observe the display screen and the data it presents (pressure, volume and flow graphics, rate, and pressure level).

6. Supplemental oxygen can be provided by selecting the "% O_2" soft key, rotating the adjustment knob to the desired FIO_2 and pressing the "Activate New Mode" soft key.

7. Alarms may be adjusted by depressing the "Alarm" hard key next to the adjustment knob. The alarm setup page is then displayed on the display screen. From this page you may adjust the following alarms:
   a. High pressure limit (cm H_2O)
   b. Low pressure limit (cm H_2O)
   c. Low pressure alarm delay (seconds)
   d. Apnea
   e. Low minute ventilation (L/min)
   f. High rate
   g. Low rate

Exercise 2: CPAP Application

Identify a laboratory partner who will act as your patient. With your laboratory instructor observing you, complete the following exercise.

1. Assemble the Respironics BiPAP Vision ventilator and attach a clean circuit.

2. Using appropriate universal precautions, select the correct nasal mask for your patient and the appropriate headgear and spacers.

3. Connect the mask to the circuit, and set the ventilator to the following settings:
   Mode: CPAP
   CPAP: 10 cm H_2O
   % O_2: 21%

4. Fit the mask to your patient, using the spacer(s) and the headgear.

5. Observe the pressure manometer and the light-emitting diodes (LEDs) for correct operation.

6. Note the following:
   a. Graphics (pressure, volume, flow)
   b. Breath rate

c. % O_2
d. CPAP setting

7. Set the following alarms:
   a. High pressure limit: 15 cm H_2O
   b. Low pressure limit: 5 cm H_2O
   c. Low pressure alarm delay: 20 seconds
   d. Low minute ventilation: 3 L/min
   e. High rate: +8 breaths per minute above patient rate
   f. Low rate: −8 breaths per minute below patient rate

8. Have your patient hyperventilate and hypoventilate to observe the alarm functions.

9. Increase the CPAP setting to 15 cm H_2O and readjust the alarms appropriately.

Questions

A. What happened to the tidal volume when the CPAP setting was changed?
B. What happened to the inspiratory time when the CPAP setting was changed?

Exercise 3: Spontaneous/Timed (S/T) Mode

1. Assemble the ventilator's circuit and prepare the ventilator for operation as described earlier.

2. Press the "Mode" key (lower left part of the control panel), and Spontaneous/Timed mode by pressing its soft key (S/T).

3. The following are the active controls:
   - IPAP
   - EPAP
   - Rate
   - Timed Inspiration
   - % O_2
   - IPAP Rise Time

4. Set the controls to the following settings by selecting the appropriate soft key and then rotating the adjustment knob to the desired setting.
   IPAP: 15 cm H_2O
   EPAP: 5 cm H_2O
   Rate: 10 breaths per minute
   Timed Inspiration: 0.1 second
   % O_2:   21%
   IPAP Rise Time: 0.1 second

   Once the adjustments have been made, push the "Activate New Mode" soft key to initiate the new settings.

5. Connect the patient outlet port to the test lung, and observe the following:
   a. Graphics (pressure, volume, flow)
   b. Breath rate
   c. % O_2
   d. IPAP and EPAP pressures

6. Change the resistance to 50, increasing the R_{AW}.

7. Note the following:
   a. Tidal volume (digital display)
   b. Graphics (pressure, volume, and flow)
   c. Inspiratory time

Questions

A. What happened to the tidal volume delivery?
B. What happened to the inspiratory time?

8. Return the R_{AW} control to zero.

9. Decrease the compliance by adding an additional spring onto the bellows of the test lung.

10. Note the following:
   a. Tidal volume (digital display)
   b. Graphics (pressure, volume, and flow)
   c. Inspiratory time

Questions

A. What happened to the tidal volume delivery?
B. What happened to the inspiratory time?

11. Change the controls to the following:
   Breaths per minute: 10
   IPAP: 20 cm H_2O
   EPAP: 8 cm H_2O
   % IPAP: 20%

12. Repeat steps 6 through 8.

13. Note the following:
   a. Tidal volume (digital display)
   b. Graphics (pressure, volume, and flow)
   c. Inspiratory time

Questions

A. What happened to the tidal volume delivery?
B. What happened to the inspiratory time?

Exercise 4: Spontaneous/Timed (S/T) Mode Application

Identify a laboratory partner who will act as your patient. With your laboratory instructor observing you, complete the following exercise.

1. Assemble the Respironics BiPAP® Vision ventilator and attach a clean circuit.

2. Using Standard Precautions, select the correct nasal mask for your patient and the appropriate headgear and spacers.

3. Connect the mask to the circuit, and set the ventilator to the following settings:
   Mode: Spontaneous/Timed
   IPAP: 15 cm H_2O
   IPAP: 4 cm H_2O
   Breaths per minute: 10/min
   Timed Inspiration: 0.1 second
   % O_2:   21%
   IPAP Rise Time: 0.1 second
   Once the settings are established, activate the new mode.

4. Fit the mask to your patient, using the spacer(s) and the headgear.

5. Note the following:
   a. Tidal volume (digital display)
   b. Graphics (pressure, volume, and flow)
   c. Inspiratory time

6. Adjust the alarms appropriately for your patient's volumes, pressures, and rate.

7. Change the IPAP to 10 cm H_2O.

8. Note the following:
   a. Tidal volume (digital display)
   b. Graphics (pressure, volume, and flow)
   c. Inspiratory time

Questions

A. What happened to the tidal volume when the IPAP pressure was changed?
B. What happened to the inspiratory time when the IPAP pressure was changed?

Practice Activities: Respironics V60 Ventilator

CIRCUIT ASSEMBLY

The circuit for the V60 Ventilator is similar to that employed with the Respironics Vison ventilator. Figure 24-11 illustrates the Respironics V60 Ventilator circuit that is assembled and ready to attach to the ventilator. Note that the circuit consists of two pieces of tubing: the patient tubing (22 mm diameter) and the proximal pressure line. The tubing must terminate at the patient end with a Whisper Swivel. The Whisper Swivel is equivalent to an exhalation valve, allowing the patient to exhale to the ambient air, and acts as a one-way valve during inspiration. The mask (nasal or full-face) attaches to the Whisper Swivel.

USING THE GRAPHICAL USER INTERFACE

The Respironics V60 Ventilator uses a touch screen graphical user interface, a round navigation ring, and the "Accept" button to make changes or select menu options. To make a change or enter a value, select a function by touching the desired tab or button on the touch screen. Once the selection has been made, turn the navigation ring until the desired value is displayed, then press the "Accept" button integral to the navigation ring.

Alternatively, when the "increase" or "decrease" symbol appears on the touch screen, touch the desired button repeatedly until the change has been made. Once the change is made, press the "Accept" button to activate the change.

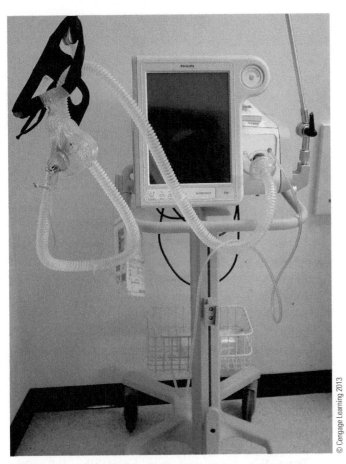

Figure 24-11 The Phillips-Respironics V60 ventilator assembled and ready for use

© Cengage Learning 2013

TABLE 24-4: Selection of Patient Interface and Exhalation Port

TYPE	DESCRIPTION
ET/Trach	Endotracheal tube or tracheostomy tube
I:1 – Intentional Leak 1	Minimal Intentional Leak Masks:
	Respironics Vinyl Nasal mask
	Respironics Contour Deluxe Nasal Mask
	Respironics PerformaTrak Mask
	Respironics Image 3 Full Mask
I:2 – Intentional Leak 2	Masks with medium intentional leaks:
	Respironics PerforMax Face Mask
Other	Other manufacturers' masks

TABLE 24-5: Selection of Exhalation Port Types

TYPE	DESCRIPTION
DEP	Respironics disposable exhalation port
Whisper Swivel	Respironics Whisper Swivel
PEV	Respironics Plateau Exhalation Valve
Other	Exhalation port from other manufacturers
None	No exhalation port in the circuit

VENTILATOR PREPARATION

1. Connect a main flow bacteria filter to the ventilator outlet. A standard bacteria filter commonly employed with acute care ventilators will work for this application.

2. Connect the large-diameter (22 mm) tubing to the bacteria filter installed at the ventilator outlet and connect the proximal pressure line to the proximal pressure port above it.

3. Connect the ventilator to a 50 psi oxygen source using a high-pressure hose and the DISS adapter located on the rear of the ventilator.

4. Connect the AC power cord to a suitable AC wall outlet.

5. Press the "On/Shutdown" soft key at the lower left front of the ventilator to turn on AC power.

6. Select the correct patient interface and exhalation port:
   a. Press the "Menu" button on the lower part of the main display screen.
   b. Select "Mask/Port" from the menu selection.
   c. Select the desired patient interface and exhalation port from the menu (refer to Tables 24-4 and 24-5).

7. Perform a preoperational check by completing the following steps:
   a. Connect to AC power and an oxygen supply.
   b. Switch the power on by pressing the "On/Shutdown" soft key.
   c. Select the mask and exhalation port.
   d. Connect the exhalation port to a test lung.
   e. Set the V60 Ventilator to the following settings:
      - S/T Mode
      - Rate: 4 breaths per minute
      - IPAP: 10 cm H_2O
      - EPAP: 6 cm H_2O

- I time: 1 second
- Rise: 1
- Ramp: Off
- O_2: 21%

Set the alarm settings to the following:

- Hi Rate: 90 breaths per minute
- Lo Rate: 1 breaths per minute
- Hi V_T: 200 mL
- Lo V_T: Off
- HIP: 50 cm H_2O
- LIP: Off
- Lo V_E: Off

f. The test lung should expand during inspiration and collapse during exhalation. A continuous flow should be noted through the exhalation port.

g. Disconnect the proximal pressure line from the front of the ventilator:
   - The "Proximal Pressure Line Disconnect" alarm should activate (audio, visual, and flashing).

h. Reconnect the proximal pressure line; the alarm should reset.

i Set the O_2 to 40% and wait for the oxygen to stablilize:
   - Oxygen should analyze between 35% and 45% using an O_2 analyzer.

j. Disconnect the ventilator from AC power while it is running. The backup battery should automatically switch on (optional accessory). The battery symbol should be displayed in the right-hand corner of the main screen.

k. Switch the power back to AC power. The battery light should go off and the battery LED will flash, indicating the battery is charging.

8. The ventilator is now ready for use.

ACTIVITIES

To complete these practice exercises, it is recommended that you use a lung analog/simulator such as an IngMar Medical Demo Lung or Quick lung, or SMS "Manley" Lung Simulator. With these units, you may easily adjust resistance (R_{AW}) and compliance for the following exercises to simulate changes in the patient's condition.

Exercise 1: Continuous Positive Airway Pressure (CPAP) Mode

CPAP mode is a spontaneous mode; there is no backup ventilatory support. If the patient fails to take a breath, the ventilator will not respond by providing one. When performing this exercise, you must provide the test lung with a spontaneous effort by expanding the bellows, simulating inspiration. Refer to Table 24-6.

1. Assemble the ventilator's circuit and prepare the ventilator for operation as described earlier.

2. Select the Modes tab from the bottom of the screen and press CPAP settings.

3. Adjust the CPAP level to 10 cm H_2O by pressing the "CPAP" soft key and rotating the Navigation ring and pressing "Accept."

TABLE 24-6: CPAP Active Controls

CPAP	4–40 cm H_2O
Ramp Time	5–45 minutes
C-Flex	1 to 3
O_2	21–100%

4. Set the O_2 percent to 21%.

5. Turn the Ramp Time Off and set C-Flex to 1.

6. Press "Activate CPAP Mode" to initiate the new mode.

7. Simulate spontaneous breathing by moving the test lung's bellows. Observe the display screen and the data it presents (pressure, volume and flow graphics, rate, and pressure level).

8. Supplemental oxygen can be provided by selecting the "% O_2" soft key, rotating the adjustment knob to the desired FIO_2 and pressing the "Activate New Mode" soft key.

9. Alarms may be adjusted by depressing the "Alarm" hard key next to the adjustment knob. The alarm setup page is then displayed on the display screen. From this page you may adjust the following alarms:
   a. High pressure limit (cm H_2O)
   b. Low pressure limit (cm H_2O)
   c. Apnea
   d. Low minute ventilation (L/min)
   e. High rate
   f. Low rate

Exercise 2: CPAP Application

Identify a laboratory partner who will act as your patient. With your laboratory instructor observing you, complete the following exercise.

1. Assemble the Respironics BiPAP Vision ventilator and attach a clean circuit.

2. Using appropriate universal precautions, select the correct nasal mask for your patient and the appropriate headgear and spacers.

3. Connect the mask to the circuit, and set the ventilator to the following settings:
   Mode: CPAP
   CPAP: 10 cm H_2O
   % O_2: 21%
   Ramp Time: Off
   C-Flex: 1

4. Fit the mask to your patient, using the spacer(s) and the headgear.

5. Observe the patient parameter displays on the upper portion of the screen and the waveform displays.

6. Note the following:
   a. Graphics (pressure, volume, flow)
   b. Breath rate
   c. % O$_2$
   d. CPAP setting

7. Set the following alarms:
   a. High pressure limit: 15 cm H$_2$O
   b. Low pressure limit: 5 cm H$_2$O
   c. Low pressure alarm delay: 20 seconds
   d. Low minute ventilation: 3 L/min
   e. High rate: +8 breaths per minute above patient rate
   f. Low rate: −8 breaths per minute below patient rate

8. Have your patient hyperventilate and hypoventilate to observe the alarm functions.

9. Increase the CPAP setting to 15 cm H$_2$O and readjust the alarms appropriately.

Questions

A. What happened to the tidal volume when the CPAP setting was changed?
B. What happened to the inspiratory time when the CPAP setting was changed?

Exercise 3: Spontaneous/Timed (S/T) Mode

1. Assemble the ventilator's circuit and prepare the ventilator for operation as described earlier.

2. Select the Modes tab from the bottom of the screen and press the "Batch S/T" button.

3. The following are the active controls:
   - IPAP
   - EPAP
   - Rate
   - Inspiratory Time
   - Rise Time
   - Ramp Time
   - % O$_2$

4. Set the controls to the following settings by selecting the appropriate soft key and then rotating the adjustment knob to the desired setting.
   IPAP: 15 cm H$_2$O
   EPAP: 5 cm H$_2$O
   Rate: 10 breaths per minute
   Inspiratory Time: 0.1 second
   % O$_2$:   21%
   Rise Time: 0.1 second
   RampTime: Off

   Once the adjustments have been made, push the "Activate S/T Mode" soft key to initiate the new settings.

5. Connect the patient outlet port to the test lung, and observe the following:
   a. Graphics (pressure, volume, flow)
   b. Breath rate
   c. % O$_2$
   d. IPAP and EPAP pressures

6. Change the resistance to 50, increasing the R$_{AW}$.

7. Note the following:
   a. Tidal volume (digital display)
   b. Graphics (pressure, volume, and flow)
   c. Inspiratory time

Questions

A. What happened to the tidal volume delivery?
B. What happened to the inspiratory time?

8. Return the R$_{AW}$ control to zero.

9. Decrease the compliance by adding an additional spring onto the bellows of the test lung.

10. Note the following:
    a. Tidal volume (digital display)
    b. Graphics (pressure, volume, and flow)
    c. Inspiratory time

Questions

A. What happened to the tidal volume delivery?
B. What happened to the inspiratory time?

11. Change the controls to the following:
    Breaths per minute: 10
    IPAP: 20 cm H$_2$O
    EPAP: 8 cm H$_2$O
    % IPAP: 20%

12. Repeat steps 6 through 8.

13. Note the following:
    a. Tidal volume (digital display)
    b. Graphics (pressure, volume, and flow)
    c. Inspiratory time

Questions

A. What happened to the tidal volume delivery?
B. What happened to the inspiratory time?

Exercise 4: Spontaneous/Timed (S/T) Mode Application

Identify a laboratory partner who will act as your patient. With your laboratory instructor observing you, complete the following exercise.

1. Assemble the Respironics BiPAP Vision ventilator and attach a clean circuit.

2. Using standard precautions, select the correct nasal mask for your patient and the appropriate headgear and spacers.

3. Connect the mask to the circuit, and set the ventilator to the following settings:
   Mode: Spontaneous/Timed
   IPAP: 15 cm H$_2$O
   IPAP: 4 cm H$_2$O
   Breaths per minute: 10/min
   Timed Inspiration: 0.1 second
   % O$_2$:   21%
   IPAP Rise Time: 0.1 second
   Ramp Time: Off

Once the settings are established, activate the new mode.

4. Fit the mask to your patient, using the spacer(s) and the headgear.

5. Note the following:
   a. Tidal volume (digital display)
   b. Graphics (pressure, volume, and flow)
   c. Inspiratory time

6. Adjust the alarms appropriately for your patient's volumes, pressures, and rate.

7. Change the IPAP to 10 cm H_2O.

8. Note the following:
   a. Tidal volume (digital display)
   b. Graphics (pressure, volume, and flow)
   c. Inspiratory time

Questions

A. What happened to the tidal volume when the IPAP pressure was changed?
B. What happened to the inspiratory time when the IPAP pressure was changed?

Exercise 5: Pressure Control Ventilation (PCV)

Pressure control ventilation (PCV) delivers mandatory (timed) or patient-initiated (spontaneous) pressure-controlled breaths. IPAP determines the maximum pressure delivered, whereas EPAP determines the baseline pressure.

1. Assemble the ventilator's circuit and prepare the ventilator for operation as described earlier.

2. Select the Modes tab from the bottom of the screen and press the "PCV" button.

3. The following are the active controls:
   - IPAP
   - EPAP
   - Rate
   - Inspiratory Time
   - Rise Time
   - Ramp Time
   - % O_2

4. Set the controls to the following settings by selecting the appropriate soft key and then rotating the adjustment knob to the desired setting.
   IPAP: 15 cm H_2O
   EPAP: 5 cm H_2O
   Rate: 10 breaths per minute
   Inspiratory Time: 0.1 second
   % O_2:   21%
   Rise Time: 0.1 second
   RampTime: Off

   Once the adjustments have been made, push the "Activate PCV Mode" soft key to initiate the new settings.

5. Connect the patient outlet port to the test lung, and observe the following:

   a. Graphics (pressure, volume, flow)
   b. Breath rate
   c. % O_2
   d. IPAP and EPAP pressures

6. Change the resistance to 50, increasing the R_{AW}.

7. Note the following:
   a. Tidal volume (digital display)
   b. Graphics (pressure, volume, and flow)
   c. Inspiratory time

Questions

A. What happened to the tidal volume delivery?
B. What happened to the inspiratory time?

8. Return the R_{AW} control to zero.

9. Decrease the compliance by adding an additional spring onto the bellows of the test lung.

10. Note the following:
    a. Tidal volume (digital display)
    b. Graphics (pressure, volume, and flow)
    c. Inspiratory time

Questions

A. What happened to the tidal volume delivery?
B. What happened to the inspiratory time?

11. Change the controls to the following:
    Breaths per minute: 10
    IPAP: 20 cm H_2O
    EPAP: 8 cm H_2O
    Inspiratory Time: 0.9 second

12. Repeat steps 6 through 8.

13. Note the following:
    a. Tidal volume (digital display)
    b. Graphics (pressure, volume, and flow)
    c. Inspiratory time

Questions

A. What happened to the tidal volume delivery?
B. What happened to the inspiratory time?

Exercise 6: Average Volume Assured Pressure Support

Average volume assured pressure support (AVAPS) delivers a target tidal volume with each pressure breath delivery. AVAPS breath delivery consists of pressure-controlled time-cycled breaths and pressure-supported spontaneous breaths. Pressure is regulated over several breaths to achieve the desired target tidal volume delivery.

1. Assemble the ventilator's circuit and prepare the ventilator for operation as described earlier.

2. Select the Modes tab from the bottom of the screen and press the "PCV" button.

3. The following are the active controls:
   - IPAP
   - EPAP

- Rate
- Inspiratory Time
- Rise Time
- Ramp Time
- % O_2

4. Set the controls to the following settings by selecting the appropriate soft key and then rotating the adjustment knob to the desired setting.

IPAP:	15 cm H_2O
EPAP:	5 cm H_2O
Rate:	10 breaths per minute
Inspiratory Time:	0.1 second
% O_2:	21%
Rise Time:	0.1 second
RampTime:	Off

Once the adjustments have been made, push the "Activate PCV Mode" soft key to initiate the new settings.

5. Connect the patient outlet port to the test lung, and observe the following:
   a. Graphics (pressure, volume, flow)
   b. Breath rate
   c. % O_2
   d. IPAP and EPAP pressures

6. Change the resistance to 50, increasing the R_{AW}.

7. Note the following:
   a. Tidal volume (digital display)
   b. Graphics (pressure, volume, and flow)
   c. Inspiratory time

Questions

A. What happened to the tidal volume delivery?
B. What happened to the inspiratory time?
C. What happened to the inspiratory pressure delivery?

8. Return the R_{AW} control to zero.

9. Decrease the compliance by adding an additional spring onto the bellows of the test lung.

10. Note the following:
    a. Tidal volume (digital display)
    b. Graphics (pressure, volume, and flow)
    c. Inspiratory time

Questions

A. What happened to the tidal volume delivery?
B. What happened to the inspiratory time?
C. What happened to the inspiratory pressure delivery?

11. Change the controls to the following:

Breaths per minute:	10
IPAP:	20 cm H_2O
EPAP:	8 cm H_2O
Inspiratory Time:	0.9 second

12. Repeat steps 6 through 8.

13. Note the following:
    a. Tidal volume (digital display)
    b. Graphics (pressure, volume, and flow)
    c. Inspiratory time

Questions

A. What happened to the tidal volume delivery?
B. What happened to the inspiratory time?
C. What happened to the inspiratory pressure delivery?

Check List: Initiation of NPPV

_____ 1. Verify the physician's order.
_____ 2. Scan the patient's chart as time permits.
_____ 3. Wash hands before seeing the patient.
4. Assess the patient:
_____ a. Respiratory rate
_____ b. Tidal volume
_____ c. Minute ventilation
_____ d. Rapid-shallow-breathing index
_____ e. Vital capacity
_____ f. SpO_2
_____ g. Arterial blood gases
5. Gather the required equipment:
_____ a. NPPV ventilator
_____ b. Circuit
_____ c. Masks and fitting guide

_____ d. Spacers and headgear
_____ e. Oxygen analyzer
_____ f. Oximeter monitor
_____ g. ECG monitor
_____ h. Noninvasive blood pressure monitor
_____ 6. Assemble the circuit and test the NPPV ventilator.
_____ 7. Adjust the ventilator to the ordered settings.
_____ 8. Fit the mask/headgear to the patient.
_____ 9. Connect the NPPV ventilator to the patient.
_____ 10. Work with the patient to promote comfort and adjustment to mask ventilation.
_____ 11. Readjust the mask/headgear as required for optimal comfort and minimal leaks.

12. Monitor the following:
  a. IPAP
  b. EPAP
  c. Rate
  d. Tidal volume
  e. Minute volume
  f. Inspiratory time
  g. Graphics (if available)
  h. SpO_2

  i. Breath sounds and work of breathing
  j. FIO_2
13. Set the alarms appropriately.
14. Record all parameters in the patient's chart.
15. Clean up the area, discarding any disposable packaging.
16. Wash hands upon leaving the area.

Self-Evaluation Post Test: Noninvasive Positive-Pressure Ventilation (NPPV)

1. Indications for NPPV include which of the following?
   I. Acute exacerbation of COPD
   II. Acute pulmonary edema
   III. Acute hypercapneic respiratory failure
   IV. Acute asthma
   a. I
   b. I, II
   c. I, II, III
   d. I, II, III, IV

2. Advantages of ventilation without intubation include which of the following?
   a. Use of lower pressures
   b. Ability to communicate better
   c. Ability to take fluids/medications orally
   d. Both b and c

3. Which of the following should be assessed prior to commitment to NPPV?
   I. SpO_2
   II. Respiratory rate and tidal volume
   III. Blood gases
   IV. Rapid-shallow-breathing index
   a. I
   b. I, II
   c. I, II, III
   d. I, II, III, IV

4. When assessing your patient, you note the following:
   Respiratory rate: 35/min
   Tidal volume: 0.27 L
   SpO_2: 85%
   FIO_2: 0.50
   The patient's rapid-shallow-breathing index is:
   a. 130.
   b. 7.7.
   c. 350.
   d. 43.

5. Advantages of the nasal mask include which of the following?
   I. Ability to communicate verbally
   II. Ability to eat or drink
   III. Less confining (to prevent claustrophobia)
   IV. Covers only the mouth
   a. I
   b. I, II
   c. I, II, III
   d. I, II, III, IV

6. The increased risks associated with use of a full-face mask include
   I. increased chance of gastric insufflation.
   II. increased risk of aspiration.
   III. perception of claustrophobia.
   IV. increased pressure required to seal the mask.
   a. I
   b. I, II
   c. I, II, III
   d. I, II, III, IV

7. Hazards and complications of NPPV include which of the following?
   I. Nasal/sinus pain or discomfort
   II. Eye irritation
   III. Barotrauma
   IV. Mucous plugging
   a. I
   b. I, II
   c. I, II, III
   d. I, II, III, IV

8. With use of NPPV, decreased compliance may result in which of the following changes?
   I. Increased tidal volume
   II. Decreased tidal volume
   III. Increased inspiratory time
   IV. Decreased inspiratory time
   a. I, III
   b. I, IV
   c. II, III
   d. II, IV

9. With use of NPPV, increased airway resistance (R_{AW}) may result in which of the following changes?
   I. Increased tidal volume
   II. Decreased tidal volume
   III. Increased inspiratory time
   IV. Decreased inspiratory time
   a. I, III
   b. I, IV
   c. II, III
   d. II, IV

10. Which of the following modes allows sensing of patient effort and delivery of assisted ventilation with a backup rate in case of apnea?
    a. Spontaneous
    b. Timed
    c. Spontaneous/timed
    d. Mandatory

PERFORMANCE EVALUATION:

Initiation of Noninvasive Positive-Pressure Ventilation (NPPV)

Date: Lab _____ Clinical _____ Agency _____

Lab: Pass _____ Fail _____ Clinical: Pass _____ Fail _____

Student name _____ Instructor name _____

No. of times observed in clinical _____

No. of times practiced in clinical _____

PASSING CRITERIA: Obtain 90% or better on the procedure. Tasks indicated by * must receive at least 1 point, or the evaluation is terminated. Procedure must be performed within the designated time, or the performance receives a failing grade.

SCORING: 2 points — Task performed satisfactorily without prompting.
1 point — Task performed satisfactorily with self-initiated correction.
0 points — Task performed incorrectly or with prompting required.
NA — Task not applicable to the patient care situation.

Tasks:	Peer	Lab	Clinical
* **1.** Verifies the physician's order	☐	☐	☐
* **2.** Reviews the patient's chart	☐	☐	☐
* **3.** Washes hands	☐	☐	☐
* **4.** Gathers the equipment	☐	☐	☐
5. Assesses the patient			
* a. Respiratory rate	☐	☐	☐
* b. Tidal volume	☐	☐	☐
* c. Minute volume	☐	☐	☐
* d. Rapid-shallow-breathing index	☐	☐	☐
* e. Vital capacity	☐	☐	☐
* f. SpO_2	☐	☐	☐
* g. Arterial blood gases	☐	☐	☐
6. Gathers the required equipment:			
* a. NPPV ventilator	☐	☐	☐
* b. Masks and fitting guide	☐	☐	☐
* c. Spacers and headgear	☐	☐	☐
* d. Oxygen analyzer	☐	☐	☐
* e. Oximeter monitor	☐	☐	☐

*	f. ECG monitor	☐ ☐ ☐
*	g. Blood pressure monitor	☐ ☐ ☐
*	**7.** Assembles the circuit and tests the NPPV ventilator	☐ ☐ ☐
*	**8.** Adjusts the ventilator to the ordered settings	☐ ☐ ☐
*	**9.** Correctly fits the mask/headgear	☐ ☐ ☐
*	**10.** Connects the patient to the NPPV ventilator	☐ ☐ ☐
*	**11.** Assists the patient with fit/comfort	☐ ☐ ☐
*	**12.** Readjusts the mask/headgear as needed	☐ ☐ ☐
	13. Monitors the patient	
*	a. IPAP	☐ ☐ ☐
*	b. EPAP	☐ ☐ ☐
*	c. Rate	☐ ☐ ☐
*	d. Tidal volume	☐ ☐ ☐
*	e. Minute volume	☐ ☐ ☐
*	f. Inspiratory time	☐ ☐ ☐
*	g. Graphics (flow, volume)	☐ ☐ ☐
*	h. SpO_2	☐ ☐ ☐
*	i. Breath sounds	☐ ☐ ☐
*	j. FIO_2	☐ ☐ ☐
*	k. Sets the alarms appropriately	☐ ☐ ☐
*	l. Records all parameters in the chart	☐ ☐ ☐
*	**14.** Cleans up the area, discarding disposable supplies	☐ ☐ ☐
*	**15.** Washes hands before leaving	☐ ☐ ☐

SCORE: Peer _____ points of possible 76; _____%

Lab _____ points of possible 76; _____%

Clinical _____ points of possible 76; _____%

TIME: _____ out of possible 40 minutes

STUDENT SIGNATURES

PEER: _____

STUDENT: _____

INSTRUCTOR SIGNATURES

LAB: _____

CLINICAL: _____

CHAPTER 25
Continuous Mechanical Ventilation

INTRODUCTION

As a respiratory care practitioner, you will work with different types of mechanical ventilators. You will be expected to assemble, test, and operate these ventilators safely and effectively.

Mechanical ventilation involves more than simply knowing how to operate the equipment safely. Mechanical ventilation may result in serious adverse effects on the pulmonary and cardiovascular systems. Knowledge of these effects and how to monitor the patient to assess them is essential.

In this chapter you will learn the concept of mechanical ventilation, the indications for mechanical ventilation, how to identify patients at risk for respiratory failure, and the complications of mechanical ventilation.

KEY TERMS

- **Assist-control mode**
- **Barotrauma**
- **Continuous mechanical ventilation**
- **Continuous positive airway pressure (CPAP)**
- **Dynamic compliance**

- **Invasive positive-pressure ventilation (IPPV)**
- **Noninvasive positive-pressure ventilation (NPPV)**
- **Pressure control ventilation**
- **Pressure limit**

- **Pressure support**
- **Static compliance**
- **Tubing compliance**
- **Volume control ventilation**

THEORY OBJECTIVES

At the end of this chapter, the reader should be able to:

- *Define the term continuous mechanical ventilation.*
  - *Volume control ventilation*
  - *Pressure control ventilation*
- *Differentiate between type I (normocapneic) and type II (hypercapneic) respiratory failure.*
- *Describe the indications for continuous mechanical ventilation, including:*
  - *Apnea*
  - *COPD exacerbation*
  - *Acute asthma*
  - *Neuromuscular disease*
  - *Acute hypoxic failure*
  - *Heart failure and cardiogenic shock*
- *Differentiate between the use of noninvasive positive-pressure ventilation (NPPV) and invasive positive-pressure ventilation (IPPV), including:*

  - *Advantages*
  - *Applications*
- *Differentiate among the following forms of ventilation:*
  - *Volume control and volume control/assist control*
  - *Pressure control and pressure control/assist control*
- *Describe the settings and alarm settings required for the following forms of ventilation:*
  - *Volume control*
  - *Pressure control*
- *Differentiate between the following spontaneous ventilation modes:*
  - *Continuous positive airway pressure (CPAP)*
  - *Pressure support*
- *List the recommended items that should be monitored when performing patient-ventilator system checks.*

CLINICAL PRACTICE GUIDELINES

AARC Clinical Practice Guideline Patient-Ventilator System Checks

MV-SC 4.0 INDICATIONS:

A patient-ventilator system check must be performed on a scheduled basis (which is institution-specific) for any patient requiring mechanical ventilation for life support. In addition, a check should be performed:

4.1 Prior to obtaining blood samples for analysis of blood gases and pH

4.2 Prior to obtaining hemodynamic or bedside pulmonary function data

4.3 Following any change in ventilator settings

4.4 As soon as possible following an acute deterioration of the patient's condition (this may or may not be heralded by a violation of ventilator-alarm thresholds)

4.5 Any time that ventilator performance is questionable (9)

MV-SC 5.0 CONTRAINDICATIONS:

There are no absolute contraindications to performance of a patient-ventilator system check. If disruption of PEEP or FDO$_2$ results in hypoxemia, bradycardia, or hypotension, portions of the check requiring disconnection of the patient from the ventilator may be contraindicated. (10,11)

MV-SC 6.0 HAZARDS/COMPLICATIONS:

6.1 Disconnecting the patient from the ventilator during a patient-ventilator system check may result in hypoventilation, hypoxemia, bradycardia, and/or hypotension. (10,11)

6.2 Prior to disconnection, preoxygenation and hyperventilation may minimize these complications. (12–19)

6.3 When disconnected from the patient, some ventilators generate a high flow through the patient circuit that may aerosolize contaminated condensate, putting both the patient and clinician at risk for nosocomial infection. (20)

MV-SC 8.0 ASSESSMENT OF NEED:

Because of the complexity of mechanical ventilators and the large number of factors that can adversely affect patient-ventilator interaction, routine checks of patient-ventilator system performance are mandatory.

MV-SC 9.0 ASSESSMENT OF OUTCOME:

Routine patient-ventilator system checks should prevent untoward incidents, warn of impending events, and ensure that proper ventilator settings, according to physician's order, are maintained.

MV-SC 11.0 MONITORING:

In order to ensure that patient-ventilator system checks are being performed according to these guidelines, an indicator should be created to monitor this activity as part of the appropriate department's quality improvement program. Specific criteria for the indicator should include at least items 2.4 and 12.0 of this guideline.

Reprinted with permission from *Respiratory Care* 1992; 37: 882–886. The complete AARC Clinical Practice Guidelines are available from the AARC Web site (http://www.aarc .org), from the AARC Executive Office, or from *Respiratory Care* journal.

AARC Clinical Practice Guideline
Care of the Ventilator Circuit and Its Relation to Ventilator–Associated Pneumonia
Summary of Recommendations

- Ventilator circuits should not be changed routinely for infection control purposes. The maximum duration of time that circuits can be used safely is unknown.
- Evidence is lacking related to ventilator-associated pneumonia (VAP) and issues of heated versus unheated circuits, type of heated humidifier, method for filling the humidifier, and technique for clearing condensate from the ventilator circuit.
- Although the available evidence suggests a lower VAP rate with passive humidification than with active humidification, other issues related to the use of passive humidifiers (resistance, dead space volume, airway occlusion risk) preclude a recommendation for the general use of passive humidifiers.
- Passive humidifiers do not need to be changed daily for reasons of infection control or technical performance. They can be safely used for at least 48 hours, and with some patient populations some devices may be able to be used for periods of up to 1 week.
- The use of closed suction catheters should be considered part of a VAP prevention strategy, and they do not need to be changed daily for infection control purposes. The maximum duration of time that closed suction catheters can be used safely is unknown.
- Clinicians caring for mechanically ventilated patients should be aware of risk factors for VAP (eg, nebulizer therapy, manual ventilation, and patient transport). [Respir Care 2003;48(9):869–879. © 2003 Daedalus Enterprises]

(Continued)

Introduction

A concern related to the care of the mechanically ventilated patient is the development of VAP. For many years this concern focused on the ventilator circuit and humidifier. Accordingly, the circuit and humidifier have been changed on a regular basis in an attempt to decrease the VAP rate. However, as the evidence evolved, it became apparent that the origin of VAP is more likely from sites other than the ventilator circuit,[1,2] and thus the prevailing practice has become one of changing circuits less frequently.[3] If this practice is safe, it will offer substantial cost savings. Other issues related to the components of the circuit and VAP have also become more important recently. For example, humidification systems can be either active or passive. Increasingly, inline suction is used, and this becomes part of the ventilator circuit.

A systematic review of the literature was conducted with the intention of making recommendations for change frequency of the ventilator circuit and additional components of the circuit. Specifically, the Writing Committee wrote these evidence-based clinical practice guidelines to address the following questions:

1. Do ventilator circuits need to be changed at regular intervals:
   a. For infection control purposes?
   b. Because of deterioration in performance?
2. What is the economic impact of decreasing the frequency of ventilator circuit changes?
3. What are the issues related to circuit type?
   a. Disposable versus reusable
   b. Cleaning techniques
   c. Site of care (acute care, long-term care, home care)
4. Does the choice of active versus passive humidification affect ventilator circuit change frequency?
5. Do passive humidifiers need to be changed at regular intervals:
   a. For infection control purposes?
   b. Because of deterioration in performance?
6. Do in-line suction catheters need to be changed at regular intervals:
   a. For infection control purposes?
   b. Because of deterioration in performance?
7. Are there specific populations for which the recommendations should be altered?
   a. Differences for age groups (neonatal, pediatric, adult)
   b. Differences for site of care (acute care, long-term care, home care)
   c. Differences for categories of patients (immunocompromised, burn)

Methods

To identify the evidence for addressing these questions, a PubMed (MEDLINE) search was conducted using the following search terms: pneumonia AND mechanical ventilation, humidifier, ventilator circuit, heated circuit, suction catheter, endotracheal suction, closed suction catheter, respiratory therapy equipment, endotracheal intubation, heat and moisture exchanger, tracheostomy, respiratory care, equipment contamination, equipment disinfection, artificial ventilation. The search was confined to human studies published in the English language. References and abstracts were retrieved into reference management software (EndNote, ISI, Berkeley, California). By inspection of these titles, references having no relevance to the study questions were eliminated. For the titles that remained, the abstracts were assessed for relevance and additional references were eliminated as appropriate. This process was conducted independently by 2 individuals, after which their reference lists were merged to provide the reference base for further analysis. Throughout the process of developing these guidelines, members of the Writing Committee surveyed cross-references to identify additional references to be added to the reference base for analysis.

Data were extracted from selected references using a standardized critique form. To validate this form and to establish the reliability of the review process, several references were evaluated by the entire committee during a face-to-face meeting. All references were then independently examined by at least 2 members of the Writing Committee. The critiques were compared and differences were resolved using an iterative process. All references were graded according to the following scheme:

Level 1: Randomized, controlled trial with statistically significant results
Level 2: Randomized, controlled trial with significant threats to validity (eg, small sample size, inappropriate blinding, weak methodology)
Level 3: Observational study with a concurrent control group
Level 4: Observational study with a historical control group
Level 5: Bench study, animal study, case series

The critique forms were submitted to the principal author of the guideline (DRH), who transferred the information into evidence tables and conducted appropriate statistical analysis.

Quantitative analysis consisted of meta-analysis and petograms. Statistical analysis was conducted using RevMan software (RevMan Analyses, Version 1.0 for Windows, in Review Manager [RevMan] 4.2,

(Continued)

Oxford, England: The Cochrane Collaboration, 2003). Relative risk was calculated using a random effect model. P = 0.05 was considered statistically significant. Following a systematic review of the literature, recommendations were drafted by the Writing Committee and assigned one of the following grades, based on the strength of the evidence:

Grade A: Scientific evidence provided by randomized, well-designed, well-conducted, controlled trials with statistically significant results that consistently support the guideline recommendation; supported by Level 1 or 2 evidence

Grade B: Scientific evidence provided by well-designed, well-conducted observational studies with statistically significant results that consistently support the guideline recommendation; supported by Level 3 or 4 evidence

Grade C: Scientific evidence from bench studies, animal studies, case studies; supported by Level 5 evidence

Grade D: Expert opinion provides the basis for the guideline recommendation, but scientific evidence either provided inconsistent results or was lacking

The draft document was then reviewed by experts on ventilator circuit care. Each of the reviewer's comments was carefully assessed and the document was further revised as appropriate.

Do Ventilator Circuits Need to Be Changed at Regular Intervals?

Based on studies published in the 1960s that showed an association between respiratory equipment and nosocomial pneumonia,[4,5] the practice of changing ventilator circuits at least daily was established. In fact, circuits were changed every 8 hours in some hospitals, in an attempt to reduce the incidence of VAP. This practice was challenged in a landmark study published by Craven et al in 1982.[6] In that study 240 cultures of inspiratory-phase gas were obtained from 95 patients. There was no significant difference in the frequency of positive cultures in circuits changed every 24 hours (30%) and in circuits changed every 48 hours (32%). Moreover, no significant increase in circuit colonization occurred between 24 and 48 hours. Based on that study, most hospitals in the United States adopted the practice of changing ventilator circuits at 48-hour intervals. Craven et al estimated that $300,000 (in 1982 dollars) would be saved at 20 Boston teaching hospitals by adopting this practice. Interestingly, Craven et al did not report VAP rates in their study.

The effect of ventilator circuit change interval on VAP rate was assessed in 4 prospective randomized, controlled trials (Table 1 and Fig. 1).[7-10] Although each of these studies evaluated different circuit change intervals, the combined effect supports the practice of less frequent circuit changes (relative risk 0.76, 95% confidence interval [CI] 0.57 to 1.00, p = 0.05). In each of these studies, the risk of VAP was decreased when circuits were changed less frequently. Ventilator circuit change interval was also assessed in 7 studies with historical control groups (Table 2 and Fig. 2).[11-17] Again, the combined effect supports the practice of less frequent circuit changes (relative risk 0.87, 95% CI 0.63 to 1.18, p = 0.37). Two well-designed randomized, controlled trials evaluated the practice of "no changes" of ventilator circuits.[8,9] However, the maximum duration of time that the circuit can be used safely is unknown. In one of those studies, the maximum duration of use of a circuit was 29 days.[8] The other study did not report the maximum duration of use of a circuit but did report that 35% of patients were ventilated for >14 days.[9]

The costs associated with ventilator circuit changes were calculated in 8 studies.[6,8,9,12-15,17] Because these studies were conducted over a span of 20 years and in different countries, direct cost comparisons are difficult. Not surprisingly, each of these studies suggests considerable savings in personnel and materials costs with less frequent ventilator circuit changes. One study evaluated equipment failure (circuit leaks) related to ventilator circuit change frequency.[9] In that study there was no significant difference in equipment failures when circuits were changed at weekly intervals and when circuits were not changed at regular intervals.

The majority of the studies were in adult patients in acute care units. One study was conducted in a subacute care unit.[13] Two studies included neonatal and pediatric mechanically ventilated patients.[10,11] Although ventilator circuit change interval has been studied less in patient groups other than adult patients in acute care units, the available evidence suggests no increased risk for VAP associated with infrequent circuit changes in these populations. There have been no studies that separately addressed special populations such as immunocompromised or burned patients.

Recommendation #1

Ventilator circuits should not be changed routinely for infection control purposes. The available evidence suggests no patient harm and considerable cost savings associated with extended ventilator circuit change intervals. The maximum duration of time that circuits can be used safely is unknown. (Grade A)

(Continued)

TABLE 1: Summary of Randomized Controlled Trials Investigating the Relationship Between Ventilator Circuit Change Frequency and the Risk of Ventilator-Associated Pneumonia

CITATION	STUDY POPULATION	BLINDING	VAP DIAGNOSIS	CONTROL GROUP	TREATMENT GROUP	CONTROL GROUP n	PNEUMONIA (%)	TREATMENT GROUP n	PNEUMONIA (%)	LEVEL	RELATIVE RISK (95% CI)
Craven 1986[7]	Adult patients requiring mechanical ventilation >48 h	VAP assessors	Clinical	Circuit changes every 24 h	Circuit changes every 48 h	106	29.2	127	14.2	1	0.48 (0.29, 0.82)
Dreyfuss 1991[8]	Adult patients requiring mechanical ventilation >48 h	VAP assessors	Quantitative cultures	Circuit changes every 48 h	No circuit changes	35	31.4	28	28.5	1	0.91 (0.42, 1.95)
Kollef 1995[9]	Adult patients requiring mechanical ventilation >5 d	VAP assessors	Clinical	Circuit changes every 7 d	No circuit changes	153	28.8	147	24.5	1	0.85 (0.58, 1.24)
Long 1996[10]	Neonatal and adult mechanically ventilated patients	None	Clinical	Circuit changes 3 times/wk	Circuit change 1/wk	213	12.7	234	11.1	2	0.88 (0.53, 1.45)
TOTAL						507	22.3	536	16.4		0.76 (0.57, 1.00)

VAP = ventilator-associated pneumonia.
CI = confidence interval.

(Continued)

TABLE 2: Summary of Observational Studies Investigating the Relationship Between Ventilator Circuit Change Frequency and the Risk of Ventilator-Associated Pneumonia

CITATION	STUDY POPULATION	VAP DIAGNOSIS	CONTROL GROUP	TREATMENT GROUP	CONTROL GROUP n	PNEUMONIA (%)	TREATMENT GROUP n	PNEUMONIA (%)	LEVEL	RELATIVE RISK (95% CI)
Lareau 1978[11]	Adult, pediatric, and neonatal mechanically ventilated patients	Clinical	Circuit changes at 8-h intervals	Circuit changes at 24-h intervals	213	7.5	271	11.8	4	1.57 (0.89, 2.79)
Hess 1995[12]	Adult mechanically ventilated patients	Clinical	Circuit changes at 2-d intervals	Circuit changes at 7-d intervals	1,708	5.6	1,715	4.6	4	0.83 (0.62, 1.11)
Thompson 1996[13]	Adult mechanically ventilated patients in a subacute care facility	Clinical	Circuit changes at 7-d intervals	Circuit changes at 14-d intervals	31	9.7	18	11.1	4	1.15 (0.21, 6.24)
Kotilainen 1997[14]	Adult mechanically ventilated patients	Clinical	Circuit changes at 3-d intervals	Circuit changes at 7-d intervals	88	9.1	146	6.2	4	0.68 (0.27, 1.69)
Fink 1998[15]	Adult mechanically ventilated patients	Clinical	Circuit changes at 2-d intervals	Circuit changes at 30-d intervals	336	10.7	157	6.4	4	0.59 (0.30, 1.17)
Han 2001[16]	Adult mechanically ventilated patients	Clinical	Circuit changes at 2-d intervals	Circuit changes at 7-d intervals	413	9.2	231	3.5	4	0.38 (0.18, 0.79)
Lien 2001[17]	Adult mechanically ventilated patients	Clinical	Circuit changes at 2-d intervals	Circuit changes at 7-d intervals	6,213	2.9	7,068	3.2	4	1.14 (0.94, 1.38)
TOTAL					9,002	4.1	9,606	3.8		0.87 (0.63, 1.18)

VAP = ventilator-associated pneumonia.
CI = confidence interval.

(Continued)

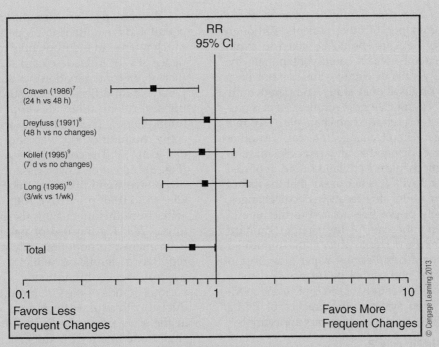

Figure 1 Randomized, controlled trials of the relationship between ventilator circuit change frequency and the risk of ventilator-associated pneumonia. RR = relative risk. CI = confidence interval

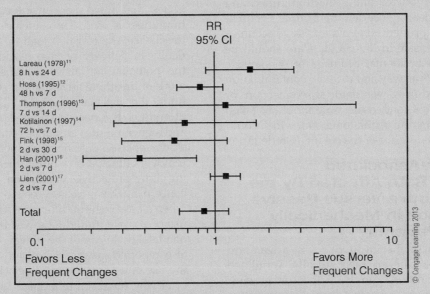

Figure 2 Observational studies of the relationship between ventilator circuit change frequency and the risk of ventilator-associated pneumonia. RR = relative risk. CI = confidence interval

Most studies used heated passover humidifiers, although several used bursting-bubble cascade-type humidifiers.[8,12,17] There is concern related to the use of bursting-bubble humidifiers because these have shown the potential to generate aerosols capable of carrying microorganisms.[18,19] However, this is not a consideration in the present day, as these devices are no longer commercially available. Moreover, bacterial levels in heated humidifiers are low and nosocomial pathogens survive poorly in this environment.[20] Although a few studies used reusable circuits,[11,17] most used disposable circuits. In several studies, heated-wire circuits were used.[10,14–16] One small study[21] compared heated-wire circuits and nonheated-wire circuits and found no difference in VAP rate (relative risk 1.57 in favor of nonheated-wire circuits, 95% CI 0.55 to 4.45). The condensate that accumulates in the ventilator circuit is

(Continued)

contaminated,[22] and care should be taken to avoid its cross-contamination of other patients. Although it makes sense that care should be taken to avoid breaking the circuit—which could contaminate the interior of the ventilator circuit—this has not been studied. One observational study compared daily with biweekly circuit changes with the use of a passive humidifier and reported no change in VAP rate with the longer circuit change interval.[23] Another study compared disposable and reusable humidifiers during mechanical ventilation, and reported no difference in VAP.[24] It is fair to say that the risk of VAP is not increased by less frequent circuit changes, despite a variety of practices related to the type of circuit used and the care of the circuit. Standard practice calls for use of sterile water in the humidifier of the ventilator circuit. Because water is an important reservoir for nosocomial pathogens and there has been no published study of this topic using modern humidification systems, the practice of filling humidifiers with sterile water appears appropriate.

Recommendation #2

Evidence is lacking related to VAP and issues of heated versus unheated circuits, type of heated humidifier, method for filling the humidifier, and technique for clearing condensate from the ventilator circuit. It is prudent to avoid excessive accumulation of condensate in the circuit. Care should be taken to avoid accidental drainage of condensate into the patient's airway and to avoid contamination of caregivers during ventilator disconnection or during disposal of condensate. Care should be taken to avoid breaking the ventilator circuit, which could contaminate the interior of the circuit. (Grade D)

Is Ventilator-Associated Pneumonia Rate Affected By the Choice of Active Versus Passive Humidification in Mechanically Ventilated Patients?

Humidification of the inspired gas is a standard practice in the care of mechanically ventilated patients. Humidifiers can be active or passive. Active humidifiers pass the inspired gas either through (bubble) or over (passover, wick) a heated water bath. Passive humidifiers (artificial nose, heat-and-moisture exchanger) trap heat and humidity from the patient's exhaled gas and return some of that to the patient on the subsequent inhalation. By its nature the ventilator circuit remains dry with the use of a passive humidifier. Passive humidifiers also have filtering characteristics, and some are constructed specifically to function as filters as well as humidifiers. The performance of humidification systems has been described in detail elsewhere.[25]

Because passive humidifiers maintain a dry circuit and have filtering properties, there has been much interest in their potential to decrease the incidence of VAP. Indeed, several studies have reported that circuit contamination is reduced with the use of passive humidifiers.[26-31] One study reported similar tracheal colonization rates with active and passive humidifiers.[32] The VAP rate with passive versus active humidification was addressed in 6 studies (Table 3).[21,33-37] The combined results of these studies (Fig. 3) indicate a lower risk of VAP with the use of passive humidification (relative risk 0.65, 95% CI 0.44 to 0.96, p = 0.03). Although the combined effect from this meta-analysis shows a statistically lower VAP for the use of passive humidifiers, it is of interest to note that only one of the studies[36] reported a significant reduction in VAP with the use of passive humidifiers. These studies used various brands of passive humidifier, all were conducted with adult patients, and all were conducted in the acute care setting. Two studies reported no significant difference in the VAP rate when comparing designs of passive humidifiers (different components, hydrophobic vs hygroscopic).[38,39]

In addition to VAP, there are other important issues that must be considered when a passive humidifier is used. These include the dead space of the device, the resistive load of the device, the difficulty in delivery of aerosolized medications, and the potential for airway occlusion. An increased work-of-breathing attributable to the use of a passive humidifier has been reported.[40] The use of a passive humidifier has been associated with higher $PaCO_2$ and higher minute ventilation requirement.[41] Another study reported significant reduction in $PaCO_2$ with removal of the passive humidifier in patients receiving lung-protective ventilation.[42] Of considerable concern is the increased risk of airway occlusion when a passive humidifier is used. In one study[33] the use of passive humidifiers was interrupted because of a fatal occlusion of the airway. Other studies have also reported greater risk of airway occlusion with the use of a passive humidifier.[34,43,44] A meta-analysis of airway occlusion associated with the use of passive humidifier reported a relative risk of 3.84 (95% CI 1.92 to 7.69, p = 0.0001), favoring the use of active humidification (ie, indicating a significantly greater risk of airway occlusion with a passive humidifier).[45] When a passive humidifier is used, it is important that one be selected that has an adequate moisture output, to minimize the risk of airway occlusion.

Recommendation #3

Although the available evidence suggests a lower VAP rate with passive humidification than with active humidification, other issues related to the use

(Continued)

TABLE 3: Summary of Randomized Controlled Trials Investigating the Relationship Between Type of Humidification and the Risk of Ventilator-Associated Pneumonia

CITATION	STUDY POPULATION	VAP DIAGNOSIS	PASSIVE HUMIDIFIER	ACTIVE HUMIDIFIER		PASSIVE HUMIDIFIER		LEVEL	RELATIVE RISK (95% CI)
				n	PNEUMONIA (%)	n	PNEUMONIA (%)		
Martin 1990[33]	Adult mechanically ventilated patients	Clinical	Pall Ultipor breathing circuit filter	42	19.0	31	6.5	2	0.34 (0.08, 1.49)
Roustan 1992[34]	Adult mechanically ventilated patients	Clinical	Pall BB 2215	61	14.8	55	9.1	1	0.62 (0.22, 1.73)
Dreyfuss 1995[35]	Adult mechanically ventilated patients	Quantitative cultures	DAR Hygrobac II	70	11.4	61	9.8	1	0.86 (0.32, 2.34)
Branson 1996[21]	Adult mechanically ventilated patients	Clinical	Baxter nonfiltered hygroscopic condenser humidifier	54	5.6	49	6.1	2	1.10 (0.23, 5.21)
Kirton 1997[36]	Adult mechanically ventilated patients	Clinical	Pall BB-100	140	15.7	140	6.4	2	0.41 (0.20, 0.86)
Kollef 1998[37]	Adult mechanically ventilated patients	Clinical	Nellcor-Puritan-Bennett hygroscopic condenser humidifier	147	10.2	163	9.2	1	0.90 (0.46, 1.78)
TOTAL				514	12.6	499	8.0		0.65 (0.44, 0.96)

VAP = ventilator-associated pneumonia.
CI = confidence interval.

(Continued)

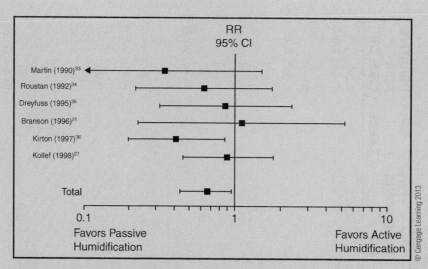

Figure 3 Randomized, controlled trials of the relationship between type of humidification and the risk of ventilator-associated pneumonia. RR = relative risk. CI = confidence interval

of passive humidifiers (resistance, dead space volume, airway occlusion risk) preclude a recommendation for the general use of these devices. The decision to use a passive humidifier should not be based solely on infection control considerations. (Grade A)

Do Passive Humidifiers Need to Be Changed at Regular Intervals?

The manufacturers of passive humidifiers typically recommend that they be changed at daily intervals. There has been interest in the safety of changing these devices less frequently, both in terms of VAP rate and device performance. Two randomized, controlled trials[46,47] and 2 observational studies compared daily versus less frequent changes of passive humidifiers (Table 4).[48,49] In 2 studies passive humidifiers were changed at 48-hour intervals,[48,49] in a separate study they were changed at 5-day intervals,[46] and in another study they were changed at 7-day intervals.[47] For the pooled results (Fig. 4), no significant difference in VAP rate was found with less frequent changes of passive humidifiers, in either the randomized, controlled studies (relative risk 0.58, 95% CI 0.24 to 1.41, p = 0.14) or the observational studies (relative risk 1.13, 95% CI 0.73 to 1.76, p = 0.9). Other studies have evaluated the technical performance of passive humidifiers used for durations up to 48 hours,[50–52] 96 hours,[53–55] and 7 days.[56] However, caution has been suggested related to prolonged use of passive humidifiers with some devices[52,57] and in some patient populations (eg, chronic obstructive pulmonary disease).[56] Based on the available evidence, it seems prudent to closely monitor the technical performance of these devices if used longer than 48 hours.

Recommendation #4

Passive humidifiers do not need to be changed daily for reasons of infection control or technical performance. They can be safely used for at least 48 hours, and with some patient populations some devices may be able to be used for up to 1 week. (Grade A)

Do In-Line Suction Catheters Need to Be Changed at Regular Intervals?

In-line closed suction systems allow mechanically ventilated patients to be suctioned without removal of ventilator support. This may decrease the complications associated with suctioning[58] and might prevent alveolar derecruitment during suctioning.[59,60] One study reported significantly less environmental contamination with closed suctioning than with open suctioning.[61] Observational studies report high levels of contamination in closed suction catheters that are in use.[62,63] However, this contamination usually arises from the endotracheal tube and the patient's lower respiratory tract. Accordingly, the patient usually contaminates the catheter, rather than vice versa. Use of closed suctioning has been recommended as part of a VAP-prevention program.[64] Two prospective, randomized, controlled trials reported similar VAP rates with closed suctioning and open suctioning.[58,65] Another study, however, reported a 3.5 times greater risk of VAP in patients randomized to receive open suctioning than those receiving closed suctioning.[66] Although the available evidence is not conclusive that closed suctioning decreases the risk of VAP, there is no high-level evidence that use of closed suction catheters increases the risk of VAP.

(Continued)

TABLE 4: Summary of Studies Investigating the Relationship Between Change Frequency for Passive Humidifiers and the Risk of Ventilator-Associated Pneumonia

CITATION	STUDY POPULATION	VAP DIAGNOSIS	CONTROL GROUP	TREATMENT GROUP	CONTROL GROUP n	CONTROL GROUP PNEUMONIA (%)	TREATMENT GROUP n	TREATMENT GROUP PNEUMONIA (%)	LEVEL	RELATIVE RISK (95% CI)
Randomized Controlled Trials										
Davis 2000[46]	Adult mechanically ventilated patients	Clinical	HME changed every 24 h	HME changed every 120 h	100	8.0	120	7.5	1	0.94 (0.38, 2.34)
Thomachot 2002[47]	Adult mechanically ventilated patients	Clinical	HME changed every 24 h	HME changed every 7 d	84	26.2	71	9.9	1	0.38 (0.17, 0.83)
TOTAL					184	16.3	191	8.4		0.58 (0.24, 1.41)
Observational Studies										
Djedaini 1995[48]	Adult mechanically ventilated patients	Quantitative cultures	HME changed every 24 h	HME changed every 48 h	61	9.8	68	11.8	4	1.20 (0.44, 3.25)
Daumal 1999[49]	Adult mechanically ventilated patients	Quantitative cultures	HME changed every 24 h	HME changed every 48 h	174	14.4	187	16.0	4	1.12 (0.68, 1.82)
TOTAL					235	13.2	255	14.9		1.13 (0.73, 1.76)

VAP = ventilator-associated pneumonia.
CI = confidence interval.

(Continued)

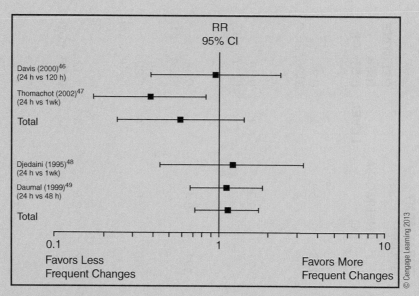

Figure 4 Studies of the relationship between passive humidifier change frequency and the risk of ventilator-associated pneumonia. RR = relative risk. CI = confidence interval

The in-line closed suction catheter might be considered an extension of the ventilator circuit. Because ventilator circuits do not need to be changed at regular intervals for infection control purposes, this might suggest that in-line suction catheters also do not need to be changed at regular intervals for infection control purposes. Although the manufacturers of in-line suction catheters recommend that these devices be changed at regular intervals, there is accumulating evidence that they might not need to be changed routinely. One observational study reported no change in VAP rate when in-line suction catheters were changed on a weekly rather than daily basis.[67] Another study reported no significant difference in VAP rate between patients randomized to receive daily changes of the in-line suction catheter and those with whom there were no routine changes of the in-line catheter (relative risk 0.99, 95% CI 0.66 to 1.50).[68] The maximum duration of use of a closed suction catheter in that study was 67 days. There were few device malfunctions when in-line catheters were changed less frequently than daily, and there were important cost savings associated with this practice.[67,68] As with ventilator circuits, the maximum duration that closed suction catheters can be used safely is not known.

Recommendation #5

The use of closed suction catheters should be considered part of a VAP prevention strategy. When closed suction catheters are used, they do not need to be changed daily for infection control purposes. The maximum duration of time that closed suction catheters can be used safely is unknown. (Grade A)

Other Issues

Other issues related to the technical aspects of mechanical ventilation may be important in relation to VAP. Medication nebulizers can be a source of contamination that could lead to VAP.[69] Accordingly, with nebulizers care must be taken to avoid contamination of the ventilator circuit and the patient's respiratory tract. It is commonly believed by respiratory therapists that the risk of ventilator circuit contamination is reduced with the use of metered-dose inhalers, but this has not been reported. Manual ventilator devices that are commonly kept at the bedside of mechanically ventilated patients have been shown to be a source of airway contamination, so care should be taken to minimize the potential infection risks associated with manual ventilator devices.[70,71] One study reported a significantly greater likelihood of VAP among patients who underwent transport out of the intensive care unit for diagnostic, surgical, or miscellaneous interventions (odds ratio 3.8, 95% CI 2.6 to 5.5, p = 0.001).[72] Because a VAP risk education program for respiratory therapists and critical care nurses decreased the incidence of VAP,[73] VAP risk education should be widely implemented.

Recommendation #6

Clinicians (respiratory therapists, nurses, and physicians) caring for mechanically ventilated patients should be aware of risk factors for VAP (eg, nebulizer therapy, manual ventilation, and patient transport). (Grade B)

(Continued)

Discussion

Substantial evidence now exists to make recommendations related to the technical practices of mechanical ventilation and the risk of VAP. However, important gaps also exist in this evidence base. For example, most of the published evidence comes from studies of adult patients. Few data have been published for neonatal and pediatric populations. In addition most studies come from the acute care setting. Finally, there has been little research done on important subgroups of patients, such as immunocompromised patients. Accordingly, much remains to be learned about important relationships between the technical aspects of mechanical ventilation and the risk of VAP. Thus, these evidence-based guidelines provide not only a basis for current practice but are also a framework for further investigation.

Reprinted with permission from *Respiratory Care* 2003; 48(9): 869–879. The complete AARC Clinical Practice Guidelines are available from the AARC Web site (http://www.aarc.org), from the AARC Executive Office, or from *Respiratory Care* journal.

AARC Clinical Practice Guideline Long-Term Invasive Mechanical Ventilation in the Home—2007 Revision & Update

HIMV 4.0 INDICATIONS:

4.1 Patients requiring invasive long-term ventilator support have demonstrated

4.1.1 An inability to be completely weaned from invasive ventilatory supportor

4.1.2 A progression of disease etiology that requires increasing ventilatory support.

4.2 Conditions that met these criteria may include but are not limited to ventilatory muscle disorders, alveolar hypoventilation syndrome, primary respiratory disorders, obstructive lung diseases, restrictive lung diseases, and cardiac disorders, including congenital anomalies[1-6,16-20]

HIMV 5.0 CONTRAINDICATIONS:

Contraindications to HIMV include:

5.1 The presence of a physiologically unstable medical condition requiring higher level of care or resources than available in the home[1-6] Examples of indicators of a medical condition too unstable for the home and long term care setting are:

5.1.1 FIO_2 requirement >0.40[1-6]

5.1.2 PEEP >10 cm H_2O[1-6]

5.1.3 Need for continuous invasive monitoring in adult patients[1-6]

5.1.4 Lack of mature tracheostomy

5.2 Patient's choice not to receive home mechanical ventilation[1-6,20-24]

5.3 Lack of an appropriate discharge plan[1-6]

5.4 Unsafe physical environment as determined by the patient's discharge planning team[1-6]

5.4.1 Presence of fire, health or safety hazards including unsanitary conditions[1-6]

5.4.2 Inadequate basic utilities (such as heat, air conditioning, electricity including adequate amperage and grounded outlets)[1-6]

5.5 Inadequate resources for care in the home

5.5.1 Financial[1-6,25-28]

5.5.2 Personnel

5.5.2.1 Inadequate medical follow-up[1-6]

5.5.2.2 Inability of VAI to care for self, if no caregiver is available[1-6]

5.5.2.3 Inadequate respite care for caregivers[21-23,29,30]

5.5.2.4 Inadequate numbers of competent caregivers[1-6] A minimum of two competent caregivers are required.

HIMV 6.0 HAZARDS AND COMPLICATIONS:

6.1 Deterioration or acute change in clinical status of VAI. Although ventilator-associated complications in the home are poorly documented, experience in other sites can be extrapolated. The following may cause death or require rehospitalization for acute treatment.

6.1.1 Medical: Hypocapnia, respiratory alkalosis hypercapnia, respiratory acidosis, hypoxemia, barotraumas, seizures hemodynamic instability, airway complications (stomal or tracheal infection, mucus plugging, tracheal erosion, or stenosis), respiratory infection (tracheobronchitis, pneumonia, bronchospasm, exacerbation of underlying disease, or natural course of the disease[1-6,14]

6.1.2 Equipment-related: Failure of the ventilator, malfunction of equipment, inadequate warming, and humidification of the inspired gases, inadvertent changes in ventilator settings, accidental disconnection from ventilator, accidental decannulation[1-6,31-36]

6.1.3 Psychosocial: Depression, anxiety, loss of resources (caregiver or financial), detrimental change in family structure or coping capacity[1-6,21-24,29,30,37,38]

HIMV 8.0 ASSESSMENT OF NEED:

8.1 Determination that indications are present and contraindications are absent

8.2 Determination that the goals listed in 2.1 can be met in the home

8.3 Determination that no continued need exists for higher level of services

(Continued)

8.4 Determination that frequent changes in the plan of care will not be needed

HIMV 9.0 ASSESSMENT OF OUTCOME:

At least the following aspects of patient management and condition should be evaluated periodically as long as the patient receives HIMV:

9.1 Implementation and adherence to the plan of care

9.2 Quality of life

9.3 Patient satisfaction

9.4 Resource utilization

9.5 Growth and development in the pediatric patient

9.6 Unanticipated morbidity, including need for higher level site of care

9.7 Unanticipated mortality

HIMV 11.0 MONITORING:

The frequency of monitoring should be determined by the ongoing individualized care plan and be based upon the patient's current medical condition. The ventilator settings, proper function of equipment, and the patient's physical condition should be monitored and verified: with each initiation of invasive ventilation to the patient, including altering the source of ventilation, as from one ventilator or resuscitation bag to another ventilator; with each ventilator setting change; after moving the patient (eg, from the bed to a chair); on a regular basis as specified by individualized plan of care.[3] All caregivers, both professional and appropriately trained lay caregivers, should follow the care plan and implement the monitoring that has been prescribed. After being trained and evaluated on their level of knowledge and ability to respond to the VAI clinical response to each intervention, lay caregivers with documented competency may operate, perform routine maintenance tasks, monitor equipment, and perform personal care required by the VAI.

11.1 After completing training, demonstrating competency and if directed in the VAI's plan of care, the lay caregivers should monitor the following

  11.1.1 Patient's physical condition (may include the following: respiratory rate, heart rate, color changes, chest excursion, diaphoresis and lethargy, blood pressure, body temperature)

  11.1.2 Ventilator settings. The frequency at which alarms and settings are to be checked should be specified in the plan of care.

    11.1.2.1 Peak pressures

    11.1.2.2 Preset tidal volume or preset pressure control

    11.1.2.3 Frequency of ventilator breaths

    11.1.2.4 Verification of oxygen concentration setting or flow rate of oxygen bled into the ventilator system

    11.1.2.5 PEEP level (if applicable)

    11.1.2.6 Appropriate humidification of inspired gases

    11.1.2.7 Temperature of inspired gases (if applicable)

    11.1.2.8 Heat-moisture exchanger (HME) function (if applicable)

  11.1.3 Equipment function[3,5]

    11.1.3.1 Appropriate configuration of ventilator circuit[3,5]

    11.1.3.2 Alarm function

    11.1.3.3 Cleanliness of filter(s)—according to manufacturer's recommendation

    11.1.3.4 Battery power level(s)—both internal and external

    11.1.3.5 Overall condition of all equipment

    11.1.3.6 Self-inflating manual resuscitator cleanliness and function

11.2 Health care professionals should perform a thorough, comprehensive assessment of the patient and the patient-ventilator system on a regular basis as prescribed by the plan of care. In addition to the variables listed in 11.1.1–11.1.3.6, the health care professional should implement, monitor, and assess results of other interventions as indicated by the clinical situation and anticipated in the care plan.

  11.2.1 Pulse oximetry—should be used to assess patients requiring a change in prescribed oxygen levels or in patients with a suspected change in condition[3,5]

    11.2.1.1 A physician's order for pulse oximetry must be obtained before oximetry testing is performed

  11.2.2 End-tidal CO_2—may be useful for establishing trends in CO_2 levels [3,20]

    11.2.2.1 A physician's order for end tidal CO_2 monitoring must be obtained before end tidal CO_2 monitoring is performed

  11.2.3 Ventilator settings

  11.2.4 Exhaled tidal volume

  11.2.5 Analysis of fraction of inspired oxygen

11.3 Health care professionals are also responsible for maintaining interdisciplinary communication concerning the plan of care

11.4 Health care professionals should integrate respiratory plan of care into the patient's total care plan.[2,3,5,6] Plan of care should include

  11.4.1 All aspects of patient's respiratory care[2,3,5,6]

  11.4.2 Ongoing assessment and education of the caregivers involved

Reprinted with permission from *Respiratory Care* 2007; 52(1): 1056–1062. The complete AARC Clinical Practice Guidelines are available from the AARC Web site (http://www.aarc.org), from the AARC Executive Office, or from *Respiratory Care* journal.

WHAT IS CONTINUOUS MECHANICAL VENTILATION?

Continuous mechanical ventilation (CMV) is the support of a patient's ventilatory needs by artificial means. A patient in respiratory failure or approaching respiratory failure may be ventilated mechanically until the disease state or underlying cause for respiratory failure has been resolved and the patient's ventilatory efforts have adequately resumed.

The mechanical ventilator applies positive pressure to the airway during inspiration until a preset pressure, volume, or time is reached. The patient is allowed to exhale passively to ambient pressure, and then the cycle is repeated.

Volume Control and Pressure Control Ventilation

Volume control ventilation (VCV) allows the respiratory care practitioner to set the volume to be delivered with each mandatory breath (Campbell, 2002). When using this form of ventilation, tidal volume remains constant while pressure varies. Volume will remain constant in the face of changes in the patient's pathophysiology (changes in resistance or compliance). Increasing airway pressures may occur in the face of decreasing compliance or increasing resistance. The advantage of VCV is the direct control of minute ventilation ($V_t \times$ rate). Figure 25-1 depicts VCV graphically using scalar waveforms.

Pressure control ventilation (PCV) allows the respiratory care practitioner to set the target pressure (inspiratory pressure) with each mandatory breath (Campbell, 2002). When using this form of ventilation, tidal volume and minute ventilation (V_E) will vary with changes in the compliance or resistance. With decreases in compliance or increases in airway resistance, tidal volume will diminish. An advantage of this form of ventilation is preventing overdistention of normal areas of the lung by application of excessive pressure. Figure 25-2 depicts PCV using scalar waveforms.

RESPIRATORY FAILURE

Respiratory failure is a syndrome in which the lungs are unable to exchange gases. The exchange of oxygen or carbon dioxide, or both, may be impaired during respiratory failure. Respiratory failure can be defined as a partial pressure of oxygen in the arterial blood (PaO_2) of 40 to 59 mm Hg while breathing room air or a partial pressure of carbon dioxide in the arterial blood ($PaCO_2$) greater than 50 mm Hg. The gas exchange abnormality may be acute or chronic. Respiratory failure may be broadly categorized into two classifications: type I and type II. Type I respiratory failure is defined as normocapneic hypoxemic respiratory failure. Although type II respiratory failure is defined as a $PaCO_2$ greater than 50 mm Hg, it is often accompanied by hypoxemia.

Type I respiratory failure, normocapneic hypoxemic respiratory failure, is defined as a PaO_2 of less than

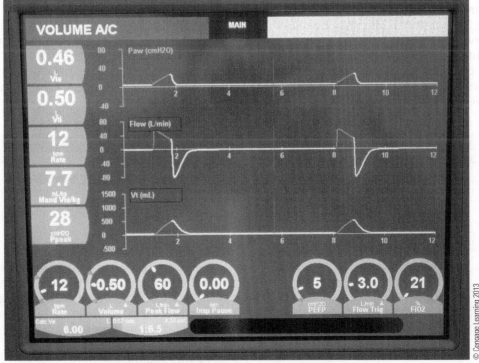

Figure 25-1   Scalar waveforms showing volume control ventilation

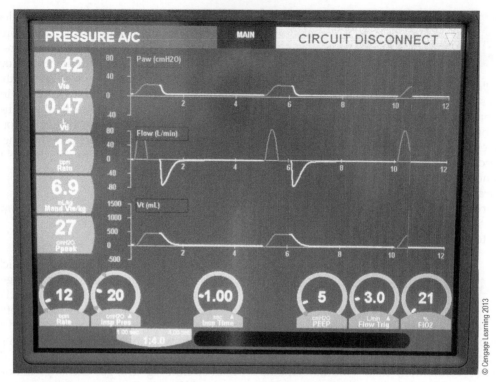

Figure 25-2 Scalar waveforms showing pressure control ventilation

PaO₂ mm Hg	Range
60 mm Hg–predicted normal	Mild
40–59 mm Hg	Moderate
<40	Server

© Cengage Learning 2013

Figure 25-3 Hypoxemia ranges based on PaO₂ values

59 mm Hg (Figure 25-3) with PaCO₂ levels within normal ranges. Type I respiratory failure may be caused by pulmonary edema, pulmonary embolism, pneumonia, pulmonary shunting, chronic obstructive pulmonary disease (COPD), or interstitial fibrosis. These conditions cause a decrease of ventilation/perfusion or increase pulmonary shunt (Neema, 2003; Pierson, 2002).

Type II respiratory failure is characterized by hypercapnia that may be accompanied by hypoxemia. It may be caused by impairment of ventilatory drive, impairment of the neuromuscular control of the ventilatory muscles, chest wall disorders, and airway obstruction (Neema, 2003). Table 25-1 summarizes the characteristics of type I and type II respiratory failure.

INDICATIONS FOR MECHANICAL VENTILATION

Mechanical ventilation can be a lifesaving modality. Commitment to mechanical ventilation usually entails the placement of an artificial airway, which with the

TABLE 25-1: Characteristics of Type I and Type II Respiratory Failure

	TYPE I RESPIRATORY FAILURE	TYPE II RESPIRATORY FAILURE
Arterial Blood Gases	pH: 7.35–7.45 PaCO₂: 25–40 mm Hg HCO₃: 22–26 mEq/L PaO₂: 40–59 mm Hg	pH: <7.35 PaCO₂: >50 mm Hg HCO₃: Normal or elevated PaO₂: <50 mm Hg
Potential Causes	• Pulmonary edema • Pulmonary embolism • Pneumonia • Pulmonary shunting • COPD • Interstitial fibrosis	• Ventilatory drive impairment (brainstem infarction or hemorrhage, brainstem trauma, drug overdose) • Neuromuscular (myasthenia gravis, amyotrophic lateral sclerosis, Guillain-Barré, spinal cord injury) • Chest wall disorders (muscular dystrophy, poliomyelitis, flail chest) • Airway obstruction (upper or lower)

application of positive pressure within the chest can cause hazards and complications. Therefore, commitment to mechanical ventilation is never taken lightly, and clear indications must be present prior to its initiation.

Apnea and Impending Respiratory Failure

The absolute indication for mechanical ventilation is apnea or impending respiratory arrest (Pierson, 2002). When caring for a patient who is apneic, bag/mask ventilation followed by intubation and mechanical ventilatory support are indicated. Only through support of ventilation by artificial means can the patient continue to survive.

Pending respiratory failure is another event in which clinicians are likely to intubate and initiate mechanical ventilation (Pierson, 2002). Clinical judgment and a clinician's assessment of the patient's pending failure play an important role in the decision to initiate mechanical ventilation. Patient appearance, degree of dyspnea, hypoxemia, and tachypnea are common indicators for impending respiratory failure or ventilatory fatigue.

Acute Exacerbation of COPD

As described in Chapter 24, Noninvasive Positive-Pressure Ventilation, positive-pressure ventilation and, specifically, noninvasive ventilation, has been applied in the treatment of exacerbation of COPD. The Global Initiative for Chronic Obstructive Lung Disease (GOLD) also specifies objective and subjective criteria to be used to initiate mechanical ventilation in the face of COPD exacerbation (Pauwels, 2001). Trending of $PaCO_2$, respiratory acidosis, and the patient's mental status is important in determining when to initiate mechanical ventilation (Pierson, 2002).

Acute Asthma

Initiation of mechanical ventilation in the treatment of acute asthma is similar to that of the treatment of exacerbation of COPD. Asthma leads to type I respiratory failure (early phases of an acute attack) and later with decompensation can result in hypoxemia, hypercarbia, and respiratory acidosis (Neema, 2003). The clinical goals while managing a patient with asthma on mechanical ventilation are to maintain the pH greater than 7.2 and to keep the oxygen saturation (SpO_2) greater than 88% to 92% while minimizing hyperinflation (Medoff, 2008). Achieving these goals requires lower tidal volumes, keeping plateau pressures less than 30 cm H_2O, and providing adequate exhalation time to minimize air trapping. Use of both pressure control and volume control breath delivery has been successful in the management of these patients (Medoff, 2008).

Neuromuscular Disease

Neuromuscular diseases such as myasthenia gravis, amyotrophic lateral sclerosis, Guillain-Barré syndrome, spinal cord injuries, and multiple sclerosis may all lead to respiratory failure. Often, this form of respiratory failure is termed *pump failure*, referring to the mechanics of ventilation. All of these disorders interrupt or interfere with the neurotransmission of signals to the ventilatory muscles. Once the muscles no longer receive signals to contract, ventilation ceases or becomes impaired. This ultimately leads to type II respiratory failure (Neema, 2003). Measuring vital capacity and maximum inspiratory pressures has been used to predict pending respiratory failure in these patients (Pierson, 2002).

Acute Hypoxemic Failure

Disorders that can lead to hypoventilation, intrapulmonary shunting, decreased cardiac output, or increased metabolic rate may lead to type I hypoxemic respiratory failure (Neema, 2003). Examples of these conditions include adult respiratory distress syndrome (ARDS), pulmonary edema, interstitial fibrosis, pneumonia, pulmonary embolism, and pulmonary hypertension. Both *noninvasive positive-pressure ventilation (NPPV)* and *invasive positive-pressure ventilation (IPPV)* have been used successfully to treat these patients (Pierson, 2002). Symptoms such as tachypnea, respiratory distress, altered mental status, hypotension, or other findings help to guide the clinician as to when to initiate ventilatory support.

Heart Failure and Cardiogenic Shock

Heart failure and cardiogenic shock can lead to type I respiratory failure (Neema, 2003). The goal of mechanical ventilatory support in these patients is to maintain adequate oxygenation when conventional oxygen therapy is inadequate. The use of continuous positive airway pressure (CPAP) and noninvasive ventilation can reduce the rate of intubation and mortality in this population (Masip, 2005).

NONINVASIVE POSITIVE-PRESSURE VENTILATION AND INVASIVE POSITIVE-PRESSURE VENTILATION

It is possible to deliver positive-pressure ventilation using two distinct methods: NPPV, sometimes referred to as just noninvasive ventilation (NIV), and IPPV, which is usually referred to as positive-pressure ventilation. NIV is the application of positive-pressure ventilation without placement of an artificial airway (usually using a mask), whereas IPPV is the application of positive-pressure ventilation through an artificial airway.

Noninvasive Ventilation

NIV is defined as the use of a mask or nasal prongs to provide positive-pressure ventilatory support through the patient's nose or mouth (Cheifetz, 2003). NIV provides a means of ventilatory support without the need to place an artificial airway (intubation with an endotracheal tube or laryngeal mask airway or tracheostomy tube placement). This form of ventilation has some unique advantages and disadvantages when compared with IPPV.

Advantages and Disadvantages of Noninvasive Ventilation

Advantages of NIV are described in Chapter 24. These include avoidance of intubation, decreased risk of hospital-acquired infections, improved comfort, improved secretion clearance, and better communication.

Disadvantages of NIV, described in Chapter 24, include complications relating to the mask or patient interface, complications related to flow or pressure delivery, complications related to aspiration and mucous plugging, complications of inadequate gas exchange, and hemodynamic compromise. Problems relating to the mask or patient interface include discomfort, skin breakdown (rash, pressure sores), increased dead space, leaks, and the risk of aspiration (Gay, 2009).

Applications of Noninvasive Ventilation

The range of applications of NIV include patients with a do not intubate (DNI) advance directive, exacerbation of COPD, pulmonary edema, obesity hypoventilation syndrome, neuromuscular diseases, and extubation failure (Pierson, 2009). In general if the patient's pathology is not severe (e.g., evidence of ARDS, acute shunting, or high oxygen demands necessitating high levels of positive end-expiratory pressure [PEEP]), NIV may be considered. However, if the patient has excessive secretions or significant infiltrates on the chest radiograph (unilateral or bilateral) or severe underlying pathology, NIV may not be the method of choice (Farha, 2006).

Invasive Positive-Pressure Ventilation

IPPV is the application of positive-pressure ventilation invasively through an endotracheal tube (Pierson, 2002). The endotracheal tube provides a secure airway and, when cuffed, minimizes loss of volume through leaks. However, as described in Chapter 20, Emergency Airway Management, there are both short-term and long-term hazards associated with the placement of the endotracheal tube. IPPV allows the utilization of more advanced modes of gas delivery, which are not possible via NIV.

Advantages of Invasive Positive-Pressure Ventilation

IPPV has several advantages when compared with NIV. These include the ability to regulate minute ventilation and tidal volumes, improved oxygen delivery, improved monitoring capability of critical care ventilators, and the availability of more advanced modes of ventilation. The ability to control and regulate minute ventilation and tidal volume delivery is a distinct advantage of IPPV. The cuffed endotracheal tube minimizes leaks and therefore ensures that what the clinician sets on the ventilator is delivered to the patient. This is especially important when employing lung protective strategies to prevent ventilator-induced lung injury (VILI) (MacIntyre, 2002). The endotracheal tube provides a secure airway and facilitates secretion removal. However, as described in Chapter 20, strategies must be employed to minimize silent aspiration and other complications associated with the placement of the endotracheal tube.

Oxygen delivery and improved gas exchange is better with IPPV when compared with NIV. The advanced intensive care unit (ICU) ventilator has better flow, pressure, and oxygen delivery capability compared with many portable ventilators employed for NIV. The advantage of a cuffed endotracheal tube also facilitates better gas exchange through the minimizing of leaks and subsequent volume or pressure loss.

Modern ICU ventilators have very advanced monitoring and alarm capabilities. These features can greatly simplify the management of acutely ill patients on ventilatory support. The use of real-time graphical waveforms; pressure, flow, and volume monitoring; and other features are important in safely applying IPPV in the management of these patients.

Advanced modes are available with IPPV such as dual control modes, closed-loop modes, and others that are not commonly applied when using NIV. These advanced modes may make significant differences in some patients who are acutely ill.

Disadvantages of Invasive Positive-Pressure Ventilation

IPPV has several disadvantages. These include decreased patient comfort, risk of ventilator-associated pneumonia (VAP), and VILI. Patient comfort is diminished through intubation. Communication is more difficult, cough effectiveness is decreased, and the patient is unable to eat or drink. Often sedation is required for patient comfort and to facilitate the use of ventilator modes with unusual patterns, such as inverse ratio ventilation.

IPPV and the placement of an endotracheal tube carry a greater risk of VAP (Gay, 2009). The endotracheal tube impairs the patient's cough and allows for accumulation of secretions above the inflated cuff. These contribute to VAP. Breaking or opening of the ventilator circuit to ambient air can also contribute to VAP.

VILI can result from the application of high pressures and volumes and delivery of increased oxygen tension. Delivery of high pressure and large volumes can lead to stretch injury or *barotrauma* (Hudson, 1998). The ARDS net data recommend that tidal volume delivery be limited to 6 mL/kg normal body weight to maintain a plateau pressure of less than 30 cm H_2O (ARDS NET, 2000).

CONTROL VARIABLE AND MODE OF VENTILATION

The microprocessor control circuit of a ventilator can control pressure, volume, flow, or time during breath delivery. The control variable is the independent variable, and that variable determines the characteristics of breath delivery along with the independent variables. The two broad categories of mechanical ventilation include the two primary control variables, pressure and volume. Often the term *mode* is used somewhat interchangeably to describe breath delivery in simpler terms.

Control Variable

The control variable refers to which variable (pressure, volume, flow, or time) is measured by the ventilator control circuit and used as a feedback signal by the ventilator to control the ventilator's output (Chatburn, 1991). The two most common control variables in adult IPPV are volume and pressure.

When volume is selected as the control variable (independent variable), this is termed *volume control*. During inspiration the ventilator measures flow (integrated over a known period to derive volume) and ends the inspiratory phase when the selected volume has been delivered (Chatburn, 1991). The majority of critical care ventilators measure flow, even though the clinician selects volume as the control variable (Campbell, 2002; Chatburn, 2001). The set volume will be delivered in the face of changing resistance or compliance (pathophysiology) and pressure will become the dependent variable. High pressures can result from worsening compliance or increasing resistance. An advantage of volume control is that both tidal volume and minute ventilation may be closely regulated. Increasing or decreasing rate (at a given tidal volume) has a direct and proportional relationship with minute ventilation. However, changes in physiologic dead space influence actual alveolar ventilation (Campbell, 2002).

When pressure is selected as the control variable (independent variable), this is termed *pressure control*. During inspiration the ventilator's control circuit measures pressure and uses it as a feedback signal to control the ventilator's output (Chatburn, 2001). The set pressure will be delivered in the face of changing resistance or compliance (pathology) and volume becomes the dependent variable. During PCV, volume will vary, resulting in changing minute ventilation and tidal breath delivery. Flow is also variable during pressure control. The ventilator increases flow output early in the breath delivery to ensure that the desired pressure target is met, and then flow decreases as the selected pressure is maintained. The typical flow pattern delivered is a decelerating flow pattern (Campbell, 2002). Advantages of PCV are that more normal areas of the lung are spared from overdistention by controlling pressure delivery and the potential of improved patient comfort for those patients with spontaneous efforts in that the variable flow delivery can more closely match their inspiratory needs (Campbell, 2002).

Mode of Ventilation

There are several modes of ventilation. For the purposes of this chapter, the discussion is limited to mandatory and spontaneous modes in either VCV or PCV. Other more advanced modes are described in Chapter 26.

Mandatory breath delivery is also referred to as continuous mandatory ventilation (CMV). During CMV, the ventilator delivers breaths at a set rate (time triggered) and a patient's spontaneous efforts to initiate a breath are ignored (Chatburn, 2001). If the patient has an intact ventilatory drive, sedation or paralysis will be required to maintain this mode of ventilation; otherwise the patient will experience dysynchrony with the ventilator.

Spontaneous triggering of ventilator breaths during VCV or PCV is termed *assist control*. Modes for the purposes of this discussion may include volume control/assist-control or pressure control/*assist-control modes* (Campbell, 2002). The clinician sets a trigger variable (pressure or flow are the most common adult trigger variables), which the ventilator measures and uses as a signal to initiate a patient-triggered breath. The control variable selected (volume or pressure) is delivered when the ventilator detects that the patient has initiated a breath. Assist-control ventilation will result in a rate and minute ventilation higher than what the clinician sets (mandatory rate), depending on how many breaths the patient triggers or initiates.

VENTILATOR SETTINGS

Once the decision has been made to commit a patient to mechanical ventilation, initial ventilator settings must be established. The selection of settings will be determined by the underlying pathology (reason for respiratory failure), the patient's ideal body weight, and other factors.

Volume Control Ventilation

Ventilator settings required for VCV include the control variable (volume control), tidal volume, rate, flow rate or inspiratory time, flow pattern, percent oxygen, and PEEP. The first step is to select the control variable, volume. Once volume control has been established, the software of the individual ventilator will prompt the clinician to select the appropriate settings.

Tidal volume is selected based on the patient's ideal body weight. Ideal body weight is based on height. The formulas for calculating ideal body weight are listed in Table 25-2.

TABLE 25-2: Ideal Body Weight Formulas (NIH, 2000)	
Males (kg)	50 + 0.91 (centimeters of height − 152.4)
Females (kg)	45.5 + 0.91 (centimeters of height − 152.4)

Tidal volume should be set in the range of 4 to 9 mL/kg (6 mL/kg) ideal body weight to attain a plateau pressure of less than 30 cm H_2O (ARDs NET, 2000). Lower tidal volumes protect the lungs from VILI.

The rate should be adjusted to maintain the desired minute ventilation. Minute ventilation will determine the patient's $PaCO_2$ and, ultimately, pH. The rate may be adjusted upward or downward to maintain the desired $PaCO_2$ and pH (MacIntyre, 2002). In some cases, it may not be possible to maintain the desired pH or $PaCO_2$ and the patient is allowed to become hypercarbic (permissive hypercapnea) with a subsequent decline in the pH.

Inspiratory flow rate or inspiratory time is adjusted to allow adequate emptying of the lungs during the expiratory phase for a given rate setting. Flow and inspiratory time should be adjusted to minimize air trapping and intrinsic PEEP (MacIntyre, 2002).

Oxygen delivery (percent oxygen) is usually set at 50% or greater initially and then titrated based on SpO_2 and arterial blood gases. In most patients, it is desirable to maintain an SpO_2 of 90% or greater with a PaO_2 of 60 mm Hg or greater. The exception would be those patients who have documented COPD. In these patients an SpO_2 of 88% to 90% is an acceptable target range for oxygen titration.

PEEP recruits lung volume by expanding the functional residual capacity (FRC), which results in an improvement in gas exchange. Application of PEEP in patients with COPD can help to unload the ventilatory muscles and improve mechanics as well as improve the patient's work of breathing (Saura, 2002). PEEP should be adjusted so that gas exchange is optimized without overdistention and increasing intrinsic PEEP. In general, a range between 5 and 24 cm H_2O should be used (NIH, 2000). It is important to monitor plateau pressures and the pressure-volume curve to prevent overdistention and VILI (Saura, 2002).

Volume Control/Assist-Control Ventilation

Settings used for volume control/assist-control ventilation are similar to the settings used for volume control except that trigger sensitivity must be added. The addition of a trigger variable allows the ventilator to detect spontaneous patient efforts and initiate a mandatory breath.

The trigger variables commonly used with adult patients include pressure and flow. Pressure triggering is set by establishing the trigger sensitivity as pressure, and then adjusting the trigger sensitivity. Pressure triggering is typically set between 1 and 3 cm H_2O. When a patient initiates a breath, subambient pressure (trigger pressure) is transmitted to the ventilator's pressure transducer, and a breath is delivered once the trigger threshold has been met. If the sensitivity is set at −2 cm H_2O, then once baseline pressure falls by 2 cm H_2O, the ventilator delivers a mandatory breath.

Flow triggering uses flow as a trigger variable to determine when a patient-triggered breath is delivered.

Flow triggering requires that a baseline flow be established (some ventilators require this to be clinician set, whereas others set the baseline flow at a multiple of the trigger sensitivity), and then the trigger sensitivity is set. A range of trigger sensitivities may be set from 0.5 L/min to as high as 20 L/min. Once the ventilator's flow sensor detects a drop in baseline flow exceeding the trigger sensitivity, a mandatory breath is delivered.

Pressure Control Ventilation

PCV is established by the clinician selecting pressure control mode and setting the pressure control level (target). Once the control variable (pressure) has been established, inspiratory time, rate, percent oxygen, and PEEP are set. Like with volume control, plateau pressures should be maintained below 30 cm H_2O.

Inspiratory time is typically ordered by the attending physician, as is the pressure target in PCV. Inspiratory time must be sufficient to allow adequate gas exchange. Lengthening inspiratory time increases mean airway pressures and may lead to hypotension, diminished cardiac output, and unwanted decline in oxygenation (Campbell, 2002). In patients with obstructive disease, allowing adequate time for lung emptying on exhalation may be more important in preventing gas trapping and intrinsic PEEP.

The rate is set to achieve adequate gas exchange and minute ventilation. Tidal volume and minute ventilation will vary during PCV because pressure is the control variable. Blood gases ($PaCO_2$ and pH), along with SpO_2, must be monitored to ensure that minute ventilation requirements are being met.

Oxygen percentage is initially set at 50% or higher. Once ventilation is established, the oxygen percentage may be titrated to maintain an SpO_2 of 90% or greater (except in COPD, in which where 88% to 90% may be acceptable).

PEEP is set to recruit the FRC and improve gas exchange. PEEP levels of between 5 and 24 cm H_2O may be used as long as plateau pressure remains below the target threshold (Saura, 2002). PEEP should be carefully titrated to avoid overdistention and to prevent VILI.

Pressure Control/Assist Control

Pressure control/assist control is similar to pressure control, except that trigger sensitivity is established. Setting the trigger variable allows the ventilator to detect the patient's spontaneous ventilation. Trigger sensitivity for adult patients includes pressure and flow.

Pressure triggering is set by establishing the trigger sensitivity as pressure, and then adjusting the trigger sensitivity. Pressure triggering is typically set between 1 and 3 cm H_2O. When a patient initiates a breath, sub-ambient pressure (trigger pressure) is transmitted to the ventilator's pressure transducer, and a breath is delivered once the trigger threshold has been met. If the sensitivity is set at -2 cm H_2O, then once baseline pressure falls by 2 cm H_2O, the ventilator delivers a mandatory breath.

Flow triggering uses flow as a trigger variable to determine when a patient-triggered breath is delivered. Flow triggering requires that a baseline flow be established (some ventilators require this to be clinician set, whereas others set the baseline flow at a multiple of the trigger sensitivity), and then the trigger sensitivity is set. A range of trigger sensitivities may be set from 0.5 L/min to as high as 20 L/min. Once the ventilator's flow sensor detects a drop in baseline flow exceeding the trigger sensitivity, a mandatory breath is delivered.

ALARM SETTINGS FOR VOLUME AND PRESSURE CONTROL VENTILATION

Once the initial ventilator settings have been established, the respiratory care practitioner (RCP) must now set the alarms. Alarms are designed to alert the clinician of changes in the patient-ventilator system that could be dangerous or harmful. Therefore, it is important to set the ventilator alarms appropriately and to adjust the alarm settings as the patient's pathology evolves.

Volume Control and Volume Control/Assist-Control Ventilation

Pressure Limit/Alarm

The *pressure limit* or alarm is one of the more important alarms to set properly during volume control and volume control/assist-control ventilation. Appropriately setting the pressure limit or alarm will protect the lungs from potential overdistention and injury (Campbell, 2002). Typically, when a pressure limit or alarm setting is reached, inspiration is terminated, a visual and audible alert/alarm is activated, and the ventilator cycles into exhalation. Typically in the adult patient, the limit/alarm should be set at 35 cm H_2O initially, and then adjusted to approximately 10 cm H_2O above the peak inspiratory pressure.

Low Minute Volume/Low Tidal Volume

The low minute volume/low tidal volume alarm will alert the clinician to tidal breath delivery below the threshold set on the alarm. Diminished tidal volumes may be caused by leaks (airway, chest tube[s], or circuit). This alarm is based on a single occurrence of a low volume breath delivery. If the patient is triggering breaths spontaneously and has variable tidal breath delivery, the use of the low minute volume alarm can minimize frequent or nuisance alarms. The low minute volume alarm averages volume delivery over a minute period. If the minute ventilation falls below the alarm threshold, the alarm will be activated.

Low Peak Pressure/Low PEEP Pressure

The low peak pressure and low PEEP pressure serve to alert the clinician to pressure levels that fall below the set alarm thresholds. These alarm thresholds may be caused by disconnects (circuit), excess leaks, or in-line suctioning.

High Rate/Low Rate

The high rate and low rate alarms are helpful when the patient is triggering breaths spontaneously. If the spontaneous ventilator rate exceeds the alarm thresholds, the clinician will be alerted to that event. High rates can be attributed to high minute ventilation demands (pathology, pain, anxiety, etc.), whereas low minute ventilation may be caused by sedation or the absence of a ventilatory drive.

Pressure Control and Pressure Control/Assist Control

Tidal volume and minute ventilation varies when applying PCV due to changes in the patient's pulmonary resistance and compliance. Therefore, alarm settings for pressure control emphasize these variables more than with VCV.

High and Low Tidal Volume

The high and low tidal volume alarms are important during PCV. These alarms alert the clinician to hypoventilation or overdistention (Campbell, 2002). Hypoventilation may lead to compromise in $PaCO_2$ elimination and difficulty in oxygenation, whereas overdistention can lead to barotrauma or lung injury. The tidal volume alarms should be set to within 100 mL of the target tidal volume.

High and Low Minute Volume

The high and low minute volume alarms like the high and low tidal volume alarms alert the clinician to hypoventilation and hyperventilation. The alarm limits should be set for within 1 liter of the desired minute ventilation.

SPONTANEOUS VENTILATION MODES

During spontaneous modes of ventilation, the primary concern to the clinician is hypoventilation. Alarm settings to alert the clinician of this condition become more important as the patient assumes more responsibility for the work of breathing in spontaneous modes.

Continuous Positive Airway Pressure (CPAP)

Continuous positive airway pressure (CPAP) is the application of positive pressure during inspiration and expiration to the airway during spontaneous breathing. CPAP may be administered to an artificial airway (endotracheal tube or tracheostomy tube) or noninvasively

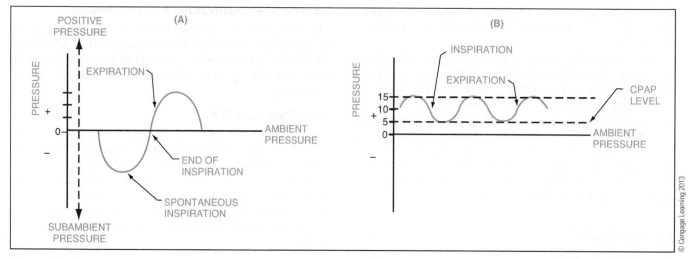

Figure 25-4 A scalar waveform showing continuous positive airway pressure (CPAP)

to a mask interface. Positive pressure is applied during CPAP both during inspiration and expiration (Figure 25-4). During spontaneous ventilation without the application of CPAP (graph A), ambient pressure or atmospheric pressure is reached at the end of exhalation. With the application of CPAP (graph B), the pressure level never falls below the CPAP level, which is 5 cm H_2O in this example. This would be termed the *application of 5 cm H_2O of CPAP*.

Pressure Support

Pressure support is a spontaneous mode of ventilation that augments a patient's spontaneous effort with positive pressure. It is a spontaneous ventilation mode whereby the patient must trigger each breath (pressure or flow triggered). This mode ensures that the spontaneous breaths are not too shallow. On initiation of a breath, a constant pressure (preset) is delivered until the flow rate reaches approximately 25% of the peak inspiratory flow (some ventilators allow selection of between 10% and 40%), and then expiration begins. In this mode, flow is variable. Whatever flow is required (within the ventilator's designed limitations) is available to maintain the selected level of pressure. This mode ensures that the patient's spontaneous breaths are large enough to maintain adequate blood gases and to reverse atelectasis. The patient demand and pathology (resistance and compliance) determine the delivered volume and ventilator rate.

PATIENT VENTILATOR SYSTEM CHECKS

Patient ventilator system checks are the evaluation and documentation of the patient's response to mechanical ventilation and the ventilator system supporting the patient's ventilation. Often, this is simply termed a *ventilator check* or *vent check*. The purpose of this evaluation is to assess the patient's response to ventilation, verify the correct operation of the ventilator, verify that the patient settings and alarms are set appropriately, verify the correct FIO_2, and ensure that the humidifier/heat and moisture exchanger (HME) is connected and functioning properly.

Patient assessment should be given the highest priority in this procedure; the ventilator can usually wait unless you are evaluating a ventilator alarm/alert occurrence. Patient assessment should include breath sounds, observation of spontaneous effort and ventilatory muscle use, chest wall motion, patient's color or pallor, SpO_2 and heart rate and rhythm, any hemodynamic data displayed on the patient's monitor, airway type (endotracheal tube, tracheostomy tube), and its size and position (endotracheal tube position relative to the teeth or gum line). If chest tube(s) are placed, verification of their correct operation, amount of drainage, and evidence of air leakage must be assessed. Much of this information can be summarized into a narrative as part of the documentation. Evaluation of the patient's chest x-ray film for pathology and confirmation of airway placement film should also be performed.

The purpose of evaluating the ventilator is to ensure that it is operating correctly and that the settings are as ordered by the physician or are in compliance with established ventilator protocols. Documentation of ventilator settings should include mode, frequency (unless spontaneous mode), peak, mean, and plateau airway pressures or pressure limit, baseline pressure if applicable, assessment for auto-PEEP, measurement of tidal volume (set or calculated), minute ventilation or minimum mandatory minute ventilation, inspiratory flow rate and waveform (if applicable), and trigger type and threshold.

PROFICIENCY OBJECTIVES

At the end of this chapter, the reader should be able to:

- *Correctly assemble and prepare a mechanical ventilator for use:*
  - *Assemble the ventilator circuit.*
  - *Correctly interface the humidifier or HME.*
  - *Perform an operational verification procedure.*
  - *Correctly document the preparation of the ventilator for use.*
- *Given a simulated physician's order or established ventilator protocol, demonstrate how to initiate*

mechanical ventilation. Establish the ordered ventilator parameters using a test lung or lung analog:
  - *Establish ordered ventilator settings.*
    - *Appropriately set all alarms depending on the mode of ventilation.*
  - *Monitor the patient-ventilator system.*
    - *Demonstrate how to remove disposable tubing and other items, disinfect, and prepare a ventilator for use.*

EQUIPMENT REQUIREMENTS

There are several pieces of equipment required for initiating mechanical ventilation. Figure 25-5 is a list of the required equipment.

Equipment Preparation

A variety of ventilators are used in the clinical setting. The assembly of the circuitry for the more common ventilators is discussed in the practice activities. The following text describes how to test the ventilator and circuit prior to initiating mechanical ventilation.

VENTILATOR OPERATIONAL VERIFICATION PROCEDURE

Performance of a ventilator operation verification procedure must be completed and documented prior to using the ventilator on a patient. One portion of ventilator operation verification procedure includes the ventilator's microprocessor verifying that the control circuit is operational and that all sensors (pressure, flow, and oxygen sensors) are functional. The other part of the procedure includes leak testing of the circuit, humidifier or HME, and filters as well as measuring the circuit

compliance. Contemporary ventilators incorporate this procedure into the ventilator's software. These tests may be termed *self test (ST)*, *short self test (SST)*, *extended systems test*, or *extended self test (EST)*. The screen display will prompt the user to perform various ventilator control settings changes with and without the patient wye occluded. Once the operational verification procedure has been completed, the display screen will indicate if the ventilator passed the test or what portion of the test the ventilator failed. If a part of the test was not successfully completed, it is important to correct any items that may be deficient (tightening circuit connections, filter assemblies, humidifier/HME connections) and repeat the verification procedure. If the ventilator continues to fail the operational verification procedure, remove the ventilator from service and have it serviced by a qualified biomedical engineer.

Documentation of completion of the ventilator operational verification procedure must also be completed prior to placing the ventilator into use on a patient. This may be part of a ventilator flow sheet, kept on the ventilator at the bedside, or it may be done electronically as a part of electronic medical recordkeeping. Basic documentation should include date, time, settings used or tests performed, the results of the test(s) (pass/fail), and the signature and credentials of the practitioner performing the procedure.

Specifics regarding how to perform these tests are described later in this chapter in the practice activities.

ESTABLISHING ORDERED VENTILATOR SETTINGS

The initiation of continuous mechanical ventilation requires a specific physician's order or by compliance with a ventilator protocol. It is the responsibility of the respiratory care practitioner to establish the settings as ordered on the ventilator. Occasionally, a physician will be unfamiliar with ventilator protocol or appropriate settings. In these instances, general guidelines are given that may be offered as suggestions.

- Ventilator
- Ventilator circuit
- Humidifer
- Oxygen analyzer
- Manual resuscitator and oxygen flowmeter
- Sterile water
- Suctioning supplies
- Ventilator flow sheets

Figure 25-5 A list of equipment requirements for the initiation of mechanical ventilation

© Cengage Learning 2013

Type of Ventilation or Control Variable

The first determination must be whether to use VCV or PCV as the control variable. The control variable (pressure or volume control) will be specified in the physician's order or the ventilator protocol. Selection and adjustment of settings will be described for each control variable.

Volume Control Ventilation

The delivered tidal volume should be the primary consideration for this form of ventilation with volume as the control variable. Volume should be set to 6 mL/kg ideal body weight, with the goal of a plateau pressure of less than 30 cm H_2O (ARDS NET, 2000). Once the volume has been established, it is important to monitor peak and plateau pressures. Inspiratory flow, inspiratory time, and flow pattern should be adjusted to optimize distribution of the volume during each breath (Campbell, 2002).

Next the rate should be set to establish an acceptable minute ventilation. Consideration must be given when setting the rate to allow for adequate expiratory time for the lungs to empty following breath delivery. Monitoring $PaCO_2$ and pH from arterial blood gases will provide guidance as to the adequacy or minute ventilation. In some cases, $PaCO_2$ will be allowed to become elevated above normal (hypercapnea) in order to minimize the risk of lung injury from higher pressures.

Oxygen percentage or FIO_2 should be set to maintain adequate SpO_2 levels (greater than 90% or PaO_2 greater than 60 mm Hg). Oxygen percentage is usually set initially at 50% and then titrated from that point based on oxygen saturations. Some patients may require a lower SpO_2 target (88% to 90%, for example), and the FIO_2 should then be adjusted to achieve the desired target range.

PEEP may be beneficial in improving oxygenation through the recruitment of FRC. PEEP should be adjusted such that gas exchange is maximized without significantly increasing airway pressures and overdistention. PEEP is typically adjusted between 5 and 24 cm H_2O and titrated to the needs of each individual patient.

Monitoring of plateau pressures is important to prevent lung injury (Saura, 2002).

Mandatory or spontaneous (assist-control) mode must then be determined. Mandatory breath delivery is purely determined by the ventilator's rate control and is time triggered. The patient's spontaneous efforts will be ignored by the ventilator's control circuitry, and the patient may require sedation to tolerate this form of ventilation. Assist control may be established by adjusting either a pressure trigger variable or a flow trigger variable to initiate a spontaneous (patient-triggered) breath. Pressure triggering is typically set between 1 and 3 cm H_2O below baseline pressure. Flow triggering may be set from 0.5 to 20 L/min; generally lower flow trigger settings (3–5 L/min) result in better ventilator response to the patient's spontaneous efforts.

Alarm settings for volume control ventilation Alarm settings for volume control ventilation are summarized in Table 25-3.

Priority should be given to the pressure limit alarm setting when using VCV. This alarm will help protect the lungs from VILI. The low tidal volume/minute volume alarms are helpful in detecting leaks.

Pressure Control Ventilation

Pressure should be the primary consideration for control adjustment when ventilating a patient using pressure control as the control variable. Pressure is usually ordered by the physician or established in the ventilator protocol. Pressure should be adjusted to maintain a plateau pressure of less than 30 cm H_2O.

Inspiratory time determines the time interval the set pressure is delivered during a breath. The inspiratory time is also usually ordered by the physician. Long inspiratory times may diminish cardiac output (Campbell, 2002). Consideration must also be given to allow adequate time for exhalation following a delivered breath.

The rate is then adjusted to achieve adequate minute ventilation. Usually the physician will also specify the rate to be set for PCV. Blood gases (pH and $PaCO_2$)

TABLE 25-3: Volume Control Ventilation Alarm Settings

ALARM	SETTING
High Pressure Limit	35 cm H_2O initial setting, then 10 cm H_2O greater than peak inspiratory pressure once the patient has been stabilized
Low Pressure Limit	Low pressure limit: 10 cm H_2O less than the inspiratory pressure setting
Low Minute Volume / Low Tidal Volume	Low minute volume: 20% or 2 L/min less than set minute ventilation Low tidal volume: 100 mL less than set tidal volume
Low Peak Pressure Low PEEP pressure	Low peak pressure: 10 cm H_2O less than peak pressure Low PEEP pressure: 5 cm H_2O below PEEP setting
High Rate	High rate: 10–15 breaths/min higher than current rate
Low Rate	Low rate: 10–15 breaths less than the current rate

can be monitored to assess the adequacy of minute ventilation.

Oxygen percentage is initially set at 50% and adjusted from that point based on oxygen saturations and blood gases. Oxygen percentage is usually titrated to maintain an SpO_2 greater than 90% and a PaO_2 greater than 60 mm Hg.

PEEP may be set to improve gas exchange through the recruitment of FRC. PEEP levels between 5 and 24 cm H_2O are common. PEEP should be adjusted so as not to increase plateau pressures significantly to avoid overdistention of the lungs.

Mandatory or spontaneous (assist-control) breath delivery must then be set. During mandatory breath delivery, the rate control determines the frequency of the breaths (time triggered). All the patient's spontaneous efforts will be ignored by the ventilator's control circuit. If assist-control ventilation is desired, then the trigger type (pressure or flow) must be determined and threshold values set. Pressure trigger levels are usually set to 1 to 3 cm H_2O below the baseline pressure. Flow trigger sensitivity is typically set between 3 and 5 L/min.

Alarm settings for pressure control ventilation The alarm settings for PCV are summarized in Table 25-4.

When using PCV, priority should be given to the setting of the low minute volume/low tidal volume alarms. These alarms will provide the most effective safety alert to hypoventilation or overdistention (Campbell, 2002).

MONITORING THE PATIENT-VENTILATOR SYSTEM

The purpose of monitoring the patient-ventilator system is to identify changes in the patient's condition and to verify that the ventilator is operating properly and maintaining the ordered settings.

The patient's position should be verified to be with the head of the bed elevated at least 30°. Elevation of the head of the bed helps to prevent silent aspiration past the airway cuff. Often, the patient will slide down toward the foot of the bed. If required, obtain assistance and move the patient up in bed such that the change in elevation occurs at the patient's waist, where one would normally bend.

The Patient

Your first and primary concern is the care of your patient. Any time the ventilator system is checked, the patient's well-being should be the first item on your agenda. A thorough assessment of your patient should be performed, and then the ventilator should be monitored.

Pulmonary

Auscultate the patient's chest. Are the airways clear or does the patient need suctioning? If suctioning is required, perform the procedure and then proceed. Listen for the distribution of breath sounds. Pay close attention when comparing sounds bilaterally. A sudden increase in inspiratory pressure combined with a localized decrease in breath sounds may signify a pneumothorax.

Check for recent results of arterial blood gas analysis. Are the PaO_2, $PaCO_2$, and pH being maintained within acceptable limits? Observe the patient's skin color and level of consciousness.

Observe for the use of accessory muscles if the patient is able to assist ventilation with spontaneous respiratory efforts. Use of accessory muscles indicates that the sensitivity may be set too high, or that there is an obstruction in the airway or circuit, increasing the effort required to initiate a breath.

Cardiac

Observe the heart monitor. Check heart rate and rhythm. Observe for any arrhythmias.

If the patient has a central venous pressure (CVP) or Swan-Ganz catheter in place, observe the monitor display for the CVP, pulmonary artery pressure, and pulmonary artery wedge pressure. If an oscilloscope is not being used, look at the nurse's flow sheet for these values.

TABLE 25-4: Pressure Control Ventilation Alarm Settings

ALARM	SETTING
High Pressure Limit	10 cm H_2O greater than peak inspiratory pressure once the patient has been stabilized
Low Pressure Limit	10 cm H_2O less than the inspiratory pressure setting
Low Minute Volume /	1 L/min less than the target minute ventilation
Low Tidal Volume	100 mL less than the target tidal volume
Low Peak Pressure	10 cm H_2O less than the set inspiratory pressure
Low PEEP Pressure	5 cm H_2O less than PEEP pressure
High Rate	High rate: 10–15 breaths/min higher than the current rate
Low Rate	Low rate: 10–15 breaths less than the current rate

Neurologic

Is the patient alert and oriented? The patient will be unable to speak owing to the presence of the artificial airway. However, you may communicate with the patient and reassure him or her that what you are doing is normal procedure. Observe the respiratory pattern for any irregularities.

The Ventilator

Monitoring the ventilator consists of verifying that the ventilator is operating within the ordered settings and also calculating some patient values.

Drain the ventilator tubing of any condensate and fill the humidifier to the proper level (if not part of an automated feed system). Attention to these small details will ensure consistency in measuring the ventilatory parameters.

DOCUMENTATION OF VENTILATOR SETTINGS

Patient ventilator system checks, sometimes referred to as ventilator checks, are the documentation of ventilator settings and the patient's response to ventilator support (AARC, 1992). In the next section, you will learn the variables to monitor and how to document the patient's response to mechanical ventilation.

Control Variable

Pressure control or volume control would be indicated to denote the control variable.

Tidal Volume or Inspiratory Pressure

Note in this space where the tidal volume or inspiratory pressure is set, depending on the control variable. If pressure control mode is being used, note the inspiratory time and any inspiratory pause.

Frequency

Note in this space where the respiratory frequency control is set. If the patient is in control mode, the frequency may be timed using your watch. However, if the patient is in assist-control mode, the frequency may vary from what is set.

FIO$_2$

Analyze the FIO$_2$ delivered from the ventilator. This is best accomplished by analyzing the gas before it enters the humidifier. Monitoring humidified gases may have detrimental effects on some oxygen analyzers. Adjust the control to the prescribed oxygen level if it is out of adjustment. The oxygen percentage should be adjusted to within 2% of the ordered FIO$_2$.

PEEP

Note the PEEP setting.

Flow Rate

Note in this space where the inspiratory flow rate is set as appropriate.

I:E Ratio

Note the displayed I:E ratio and record it.

Temperature

Measure the temperature at the patient wye or note the temperature indicated on the servocontroller.

Alarms

Note all alarm and limit settings.

DOCUMENTATION OF PATIENT VALUES

The patient variables that should be monitored during a system check include pressures, volumes, compliance, resistance, rate, and arterial blood gases. In addition, breath sounds, oximetry, artificial airway type and placement, cuff pressures, and the patient's status should be documented.

Peak Pressure

Note in this space the peak inspiratory pressure delivered during each machine breath.

End-Expiratory Pressure

If the patient is not on PEEP, this should be zero.

Plateau Pressure

The plateau pressure or static pressure is measured when there is no airflow in the patient-ventilator circuit. Explain to the patient what you are doing and that a momentary period of holding the breath will be required. Plateau pressure may be measured by the addition of a temporary inspiratory pause (0.5 second) or by depressing the manual inspiratory hold control. This will cease gas flow at the end of inspiration, holding the airway/circuit pressure and not opening the exhalation valve. Once peak pressure is reached, the lungs/chest wall will recoil slightly, which then results in a plateau in pressure at zero flow.

Measured Tidal Volume

Using the ventilator's monitoring system, record the measured tidal volume.

Dynamic Compliance

Dynamic compliance is the compliance of the lungs, thorax, and the patient-ventilator circuit. It is measured during gas flow conditions. To measure this value, divide the corrected tidal volume by the peak inspiratory pressure minus PEEP: dynamic compliance = V_t corr/(PIP − PEEP).

Static Compliance

Static compliance is an indicator of the compliance of the lungs and thorax. It is calculated by dividing the corrected tidal volume by the plateau pressure minus PEEP: static compliance = V_t corr/(plateau pressure − PEEP).

Airway Resistance

Airway resistance may be easily calculated once the peak and plateau pressures are known. The formula to calculate the airway resistance is as follows:

$$R_{AW} = \frac{\text{peak pressure} - \text{plateau pressure}}{\text{flow}}$$

where

R_{AW} = airway resistance
peak pressure = peak airway pressure
plateau pressure = plateau pressure
flow = flow rate setting in liters per second

As the pressure difference becomes greater, airway resistance increases. Airway resistance may be lowered by administering bronchodilators or anti-inflammatory agents and by keeping the airway suctioned.

Frequency

Note in this space the respiratory rate that you counted when you measured the minute volume.

Arterial Blood Gases and SpO_2

When arterial blood gases are drawn, the results should be noted on the ventilator flow sheet. Note the date, time, FIO_2, and ventilator settings. If the ventilator settings are changed, 20 minutes should be allowed for the patient to equilibrate to the new settings before arterial blood gases are drawn.

Note the patient's oxygen saturation. Compare the monitor's heart rate with the ECG monitor and note the quality of the plethysmographic signal.

VENTILATOR DISINFECTION AND PREPARATION FOR USE

The ventilator circuit should not be routinely changed for the purposes of infection control (AARC, 2003). Upon ventilator discontinuance, the patient circuit should be aseptically removed and discarded using biohazard precautions. Any disposable parts of the circuit (in-line suction catheter) or disposable probes should also be discarded at that time. If a heated humidifier platen was used, it should be safely and aseptically drained of liquid and discarded. Once the ventilator circuit is removed and all reusable components (expiratory condensate trap and connectors) have been removed, wipe all surfaces of the ventilator with a manufacturer-approved disinfectant. Once the disinfectant has dried, a new circuit and humidification platen may be reinstalled. The ventilator should then go through a ventilator operational verification procedure as described earlier.

References

Acute Respiratory Distress Syndrome Network. (2000). Ventilation with lower tidal volumes as compared with traditional tidal volumes for acute lung injury and the acute respiratory distress syndrome. *New England Journal of Medicine, 342*(18), 1301–1308.

American Association for Respiratory Care (AARC). (1992). AARC clinical practice guidelines: Patient-ventilator system checks. *Respiratory Care, 37*(8), 882–886.

American Association for Respiratory Care (AARC). (2003). AARC clinical practice guideline: Care of the ventilator circuit and its relation to ventilator associated pneumonia. *Respiratory Care, 48*(9), 869–879.

American Association for Respiratory Care (AARC). (2007). AARC clinical practice guidelines: Long-term invasive mechanical ventilation in the home—2007 revision & update. *Respiratory Care, 52*(1), 1056–1062.

Campbell, R. S. (2002). Pressure-controlled versus volume-controlled ventilation: Does it matter? *Respiratory Care, 47*(4), 416–426.

Chatburn, R. L. (2001). A new system for understanding mechanical ventilators. *Respiratory Care, 36*(10), 1123–1155.

Cheifetz, I. M. (2003). Invasive and noninvasive pediatric mechanical ventilation. *Respiratory Care, 48*(4), 442–453.

Farha, S., Ziad, W., Ghamra, M. D., Hisington, E. R., Butler, R. S., & Stoller, J. K., (2006). Use of noninvasive positive-pressure ventilation on the regular hospital ward: experience and correlates of success. *Respiratory Care, 51* (11), 1237–1243.

Gay, P. C. (2009). Complications of noninvasive ventilation in acute care. *Respiratory Care, 54*(2), 246–257.

Hudson, L. D. (1998). Protective ventilation for patients with acute respiratory distress syndrome. *New England Journal of Medicine, 338*(6), 347–354.

MacIntyre, N. R. (2002). Setting the frequency-tidal volume pattern. *Respiratory Care, 47*(3), 266–274.

Masip, J. (2005). Noninvasive ventilation in acute cardiogenic pulmonary edema: Systematic review and meta-analysis. *Journal of the American Medical Association, 294*(24), 3124.

Medoff, B. D. (2008). Invasive and noninvasive ventilation in patients with asthma. *Respiratory Care, 35*(3), 740.

Neema, P. K. (2003). Respiratory failure. *Indian Journal of Anesthesia, 47*(5), 360–366.

Pauwels, R. A. (2001). Global strategy for the diagnosis, management and prevention of chronic obstructive pulmonary disease. NHLBI/WHO Global Initiative for Chronic Obstructive Lung Disease (GOLD) Workshop Summary. *American Journal of Respiratory and Critical Care Medicine, 17*(6), 1256–1276.

Pierson, D. J. (2002). Indications for mechanical ventilation. *Respiratory Care, 47*(3), 249–262.

Pierson, D. J. (2009). History and epidemiology of noninvasive ventilation in the acute-care setting. *Respiratory Care, 54*(1), 40–32.

Saura, P. (2002). How to set positive end-expiratory pressure. *Respiratory Care, 47*(3), 279–292.

Additional Resources

BEAR 1000 ventilator instruction manual. (1994). Riverside, CA: Bear Medical Systems.

8400ST volume ventilator instruction manual. (1990). Palm Springs, CA: Bird Products.

Demers, R. R., Pratter, M. R., & Irwin, R. S. (1981). Use of the concept of ventilator compliance in the determination of static total compliance. *Respiratory Care, 26*(7), 644.

840 operator's and technical reference manual. (2003). Carlsbad, CA : Nellcor Puritan-Bennett.

Gillette, M. A., & Hess, D. R. (2001). Ventilator-induced lung injury and the evolution of lung-protective strategies in acute respiratory distress syndrome. *Respiratory Care, 46*(2), 130–148.

Nelson, E. J., Hunter, P. M., & Morton, E. (1983). *Critical care respiratory therapy: A laboratory and clinical manual.* Boston: Little, Brown.

Operator's manual AVEA™ ventilator systems. (2005). Palm Springs, CA : Viasys.

SERVO-i Ventilator 300—operating manual. (1993). Solona, Sweden: Siemens-Elema AB.

User's manual SERVO-i ventilator system. (2006). Solna, Sweden: Maquet.

Practice Activities: BEAR 1000

Circuit Assembly

Figure 25-6 shows the BEAR-1000 with the optional graphics display module assembled and ready for initiation of mechanical ventilation.

1. Attach the two high-pressure hoses, one to 50 psi air and the other to 50 psi oxygen.

2. Connect the power cord to a suitable alternating current (AC) grounded outlet.

3. Attach the exhalation valve diaphragm to the exhalation valve assembly and check it for leaks. Install the exhalation valve diaphragm assembly into its seat by rotating the mounting to lock it into place. Attach the condensate collection jar assembly and the expiratory flow sensor.

4. Connect a bacteria filter to the ventilator outlet and connect it to the humidifier using a short length of 22 mm diameter aerosol tubing.

5. Connect the inspiratory limb of the patient circuit to the humidifier and the expiratory limb to the condensate collection jar assembly.

6. Connect the proximal airway line to the proximal pressure fitting on the front of the ventilator.

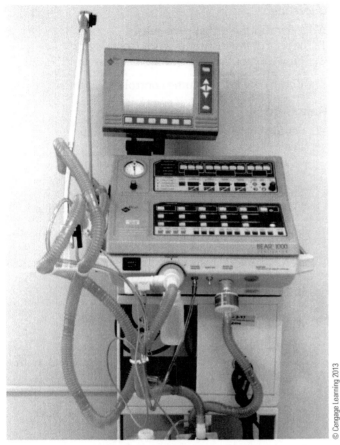

Figure 25-6 A photograph of the BEAR® 1000 ventilator with the optional graphics display module

© Cengage Learning 2013

Testing the Ventilator before Use (Quick Checkout)

Prior to using the ventilator for patient care, the quick checkout procedure should be performed to verify that all major subsystems are operational. This test takes approximately 2.5 minutes.

1. Turn the optional graphics display module off. Failure to do so will result in an error code d2, which may be a false indication.

2. With an adult circuit attached, press and hold the "Test" key on the control panel located on the front panel in the lower right-hand corner while simultaneously turning on the power switch located on the right rear of the ventilator.

3. Verify that the operator diagnostics mode has been activated by observing that the RUN DIAGNOSTICS LED is illuminated.

4. Adjust the PEEP pressure to zero by rotating the PEEP control located adjacent to the pressure manometer fully counterclockwise.

5. Observe that ALL appears in the Pres Sup/Insp Press display window; this indicates that all seven diagnostics tests will be performed.
   a. If ALL does not appear, depress the "Pres Sup/ Insp Pres" key and rotate the green SET knob until ALL appears.

6. Plug the patient wye using a cap or other secure occlusion device.

7. Depress the "Manual Breath" key located at the lower center part of the control panel. The automated self test will begin and will take approximately 2.5 minutes.

8. When all diagnostics tests have been passed, a "P" will be displayed in the Assist Sensitivity display window.

System Leak Test

1. Set the controls to the following settings:

Mode	Assist CMV
Peak Flow	20 L/min
Inspiratory Pause	2 seconds
Tidal Volume	200 mL
Peak Insp Pressure	140 cm H_2O
Rate	10/min

2. Using a sterile gauze or a sterile plastic wrap, occlude the patient wye completely.

3. Observe the pressure manometer. The pressure should read between 60 and 80 cm H_2O. The pressure should fall no more than 10 cm H_2O.

4. In the event of a leak, check all tubing connections, the humidifier, and exhalation valve diaphragm.

5. Repeat steps 1 through 4 until pressure remains steady.

Tubing Compliance

1. Set the controls to the values listed in the system leak test, and occlude the patient wye as described previously.

2. Observe and record the pressure and exhaled tidal volume readings during inspiration.

3. Divide the exhaled volume by the peak pressure.

4. Depress the "Compliance Comp" key located at the lower center of the control panel and enter the calculated value by rotating the SET knob and depressing the key once again.

Activities

To complete these practice activities, it is recommended that you use a lung analog/simulator such as a Medishield Lung Ventilator Performance Analyzer or other similar device in which resistance and compliance may be easily controlled and altered.

Initial Settings

Mode	Assist CMV
Peak Flow	40 L/min
Assist Sensitivity	2 cm H_2O
High Pressure Limit	120 cm H_2O
Tidal Volume	500 mL
Rate	12/min
O_2%	21%
Waveform	square

Nebulizer	off
Inspiratory Pause	0.0 second
PEEP	0.0 cm H_2O
Alarms	off

Manipulate only one control at a time and record your results on a sheet of paper. Answer the questions that follow each activity, recording each answer on your paper. If you have difficulty, ask your laboratory instructor for assistance.

Peak Flow Control

1. Set the peak flow to 20 L/min.
   a. Measure the inspiratory time using a watch with a second hand or a stopwatch.
   b. Measure the peak pressure by depressing the "Peak Pressure" key on the monitoring panel.
   c. Record the corrected tidal volume (exhaled tidal volume).
   d. Record the I:E ratio by depressing the "I:E ratio" key and observing the display.

2. Adjust the peak flow to 100 L/min.
   a. Measure the inspiratory time using a watch with a second hand or a stopwatch.
   b. Measure the peak pressure by depressing the "Peak Pressure" key on the monitoring panel.
   c. Record the corrected tidal volume (exhaled tidal volume).
   d. Record the I:E ratio by depressing the "I:E ratio" key and observing the display.

Questions

A. How do you account for the differences in inspiratory time?
B. Why were there differences in peak inspiratory pressure?
C. Why did the corrected tidal volume vary?
D. Why did the I:E ratio vary between the two activities?

3. Return the peak flow control to 40 L/min.

Tidal Volume Control

1. Set the controls to the following settings:

Peak Flow	40 L/min
Tidal Volume	500 mL
Rate	12/min

Leave all other controls set at the same values you established for the peak flow activity.
   a. Measure the inspiratory time using a watch with a second hand or a stopwatch.
   b. Measure the peak inspiratory pressure.
   c. Record the exhaled tidal volume.
   d. Record the I:E ratio.

2. Adjust the tidal volume to 1200 mL.
   a. Measure the inspiratory time using a watch with a second hand or a stopwatch.
   b. Measure the peak inspiratory pressure.
   c. Record the exhaled tidal volume.
   d. Record the I:E ratio.

Questions

A. Why did the pressure increase?
B. Why did the inspiratory time increase?
C. How do you account for the decrease in I:E ratio?

3. Return the tidal volume control to 500 mL.

Rate Control

1. Set the controls to the following settings:

Peak Flow	40 L/min
High Pressure Limit	120 cm H_2O
Tidal Volume	500 mL
Rate	12/min
I:E Override	depressed and activated

2. With the controls as set above, perform the following:
   a. Measure the inspiratory time using a watch with a second hand or a stop watch.
   b. Measure the peak inspiratory pressure.
   c. Record the exhaled tidal volume.
   d. Record the I:E ratio.

3. Adjust the rate control to 40 breaths/min.
   a. Measure the inspiratory time using a watch with a second hand or a stopwatch.
   b. Measure the peak inspiratory pressure.
   c. Record the exhaled tidal volume.
   d. Record the I:E ratio.

Questions

A. What was the I:E ratio?
B. Why was the I:E ratio so low?

Triggering

In this section you will explore both pressure and flow triggering. It is helpful to use the graphics display panel and to select the pressure volume loop to view how changes affect inspiratory work.

Pressure Triggering

Adjust the ventilator to the following settings:

Mode	Assist CMV
Peak Flow	40L/min
Assist Sensitivity	5 cm H_2O
Peak Insp Pressure	10 cm H_2O greater than PIP
Tidal Volume	500 mL
Rate	8 breaths/min
$O_2\%$	21%
Inspiratory Pause	0.0 second
PEEP	0.0 cm H_2O

1. Attach a mouthpiece to the patient wye and attempt to initiate a breath. Observe both the pressure manometer and the pressure volume loop on the graphics display panel.

2. Set the assist sensitivity to 0.2 cm H_2O. Again using a mouthpiece, initiate a breath while observing the pressure manometer and the pressure volume loop.

Questions

A. When were you able to initiate a breath most easily?
B. Where would you prefer, as a patient, to have the assist sensitivity control set?
C. What changes did you observe on the pressure volume loop between the two settings?

Flow Triggering

Adjust the ventilator to the following settings:

Mode	Assist CMV
Peak Flow	40 L/min
Base Flow	10 L/min
Flow Trigger	3 L/min
Peak Insp Pressure	10 cm H_2O greater than PIP
Tidal Volume	500 mL
Rate	8 breaths/min
O_2%	21%
Inspiratory Pause	0.0 second
PEEP	0.0 cm H_2O

1. Attach a mouthpiece to the patient wye and attempt to initiate a breath. Observe both the pressure manometer and the pressure volume loop on the graphics display panel.

2. Adjust the base flow to 18 L/min. Again initiate a breath using a mouthpiece and observe the pressure manometer and the pressure volume loop.

3. Return the base flow to 10 L/min and adjust the flow trigger level to 8 L/min. Initiate a breath using a mouthpiece and observe the pressure manometer and the pressure volume loop on the graphics display panel.

Questions

A. Which setting would you prefer as a patient?
B. Which setting was easiest for you?
C. What changes did you observe on the graphics display panel?
D. How can you use the pressure volume loop and the graphics display panel to minimize inspiratory work?

Pressure Control Ventilation

Set the controls to the following settings and attach the ventilator to the test lung:

Mode	Pressure Control
Inspiratory Pressure	30 cm H_2O
Inspiratory Time	1 second
Assist Sensitivity	5 cm H_2O
Rate	12 breaths/min
O_2%	21%
PEEP	0.0 cm H_2O

Inspiratory Pressure Control

1. Measure and record the following using the display panel:
   a. Exhaled tidal volume
   b. I:E ratio
   c. Peak pressure
   d. Mean pressure

2. Adjust the inspiratory pressure level to 50 cm H_2O. Measure the following using the display panel:
   a. Exhaled tidal volume
   b. I:E ratio
   c. Peak pressure
   d. Mean pressure

Questions

A. How did the change in pressure affect the I:E ratio?
B. How did the change in pressure affect the exhaled tidal volume?

Inspiratory Time Control

1. Set the ventilator to the following settings:

Mode	Pressure Control
Inspiratory Pressure	30 cm H_2O
Inspiratory Time	1 second
Assist Sensitivity	5 cm H_2O
Rate	6 breaths/min
O_2%	21%
PEEP	0.0 cm H_2O

2. Measure the following using the display panel:
   a. Exhaled tidal volume
   b. I:E ratio
   c. Peak pressure
   d. Mean pressure

3. Change the inspiratory time to 3 seconds, and measure and record the following:
   a. Exhaled tidal volume
   b. I:E ratio
   c. Peak pressure
   d. Mean pressure

Questions

A. How did the inspiratory time change affect the I:E ratio?
B. How did the inspiratory time change affect tidal volume delivery?
C. How did the inspiratory time change affect the inspiratory pressure?

Alarm Systems

Total Minute Volume

Set the ventilator to the following settings:

Mode	Assist CMV
Peak Flow	40 L/min
Assist Sensitivity	2 cm H_2O
Tidal Volume	500 mL
Rate	8 breaths/min
O_2%	21%
Inspiratory Pause	0.0 second
PEEP	0.0 cm H_2O

1. Depress the Up arrow below the total minute volume alarm indicator and adjust the control to 6 L/min.

2. Using the test lung, simulate a respiratory rate of 20/min.

Questions

A. What occurred?
B. How could you set the alarm appropriately for a patient rate of 20/min?

3. Set the alarm's upper limit to 6 L/min and lower limit to 4 L/min.

Total Breath Rate

1. Depress the Up arrow below the total breath rate alarm display and set the rate to 10 breaths/min.

2. Using the test lung, simulate a rate of 20 breaths/min.

Questions

A. What occurred?
B. How could you set the alarm appropriately for a patient rate of 20/min?

3. Set the alarm's upper limit to 12 breaths/min and lower limit to 6 breaths/min.

Peak Inspiratory Pressure

1. Depress the Up arrow below the peak inspiratory pressure display and set it for 15 cm H_2O above the peak inspiratory pressure. Depress the Down arrow, and set its limit 15 cm H_2O below the peak inspiratory pressure.

2. Simulate a cough by rapidly squeezing the test lung.

Questions

A. What occurred?
B. Was the alarm set appropriately?
C. What other conditions might cause this alarm to be activated?

Baseline Pressure

Set the controls to the following values:

Mode	Assist CMV
Peak Flow	40 L/min
Assist Sensitivity	4 cm H_2O
Tidal Volume	500 mL
Rate	8 breaths/min
O_2%	21%
Inspiratory Pause	0.0 second
PEEP	5 cm H_2O

1. Depress the Down arrow key below the baseline pressure display and set it for 3 cm H_2O.

2. Simulate a patient effort by expanding the test lung's bellows to trigger a breath.

Questions

A. What occurred?
B. How could you change the control settings to prevent this?
C. Is the alarm set appropriately for this level of PEEP?

3. Readjust your baseline pressure alarm to bracket the PEEP level by 3 cm H_2O.

Practice Activities: Bird 8400ST

Circuit Assembly

Figure 25-7A and B shows the Bird 8400ST ventilator and a drawing of its control panel.

1. Attach the two high-pressure hoses, one to 50 psi air and the other to 50 psi oxygen to the external blender located below the ventilator. Ensure that the blender outlet is connected to the gas inlet on the back of the ventilator.

2. Connect the power cord to a suitable AC grounded outlet.

3. Install the exhalation valve diaphragm onto the ventilator exhalation valve port. Next install the exhalation valve body onto the port, ensuring that the spring-loaded safety tab is engaged.

4. Connect a bacteria filter to the ventilator outlet and connect it to the humidifier using a short length of 22 mm diameter aerosol tubing.

5. Connect the inspiratory limb of the patient circuit to the humidifier and the expiratory limb to the exhalation valve body assembly.

6. Attach the exhalation flow transducer assembly to the ventilator's right front panel by inserting the gray fitting into the female receptacle and rotating it clockwise, locking it in place. Connect the opposite end to the exhalation valve body.

Preoperational Performance Check

Prior to using the ventilator for patient care, you should complete a performance check. This will ensure that all systems and subsystems are operational before patient use.

Power-up Self Test

1. Turn the power switch on the rear of the ventilator to the ON position.

2. The ventilator will perform a 5-second test when powered up.
   a. The Power LED on the front panel illuminates and a brief audible alarm can be heard.
   b. The front panel LEDs will display segmentally in unison.
   c. The microprocessors will confirm communication links.

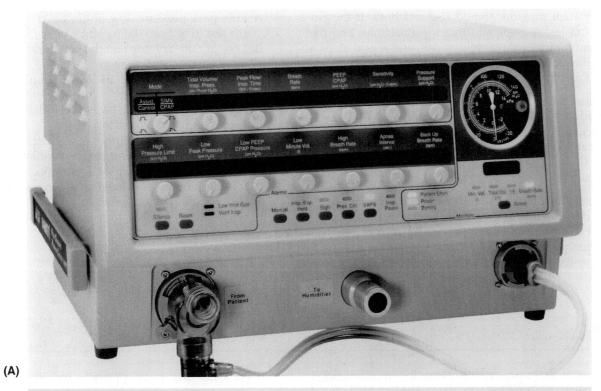

(A)

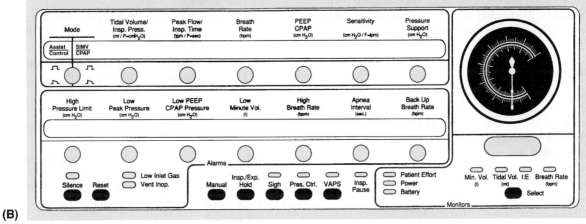

(B)

Figure 25-7 A photograph of the Bird 8400ST ventilator (A); a drawing of the control panel (B). *(Courtesy of Bird Products Corporation, Plam Springs, CA)*

d. The exhalation and flow control valves perform checks.

e. A second audible alarm will briefly sound.

f. Front panel LEDs will illuminate and the ventilator is ready for use.

Performance Check

Set the ventilator to the following settings.

Ventilator Settings

Mode	Assist-control (Square Wave)
Tidal Volume	500 mL
Peak Flow	60 L/min
Breath Rate	12/min
PEEP/CPAP	5 cm H_2O
Assist Sensitivity	off
Pressure Support	off

Alarm Settings

High Pressure Limit	5 cm H_2O above peak inspiratory pressure
Low Peak Pressure	10 cm H_2O below peak inspiratory pressure
Low PEEP/CPAP	2 cm H_2O below baseline pressure
High Breath Rate	14/min
Low Minute Volume	4 L/min
Apnea Interval	20 seconds
Backup Breath Rate	12/min

1. Complete a circuit pressure test:
   a. Set the breath rate to zero.
   b. Attach a test lung to the patient wye.
   c. Press and hold the "Inspiratory Hold" button.
   d. Press the "Manual Breath" button.

e. Circuit pressure should rise and hold. If the circuit leaks, check all fittings, connections, and the humidifier for possible causes, and repeat steps a through d.

f. Reset the breath rate control to 12/min.

2. Allow the ventilator to run for about 2 minutes and verify the following monitor values:

Minute Volume	6 L ± 0.6 L
Tidal Volume	500 mL ± 7.5 mL
I:E Ratio	1:5.7 ± 5%
Breath Rate	12/min ± 2/min

3. Verify the following alarms and their function:
   a. Power failure (Disconnect the power cord.)
   b. High pressure limit (Manually restrict the test lung.)
   c. Low peak pressure, low PEEP/CPAP (Disconnect the test lung from the patient wye.)
   d. Low minute volume (Set the breath rate control at 6/min.)
   e. High breath rate (Set the breath rate control at 15/min.)
   f. Apnea interval/apnea backup ventilation (Set the breath rate control at zero.)
   g. Flow transducer alarm (Disconnect the flow transducer from the front of the ventilator.)
   h. "CIRC" alarm and display (Disconnect the expiratory limb from the exhalation valve assembly and occlude it with your hand.)

Practice Activities:

To complete these practice activities, it is recommended that you use a lung analog/simulator such as a Medishield Lung Ventilator Performance Analyzer or other similar device in which resistance and compliance may be easily controlled and altered.

Initial Settings

Mode	Assist-control
Peak Flow	40 L/min
Sensitivity	2 cm H_2O
High Peak Pressure	120 cm H_2O
Tidal Volume	500 mL
Breath Rate	12/min
$O_2\%$	21%
Waveform	square
PEEP	0.0 cm H_2O
Alarms	off

Manipulate only one control at a time and record your results on a sheet of paper. Answer the questions that follow each activity, recording each answer on your paper. If you have difficulty, ask your laboratory instructor for assistance.

Peak Flow Control

1. Set the peak flow to 20 L/min.
   a. Measure the inspiratory time using a watch with a second hand or a stopwatch.
   b. Measure the peak pressure by observing the pressure manometer.
   c. Record the exhaled tidal volume. (Depress the "Tidal Volume" button below the pressure manometer.)
   d. Record the I:E ratio by depressing the "I:E ratio" key and observing the display.

2. Adjust the peak flow to 100 L/min.
   a. Measure the inspiratory time using a watch with a second hand or a stopwatch.
   b. Measure the peak pressure by observing the pressure manometer.
   c. Record the exhaled tidal volume. (Depress the "Tidal Volume" button below the pressure manometer.)
   d. Record the I:E ratio by depressing the "I:E ratio" key and observing the display.

Questions

A. How do you account for the differences in inspiratory time?
B. Why were there differences in peak inspiratory pressure?
C. Why did the corrected tidal volume vary?
D. Why did the I:E ratio vary between the two activities?

3. Return the peak flow control to 40 L/min.

Tidal Volume Control

1. Set the controls to the following settings:

Peak Flow	40 L/min
Tidal Volume	500 mL
Breath Rate	12/min

Leave all other controls set at the same values you established for the peak flow activity.
   a. Measure the inspiratory time using a watch with a second hand or a stop watch.
   b. Measure the peak inspiratory pressure.
   c. Record the exhaled tidal volume.
   d. Record the I:E ratio.

2. Adjust the tidal volume to 1200 mL.
   a. Measure the inspiratory time using a watch with a second hand or a stop watch.
   b. Measure the peak inspiratory pressure.
   c. Record the exhaled tidal volume.
   d. Record the I:E ratio.

Questions

A. Why did the pressure increase?
B. Why did the inspiratory time increase?
C. How do you account for the decrease in I:E ratio?

3. Return the tidal volume control to 500 mL.

Rate Control

1. Set the controls to the following settings:

Peak Flow	40 L/min
High Peak Pressure	120 cm H$_2$O
Tidal Volume	500 mL
Breath Rate	12/min

2. With the controls as set above, perform the following:
   a. Measure the inspiratory time using a watch with a second hand or a stopwatch.
   b. Measure the peak inspiratory pressure.
   c. Record the exhaled tidal volume.
   d. Record the I:E ratio.

3. Adjust the rate control to 25 breaths/min.
   a. Measure the inspiratory time using a watch with a second hand or a stop watch.
   b. Measure the peak inspiratory pressure.
   c. Record the exhaled tidal volume.
   d. Record the I:E ratio.

Questions

A. What was the I:E ratio?
B. Why was the I:E ratio so low?

Triggering

In this section you will explore how the Bird 8400ST triggers breaths when the patient has a spontaneous effort.

Pressure Triggering

Adjust the ventilator to the following settings:

Mode	Assist-control
Peak Flow	40 L/min
Sensitivity	10 cm H$_2$O
High Peak Pressure	10 cm H$_2$O greater than PIP
Tidal Volume	500 mL
Breath Rate	8 breaths/min
O$_2$%	21%
PEEP	0.0 cm H$_2$O

1. Attach a mouthpiece to the patient wye and attempt to initiate a breath. Observe the pressure manometer.

2. Set the assist sensitivity to 1 cm H$_2$O. Again using a mouthpiece, initiate a breath while observing the pressure manometer and the pressure volume loop.

Questions

A. When were you able to initiate a breath most easily?
B. Where would you prefer as a patient to have the assist sensitivity control set?
C. What changes did you observe on the pressure volume loop between the two settings?

Flow Triggering

To complete the practice activities on flow triggering, you must install the special flow triggering flow sensor. When

the sensor is installed, a bias flow of 10 L/min will pass through the circuit and flow sensitivities of 1 to 10 L/min may be set.

Adjust the ventilator to the following settings:

Mode	Assist-control
Peak Flow	40 L/min
Flow Sensitivity	3 L/min
High Peak Pressure	10 cm H$_2$O greater than PIP
Tidal Volume	500 mL
Rate	8 breaths/min
O$_2$%	21%
PEEP	0.0 cm H$_2$O

1. Attach a mouthpiece to the patient wye and attempt to initiate a breath. Observe the pressure manometer.

2. Adjust the flow sensitivity level to 8 L/min. Initiate a breath using a mouthpiece and observe the pressure manometer.

Questions

A. Which setting would you prefer as a patient?
B. Which setting was easiest for you?
C. What changes did you observe on the graphics display panel?
D. How can you use the pressure volume loop and the graphics display panel to minimize inspiratory work?

Pressure Control Ventilation

Set the controls to the following settings and attach the ventilator to the test lung:

Mode	Assist-control (Depress the "Pres. Ctrl." button.)
Inspiratory Pressure	30 cm H$_2$O (Tidal Volume/Insp. Pres.)
Inspiratory Time	1 second (Peak Flow/Insp. Time)
Sensitivity	5 cm H$_2$O
Breath Rate	12 breaths/min
O$_2$%	21%
PEEP	0.0 cm H$_2$O

Inspiratory Pressure Control

1. Using a test lung, measure and record the following using the display panel and manometer:
   a. Exhaled tidal volume
   b. I:E ratio
   c. Peak pressure

2. Adjust the inspiratory pressure level to 50 cm H$_2$O. Measure the following using the display panel and manometer:
   a. Exhaled tidal volume
   b. I:E ratio
   c. Peak pressure

Questions

A. How did the change in pressure affect the I:E ratio?
B. How did the change in pressure affect the exhaled tidal volume?

Inspiratory Time Control

1. Set the ventilator to the following settings:

Mode	Assist-control (Depress the "Pres. Ctrl." button.)
Inspiratory Pressure	30 cm H_2O (Tidal Volume/Insp. Pres. control)
Inspiratory Time	1 second (Peak Flow/Insp. Time control)
Sensitivity	5 cm H_2O
Rate	6 breaths/min
O_2%	21%
PEEP	0.0 cm H_2O

2. Using a test lung, measure the following using the display panel and manometer:
   a. Exhaled tidal volume
   b. I:E ratio
   c. Peak pressure

3. Change the inspiratory time to 3 seconds, and measure and record the following:
   a. Exhaled tidal volume
   b. I:E ratio
   c. Peak pressure

Questions

A. How did the inspiratory time change affect the I:E ratio?
B. How did the inspiratory time change affect tidal volume delivery?
C. How did the inspiratory time change affect the inspiratory pressure?

Alarm Systems

Set the ventilator to the following settings:

Mode	Assist-control
Peak Flow	40 L/min
Sensitivity	2 cm H_2O
Tidal Volume	500 mL
Breath Rate	8 breaths/min
O_2 %	21%
PEEP	0.0 cm H_2O

High Pressure Limit an\d Low Peak Pressure

1. Set the pressure limit for 15 cm H_2O above the peak inspiratory pressure.

2. Set the low peak pressure control to 15 cm H_2O below the peak inspiratory pressure.

3. Simulate a cough by rapidly squeezing the test lung.

Questions

A. What occurred?
B. Was the alarm set appropriately?
C. What other conditions might cause this alarm to be activated?

4. Decrease the tidal volume to 250 mL.

Questions

A. What occurred?
B. Was the alarm set appropriately?
C. What other conditions might cause this alarm to be activated?

Baseline Pressure

Set the controls to the following values:

Mode	Assist-control
Peak Flow	40 L/min
Sensitivity	4 cm H_2O
Tidal Volume	500 mL
Rate	8 breaths/min
O_2%	21%
PEEP	5 cm H_2O

1. Set the Low PEEP/CPAP pressure alarm for 3 cm H_2O.

2. Simulate a patient effort by expanding the test lung's bellows to trigger a breath.

Questions

A. What occurred?
B. How could you change the control settings to prevent this?
C. Is the alarm set appropriately for this level of PEEP?

3. Readjust your baseline pressure alarm to 3 cm H_2O.

Low Minute Volume

1. Set the low minute volume alarm indicator and adjust the control to 3 L/min.

Questions

A. What occurred?
B. How could you set the alarm appropriately for the current ventilator settings?

2. Set the alarm's upper limit to 6 L/min and lower limit to 4 L/min.

High Breath Rate

1. Set the high breath rate alarm to 10 breaths/min.

2. Using the test lung, simulate a rate of 20 breaths/min.

Questions

A. What occurred?
B. How could you set the alarm appropriately for a patient rate of 20/min?
C. Set the alarm's upper limit to 12 breaths/min and lower limit to 6 breaths/min.

Practice Activities: Nellcor Puritan Bennett 840

Circuit Assembly

Figure 25-8 shows the Nellcor Puritan Bennett 840 assembled and ready for use. To prepare the ventilator for use, follow these steps:.

1. Install a bacteria inspiratory filter on the patient outlet located on the upper right portion of the breath delivery unit (BDU).

2. Lift the expiratory filter latch to the Up position.

3. Install an expiratory filter and collector vial by positioning the upper filter rim into the tracks on the upper part of the patient port on the BDU. Once the expiratory filter has been correctly positioned, push the latch down to lock it in place.

4. Install a 12- to 18-inch length of 22 mm tubing between the inspiratory filter and the ventilator's humidifier inlet.

5. Connect the inspiratory limb of the patient circuit to the humidifier outlet.

6. Connect the expiratory limb of the patient circuit to the expiratory filter and collection vial's 22 mm fitting.

7. Attach the patient circuit to the flex arm at its midpoint by clamping the ball fitting on the circuit to the flex arm.

Testing the Ventilator before Use

Power-on Self Test (POST)

Each time the power switch is turned on or if the ventilator microprocessor detects selected fault conditions, a power-on self test (POST) is automatically executed. The POST takes approximately 10 seconds. The test verifies the integrity of the BDU and the graphic user interface (GUI) and their subsystems.

The POST does not check the ventilator's pneumatic systems. To check the operation of the pneumatic systems, do a short self test (SST).

Short Self Test (SST)

The SST is a short 2- to 3-minute test that will verify the operation of the BDU hardware including the pressure and flow sensors, the patient circuit, and its compliance and resistance. The test also measures the exhalation filter's resistance. It is recommended that the SST be performed every 15 days, between patients, or when the

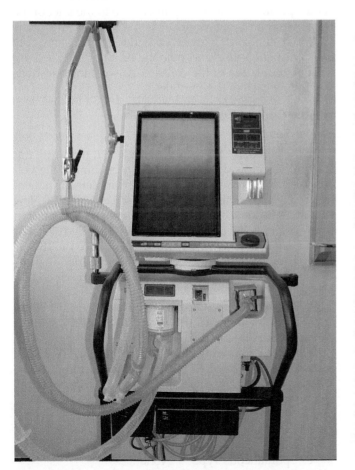
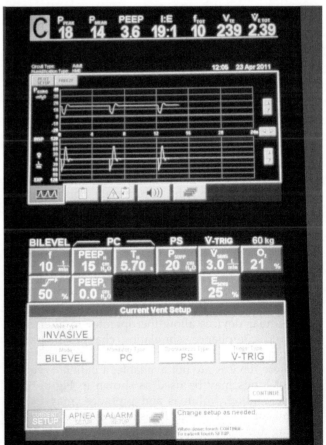

Figure 25-8 A photograph of the Nellcor Puritan-Bennett 840 ventilator and the GUI screen

patient circuit is changed. To complete an SST, perform the following steps:

1. The SST will prompt you to verify that a patient is not connected to the circuit.

2. Turn the ventilator's power switch on. Upon ventilator start-up, touch the "SST" prompt on the lower GUI screen and then press the "Test" button on the left side of the ventilator within 5 seconds of start-up.

3. Follow the prompts on the GUI screen. The microprocessor will then verify that the patient wye is blocked and the SST test will automatically begin.

4. The SST measures the following:
   a. Tests the accuracy of expiratory flow sensors
   b. Verifies the proper function of the pressure sensors
   c. Tests the patient circuit for leaks
   d. Calculates the compliance compensation for the patient circuit
   e. Measures the pressure drop across the expiratory filter
   f. Measures the resistance of the inspiratory and expiratory limbs of the circuit
   g. Checks the pressure drop across the inspiratory limb of the circuit

Using the Keyboard Entry System

All functions of the Nellcor Puritan Bennett 840 ventilator are controlled from the GUI screen (see Figure 25-8). The upper screen displays monitored information including patient data, graphics, and an alarm log. The lower screen displays ventilator setup, alarm settings, and breath timing information. To enter ventilator or alarm settings, follow the "touch–turn–touch" method for entering new settings. Touch the desired value or setting you wish to change (e.g., tidal volume), and then turn the knob on the lower right side of the GUI interface until the desired value is displayed (clockwise increases, counterclockwise decreases). Touch or press "Accept" to apply the new setting. The new setting will now be displayed on the appropriate portion of the upper or lower GUI screen.

Activities

To complete these practice activities, it is recommended that you use a lung analog/simulator such as an SMS "Manley" lung simulator or an IngMar Medical Quick Lung or Demonstration Lung Model. These devices or other similar devices allow the operator to alter resistance and compliance, simulating changes in patient condition.

If these devices are not available, a patient wye and two test lungs may be used as shown in Figure 25-9. Exercise caution. Volumes and pressures may exceed the limits of the test lungs. Resistance may be altered by adapting different sizes of endotracheal tubes, and compliance may be altered by the addition of rubber bands to the test lungs.

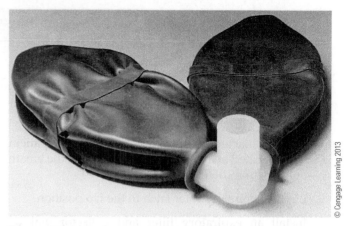

© Cengage Learning 2013

Figure 25-9 Two test lungs assembled for use during the practice procedures

Lung Simulator Setup

If you are using an SMS ("Manley") lung simulator, connect one spring for compliance, set the resistance control to zero, and rotate the leak control fully clockwise, eliminating any leaks. Attach the patient wye to the inlet of the SMS lung simulator.

If you are using an IngMar Medical Demonstration Lung Model, rotate all of the compliance springs fully clockwise, adjust the resistance controls to "OFF," and adjust both the ET Leak and System Leak controls to the "OFF" position. Attach the patient wye to the inlet of the Demonstration Lung Model.

When completing these activities, manipulate only one control at a time and note the result of each activity with manipulation of the controls. Answer the questions that follow each of the activities.

Volume Control Exercises

Patient Setup

Once the ventilator has completed a POST, the Ventilator Start-up screen is displayed. Prior to beginning the volume control exercises, you must first complete the patient setup. At the Ventilator Start-up screen, select "New Patient." The ideal body weight input screen appears and you must enter the patient's ideal body weight (IBW). For these exercises, enter 70 kg as the IBW. Once the IBW is entered, press "Continue" to accept the value, or press "Restart" to return to the Ventilator Start-up screen and reenter the IBW.

A new Ventilator Start-up screen will appear following entry of the patient's IBW. Table 25-5 lists the settings that appear on this screen.

Make the following selections from the Ventilator Start-up Settings screen. Press the desired setting (Mode, Mandatory Type, Spontaneous Type, or Trigger Type), and rotate the knob on the lower right side of the GUI to change the settings.
   a. Mode   A/C
   b. Mandatory Type   VC
   c. Spontaneous Type   None
   d. Trigger Type   P Trigger (pressure)

TABLE 25-5: Ventilator Start-Up Settings

Mode	Assist-Control (A/C)
	SIMV
	Spontaneous (SPONT)
	BILEVEL
Mandatory Type	Pressure Control (PC)
	Volume Control (VC)
Spontaneous Type	Pressure Support
	None (CPAP)
Trigger Type	Pressure Trigger (P-Trig)
	Flow Trigger (V-Trig)

If you make an error, simply touch the desired button to change the setting (i.e., Mode, Mandatory Type, Spontaneous Type, or Trigger Type), make the change by rotating the knob on the lower right of the GUI, and press "Continue." Once the initial settings are complete, a new Ventilator Settings screen will appear.

Ventilator Settings Screen (Volume Control)	
Frequency (f)	Adjustable from 1 to 100 breaths/min
Tidal Volume (V_t)	Adjustable from 25 to 2500 mL
Flow (V_{max})	Adjustable from 3 to 150 L/min
Pressure Trigger (P_{SENS})	Adjustable from 0.1 to 20 cm H_2O below baseline
Oxygen Percent	Adjustable from 21% to 100%
Flow Sensitivity ($\dot{V}_{SENS}$)	Adjustable from 0.5 to 20 L/min
Plateau time (T_{PL})	Adjustable from 0 to 2 seconds
Flow Pattern	Square Decelerating ramp
PEEP	Adjustable from 0 to 45 cm H_2O

© Cengage Learning 2013

From the Ventilator Settings screen, make the following selections by touching the appropriate button, rotating the knob, and touching the button once again. Simply follow the "touch–turn–touch" sequence to make your selection.

a.	Respiratory Rate	12/min
b.	Tidal Volume	500 mL
c.	Peak Flow	40 L/min
d.	P-Trigger	−2 cm H_2O
e.	Oxygen Percent	21%
f.	Plateau Time	0 second
g.	Flow Pattern	square
h.	PEEP	0 cm H_2O

If you make an error, simply touch the button you wish to change, rotate the knob to enter the correct setting, and complete the change by touching the button once again.

Patient Monitoring

The GUI screen is divided into two large sections. The lower section is devoted to ventilator settings, and you have already been making entries and using this portion of the screen. The upper screen is devoted to "Monitored Data" or patient data and alarms. Pressing the Graphics symbol at the lower left edge of the monitored data allows you to select between two scalar graphics (pressure time or flow time) or pressure volume. Using the "Plot Setup" button and the control knob, scroll through the options and press "Continue" to make your selection. Should you select pressure volume, it will occupy the entire screen. Pressure time and flow time scalars can be displayed simultaneously.

Above the graphics display, patient data are displayed numerically. In the upper left corner of the display, breath type (type and phase) will be displayed. Display of types include control, assist, or spontaneous, while phase includes inspiration or expiration. Other monitored patient data include pressure at the end of inspiration (P_{IEND}), rate (f_{TOT}), exhaled volume (V_{TE}), maximum circuit pressure during inspiration ($P_{CIRC\ MAX}$), end-expiratory pressure ($P_{E\ END}$), I:E ratio, and exhaled minute volume ($V_{E\ TOT}$).

Between the monitored patient data and the graphics display on the GUI is an alarm area. This section of the screen displays the two highest priority alarms and suggested remedies to correct the alarm condition. You may also press the "Alarm Log" button (clipboard with a speaker), and a list of alarm events, time, and urgency will be displayed.

Peak Flow Control

From the initial settings you have previously set, note the following ventilatory (patient) parameters before you make the next changes:
1. I:E ratio
2. Peak pressure
3. Inspiratory time (note the time using your watch and a sweep second hand)

1. Set the peak flow to 20 L/min.
   a. Measure the inspiratory time.
   b. Measure the peak pressure.
   c. Record the I:E ratio.

2. Adjust the peak flow to 60 L/min.
   a. Measure the inspiratory time.
   b. Measure the peak pressure.
   c. Record the I:E ratio.

Questions

A. How do you account for the differences in inspiratory time?
B. Why were their differences in peak inspiratory pressure?
C. Why did the I:E ratio vary between the two activities?

Tidal Volume Control

1. Set the controls to the following settings:
   a. Respiratory Rate   12/min
   b. Tidal Volume   500 mL
   c. Peak Flow   60 L/min
   d. P-Trigger   −2 cm H_2O
   e. Oxygen Percent   21%
   f. Plateau Time   0 second
   g. Flow Pattern   square
   h. PEEP   0 cm H_2O

   Once these settings have been established, record the following ventilatory (patient) parameters.
   a. Measure the inspiratory time (estimate using your watch and a sweep second hand)
   b. Measure the peak inspiratory pressure.
   c. Record the tidal volume.
   d. Record the I:E ratio.

2. Set the normal tidal volume control to 1000 mL.
   a. Measure the inspiratory time.
   b. Measure the peak inspiratory pressure.
   c. Record the corrected tidal volume.
   d. Record the I:E ratio.

Questions

A. Why did the pressure increase?
B. Why did the inspiratory time increase?
C. How do you account for the change in I:E ratio?

Normal Rate Control (Cycles or Breaths per Minute)

Set the controls to the following settings:
   a. Respiratory Rate   12/min
   b. Tidal Volume   500 mL
   c. Peak Flow   60 L/min
   d. P-Trigger   −2 cm H_2O
   e. Oxygen Percent   21%
   f. Plateau Time   0 second
   g. Flow Pattern   square
   h. PEEP   0 cm H_2O

   Go to the alarm settings screen and adjust the peak pressure alarm to 100 cm H_2O.

1. With the controls set as above, perform the following:
   a. Measure the peak inspiratory pressure.
   b. Measure the inspiratory time.
   c. Record the corrected tidal volume.
   d. Record the I:E ratio.

2. Adjust the rate control to 30 breaths/min.
   a. Measure the peak inspiratory pressure.
   b. Measure the inspiratory time.
   c. Record the corrected tidal volume.
   d. Record the I:E ratio.

Questions

A. What alarm was triggered and why?
B. What was the I:E ratio?
C. Why was the I:E ratio so high?

Changes in Resistance and Compliance

1. Set the controls to the following settings:
   a. Respiratory Rate   12/min
   b. Tidal Volume   500 mL
   c. Peak Flow   60 L/min
   d. P-Trigger   −2 cm H_2O
   e. Oxygen Percent   21%
   f. Plateau Time   0 second
   g. Flow Pattern   square
   h. PEEP   0 cm H_2O

   Go to the alarm settings screen and adjust the peak pressure alarm to 100 cm H_2O.

   Once the settings are established, measure and record the following ventilatory (patient) parameters from the monitoring screen.
   a. Measure the peak inspiratory pressure.
   b. Measure the inspiratory time.
   c. Record the tidal volume.
   d. Record the I:E ratio.

2. Decrease the compliance by 1/3 by adjusting the spring tension on the test lung.
   a. Measure the peak inspiratory pressure.
   b. Measure the inspiratory time (estimate the time using your watch and a second hand).
   c. Record the tidal volume.
   d. Record the I:E ratio.

Questions

A. Why did the corrected tidal volume decrease?
B. Why did the I:E ratio vary?
C. Why did the peak inspiratory pressure increase?

3. Increase the resistance by 2/3 by adjusting the resistance control on the lung analog.
   a. Measure the peak inspiratory pressure.
   b. Measure the inspiratory time.
   c. Record the corrected tidal volume.
   d. Record the I:E ratio.

Questions

A. Why did the inspiratory pressure increase?
B. Why did the I:E ratio vary?
C. How do you account for differences in the corrected tidal volume?
D. Can you think of human physiologic conditions that could produce similar results?

Return the resistance control to its original setting on the lung analog. Set the ventilator to the following settings:
   a. Respiratory Rate   12/min
   b. Tidal Volume   500 mL
   c. Peak Flow   60 L/min
   d. P-Trigger   −2 cm H_2O
   e. Oxygen Percent   21%
   f. Plateau Time   0 second
   g. Flow Pattern   square
   h. PEEP   0 cm H_2O

Set the peak pressure to 10 cm H_2O greater than the current peak pressure setting. Now decrease the compliance by

1/3 by adjusting the spring tension or adjusting the compliance control on the lung analog (1/3 greater than its normal setting without adjustment). Once the settings are established, answer the following questions.

Questions

A. What event(s) occurred?
B. Can you think of a patient situation that could cause this?
C. What is the purpose of the normal pressure limit control?

Triggering Adjustment

Pressure Triggering

Touch the "Vent Setup" soft key, and from "Trigger Type" select "P–Trigger." Set the ventilator to the following settings:

a.	Respiratory Rate	12/min
b.	Tidal Volume	500 mL
c.	Peak Flow	60 L/min
d.	P-Trigger	−2 cm H_2O
e.	Oxygen Percent	21%
f.	Plateau Time	0 second
g.	Flow Pattern	square
h.	PEEP	0 cm H_2O

1. Attach a mouthpiece to the patient wye and attempt to initiate a breath.

2. With the sensitivity control at −2 cm H_2O, initiate a breath. Observe the pressure time curve on the monitoring screen or the pressure volume loop. Adjust the screen scale to expand the scale, making it easier to observe pressure changes. Note the display in the upper left corner of the "Monitored Data" section of the display screen.

3. Adjust the sensitivity control to –20 cm H_2O and initiate a breath. Observe the pressure time curve on the monitoring screen or the pressure volume loop. Adjust the screen scale to expand the scale, making it easier to observe pressure changes. Note the display in the upper left corner of the "Monitored Data" section of the display screen.
   a. Record the negative pressure when the ventilator cycled on.
   b. Observe the monitoring screen for any changes in ventilatory (patient) parameters.

Questions

A. When you were able to initiate an assisted breath, what event(s) occurred?
B. What breath type was momentarily displayed when you triggered a breath?
C. Where would you want to set the sensitivity control for assist-control mode?

Flow Triggering

Touch the "Vent Setup" soft key and select "Flow Triggering" ($\dot{V}$ Trigger).

Adjust the ventilator to the following settings in volume control mode:

a.	Respiratory Rate	12/min
b.	Tidal Volume	500 mL

c.	Peak Flow	60 L/min
d.	$\dot{V}$ Trigger	4 L/min
e.	Oxygen Percent	21%
f.	Plateau Time	0 second
g.	Flow Pattern	square
h.	PEEP	0 cm H_2O

1. Attach a mouthpiece to the patient wye and attempt to initiate a breath.

2. Set the sensitivity control to 4 L/min and initiate a breath. Observe the flow time curve on the monitoring screen or the pressure volume loop. Adjust the screen scale to expand the scale, making it easier to observe pressure changes. Note the display in the upper left corner of the "Monitored Data" section of the display screen.

3. Adjust the sensitivity control to 8 L/min and initiate a breath. Observe the flow time curve on the monitoring screen or the pressure volume loop. Adjust the screen scale to expand the scale, making it easier to observe pressure changes. Note the display in the upper left corner of the "Monitored Data" section of the display screen.
   a. Record what threshold is met when the ventilator cycled on.
   b. Observe the monitoring screen for any changes in ventilatory (patient) parameters.

Questions

A. When you were able to initiate an assisted breath, what event(s) occurred?
B. What breath type was momentarily displayed when you triggered a breath?
C. Where would you want to set the sensitivity control for assist-control mode?

Pressure Control Ventilation

Test Lung Setup

If you are using an SMS ("Manley") lung simulator, connect one spring for compliance, set the resistance control to zero, and rotate the leak control fully clockwise, eliminating any leaks. Attach the patient wye to the inlet of the SMS lung simulator.

If you are using an IngMar Medical Demonstration Lung Model, rotate all of the compliance springs fully clockwise, adjust the resistance controls to "OFF," and adjust both the ET Leak and System Leak controls to the "OFF" position. Attach the patient wye to the inlet of the Demonstration Lung Model.

When completing these activities, manipulate only one control at a time and note the result of each activity with manipulation of the controls. Answer the questions that follow each of the activities.

Initial Ventilator Settings

Begin this section by setting the ventilator to the following settings. Touch the "Vent Setup" soft key. From the "Mode" key, select "A/C" (assist-control) mode. Press the "Mandatory Type" soft key, and select "PC" for Pressure Control mode. Touch the "Trigger Type" key, and select "P-Trigger" for pressure triggering.

Adjust the ventilator to the following settings in pressure control mode:

a. A/C	12/min
b. P_I	15 cm H_2O
c. T_I	0.76
d. Rise Time %	50%
e. P-Trigger	–2 cm H_2O
f. Oxygen Percent	21%
g. PEEP	0 cm H_2O

Inspiratory Pressure Control

1. Using a test lung, measure and record the following using the monitoring screen:
   a. Peak inspiratory pressure
   b. I:E ratio
   c. Tidal volume
   d. Minute ventilation

2. Adjust the inspiratory pressure level to 25 cm H_2O. Measure the following using the display panel and manometer:
   a. Peak inspiratory pressure
   b. I:E ratio
   c. Tidal volume
   d. Minute ventilation

3. Adjust the inspiratory pressure level to 5 cm H_2O. Using the monitoring screen, measure the following:
   a. Peak inspiratory pressure
   b. I:E ratio
   c. Tidal volume
   d. Minute ventilation

Questions

A. How did the change in inspiratory pressure affect the I:E ratio?
B. How did the change in inspiratory pressure affect the exhaled tidal volume?
C. How did the change in inspiratory pressure affect the exhaled minute volume?

Inspiratory Time Control

Begin this section by setting the ventilator to the following settings. Touch the "Vent Setup" soft key. From the "Mode" key, select "A/C" (assist-control) mode. Press the "Mandatory Type" soft key, and select "PC" for pressure control mode. Touch the "Trigger Type" key, and select "P-Trigger" for pressure triggering.

Adjust the ventilator to the following settings in pressure control mode:

a. A/C	12/min
b. P_I	15 cm H_2O
c. T_I	0.76
d. Rise Time %	50%
e. P-Trigger	–2 cm H_2O
f. Oxygen Percent	21%
g. PEEP	0 cm H_2O

1. Using a test lung, measure the following using the display panel and manometer:
   a. Peak inspiratory pressure
   b. I:E ratio
   c. Exhaled tidal volume
   d. Exhaled minute volume

2. Change the inspiratory time to 1 second, and measure and record the following:
   a. Peak inspiratory pressure
   b. I:E ratio
   c. Exhaled tidal volume
   d. Exhaled minute volume

3. Change the inspiratory time to 3 seconds, and measure and record the following:
   a. Peak inspiratory pressure
   b. I:E ratio
   c. Exhaled tidal volume
   d. Exhaled minute volume

Questions

A. How did the inspiratory time change affect the I:E ratio?
B. How did the inspiratory time change affect tidal volume delivery?
C. How did the inspiratory time change affect the inspiratory pressure?

Rate Control

Adjust the ventilator to the following settings in pressure control mode:

a. A/C	12/min
b. P_I	15 cm H_2O
c. T_I	0.76
d. Rise Time %	50%
e. P-Trigger	–2 cm H_2O
f. Oxygen Percent	21%
g. PEEP	0 cm H_2O

1. Using a test lung, measure the following using the monitoring screen:
   a. Peak inspiratory pressure
   b. I:E ratio
   c. Exhaled tidal volume
   d. Exhaled minute volume

2. Change the rate control to 24 breaths/min, and measure and record the following:
   a. Peak inspiratory pressure
   b. I:E ratio
   c. Exhaled tidal volume
   d. Exhaled minute volume

3. Change the rate control to 6 breaths/min, and measure and record the following:
   a. Peak inspiratory pressure
   b. I:E ratio
   c. Exhaled tidal volume
   d. Exhaled minute volume

Questions

A. What happened to the I:E ratio when you changed the rate?
B. What happened to the minute ventilation when you changed the rate?

Spontaneous Ventilation

The Nellcor-Puritan Bennett 840 may be set up in spontaneous ventilation without pressure support (CPAP) or with pressure support. To initiate spontaneous ventilation modes, complete the following steps.

Spontaneous (CPAP)
1. Touch the "Vent Setup" soft key.
2. Touch the "Mode" soft key and select "Spont" for spontaneous mode.
3. Touch the "Spont Type" soft key. Using the adjustment knob, scroll down to select "None."
4. Touch the "Continue" soft key and press "Accept."

From the displayed screen, you may now enter a PEEP (CPAP) level.
1. Touch the "PEEP" button on the right side of the spontaneous settings screen.
2. Turn the knob to adjust the PEEP (CPAP) level to 5 cm H_2O.
3. Touch the "PEEP" (CPAP) button again. The setting will now be displayed with a light blue background.
4. Press the "Accept" button. The PEEP (CPAP) setting will now change to a dark blue background and the setting will become the active or set CPAP level.

PEEP (CPAP Level)

Test Lung Setup

1. If you are using an SMS ("Manley") lung simulator, connect one spring for compliance, set the resistance control to zero, and rotate the leak control fully clockwise, eliminating any leaks. Attach the patient wye to the inlet of the SMS lung simulator.
2. If you are using an IngMar Medical Demonstration Lung Model, rotate all of the compliance springs fully clockwise, adjust the resistance controls to "OFF," and adjust both the ET Leak and System Leak controls to the "OFF" position. Attach the patient wye to the inlet of the Demonstration Lung Model.
3. When completing these activities, manipulate only one control at a time and note the result of each activity with manipulation of the controls. Answer the questions that follow each of the activities.

Set the controls to the following settings:
a. Mode — Spont
b. SPONT Type — None
c. E_{SENS} — 25%
d. PEEP (CPAP level) — 5 cm H_2O

Once the settings have been established, simulate a spontaneous breath by moving the test lung's bellows. Repeat the process, simulating a spontaneous rate and tidal volume. Observe the pressure time curve on the monitoring screen or the pressure volume loop. Adjust the screen scale to expand the scale, making it easier to observe pressure changes. Note the display in the upper left corner of the "Monitored Data" section of the display screen.

Questions

A. What breath type was displayed momentarily during your spontaneous breathing efforts?
B. What did you observe as the baseline pressure on the pressure time scalar waveform?
C. What happened when you stopped your simulated breathing?
D. What was an average inspiratory pressure during your spontaneous efforts?

Change the ventilator controls to the following settings:
a. Mode — Spont
b. SPONT Type — None
c. E_{SENS} — 25%
d. PEEP (CPAP level) — 15 cm H_2O

Once the settings have been established, simulate a spontaneous breath by moving the test lung's bellows. Repeat the process, simulating a spontaneous rate and tidal volume. Observe the pressure time curve on the monitoring screen or the pressure volume loop. Adjust the screen scale to expand the scale, making it easier to observe pressure changes. Note the display in the upper left corner of the "Monitored Data" section of the display screen.

Questions

A. What breath type was displayed momentarily during your spontaneous breathing efforts?
B. What did you observe as the baseline pressure on the pressure time scalar waveform?
C. What happened when you stopped your simulated breathing?
D. What was an average inspiratory pressure during your spontaneous efforts?

Pressure Support

Spontaneous–Pressure Support

5. Touch the "Vent Setup" soft key.
6. Touch the "Mode" soft key and select "Spont" for spontaneous mode.
7. Touch the "Spont Type" soft key. Using the adjustment knob, scroll down to select "P_{SUPP}" for pressure support.
8. Touch the "Continue" soft key and press "Accept."

From the displayed screen, you may now enter a PEEP (CPAP) level and pressure support level.
1. Touch the "PEEP" button on the right side of the spontaneous settings screen.
2. Turn the knob to adjust the PEEP (CPAP) level to 5 cm H_2O.
3. Touch the "PEEP" (CPAP) button again. The setting will now be displayed with a light blue background.
4. Press the "Accept" button. The PEEP (CPAP) setting will now change to a dark blue background and the setting will become the active or set CPAP level.

5. Touch the "P$_{SUPP}$" key, turn the knob until 5 cm H$_2$O is displayed, touch the "P$_{SUPP}$" key again, and press "Accept."

Test Lung Setup

1. If you are using an SMS ("Manley") lung simulator, connect one spring for compliance, set the resistance control to zero, and rotate the leak control fully clockwise, eliminating any leaks. Attach the patient wye to the inlet of the SMS lung simulator.
2. If you are using an IngMar Medical Demonstration Lung Model, rotate all of the compliance springs fully clockwise, adjust the resistance controls to "OFF," and adjust both the ET Leak and System Leak controls to the "OFF" position. Attach the patient wye to the inlet of the Demonstration Lung Model.
3. When completing these activities, manipulate only one control at a time and note the result of each activity with manipulation of the controls. Answer the questions that follow each of the activities.
   Set the controls to the following settings:
   a. Mode   Spont
   b. SPONT Type   PS (pressure support)
   c. E$_{SENS}$ 25%
   d. PEEP (CPAP level)   5 cm H$_2$O
   e. Pressure Support   5 cm H$_2$O

Once the settings have been established, simulate a spontaneous breath by moving the test lung's bellows. Repeat the process, simulating a spontaneous rate and tidal volume. Observe the pressure time curve on the monitoring screen or the pressure volume loop. Adjust the screen scale to expand the scale, making it easier to observe pressure changes. Note the display in the upper left corner of the "Monitored Data" section of the display screen.

Questions

A. What breath type was displayed momentarily during your spontaneous breathing efforts?
B. What did you observe as the baseline pressure on the pressure time scalar waveform?
C. What happened when you stopped your simulated breathing?
D. What was an average inspiratory pressure during your spontaneous efforts?

Set the controls to the following settings:
   a. Mode   Spont
   b. SPONT Type   PS (pressure support)
   c. E$_{SENS}$ 25%
   d. PEEP (CPAP level)   5 cm H$_2$O
   e. Pressure Support   10 cm H$_2$O

Repeat your spontaneous efforts with the test lung, simulating a rate and a tidal volume. Observe the pressure time curve on the monitoring screen or the pressure volume loop. Adjust the screen scale to expand the scale,

making it easier to observe pressure changes. Note the display in the upper left corner of the "Monitored Data" section of the display screen.

Questions

A. What breath type was displayed momentarily during your spontaneous breathing efforts?
B. What did you observe as the baseline pressure on the pressure time scalar waveform?
C. What happened when you stopped your simulated breathing?
D. What was an average inspiratory pressure during your spontaneous efforts?

Alarm Functions

Input Power and Control Circuit Alarms

Input power alarms alert the clinician to loss of electrical power or pneumatic sources, rendering the ventilator inoperative. Control circuit alarms alert the clinician to incompatible settings or settings that are out of range as well as potential faults in the microprocessor control circuitry. These alarms are summarized in Table 25-6.

Output Alarms

Output alarms are triggered when the alarm limits of the ventilator's output have been exceeded. Examples of typical output alarms include pressure, volume, flow, and time. The output alarms for the Puritan Bennett 840 are summarized in the Table 25-7.

To set the alarms, press the "Alarm Setup" tab at the bottom of the screen. A presentation of the alarms appears in a bar graph format. To set an alarm, touch the desired setting, turn the adjustment knob, touch the setting again or press "Accept." The current parameter is displayed as an arrow to the left of the bar graph display. Both high and low limits may be set in reference to the current patient parameter.

Apnea Ventilation

In the event the patient becomes apneic, the Puritan Bennett 840 ventilator will automatically deliver a rate, tidal volume or pressure, and a set FIO$_2$. To set the Apnea Ventilation parameters, complete the following steps:

1. Touch the "Apnea Setup" key at the bottom of the screen.
2. You have the option of delivering volume control or pressure control breaths. Select either "VC" or "PC" by pressing the "Change VC/PC" key.
3. Once VC or PC modes have been selected, select the appropriate keys for rate, volume (or pressure and Insp time), and the desired FIO$_2$. To make your selections, touch the key, turn the knob, and touch the key again. Once all of your selections are made, press "Accept" to apply the new settings.

TABLE 25-6: Puritan Bennett 840 Input Power Alarms

ALARM	CAUSE	CORRECTIVE ACTION
AC Power Loss	Power switch is in "ON" position, but AC power is not available.	1. Manually ventilate the patient. 2. Check the integrity of the AC power source. 3. If the ventilator is operating on internal battery, prepare for alternative ventilation.
Device Alert	POST has detected a problem.	1. Manually ventilate the patient if needed. 2. Remove the ventilator from service and contact the biomedical department for service.
Inoperative Battery	The backup battery power system is installed but not functioning.	1. Remove the ventilator from service and contact the biomedical department for service.
Loss of Power	The power switch is in the "ON" position, and both AC power and internal battery backup power are not sufficient.	1. Manually ventilate the patient. 2. Check the integrity of power sources.
Low AC Power	AC voltage has dropped to 80% of nominal voltage for at least 1 second. AC power has dropped significantly, and there is a potential for total power failure.	1. Check the AC power connections. 2. Check the integrity of the AC power. 3. Prepare to manually ventilate the patient.
Low Battery	The backup battery has less than 2 minutes of operational time remaining.	1. Replace the battery if needed. 2. Allow the battery to recharge while operating the ventilator on AC power.
Low Delivered O_2%	The measured O_2% is 7% or more below the O_2% setting.	1. Check the patient's SpO_2 to ensure patient safety. 2. Check both air and O_2 gas connections. 3. Recalibrate the oxygen sensor (100% O_2/CAL 2 min key).
No Air Supply	Air supply pressure is less than the minimum required. Oxygen delivery may be compromised.	1. Manually ventilate the patient if required. 2. Check both air and oxygen pneumatic sources.
No O_2 Supply	Oxygen supply pressure is less than the minimum required. Accuracy of O_2% may be compromised.	1. Manually ventilate the patient if required. 2. Check both air and oxygen pneumatic sources.
Procedure Error	Patient is attached before the ventilator start-up is complete.	1. Manually ventilate the patient if required. 2. Complete the ventilator start-up procedure.
Screen Block	Potential blocked beam or touch screen fault.	1. Manually ventilate the patient if required. 2. Contact biomedical for service.

TABLE 25-7: Puritan Bennett 840 Output Alarms

ALARM	CAUSE	CORRECTIVE ACTION
P_{CIRC} (Mean Circuit Pressure)	The measured airway pressure is greater or lower than the alarm setting.	Evaluate the patient: 1. Suctioning needed? 2. Bronchospasm? 3. Circuit disconnect/leaks? 4. Airway secure?
f_{TOT} (Respiratory Rate)	The respiratory rate exceeds the limit of the alarm setting.	Evaluate the patient and the ventilator settings.
$\dot{V}_{E\,TOT}$ (Exhaled Minute Volume)	The patient's exhaled minute volume is greater or less than the alarm setting.	Evaluate the patient and the ventilator settings.
$V_{TE\,MAND}$ (Mandatory Exhaled Tidal Volume)	The patient's exhaled mandatory tidal volume is greater or less than the alarm setting.	Evaluate the patient and the ventilator settings.
$V_{TE\,SPONT}$ (Spontaneous Exhaled Tidal Volume)	The patient's spontaneous exhaled tidal volume is greater or less than the alarm setting.	Evaluate the patient and the ventilator settings.
$O_2\%$	Delivered $O_2\%$ is greater or less than the $O_2\%$ setting for more than 30 seconds.	Evaluate the patient. Check the air and oxygen supply lines. Check the oxygen analyzer cell. Press the "100% O_2/CAL 2 min" key.

Practice Activities: Maquet SERVO-i Ventilator

Circuit Assembly

Figure 25-10 shows the Maquet SERVO-i ventilator assembled and ready for use. To prepare the ventilator for use, follow the steps listed next.

1. Install a bacteria inspiratory filter on the patient outlet located on the right side of the patient unit.
2. Connect a short length of 22 mm tubing (18 inches) between the bacteria filter and the humidifier.
3. Connect the inpsiratory limb of the patient circuit to the humidifier outlet.
4. Connect the expiratory limb of the patient circuit to the expiratory port on the right side of the patient unit.
5. Attach the patient circuit to the flex arm at its midpoint by clamping the ball fitting on the circuit to the flex arm.

Testing the Ventilator before Use

Pre-use Check

The pre-use check tests the function of the microprocessor control system; measures internal leakage; tests the pressure transducers, O_2 cell/sensor, flow transducers, and safety valve; measures circuit leakage; and calculates circuit compliance. It is recommended to perform a pre-use check prior to connecting the ventilator to a patient or whenever a patient circuit is changed. To perform the pre-use check, complete the following steps:

1. Connect the power cord to a 110 volt 60 Hz outlet.
2. Connect the air and oxygen supply lines to 50 psi sources.
3. Turn the ventilator power switch to the "ON" position.
4. From the Standby screen, select "Yes" to the question "Do you want to start Pre-use check?"
5. Connect the blue 22 mm test tube between the ventilator outlet and exhalation inlet on the right side of the patient unit.
6. Follow the onscreen prompts. You will be asked to perform the following:
   a. Disconnect the ventilator from AC power.
   b. Reconnect the ventilator to AC power.
   c. Connect a patient circuit, including the humidifier.
   d. Block and unblock the patient wye.
7. Once the circuit compliance is calculated, you will have the option to add compliance compensation (answer Yes) or not add it (answer No).
8. The outcome of the pre-use check will be displayed on the user interface screen.
9. Once the test is complete, press "OK" to log the pre-use check and to switch the ventilator back to Standby mode.

Using the Maquet SERVO-i User Interface

The Maquet SERVO-i user interface consists of a large screen, four direct access knobs below the screen, several fixed soft keys, and a rotary dial located at the

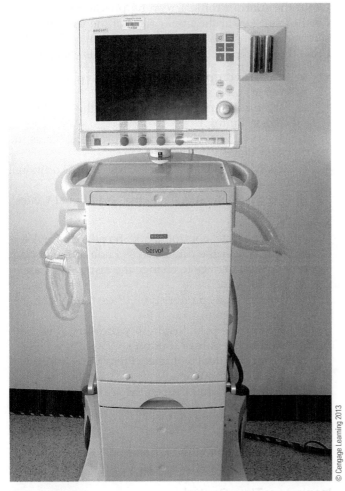

Figure 25-10 A photograph of the Maquet SERVO-i ventilator with a circuit attached

© Cengage Learning 2013

lower right of the user interface that can be turned clockwise, turned counterclockwise (to increase or decrease values), and then pushed to select the desired value.

Activities

To complete these practice activities, it is recommended that you use a lung analog/simulator such as an SMS "Manley" lung simulator or an IngMar Medical Quick Lung or Demonstration Lung Model. These devices or other similar devices allow the operator to alter resistance and compliance, simulating changes in patient condition.

If these devices are not available, a patient wye and two test lungs may be used as shown in Figure 25-10. Exercise caution. Volumes and pressures may exceed the limits of the test lungs. Resistance may be altered by adapting different sizes of endotracheal tubes, and compliance may be altered by the addition of rubber bands to the test lungs.

Lung Simulator Setup

If you are using an SMS ("Manley") lung simulator, connect one spring for compliance, set the resistance control to zero, and rotate the leak control fully clockwise, eliminating any leaks. Attach the patient wye to the inlet of the SMS lung simulator.

If you are using an IngMar Medical Demonstration Lung Model, rotate all of the compliance springs fully clockwise, adjust the resistance controls to "OFF," and adjust both the ET Leak and System Leak controls to the "OFF" position. Attach the patient wye to the inlet of the Demonstration Lung Model.

When completing these activities, manipulate only one control at a time and note the result of each activity with manipulation of the controls. Answer the questions that follow each of the activities.

Volume Control Exercises

Patient Setup

Once the ventilator pre-use check has been completed, select "Adult" from the Standby screen by pressing the "Adult" button. Once the "Adult" button is selected, press the "Volume Control" button on the upper left part of the screen. Table 25-8 lists the settings for this ventilator.

Make the following selections from the Set Ventilation Mode screen. Press the desired setting and rotate the knob on the lower right side of the user interface to change the settings. Then press the button again to capture the desired change.

a.	Tidal Volume	500 mL
b.	Resp. Rate	12/min
c.	PEEP	0 cm H_2O
d.	$O_2\%$	21%
e.	Ti	0.6 second
f.	T pause	0.0 second
g.	T insp. Rise	0.2 second
h.	Trigg. Pressure	−2 cm H_2O

If you make an error, simply touch the button you wish to change, rotate the knob to enter the correct setting, and complete the change by touching the button once again. Once the settings are complete, press the "Accept" button on the lower right of the user interface screen. Then press the "Start/Stop (Standby)" soft key located at the lower left of the user interface adjacent to the four direct access knobs on the lower part of the interface.

TABLE 25-8: SERVO-i Settings Volume Control A/C	
BASIC SETTINGS	
Tidal Volume	100 to 4000 mL
Respiratory Rate	4 to 150 breaths/min
PEEP	0 to 50 cm H_2O
O_2 Concentration	21 to 100%
Inspiratory Time (Ti)	0.1 to 5 seconds
Pause Time (Tpause)	0 to 1.5 seconds
Inspiratory Rise Time (T insp. rise)	0 to 0.4 second
Trigger Sensitivity	Pressure 0 to −20 cm H_2O Flow 0 to 10 L/min

Patient Monitoring

The user interface screen is divided into two large sections. Scalar waveforms from pressure, flow, and volume occupy the majority of the screen display. To the right of the waveform display is a section devoted to patient-monitored parameters. The basic screen includes Peak pressure, respiratory rate, and minute volume with inspired and expired tidal volumes being displayed in the same window.

Pressing the "Additional Values" button at the lower right of the screen opens additional monitoring parameters, including peak, plateau, mean and PEEP pressures, respiratory rate, O_2%, inspiratory time, I:E ratio, minute volumes (inspired and exhaled), and tidal volumes (inspired and exhaled).

Tidal Volume Control

1. Once these settings have been established and the ventilator is operating in volume control A/C mode, record the following ventilatory (patient) parameters:
   a. Measure the inspiratory time. (Press the "Additional Values" button.)
   b. Measure the peak inspiratory pressure. (Press the "Additional Values" button.)
   c. Record the tidal volume. (Press the "Additional Values" button.)
   d. Record the I:E-ratio. (Press the "Additional Values" button.)

2. Press the "Volume Control" button at the top left of the user interface screen. Set normal tidal volume control to 1000 mL and press the "Accept" button. Alternatively, adjust the Tidal Volume direct-access knob at the lower right of the user interface screen to adjust the tidal volume to 1000 mL.
   a. Measure the inspiratory time. (Press the "Additional Values" button.)
   b. Measure the peak inspiratory pressure. (Press the "Additional Values" button.)
   c. Record the tidal volume. (Press the "Additional Values" button.)
   d. Record the I:E ratio. (Press the "Additional Values" button.)

Questions

A. Why did the pressure increase?
B. Why did the inspiratory time increase?
C. How do you account for the change in I:E ratio

Respiratory Rate Control

Set the controls to the following settings:

a. Tidal Volume	500 mL
b. Resp. Rate	12/min
c. PEEP	0 cm H_2O
d. O_2%	21%
e. Ti	0.6 second
f. T pause	0.0 second
g. T insp. Rise	0.2 second
h. Trigg. Pressure	−2 cm H_2O

Go to the Alarm Profile screen by pressing the "Alarm Profile" soft key at the upper right of the user interface screen and adjust the peak pressure alarm to 75 cm H_2O. Press the "Accept" button to complete this change.

1. With the controls set as above, perform the following:
   a. Measure the inspiratory time. (Press the "Additional Values" button.)
   b. Measure the peak inspiratory pressure. (Press the "Additional Values" button.)
   c. Record the tidal volume. (Press the "Additional Values" button.)
   d. Record the I:E ratio. (Press the "Additional Values" button.)

2. Adjust the rate control to 30 breaths/min. Alternatively, adjust the direct-access knob at the bottom of the user interface to change the respiratory rate to 30 breaths/min.
   a. Measure the inspiratory time. (Press the "Additional Values" button.)
   b. Measure the peak inspiratory pressure. (Press the "Additional Values" button.)
   c. Record the tidal volume. (Press the "Additional Values" button.)
   d. Record the I:E ratio. (Press the "Additional Values" button.)

Questions

A. What happened to the I:E ratio?
B. What happened to the minute volume?

Inspiratory Time Control

Set the ventilator to the following settings:

a. Tidal Volume	500 mL
b. Resp. Rate	12/min
c. PEEP	0 cm H_2O
d. O_2%	21%
e. Ti	0.6 second
f. T pause	0.0 second
g. T insp. Rise	0.2 second
h. Trigg. Pressure	−2 cm H_2O

Measure the following:
   a. Measure the inspiratory time. (Press the "Additional Values" button.)
   b. Measure the peak inspiratory pressure. (Press the "Additional Values" button.)
   c. Record the tidal volume. (Press the "Additional Values" button.)
   d. Record the I:E ratio. (Press the "Additional Values" button.)

Adjust the ventilator to the following settings:

a. Tidal Volume	500 mL
b. Resp. Rate	12/min
c. PEEP	0 cm H_2O
d. O_2%	21%
e. Ti	0.45 second
f. T pause	0.0 second
g. T insp. Rise	0.2 second
h. Trigg. Pressure	−2 cm H_2O

Record the following once the change is complete:
   a. Measure the inspiratory time. (Press the "Additional Values" button.)
   b. Measure the peak inspiratory pressure. (Press the "Additional Values" button.)
   c. Record the tidal volume. (Press the "Additional Values" button.)
   d. Record the I:E ratio. (Press the "Additional Values" button.)

Change the ventilator settings to the following:
   a. Tidal Volume   500 mL
   b. Resp. Rate   12/min
   c. PEEP   0 cm H_2O
   d. O_2%   21%
   e. Ti   1.5 seconds
   f. T pause   0.0 second
   g. T insp. Rise   0.2 second
   h. Trigg. Pressure   −2 cm H_2O

Record the following once the change is complete:
   a. Measure the inspiratory time. (Press the "Additional Values" button.)
   b. Measure the peak inspiratory pressure. (Press the "Additional Values" button.)
   c. Record the tidal volume. (Press the "Additional Values" button.)
   d. Record the I:E ratio. (Press the "Additional Values" button.)

Questions

A. What happened to the I:E ratio?
B. What happened to the minute volume?
C. What happened to the flow rate? (Look on the upper right portion of the Volume Control screen.)

Inspiratory Pause Control

Establish the following settings in volume control A/C ventilation:
   a. Tidal Volume   500 mL
   b. Resp. Rate   12/min
   c. PEEP   0 cm H_2O
   d. O_2%   21%
   e. Ti   0.6 second
   f. T pause   0.0 second
   g. T insp. Rise   0.2 second
   h. Trigg. Pressure   −2 cm H_2O

Record the following once the change is complete:
   a. Measure the inspiratory time. (Press the "Additional Values" button.)
   b. Measure the peak inspiratory pressure. (Press the "Additional Values" button.)
   c. Record the tidal volume. (Press the "Additional Values" button.)
   d. Record the I:E ratio. (Press the "Additional Values" button.)

Press the "Additional Settings" button at the lower left of the user interface screen. Press the "Inspiratory Times" button and select the "T pause" button (inspiratory pause). Set the inspiratory pause to 1 second. Press the "Close" button to close that screen.

Record the following once the change is complete:
   a. Measure the inspiratory time. (Press the "Additional Values" button.)
   b. Measure the peak inspiratory pressure. (Press the "Additional Values" button.)
   c. Measure the mean inspiratory pressure. (Press the "Additional Values" button.)
   d. Record the I:E ratio. (Press the "Additional Values" button.)

Questions

A. What happened to the I:E ratio?
B. What happened to the mean pressure?
C. What changes did you see on the waveforms display?

Inspiratory Rise Time

Establish the following settings in volume control A/C ventilation:
   a. Tidal Volume   500 mL
   b. Resp. Rate   12/min
   c. PEEP   0 cm H_2O
   d. O_2%   21%
   e. Ti   0.6 second
   f. T pause   0.0 second
   g. T insp. Rise   0.2 second
   h. Trigg. Pressure   −2 cm H_2O

Record the following once the change is complete:
   a. Measure the inspiratory time. (Press the "Additional Values" button.)
   b. Measure the peak inspiratory pressure. (Press the "Additional Values" button.)
   c. Record the I:E ratio. (Press the "Additional Values" button.)
   d. Observe the shape of the flow waveform.

Change the ventilator settings to the following:
   a. Tidal Volume   500 mL
   b. Resp. Rate   12/min
   c. PEEP   0 cm H_2O
   d. O_2%   21%
   e. Ti   0.6 second
   f. T pause   0.0 second
   g. T insp. Rise   0.0 second
   h. Trigg. Pressure   −2 cm H_2O

Record the following once the change is complete:
   a. Measure the inspiratory time. (Press the "Additional Values" button.)
   b. Measure the peak inspiratory pressure. (Press the "Additional Values" button.)
   c. Record the I:E ratio. (Press the "Additional Values" button.)
   d. Observe the shape of the flow waveform.

Change the ventilator settings to the following:
   a. Tidal Volume   500 mL
   b. Resp. Rate   12/min
   c. PEEP   0 cm H_2O
   d. O_2%   21%
   e. Ti   0.6 second
   f. T pause   0.0 second
   g. T insp. Rise   0.4 second
   h. Trigg. Pressure   −2 cm H_2O

Record the following once the change is complete:
   a. Measure the inspiratory time. (Press the "Additional Values" button.)
   b. Measure the peak inspiratory pressure. (Press the "Additional Values" button.)
   c. Record the I:E ratio. (Press the "Additional Values" button.)
   d. Observe the shape of the flow waveform.

Questions

A. What happened to the inspiratory time?
B. Did you observe any changes in the peak pressure?
C. What happened to the I:E ratio?
D. What changes did you observe in flow waveform?

Trigger Sensitivity

Pressure Triggering

Change the ventilator settings to the following:

a. Tidal Volume	500 mL
b. Resp. Rate	12/min
c. PEEP	0 cm H_2O
d. O_2%	21%
e. Ti	0.6 second
f. T pause	0.0 second
g. T insp. Rise	0.2 second
h. Trigg. Pressure	−2 cm H_2O

1. Attach a mouthpiece to the patient wye and attempt to initiate a breath.

2. With the sensitivity control at −2 cm H_2O, initiate a breath. Observe the pressure time curve on the monitoring screen. Adjust the screen scale to expand the scale, making it easier to observe pressure changes.

3. Observe the upper portion of the user interface screen. Observe for any new displays when a breath is initiated.

4. Adjust the sensitivity control to −20 cm H_2O and initiate a breath. Observe the pressure time curve on the monitoring screen. Adjust the screen scale to expand the scale, making it easier to observe pressure changes.
   a. Record the negative pressure when the ventilator cycled on.
   b. Observe the monitoring screen for any changes in ventilatory (patient) parameters.

Questions

A. When you were able to initiate an assisted breath, what event(s) occurred?
B. What was momentarily displayed when you triggered a breath?
C. Where would you want to set the sensitivity control for assist-control mode?

Flow Triggering

Touch the "Volume Control" button at the upper left portion of the user interface screen. Touch the "Pressure Trigger" button, and rotate the main rotary dial clockwise until "Trigg. Flow" appears on the button. Continue to rotate the rotary dial until 4 L/min is in the display. Touch the button

once again to accept the change and press "Accept" on the lower right portion of the user interface screen. Establish the following ventilator settings:

a. Tidal Volume	500 mL
b. Resp. Rate	12/min
c. PEEP	0 cm H_2O
d. O_2%	21%
e. Ti	0.6 second
f. T pause	0.0 second
g. T insp. Rise	0.2 second
h. Trigg. Flow	4 L/min

1. Attach a mouthpiece to the patient wye and attempt to initiate a breath.

2. Set the sensitivity control to 4 L/min and initiate a breath. Observe the flow time curve on the monitoring screen or the pressure volume loop. Observe for any changes in the user interface display screen.

3. Adjust the sensitivity control to 8 L/min and initiate a breath. Observe the flow time curve on the monitoring screen. Note any changes in the user interface display in the upper portion of the display screen.
   a. Record what threshold is met when the ventilator cycled on.
   b. Observe the monitoring screen for any changes in ventilatory (patient) parameters.

Questions

A. When you were able to initiate an assisted breath, what event(s) occurred?
B. What was momentarily displayed when you triggered a breath?
C. Where would you want to set the sensitivity control for assist-control mode?

Changes in Resistance and Compliance

Set controls to the following settings:

a. Tidal Volume	500 mL
b. Resp. Rate	12/min
c. PEEP	0 cm H_2O
d. O_2%	21%
e. Ti	0.6 second
f. T pause	0.0 second
g. T insp. Rise	0.2 second
h. Trigg. Pressure	−2 cm H_2O

Go to the alarm settings screen and adjust the peak pressure alarm to 100 cm H_2O.

1. Once the settings are established, measure and record the following ventilatory (patient) parameters from the monitoring screen:
   a. Measure the peak inspiratory pressure.
   b. Measure the inspiratory time.
   c. Record the tidal volume.
   d. Record the I:E ratio.

2. Decrease the compliance by 1/3 by adjusting the spring tension on the test lung.
   a. Measure the peak inspiratory pressure.
   b. Measure the inspiratory time (estimate the time using your watch and a second hand).

c. Record the tidal volume.

d. Record the I:E ratio.

Questions

A. Why did the corrected tidal volume decrease?

B. Why did the I:E ratio vary?

C. Why did the peak inspiratory pressure increase?

3. Increase the resistance by 1/3 by adjusting the resistance control on the lung analog.

a. Measure the peak inspiratory pressure.

b. Measure the inspiratory time.

c. Record the corrected tidal volume.

d. Record the I:E ratio.

Questions

A. Why did the inspiratory pressure increase?

B. Why did the I:E ratio vary?

C. How do you account for differences in the corrected tidal volume?

D. Can you think of human physiologic conditions that could produce similar results?

Return the resistance control to its original setting on the lung analog. Set the ventilator to the following settings:

a. Tidal Volume   500 mL

b. Resp. Rate   12/min

c. PEEP   0 cm H_2O

d. O_2%   21%

e. Ti   0.6 second

f. T pause   0.0 second

g. T insp. Rise   0.2 second

h. Trigg. Pressure   −2 cm H_2O

Set the pressure alarm to 10 cm H_2O greater than the current peak pressure setting by pressing the "Alarm Profile" soft key and pressing the "Upper Pressure Alarm" button and adjusting it using the rotary dial. Now decrease the compliance by 1/3 by adjusting the spring tension or adjusting the compliance control on the lung analog (1/3 greater than its normal setting without adjustment). Once the settings are established, answer the following questions.

Questions

A. What event(s) occurred?

B. Can you think of a patient situation that could cause this?

C. What is the purpose of the normal pressure limit control?

Pressure Control Ventilation

Test Lung Setup

If you are using an SMS ("Manley") lung simulator, connect one spring for compliance, set the resistance control to zero, and rotate the leak control fully clockwise, eliminating any leaks. Attach the patient wye to the inlet of the SMS lung simulator.

If you are using an IngMar Medical Demonstration Lung Model, rotate all of the compliance springs fully clockwise, adjust the resistance controls to "OFF," and adjust both the ET Leak and System Leak controls to the "OFF" position. Attach the patient wye to the inlet of the Demonstration Lung Model.

When completing these activities, manipulate only one control at a time and note the result of each activity with manipulation of the controls. Answer the questions that follow each of the activities.

Initial Ventilator Settings

Begin this section by pressing the "Volume Control" button on the upper left portion of the user interface screen. Press the "Volume Control" (mode button) in the new display at the upper left corner of the display. Select the "Pressure Control" button (pressure control mode) by pressing it. The following settings are available in pressure control mode (Table 25-9).

Adjust the ventilator to the following settings in pressure control mode. Touch the "Vent Setup" soft key. From the "Mode" key, select "A/C" (assist-control) mode. Press the "Mandatory Type" soft key, and select "PC" for pressure control mode. Touch the "Trigger Type" key, and select "P-Trigger" for pressure triggering.

Adjust the ventilator to the following settings in pressure control mode:

a. PC above PEEP   15 cm H_2O

b. Resp. Rate   12/min

c. PEEP   0 cm H_2O

d. Oxygen Percent   21%

e. T_i 0.60

f. Rise Time %   0.2

g. P-Trigger   −2 cm H_2O

Once all settings are complete, press the "Accept" button at the lower right of the user interface screen.

PC above PEEP (Pressure)

1. Using a test lung, measure and record the following using the monitoring screen:

a. Peak inspiratory pressure

b. I:E ratio

c. Tidal volume

d. Minute ventilation

2. Adjust the PC above PEEP to 25 cm H_2O. Measure the following using the monitoring screen:

a. Peak inspiratory pressure

b. I:E ratio

c. Tidal volume

d. Minute ventilation

TABLE 25-9: SERVO-i Settings for Pressure Control A/C	
Pressure Control above PEEP	0 to 120 cm H_2O
Respiratory Rate	0 to 150 breaths/min
PEEP	0 to 50 cm H_2O
O_2% Concentration	21 to 100%
Inspiratory Time	0.1 to 5 seconds
Inspiratory Rise Time	0.0 to 0.4 second
Trigger	Pressure −20 to 0.0 cm H_2O Flow 1 to 10 L/min

3. Adjust the inspiratory pressure level to 5 cm H_2O. Using the monitoring screen, measure the following:
   a. Peak inspiratory pressure
   b. I:E ratio
   c. Tidal volume
   d. Minute ventilation

Questions

A. How did the change in inspiratory pressure affect the I:E ratio?
B. How did the change in inspiratory pressure affect the exhaled tidal volume?
C. How did the change in inspiratory pressure affect the exhaled minute volume?

Inspiratory Time Control

Begin this section by setting the ventilator to the following settings. Touch the "Vent Setup" soft key. From the "Mode" key, select "A/C" (assist-control) mode. Press the "Mandatory Type" soft key, and select "PC" for pressure control mode. Touch the "Trigger Type" key, and select "P-Trigger" for pressure triggering.

Adjust the ventilator to the following settings in pressure control mode:

a. A/C	12/min
b. P_I	15 cm H_2O
c. T_I	0.6 second
d. Rise Time %	0.2 second
e. P-Trigger	−2 cm H_2O
f. Oxygen Percent	21%
g. PEEP	0 cm H_2O

1. Using a test lung, measure the following using the monitoring screens:
   a. Peak inspiratory pressure
   b. I:E ratio
   c. Exhaled tidal volume
   d. Exhaled minute volume

2. Change the inspiratory time to 1 second, and press the "Accept" button. Measure and record the following:
   a. Peak inspiratory pressure
   b. I:E ratio
   c. Exhaled tidal volume
   d. Exhaled minute volume

3. Change the inspiratory time to 2.5 seconds, and measure and record the following:
   a. Peak inspiratory pressure
   b. I:E ratio
   c. Exhaled tidal volume
   d. Exhaled minute volume

Questions

A. How did the inspiratory time change affect the I:E ratio?
B. How did the inspiratory time change affect tidal volume delivery?
C. How did the inspiratory time change affect the inspiratory pressure?

Rate Control

Adjust the ventilator to the following settings in pressure control mode:

a. A/C	12/min
b. P_I	15 cm H_2O
c. T_I	0.6 second
d. Rise Time %	0.2 second
e. P-Trigger	−2 cm H_2O
f. Oxygen Percent	21%
g. PEEP	0 cm H_2O

1. Using a test lung, measure the following using the monitoring screen:
   a. Peak inspiratory pressure
   b. I:E ratio
   c. Exhaled tidal volume
   d. Exhaled minute volume

2. Change the rate control to 24 breaths/min, and measure and record the following:
   a. Peak inspiratory pressure
   b. I:E ratio
   c. Exhaled tidal volume
   d. Exhaled minute volume

3. Change the rate control to 9 breaths/min, and measure and record the following:
   a. Peak inspiratory pressure
   b. I:E ratio
   c. Exhaled tidal volume
   d. Exhaled minute volume

Questions

A. What happened to the I:E ratio when you changed the rate?
B. What happened to the minute ventilation when you changed the rate?

Inspiratory Rise Time Control

Adjust the ventilator to the following settings in pressure control mode:

a. A/C	12/min
b. P_I	15 cm H_2O
c. T_I	0.6 second
d. Rise Time %	0.2 second
e. P-Trigger	−2 cm H_2O
f. Oxygen Percent	21%
g. PEEP	0 cm H_2O

Observe the monitoring screen for the following:
   a. Measure the inspiratory time. (Press the "Additional Values" button.)
   b. Measure the peak inspiratory pressure. (Press the "Additional Values" button.)
   c. Record the I:E ratio. (Press the "Additional Values" button.)
   d. Observe the shape of the flow waveform.

Change the ventilator settings to the following:

a. A/C	12/min
b. P_I	15 cm H_2O
c. T_I	0.6 second
d. Rise Time %	0.0 second

e. P-Trigger   −2 cm H_2O
f. Oxygen Percent   21%
g. PEEP   0 cm H_2O

Observe the monitoring screen for the following:

a. Measure the inspiratory time. (Press the "Additional Values" button.)
b. Measure the peak inspiratory pressure. (Press the "Additional Values" button.)
c. Record the I:E ratio. (Press the "Additional Values" button.)
d. Observe the shape of the flow waveform.

Change the ventilator settings to the following:

a. A/C   12/min
b. P_I 15 cm. H_2O
c. T_I 0.6 second
d. Rise Time %   0.4 second
e. P-Trigger   −2 cm H_2O
f. Oxygen Percent   21%
g. PEEP   0 cm H_2O

Observe the monitoring screen for the following:

a. Measure the inspiratory time. (Press the "Additional Values" button.)
b. Measure the peak inspiratory pressure. (Press the "Additional Values" button.)
c. Record the I:E ratio. (Press the "Additional Values" button.)
d. Observe the shape of the flow waveform.

Questions

A. What happened to the inspiratory time?
B. Did you observe any changes in peak pressure?
C. What changes did you see in the I:E ratio?
D. How did the inspiratory flow waveform change?

Trigger Sensitivity

Pressure Triggering

Change the ventilator settings to the following:

a. A/C   12/min
b. P_I 15 cm H_2O
c. T_I 0.6 second
d. Rise Time %   0.2 second
e. P-Trigger   −2 cm H_2O
f. Oxygen Percent   21%
g. PEEP   0 cm H_2O

1. Attach a mouthpiece to the patient wye and attempt to initiate a breath.

2. With the sensitivity control at −2 cm H_2O, initiate a breath. Observe the pressure time curve on the monitoring screen. Adjust the screen scale to expand the scale, making it easier to observe pressure changes.

3. Observe the upper portion of the user interface screen. Observe for any new displays when a breath is initiated.

4. Adjust the sensitivity control to −20 cm H_2O and initiate a breath. Observe the pressure time curve on the monitoring screen. Adjust the screen scale to expand the scale, making it easier to observe pressure changes.

a. Record the negative pressure when the ventilator cycled on.
b. Observe the monitoring screen for any changes in ventilatory (patient) parameters.

Questions

A. When you were able to initiate an assisted breath, what event(s) occurred?
B. What was momentarily displayed when you triggered a breath?
C. Where would you want to set the sensitivity control for assist-control mode?

Flow Triggering

Touch the "Volume Control" button at the upper left portion of the user interface screen. Touch the "Pressure Trigger" button, and rotate the main rotary dial clockwise until "Trigg. Flow" appears on the button. Continue to rotate the rotary dial until 4 L/min is in the display. Touch the button once again to accept the change and press "Accept" on the lower right portion of the user interface screen.

Establish the following ventilator settings:

a. A/C   12/min
b. P_I 15 cm H_2O
c. T_I 0.6 second
d. Rise Time %   0.2 second
e. FlowTrigger   4 L/min
f. Oxygen Percent   21%
g. PEEP   0 cm H_2O

1. Attach a mouthpiece to the patient wye and attempt to initiate a breath.

2. Set the sensitivity control to 4 L/min and initiate a breath. Observe the flow time curve on the monitoring screen or the pressure volume loop. Observe for any changes in the user interface display screen.

3. Adjust the sensitivity control to 8 L/min and initiate a breath. Observe the flow time curve on the monitoring screen. Note any changes in the user interface display in the upper portion of the display screen.

a. Record what threshold is met when the ventilator cycled on.
b. Observe the monitoring screen for any changes in ventilatory (patient) parameters.

Questions

A. When you were able to initiate an assisted breath, what event(s) occurred?
B. What was momentarily displayed when you triggered a breath?
C. Where would you want to set the sensitivity control for assist-control mode?

Spontaneous Ventilation

Test Lung Setup

If you are using an SMS ("Manley") lung simulator, connect one spring for compliance, set the resistance control to zero, and rotate the leak control fully clockwise, eliminating any leaks. Attach the patient wye to the inlet of the SMS lung simulator.

If you are using an IngMar Medical Demonstration Lung Model, rotate all of the compliance springs fully clockwise, adjust the resistance controls to "OFF," and adjust both the ET Leak and System Leak controls to the "OFF" position. Attach the patient wye to the inlet of the Demonstration Lung Model.

When completing these activities, manipulate only one control at a time and note the result of each activity with manipulation of the controls. Answer the questions that follow each of the activities.

Initial Ventilator Settings

Begin this section by pressing the "Pressure Control" button on the upper left portion of the user interface screen. Press the "Pressure Control" (mode button) in the new display at the upper left corner of the display. Select the "Pressure Support/CPAP" (spontaneous modes) by pressing it. The following settings are available in pressure support/CPAP mode (Table 25-10).

CPAP Mode

Test Lung Setup

a. If you are using an SMS ("Manley") lung simulator, connect one spring for compliance, set the resistance control to zero, and rotate the leak control fully clockwise, eliminating any leaks. Attach the patient wye to the inlet of the SMS lung simulator.

b. If you are using an IngMar Medical Demonstration Lung Model, rotate all of the compliance springs fully clockwise, adjust the resistance controls to "OFF," and adjust both the ET Leak and System Leak controls to the "OFF" position. Attach the patient wye to the inlet of the Demonstration Lung Model.

c. When completing these activities, manipulate only one control at a time and note the result of each activity with manipulation of the controls. Answer the questions that follow each of the activities.

TABLE 25-10: SERVO-i Settings for Pressure Support/CPAP Modes

PS above PEEP	0 to 120 cm H_2O
PEEP	0 to 50 cm H_2O
O_2% Concentration	21 to 100%
Inspiratory Rise Time	0.0 to 4 seconds
Trigger Sensitivity	Pressure −20 to 0 cm H_2O Flow 0 to 10 L/min
Inspiratory Cycle Off	1 to 70% of measured peak flow

Set the controls to the following settings:
a. PS above PEEP   0 cm H_2O
b. PEEP   5 cm H_2O
c. O_2%   21%
d. Insp. Rise Time   0.4 second
e. Trigger   −2 cm H_2O
f. Insp. Cycle off   25%

Once the settings have been established, simulate a spontaneous breath by moving the test lung's bellows. Repeat the process, simulating a spontaneous rate and tidal volume. Observe the pressure time curve on the monitoring screen. Adjust the screen scale to expand the scale, making it easier to observe pressure changes. Note the display in the upper portion of the display screen.

Questions

A. What change did you observe on the display screen during your spontaneous breathing efforts?
B. What did you observe as the baseline pressure on the pressure time scalar waveform?
C. What happened when you stopped your simulated breathing?
D. What was an average inspiratory pressure during your spontaneous efforts?

Change the ventilator controls to the following settings:
a. PS above PEEP   0 cm H_2O
b. PEEP   10 cm H_2O
c. O_2%   21%
d. Insp. Rise Time   0.4 second
e. Trigger   −2 cm H_2O
f. Insp. Cycle off   25%

Once the settings have been established, simulate a spontaneous breath by moving the test lung's bellows. Repeat the process, simulating a spontaneous rate and tidal volume. Observe the pressure time curve on the monitoring screen. Adjust the screen scale to expand the scale, making it easier to observe pressure changes. Note the display in the upper portion of the display screen.

Questions

A. What breath type was displayed momentarily during your spontaneous breathing efforts?
B. What did you observe as the baseline pressure on the pressure time scalar waveform?
C. What happened when you stopped your simulated breathing?
D. What was an average inspiratory pressure during your spontaneous efforts?

Pressure Support

Touch the "Pressure Support/CPAP" button at the top left of the user interface screen. Make the following changes in the ventilator settings:
a. PS above PEEP   10 cm H_2O
b. PEEP   5 cm H_2O
c. O_2%   21%
d. Insp. Rise Time   0.4 second
e. Trigger   −2 cm H_2O
f. Insp. Cycle off   25%

Once the changes have been made, press the "Accept" button at the lower right of the display screen.

Test Lung Setup

a. If you are using an SMS ("Manley") lung simulator, connect one spring for compliance, set the resistance control to zero, and rotate the leak control fully clockwise, eliminating any leaks. Attach the patient wye to the inlet of the SMS lung simulator.

b. If you are using an IngMar Medical Demonstration Lung Model, rotate all of the compliance springs fully clockwise, adjust the resistance controls to "OFF," and adjust both the ET Leak and System Leak controls to the "OFF" position. Attach the patient wye to the inlet of the Demonstration Lung Model.

c. When completing these activities, manipulate only one control at a time and note the result of each activity with manipulation of the controls. Answer the questions that follow each of the activities.

Once the settings have been established, simulate a spontaneous breath by moving the test lung's bellows. Repeat the process, simulating a spontaneous rate and tidal volume. Observe the pressure time curve on the monitoring screen. Adjust the screen scale to expand the scale, making it easier to observe pressure changes. Note the display in the upper portion of the display screen.

Questions

A. What did you observe in the upper portion of the screen?
B. What did you observe as the baseline pressure on the pressure time scalar waveform?
C. What was the peak pressure observed on the screen and the monitoring section of the display?
D. What happened when you stopped your simulated breathing?
E. What was an average inspiratory pressure during your spontaneous efforts?

Set the controls to the following settings:

a. PS above PEEP   5 cm H_2O
b. PEEP   5 cm H_2O
c. O_2%   21%
d. Insp. Rise Time   0.4 second
e. Trigger   −2 cm H_2O
f. Insp. Cycle off   25%

Repeat your spontaneous efforts with the test lung, simulating a rate and a tidal volume. Observe the pressure time curve on the monitoring screen or the pressure volume loop. Adjust the screen scale to expand the scale, making it easier to observe pressure changes. Note the display in the upper portion of the display screen.

Questions

A. What did you observe in the upper portion of the screen?
B. What did you observe as the baseline pressure on the pressure time scalar waveform?
C. What happened when you stopped your simulated breathing?
D. What was an average inspiratory pressure during your spontaneous efforts?

BACKUP VENTILATION

Alarm Functions

Input Power and Control Circuit Alarms

Input power alarms alert the clinician to loss of electrical power or pneumatic sources, rendering the ventilator inoperative. Control circuit alarms alert the clinician to incompatible settings or settings that are out of range as well as potential faults in the microprocessor control circuitry. These alarms are summarized in Table 25-11.

Output Alarms

Output alarms are triggered when the alarm limits of the ventilator's output have been exceeded. Examples of typical output alarms include pressure, volume, flow, and time. The output alarms for the Puritan Bennett 840 are summarized in Table 25-12.

To set the alarms, press the "Alarm Profile" soft key at the top right of the user interface. A presentation of the alarms appears on the user interface screen. To set an alarm, touch the desired setting, turn the adjustment knob, and touch the setting again or press "Accept." The current parameter is displayed as an arrow to the left of the bar graph display. Both high and low limits may be set in reference to the current patient parameter.

TABLE 25-11: Maquet SERVO-i Input Power Alarms

ALARM	CAUSE	CORRECTIVE ACTION
Technical error	Power failure.	1. Manually ventilate the patient. 2. Check the integrity of the power source. 3. Contact a biomedical technician.
Check battery status	There is a problem with one or more battery modules.	Replace the battery module(s).
Limited battery capacity	Battery capacity is limited to no more than 10 minutes of operation.	1. Connect to AC power. 2. Replace the battery module(s).
Gas supply pressure: low	Air or oxygen supply pressures are low.	Check gas connections.
No air supply	Air supply pressure is less than the minimum required. Oxygen delivery may be compromised.	1. Manually ventilate the patient if required. 2. Check both air and oxygen pneumatic sources.
O_2 cell/sensor failure	O_2 cell is missing or disconnected.	1. Check the O_2 cell connection. 2. Replace the O_2 cell.
Restart ventilator	Software error.	1. Restart the ventilator and perform a pre-use check. 2. Contact a biomedical technician.
Technical error in the expiratory cassette	Technical problem is in the expiratory cassette.	1. Replace the cassette and perform a pre-use check. 2. Contact a biomedical technician for repair.
Technical error: Restart ventilator	Ventilator settings are lost.	1. Restart the ventilator and perform a pre-use check. 2. Contact a biomedical technician for repair.

TABLE 25-12: Maquet SERVO-i Ventilator Output Alarms

ALARM	CAUSE	CORRECTIVE ACTION
Airway Pressure (upper)	The measured airway pressure is greater than the alarm setting.	Evaluate the patient: 1. Suctioning needed? 2. Bronchospasm? 3. Circuit disconnect/leaks? 4. Airway secure?
Respiratory Rate	The respiratory rate exceeds the limit of the alarm setting.	Evaluate the patient and the ventilator settings.
Expired Minute Ventilation (upper)	The patient's exhaled minute volume exceeds the setting on the alarm.	Evaluate the patient and the ventilator settings.
Exhaled Minute Ventilation (lower)	The patient's exhaled minute ventilation is less than the alarm setting.	Evaluate the patient and the ventilator settings.
CPAP (upper limit)	The patient's CPAP pressure exceeds the alarm setting.	Evaluate the patient and the ventilator settings.
CPAP (lower limit)	The patient's CPAP pressure is lower than the alarm setting.	Evaluate the patient and the ventilator settings.

Circuit Assembly

Figure 25-11 shows the Viasys Avea ventilator assembled and ready for use. To prepare the ventilator for use, follow the steps listed next.

1. Attach the collection bottle to the water trap by screwing it clockwise into the receptacle in the water trap (Figure 25-12).
2. Install an exhalation filter to the upper portion of the water trap by pushing it onto the seal at the top of the water trap (Figure 25-13).
3. Align the ridge on the water trap assembly with the slot on the exhalation filter cartridge.
4. Slide the water trap/exhalation filter assembly upward into the lower right front portion of the ventilator body and rotate the locking lever to the left, holding the assembly in place (Figure 25-14).
5. Connect the expiratory limb of the patient circuit to the expiratory filter and collection vial's 22 mm fitting.
6. Attach the patient circuit to the flex arm at its midpoint by clamping the ball fitting on the circuit to the flex arm.

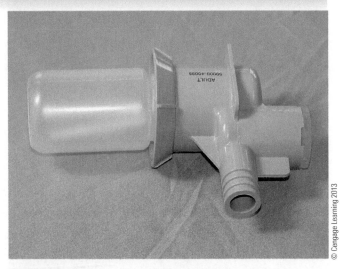

Figure 25-12 Attachment of the collection bottle to the water trap

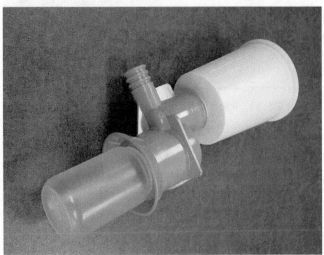

Figure 25-13 Installation of the exhalation filter onto the upper portion of the water trap

7. Connect an 18-inch length of 22 mm tubing between the ventilator outlet located to the right of the water trap/exhalation filter assembly and the humidifier.
8. Connect the inspiratory limb of the patient circuit to the outlet of the humidifier.
9. Connect the 50 psi air and oxygen supply lines to appropriate gas connections.
10. Connect the electrical power cord to a 115 volt 60 Hz outlet.

Testing the Ventilator before Use

Power-on Self Test (POST)

Each time the power switch is turned on or if the ventilator microprocessor detects selected fault conditions, a POST is automatically executed. The POST takes only a few seconds and is transparent to the clinician.

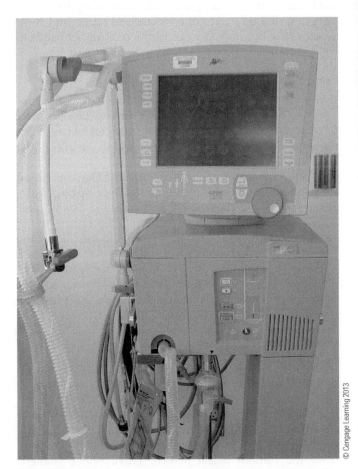

Figure 25-11 A photograph of the Viasys AVEA ventilator with a circuit attached

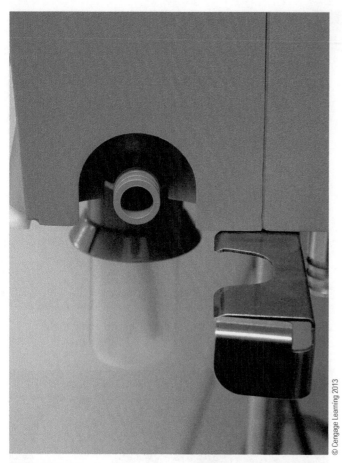

© Cengage Learning 2013

Figure 25-14 Insertion of the water trap/exhalation filter into the ventilator

The test verifies the integrity of the microprocessor, read-only memory (ROM) and random access memory (RAM). Only if a problem is detected will a message be displayed.

Extended Systems Test (EST)

The extended systems test (EST) should only be performed prior to connecting the ventilator to a patient. The EST will perform a leak test of the patient circuit, determine circuit compliance, and perform a two-point calibration of the oxygen sensor. To perform an EST, complete the following steps:

1. Access the EST test by pressing the "EST" button on the Setup screen.
2. When instructed to remove the ventilator from the patient and block the patient wye, do so.
3. Confirm that the ventilator is off the patient and that the wye is blocked by pressing "Cont" (continue).
4. The ventilator will perform the EST and a countdown timer will be displayed. The first portion of the test will check the circuit for leaks, calculate circuit compliance, and perform a two-point calibration of the oxygen sensor. The maximum time for this test is 90 seconds.
5. Following each test, a PASSED or FAILED message will be displayed. Once the first portion of the test is complete, will all tests PASSED, press the "Continue" button on the screen.

6. From the Setup screen, press "Setup Accept" to capture and retain the circuit compliance measurement.

Using the Keyboard Entry System

All functions of the Viasys Avea ventilator are controlled from the user interface module (UIM) shown in Figure 25-15. To enter ventilator or alarm settings, follow the "touch–turn–touch" method for entering new settings. Touch the desired value or setting you wish to change (e.g., tidal volume), and then turn the knob on the lower right side of the UIM until the desired value is displayed (clockwise increases, counterclockwise decreases). Touch the desired setting again or press the "Accept" button to apply the new setting. The new setting will now be displayed on the appropriate portion of the UIM screen.

Activities

To complete these practice activities, it is recommended that you use a lung analog/simulator such as an SMS "Manley" lung simulator or an IngMar Medical Quick Lung or Demonstration Lung Model. These devices or other similar devices allow the operator to alter resistance and compliance, simulating changes in patient condition.

If these devices are not available, a patient wye and two test lungs may be used as shown in Figure 25-9. Exercise caution. Volumes and pressures may exceed the limits of the test lungs. Resistance may be altered by adapting different sizes of endotracheal tubes, and compliance may be altered by the addition of rubber bands to the test lungs.

Lung Simulator Setup

If you are using an SMS ("Manley") lung simulator, connect one spring for compliance, set the resistance control to zero, and rotate the leak control fully clockwise, eliminating any leaks. Attach the patient wye to the inlet of the SMS lung simulator.

If you are using an IngMar Medical Demonstration Lung Model, rotate all of the compliance springs fully clockwise, adjust the resistance controls to "OFF," and adjust both the ET Leak and System Leak controls to the "OFF" position. Attach the patient wye to the inlet of the Demonstration Lung Model.

When completing these activities, manipulate only one control at a time and note the result of each activity with manipulation of the controls. Answer the questions that follow each of the activities.

Volume Control Exercises

Patient Setup

Once the ventilator has completed a POST and an EST has been performed, select "New Patient Setup" from the UIM screen. Prior to beginning the volume control exercises, you must first complete the patient setup. At the Ventilator Start-up screen, select "New Patient" from the Patient Select screen. Next, select "Patient size." For these exercises, press the "Adult" key on the screen. Press the "Size Accept" button to enter the desired patient size.

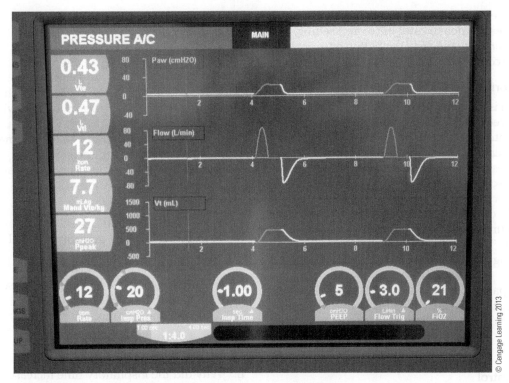

Figure 25-15 A photograph of the user interface module (UIM)

Enter the endotracheal tube size and length (8.5 and 30 cm), turn the Leak Compensation off, and enter the patient weight at 80 kg. Once the setup is complete, press "Setup Accept" to capture and store these values.

Breath Type and Mode

Press the "Mode" soft key located on the lower left portion of the UIM next to the screen (Table 25-13).

Make the following selections from the Breath Type and Mode screen. Press the desired setting and rotate the knob on the lower right side of the screen to change the settings.

    a. Mode   Volume A/C
    b. Trigger Type P Trigger (pressure)

If you make an error, simply touch the desired button to change the setting (Mode, Mandatory Type, Spontaneous Type, or Trigger Type). Make the change by rotating the

knob on the lower right of the GUI and press "Continue." Once the initial settings are complete, a new Ventilator Settings screen will appear (Table 25-14).

From the Ventilator Settings screen, make the following selections by touching the appropriate button, rotating the knob, and touching the button once again. Simply follow the touch–turn–touch sequence to make your selection.

    a. Respiratory Rate   12/min
    b. Tidal Volume   500 mL
    c. Peak Flow   40 L/min
    d. P-Trigger   –2 cm H_2O
    e. Oxygen Percent   21%
    f. Inspiratory Pause   0 second
    g. PEEP   0 cm H_2O

TABLE 25-13: Mode Select Settings

Volume Modes	Volume A/C
	Volume SIMV
Pressure Modes	Pressure A/C
	Pressure SIMV
	Pressure regulated volume control
	Pressure regulated volume control SIMV
	Airway pressure release ventilation/BiPhasic
Spontaneous Type	CPAP/pressure support

TABLE 25-14: Ventilator Settings Screen (Volume A/C)

Rate	Adjustable from 1 to 120 breaths/min
Volume	Adjustable from 10 to 2500 mL
Peak Flow	Adjustable from 3 to 150 L/min
Inspiratory Pause	Adjustable from 0.0 to 3 seconds
PEEP	Adjustable from 0 to 50 cm H_2O
Pressure Trigger (Advanced Settings)	Adjustable from 0.1 to 20 cm H_2O below baseline

If you make an error, simply touch the button you wish to change, rotate the knob to enter the correct setting, and complete the change by touching the button once again or pressing the "Accept" key.

Patient Monitoring

The UIM screen is divided into sections. The lower section is devoted to ventilator settings, and you have already been making entries and using this portion of the screen. The upper center part of the screen is devoted to scalar waveforms (pressure, volume, and flow). These waveforms may be scaled to be larger or smaller as well as "frozen" to observe specific changes one might observe.

The left side of the screen displays the values for the patient's measured peak pressure, tidal volume, rate, PEEP, and FIO_2. These values are those measured by the ventilator during either a mandatory or patient-triggered volume breath.

The lower part of the screen displays the ventilator control settings that are active for this mode of ventilation. Volume A/C settings include rate, volume, peak flow, inspiratory pause, PEEP, flow triggering, and oxygen percent.

Peak Flow Control

From the initial settings you have previously set, note the following ventilatory (patient) parameters before you make the next changes. Press the "Screens" soft key at the upper left of the UIM. The "Screen Select" menu will appear. Press the "Monitor" button and a display measured parameters will appear. From the Monitor screen, note the following initial parameters prior to making any changes.

1. I:E ratio
2. Peak pressure
3. Inspiratory time (note the time using your watch and a sweep second hand)

1. Set the peak flow to 20 L/min. Using the Monitor screen, perform the following:
   a. Measure the inspiratory time.
   b. Measure the peak pressure.
   c. Record the I:E ratio.

2. Adjust the peak flow to 60 L/min. Using the Monitor screen, perform the following:
   a. Measure the inspiratory time.
   b. Measure the peak pressure.
   c. Record the I:E ratio.

Questions

A. How do you account for the differences in inspiratory time?
B. Why were there differences in peak inspiratory pressure?
C. Why did the I:E ratio vary between the two activities?

Tidal Volume Control

1. Set the controls to the following settings:
   a. Respiratory Rate   12/min
   b. Tidal Volume   500 mL

c.	Peak Flow	60 L/min
d.	P-Trigger	−2 cm H_2O
e.	Oxygen Percent	21%
f.	Plateau Time	0 second
g.	PEEP	0 cm H_2O

Once these settings have been established, select the Monitoring screen and perform the following ventilatory (patient) parameters:
   a. Measure the inspiratory time (estimate using your watch and a sweep second hand).
   b. Measure the peak inspiratory pressure.
   c. Record the tidal volume.
   d. Record the I:E ratio.

2. Set the tidal volume control to 1000 mL. Using the Monitoring screen, perform the following parameters:
   a. Measure the inspiratory time.
   b. Measure the peak inspiratory pressure.
   c. Record the corrected tidal volume.
   d. Record the I:E ratio.

Questions

A. Why did the pressure increase?
B. Why did the inspiratory time increase?
C. How do you account for the change in I:E ratio?

Rate Control

Set the controls to the following settings:
   a. Respiratory Rate   12/min
   b. Tidal Volume   500 mL
   c. Peak Flow   60 L/min
   d. P-Trigger   −2 cm H_2O
   e. Oxygen Percent   21%
   f. Plateau Time   0 second
   g. PEEP   0 cm H_2O

Go to the alarm settings screen and adjust the peak pressure alarm to 100 cm H_2O.

1. With the controls set as above, perform the following, using the Monitoring screen:
   a. Measure the peak inspiratory pressure.
   b. Measure the inspiratory time.
   c. Record the corrected tidal volume.
   d. Record the I:E ratio.

2. Adjust the rate control to 30 breaths/min, and perform the following using the Monitoring screen:
   a. Measure the peak inspiratory pressure.
   b. Measure the inspiratory time.
   c. Record the corrected tidal volume.
   d. Record the I:E ratio.

Questions

A. What alarm was triggered and why?
B. What was the I:E ratio?
C. Why was the I:E ratio so high?

Changes in Resistance and Compliance

Set controls to the following settings:
   a. Respiratory Rate   12/min
   b. Tidal Volume   500 mL

c. Peak Flow   60 L/min
d. P-Trigger   −2 cm H$_2$O
e. Oxygen Percent   21%
f. Plateau Time   0 second
g. PEEP   0 cm H$_2$O

Go into the alarm settings screen and adjust the peak pressure alarm to 100 cm H$_2$O.

1. Once the settings are established, measure and record the following ventilatory (patient) parameters from the Monitoring screen:
   a. Peak inspiratory pressure
   b. Inspiratory time
   c. Tidal volume
   d. I:E ratio

2. Decrease the compliance by 1/3 by adjusting the spring tension on the test lung. Measure and record the following from the Monitoring screen:
   a. Inspiratory pressure
   b. Inspiratory time (estimate the time using your watch and a second hand)
   c. Tidal volume
   d. I:E ratio

Questions

A. Why did the corrected tidal volume decrease?
B. Why did the I:E ratio vary?
C. Why did the peak inspiratory pressure increase?

3. Increase the resistance by 1/3 by adjusting the resistance control on the lung analog. Using the MONITORING screen, measure and record the following parameters:
   a. Inspiratory pressure
   b. Inspiratory time
   c. Corrected tidal volume
   d. I:E ratio

Questions

A. Why did the inspiratory pressure increase?
B. Why did the I:E ratio vary?
C. How do you account for differences in the corrected tidal volume?
D. Can you think of human physiologic conditions that could produce similar results?

Return the resistance control to its original setting (lowest setting) on the lung analog. Set the ventilator to the following settings:
   a. Respiratory Rate   12/min
   b. Tidal Volume   500 mL
   c. Peak Flow   60 L/min
   d. P-Trigger   −2 cm H$_2$O
   e. Oxygen Percent   21%
   f. Plateau Time   0 second
   g. PEEP   0 cm H$_2$O

Set the peak pressure to 10 cm H$_2$O greater than the current peak pressure setting as measured on the left side of the UIM. Now decrease the compliance by 1/3 by adjusting the spring tension or adjusting the compliance control on the lung analog (1/3 greater than its normal

setting without adjustment). Once the settings are established, answer the following questions.

Questions

A. What event(s) occurred?
B. Can you think of a patient situation that could cause this?
C. What is the purpose of the normal pressure limit control?

Triggering Adjustment

Pressure Triggering

Touch the "Advanced Settings" soft key at the lower left side of the UIM. This will open the advanced settings screen and present a menu of advanced settings specific to this mode/type of ventilation (Volume A/C). Press the "Pres Trig" key and set pressure triggering to −2 cm H$_2$O. Return to the main screen by pressing the "Screens" soft key, and then pressing "Main." Set the ventilator to the following settings:
   a. Respiratory Rate   12/min
   b. Tidal Volume   500 mL
   c. Peak Flow   60 L/min
   d. P-Trigger   −2 cm H$_2$O
   e. Oxygen Percent   21%
   f. Plateau Time   0 second
   g. PEEP   0 cm H$_2$O

1. Attach a mouthpiece to the patient wye and attempt to initiate a breath.

2. With the sensitivity control at −2 cm H$_2$O, initiate a breath. Observe the pressure time curve on the monitoring screen. Adjust the screen scale to expand the scale, making it easier to observe pressure changes. Note any changes that appear on the screen display in the upper left portion of the screen.

3. Adjust the sensitivity control to −20 cm H$_2$O and initiate a breath. Observe the pressure time curve on the monitoring screen. Adjust the screen scale to expand the scale, making it easier to observe pressure changes. Note the display in the upper left corner of the display screen.
   a. Record the negative pressure when the ventilator cycled on.
   b. Observe the monitoring screen for any changes in ventilatory (patient) parameters.

Questions

A. When you were able to initiate an assisted breath, what event(s) occurred?
B. What did you observe on the display screen during a spontaneous breath?
C. As a patient, where would you want to set the sensitivity control for assist-control mode?

Flow Triggering

Touch the "Screens" soft key and press the "Main" button. This will return the display to the scalar waveforms and primary controls available for Volume A/C mode. Press the "Flow Trig" button and rotate the adjustment knob until 4 L/min is displayed. Touch the "Flow Trig" button again or press "Accept."

Adjust the ventilator to the following settings in volume control mode:

a.	Respiratory Rate	12/min
b.	Tidal Volume	500 mL
c.	Peak Flow	60 L/min
d.	Flow Trigger	4 L/min
e.	Oxygen Percent	21%
f.	Plateau Time	0 second
g.	PEEP	0 cm H_2O

1. Attach a mouthpiece to the patient wye and attempt to initiate a breath.

2. With the sensitivity control to 4 L/min, attempt to initiate a breath. Observe the flow time curve on the monitoring screen. Adjust the screen scale to expand the scale, making it easier to observe pressure changes. Note the display in the upper left corner of the of the display screen.

3. Adjust the Flow Trig control to 8 L/min and initiate a breath. Observe the flow time curve on the monitoring screen. Adjust the screen scale to expand the scale, making it easier to observe pressure changes. Note the display in the upper left corner of the display screen.
   a. Record what threshold is met when the ventilator cycled on.
   b. Observe the monitoring screen for any changes in ventilatory (patient) parameters.

Questions

A. When you were able to initiate an assisted breath, what event(s) occurred?
B. What did you observe in the upper left portion of the screen?
C. As a patient, where would you want to set the sensitivity control for assist-control mode?

Pressure Control Ventilation

Test Lung Setup

If you are using an SMS ("Manley") lung simulator, connect one spring for compliance, set the resistance control to zero, and rotate the leak control fully clockwise, eliminating any leaks. Attach the patient wye to the inlet of the SMS lung simulator.

If you are using an IngMar Medical Demonstration Lung Model, rotate all of the compliance springs fully clockwise, adjust the resistance controls to "OFF," and adjust both the ET Leak and System Leak controls to the "OFF" position. Attach the patient wye to the inlet of the Demonstration Lung Model.

When completing these activities, manipulate only one control at a time and note the result of each activity with manipulation of the controls. Answer the questions that follow each of the activities.

Initial Ventilator Settings

Press the "Mode" soft key located to the lower left of the display screen. Once the mode options appear on the

screen, select "Pressure A/C" by pressing that button. Then press the "Mode Accept" key.

Adjust the ventilator to the following settings in pressure control mode:

a.	Rate	12/min
b.	P_I	15 cm H_2O
c.	T_I	0.76 second
d.	P-Trigger	−2 cm H_2O (access through the "Advanced Settings" soft key)
e.	Oxygen Percent	21%
f.	PEEP	0 cm H_2O

Inspiratory Pressure Control

1. Using a test lung, measure and record the following using the monitoring screen:
   a. Peak inspiratory pressure
   b. I:E ratio
   c. Tidal volume
   d. Minute ventilation

2. Adjust the inspiratory pressure level to 25 cm H_2O. Measure the following using the display panel and manometer:
   a. Peak inspiratory pressure
   b. I:E ratio
   c. Tidal volume
   d. Minute ventilation

3. Adjust the inspiratory pressure level to 5 cm H_2O. Using the monitoring screen, measure the following:
   a. Peak inspiratory pressure
   b. I:E ratio
   c. Tidal volume
   d. Minute ventilation

Questions

A. How did the change in inspiratory pressure affect the I:E ratio?
B. How did the change in inspiratory pressure affect the exhaled tidal volume?
C. How did the change in inspiratory pressure affect the exhaled minute volume?

Inspiratory Time Control

Using the primary controls located at the bottom of the screen, adjust the ventilator to the following settings:

a.	A/C	12/min
b.	P_I	15 cm H_2O
c.	T_I	0.76
d.	P-Trigger	−2 cm H_2O (access through the "Advanced Settings" soft key)
e.	Oxygen Percent	21%
f.	PEEP	0 cm H_2O

1. Using a test lung, measure the following using the display panel and manometer:
   a. Peak inspiratory pressure
   b. I:E ratio
   c. Exhaled tidal volume
   d. Exhaled minute volume

2. Change the inspiratory time to 1 second, and measure and record the following:
   a. Peak inspiratory pressure
   b. I:E ratio
   c. Exhaled tidal volume
   d. Exhaled minute volume

3. Change the inspiratory time to 3 seconds, and measure and record the following:
   a. Peak inspiratory pressure
   b. I:E ratio
   c. Exhaled tidal volume
   d. Exhaled minute volume

Questions

A. How did the inspiratory time change affect the I:E ratio?
B. How did the inspiratory time change affect tidal volume delivery?
C. How did the inspiratory time change affect the inspiratory pressure?

Rate Control

Adjust the ventilator to the following settings in pressure control A/C mode:

a. A/C	12/min
b. P_I	15 cm H_2O
c. T_I	0.76
d. P-Trigger	−2 cm H_2O
e. Oxygen Percent	21%
f. PEEP	0 cm H_2O

1. Using a test lung, measure the following using the monitoring screen:
   a. Peak inspiratory pressure
   b. I:E ratio
   c. Exhaled tidal volume
   d. Exhaled minute volume

2. Change the rate control to 24 breaths/min, and measure and record the following:
   a. Peak inspiratory pressure
   b. I:E ratio
   c. Exhaled tidal volume
   d. Exhaled minute volume

3. Change the rate control to 6 breaths/min, and measure and record the following:
   a. Peak inspiratory pressure
   b. I:E ratio
   c. Exhaled tidal volume
   d. Exhaled minute volume

Questions

A. What happened to the I:E ratio when you changed the rate?
B. What happened to the minute ventilation when you changed the rate?

Spontaneous Ventilation

The Viasys Avea ventilator is able to provide two spontaneous ventilation modes: CPAP and CPAP with Pressure Support. To access these spontaneous modes, press the "Mode" soft key located at the lower left of the display screen.

Spontaneous (CPAP)

1. Touch the "Mode" soft key.
2. Select "CPAP PSV" for spontaneous mode.
3. Press the "Mode Accept" button to activate the spontaneous modes.
4. Touch the "Accept" soft key.

From the displayed screen, you may now enter a PEEP (CPAP) level.
   a. Touch the "PEEP" button.
   b. Turn the knob to adjust the PEEP (CPAP) level to 5 cm H_2O.
   c. Touch the "PEEP" (CPAP) button again or press "Accept."

PEEP (CPAP Level)

Test Lung Setup

a. If you are using an SMS ("Manley") lung simulator, connect one spring for compliance, set the resistance control to zero, and rotate the leak control fully clockwise, eliminating any leaks. Attach the patient wye to the inlet of the SMS lung simulator.

b. If you are using an IngMar Medical Demonstration Lung Model, rotate all of the compliance springs fully clockwise, adjust the resistance controls to "OFF," and adjust both the ET Leak and System Leak controls to the "OFF" position. Attach the patient wye to the inlet of the Demonstration Lung Model.

c. When completing these activities, manipulate only one control at a time and note the result of each activity with manipulation of the controls. Answer the questions that follow each of the activities.

Set the controls to the following settings:

a. Mode	CPAP/PSV
b. Flow Trig	4 L/min
c. PEEP (CPAP level)	5 cm H_2O

Once the settings have been established, simulate a spontaneous breath by moving the test lung's bellows. Repeat the process, simulating a spontaneous rate and tidal volume. Observe the pressure time curve on the monitoring screen or the pressure volume loop. Adjust the screen scale to expand the scale, making it easier to observe pressure changes. Note the display in the upper left corner of the display screen.

Questions

A. What did you observe in the upper left portion of the display screen?
B. What did you observe as the baseline pressure on the pressure time scalar waveform?
C. What happened when you stopped your simulated breathing?
D. What was an average inspiratory pressure during your spontaneous efforts?

Change the ventilator controls to the following settings:
 a. Mode   CPAP/PSV
 b. Flow Trigger   4 L/min
 c. PEEP (CPAP level)   15 cm H_2O

Once the settings have been established, simulate a spontaneous breath by moving the test lung's bellows. Repeat the process, simulating a spontaneous rate and tidal volume. Observe the pressure time curve on the monitoring screen or the pressure volume loop. Adjust the screen scale to expand the scale, making it easier to observe pressure changes. Note the display in the upper left corner of the display screen.

Questions

A. What did you observe in the upper left corner of the display screen?
B. What did you observe as the baseline pressure on the pressure time scalar waveform?
C. What happened when you stopped your simulated breathing?
D. What was an average inspiratory pressure during your spontaneous efforts?

Pressure Support

Spontaneous–Pressure Support

1. Touch the "PSV" (pressure support) key.

2. Using the adjustment knob, set the pressure support level to 5 cm H_2O.

3. Touch the "Accept" soft key or press the "PSV" key once again.

From the displayed screen, you may now enter a PEEP (CPAP) level and pressure support level.
 1. Touch the "PEEP" button on the spontaneous settings screen.
 2. Turn knob to adjust the PEEP (CPAP) level to 5 cm H_2O.
 3. Touch the "PEEP" (CPAP) button again or press the "Accept" soft key.

Test Lung Setup

1. If you are using an SMS ("Manley") lung simulator, connect one spring for compliance, set the resistance control to zero, and rotate the leak control fully clockwise, eliminating any leaks. Attach the patient wye to the inlet of the SMS lung simulator.
2. If you are using an IngMar Medical Demonstration Lung Model, rotate all of the compliance springs fully clockwise, adjust the resistance controls to "OFF," and adjust both the ET Leak and System Leak controls to the "OFF" position. Attach the patient wye to the inlet of the Demonstration Lung Model.
3. When completing these activities, manipulate only one control at a time and note the result of each activity with manipulation of the controls. Answer the questions that follow each of the activities.
 Set the controls to the following settings:
 a. Mode   CPAP/PSV
 b. Flow Trig   4 L/min
 c. PEEP (CPAP level)   5 cm H_2O
 d. Pressure Support   5 cm H_2O

Once the settings have been established, simulate a spontaneous breath by moving the test lung's bellows. Repeat the process, simulating a spontaneous rate and tidal volume. Observe the pressure time curve on the monitoring screen or the pressure volume loop. Adjust the screen scale to expand the scale, making it easier to observe pressure changes. Note the display in the upper left corner of the display screen.

Questions

A. What did you observe in the upper left portion of the display screen?
B. What did you observe as the baseline pressure on the pressure time scalar waveform?
C. What happened when you stopped your simulated breathing?
D. What was an average inspiratory pressure during your spontaneous efforts?

Set the controls to the following settings:
 a. Mode   CPAP/PSV
 b. Flow Trig   4 L/min
 c. PEEP (CPAP level)   5 cm H_2O
 d. Pressure Support   10 cm H_2O

Repeat your spontaneous efforts with the test lung, simulating a rate and a tidal volume. Observe the pressure time curve on the monitoring screen or the pressure volume loop. Adjust the screen scale to expand the scale, making it easier to observe pressure changes. Note the display in the upper left corner of the display screen.

Questions

A. What did you observe in the upper left corner of the display screen?
B. What did you observe as the baseline pressure on the pressure time scalar waveform?
C. What happened when you stopped your simulated breathing?
D. What was an average inspiratory pressure during your spontaneous efforts?

Alarm Functions

Input Power and Control Circuit Alarms

Input power alarms alert the clinician to loss of electrical power or pneumatic sources rendering the ventilator inoperative. Control circuit alarms alert the clinician to incompatible settings or settings that are out of range as well as potential faults in the microprocessor control circuitry. These alarms are summarized in Table 25-15.

TABLE 25-15: Viasys Avea Input Power and Control Circuit Alarms

ALARM	CAUSE	CORRECTIVE ACTION
Loss AC Power	Power switch is in the "ON" position but AC power is not available.	1. Manually ventilate the patient. 2. Check the integrity of the AC power source. 3. If the ventilator is operating on internal battery, prepare for alternative ventilation.

Vent Inop	Internal microprocessor failure
	    1. Safety valve opens.
	    2. PEEP is not maintained.
		1. Manually ventilate the patient if needed.
		2. Remove the ventilator from service and contact the biomedical department for service.

Low Battery	The backup battery power is depleted and can only provide 2 minutes of ventilation.	1. Connect the ventilator to AC power. 2. Verify that the internal battery is charging.
Low FIO$_2$ O$_2$	The measured O$_2$% is 6% or 18%.	1. Check the patient's SpO$_2$ to ensure patient safety. 2. Check both air and O$_2$ gas connections.
Loss Air Supply	Air supply pressure is less than the minimum required. Oxygen delivery may be compromised.	1. Manually ventilate the patient if required. 2. Check both air and oxygen pneumatic sources.
Loss O$_2$ Supply	Oxygen supply pressure is less than the minimum required. Accuracy of O$_2$% may be compromised.	1. Manually ventilate the patient if required. 2. Check both air and oxygen pneumatic sources.

Safety Valve Open	The safety valve has been opened.
	    1. Patient can breathe room air.
	    2. No PEEP level is provided.
		1. Manually ventilate the patient.
		2. Remove the ventilator from service.
		3. Contact a biomedical technician.

Loss of Gas Supply	All gas supplies have been lost.	1. Manually ventilate the patient if required. 2. Contact biomedical for service.

Output Alarms

Output alarms are triggered when the alarm limits of the ventilator's output have been exceeded. Examples of typical output alarms include pressure, volume, flow, and time. The output alarms for the Puritan Bennett 840 are summarized in the Table 25-16.

To set the alarms, press the "Alarm Limits" soft key located next to the upper right portion of the display screen. A presentation of the alarms appears in the lower portion of the screen. To set an alarm, touch the desired setting, turn the adjustment knob, and touch the setting again or press "Accept."

Apnea Backup

In the event the patient becomes apneic, the Viasys Avea ventilator will automatically deliver a rate, tidal volume or pressure, and a set FIO$_2$. Apnea Backup parameters are available in CPAP/PSV modes. To set the Apnea Backup parameters, complete the following steps:

1. Touch the "Apnea Setup" key at the bottom of the screen.

2. You have the option of delivering volume control or pressure control breaths. Select either "VC" or "PC" by pressing the "Change VC/PC" key.

3. Once VC or PC modes have been selected, select the appropriate keys for rate, volume (or pressure and Insp time), and the desired FIO$_2$ To make your selections touch, turn the knob and touch the key again. Once all of your selections are made, press "Accept" to apply the new settings.

TABLE 25-16: Viasys Avea Output Alarms

ALARM	CAUSE	CORRECTIVE ACTION
High Peak	The measured airway pressure is greater than the alarm setting.	Evaluate the patient: 1. Suctioning needed? 2. Bronchospasm? 3. Circuit disconnect/leaks? 4. Airway secure?
Low Peak	The measured airway pressure is lower than the alarm setting.	Evaluate the patient: 1. Circuit disconnected/leaks? 2. Airway secure?
Low $\dot{V}^E$	The patient's exhaled minute volume is less than the alarm setting.	Evaluate the patient and the ventilator settings.
High $\dot{V}^E$	The patient's exhaled minute volume is greater than the alarm setting.	Evaluate the patient and the ventilator settings.
High Vt	The patient's exhaled tidal volume is greater than the alarm setting.	Evaluate the patient and the ventilator settings.
Low Vt	The patient's exhaled tidal volume is less than the alarm setting.	Evaluate the patient and the ventilator settings.
High Rate	The monitored total breath rate exceeds the alarm setting.	Evaluate the patient and the ventilator settings.
I-Time Limit	The inspiratory time exceeds the alarm setting.	Evaluate the patient and the ventilator settings.
I:E Limit	The I:E ratio for a mandatory breath exceeds 4:1.	Evaluate the patient and the ventilator settings.
Low FIO_2	Delivered O_2% is less than 6% or 18% from the setting.	Evaluate the patient. Check the air and oxygen supply lines. Check the oxygen analyzer cell.

Check List: Initiation of Volume Control Ventilation

_____ 1. Verify the order or protocol.

_____ 2. Scan the patient's chart as time permits.

_____ 3. Assess oxygenation, ventilation, and cardiac status.

_____ 4. Gather the required equipment.

_____ 5. Assemble the ventilator and perform an operational verification procedure.

6. Adjust the ventilator to the appropriate settings.

_____ a. Tidal volume

_____ b. Rate

_____ c. FIO_2

_____ d. PEEP

_____ e Trigger sensitivity

_____ f Alarm settings

_____ 7. Connect the patient.

8. Monitor all ventilator parameters.

_____ a. Corrected tidal volume

_____ b. Rate

_____ c. FIO_2

_____ d. Adjust the trigger sensitivity.

_____ e. Set the pressure limit.

_____ f. Set all alarms.

9. Document the patient's physiologic response.

_____ a. Heart rate

_____ b. SpO_2

_____ c. Breath sounds

_____ d. Hemodynamic changes

_____ 10. Clean up the area.

_____ 11. Document the procedure on the patient's record.

_____ 12. Maintain aseptic technique.

Check List: Initiation of Pressure Control Ventilation

_____ 1. Verify the order or protocol.

_____ 2. Scan the patient's chart as time permits.

_____ 3. Assess oxygenation, ventilation, and cardiac status.

_____ 4. Gather the required equipment.

_____ 5. Assemble the ventilator and perform an operational verification procedure.

6. Adjust the ventilator to the appropriate settings.

_____   a. Inspiratory pressure

_____   b. Inspiratory time

_____   c. Rate

_____   d. FIO$_2$

_____   e. PEEP

_____   f. Trigger sensitivity

_____   g. Alarm settings

_____ 7. Connect the patient.

8. Monitor all ventilator parameters.

_____   a. Inspiratory pressure

_____   b. Inspiratory time

_____   c. Rate

_____   d. FIO$_2$

_____   e. PEEP

_____   f. Trigger sensitivity

_____   g. Set all alarms.

9. Document the patient's physiologic response.

_____   a. Heart rate

_____   b. SpO$_2$

_____   c. Breath sounds

_____   d. Hemodynamic changes

_____ 10. Clean up the area.

_____ 11. Document the procedure on the patient's record.

_____ 12. Maintain aseptic technique.

Check List: Initiation of CPAP or Pressure Support Ventilation

_____ 1. Verify the order or protocol.

_____ 2. Scan the patient's chart as time permits.

_____ 3. Assess oxygenation, ventilation, and cardiac status.

_____ 4. Gather the required equipment.

_____ 5. Assemble the ventilator and perform an operational verification procedure.

6. Adjust the ventilator to the appropriate settings.

_____   a. CPAP pressure

_____   b. Pressure support level

_____   c. FIO$_2$

_____   d. Trigger sensitivity

_____   e. Alarm settings

_____   f. Backup ventilation settings

_____ 7. Connect the patient.

8. Monitor all ventilator parameters.

_____   a. CPAP pressure

_____   b. Pressure support level

_____   c. Patient's rate

_____   d. FIO$_2$

_____   e. Trigger sensitivity

_____   f. Alarms

9. Document the patient's physiologic response.

_____   a. Heart rate

_____   b. SpO$_2$

_____   c. Breath sounds

_____   d. Hemodynamic changes

_____ 10. Clean up the area.

_____ 11. Document the procedure on the patient's record.

_____ 12. Maintain aseptic technique.

Check List: Monitoring Ventilation

_____ 1. Verify the physician's order or ventilation protocol.

_____ 2. Review the patient's record.

3. Assemble the needed equipment.

_____   a. Cuff pressure manometer

_____   b. Stethoscope

4. Assess the patient.

_____   a. Color

_____   b. Work of breathing

_____   c. Heart rate

_____   d. ECG and rhythm

_____   e. SpO$_2$

_____   f. Level of consciousness and response to stimuli

_____   g. Breath sounds

_____   h. Verify elevation of the head of the bed

_____ 5. Suction the patient as needed.

_____ 6. Appropriately drain any condensate from the ventilator tubing.

7. Monitor all ventilator settings.

_____   a. Tidal volume
_____   b. Inspiratory pressure
_____   c. Inspiratory time
_____   d. Rate
_____   e. FIO_2

_____   f. PEEP
_____   g. Trigger sensitivity
_____   h. Alarm settings
_____   8. Appropriately document the procedure in the patient record.
_____   9. Maintain aseptic technique.

Self-Evaluation Post Test: Continuous Mechanical Ventilation

1. Which of the following are characteristics of type I respiratory failure?
   I.   pH 7.35–7.45
   II. pH < 7.35
   III. $PaCO_2$ 25–40 mm Hg
   IV. PaO_2 40–59 mm Hg
   a. I, III   c. II, III
   b. I, IV   d. II, IV

2. Which of the following are characteristics of type II respiratory failure?
   I.   pH 7.35–7.45
   II. pH < 7.35
   III. $PaCO_2$ > 50 mm Hg
   IV. PaO_2 40–59 mm Hg
   a. I, III   c. II, III
   b. I, IV   d. II, IV

3. Which of the following are indications for mechanical ventilation?
   I.   Apnea
   II. Acute asthma
   III. Exacerbation of neuromuscular disease
   IV. Acute hypoxemic failure
   a. I   c. I, II, III
   b. I, II   d. I, II, III, IV

4. Which of the following are common patient interface(s) for noninvasive ventilation?
   I.   Mask
   II. Nasal prongs
   III. Nasal pillows
   IV. Nasal mask
   a. I   c. I, II, III
   b. I, II   d. I, II, III, IV

5. Which of the following are advantages of noninvasive mechanical ventilation?
   I.   Improved patient communication
   II. Improved ability to regulate minute ventilation
   III. Increased patient tolerance
   IV. Improved gas exchange
   a. I, II   c. II, III
   b. I, III   d. II, IV

6. Which of the following may be cause to consider invasive positive-pressure ventilation over noninvasive mechanical ventilation?
   I.   Increased secretions
   II. Infiltrates on chest x-ray
   III. Severe pathology
   a. I   c. II, III
   b. I, II   d. I, II, III

7. Which of the following are advantages of invasive positive-pressure ventilation?
   I.   Improved patient communication
   II. Improved ability to regulate minute ventilation
   III. Increased patient tolerance
   IV. Improved gas exchange
   a. I, II   c. II, III
   b. I, III   d. II, IV

8. Which of the following are required settings for volume control ventilation?
   I.   Tidal volume
   II. Inspiratory pressure
   III. Inspiratory time
   IV. Rate
   a. I, IV   c. II, III
   b. I, II   d. III, IV

9. Which of the following are required settings for pressure control ventilation?
   I.   Tidal volume
   II. Inspiratory pressure
   III. Inspiratory time
   IV. Rate
   a. I, IV   c. II, III, IV
   b. I, II   d. III, IV

10. Which of the following patient parameters should be trended during routine patient-ventilator system checks?
    I.   Pressures
    II. Tidal volume
    III. Airway resistance
    IV. Compliance
    a. I   c. I, II, III
    b. I, II   d. I, II, III, IV

PERFORMANCE EVALUATION:

Initiation of Volume Control Ventilation

Date: Lab _____ Clinical _____ Agency _____

Lab: Pass _____ Fail _____ Clinical: Pass _____ Fail _____

Student name _____ Instructor name _____

No. of times observed in clinical _____

No. of times practiced in clinical _____

PASSING CRITERIA: Obtain 90% or better on the procedure. Tasks indicated by * must receive at least 1 point, or the evaluation is terminated. Procedure must be performed within the designated time, or the performance receives a failing grade.

SCORING:
2 points — Task performed satisfactorily without prompting.
1 point — Task performed satisfactorily with self-initiated correction.
0 points — Task performed incorrectly or with prompting required.
NA — Task not applicable to the patient care situation.

Tasks:	Peer	Lab	Clinical
* 1. Verifies the physician's order or protocol	☐	☐	☐
2. Reviews the patient's record	☐	☐	☐
* 3. Gathers the equipment	☐	☐	☐
* 4. Assembles the ventilator and performs operational verification tests	☐	☐	☐
* 5. Assesses oxygenation and cardiac status	☐	☐	☐
6. Adjusts the ventilator to the ordered settings			
* a. Tidal volume	☐	☐	☐
* b. Rate	☐	☐	☐
* c. FIO_2	☐	☐	☐
* d. PEEP	☐	☐	☐
* e. Trigger sensitivity	☐	☐	☐
* f. Alarm settings	☐	☐	☐
* 7. Connects the patient	☐	☐	☐
8. Monitors the ventilator parameters			
* a. Rate	☐	☐	☐
* b. Tidal volume	☐	☐	☐
* c. FIO_2	☐	☐	☐
* d. Trigger sensitivity	☐	☐	☐

*   e. Circuit temperature ☐ ☐ ☐

*   f. Adjusts all alarms ☐ ☐ ☐

   9. Documents the patient's physiologic response ☐ ☐ ☐

*   a. Heart rate ☐ ☐ ☐

*   b. SpO$_2$ ☐ ☐ ☐

*   c. Breath sounds ☐ ☐ ☐

*   d. Hemodynamic changes ☐ ☐ ☐

  10. Cleans up the area ☐ ☐ ☐

* **11.** Records the procedure in the patient record ☐ ☐ ☐

* **12.** Maintains aseptic technique ☐ ☐ ☐

SCORE: Peer _____ points of possible 52; _____%

                  Lab _____ points of possible 52; _____%

                  Clinical _____ points of possible 52; _____%

TIME: _____ out of possible 30 minutes

STUDENT SIGNATURES

PEER: _____

STUDENT: _____

INSTRUCTOR SIGNATURES

LAB: _____

CLINICAL: _____

Date: Lab _____ Clinical _____ Agency _____

Lab: Pass _____ Fail _____ Clinical: Pass _____ Fail _____

Student name _____ Instructor name _____

No. of times observed in clinical _____

No. of times practiced in clinical _____

PASSING CRITERIA: Obtain 90% or better on the procedure. Tasks indicated by * must receive at least 1 point, or the evaluation is terminated. Procedure must be performed within the designated time, or the performance receives a failing grade.

SCORING:
2 points — Task performed satisfactorily without prompting.
1 point — Task performed satisfactorily with self-initiated correction.
0 points — Task performed incorrectly or with prompting required.
NA — Task not applicable to the patient care situation.

Tasks:	Peer	Lab	Clinical
* **1.** Verifies the physician's order or protocol	☐	☐	☐
2. Reviews the patient's record	☐	☐	☐
* **3.** Gathers the equipment	☐	☐	☐
* **4.** Assembles the ventilator and performs operational verification tests	☐	☐	☐
* **5.** Assesses oxygenation and cardiac status	☐	☐	☐
6. Adjusts the ventilator to the ordered settings			
* a. Inspiratory pressure	☐	☐	☐
* b. Inspiratory time	☐	☐	☐
* c. Rate	☐	☐	☐
* d. FIO$_2$	☐	☐	☐
* e. PEEP	☐	☐	☐
* f. Trigger sensitivity	☐	☐	☐
* g. Alarm settings	☐	☐	☐
* **7.** Connects the patient	☐	☐	☐
8. Monitors the ventilator parameters			
* a. Inspiratory pressure	☐	☐	☐
* b. Inspiratory time	☐	☐	☐
* c. Rate	☐	☐	☐

*   d. FIO$_2$ ☐ ☐ ☐

*   e. PEEP   ☐ ☐ ☐

*   f. Trigger sensitivity   ☐ ☐ ☐

*   g. Circuit temperature   ☐ ☐ ☐

*   h. Adjusts all alarms   ☐ ☐ ☐

*   **9.** Documents the patient's physiologic response   ☐ ☐ ☐

*   a. Heart rate   ☐ ☐ ☐

*   b. SpO$_2$ ☐ ☐ ☐

*   c. Breath sounds   ☐ ☐ ☐

*   d. Hemodynamic changes   ☐ ☐ ☐

* **10.** Cleans up the area   ☐ ☐ ☐

* **11.** Records the procedure in the patient record   ☐ ☐ ☐

* **12.** Maintains aseptic technique   ☐ ☐ ☐

SSCORE: Peer _____ points of possible 56; _____%

                 Lab _____ points of possible 56; _____%

                 Clinical _____ points of possible 56; _____%

TIME: _____ out of possible 30 minutes

STUDENT SIGNATURES   **INSTRUCTOR SIGNATURES**

PEER: _____   LAB: _____

STUDENT: _____   CLINICAL: _____

PERFORMANCE EVALUATION:

Initiation of CPAP or Pressure Support Ventilation

Date: Lab _____ Clinical _____ Agency _____

Lab: Pass _____ Fail _____ Clinical: Pass _____ Fail _____

Student name _____ Instructor name _____

No. of times observed in clinical _____

No. of times practiced in clinical _____

PASSING CRITERIA: Obtain 90% or better on the procedure. Tasks indicated by * must receive at least 1 point, or the evaluation is terminated. Procedure must be performed within the designated time, or the performance receives a failing grade.

SCORING:
2 points — Task performed satisfactorily without prompting.
1 point — Task performed satisfactorily with self-initiated correction.
0 points — Task performed incorrectly or with prompting required.
NA — Task not applicable to the patient care situation.

Tasks:	Peer	Lab	Clinical
* **1.** Verifies the physician's order or protocol	☐	☐	☐
2. Reviews the patient's record	☐	☐	☐
* **3.** Gathers the equipment	☐	☐	☐
* **4.** Assembles the ventilator and performs operational verification tests	☐	☐	☐
* **5.** Assesses oxygenation and cardiac status	☐	☐	☐
6. Adjusts the ventilator to the ordered settings			
* a. CPAP pressure	☐	☐	☐
* b. Pressure support level	☐	☐	☐
* c. FIO$_2$	☐	☐	☐
* d. Trigger sensitivity	☐	☐	☐
* e. Alarm settings	☐	☐	☐
* f. Backup ventilation settings	☐	☐	☐
* **7.** Connects the patient	☐	☐	☐
8. Monitors the ventilator parameters			
* a. CPAP pressure	☐	☐	☐
* b. Pressure support level	☐	☐	☐
* c. Patient's rate	☐	☐	☐
* d. FIO$_2$	☐	☐	☐

*   e. PEEP ☐ ☐ ☐

*   f. Trigger sensitivity ☐ ☐ ☐

*   g. Circuit temperature ☐ ☐ ☐

*   h. Adjusts all alarms ☐ ☐ ☐

  9. Documents the patient's physiologic response ☐ ☐ ☐

*   a. Heart rate ☐ ☐ ☐

*   b. SpO$_2$ ☐ ☐ ☐

*   c. Breath sounds ☐ ☐ ☐

*   d. Hemodynamic changes ☐ ☐ ☐

  10. Cleans up the area ☐ ☐ ☐

* **11.** Records the procedure in the patient record ☐ ☐ ☐

* **12.** Maintains aseptic technique ☐ ☐ ☐

SCORE: Peer _____ points of possible 54; _____%

                     Lab _____ points of possible 54; _____%

                     Clinical _____ points of possible 54; _____%

TIME: _____ out of possible 30 minutes

STUDENT SIGNATURES   **INSTRUCTOR SIGNATURES**

PEER: _____   LAB: _____

STUDENT: _____   CLINICAL: _____

PERFORMANCE EVALUATION:
Monitoring Mechanical Ventilation

Date: Lab _____ Clinical _____ Agency _____

Lab: Pass _____ Fail _____ Clinical: Pass _____ Fail _____

Student name _____ Instructor name _____

No. of times observed in clinical _____

No. of times practiced in clinical _____

PASSING CRITERIA: Obtain 90% or better on the procedure. Tasks indicated by * must receive at least 1 point, or the evaluation is terminated. Procedure must be performed within the designated time, or the performance receives a failing grade.

SCORING:
2 points — Task performed satisfactorily without prompting.
1 point — Task performed satisfactorily with self-initiated correction.
0 points — Task performed incorrectly or with prompting required.
NA — Task not applicable to the patient care situation.

Tasks:	Peer	Lab	Clinical
* **1.** Verifies the physician's order or ventilation protocol	☐	☐	☐
2. Reviews the patient's record	☐	☐	☐
3. Assembles needed equipment			
* a. Cuff pressure manometer	☐	☐	☐
* b. Stethoscope	☐	☐	☐
* **4.** Explains the procedure to the patient	☐	☐	☐
5. Assesses the patient			
* a. Color	☐	☐	☐
* b. Work of breathing	☐	☐	☐
* c. Cardiac rate/rhythm/blood pressure	☐	☐	☐
* d. Level of consciousness	☐	☐	☐
* e. SpO$_2$	☐	☐	☐
* f. Breath sounds	☐	☐	☐
* g. Verifies elevation of the head of the bed	☐	☐	☐
* h. Artificial airway type and placement	☐	☐	☐
* **6.** Suctions the patient as required	☐	☐	☐
* **7.** Empties the condensate from the tubing	☐	☐	☐

8. Monitors the ventilator parameters

* a. Tidal volume ☐ ☐ ☐

* b. Inspiratory pressure ☐ ☐ ☐

* c. Inspiratory time ☐ ☐ ☐

* d. Rate ☐ ☐ ☐

* e. FIO_2 ☐ ☐ ☐

* f. PEEP ☐ ☐ ☐

* g. Trigger sensitivity ☐ ☐ ☐

* h. Alarm settings ☐ ☐ ☐

9. Cleans up the area ☐ ☐ ☐

* **10.** Records the procedure on the chart ☐ ☐ ☐

* **11.** Maintains aseptic technique ☐ ☐ ☐

SCORE: Peer _____ points of possible 52; _____%

       Lab _____ points of possible 52; _____%

       Clinical _____ points of possible 52; _____%

TIME: _____ out of possible 30 minutes

STUDENT SIGNATURES   **INSTRUCTOR SIGNATURES**

PEER: _____ LAB: _____

STUDENT: _____ CLINICAL: _____

CHAPTER 26

Advanced Modes of Mechanical Ventilation

INTRODUCTION

As a respiratory care practitioner, you will be required to understand the various modes of mechanical ventilation and how each mode functions. More importantly, you must understand how best to interface the ventilator with the patient to minimize patient discomfort and dysynchrony and to optimize breath delivery (Chatburn, 2007).

In this chapter you will learn a basic classification scheme by which different ventilators from different manufacturers may be compared with one another more easily. Once a framework of understanding is developed, you may then better understand how each mode functions and how best to apply it clinically.

KEY TERMS

- **Airway pressure release ventilation (APRV)**
- **Automatic tube compensation**
- **Automode**
- **Control variable**
- **Dual control within a breath mode**
- **Dual control breath-to-breath mode**
- **Intermittent mandatory ventilation (IMV)**
- **Inverse ratio ventilation**
- **Mandatory minute volume (MMV)**
- **Pressure augmentation**

- **Pressure control inverse ratio ventilation (PCIRV)**
- **Pressure limited**
- **Pressure regulated volume control (PRVC)**
- **Proportional assist ventilation (PAV)**
- **Set-point**
- **Time cycled**
- **Volume assured pressure support (VAPS)**
- **Volume control plus**
- **Volume support ventilation (VSV)**

THEORY OBJECTIVES

- *Describe the term control variable and the conditions that must be met for a ventilator to be classified as:*
  - *Primary volume controller*
  - *Primary pressure controller*
  - *Dual controller*
- *Describe the dual control within breath modes and their application.*
  - *Pressure augmentation*
  - *Volume assured pressure support (VAPS)*
- *Describe the dual control breath-to-breath, pressure-limited, time-cycled modes and their application.*
  - *Pressure regulated volume control (PRVC)*
  - *Volume control plus (VC +)*
- *Describe the dual control breath-to-breath, pressure-limited, flow-cycled modes and their application.*
  - *Volume support ventilation (VSV)*

- *Describe inverse ratio ventilation and its application.*
  - *Pressure control inverse ratio ventilation*
  - *Volume control inverse ratio ventilation*
- *Describe airway pressure release ventilation (APRV) and its application.*
- *Describe intermittent mandatory ventilation (IMV) and its application.*
- *Describe the following ventilation modes and their application.*
  - *Mandatory minute ventilation (MMV)*
  - *Automatic tube compensation*
  - *Proportional assist ventilation (PAV)*
  - *Automode*

THE CONTROL VARIABLE

The *control variable* describes what the ventilator measures and uses as a feedback signal within a breath to regulate its output (Chatburn, 1992, 2007). Control variables may include pressure, volume, flow, or time. Most commonly, ventilators are primary pressure or primary volume controllers.

When pressure is the primary control variable, pressure is increased during inspiration to a preset level (set-point) and remains constant through the remainder of the breath delivery. The *set-point* describes the variable (pressure, volume, flow, or time) that the clinician establishes using the ventilator's controls to regulate how the ventilator delivers a breath. A *primary pressure controller* maintains a constant pressure during inspiration, and volume and flow will vary depending on the compliance and resistance of the patient's lungs (Chatburn, 1992, 2007).

When volume is used as a primary control variable, the ventilator measures volume and delivers a fixed volume (tidal volume) with each breath delivery (Chatburn, 2007). Both pressure and flow vary during inspiration depending on the resistance and compliance of the patient's lungs. The set-point for a *primary volume* controller is volume and is preset by the clinician using the ventilator's controls.

A *primary flow* controller is where flow becomes the set-point, and pressure and volume vary depending on the resistance and compliance of the patient's lungs. Flow increases to a pre-set level and remains constant during inspiration. The ventilator measures flow and uses it as a feedback signal to regulate breath delivery.

Time may also be a set-point and used as a control variable. Early infant ventilators used a set flow rate (established using a built-in flowmeter), and inspiratory time became the set-point used by the clinician (Chatburn, 2001). The ventilator measures and uses time (constant inspiratory time) as the control variable. These ventilators also incorporate a high-pressure pop-off valve to prevent excessive pressure delivery in the event of worsening compliance or resistance.

A ventilator may only regulate one control variable at one time (pressure, volume, flow, or time) (Chatburn, 2007). However, during the delivery of a breath, the ventilator can switch from one variable to another.

DUAL CONTROL WITHIN A BREATH

Dual control within a breath mode implies that two variables become control variables during inspiration. However, as described earlier, a ventilator can only regulate (control) one variable at any one time. During dual control within a breath mode, the ventilator switches from pressure control to volume control. The clinician sets a desired tidal volume, which becomes a volume guarantee during the breath. The ventilator begins the breath as a pressure controller, delivering a constant pressure initially during the breath. During breath delivery, tidal volume is measured and the pressure is adjusted automatically by the ventilator to maintain the guaranteed tidal volume (volume control). Dual control within a breath mode establishes a high initial inspiratory flow (pressure-controlled breath) and a taper or plateau in flow as the volume target is met. Examples of dual control within a breath mode are summarized in Figure 26-1.

Application

The application of dual control within a breath mode of ventilation is to reduce the work of breathing while maintaining a constant minute volume and tidal volume (Chatburn, 2007). Work of breathing reduction is thought to occur by providing higher inspiratory flows and better patient-ventilator synchrony (Amato, 1992). The evidence suggests that the application of this mode accomplishes the above goals in the short term, but long-term studies have not been performed (Branson & Johannigman, 2004).

DUAL CONTROL BREATH TO BREATH

Selecting a *dual control breath-to-breath mode* allows the clinician to set a volume target. The ventilator delivers pressure-controlled breaths, attempting to achieve the desired target tidal volume. The ventilator may operate in either pressure support or pressure control mode with the pressure limit increasing or decreasing to achieve the desired volume target (Branson & Johannigman, 2004).

Pressure Limited, Time Cycled

Dual control breath-to-breath modes begin inspiration as *pressure-limited* breaths (pressure increases to a set value or target) and are *time cycled* (inspiration ends at a specified time interval). The clinician sets a desired tidal volume and maximum pressure. The ventilator delivers a test breath and calculates the patient's lung resistance and compliance. Once resistance and compliance have been determined, pressure is adjusted automatically to reach the desired tidal volume. Pressure is adjusted in increments of 1 to 3 cm H_2O at a time between breaths until the maximum pressure is reached or a set level below the upper pressure limit. If the desired volume is not met, an alarm alerts the clinician to the fact and the upper pressure limit is never exceeded. Examples of dual control breath-to-breath pressure-limited, time-cycled modes are summarized in Figure 26-2.

Ventilator	Mode
BEAR 1000	Pressure Augmentation
Bird 8400 STi	Volume Assured Pressure support

Figure 26-1 Examples of dual control within a breath mode

Ventilator	Mode
Puritan Bennett 840	Volume Control Plus (VC+)
Maquet SERVO-i	Pressure Regulated Volume Control
Viasys AVEA	Pressure Regulated Volume Control

Figure 26-2 Examples of dual control breath-to-breath, pressure-limited, time-cycled modes

Application

The application of dual control breath-to-breath, pressure-limited, time-cycled ventilation is to provide the positive aspects of pressure control ventilation with a constant minute ventilation and tidal volume, while automatically reducing the pressure as the patient's lung compliance and resistance improve (Chatburn, 2007). The evidence supports reduction in peak inspiratory pressure when compared with volume control ventilation at a constant flow waveform. Improvement in patient-ventilator synchrony, reduction in ventilator days, or improved survival has not been demonstrated in long-term studies (Branson & Johannigman, 2004).

Pressure Limited, Flow Cycled

Each breath is delivered as pressure support breath, with a targeted volume set by the clinician. Inspiration is *flow cycled* (inspiration ends when inspiratory flow falls to the predetermined value). The clinician sets a tidal volume (target), positive end-expiratory pressure (PEEP), and pressure limit. The breath begins as a pressure-controlled breath and the ventilator measures the tidal volume delivered. If the tidal volume falls below the target level, inspiratory pressure is increased on the next breath to attempt to achieve the target. As in pressure support, the breath ends when inspiratory flow decays to a percentage of the peak flow. If the patient becomes apneic, the ventilator switches to a volume control backup ventilation mode. This mode is available on the Maquet SERVO-i as volume support ventilation.

Application

Volume support ventilation (VSV) provides a means of delivering pressure support breaths with a volume guarantee or target. The ventilator will increase or decrease the pressure limit, depending on changes in resistance and compliance (Branson & Johannigman, 2004). In the event of apnea, the ventilator will automatically switch to volume control and sound an alarm to alert the clinician.

INVERSE RATIO VENTILATION

Inverse ratio ventilation describes ventilator modes in which the inspiratory phase is longer than the expiratory phase, exceeding 1:1. Inverse ratio ventilation may be pressure controlled or volume controlled. The goal of inverse ratio ventilation is to decrease mean airway pressures and to improve oxygenation in acute respiratory distress syndrome (ARDS). Air trapping may occur, causing auto-PEEP, which should be monitored. The auto-PEEP may prevent alveoli from collapsing during exhalation, further improving the patient's functional residual capacity (FRC) and improving oxygenation. Current guidelines recommend keeping inspiratory pressures less than 30 cm H_2O to reduce the likelihood of ventilator-induced lung injury (VILI) (National Institutes of Health [NIH], 2000).

Pressure Control Inverse Ratio Ventilation

Pressure control inverse ratio ventilation (PCIRV) is inverse ratio ventilation where pressure is used as the control variable. A pressure limit is set by the clinician (as well as PEEP), and inspiratory time is adjusted to maintain an inspiratory-to-expiratory ratio of greater than 1:1. The presence of auto PEEP should be monitored and pressures and inspiratory time adjusted to maintain pressures of less than 30 cm H_2O.

Volume Control Inverse Ratio Ventilation

Inverse ratio ventilation may also be accomplished using volume as the control variable. Ways to lengthen inspiratory time when volume breaths are not normally time cycled include reducing inspiratory flow or adding an inspiratory pause. Both of these strategies will increase inspiratory time. As stated previously, pressures should be monitored and maintained at less than 30 cm H_2O.

Application

Inverse ratio ventilation is thought to improve the patient's FRC, recruiting alveoli and improving oxygenation. This technique is typically not well tolerated by most patients, and, therefore, sedation may be required.

AIRWAY PRESSURE RELEASE VENTILATION

Airway pressure release ventilation (APRV) is a form of continuous positive airway pressure (CPAP) with two distinct pressure levels. APRV maintains spontaneous breathing throughout the entire ventilatory cycle at both pressure levels (Figure 26-3). APRV is a time-triggered, pressure-limited, and time-cycled mode that allows spontaneous breathing. It is similar to PCIRV, except that the patient may breathe spontaneously at any point in the ventilatory cycle (Branson & Johannigman, 2004).

The clinician sets the high and low pressures and the inspiratory times at each pressure level. Typically the higher pressure is set above the lower inflection point of the lung's pressure volume curve, close to what the mean airway pressure would be during pressure control ventilation (Myers & MacIntyre, 2007). The higher pressure

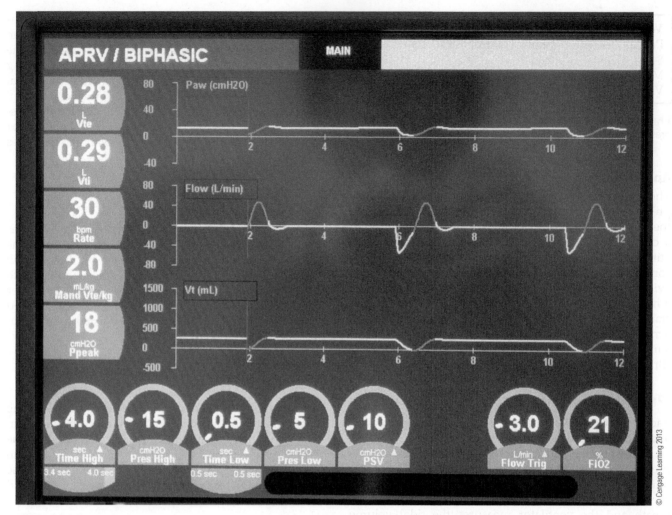

Figure 26-3   Airway pressure release ventilation showing spontaneous breathing at two separate pressure levels

keeps the alveoli recruited and inflated. The time interval at the higher pressure (T_{high}) is longer than the time spent at the lower pressure (T_{low}). Release of the pressure to the lower setting helps to facilitate removal of CO_2 (Myers & MacIntyre, 2007). Time triggering is established using set time intervals for T_{high} and T_{low}. Additionally most ventilators allow patient triggering of a breath (pressure or flow). Some manufacturers also permit the application of pressure support during the spontaneous portion at the higher CPAP level (Figure 26-4).

Figure 26-5 summarizes the availability of APRV on the ventilators highlighted in this chapter

Application

APRV provides improved gas exchange, reduces dead space, and may require less sedation when compared with pressure control ventilation (Myers & MacIntyre, 2007). APRV may result in less VILI when compared with other more conventional modes because the peak inspiratory pressure does not exceed the CPAP (P_{high}) pressure. Another advantage of APRV is that it allows spontaneous ventilation, which may help with gas distribution, especially to the bases of the lungs.

INTERMITTENT MANDATORY VENTILATION (IMV)

Intermittent mandatory ventilation (IMV) allows spontaneous breathing between time-triggered ventilator breaths that may be volume or pressure controlled. The patient breathes through the ventilator circuit spontaneously without triggering the set volume or pressure delivery during ventilator (mandatory) breaths (Figure 26-6). The set baseline pressure (PEEP) during mandatory breaths determines the baseline pressure during spontaneous breathing (CPAP). Spontaneous breaths may also be augmented using pressure support to increase the patient's spontaneous tidal volume and to reduce some of the inspiratory work associated with the endotracheal tube's resistance.

Application

IMV shifts some of the work of breathing onto the patient (spontaneous breaths). When used for weaning from mechanical ventilation, the mandatory rates (ventilator

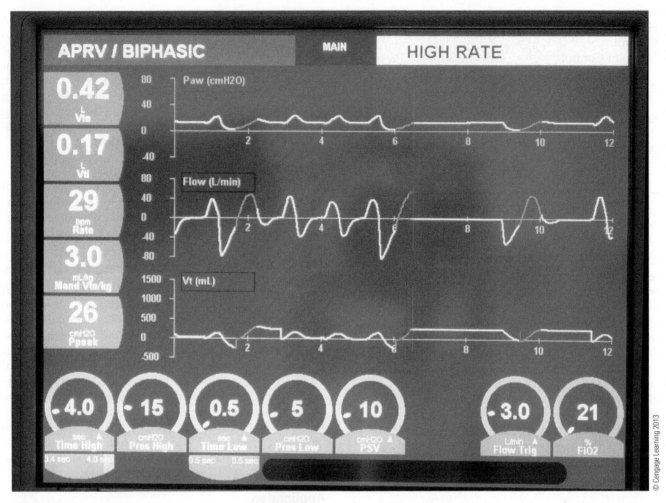

Figure 26-4   Application of pressure support during APRV

Ventilator	Mode
Puritan Bennett 840	BiLevel with Pressure Support
Maquet SERVO-i	Bi-Vent with Pressure Support
Viasys AVEA	APRV/BiPhasic with pressure support

© Cengage Learning 2013

Figure 26-5   Examples of airway pressure release ventilation

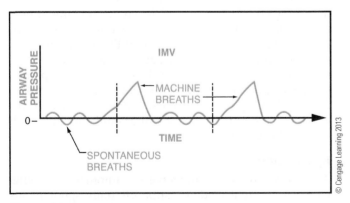

Figure 26-6   SIMV mode showing mandatory and spontaneous breaths

breaths) are gradually reduced, increasing the ventilatory work assumed by the patient. Once the majority of breaths are spontaneous, the patient is given a spontaneous breathing trial, and readiness for ventilator discontinuance is determined.

ADDITIONAL MECHANICAL VENTILATION MODES

The additional modes of mechanical ventilation described in this chapter include mandatory minute ventilation (MMV), automatic tube compensation, proportional assist ventilation (PAV), and automode. All of these modes share commonalities with the modes previously discussed in that they are closed-loop mechanical ventilation modes (Branson, 2002). In a closed-loop mechanical ventilation, the ventilator measures an output signal (pressure, volume, or flow) and uses that signal to modify or control the ventilator's output to more closely match the set-point established by the clinician (Chatburn, 2004).

The different closed-loop ventilator modes are summarized in Figure 26-7. The hierarchy or complexity increases as one moves from set-point control to adaptive

Hierarchy of Ventilator Control	Examples
Set-Point Control	Pressure Support, Pressure Control, Volume Control
Auto-Set-Point Control	Volume Assured Pressure Support
Servo Control	Proportional Assist Ventilation
Adaptive Control	Dual Control Modes (i.e. pressure regulated volume control)

© Cengage Learning 2013

Figure 26-7 Examples of closed-loop mechanical ventilation modes

control. Auto set-point control describes modes in which the ventilator may switch from pressure control to flow control during a breath based on the clinician's set priorities (desired tidal volume as an example). Servo-control increases the sophistication of the control hierarchy. An example of servo-control is where the ventilator attempts to maintain a constant output to match a changing input. For example, in PAV, airway pressure is increased or decreased depending on the patient's inspiratory effort. Adaptive control hierarchy is a system in which the ventilator automatically adjusts a set-point to maintain a different clinician-determined set-point. PRVC is an example of this hierarchical control.

Mandatory Minute Volume

Mandatory minute volume (MMV) may be either volume control or pressure control ventilation. MMV is a mode in which the patient assumes a portion of the ventilatory work (spontaneous breathing) and the clinician sets guaranteed minimum minute ventilation that will be provided in the event the patient's spontaneous efforts may change. The ventilator measures the patient's minute volume over a series of breaths or time interval. If the patient's spontaneous efforts do not meet the desired minute ventilation, the ventilator delivers volume- or pressure-controlled breaths until the minimum minute ventilation is met. MMV is available on the BEAR 1000 or the SERVO-i as VSV.

Application

MMV is commonly applied as patients are progressing toward weaning (Branson, 2002). MMV provides a safety net or backup in the event the patient's spontaneous efforts (workload) fall below the desired minute ventilation level. However, this mode may not prevent rapid-shallow breathing, breath stacking (intrinsic PEEP), or higher than desired tidal volumes (Branson, 2002).

Automatic Tube Compensation

Automatic tube compensation is a mode of ventilation that will automatically compensate for the resistance of the endotracheal tube. The pressure applied is based on the size and type of artificial airway (endotracheal tube

or tracheostomy tube) and how much support is desired by the clinician. Automatic tube compensation can eliminate the resistance imposed by the artificial airway. The ventilator adjusts the pressure to compensate for airway size or flow demands (Branson & Johannigman, 2004). Automatic tube compensation is active both during inspiration and exhalation and may reduce air trapping and intrinsic PEEP. Automatic tube compensation is available on the Puritan-Bennett 840 ventilator.

Application

Automatic tube compensation may reduce the work of breathing imposed by the resistance of the artificial airway, improve patient-ventilator synchrony, and reduce air trapping on exhalation (Branson & Johannigman, 2004).

Proportional Assist Ventilation

Proportional assist ventilation (PAV) is a mode in which the ventilator will proportionally assist the patient's spontaneous ventilation. The ventilator does so by proportionally amplifying the delivered pressure (pressure support) in proportion to the measured inspiratory flow and volume (Branson & Johannigman, 2004). The amount of support provided by the ventilator is tailored or adjusted to the patient's spontaneous effort increasing or decreasing pressure support relative to the patient's work of breathing. PAV may be pressure or flow triggered and is cycled when the patient's volume or flow demands are met. PAV is available on the Puritan-Bennett 840 ventilator.

Application

PAV is an alternative mode of ventilation for spontaneously breathing patients. Studies have compared PAV with noninvasive pressure support. These studies show an improved patient tolerance and comfort level with PAV when compared with pressure support. However, there was no significant difference in intubation rates or outcomes.

Automode

Automode combines PRVC and volume support (VS) into a single mode (Branson, 2004). In the absence of spontaneous patient effort, the ventilator delivers mandatory breaths using a time-triggered, pressure-limited, time-cycled mode, adjusting the pressure limit to maintain the clinician-set tidal volume. If the patient breathes spontaneously for two consecutive breaths, the ventilator will switch to VSV in which the breaths are patient triggered (pressure or flow), pressure limited, and flow cycled. If the patient becomes apneic (12 seconds for adults, 8 seconds for pediatrics), the ventilator will switch back to PRVC mode.

Application

Automode provides a potential for automatic weaning. However, current evidence supports daily spontaneous breathing trials to determine readiness for liberation from mechanical ventilation rather than slower techniques (Branson & Johannigman, 2004).

PROFICIENCY OBJECTIVES

At the end of this chapter, the reader should be able to:

- *Identify the baseline physiologic data that should be assessed and monitored during the application of spontaneous ventilation modes.*
- *Demonstrate how to establish the following modes of ventilation:*
  - *Airway pressure release ventilation*
  - *Automatic tube compensation*
  - *Automode*
  - *Intermittent mandatory ventilation (SIMV)*
  - *Inverse ratio ventilation*
  - *Pressure regulated volume control (PRVC)*
  - *Proportional assist ventilation (PAV)*
  - *Volume support ventilation (VSV)*
- *Describe the potential hazards of spontaneous ventilation modes and how alarms or backup ventilation modes should be set.*

PATIENT ASSESSMENT AND MONITORING

The majority of the advanced ventilation modes are intended to supplement or augment the patient's spontaneous breathing efforts. Several modes are self-adjusting or regulating such that mechanical (ventilator) support is automatically reduced as the patient's effort (tidal volume and minute ventilation) improves. A clinician employing these modes should be aware that these modes may place additional ventilatory work on the patient and may result in fatigue, manifesting changes in monitored data.

Ventilation

The key indicator of ventilation is partial pressure of carbon dioxide in the arterial blood ($PaCO_2$). Increased minute ventilation will decrease $PaCO_2$ and vice versa. CO_2 production via metabolism is relatively constant moment by moment; much of the CO_2 produced is eliminated through the lungs. An increase in CO_2 is a direct indicator of a decrease in minute ventilation.

Other signs of ventilation are respiratory rate, tidal volume, minute volume, and the rapid-shallow-breathing index (RSBI). When a patient begins to fatigue, often the respiratory rate increases more than the tidal volume increases. It takes more energy to increase volume (especially if resistance is high or compliance is low) than it does to pick up the rate. Minute volume being the product of tidal volume and respiratory rate may not change initially as a patient fatigues. However, with prolonged ventilatory work, the minute ventilation will fall as the patient becomes more fatigued. The RSBI is one means of attempting to quantify the relationship between tidal volume and respiratory rate.

$$RSBI = \frac{Respiratory\ Rate}{V_T\ (in\ Liters)}$$

An RSBI of greater than 105 indicates that the patient may become more fatigued and his or her work of breathing is increasing.

Oxygenation

Oxygenation can be assessed both noninvasively and invasively. Noninvasive oxygen assessment is accomplished through pulse oximetry. Maintenance of oxygen saturation (SpO_2) of greater than 88% to 90% is a desired goal for the majority of mechanically ventilated patients. As described in a previous chapter, oxygen saturation monitoring accuracy is subject to abnormal circulation and temperature changes in the periphery. The partial pressure of oxygen in the arterial blood (PaO_2) and CaO_2 are the invasive indices of oxygenation and require the collection of an arterial blood sample (invasive) to perform the assessment. A PaO_2 of greater or equal to 60 mm Hg is the typical goal for most patients on mechanical ventilation.

Cardiovascular

Heart rate, blood pressure, and electrocardiogram (ECG) monitoring is the standard of care for every patient in the intensive care unit (ICU). An increase in heart rate is the first clinical sign of hypoxemia. If an increase in heart rate is noted shortly following a change in ventilator settings or modes, and nothing else has changed (medication, pain, etc.), one should be suspect of oxygenation changes. Blood pressure will also change with fatigue or an increase in ventilatory work. ECG changes, such as an increase in arrhythmias as with tachycardia, may signal changes in oxygenation and an increasing ventilatory workload.

Work of Breathing

Physical inspection, the observational assessment that can be performed from the patient's doorway, is just as valuable as the most high-tech monitoring equipment. Observation of the use of accessory muscles is an indicator of increased ventilatory work. Use of scalene muscles, retractions, elevation of the shoulders during inspiration, or see-saw motion between the chest wall and abdomen are all signs of increased work. Facial appearance is also important. Does the patient appear to be in distress? Check the patient for diaphoresis, also an indicator of increased work.

SETTING VENTILATOR MODES

Often ventilator modes are released as a means to market a specific ventilator, making it unique compared with other manufacturers' ventilators. The modes are developed and released without sound evidence-based trials or extensive bench testing (Branson & Johannigman, 2004). Therefore, it is up to the physician and clinician to apply past experience and successes in the selection of modes or to rely on smaller trials or observational studies to guide their practice.

Airway Pressure Release Ventilation

APRV provides improved gas exchange, reduces dead space, and may require less sedation when compared with pressure control ventilation (Myers & MacIntyre, 2007). APRV allows spontaneous ventilation, which may help with gas distribution especially to the bases of the lungs. Spontaneous ventilation is possible at both the high-pressure (P_{high}) and low-pressure (P_{low}) levels. The spontaneous breaths may also be augmented by pressure support, with some ventilators being capable of providing pressure support at both P_{high} and P_{low}.

Tidal volume delivery during APRV is dependent on lung compliance, resistance, and the pressure applied ($P_{high} - P_{low}$), along with the time pressure applied (Branson & Johannigman, 2004). The patient's spontaneous effort may also augment tidal volume delivery, along with the application of pressure support (PS above P_{high} or P_{low}).

The duration of the time spent at low pressure (T_{low}) is proportional to the amount of CO_2 eliminated through ventilation. In general, as T_{low} shortens, $PaCO_2$ increases (Myers & MacIntyre, 2007). Adequate expiratory time must be established to maintain $PaCO_2$ levels within the desired physiologic range.

APRV Setup

- Establish P_{high}.
- Establish P_{low}.
- Establish T_{high}.
- Establish T_{low}.
- Establish fraction of inspired oxygen (FIO_2).
- Establish trigger level (flow/pressure).
- Establish pressure support.

Automatic Tube Compensation

Automatic tube compensation can eliminate the resistance imposed by the artificial airway, may reduce air trapping during exhalation, and may improve ventilator synchrony (Branson & Johannigman, 2004). The applied pressure is based on the size and type of artificial airway (endotracheal or tracheostomy tube) and how much support is desired by the clinician.

Tube Compensation Setup
- Select the "Tube Compensation" button on the graphic user interface (GUI) screen.
- Select the tube type (endotracheal or tracheostomy).
- Select the tube inner diameter in mm.
- Set the desired % support (10 to 100%).
- Set the trigger sensitivity (pressure or flow).
- Set the expiratory sensitivity (1 to 45%).
- Set the desired FIO_2.

Automode

Automode combines PRVC and VS into a single mode. During spontaneous ventilation the ventilator operates in VSV. If the patient becomes apneic for more than 12 seconds (8 seconds for pediatric patients), the ventilator will automatically change the PRVC mode. In automode, the pressure will be adjusted upward to compensate for worsening patient condition or effort or adjusted downward as the patient's condition improves.

Automode Setup
- Select "Automode" by pressing the button on the Ventilator Settings screen.
- Set the desired tidal volume or pressure (volume control or pressure control mode).
- Set the desired rate.
- Set the desired FIO_2.
- Set the desired baseline pressure (PEEP).
- Set the inspiratory rise time or inspiratory time (volume control or pressure control).
- Set the trigger sensitivity (pressure or flow).
- Set the inspiratory cycle off percent (1 to 70%).
- Set the trigger time out (3 to 7 seconds, infant; 7 to 12 seconds, adult).

Synchronized Intermittent Mandatory Ventilation

Synchronized intermittent mandatory ventilation (SIMV) allows the patient to spontaneous breathe between mandatory (ventilator) breaths. The spontaneous breaths can be delivered with elevated baseline pressures (CPAP) or pressure support. Frequently, a small amount of pressure support (5 to 8 cm H_2O) is added when using spontaneous modes to help compensate for the resistance of the artificial airway.

SIMV Setup

- Select the volume control or pressure control SIMV modes from the Mode Settings screen.
- Establish the appropriate mandatory (ventilator) settings for volume or pressure control modes.
- Set the desired baseline pressure, PEEP delivery during mandatory breaths, and CPAP during spontaneous breaths.
- Set the rate control such that a minimum minute ventilation will be ensured, yet spontaneous breathing will occur.
- Set the desired F_iO_2.
- Set the trigger sensitivity (pressure or flow).
- Set the desired pressure support level.

Inverse Ratio Ventilation

Inverse ratio ventilation establishes an inspiratory time that exceeds expiratory time (inverse I:E ratio). The goal of this mode of ventilation is to improve oxygenation (air trapping and alveolar recruitment) while attempting to reduce mean airway pressures. This mode may be achieved in pressure control or volume control modes, depending on the ventilator's software.

PCIRV Setup

- Select and enter the Pressure Control Ventilator Setup screen.
- Establish the desired pressure control above baseline pressure.
- Set the desired rate.
- Set the desired FIO$_2$.
- Set the inspiratory time to exceed expiratory time, establishing a desired I:E ratio.
- Set the desired inspiratory rise time.
- Set the trigger sensitivity (pressure or flow).

Pressure Regulated Volume Control

Pressure regulated volume control (PRVC) provides the advantages of pressure control ventilation with a constant tidal volume and minute ventilation (Branson, 2004). Pressure application is automatically reduced as the patient's condition or effort improves. The clinician sets a desired tidal volume and maximum pressure. Then over a series of breaths the ventilator determines the pressure required to maintain the desired tidal volume and minute ventilation.

PRVC Setup

- Select and enter the volume control mode and select "PRVC or VC+" depending on the ventilator's software.
- Establish a desired rate.
- Set the desired tidal volume.
- Set the desired FIO$_2$.
- Set the desired inspiratory time.
- Set the desired baseline pressure (PEEP).
- Set the trigger sensitivity (pressure or flow).

Proportional Assist Ventilation

PAV is a mode in which the ventilator will proportionally assist the patient's spontaneous ventilation. The pressure support is adjusted relative to the patient's effort, increasing or decreasing with patient effort. This may allow PAV to provide better synchrony and a more physiologic application of pressure (Branson & Johannigman, 2004).

PAV Setup

- Enter the spontaneous modes selection, and select "Proportional Assist" ventilation (Proportional Assist).

- Set the desired tidal volume and peak inspiratory flow.
- Set the FIO$_2$.
- Set the desired baseline pressure (PEEP/CPAP).
- Set the percentage of desired proportional assist.
- Set the trigger sensitivity.
- Set the expiratory flow sensitivity.
- Set the artificial airway type and diameter.
- Set the inspired tidal volume alarm and peak pressure alarm.

Volume Support Ventilation

VSV is a form of pressure support ventilation with a guaranteed delivery of a desired tidal volume. The ventilator automatically adjusts the pressure limit to achieve the desired tidal volume target.

VSV Setup

- Set the desired tidal volume target.
- Set the baseline pressure (PEEP).
- Set the desired FIO$_2$.
- Set the inspiratory rise time.
- Set the trigger sensitivity (pressure or flow).
- Set the inspiratory cycle off percent.

HAZARDS AND PRECAUTIONS

Many of these modes involve spontaneous ventilation. Therefore, appropriate alarm settings and, when possible, backup ventilation settings are important to alert the clinician to adverse changes in the patient's condition.

A decline in minute ventilation, tidal volume, and respiratory rate are often the first signs of an adverse change in the patient's condition. Therefore, minute ventilation, tidal volume, and low respiratory rate alarms are important in alerting the clinician to these changes. Setting these alarms appropriately and not making them too wide is critical.

Most ventilators provide backup ventilation settings either in volume control or pressure control in the event of apnea. When spontaneous ventilation modes are initiated, it is important to enter the backup ventilation settings screen to evaluate and change these settings as needed. It is important to provide the patient with a safety margin in backup ventilation in the event that the spontaneous mode imposes too much work on the patient and the patient fatigues.

References

Amato, M. B., Barbas, C. S., Bonassa, J., Saldiva, P. H., Zin, W. A., de Carvalho, C. R. (1992). Volume-assured pressure support ventilation (VAPSV): A new approach for reducing muscle workload during acute respiratory failure. *Chest, 102*(4), 1225–1234.

Acute Respiratory Distress Syndrome Network. (2000). Ventilation with lower tidal volumes as compared with traditional tidal volumes for acute lung injury and the acute respiratory distress syndrome. *New England Journal of Medicine, 342*(18), 1301–1308.

Branson, R. D. (2002). Closed-loop mechanical ventilation. *Respiratory Care, 47*(4), 427–453.

Branson, R. D., & Johannigman, J. A. (2004). What is the evidence base for the newer ventilation modes? *Respiratory Care, 49*(7), 742–760.

Chatburn, R. L. (1992). Classification of mechanical ventilators. *Respiratory Care, 37*(9), 1009–1025.

Chatburn, R.L. (2004). Computer control of mechanical ventilation. *Respiratory Care, 49*(5), 507–517.

Chatburn, R. L. (2007). Classification of ventilator modes: Update and proposal for implementation. *Respiratory Care, 52*(3), 301–323.

Myers, T. R., & MacIntyre, N. R. (2007). Does airway pressure release ventilation offer important new advantages in mechanical ventilator support? *Respiratory Care, 52*(4), 452–460.

Operator's and technical reference manual 840 ventilator system. Pleasanton, CA: Nellcor Puritan Bennett.

Operator's manual Avea ventilator systems. (2005). Yorba Linda, CA: Viasys Healthcare.

User's manual SERVO-i ventilator system. (2004). Wayne, NJ: Maquet.

Practice Activities: Nellor Puritan Bennett 840

Circuit Assembly

Figure 26-8 shows the Nellcor Puritan Bennett 840 assembled and ready for use. To prepare the ventilator for use, follow the steps listed next.

1. Install a bacteria inspiratory filter on the patient outlet located on the upper right portion of the breath delivery unit (BDU).
2. Lift the expiratory filter latch into the up position.
3. Install an expiratory filter and collector vial by positioning the upper filter rim into the tracks on the upper part of the from-patient port on the BDU. Once the expiratory filter has been correctly positioned, push the latch down to lock it into place.
4. Install a 12- to 18-inch length of 22 mm tubing between the inspiratory filter and the ventilator's humidifier inlet.
5. Connect the inspiratory limb of the patient circuit to the humidifier outlet.
6. Connect the expiratory limb of the patient circuit to the expiratory filter and collection vial's 22 mm fitting.
7. Attach the patient circuit to the flex arm at its midpoint by clamping the ball fitting on the circuit to the flex arm.

Testing the Ventilator before Use

Power-on Self Test (POST)

Each time the power switch is turned on or if the ventilator microprocessor detects selected fault conditions, a power-on self test (POST) is automatically executed. The POST takes approximately 10 seconds. The test verifies the integrity of the breath delivery unit (BDU) and the GUI and their subsystems.

The POST does not check the ventilator's pneumatic systems. To check the operation of the pneumatic systems, a short self test (SST) is conducted.

Short Self Test (SST)

The SST is a short 2- to 3-minute test that will verify the operation of the BDU hardware including the pressure and flow sensors, the patient circuit, and its compliance and resistance. The test also measures exhalation filter's resistance. It is recommended that the SST be performed every 15 days, between patients, or when the patient circuit is changed. To complete an SST, perform the following steps:

1. The SST will prompt you to verify that a patient is not connected to the circuit.

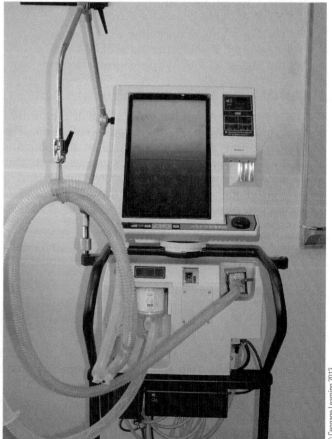

Figure 26-8 The Nellcor Puritan Bennett 840 ventilator assembled and ready for use

2. Turn the ventilator's power switch on. Upon ventilator start-up, touch the "SST" prompt on the lower GUI screen and then press the "Test" button on the left side of the ventilator within 5 seconds of start-up.

3. Follow the prompts on the GUI screen. The microprocessor will then verify that the patient wye is blocked and the SST test will automatically begin.

4. The SST measures the following:
   a. Tests the accuracy of expiratory flow sensors
   b. Verifies the proper function of the pressure sensors
   c. Tests the patient circuit for leaks
   d. Calculates the compliance compensation for the patient circuit
   e. Measures the pressure drop across the expiratory filter
   f. Measures the resistance of the inspiratory and expiratory limbs of the circuit
   g. Checks the pressure drop across the inspiratory limb of the circuit

USING THE KEYBOARD ENTRY SYSTEM

All functions of the Nellcor Puritan Bennett 840 ventilator are controlled from the GUI screen (Figure 26-9). The upper screen displays monitored information, including patient data, graphics, and an alarm log. The lower screen displays ventilator setup, alarm settings, and breath timing information. To enter ventilator or alarm settings, follow the "touch–turn–touch" method for entering new settings. Touch the desired value or setting you wish to change (e.g., tidal volume), and then turn the knob on the lower right side of the GUI interface until the desired value is displayed (clockwise increases, counterclockwise decreases). Touch or press "Accept" to apply the new setting. The new setting will now be displayed on the appropriate portion of the upper or lower GUI screen.

Activities

To complete these practice activities, it is recommended that you use a lung analog/simulator such as an SMS "Manley" lung simulator or an IngMar Medical Quick Lung or Demonstration Lung Model. These devices or other similar devices allow the operator to alter resistance and compliance simulating changes in patient condition.

If these devices are not available, a patient wye and two test lungs may be used as shown in Figure 26-10. Exercise caution. Volumes and pressures may exceed the limits of the test lungs. Resistance may be altered by adapting different sizes of endotracheal tubes, and compliance may be altered by the addition of rubber bands to the test lungs.

Lung Simulator Setup

If you are using an SMS ("Manley") lung simulator, connect one spring for compliance, set the resistance control to zero, and rotate the leak control fully clockwise, eliminating any leaks. Attach the patient wye to the inlet of the SMS lung simulator.

If you are using an IngMar Medical Demonstration Lung Model, rotate all of the compliance springs fully clockwise, adjust the resistance controls to "OFF," and adjust both the ET Leak and System Leak controls to the "OFF" position. Attach the patient wye to the inlet of the Demonstration Lung Model.

When completing these activities, manipulate only one control at a time and note the result of each activity with manipulation of the controls. Answer the questions that follow each of the activities.

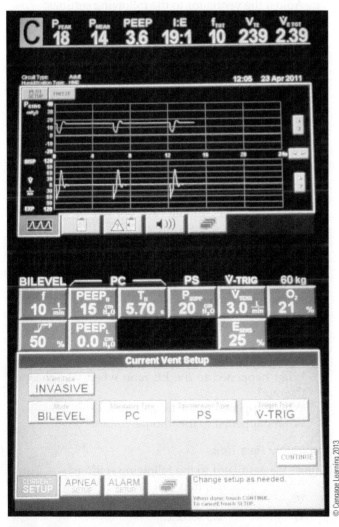

Figure 26-9 The Nellcor Puritan Bennett 840 GUI screen

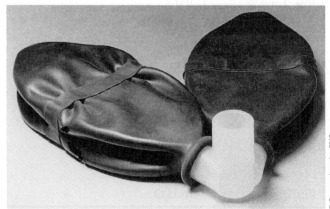

Figure 26-10 Two test lungs assembled for use during the practice procedures

Volume Control Plus (VC+)

To complete the volume control plus (VC+) practice activities, perform the following steps:

1. From the Patient Setup screen, enter an ideal body weight (IBW) of 50 kg, and press "Continue."
2. From the "New Patient Setup" screen, touch "Volume Control" (VC) and turn the adjustment knob clockwise until "VC+" is highlighted, then press "Continue."
3. The VC+ setup screen allows you to select the settings listed in Figure 26-11.

Using the upper monitoring portion of the screen, record the following: peak pressure, PEEP, I:E ratio, rate, exhaled tidal volume, minute volume.

Rate Control

1. Increase the rate to 20 breaths per minute, and press "Accept."

Using the upper monitoring portion of the screen, record the following: peak pressure, PEEP, I:E ratio, rate, exhaled tidal volume, minute volume.

2. Decrease the rate to 5 breaths per minute, and press "Accept."

Using the upper monitoring portion of the screen, record the following: peak pressure, PEEP, I:E ratio, rate, exhaled tidal volume, minute volume.

Questions

A. What happened to the peak pressure?
B. What happened to the I:E ratio when you changed the rate?
C. What happened to the tidal volume?
D. What happened to the minute volume?

Tidal Volume Control

Set the ventilator to the following settings:

f	12/min
V_T	400 mL

Parameter	Setting
f(rate)	1–33 breaths/min
Tidal Vol (V_T)	150–750 mL
Rise Time %	1–100%
Insp Time (T_I)	0.9–2.5 seconds
Flow sensitivity	0.2–20 L/min
O_2	21–100%
PEEP	0–33 cm H_2O

Set the ventilator to the following settings:

f	12/min
V_T	400 mL
T_I	0.8 seconds
Rise Time %	50%
Flow Sens	3 L/min
O_2%	21%
PEEP	5 cm H_2O

Figure 26-11   Volume control plus (VC+) settings

T_I	0.8 second
Rise Time %	50%
Flow Sens	3 L/min
O_2%	21%
PEEP	5 cm H_2O

Complete the following steps:

1. Set the tidal volume control to 700 mL.

Using the upper monitoring portion of the screen, record the following: peak pressure, PEEP, I:E ratio, rate, exhaled tidal volume, minute volume.

2. Decrease the tidal volume to 300 mL.

Using the upper monitoring portion of the screen, record the following: peak pressure, PEEP, I:E ratio, rate, exhaled tidal volume, minute volume.

Questions

A. What happened to the peak pressure?
B. What happened to the I:E ratio when you changed the rate?
C. What happened to the tidal volume?
D. What happened to the minute volume?

Inspiratory Time

1. Adjust the ventilator to the following settings:

f	12/min
V_T	400 mL
T_I	0.4 second
Rise Time %	50%
Flow Sens	3 L/min
O_2%	21%
PEEP	5 cm H2O

Using the upper monitoring portion of the screen, record the following: peak pressure, PEEP, I:E ratio, rate, exhaled tidal volume, minute volume.

2. Change the inspiratory time to 0.8 second.

Using the upper monitoring portion of the screen, record the following: peak pressure, PEEP, I:E ratio, rate, exhaled tidal volume, minute volume.

3. Change the inspiratory time to 2.3 seconds.

Using the upper monitoring portion of the screen, record the following: peak pressure, PEEP, I:E ratio, rate, exhaled tidal volume, minute volume.

Questions

A. What happened to the peak pressure?
B. What happened to the I:E ratio when you changed the rate?
C. What happened to the tidal volume?
D. What happened to the minute volume?

Inspiratory Rise Time

Adjust the ventilator to the following settings:

f	12/min
V_T	400 mL
T_I	0.8 second

Rise Time %   50%
Flow Sens   3 L/min
O_2%   21%
PEEP   5 cm H_2O

Complete the following steps:

1. Set the inspiratory rise time to 25%.

Using the upper monitoring portion of the screen, record the following: peak pressure, PEEP, I:E ratio, rate, exhaled tidal volume, minute volume.

2. Set the inspiratory rise time to 50%.

Using the upper monitoring portion of the screen, record the following: peak pressure, PEEP, I:E ratio, rate, exhaled tidal volume, minute volume.

3. Set the inspiratory rise time to 75%.

Question:

What did you notice about breath delivery as the rise time % changed?

Flow Triggering

Touch the "Vent Setup" soft key and select "Flow triggering" ($\dot{V}$ Trigger).

Adjust the ventilator to the following settings in volume control mode:

f   12/min
V_T 400 mL
T_I 0.8 second
Rise Time %   50%
Flow Sens   3 L/min
O_2%   21%
PEEP   5 cm H_2O

1. Attach a mouthpiece to the patient wye and attempt to initiate a breath.

2. Set the sensitivity control to 4 L/min and initiate a breath. Observe the flow time curve on the monitoring screen or the pressure volume loop. Adjust the screen scale to expand the scale, making it easier to observe pressure changes. Note the display in the upper left corner of the "Monitored Data" section of the display screen.

3. Adjust the sensitivity control to 8 L/min and initiate a breath. Observe the flow time curve on the monitoring screen or the pressure volume loop. Adjust the screen scale to expand the scale, making it easier to observe pressure changes. Note the display in the upper left corner of the "Monitored Data" section of the display screen.
    a. Record what threshold is met when the ventilator cycled on.
    b. Observe the monitoring screen for any changes in ventilatory (patient) parameters.

Questions

A. When you were able to initiate an assisted breath, what event(s) occurred?
B. What breath type was momentarily displayed when you triggered a breath?

C. Where would you want to set the sensitivity control for assist-control mode?

BILEVEL VENTILATION

From the Ventilator Setup screen, touch the "Mode" button and rotate the knob on the lower right of the GUI interface until "Bilevel" has been selected. Press "Continue," and the Bilevel Setup screen will appear. Adjust the ventilator to the following settings:

Rate (f)   12/min
Inspiratory Rise Time   50%
High PEEP ($PEEP_H$)   15 cm H_2O
Low PEEP ($PEEP_L$)   5 cm H_2O
Time High (T_H)   1 second
Pressure Support   0 cm H_2O
Flow Sensitivity   3 L/min
Expiratory Sensitivity   25%
Oxygen Percent   21%

Once you have established these settings, using the upper monitoring portion of the screen, record the following: peak pressure, PEEP, I:E ratio, rate, exhaled tidal volume, minute volume.

Rate Control

1. Adjust the rate control to 5 breaths per minute.

Using the upper monitoring portion of the screen, record the following: peak pressure, PEEP, I:E ratio, rate, exhaled tidal volume, minute volume.

2. Adjust the rate control to 10 breaths per minute.

Using the upper monitoring portion of the screen, record the following: peak pressure, PEEP, I:E ratio, rate, exhaled tidal volume, minute volume.

3. Adjust the rate control to 15 breaths per minute.

Using the upper monitoring portion of the screen, record the following: peak pressure, PEEP, I:E ratio, rate, exhaled tidal volume, minute volume. Once these have been recorded, change the rate control to 10 breaths per minute.

Questions

A. What happened to the peak pressure?
B. What happened to the I:E ratio when you changed the rate?
C. What happened to the minute volume?

High PEEP ($PEEP_H$) Control

Set the ventilator to the following settings:

Rate (f)   12/min
Inspiratory Rise Time   50%
High PEEP ($PEEP_H$)   15 cm H_2O
Low PEEP ($PEEP_L$)   5 cm H_2O
Time High (T_H)   1 second
Pressure Support   0 cm H_2O
Flow Sensitivity   3 L/min
Expiratory Sensitivity   25%
Oxygen Percent   21%

Using the upper monitoring portion of the screen, record the following: peak pressure, PEEP, I:E ratio, rate, exhaled tidal volume, minute volume.

1. Adjust the $PEEP_H$ control to 5 cm H_2O.

Using the upper monitoring portion of the screen, record the following: peak pressure, PEEP, I:E ratio, rate, exhaled tidal volume, minute volume.

2. Adjust the $PEEP_H$ control to 20 cm H_2O.

Using the upper monitoring portion of the screen, record the following: peak pressure, PEEP, I:E ratio, rate, exhaled tidal volume, minute volume.

Questions

A. What happened to the peak pressure?
B. What happened to the mean pressure?
C. What happened to the tidal volume as you increased $PEEP_H$?
D. What happened to the minute volume as you increased $PEEP_H$?

Time $PEEP_H$ Control

Set the ventilator to the following settings:

Rate (f)	12/min
Inspiratory Rise Time	50%
High PEEP ($PEEP_H$)	15 cm H_2O
Low PEEP ($PEEP_L$)	5 cm H_2O
Time High (T_H)	1 second
Pressure Support	0 cm H_2O
Flow Sensitivity	3 L/min
Expiratory Sensitivity	25%
Oxygen Percent	21%

Using the upper monitoring portion of the screen, record the following: peak pressure, PEEP, I:E ratio, rate, exhaled tidal volume, minute volume.

1. Adjust the $PEEP_H$ control to 0.5 second.

Using the upper monitoring portion of the screen, record the following: peak pressure, PEEP, I:E ratio, rate, exhaled tidal volume, minute volume.

2. Adjust the $PEEP_H$ control to 2 seconds.

Using the upper monitoring portion of the screen, record the following: peak pressure, PEEP, I:E ratio, rate, exhaled tidal volume, minute volume.

3. Adjust the T_H control and rotate the black knob until you hear a multiple high-pitched sound. Press "Accept."

Using the upper monitoring portion of the screen, record the following: peak pressure, PEEP, I:E ratio, rate, exhaled tidal volume, minute volume.

Questions

A. What happened to the peak pressure?
B. What happened to the mean pressure?
C. What happened to the tidal volume as you increased T_H?
D. What happened to the minute volume as you increased T_H?

E. What does the software prevent you from doing when adjusting the T_H control?

Low PEEP ($PEEP_L$) Control

Set the ventilator to the following parameters:

Rate (f)	12/min
Inspiratory Rise Time	50%
High PEEP ($PEEP_H$)	20 cm H_2O
Low PEEP ($PEEP_L$)	5 cm H_2O
Time High (T_H)	1 second
Pressure Support	0 cm H_2O
Flow Sensitivity	3 L/min
Expiratory Sensitivity	25%
Oxygen Percent	21%

Using the upper monitoring portion of the screen, record the following: peak pressure, mean airway pressure, PEEP, I:E ratio, rate, exhaled tidal volume, minute volume.

1. Change the low PEEP ($PEEP_L$) to 10 cm H_2O.

Using the upper monitoring portion of the screen, record the following: peak pressure, mean airway pressure, PEEP, I:E ratio, rate, exhaled tidal volume, minute volume.

2. Change the low PEEP ($PEEP_L$) to 15 cm H_2O.

Using the upper monitoring portion of the screen, record the following: peak pressure, mean airway pressure, PEEP, I:E ratio, rate, exhaled tidal volume, minute volume.

Questions

A. What happened to the peak pressure?
B. What happened to the mean pressure?
C. What happened to the tidal volume as you increased T_L?
D. What happened to the minute volume as you increased T_L?

Pressure Support

Set the ventilator to the following parameters:

Rate (f)	12/min
Inspiratory Rise Time	50%
High PEEP ($PEEP_H$)	15 cm H_2O
Low PEEP ($PEEP_L$)	5 cm H_2O
Time High (T_H)	1 second
Pressure Support	0 cm H_2O
Flow Sensitivity	3 L/min
Expiratory Sensitivity	25%
Oxygen Percent	21%

Using the upper monitoring portion of the screen, record the following: peak pressure, mean airway pressure, PEEP, I:E ratio, rate, exhaled tidal volume, minute volume.

1. Add 5 cm H_2O of pressure support.
2. Simulate a spontaneous breath by expanding the test lung to create subambient pressure.

Using the upper monitoring portion of the screen, record the following: peak pressure, mean airway pressure, PEEP, I:E ratio, rate, exhaled tidal volume, minute volume. Observe the pressure-time scalar waveform.

Questions

A. What happened to the peak pressure?
B. What happened to the mean airway pressure?
C. What happened to the minute volume?
D. When did you see pressure support applied?
E. What did you observe in the upper left portion of the GUI screen during your spontaneous efforts?

Practice Activities: SIMV

To perform the SIMV practice activities, complete the following steps:

1. Touch the "Vent Setup" button at the lower left of the GUI screen.

2. Touch the "Mode" button, and then rotate the black knob at the lower right of the control panel until "SIMV" is highlighted.

3. Press "Continue" then press "Accept."

4. Touch the "Mandatory Type" button, and then rotate the black knob until "Volume Control" (VC) is highlighted. Press "Continue" and then press "Accept." Set the ventilator to the following parameters:

Rate	10/min
Tidal Volume	400 mL
Flow (V_{MAX})	60 L/min
Insp. Rise Time	40%
Insp. Plateau	0.0 second
Pressure Support	0 cm H_2O
Flow Sensitivity	3 L/min
Expiratory Sensitivity	25%
Oxygen Percent	21%
PEEP	0 cm H_2O

Using the upper monitoring portion of the screen, record the following: peak pressure, mean airway pressure, PEEP, I:E ratio, rate, exhaled tidal volume, minute volume.

1. Simulate spontaneous breathing by expanding the test lung's bellows to simulate inspiratory efforts. Observe the pressure-time and flow-time scalar waveforms.

2. Set the rate control to 5 breaths per minute. Simulate a respiratory rate of 20 by expanding the test lung's bellows.

Using the upper monitoring portion of the screen, record the following: peak pressure, mean airway pressure, PEEP, I:E ratio, rate, exhaled tidal volume, minute volume. Observe the pressure-time and flow-time scalar waveforms.

Questions

A. What happened to the peak pressure?
B. What happened to the tidal volume (spontaneous)?
C. What happened to the minute volume?
D. What did you observe in the upper left portion of the GUI screen during your spontaneous efforts?

3. Add 10 cm H_2O of pressure support and simulate spontaneous breathing.

Using the upper monitoring portion of the screen, record the following: peak pressure, mean airway pressure, PEEP, I:E ratio, rate, exhaled tidal volume, minute volume. Observe the pressure-time and flow-time scalar waveforms.

Questions

A. What happened to the peak pressure?
B. What happened to the tidal volume (spontaneous)?
C. What happened to the minute volume?
D. When did you see the application of pressure support?
E. What did you observe in the upper left portion of the GUI screen during your spontaneous efforts?

4. Add 5 cm H_2O of PEEP.

Using the upper monitoring portion of the screen, record the following: peak pressure, mean airway pressure, PEEP, I:E ratio, rate, exhaled tidal volume, minute volume. Observe the pressure-time and flow-time scalar waveforms.

Question:

A. What happened to the baseline pressure?

Pressure Control with SIMV

Make the following settings changes on the ventilator:

1. Touch the "Vent Setup" button at the lower left of the GUI screen.

2. Touch the "Mode" button, and then rotate the black knob at the lower right of the control panel until "SIMV" is highlighted.

3. Press "Continue" then press "Accept."

4. Touch the "Mandatory Type" button, and then rotate the black knob until "Pressure Control" (PC) is highlighted. Press "Continue" and then press "Accept." Set the ventilator to the following settings:

Rate	10 breaths per minute
Inspiratory Pressure	15 cm H_2O
Inspiratory Time	0.8 second
Inspiratory Rise Time	40%
Pressure Support	0 cm H_2O
Flow Sensitivity	3 L/min
Expiratory Sensitivity	25%
Oxygen Percent	21%
PEEP	0 cm H_2O

1. Simulate spontaneous breathing by expanding the test lung's bellows to simulate inspiratory efforts.

Using the upper monitoring portion of the screen, record the following: peak pressure, mean airway pressure, PEEP, I:E ratio, rate, exhaled tidal volume, minute volume. Observe the pressure-time and flow-time scalar waveforms.

2. Set the rate control to 5 breaths per minute. Simulate a respiratory rate of 20 by expanding the test lung's bellows.

Using the upper monitoring portion of the screen, record the following: peak pressure, mean airway pressure, PEEP, I:E ratio, rate, exhaled tidal volume, minute volume. Observe the pressure-time and flow-time scalar waveforms.

Questions

A. What happened to the peak pressure?
B. What happened to the tidal volume (spontaneous)?
C. What happened to the minute volume?
D. What did you observe in the upper left portion of the GUI screen during your spontaneous efforts?

3. Add 10 cm H_2O of pressure support and simulate spontaneous breathing.

Using the upper monitoring portion of the screen, record the following: peak pressure, mean airway pressure, PEEP, I:E ratio, rate, exhaled tidal volume, minute volume. Observe the pressure-time and flow-time scalar waveforms.

Questions

A. What happened to the peak pressure?
B. What happened to the tidal volume (spontaneous)?
C. What happened to the minute volume?
D. When did you see the application of pressure support?
E. What did you observe in the upper left portion of the GUI screen during your spontaneous efforts?

4. Add 5 cm H_2O of PEEP.

Using the upper monitoring portion of the screen, record the following: peak pressure, mean airway pressure, PEEP, I:E ratio, rate, exhaled tidal volume, minute volume. Observe the pressure-time and flow-time scalar waveforms.

Question:

A. What happened to the baseline pressure?

TUBE COMPENSATION

Make the following settings changes on the ventilator:

1. Touch the "Vent Setup" button at the lower left of the GUI screen.
2. Touch the "Mode" button, and then rotate the black knob at the lower right of the control panel until "SIMV" is highlighted.

3. Press "Continue" then press "Accept."
4. Touch the "Mandatory Type" button, and then rotate the black knob until "Pressure Control" (PC) is highlighted. Press "Continue" and then press "Accept."
5. Touch the "Spontaneous Type" button and rotate the knob until "Tube Compensation" (TC) is highlighted then press "Continue" and press "Accept."

Set the ventilator to the following settings:

Rate	10 breaths per minute
Inspiratory Pressure	15 cm H_2O
Inspiratory Time	0.8 second
Inspiratory Rise Time	40%
% Support	75%
Flow Sensitivity	3 L/min
Expiratory Sensitivity	25%
Oxygen Percent	21%
PEEP	0 cm H_2O
Tube ID	8 mm
Tube Type	ET (Rotate the knob until "ET" is highlighted, then touch the button again.)
Inspired V_T Alarm	Touch the lower right "V_{TI}" button and rotate to 1000 mL, then touch the button once again.
Peak Pressure Alarm	Touch the "P_{PEAK}" button and rotate it until 35 cm H_2O is displayed, then touch the button again.

Once all settings have been completed, press "Accept."

1. Simulate spontaneous breathing by expanding the test lung's bellows to simulate inspiratory efforts.

Using the upper monitoring portion of the screen, record the following: peak pressure, mean airway pressure, PEEP, I:E ratio, rate, exhaled tidal volume, minute volume. Observe the pressure-time and flow-time scalar waveforms.

2. Change the % support to 25%.

Using the upper monitoring portion of the screen, record the following: peak pressure, mean airway pressure, PEEP, I:E ratio, rate, exhaled tidal volume, minute volume. Observe the pressure-time and flow-time scalar waveforms.

Question:

A. What did you observe on the scalar waveforms and numerical data?

PROPORTIONAL ASSIST VENTILATION (PAV) PRACTICE ACTIVITIES

Make the following settings changes on the ventilator:

1. Touch the "Vent Setup" button at the lower left of the GUI screen.

2. Touch the "Mode" button, and then rotate the black knob at the lower right of the control panel until "Spont" is highlighted.
3. Touch the "Mandatory Type" button, and then rotate the black knob until "Proportional Assist Ventilation" (PA) is highlighted. Press "Continue."

Tidal Volume (Mandatory)	400 mL
Peak Flow	60 L/min
Inspiratory Plateau	0 second
Waveform	Ramp
PA % Support	75%
Flow Sensitivity	3 L/min
Expiratory Sensitivity	3 L/min
Oxygen Percent	21%
PEEP	0 cm H_2O
Tube ID	8 mm
Tube Type	ET (Rotate the knob until "ET" is highlighted, then touch the button again.)
Inspired V_T Alarm	Touch the lower right "V_{TI}" button and rotate to 1000 mL, then touch the button once again.
Peak Pressure Alarm	Touch the "P_{PEAK}" button and rotate it until 35 cm H_2O is displayed, then touch the button again.

Once all settings have been completed, press "Accept."

1. Simulate spontaneous breathing by expanding the test lung's bellows, simulating spontaneous efforts. The inspired tidal volume and peak pressure alarms may need to be readjusted as well as minute ventilation and tidal volume alarms from the alarm setup page.

Using the upper monitoring portion of the screen, record the following: peak pressure, mean airway pressure, PEEP, I:E ratio, rate, exhaled tidal volume, minute volume. Observe the pressure-time and flow-time scalar waveforms.

2. Change the % support to 25%.

Using the upper monitoring portion of the screen, record the following: peak pressure, mean airway pressure, PEEP, I:E ratio, rate, exhaled tidal volume, minute volume. Observe the pressure-time and flow-time scalar waveforms.

Questions

A. What did you observe on the screen when the support was changed?
B. As a patient, which do you think would be the most comfortable? You might wish to attach a mouthpiece and bacteria filter to experience the difference.

VOLUME SUPPORT PRACTICE ACTIVITIES

Make the following settings changes on the ventilator:

1. Touch the "Vent Setup" button at the lower left of the GUI screen.
2. Touch the "Mode" button, and then rotate the black knob at the lower right of the control panel until "Spont" is highlighted.
3. Touch the "Mandatory Type" button, and then rotate the black knob until "Proportional Assist Ventilation" (PA) is highlighted. Press "Continue."

Tidal Volume (Mandatory)	500 mL
Peak Flow	60 L/min
Rise Time %	50%
Waveform	Ramp
$V_{T SUPP}$	300 mL
Flow Sensitivity	3 L/min
Expiratory Sensitivity	25%
Oxygen Percent	21%
PEEP	0 cm H_2O
Inspired V_T Alarm	Touch the lower right "V_{TI}" button and rotate to 1000 mL, then touch the button once again.
Peak Pressure Alarm	Touch the "P_{PEAK}" button and rotate it until 35 cm H_2O is displayed, then touch the button again.

1. Simulate spontaneous breathing by expanding the bellows of the test lung, simulating inspiratory efforts over several breaths.
2. Observe the measured parameters (top line) and the graphical waveform display.
3. Increase the $V_{T SUPP}$ to 500 mL, and observe the measured parameters and the graphical waveform display.

Questions

A. What happened to the tidal volume delivery over several breaths?
B. What happened to the tidal volume when you increased the $V_{T SUPP}$ from 300 to 500 mL?
C. What did you observe on the graphics display?

Practice Activities: Maquet SERVO-i Ventilator

Circuit Assembly

Figure 26-12 shows the Maquet SERVO-i ventilator assembled and ready for use. To prepare the ventilator for use, follow the steps listed next.

1. Install a bacteria inspiratory filter on the patient outlet located on the right side of the patient unit.
2. Connect a short length of 22 mm tubing (18 inches) between the bacteria filter and the humidifier.
3. Connect the inspiratory limb of the patient circuit to the humidifier outlet.
4. Connect the expiratory limb of the patient circuit to the expiratory port on the right side of the patient unit.
5. Attach the patient circuit to the flex arm at its midpoint by clamping the ball fitting on the circuit to the flex arm.

Testing the Ventilator before Use

Pre-use Check

The pre-use check tests the function of the microprocessor control system; measures internal leakage; tests the pressure transducers, O_2 cell/sensor, flow transducers, and safety valve; measures circuit leakage; and calculates circuit compliance. It is recommended to perform a pre-use check prior to connecting the ventilator to a patient or whenever a patient circuit is changed. To perform the pre-use check, complete the following steps:

1. Connect the power cord to a 110 volt 60 Hz outlet.
2. Connect the air and oxygen supply lines to 50 psi sources.
3. Turn the ventilator power switch to the "ON" position.
4. From the Standby screen, select "Yes" to the question "Do you want to start Pre-use check?"
5. Connect the blue 22 mm test tube between the ventilator outlet and exhalation inlet on the right side of the patient unit.
6. Follow the onscreen prompts. You will be asked to perform the following:
   a. Disconnect the ventilator from AC power.
   b. Reconnect the ventilator to AC power.
   c. Connect a patient circuit including the humidifier.
   d. Block and unblock the patient wye.
7. Once the circuit compliance is calculated, you will have the option to add compliance compensation (answer Yes) or not add it (answer No).
8. The outcome of the pre-use check will be displayed on the user interface screen.
9. Once the test is complete, press "OK" to log the pre-use check and to switch the ventilator back to Standby mode.

Using the Maquet SERVO-i User Interface

The Maquet SERVO-i user interface consists of a large screen, four direct access knobs below the screen, several fixed soft keys, and a rotary dial located at the lower right of the user interface that can be turned clockwise, turned counterclockwise (to increase or decrease values), and then pushed to select the desired value.

Activities

To complete these practice activities, it is recommended that you use a lung analog/simulator such as an SMS "Manley" lung simulator or an IngMar Medical Quick Lung or Demonstration Lung Model. These devices or other similar devices allow the operator to alter resistance and compliance, simulating changes in patient condition.

If these devices are not available, a patient wye and two test lungs may be used as shown in Figure 26-10. Exercise caution. Volumes and pressures may exceed the limits of the test lungs. Resistance may be altered by adapting different sizes of endotracheal tubes, and compliance may be altered by the addition of rubber bands to the test lungs.

Lung Simulator Setup

If you are using an SMS ("Manley") lung simulator, connect one spring for compliance, set the resistance control to zero, and rotate the leak control fully clockwise, eliminating any leaks. Attach the patient wye to the inlet of the SMS lung simulator.

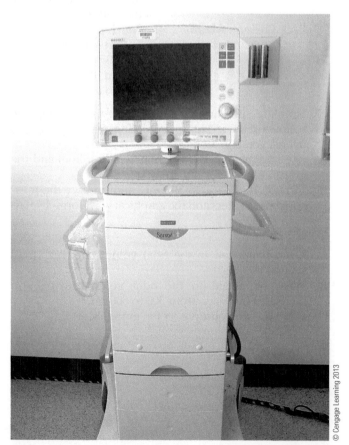

Figure 26-12 The Maquet SERVO-i assembled and ready for use

© Cengage Learning 2013

If you are using an IngMar Medical Demonstration Lung Model, rotate all of the compliance springs fully clockwise, adjust the resistance controls to "OFF," and adjust both the ET Leak and System Leak controls to the "OFF" position. Attach the patient wye to the inlet of the Demonstration Lung Model.

When completing these activities, manipulate only one control at a time and note the result of each activity with manipulation of the controls. Answer the questions that follow each of the activities.

Pressure Regulated Volume Control

Set the ventilator to the following settings:

1. Press the "Adult" button at the bottom center of the screen.
2. Press the "Volume Control" button at the top left of the screen.
3. A new screen will open. Press the "Volume Control" button on the upper left portion of the new screen.
4. Select "Pressure Regulated Volume Control (PRVC)." A new window will open showing the available ventilator settings.
5. Make the following selections from the Set Ventilation Mode screen. Press the desired setting, and rotate the knob on the lower right side of the user interface to change the settings. Then press the button again to capture the desired change.

a.	Tidal Volume	450 mL
b.	Resp. Rate	10/min
c.	PEEP	0 cm H_2O
d.	O_2 %	21%
e.	Ti	0.9 second
f.	T insp. Rise	0.2 second
g.	Trigg. Sensitivity	3 L/min

If you make an error, simply touch the button you wish to change, rotate the knob to enter the correct setting, and complete the change by touching the button once again. Once the settings are complete, press the "Accept" button on the lower right of the user interface screen. Then press the "Start/Stop (Standby)" soft key located at the lower left of the user interface adjacent to the four direct access knobs on the lower part of the interface.

Patient Monitoring

The user interface screen is divided into two large sections. Scalar waveforms for pressure, flow, and volume occupy most of the screen display. To the right of the waveform display is a section devoted to patient-monitored parameters. The basic screen includes peak pressure, respiratory rate, and minute volume with inspired and expired tidal volumes being displayed in the same window.

Pressing the "Additional Values" button at the lower right of the screen opens additional monitoring parameters including peak, plateau, mean and PEEP pressures, respiratory rate, O_2%, inspiratory time, I:E ratio, minute volumes (inspired and exhaled), and tidal volumes (inspired and exhaled).

Tidal Volume Control

1. Simulate spontaneous breathing by expanding the bellows of the test lung, simulating spontaneous efforts. Observe the graphics screen.

Once these settings have been established and the ventilator is operating in PRVC mode, record the following ventilatory (patient) parameters.
   a. Measure the inspiratory time. (Press the "Additional Values" button.)
   b. Measure the peak inspiratory pressure.
   c. Record the tidal volume.
   d. Record the minute ventilation.
   e. Record the I:E ratio. (Press the "Additional Values" button.)
2. Increase the tidal volume to 700 mL.
3. Simulate spontaneous ventilation again and observe the graphics display.

Once these settings have been established and the ventilator is operating in PRVC mode, record the following ventilatory (patient) parameters:
   a. Measure the inspiratory time. (Press the "Additional Values" button.)
   b. Measure the peak inspiratory pressure.
   c. Record the tidal volume.
   d. Record the minute ventilation.
   e. Record the I:E ratio. (Press the "Additional Values" button.)

Questions

A. How did tidal volume, pressures, and minute ventilation change?
B. What did you observe on the screen when you simulated spontaneous breathing?
C. How did the ventilator respond to your spontaneous efforts?
D. How did the ventilator increase the tidal volume?

Volume Support Ventilation (VSV)

To complete the VSV activities, complete the following steps:

1. Press the "PRVC" button at the top left of the screen.
2. A new screen will open. Press the "PRVC" button at the upper left portion of the new screen, and a drop down menu will appear.
3. Press the "Volume Support" button at the lower left part of the new screen.
4. A window will open providing the settings that can be made in this mode. Set the ventilator to the following settings:

Tidal Volume	500 mL
PEEP	0 cm H_2O
O_2 Conc.	21%
Inspiratory Rise Time	0.2 second
Trigger Flow	3 L/min
Insp. Cycle Off	25%

Once you have completed the ventilator setup, press "Accept" at the lower right portion of the screen.

5. Simulate spontaneous ventilation by expanding the bellows of the test lung, simulating spontaneous efforts.
6. Using the user interface screen, monitor the following:
   a. Measure the inspiratory time. (Press the "Additional Values" button.)
   b. Measure the peak inspiratory pressure.
   c. Record the tidal volume.
   d. Record the minute ventilation.
7. Increase the tidal volume to 700 mL.
8. Using the user interface screen, measure the following:
   a. Measure the inspiratory time. (Press the "Additional Values" button.)
   b. Measure the peak inspiratory pressure.
   c. Record the tidal volume.
   d. Record the minute ventilation.

Questions

A. How did tidal volume, pressures, and minute ventilation change?
B. What did you observe on the screen when you simulated spontaneous breathing?
C. How did the ventilator respond to your spontaneous efforts?
D. How did the ventilator increase the tidal volume?

Pressure Control Inverse Ratio Ventilation (PCIRV)

Test Lung Setup

If you are using an SMS ("Manley") lung simulator, connect one spring for compliance, set the resistance control to zero, and rotate the leak control fully clockwise, eliminating any leaks. Attach the patient wye to the inlet of the SMS lung simulator.

If you are using an IngMar Medical Demonstration Lung Model, rotate all of the compliance springs fully clockwise, adjust the resistance controls to "OFF," and adjust both the ET Leak and System Leak controls to the "OFF" position. Attach the patient wye to the inlet of the Demonstration Lung Model.

When completing these activities, manipulate only one control at a time and note the result of each activity with manipulation of the controls. Answer the questions that follow each of the activities.

Initial Ventilator Settings

Once you have completed a pre-use check and patient circuit test, complete the following steps:

1. Press the "Adult" icon on the lower portion of the user interface screen.
2. Press the "Volume Control" button at the top left of the user interface screen.
3. A new screen will open; press the "Volume Control" button at the top left of the newly opened screen.
4. Press "Pressure Control" and a new screen will open with the allowed settings. Set the ventilator to the following settings:

PC above PEEP	20 cm H$_2$O
Resp. Rate	10 per minute
PEEP	5 cm H$_2$O
Insp. Time	1 second
Insp. Rise Time	0.2 second
Trigger Flow	3 L/min

5. Once these settings have been established, press the "Start/Stop" (Standby) soft key at the lower left of the user interface module.

Using the monitoring screen, press "Additional Values" and record the following:
   a. Peak pressure
   b. Mean airway pressure
   c. Inspiratory time
   d. I:E ratio
   e. Tidal volume (exhaled)
   f. Minute ventilation

6. Press the "Pressure Control" button at the top left of the screen to open the window to adjust the ventilator settings.
7. Set the inspiratory time to 2 seconds, and press "Accept."

Using the monitoring screen, press "Additional Values" and record the following:
   a. Peak pressure
   b. Mean airway pressure
   c. Inspiratory time
   d. I:E ratio
   e. Tidal volume (exhaled)
   f. Minute ventilation

8. Press the "Pressure Control" button at the top left of the screen to open the window to adjust the ventilator settings.
9. Set the inspiratory time to 4 seconds, and press "Accept." You will need to touch the "Inspiratory Time" button once again after the ventilator beeps to set the time to 4 seconds.

Using the monitoring screen, press "Additional Values" and record the following:
   a. Peak pressure
   b. Mean airway pressure
   c. Inspiratory time
   d. I:E ratio
   e. Tidal volume (exhaled)
   f. Minute ventilation

Questions

A. What happened to the peak pressure?
B. What happened to the mean airway pressure?
C. What happened to the I:E ratio?
D. What happened to the minute ventilation?

Bi-Vent

Initial Ventilator Settings

Once you have completed a pre-use check and patient circuit test, complete the following steps:

1. Press the "Adult" icon on the lower portion of the user interface screen.

2. Press the "Volume Control" button at the top left of the user interface screen.

3. A new screen will open; press the "Volume Control" button at the top left of the newly opened screen.

4. Press "Bi-Vent" and a new screen will open with the allowed settings. Set the ventilator to the following settings:

P High	12 cm H_2O
PEEP Low	6 cm H_2O
O_2 Conc	21%
Time High	4 seconds
Time PEEP	2 seconds
Insp. Rise Time	1 second
Insp. Cycle Off	25%
P High +	0 cm H_2O
PS +	0 cm H_2O

Once the settings are established, press "Accept" in the lower right part of the user interface screen.

Using the monitoring screen, press "Additional Values" and record the following:
   a. Peak pressure
   b. Mean airway pressure
   c. Inspiratory time
   d. I:E ratio
   e. Tidal volume (exhaled)
   f. Minute ventilation

Time High Control

1. Set the Time High to 2 seconds.

Using the monitoring screen, press "Additional Values" and record the following:
   a. Peak pressure
   b. Mean airway pressure
   c. Inspiratory time
   d. I:E ratio
   e. Tidal volume (exhaled)
   f. Minute ventilation

2. Set the Time High to 6 seconds.

Using the monitoring screen, press "Additional Values" and record the following:
   a. Peak pressure
   b. Mean airway pressure
   c. Inspiratory time
   d. I:E ratio
   e. Tidal volume (exhaled)
   f. Minute ventilation

Questions

A. What happened to the peak pressure?
B. What happened to the I:E ratio when you changed the Time High control?
C. What happened to the minute volume?
D. What happened to the rate when the Time High control decreased?

P High Control

Press the "Bi-Vent" button to access the Settings screen. Set the ventilator to the following settings:

P High	12 cm H_2O
PEEP Low	6 cm H_2O
O_2 Conc	21%
Time High	4 seconds
Time PEEP	2 seconds
Insp. Rise Time	1 second
Insp. Cycle Off	25%
P High +	0 cm H_2O
PS +	0 cm H_2O

Using the monitoring screen, press "Additional Values" and record the following:
   a. Peak pressure
   b. Mean airway pressure
   c. Inspiratory time
   d. I:E ratio
   e. Tidal volume (exhaled)
   f. Minute ventilation

1. Set the P High control to 8 cm H_2O.

Using the monitoring screen, press "Additional Values" and record the following:
   a. Peak pressure
   b. Mean airway pressure
   c. Inspiratory time
   d. I:E ratio
   e. Tidal volume (exhaled)
   f. Minute ventilation

2. Set the P High control to 20 cm H_2O.

Using the monitoring screen, press "Additional Values" and record the following:
   a. Peak pressure
   b. Mean airway pressure
   c. Inspiratory time
   d. I:E ratio
   e. Tidal volume (exhaled)
   f. Minute ventilation

Questions

A. What happened to the peak pressure?
B. What happened to the mean pressure?
C. What happened to the tidal volume as you increased the P High control?
D. What happened to the minute volume as you increased P High control?

Time PEEP Control

Press the "Bi-Vent" button to access the Settings screen. Set the ventilator to the following settings:

P High	15 cm H_2O
PEEP Low	5 cm H_2O
O_2 Conc	21%
Time High	4 seconds
Time PEEP	2 seconds
Insp. Rise Time	1 second
Insp. Cycle Off	25%
P High +	0 cm H_2O
PS +	0 cm H_2O

1. Set the Time PEEP to 1 second.

Using the monitoring screen, press "Additional Values" and record the following:
   a. Peak pressure
   b. Mean airway pressure

c. Inspiratory time
d. I:E ratio
e. Tidal volume (exhaled)
f. Minute ventilation

2. Set the Time PEEP control to 4 seconds.

Using the monitoring screen, press "Additional Values" and record the following:
   a. Peak pressure
   b. Mean airway pressure
   c. Inspiratory time
   d. I:E ratio
   e. Tidal volume (exhaled)
   f. Minute ventilation

Questions

A. What happened to the peak pressure?
B. What happened to the mean pressure?
C. What happened to the tidal volume as you increased the Time PEEP?
D. What happened to the minute volume as you increased the Time PEEP?
E. What happened to the rate as you adjusted the Time PEEP?

PEEP Low Control

Press the "Bi-Vent" button to access the Settings screen. Set the ventilator to the following settings:

P High	20 cm H$_2$O
PEEP Low	5 cm H$_2$O
O$_2$ Conc	21%
Time High	4 seconds
Time PEEP	2 seconds
Insp. Rise Time	1 second
Insp. Cycle Off	25%
P High +	0 cm H$_2$O
PS +	0 cm H$_2$O

Using the monitoring screen, press "Additional Values" and record the following:
   a. Peak pressure
   b. Mean airway pressure
   c. Inspiratory time
   d. I:E ratio
   e. Tidal volume (exhaled)
   f. Minute ventilation

1. Change the PEEP Low pressure to 10 cm H$_2$O.

Using the monitoring screen, press "Additional Values" and record the following:
   a. Peak pressure
   b. Mean airway pressure
   c. Inspiratory time
   d. I:E ratio
   e. Tidal volume (exhaled)
   f. Minute ventilation

2. Change the PEEP Low pressure to 15 cm H$_2$O.

Using the monitoring screen, press "Additional Values" and record the following:
   a. Peak pressure
   b. Mean airway pressure

c. Inspiratory time
d. I:E ratio
e. Tidal volume (exhaled)
f. Minute ventilation

Questions

A. What happened to the peak pressure?
B. What happened to the mean pressure?
C. What happened to the tidal volume as you changed the PEEP Low control?
D. What happened to the minute volume as you changed the PEEP Low control?

Pressure Support

The SERVO-i can provide pressure-supported breaths during spontaneous breathing at both the high- and low-pressure levels. Press the "Bi-Vent" button to access the Settings screen. Set the ventilator to the following settings:

P High	15 cm H$_2$O
PEEP Low	5 cm H$_2$O
O$_2$ Conc	21%
Time High	4 seconds
Time PEEP	2 seconds
Insp. Rise Time	1 second
Insp. Cycle Off	25%
P High +	0 cm H$_2$O
PS +	0 cm H$_2$O

1. Simulate spontaneous ventilation by expanding the test lung's bellows, simulating inspiratory efforts.

Using the monitoring screen, press "Additional Values" and record the following:
   a. Peak pressure
   b. Mean airway pressure
   c. Inspiratory time
   d. I:E ratio
   e. Tidal volume (exhaled)
   f. Minute ventilation

2. Set the P High + to 8 cm H$_2$O, and simulate spontaneous breathing.

Using the monitoring screen, press "Additional Values" and record the following:
   a. Peak pressure
   b. Mean airway pressure
   c. Inspiratory time
   d. I:E ratio
   e. Tidal volume (exhaled)
   f. Minute ventilation

3. Return the P High + control to 0 cm H$_2$O.
4. Set the PS + control to 5 cm H$_2$O and simulate spontaneous breathing.

Using the monitoring screen, press "Additional Values" and record the following:
   a. Peak pressure
   b. Mean airway pressure
   c. Inspiratory time
   d. I:E ratio
   e. Tidal volume (exhaled)
   f. Minute ventilation

Questions

A. How did the values change with the addition of pressure support?
B. What did you observe on the graphical display during spontaneous breathing?

Volume SIMV Practice Activities

Initial Ventilator Settings

Once you have completed a pre-use check and patient circuit test, complete the following steps:

1. Press the "Adult" icon on the lower portion of the user interface screen.
2. Press the "Volume Control" button at the top left of the user interface screen.
3. A new screen will open. Press the "Volume Control" button at the top left of the newly opened screen.
4. Press the "SIMV (Vol. Contr.) + Pressure Support" button. A new window will open, providing you with the allowed ventilator settings for this mode.

Volume	400 mL
SIMV Rate	8 per minute
PEEP	5 cm H_2O
O_2 Conc	21%
Inspiratory Time	1 second
Time Pause	0.0 second
Inspiratory Pause	0.2 second
Trigger Flow	3 L/min
Insp. Cycle Off	25%
PS above PEEP	0 cm H_2O
PEEP	0 cm H_2O
Flow Trigger	1 L/min
FIO_2	21%

Once the settings have been established, press "Accept" at the lower right part of the user interface screen. Then press the "Start/Stop Standby" soft key at the lower left part of the user interface.

Using the monitoring screen, press "Additional Values" and record the following:
   a. Peak pressure
   b. Mean airway pressure
   c. Inspiratory time
   d. I:E ratio
   e. Tidal volume (exhaled)
   f. Minute ventilation

1. Simulate spontaneous breathing by expanding the bellows of the test lung, simulating spontaneous efforts. Observe the graphics screen.
2. Increase the tidal volume to 600 mL.

Using the monitoring screen, press "Additional Values" and record the following:
   a. Peak pressure
   b. Mean airway pressure
   c. Inspiratory time
   d. I:E ratio
   e. Tidal volume (exhaled)
   f. Minute ventilation

3. Simulate spontaneous ventilation again and observe the graphics display.

Questions

A. How did tidal volume, pressures, and minute ventilation change?
B. What did you observe on the user interface module (UIM) screen when you simulated spontaneous breathing?
C. How did the ventilator respond to your spontaneous efforts?

4. Add 10 cm H_2O of pressures support, and simulate spontaneous ventilation.

Using the monitoring screen, press "Additional Values" and record the following:
   a. Peak pressure
   b. Mean airway pressure
   c. Inspiratory time
   d. I:E ratio
   e. Tidal volume (exhaled)
   f. Minute ventilation

5. Add 8 cm H_2O of PEEP, and simulate spontaneous ventilation.

Using the monitoring screen, press "Additional Values" and record the following:
   a. Peak pressure
   b. Mean airway pressure
   c. Inspiratory time
   d. I:E ratio
   e. Tidal volume (exhaled)
   f. Minute ventilation

Questions

A. How did the ventilator respond to your spontaneous efforts?
B. What happened when you added PEEP?
C. What happened when you added pressure support?

Pressure SIMV Practice Activities

Initial Ventilator Settings

Once you have completed a pre-use check and patient circuit test, complete the following steps:

1. Press the "Adult" icon on the lower portion of the user interface screen.
2. Press the "Volume Control" button at the top left of the user interface screen.
3. A new screen will open. Press the "Volume Control" button at the top left of the newly opened screen.
4. Press the "SIMV (Press. Contr.) + Pressure Support" button. A new window will open, providing you with the allowed ventilator settings for this mode.

PC above PEEP	20 cm H_2O
SIMV Rate	8 per minute
Inspiratory Pressure	15 cm H_2O
Inspiratory Time	1 second

Inspiratory Rise Time 0.2 second
PS above PEEP 0 cm H_2O
Insp. Cycle Off 25%
PEEP 0 cm H_2O
Flow Trigger 3 L/min
FIO_2 21%

Using the monitoring screen, press "Additional Values" and record the following:

   a. Peak pressure
   b. Mean airway pressure
   c. Inspiratory time
   d. I:E ratio
   e. Tidal volume (exhaled)
   f. Minute ventilation

1. Simulate spontaneous breathing by expanding the bellows of the test lung, simulating spontaneous efforts. Observe the Graphics screen.
2. Increase the PC above PEEP to 25 cm H_2O.

Using the monitoring screen, press "Additional Values" and record the following:

   a. Peak pressure
   b. Mean airway pressure
   c. Inspiratory time
   d. I:E ratio
   e. Tidal volume (exhaled)
   f. Minute ventilation

3. Simulate spontaneous ventilation again and observe the graphics display.

Questions

A. How did tidal volume, pressures, and minute ventilation change?
B. What did you observe on the UIM screen when you simulated spontaneous breathing?
C. How did the ventilator respond to your spontaneous efforts?

4. Add 10 cm H_2O of PS above PEEP, and simulate spontaneous ventilation.

Using the monitoring screen, press "Additional Values" and record the following:

   a. Peak pressure
   b. Mean airway pressure
   c. Inspiratory time
   d. I:E ratio
   e. Tidal volume (exhaled)
   f. Minute ventilation

5. Add 8 cm H_2O of PEEP, and simulate spontaneous ventilation.

Using the monitoring screen, press "Additional Values" and record the following:

   a. Peak pressure
   b. Mean airway pressure
   c. Inspiratory time
   d. I:E ratio
   e. Tidal volume (exhaled)
   f. Minute ventilation

Questions

A. How did the ventilator respond to your spontaneous efforts?
B. What happened when you added PEEP?
C. What happened when you added pressure support?

Automode

Initial Ventilator Settings

Once you have completed a pre-use check and patient circuit test, complete the following steps:

1. Press the "Adult" icon on the lower portion of the user interface screen.
2. Press the "Volume Control" button at the top left of the user interface screen.
3. A new screen will open. Press the "Volume Control" button at the top left of the newly opened screen.
4. Press the "Automode" button to the right of the "Volume Control" button. A new selection of settings will be displayed. Set the ventilator to the following settings:

Tidal Volume 500 mL
Resp Rate 6/min
PEEP 5 cm H_2O
O_2 Conc 21%
Inspiratory Time 1 second
Inspiratory Pause 0.0 second
Inspiratory Rise Time 0.2 second
Trigger Flow 3 L/min
Inspiratory Cycle Off 25%
Trigger Timeout 7 seconds

Using the monitoring screen, press "Additional Values" and record the following:

   a. Peak pressure
   b. Mean airway pressure
   c. Inspiratory time
   d. I:E ratio
   e. Tidal volume (exhaled)
   f. Minute ventilation

1. Simulate spontaneous ventilation by expanding the bellows of the test lung, simulating spontaneous efforts.
2. Establish a spontaneous rate of 12 breaths per minute.

Using the monitoring screen, press "Additional Values" and record the following:

   a. Peak pressure
   b. Mean airway pressure
   c. Inspiratory time
   d. I:E ratio
   e. Tidal volume (exhaled)
   f. Minute ventilation

3. Stop your spontaneous efforts for 45 seconds. During this time:

Using the monitoring screen, press "Additional Values" and record the following:

   a. Peak pressure
   b. Mean airway pressure

c. Inspiratory time
d. I:E ratio
e. Tidal volume (exhaled)
f. Minute ventilation

4. Change the Trigger timeout setting to 10 seconds.

Using the monitoring screen, press "Additional Values" and record the following:
a. Peak pressure
b. Mean airway pressure
c. Inspiratory time
d. I:E ratio
e. Tidal volume (exhaled)
f. Minute ventilation

5. Establish a spontaneous rate of 12 breaths per minute.

Using the monitoring screen, press "Additional Values" and record the following:
a. Peak pressure
b. Mean airway pressure
c. Inspiratory time

d. I:E ratio
e. Tidal volume (exhaled)
f. Minute ventilation

6. Stop your spontaneous efforts for 45 seconds. During this time:

Using the monitoring screen, press "Additional Values" and record the following:
a. Peak pressure
b. Mean airway pressure
c. Inspiratory time
d. I:E ratio
e. Tidal volume (exhaled)
f. Minute ventilation

Questions

A. What changes did you see in pressures, minute ventilation, and tidal volume?
B. How did the ventilator respond to the apneic periods at the two different trigger timeout settings?

Practice Activities: Viasys Avea Ventilator

Circuit Assembly

Figure 26-13 shows the Viasys Avea ventilator assembled and ready for use. To prepare the ventilator for use, follow the steps listed next.

1. Attach the collection bottle to the water trap by screwing it clockwise into the receptacle in the water trap (Figure 26-14).
2. Install an exhalation filter to the upper portion of the water trap by pushing it onto the seal at the top of the water trap (Figure 26-15).
3. Align the ridge on the water trap assembly with the slot on the exhalation filter cartridge (Figure 26-16).
4. Slide the water trap/exhalation filter assembly upward into the lower right front portion of the ventilator body and rotate the locking lever to the left, holding the assembly in place (Figure 26-17).
5. Connect the expiratory limb of the patient circuit to the expiratory filter and collection vial's 22 mm fitting.
6. Attach the patient circuit to the flex arm at its midpoint by clamping the ball fitting on the circuit to the flex arm.
7. Connect an 18 inch length of 22 mm tubing between the ventilator outlet located to the right of the water trap/exhalation filter assembly and the humidifier.
8. Connect the inspiratory limb of the patient circuit to the outlet of the humidifier.
9. Connect the 50 psi air and oxygen supply lines to appropriate gas connections.
10. Connect the electrical power cord to a 115 volt 60 Hz outlet.

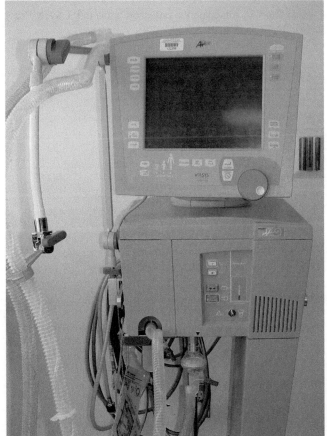

Figure 26-13 The Viasys Avea ventilator assembled and ready for use

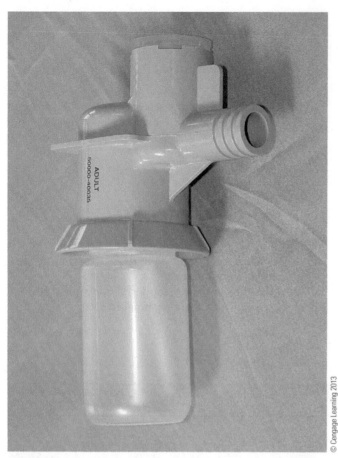

Figure 26-14 Attaching the collection bottle to the water trap assembly

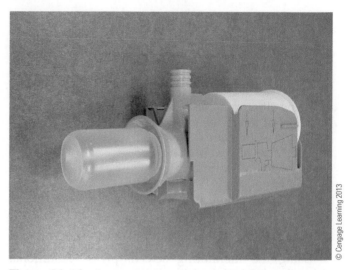

Figure 26-16 Connecting the water trap/filter assembly to the exhalation cartridge

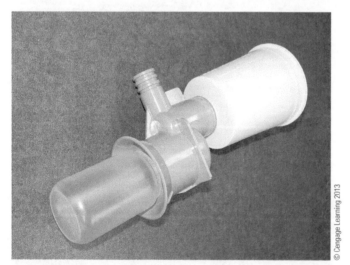

Figure 26-15 Attaching the water trap assembly to the exhalation filter

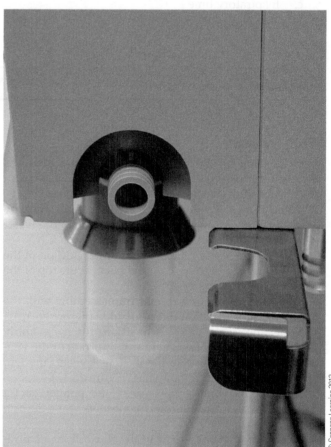

Figure 26-17 Attaching the exhalation water trap/filter assembly to the ventilator

Testing the Ventilator before Use

Power-on Self Test (POST)

Each time the power switch is turned on or if the ventilator microprocessor detects selected fault conditions, a POST is automatically executed. The POST takes only a few seconds and is transparent to the clinician. The test verifies the integrity of the microprocessor, read-only memory (ROM) and random access memory (RAM). Only if a problem is detected will a message be displayed.

Extended Systems Test (EST)

The extended systems test (EST) should only be performed prior to connecting the ventilator to a patient. The EST will perform a leak test of the patient circuit, determine circuit compliance, and perform a two-point calibration of the oxygen sensor. To perform an EST, complete the following steps:

1. Access the EST test by pressing the "EST" button on the Setup screen.
2. When instructed to remove the ventilator from the patient and block the patient wye, do so.
3. Confirm that the ventilator is off the patient and that the wye is blocked by pressing "Cont" (continue).
4. The ventilator will perform the EST, and a countdown timer will be displayed. The first portion of the test will check the circuit for leaks, calculate circuit compliance, and perform a two-point calibration of the oxygen sensor. The maximum time for this test is 90 seconds.
5. Following each test, a PASSED or FAILED message will be displayed. Once the first portion of the test is complete, When "ALL TESTS PASSED" is displayed, press the "Continue" button on the screen.
6. From the Setup screen, press "Setup Accept" to capture and retain the circuit compliance measurement.

Using the Keyboard Entry System

All functions of the Viasys Avea ventilator are controlled from the UIM shown in Figure 26-18. To enter ventilator or alarm settings, follow the "touch–turn–touch" method for entering new settings. Touch the desired value or setting you wish to change (e.g., tidal volume), and then turn the knob on the lower right side of the UIM interface until the desired value is displayed (clockwise increases, counterclockwise decreases). Touch the desired setting again or press the "Accept" button to apply the new setting. The new setting will now be displayed on the appropriate portion of the UIM screen.

Activities

To complete these practice activities, it is recommended that you use a lung analog/simulator such as an SMS "Manley" lung simulator or an IngMar Medical Quick Lung or Demonstration Lung Model. These devices or other similar devices allow the operator to alter resistance and compliance, simulating changes in patient condition.

If these devices are not available, a patient wye and two test lungs may be used as shown in Figure 26-10. Exercise caution. Volumes and pressures may exceed the limits of the test lungs. Resistance may be altered by adapting different sizes of endotracheal tubes, and compliance may be altered by the addition of rubber bands to the test lungs.

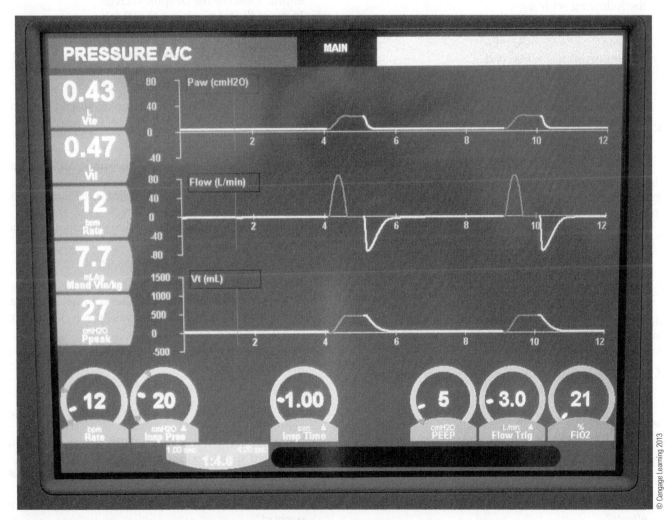

Figure 26-18 The Viasys AVEA user interface module (UIM)

Lung Simulator Setup

If you are using an SMS ("Manley") lung simulator, connect one spring for compliance, set the resistance control to zero, and rotate the leak control fully clockwise, eliminating any leaks. Attach the patient wye to the inlet of the SMS lung simulator.

If you are using an IngMar Medical Demonstration Lung Model, rotate all of the compliance springs fully clockwise, adjust the resistance controls to "OFF," and adjust both the ET Leak and System Leak controls to the "OFF" position. Attach the patient wye to the inlet of the Demonstration Lung Model.

When completing these activities, manipulate only one control at a time and note the result of each activity with manipulation of the controls. Answer the questions that follow each of the activities.

PRESSURE REGULATED VOLUME CONTROL A/C (PRVC A/C)

Set the ventilator to the following settings:

1. Press the "Mode" soft key, located at the lower left side of the UIM screen.
2. The Mode Select screen will appear. Press "PRVC A/C," and then press "Mode Accept."
3. Using the touch-turn-touch methodology, establish the following settings:

Rate	10 per minute
Volume	450 mL
Inspiratory Time	1 second
PEEP	0 cm H_2O
Flow Trigger	3 L/min
FIO_2	21%

4. Press the "Screens" soft key at the upper right of the UIM screen. Select "Monitors."

Using the Monitors screen, record the peak pressure, tidal volume, mean pressure, minute volume, and rate. Once you have recorded the values, press "Main" to return to the graphics display.

5. Simulate spontaneous breathing by expanding the bellows of the test lung, simulating spontaneous efforts. Observe the Graphics screen.
6. Increase the tidal volume to 700 mL.

Using the Monitors screen, record the peak pressure, tidal volume, mean pressure, minute volume, and rate. Once you have recorded the values, press "Main" to return to the graphics display.

7. Simulate spontaneous ventilation again and observe the graphics display.

Questions

A. How did the tidal volume, pressures, and minute ventilation change?
B. What did you observe on the UIM screen when you simulated spontaneous breathing?
C. How did the ventilator respond to your spontaneous efforts?

Pressure Regulated Volume Control SIMV (PRVC SIMV)

Set the ventilator to the following settings:
1. Press the "Mode" soft key located at the lower left side of the UIM screen.
2. The Mode Select screen will appear. Press "PRVC SIMV," and then press "Mode Accept."
3. Using the touch-turn-touch methodology, establish the following settings:

Rate	8 per minute
Volume	350 mL
Inspiratory Time	1 second
Pressure Support	0 cm H_2O
PEEP	0 cm H_2O
Flow Trigger	1 L/min
FIO_2	21%

4. Press the "Screens" soft key at the upper right of the UIM screen. Select "Monitors."

Using the Monitors screen, record the peak pressure, tidal volume, mean pressure, minute volume, and rate. Once you have recorded the values, press "Main" to return to the graphics display.

5. Simulate spontaneous breathing by expanding the bellows of the test lung, simulating spontaneous efforts. Observe the Graphics screen.
6. Increase the tidal volume to 600 mL.

Using the Monitors screen, record the peak pressure, tidal volume, mean pressure, minute volume, and rate. Once you have recorded the values, press "Main" to return to the graphics display.

7. Simulate spontaneous ventilation again and observe the graphics display.

Questions

A. How did the tidal volume, pressures, and minute ventilation change?
B. What did you observe on the UIM screen when you simulated spontaneous breathing?
C. How did the ventilator respond to your spontaneous efforts?

8. Add 10 cm H_2O of pressure support.

Using the Monitors screen, record the peak pressure, tidal volume, mean pressure, minute volume, and rate. Once you have recorded the values, press "Main" to return to the graphics display.

9. Simulate spontaneous ventilation again and observe the graphics display.

Questions

A. How did the tidal volume, pressures, and minute ventilation change?
B. What did you observe on the UIM screen when you simulated spontaneous breathing?
C. How did the ventilator respond to your spontaneous efforts?
D. What happened with the addition of pressure support?

Volume SIMV Practice Activities

Set the ventilator to the following settings:

6. Press the "Mode" soft key located at the lower left side of the UIM screen.
7. The Mode Select screen will appear. Press "Volume SIMV," and then press "Mode Accept."
8. Using the touch-turn-touch methodology, establish the following settings:

Rate	8 per minute
Volume	350 mL
Peak Flow	60 L/min
Inspiratory Pause	0 second
Pressure Support	0 cm H_2O
PEEP	0 cm H_2O
Flow Trigger	1 L/min
FIO_2	21%

1. Press the "Screens" soft key at the upper right of the UIM screen. Select "Monitors."

Using the Monitors screen, record the peak pressure, tidal volume, mean pressure, minute volume, and rate. Once you have recorded the values, press "Main" to return to the graphics display.

2. Simulate spontaneous breathing by expanding the bellows of the test lung, simulating spontaneous efforts. Observe the graphics screen.
3. Increase the tidal volume to 600 mL.

Using the Monitors screen, record the peak pressure, tidal volume, mean pressure, minute volume, and rate. Once you have recorded the values, press "Main" to return to the graphics display.

4. Simulate spontaneous ventilation again and observe the graphics display.

Questions

A. How did the tidal volume, pressures, and minute ventilation change?
B. What did you observe on the UIM screen when you simulated spontaneous breathing?
C. How did the ventilator respond to your spontaneous efforts?

5. Add 10 cm H_2O of pressures support, and simulate spontaneous ventilation.

Using the Monitors screen, record the peak pressure, tidal volume, mean pressure, minute volume, and rate. Once you have recorded the values, press "Main" to return to the graphics display.

6. Add 8 cmH_2O of PEEP, and simulate spontaneous ventilation.

Using the Monitors screen, record the peak pressure, tidal volume, mean pressure, minute volume, and rate. Once you have recorded the values, press "Main" to return to the graphics display.

Questions

A. How did the ventilator respond to your spontaneous efforts?

B. What happened when you added PEEP?
C. What happened when you added pressure support?

Pressure SIMV Practice Activities

Set the ventilator to the following settings:

1. Press the "Mode" soft key located at the lower left side of the UIM screen.
2. The Mode Select screen will appear. Press "Pressure SIMV," and then press "Mode Accept."
3. Using the touch-turn-touch methodology, establish the following settings:

Rate	8 per minute
Inspiratory Pressure	15 cm H_2O
Inspiratory Time	1 second
Pressure Support	0 cm H_2O
PEEP	0 cm H_2O
Flow Trigger	1 L/min
FIO_2	21%

4. Press the "Screens" soft key at the upper right of the UIM screen. Select "Monitors."

Using the Monitors screen, record the peak pressure, tidal volume, mean pressure, minute volume, and rate. Once you have recorded the values, press "Main" to return to the graphics display.

5. Simulate spontaneous breathing by expanding the bellows of the test lung, simulating spontaneous efforts. Observe the graphics screen.
6. Increase the inspiratory pressure to 25 cm H_2O.

Using the Monitors screen, record the peak pressure, tidal volume, mean pressure, minute volume, and rate. Once you have recorded the values, press "Main" to return to the graphics display.

7. Simulate spontaneous ventilation again and observe the graphics display.

Questions

A. How did the tidal volume, pressures, and minute ventilation change?
B. What did you observe on the UIM screen when you simulated spontaneous breathing?
C. How did the ventilator respond to your spontaneous efforts?

8. Add 10 cm H_2O of pressures support, and simulate spontaneous ventilation.

Using the Monitors screen, record the peak pressure, tidal volume, mean pressure, minute volume, and rate. Once you have recorded the values, press "Main" to return to the graphics display.

9. Add 8 cm H_2O of PEEP, and simulate spontaneous ventilation.

Using the Monitors screen, record the peak pressure, tidal volume, mean pressure, minute volume, and rate. Once you have recorded the values, press "Main" to return to the graphics display.

Questions

A. How did the ventilator respond to your spontaneous efforts?
B. What happened when you added PEEP?
C. What happened when you added pressure support?

Airway Pressure Release Ventilation Biphasic

Set the ventilator to the following settings:
1. Press the "Mode" soft key located at the lower left side of the UIM screen.
2. The Mode Select screen will appear. Press "APRV BiPhasic," and then press "Mode Accept."
3. Using the touch-turn-touch methodology, establish the following settings:

Time High	4 seconds
Pressure High	12 cm H_2O
Time Low	2 seconds
Pressure Low	6 cm H_2O
Pressure Support	0 cm H_2O
Flow Trigger	1 L/min
FIO_2	21%

4. Press the "Screens" soft key at the upper right of the UIM screen. Select "Monitors."

Using the Monitors screen, record the peak pressure, tidal volume, mean pressure, minute volume, and rate. Once you have recorded the values, press "Main" to return to the graphics display.

5. Simulate spontaneous breathing by expanding the bellows of the test lung, simulating spontaneous efforts. Observe the graphics screen.

Time High Control

1. Adjust the time high control to 6 seconds.

Using the Monitors screen, record the peak pressure, tidal volume, mean pressure, minute volume, and rate. Once you have recorded the values, press "Main" to return to the graphics display.

2. Adjust the time high control to 2 seconds.

Using the Monitors screen, record the peak pressure, tidal volume, mean pressure, minute volume, and rate. Once you have recorded the values, press "Main" to return to the graphics display.

Questions

A. What happened to the peak pressure?
B. What happened to the I:E ratio when you changed the time high control?
C. What happened to the minute volume?
D. What happened to the rate when the time high control decreased?

High Pressure Control

Set the ventilator to the following settings:
1. Press the "Mode" soft key located at the lower left side of the UIM screen.
2. The Mode Select screen will appear. Press "APRV BiPhasic," and then press "Mode Accept."

3. Using the touch-turn-touch methodology, establish the following settings:

Time High	4 seconds
Pressure High	12 cm H_2O
Time Low	2 seconds
Pressure Low	6 cm H_2O
Pressure Support	0 cm H_2O
Flow Trigger	1 L/min
FIO_2	21%

Using the Monitors screen, record the peak pressure, tidal volume, mean pressure, minute volume, and rate. Once you have recorded the values, press "Main" to return to the graphics display.

4. Adjust the Pres High control to 8 cm H_2O.

Using the Monitors screen, record the peak pressure, tidal volume, mean pressure, minute volume, and rate. Once you have recorded the values, press "Main" to return to the graphics display.

5. Adjust the $PEEP_H$ control to 20 cm H_2O.

Using the Monitors screen, record the peak pressure, tidal volume, mean pressure, minute volume, and rate. Once you have recorded the values, press "Main" to return to the graphics display.

Questions

A. What happened to the peak pressure?
B. What happened to the mean pressure?
C. What happened to the tidal volume as you increased the Pres High control?
D. What happened to the minute volume as you increased High control?

Time Low Control

Set the ventilator to the following settings:

Time High	4 seconds
Pressure High	15 cm H_2O
Time Low	2 seconds
Pressure Low	6 cm H_2O
Pressure Support	0 cm H_2O
Flow Trigger	1 L/min
FIO_2	21%

Using the Monitors screen, record the peak pressure, tidal volume, mean pressure, minute volume, and rate. Once you have recorded the values, press "Main" to return to the graphics display.

1. Adjust the Time Low control to 1 second.

Using the Monitors screen, record the peak pressure, tidal volume, mean pressure, minute volume, and rate. Once you have recorded the values, press "Main" to return to the graphics display.

2. Adjust the Time Low control to 4 seconds.

Using the Monitors screen, record the peak pressure, tidal volume, mean pressure, minute volume, and rate. Once you have recorded the values, press "Main" to return to the graphics display.

Questions

A. What happened to the peak pressure?
B. What happened to the mean pressure?
C. What happened to the tidal volume as you increased T_H?
D. What happened to the minute volume as you increased T_H?
E. What happened to the rate as you adjusted the Time Low control?

Pres Low Control

Set the ventilator to the following parameters:

Time High	4 seconds
Pressure High	20 cm H_2O
Time Low	2 seconds
Pressure Low	5 cm H_2O
Pressure Support	0 cm H_2O
Flow Trigger	1 L/min
FIO$_2$	21%

Using the Monitors screen, record the peak pressure, tidal volume, mean pressure, minute volume, and rate. Once you have recorded the values, press "Main" to return to the graphics display.

1. Change the low Pres Low control to 10 cm H_2O.

Using the Monitors screen, record the peak pressure, tidal volume, mean pressure, minute volume, and rate. Once you have recorded the values, press "Main" to return to the graphics display.

2. Change the Pres Low control to 15 cm H_2O.

Using the Monitors screen, record the peak pressure, tidal volume, mean pressure, minute volume, and rate. Once you have recorded the values, press "Main" to return to the graphics display.

Questions

A. What happened to the peak pressure?
B. What happened to the mean pressure?
C. What happened to the tidal volume as you changed the Pres Low control?
D. What happened to the minute volume as you changed the Pres Low control?

Pressure Support

Set the ventilator to the following parameters:

Time High	4 seconds
Pressure High	15 cm H_2O
Time Low	2 seconds
Pressure Low	5 cm H_2O
Pressure Support	0 cm H_2O
Flow Trigger	1 L/min
FIO$_2$	21%

Using the Monitors screen, record the peak pressure, tidal volume, mean pressure, minute volume, and rate. Once you have recorded the values, press "Main" to return to the graphics display.

1. Add 5 cm H_2O of pressure support.
2. Simulate a spontaneous breath by expanding the test lung to create subambient pressure.

Using the Monitors screen, record the peak pressure, tidal volume, mean pressure, minute volume, and rate. Once you have recorded the values, press "Main" to return to the graphics display.

Questions

A. What happened to the peak pressure?
B. What happened to the mean airway pressure?
C. What happened to the minute volume?
D. When did you see pressure support applied?
E. What did you observe in the upper left portion of the GUI screen during your spontaneous efforts?

Check List: Advanced Ventilation Modes

_____ 1. Verify the physician's order or protocol.
_____ 2. Follow standard precautions including hand hygiene.
_____ 3. Auscultate the patient's chest and suctions as needed.
_____ 4. Assess the patient's baseline data:
_____   a. Ventilation
_____   b. Oxygenation
_____   c. Circulation
_____   d. Work of breathing
_____ 5. Initiate the ventilation mode:
_____   a. Set the volume or pressure.
_____   b. Set the FIO$_2$.
_____   c. Set the rate or inspiratory time.

_____   d. Set the baseline pressure.
_____   e. Set the trigger sensitivity.
       6. Set the alarm parameters.
_____   a. Tidal volume
_____   b. Minute ventilation
_____   c. Low respiratory rate
_____   d. Set other alarms appropriately.
_____ 7. Set backup ventilation parameters.
_____ 8. Monitor pulmonary and cardiovascular parameters.
_____ 9. Follow standard precautions including hand hygiene.
_____ 10. Document the procedure.

Self-Evaluation Post Test: Advanced Ventilator Modes

1. When a mandatory breath is delivered, pressure increases to a preset level and is maintained at that level. This best describes:
   a. pressure control.
   b. volume control.
   c. SIMV.
   d. pressure support.

2. Dual control within a breath modes include which of the following modes?
   I. Volume assured pressure support (VAPS)
   II. Pressure regulated volume control (PRVC)
   III. Pressure augmentation
   IV. Volume control plus (VC+)
   a. I, II   c. II, III
   b. I, III   d. II, IV

3. Dual control breath-to-breath modes include which of the following modes?
   I. Volume assured pressure support (VAPS)
   II. Pressure regulated volume control (PRVC)
   III. Pressure augmentation
   IV. Volume control plus (VC+)
   a. I, II   c. II, III
   b. I, III   d. II, IV

4. A mode of ventilation that automatically regulates pressure support based on the patient's effort is:
   a. volume assured pressure support (VAPS).
   b. volume support ventilation (VSV).
   c. proportional assist ventilation (PAV).
   d. pressure regulated volume control (PRVC).

5. Which of the following modes are breath-to-breath dual control and flow cycled?
   a. Volume assured pressure support (VAPS)
   b. Volume support ventilation (VSV)
   c. Proportional assist ventilation (PAV)
   d. Pressure regulated volume control (PRVC)

6. Which of the following are true regarding inverse ratio ventilation?
   I. Inspiration is longer than expiration.
   II. Expiration is longer than inspiration.
   III. Removal of CO_2 is the primary goal.
   IV. Improvement of oxygenation is the primary goal.
   a. I, III   c. II, III
   b. I, IV   d. II, IV

7. Which of the following are characteristics of airway pressure release ventilation?
   I. There are two set pressure levels.
   II. Spontaneous ventilation is possible throughout the ventilatory cycle.
   III. Pressure support may be provided.
   IV. Two inspiratory times must be set.
   a. I   c. I, II, III
   b. I, II   d. I, II, III, IV

8. Which of the following modes attempts to overcome the resistance of the artificial airway?
   a. Pressure support
   b. Pressure regulated volume control
   c. Automatic tube compensation
   d. Volume support ventilation

9. A mode of ventilation that permits spontaneous breathing between mandatory (ventilator) breaths is:
   a. pressure support.
   b. SIMV.
   c. pressure augmentation.
   d. volume assured pressure support.

10. An example of autoregulating servo-controlled ventilation would be:
    a. pressure support.
    b. proportional assist ventilation.
    c. pressure regulated volume control (PRVC).
    d. SIMV.

PERFORMANCE EVALUATION:
Advanced Ventilation Modes

Mode Initiated: _____

Date: Lab _____ Clinical _____ Agency _____

Lab: Pass _____ Fail _____ Clinical: Pass _____ Fail _____

Student name _____ Instructor name _____

No. of times observed in clinical _____

No. of times practiced in clinical _____

PASSING CRITERIA: Obtain 90% or better on the procedure. Tasks indicated by * must receive at least 1 point, or the evaluation is terminated. Procedure must be performed within the designated time, or the performance receives a failing grade.

SCORING: 2 points — Task performed satisfactorily without prompting.
1 point — Task performed satisfactorily with self-initiated correction.
0 points — Task performed incorrectly or with prompting required.
NA — Task not applicable to the patient care situation.

Tasks:	Peer	Lab	Clinical
* 1. Verifies the physician's order or protocol	☐	☐	☐
* 2. Follows standard precautions, including hand hygiene	☐	☐	☐
3. Auscultates and suctions the patient as required	☐	☐	☐
* 4. Obtains the patient's baseline data			
a. Assesses ventilatory status ($PaCO_2$, rate, RSBI)	☐	☐	☐
b. Assesses oxygenation status (PaO_2, SpO_2)	☐	☐	☐
c. Assesses circulatory status (BP, HR, ECG)	☐	☐	☐
d. Assesses work of breathing	☐	☐	☐
5. Initiates the ventilation mode			
* a. Sets the pressure/volume appropriately	☐	☐	☐
* b. Sets the FIO_2 level	☐	☐	☐
* c. Sets the rate/inspiratory time(s)	☐	☐	☐
* d. Sets the baseline pressure	☐	☐	☐
* e. Sets the trigger sensitivity	☐	☐	☐
6. Sets the alarm parameters			
* a. Minute ventilation	☐	☐	☐
* b. Tidal volume	☐	☐	☐

*   c. Low respiratory rate

*   d. Adjusts and sets other alarms as appropriate

*   **7.** Sets backup ventilation parameters

*   **8.** Monitors the cardiovascular and pulmonary parameters

*   **9.** Follows standard precautions, including hand hygiene

* **10.** Documents the procedure

SCORE: Peer _____ points of possible 40; _____%

                        Lab _____ points of possible 40; _____%

                        Clinical _____ points of possible 40; _____%

TIME: _____ out of possible 30 minutes

STUDENT SIGNATURES   **INSTRUCTOR SIGNATURES**

PEER: _____   LAB: _____

STUDENT: _____   CLINICAL: _____

CHAPTER 27

Waveform Analysis

INTRODUCTION

The capability to track airway pressures, volumes, and flows graphically during mechanical ventilation of the patient has been available for some time (BEAR, 1987). The most recent acute care ventilators have expanded this graphical monitoring capability beyond pressure, volume, and flow to include combinations of these reflecting air trapping, work of breathing, airway resistance, and other clinical problems and variables relating to ventilation. The method of waveform analysis can be applied for rapid, real-time assessment of the patient-ventilator system, providing important information regarding changes in the patient's status. As a respiratory care practitioner, you must be able to use this information at the bedside in the care of your patients.

In this chapter you will learn how to interpret pressure, volume, flow, pressure-volume, and flow-volume waveforms. You will learn how this information can assist you in adjusting ventilator flow, sensitivity, and pressure and in determining the patient's work of breathing, airway resistance, compliance, and other clinical variables.

KEY TERMS

- **Air trapping**
- **Plateau pressure**
- **Static pressure**

THEORY OBJECTIVES

At the end of this chapter, the reader should be able to:

- *Differentiate among the following waveforms:*
  - *Pressure versus time*
  - *Volume versus time*
  - *Flow versus time*
  - *Pressure versus volume*
  - *Flow versus volume*
- *Differentiate among the following waveform morphologies:*
  - *Rectangular*
  - *Accelerating*
  - *Decelerating*
  - *Sinusoidal*
  - *Oscillating*
- *Analyze a pressure versus time waveform and identify the following:*
  - *Inspiration and expiration*
  - *PEEP*
  - *Patient effort*
  - *Peak pressure*
  - *Plateau or static pressure*
  - *Inadequate inspiratory flow*
  - *Spontaneous breaths and inspiratory effort*
  - *Ventilator or mandatory breaths*

- *Analyze a flow versus time waveform and identify the following:*
  - *Inspiratory flow pattern*
  - *Inspiration and expiration*
  - *Air trapping*
  - *Increased airway resistance*
- *Analyze a volume versus time waveform and identify the following:*
  - *Inspiration versus expiration*
  - *Tidal volume*
  - *Air trapping*
  - *Spontaneous and ventilator or mandatory breaths*
- *Analyze a volume versus pressure waveform and identify the following:*
  - *Inspiration versus expiration*
  - *Tidal volume*
  - *Inspiratory work*
  - *Overdistention*
  - *Increases or decreases in compliance*
  - *Increases or decreases in airway resistance*
- *Analyze a flow versus volume waveform and identify changes in airway resistance.*

COMMON WAVEFORMS

Three waveforms are typically presented together on the same screen or page with most acute care ventilators. These waveforms include pressure, flow, and volume (Figure 27-1). All of these waveforms plot the variable—pressure, flow, or volume—versus time. At any point along the time axis, a vertical line can be projected through all three waveforms to analyze what occurred at that moment in time (see Figure 27-1). This information is presented by most ventilators on a real-time, breath-by-breath basis.

Other waveforms are pressure versus volume and flow versus volume waveforms.

The *pressure versus volume* waveform is illustrated in Figure 27-2. Notice that the volume versus pressure waveform makes a loop. This presentation of data is helpful in assessing compliance, airway resistance, and work of breathing. Interpretation of these specifics is described later in this chapter.

The *flow versus volume* waveform also makes a loop, as illustrated in Figure 27-3. Flow-volume loops are common in pulmonary function application. The flow-volume loop is helpful in detecting changes in airway resistance. Changes in this graphical display may be observed before and after administration of bronchodilators.

WAVEFORM MORPHOLOGIES

The shape of a waveform may be classified as rectangular, accelerating, decelerating, sinusoidal, or oscillating (Chatburn, 1991; Lucangelo, 2005). These waveform

morphologies are illustrated in Figure 27-4. These waveform shapes are usually observed in evaluating the flow versus time graphic. The shape is often determined by the drive mechanism of the ventilator, or the flow pattern setting (White, 1999).

IngMar Medical Adult/Pediatric Lung Model: Settings C=n/s, R=1, no leaks

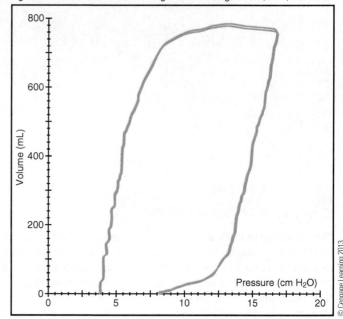

Figure 27-2　Volume versus pressure waveform. Volume is plotted on the vertical axis while pressure is plotted on the horizontal axis

IngMar Medical Adult/Pediatric Lung Model: Settings C=n/s, R=1, no leaks

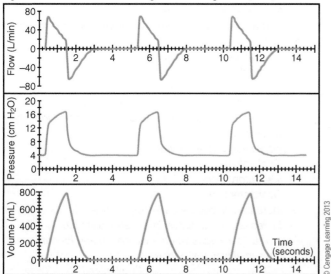

Figure 27-1　The standard display of pressure, flow, and volume versus time. Note how a vertical line projected through each waveform allows one to see what occurred at that moment

IngMar Medical Adult/Pediatric Lung Model: Settings C=n/s, R=1, no leaks

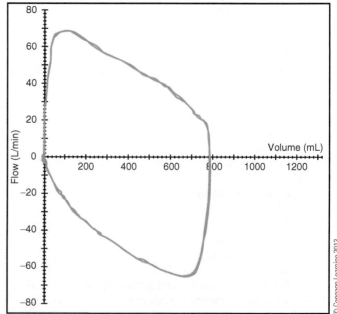

Figure 27-3　The flow versus volume loop. Flow is plotted on the vertical axis while pressure is plotted on the horizontal axis

© Cengage Learning 2013

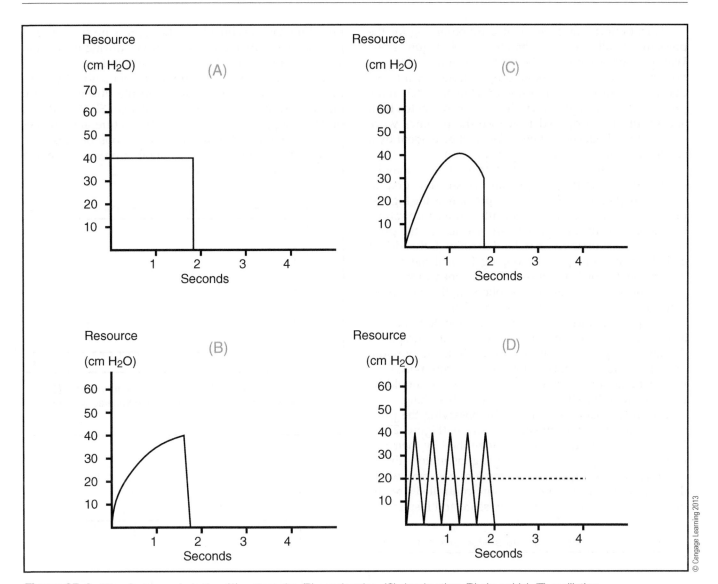

Figure 27-4 Waveform morphologies: (A) rectangular, (B) accelerating, (C) decelerating, (D) sinusoidal, (E) oscillating

© Cengage Learning 2013

ANALYSIS OF SPECIFIC WAVEFORMS

Specific waveforms (scalar or loops) are helpful to analyze changes in the patient's pathology and to assess the patient's response to positive-pressure ventilation. Airway resistance, lung compliance, overdistention, and other key information may be readily assessed by observing the morphology of the correct waveform on the graphics display. This section discusses the use of the different waveforms and their specific applications.

Pressure versus Time

The pressure versus time graphical display is very helpful in answering many clinical questions. Pressure rises from baseline to the peak pressure value during inspiration and then falls to baseline again during exhalation (Figure 27-5). Addition of positive end-expiratory

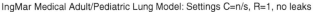

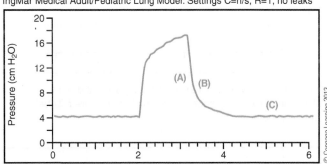

Figure 27-5 The pressure versus time graphic. Note inspiration (A) and expiration (B). With the addition of PEEP (C), the baseline pressure changes, reflecting the PEEP level

© Cengage Learning 2013

pressure (PEEP) raises the baseline pressure to the PEEP level. Observation of this graphical display allows determination of patient effort, peak and plateau pressures, adequacy of inspiratory flow, and mandatory (ventilator) versus spontaneous breath types.

Patient effort may be evaluated by observing for the pressure to fall below the baseline level (Figure 27-6). With pressure triggering, the ventilator initiates inspiration in response to a pressure drop detected by a transducer (Chatburn, 1991; Nilsestuen & Hargett, 2005). If the pressure drop is large, the sensitivity may be set too high and should be readjusted to reduce the patient's work of breathing. Reduced patient effort will be evident by a smaller pressure drop to initiate inspiration.

Peak pressure and *static* or *plateau pressure* may be evaluated by assessing the pressure versus time graphical display (Figure 27-7). The peak pressure is the highest pressure attained for a given breath during inspiration. By reading the maximum pressure reached on the pressure scale, this pressure may be determined. By adding a slight inspiratory pause, stopping flow at the end of inspiration, the plateau pressure may be measured.

The plateau pressure occurs following the peak pressure and is usually lower (see Figure 27-7).

Adequacy of inspiratory flow may be determined by assessing the rise on the pressure versus time graphical display during inspiration (Figure 27-8). If the pressure rises slowly, or if the curve shows signs of concavity, flow is inadequate for the patient's demand. Flow should be increased to reduce the patient's work of breathing.

Breath type can be identified by observing the pressure versus time morphology or shape (Figure 27-9). Pressure support breaths may be identified by their rise to a set plateau pressure with varying inspiratory times. The pressure level (peak value) remains constant, while the inspiratory time varies. Pressure-controlled breaths maintain a constant inspiratory pressure and inspiratory

time. Spontaneous breaths without pressure support display smaller variable pressure curves during exhalation and shorter pressure drops during inspiration.

Figure 27-10 shows a combination of mandatory (ventilator) breaths with spontaneous breaths during synchronized intermittent mandatory ventilation (SIMV) without pressure support. Note the variable nature and smaller pressure changes during the spontaneous breaths. The mandatory breaths display a smoother pressure rise to a much higher pressure level.

IngMar Medical Adult/Pediatric Lung Model: Settings C=n/s, R=1, no leaks

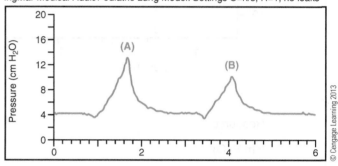

Figure 27-8 Note how the change in peak flow setting (B) caused the pressure to rise quicker when compared with (A)

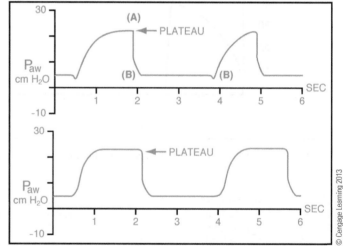

Figure 27-9 The type of breath may be determined by observing the pressure versus time morphology: (A) pressure-supported breaths, (B) pressure-controlled breaths, (C) spontaneous breaths without pressure support

IngMar Medical Adult/Pediatric Lung Model: Settings C=n/s, R=1, no leaks

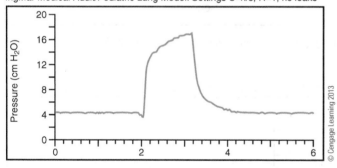

Figure 27-6 A pressure versus time graphical display illustrating inspiraotry effort. Note how the pressure falls below the baseline level

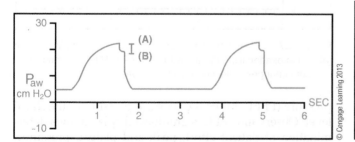

Figure 27-7 The peak (A) and plateau (B) pressures may be interpreted by assessing the pressure versus time graphic

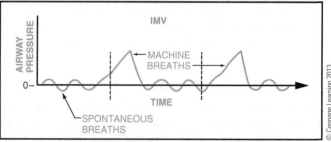

Figure 27-10 Spontaneous and mandatory breath delivery during SIMV

Flow versus Time

The flow versus time graphical display is helpful in assessing the inspiratory flow pattern, air trapping, and airway resistance. Flow rises above baseline during inspiration and falls below baseline during exhalation (Figure 27-11). Careful study of this waveform will help in assessing many different clinical situations.

IngMar Medical Adult/Pediatric Lung Model: Settings C=n/s, R=1, no leaks

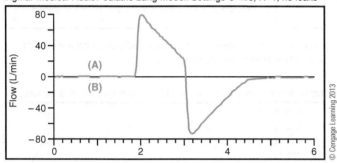

Figure 27-11 Flow versus time graphic. Inspiration (A) is above baseline, while expiration (B) is below baseline

The inspiratory flow pattern or morphology may be easily assessed using the flow versus time graphical display. Figure 27-12 illustrates the different types of inspiratory flow patterns. Many of these flow patterns are generated according to the drive mechanism for the particular ventilator (sinusoidal, for example). Most contemporary ventilators allow the operator to select the desired inspiratory flow pattern, and then the microprocessor alters the ventilator's output to match the selected flow pattern.

Air trapping, or "auto-PEEP," may be detected by failure of the expiratory flow pattern to reach baseline (zero) prior to delivery of the next breath (Figure 27-13). Failure of the lungs to empty prior to delivery of the next breath causes an increased baseline pressure or PEEP. Sometimes, air trapping is intentional—for example, during pressure-controlled inverse ratio ventilation (PCIRV). Other times, the presence of auto-PEEP is not intentional. Reducing the ventilatory rate (allowing for more expiratory time) may resolve the air trapping and allow flow to reach zero before the next breath is delivered.

Airway resistance may be assessed by observing the slope of the expiratory flow tracing. A lower slope (smaller

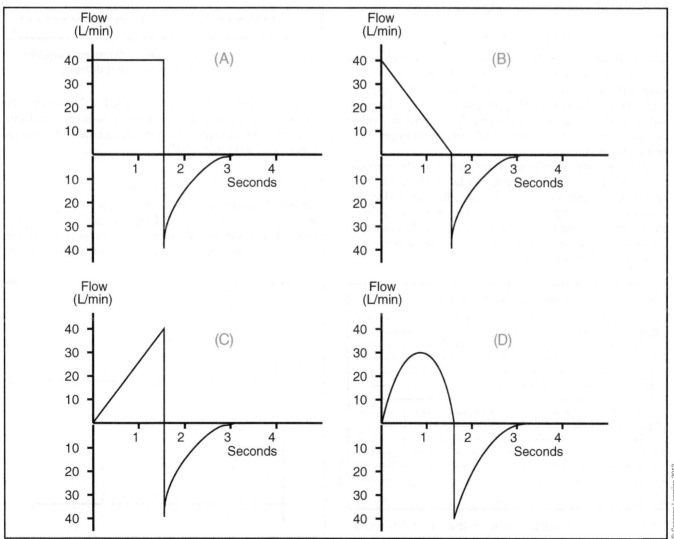

Figure 27-12 Inspiratory flow patterns: (A) rectangular, (B) accelerating, (C) decelerating, and (D) sinusoidal

IngMar Medical Adult/Pediatric Lung Model: Settings C=n/s, R=3, no leaks

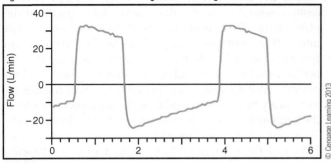

Figure 27-13 Air trapping or auto PEEP. Notice how the expiratory flow never reaches zero prior to the next breath being delivered

angle) is indicative of higher resistance to expiratory flow, while a steeper slope (greater angle) is indicative of lower resistance to expiratory flow (Figure 27-14). The patient's response to bronchodilators may be assessed by observing the flow versus time graphical display before and after bronchodilator administration. If the slope changes (increases) and expiratory time decreases, the patient has responded positively with decreased airway resistance (Puritan-Bennett Corporation, 1990).

Volume versus Time

The volume versus time waveform is illustrated in Figure 27-15. Analysis of this graphical display allows the determination of tidal volume, detection of air trapping, and identification of breath type. Tidal volume is the peak value reached during inspiration. By reading the value on the vertical axis in liters, tidal volume delivery may be determined.

Air trapping is evident from failure of the volume waveform to reach zero during exhalation (Figure 27-16). Insufficient expiratory time has been allowed, and gas is trapped in the lungs. Decreasing the ventilatory rate or increasing inspiratory flow may allow for sufficient exhalation time, returning the expiratory volume to zero prior to delivery of the next breath.

IngMar Medical Adult/Pediatric Lung Model: Settings C=n/s, R=1, no leaks

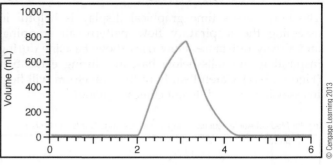

Figure 27-15 Volume versus time. Volume is on the vertical axis, while time is on the horizontal axis

IngMar Medical Adult/Pediatric Lung Model: Settings C=1, R=3, no leaks

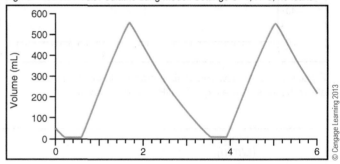

Figure 27-16 Air trapping, shown by the volume waveform failing to reach zero before the next breath is delivered

Spontaneous and mandatory breath delivery may be assessed by observing the volume versus time waveform. Mandatory breaths have larger volumes than do spontaneous breaths (Figure 27-17).

Combined Waveforms

Combined waveforms are combination displays of two *scalar* waveforms that form a loop (Nilsestuen & Hargett, 1996). The two most common combined waveforms are pressure versus volume and flow versus volume loops.

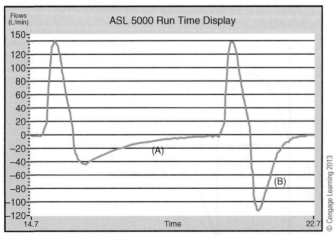

Figure 27-14 Differences in airway resistance. (A) Note where the slope is less and expiratory time is greater. (B) illustrates decreased resistance with a greater slope and shorter expiratory time

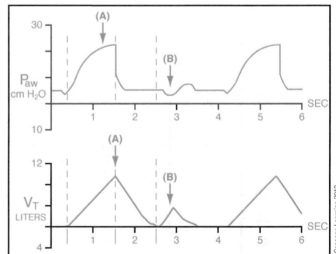

Figure 27-17 Mandatory breaths (A) have large volumes when compared with spontaneous breaths (B)

The graphical display presents information for each scalar relative to each other and to time.

Pressure versus Volume

The pressure versus volume loop is shown in Figure 27-18. Volume is on the vertical axis, while pressure is on the horizontal axis. Positive pressure is displayed to the right of the volume scale, while subambient pressure is displayed to the left of it. Inspiration progresses from the zero point to the right, while exhalation moves from right to left. This graphical display is helpful in determining tidal volume and inspiratory work and in detecting overdistention and changes in compliance and resistance.

Tidal volume delivery during both spontaneous and mandatory breaths is reflected by the maximum value attained on the vertical (volume) axis. Tidal breath delivery may be measured directly using this technique. The maximal point on the loop for tidal volume and peak inspiratory pressure represents the dynamic compliance of the thorax and lungs. If the patient's compliance worsens (fibrotic disease or severe atelectasis), the loop will shift right and flatten out.

With spontaneous breath, the graphical loop progresses clockwise from the zero point (moving into subambient pressures) until the tidal volume is reached; with exhalation it continues clockwise, displaying positive pressures (Figure 27-19).

Inspiratory work is reflected by the portion of the loop that remains in the subambient pressure range. Inspiratory work is generated by the primary muscles of ventilation. By making ventilator adjustments to minimize the area of the loop in the subambient pressure range, work may be minimized. Adjustments may

include sensitivity (pressure or flow triggering), inspiratory flow, and baseline flow settings. Figure 27-20 illustrates two mandatory breaths delivered at different inspiratory work levels.

Overdistention occurs when pressure continues to rise without concomitant volume delivery (Figure 27-21). This phenomenon results in a graph feature referred to as "beaking" because the curve looks similar to a bird's beak. Overdistention causes the lungs to be stretched,

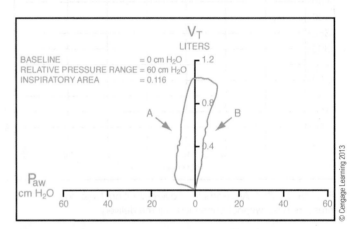

Figure 27-19 A spontaneous pressure versus volume loop. Note how inspiration is in the subambient pressure range, while expiration is positive. The loop progresses clockwise from left to right. Inspiration is displayed on the lower part of the tracing (A), while expiration (B) is on the upper part

IngMar Medical Adult/Pediatric Lung Model: Settings C=n/s, R=1, no leaks

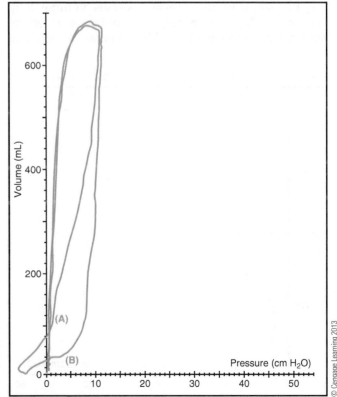

Figure 27-20 Two different mandatory breaths with differing inspiratory work levels. Loop (A) shows the same volume delivery at a reduced level of work; loop (B)O represents greater work (larger area in the subambient range)

IngMar Medical Adult/Pediatric Lung Model: Settings C=n/s, R=1, no leaks

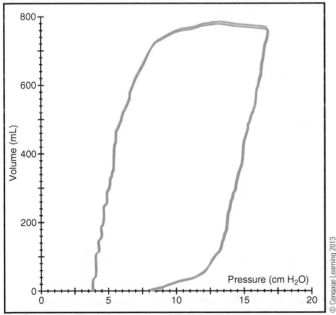

Figure 27-18 Pressure versus volume graphic. Volume is displayed on the vertical axis, while pressure is displayed on the horizontal axis

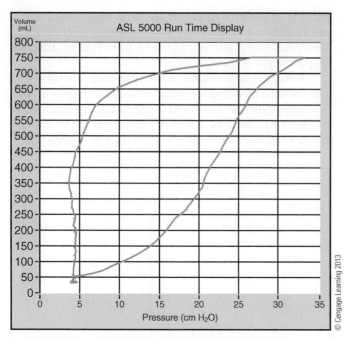

Figure 27-21   An example of overdistention. Note how pressure rises without continued volume delivery

being subjected to higher pressures with little or no change in volume. To minimize this effect, pressure or volume should be lowered (depending on which is a control variable) to match more closely the compliance of the lung/thoracic system.

Changes in compliance may be assessed by observing the slope of the pressure versus volume loop (Figure 27-22). An increased compliance is represented by a steeper slope. More volume is attained at a lower pressure, whereas decreased compliance is represented by a lower slope (smaller volume change for a given pressure).

Changes in airway resistance may be assessed by observing the hysteresis displayed in the loop. *Hysteresis* is the space between the inspiratory and expiratory loops. Two loops of differing airway resistances are shown in Figure 27-23. The loop with greater resistance—loop (B)—is referred to as "bowed"—that is, the inspiratory portion is more rounded and distends toward the pressure axis.

Flow versus Volume

Flow-volume loops are commonly used in the evaluation of spirometry readings (Fitzgerald, Speir, & Callahan, 1996). This graphical display plots flow on the vertical axis and volume on the horizontal axis (Figure 27-24). Flow-volume loops are helpful in assessing changes in airway resistance, which may often be detected after bronchodilator administration. When airway resistance is improved, expiratory flows are greater and the slope of the tracing is also steeper (Nilsestuen & Hargett, 1996).

Waveform selection will vary depending on the ventilator being used. Graphics may be selected by depressing soft or hard keys on the display and function keys on the control panel or by scrolling through menu options. You should learn how to use the graphical display monitors for each of the ventilators used in your institution (whether a college or a clinical facility). Graphical analysis is important in patient assessment, and your ability to use these systems quickly and comfortably will enable you to deliver good patient care.

IngMar Medical Adult/Pediatric Lung Model: C=n/s, R=1; and C=1+2, R=1

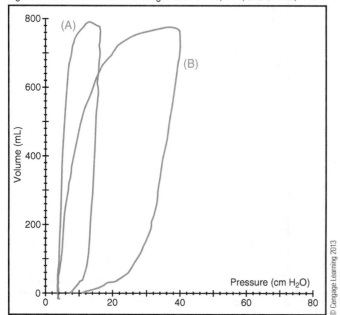

Figure 27-22   Two pressure-volume loops with differing compliance. (A) represents a higher compliance (more volume change for a given pressure), while (B) represents a lower compliance

IngMar Medical Adult/Pediatric Lung Model: C=n/s, R=3; and C=n/s, R=1

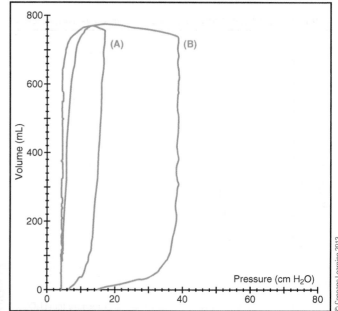

Figure 27-23   Two pressure-volume loops with different airway resistances. Loop (A) shows the same volume and compliance at a lower resistance; loop (B) displays a greater hysteresis (space between inspiratory and expiratory traces) and resistance

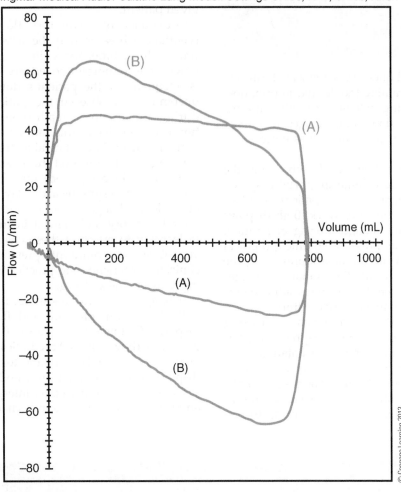

IngMar Medical Adult/Pediatric Lung Model: Settings C=n/s, R=1; C=n/s, R=3

Figure 27-24 A flow-volume loop display. Part (A) indicates greater R_{AW} while (B) reflects a decrease in R_{AW}

PROFICIENCY OBJECTIVES

At the end of this chapter, the reader should be able to:

- *Demonstrate how to select the desired waveform for display:*
  - *Pressure-time*
  - *Flow-time*
  - *Volume-time*
  - *Pressure-volume*
  - *Flow-volume*

- *Demonstrate how to interpret a selected waveform.*
- *Demonstrate how to select an appropriate waveform to assess:*
  - *Patient effort*
  - *Air trapping or auto-PEEP*
  - *Inspiratory flow*
  - *Airway resistance*

WAVEFORM INTERPRETATION

Once the desired waveform is selected, you must be able to interpret the it. Common clinical variables and problems that graphical analysis helps to assess include volume delivery, inspiratory work, overdistention, and compliance and resistance changes. Your laboratory and clinical instructors can assist you in learning how to interpret changes in the waveforms displayed on the ventilator monitor. Using the theoretical concepts presented earlier in this chapter, practice interpreting waveforms every time you are at the bedside caring for patients. Only through repeated practice can you become proficient at this new skill.

CLINICAL CRITERIA FOR APPROPRIATE WAVEFORM SELECTION

Depending on the clinical question, some waveforms are better than others for obtaining the desired information. Clinical scenarios involving patient effort, air trapping, adequacy of inspiratory flow, and changes in airway resistance and compliance are commonly assessed using ventilator graphics.

Patient effort may be determined by observing the pressure-time and pressure-volume graphical displays. Subambient pressure generated by the patient in initiating a breath represents ventilatory work. Both displays show subambient pressure changes during inspiration. Some ventilators use the pressure-volume graphical display and actually measure the area representing the subambient portion of the breath. By comparing changes in this area with different ventilator settings, adjustments can be made to minimize patient work or effort.

Air trapping, or auto-PEEP, may be assessed using either the flow-time or volume-time graphical display. For either display, determine whether exhalation (flow or volume) reaches zero prior to delivery of the next breath. If air trapping or auto-PEEP is not desired, make ventilator adjustments to minimize it. Your laboratory or clinical instructor can assist you in learning to rec-ognize this and when it is and is not appropriate for a given patient.

Adequacy of inspiratory flow during mandatory (ventilator) breaths may be assessed using pressure-time, volume-time, and volume-pressure graphical displays. It is important to ensure that the flow setting is adequate for the patient's flow demands. It is not uncommon to observe the patient actively working during a mandatory breath (volume-pressure or flow-time). If you detect this, adjust the flow to meet the patient's needs. Your clinical instructor can assist you in learning how to interpret this event.

Changes in compliance may be assessed using the pressure-volume graphical display. By assessing the slope of the loop, changes in compliance may be determined. Your laboratory and clinical instructors can assist you in learning to interpret these changes. Sometimes they are subtle and require interpretation by an experienced clinician. Experience and practice will help you in learning to assess these changes.

Changes in airway resistance may be assessed using both the volume-pressure and flow-volume graphical displays. Changes in hysteresis (volume-pressure) and peak flow (flow-volume) are indicative of changes in airway resistance. Make it a habit to assess these graphical displays before and after bronchodilator administration. With your clinical instructor, interpret these waveforms and learn to assess these subtle changes.

References

Bear Medical Systems, Inc. (1987). *BEAR 5 ventilator instruction manual*. Riverside, CA: Author.

Chatburn, R. L. (1991) A new system for understanding mechanical ventilators. *Respiratory Care, 36*(10), 1123–1155.

Fitzgerald, D. J., Speir, W. A., & Callahan, L. A. (1996). Office evaluation of pulmonary function: Beyond the numbers. *American Family Physician, 54*(2), 525–534.

Lucangelo, U., Bernabe, F., Blanch, L. (2005). Respiratory mechanics derived from signals in the ventilator circuit, *Respiratory Care, 50*(1), 55–67.

Nilsestuen, J. O., & Hargett, K. (1996). Managing the patient-ventilator system using graphic analysis: An overview and introduction to *Graphics Corner. Respiratory Care, 41*(12), 1105–1122.

Nilsestuen, J. O., & Hargett, K. D. (2005). Using ventilator graphics to identify patient-ventilator asynchrony. *Respiratory Care, 50*(2), 202–234.

Puritan-Bennett Corporation. (1990). Waveforms: The graphical presentation of ventilatory data, Form AA-1594. Carlsbad, CA: Author.

White, G. (1999). *Equipment theory for respiratory care* (3rd ed.). Clifton Park, NY: Delmar Cengage Learning.

Practice Activities: Waveform Analysis

1. Using a test lung, set up the ventilator(s) used at your institution and practice selecting the following wave-forms:
   a. Pressure-time
   b. Flow-time
   c. Volume-time
   d. Pressure-volume
   e. Flow-volume

2. Using a lung analog (Retec or Manley) in which compliance and resistance may be altered, change the compliance, the resistance, and then both, and observe the changes in the following waveform graphical displays:
   a. Flow-time
   b. Volume-time
   c. Pressure-volume
   d. Flow-volume

3. Using a lung analog (Retec or Manley), establish routine continuous mechanical ventilation settings. Have your laboratory partner change compliance or resistance, or both, without your being able to see the lung analog. Assess the ventilator graphics and state what has been changed.

Check List: Waveform Analysis

_____ 1. Verify the physician's order.
_____ 2. Scan the patient's chart as time permits.
_____ 3. Wash hands before seeing the patient.
4. Select the desired waveform:
_____ a. Pressure-time
_____ b. Flow-time
_____ c. Volume-time
_____ d. Pressure-volume
_____ e. Flow-volume

5. Interpret the waveform for:
_____ a. Inspiratory flow
_____ b. Inspiratory work
_____ c. Overdistention
_____ d. Changes in compliance
_____ e. Changes in resistance
_____ 6. Adjust the ventilator as required.
_____ 7. Chart appropriately on the patient record.
_____ 8. Wash hands upon leaving the area.

Self-Evaluation Post Test: Waveform Analysis

1. Which of the following waveform displays are scalars?
   I.   Pressure-time
   II. Pressure-volume
   III. Flow-time
   IV. Flow-volume
   a. I, III   c. II, III
   b. I, IV   d. II, IV

2. Which of the following waveforms may be used to assess adequacy of inspiratory flow?
   I.   Pressure-time
   II. Flow-time
   III. Pressure-volume
   IV. Flow-volume
   a. I   c. I, II, III
   b. I, II   d. I, II, III, IV

3. Which of the following waveforms may be used to assess inspiratory work?
   I.   Pressure-time
   II. Pressure-volume
   III. Flow-time
   IV. Flow-volume
   a. I, II   c. II, III
   b. I, III   d. III, IV

4. In assessing the pressure-volume waveform, which of the following would indicate a change in airway resistance?
   a. Increased hysteresis
   b. Increased slope
   c. Decreased slope
   d. Increased volume

5. In assessing the pressure-volume waveform for changes in compliance, which of the following reflects an increase in lung/thoracic compliance?
   a. Increased hysteresis
   b. Increased slope
   c. Decreased slope
   d. Increased volume

6. In assessing the pressure-volume waveform for changes in compliance, which of the following reflects a decrease in lung/thoracic compliance?
   a. Increased hysteresis
   b. Increased slope
   c. Decreased slope
   d. Increased volume

7. In assessing the flow-time waveform, air trapping is manifested by:
   a. an increased slope.
   b. lower flow rates.
   c. shorter inspiratory times.
   d. flow not reaching zero.

8. Which of the following is indicated when volume fails to reach zero during exhalation in assessing the volume-time graphical display?
   a. Increased compliance
   b. Decreased compliance
   c. Increased resistance
   d. Air trapping

9. "Bowing" of the pressure-volume curve toward the pressure axis is indicative of:
   a. increased compliance.
   b. decreased compliance.
   c. increased resistance.
   d. air trapping.

10. A positive response to bronchodilator therapy is indicated by which of the following changes in the flow-volume graphical display?
    I.   Increased slope
    II. Increased peak flow
    III. Decreased slope
    IV. Decreased peak flow
    a. I, II   c. II, III
    b. I, III   d. III, IV

PERFORMANCE EVALUATION:
Waveform Analysis

Date: Lab _____ Clinical _____ Agency _____

Lab: Pass _____ Fail _____ Clinical: Pass _____ Fail _____

Student name _____ Instructor name _____

No. of times observed in clinical _____

No. of times practiced in clinical _____

PASSING CRITERIA: Obtain 90% or better on the procedure. Tasks indicated by * must receive at least 1 point, or the evaluation is terminated. Procedure must be performed within the designated time, or the performance receives a failing grade.

SCORING: 2 points — Task performed satisfactorily without prompting.
1 point — Task performed satisfactorily with self-initiated correction.
0 points — Task performed incorrectly or with prompting required.
NA — Task not applicable to the patient care situation.

Tasks:	Peer	Lab	Clinical
* 1. Verifies the physician's order	☐	☐	☐
* 2. Reviews the patient's chart	☐	☐	☐
* 3. Washes hands	☐	☐	☐
4. Selects the desired waveform			
* a. Pressure-time	☐	☐	☐
* b. Flow-time	☐	☐	☐
* c. Volume-time	☐	☐	☐
* d. Pressure-volume	☐	☐	☐
* e. Flow-volume	☐	☐	☐
5. Interprets the waveform for			
* a. Inspiratory flow	☐	☐	☐
* b. Inspiratory work	☐	☐	☐
* c. Overdistention	☐	☐	☐
* d. Changes in compliance	☐	☐	☐
* e. Changes in resistance	☐	☐	☐
* 6. Adjusts the ventilator as required	☐	☐	☐
* 7. Charts appropriately on the patient record	☐	☐	☐
* 8. Washes hands upon leaving the area	☐	☐	☐

SCORE: Peer _____ points of possible 26; _____%

Lab _____ points of possible 26; _____%

Clinical _____ points of possible 26; _____%

TIME: _____ out of possible 15 minutes

STUDENT SIGNATURES

PEER: _____

STUDENT: _____

INSTRUCTOR SIGNATURES

LAB: _____

CLINICAL: _____

CHAPTER 28

Weaning and Discontinuation of Mechanical Ventilation

Scott J. Mahoney

INTRODUCTION

In critical care units across the country, mechanical ventilation is regularly employed to support critically ill patients. Technology in the field of mechanical ventilation has increased dramatically over recent years, giving clinicians a multitude of modes, protocols, and techniques with which to help achieve stable cardiopulmonary status for their patients. Yet, with all of these advances and improvements, there are many hazards and complications associated with being supported by a mechanical ventilator. The likelihood of ventilator-associated pneumonia and complications associated with having an artificial airway in place continue to increase so long as the patient remains intubated and ventilated. With this being the case, it is imperative that the expert clinician have an established, standardized method to routinely assess the critically ill patient to determine when the patient is ready to be weaned and extubated.

KEY TERMS

- **Automatic tube compensation (ATC)**
- **Closed-loop ventilation**
- **Continuous positive airway pressure (CPAP)**
- **Pressure support (PS)**
- **Rapid-shallow-breathing index (RSBI)**
- **Spontaneous breathing trial (SBT)**
- **Ventilator dependence**

THEORY OBJECTIVES

At the end of this chapter, the reader should be able to:

- *Describe respiratory, cardiovascular, neurologic, and psychological reasons for ventilator dependence.*
- *Identify signs that point toward resolution of a ventilator-dependent patient's disease process.*
- *Describe how to correctly perform a spontaneous breathing trial.*
- *Given a set of clinical data, determine if a patient qualifies for a spontaneous breathing trial.*
- *Determine if a patient is tolerating a spontaneous breathing trial.*
- *Calculate and interpret a rapid-shallow-breathing index (RSBI).*

AARC Clinical Practice Guideline
Evidence-Based Guidelines
for Weaning and Discontinuing
Ventilatory Support

A Collective Task Force Facilitated by the American College of Chest Physicians, the American Association for Respiratory Care, and the American College of Critical Care Medicine

RECOMMENDATION 1

In patients requiring mechanical ventilation for >24 hours, a search for all the causes that may be contributing to ventilator dependence should be undertaken. This is particularly true in the patient who has failed attempts at withdrawing the mechanical ventilator. Reversing all possible ventilatory and nonventilatory issues should be an integral part of the ventilator discontinuation process.

Evidence (Grade B)

RECOMMENDATION 2

Patients receiving mechanical ventilation for respiratory failure should undergo a formal assessment of discontinuation potential if the following criteria are satisfied:

1. Evidence for some reversal of the underlying cause of respiratory failure;
2. Adequate oxygenation (eg, $P_{aO_2}/F_{IO_2} > 150$–200; requiring positive end-expiratory pressure [PEEP] < or = 5–8 cm H_2O; F_{IO_2} < or = 0.4–0.5) and pH (eg, > or = 7.25);
3. Hemodynamic stability as defined by the absence of active myocardial ischemia and the absence of clinically important hypotension (ie, a condition requiring no vasopressor therapy or therapy with

only low-dose vasopressors such as dopamine or dobutamine <5 micro g/kg/min); and
4. The capability to initiate an inspiratory effort.

The decision to use these criteria must be individualized. Some patients not satisfying all of the above the criteria (eg, patients with chronic hypoxemia below the thresholds cited) may be ready for attempts at discontinuation of mechanical ventilation.

Rationale and Evidence (Grade B)

RECOMMENDATION 3

Formal discontinuation assessments for patients receiving mechanical ventilation for respiratory failure should be done during spontaneous breathing rather than while the patient is still receiving substantial ventilatory support. An initial brief period of spontaneous breathing can be used to assess the capability of continuing on to a formal SBT. The criteria with which to assess patient tolerance during SBTs are the respiratory pattern, adequacy of gas exchange, hemodynamic stability, and subjective comfort. The tolerance of SBTs lasting 30 to 120 minutes should prompt consideration for permanent ventilator discontinuation.

Rationale and Evidence (Grade A)

RECOMMENDATION 4

The removal of the artificial airway from a patient who has successfully been discontinued from ventilatory support should be based on assessments of airway patency and the ability of the patient to protect the airway.

Rationale and Evidence (Grade C)

RECOMMENDATION 5

Patients receiving mechanical ventilation for respiratory failure who fail an SBT should have the cause for the failed SBT determined. Once reversible causes for failure are corrected, and if the patient still meets the criteria listed in Table 28-2, subsequent SBTs should be performed every 24 hours.

Rationale and Evidence (Grade A)

RECOMMENDATION 6

Patients receiving mechanical ventilation for respiratory failure who fail an SBT should receive a stable, nonfatiguing, comfortable form of ventilatory support.

Rationale and Evidence (Grade B)

RECOMMENDATION 7

Anesthesia/sedation strategies and ventilator management aimed at early extubation should be used in postsurgical patients.

Rationale and Evidence (Grade A)

TABLE 28-1: Grades of Evidence	
GRADE	**DESCRIPTION**
A.	Scientific evidence provided by well-designed, well-conducted, controlled trials (randomized and nonrandomized) with statistically significant results that consistently support the guideline recommendation.
B.	Scientific evidence provided by observational studies or by controlled trials with less consistent results to support the guideline recommendation.
C.	Expert opinion supported the guideline recommendation, but scientific evidence either provided inconsistent results or was lacking.

(Continued)

TABLE 28-2: Criteria Used in Weaning/Discontinuation Studies to Determine Whether Patients Receiving High Levels of Ventilatory Support Can Be Considered for Discontinuation (ie, Entered into Trials)

Objective measurements	• Adequate oxygenation (eg, $P_{O_2} \geq 60$ mmHg on $F_{IO_2} \leq 0.4$; PEEP $\leq 5–10$ cm H_2O; $P_{O_2}/F_{IO_2} \geq 150–300$)
	• Stable cardiovascular system (eg, HR ≤ 140 beats/min; stable blood pressure; no or minimal vasopressors)
	• Afebrile (eg, temperature $< 38°C$)
	• No significant respiratory acidosis
	• Adequate hemoglobin (eg, Hgb $\geq 8–10$ g/dL)
	• Adequate mentation (eg, arousable, GCS ≥ 13, no continuous sedative infusions)
	• Stable metabolic status (eg, acceptable electrolytes)
Subjective clinical assessments	Resolution of disease acute phase; physician believes discontinuation possible; adequate cough

RECOMMENDATION 8

Weaning/discontinuation protocols designed for nonphysician health care professionals (HCPs) should be developed and implemented by ICUs. Protocols aimed at optimizing sedation should also be developed and implemented.

Rationale and Evidence (Grade A)

RECOMMENDATION 9

Tracheotomy should be considered after an initial period of stabilization on the ventilator when it becomes apparent that the patient will require prolonged ventilator assistance. Tracheotomy should then be performed when the patient appears likely to gain one or more of the benefits ascribed to the procedure. Patients who may derive particular benefit from early tracheotomy are the following:

- Those requiring high levels of sedation to tolerate translaryngeal tubes
- Those with marginal respiratory mechanics (often manifested as tachypnea) in whom a tracheostomy tube having lower resistance might reduce the risk of muscle overload
- Those who may derive psychological benefit from the ability to eat orally, communicate by articulated speech, and experience enhanced mobility; and
- Those in whom enhanced mobility may assist physical therapy efforts

Rationale and Evidence (Grade B)

RECOMMENDATION 10

Unless there is evidence for clearly irreversible disease (eg, high spinal cord injury or advanced amyotrophic lateral sclerosis), a patient requiring prolonged mechanical ventilatory support for respiratory failure should not be considered permanently ventilator dependent until 3 months of weaning attempts have failed.

Rationale and Evidence (Grade B)

RECOMMENDATION 11

Critical-care practitioners should familiarize themselves with facilities in their communities, or units in hospitals they staff, that specialize in managing patients who require prolonged dependence on mechanical ventilation. Such familiarization should include reviewing published peer-reviewed data from those units, if available. When medically stable for transfer, patients who have failed ventilator discontinuation attempts in the ICU should be transferred to those facilities that have demonstrated success and safety in accomplishing ventilator discontinuation.

Rationale and Evidence (Grade C)

RECOMMENDATION 12

Weaning strategy in the prolonged mechanical ventilation (PMV) patient should be slow-paced and should include gradually lengthening self-breathing trials.

Rationale and Evidence (Grade C)

Reprinted with permission from *Respiratory Care* 2002; 47(1): 69–90. The complete AARC Clinical Practice Guidelines are available from the AARC Web site (http://www.aarc.org), from the AARC Executive Office, or from *Respiratory Care* journal.

REASONS FOR VENTILATOR DEPENDENCE

Before any attempt is made to wean and discontinue mechanical ventilatory support, it is crucial that the clinician determine whether or not the circumstances that caused the patient to be placed on mechanical support in the first place have resolved. Knowing the reasons for a patient's intubation is very important. For example, if a patient with chronic obstructive pulmonary disease (COPD) was intubated for respiratory failure secondary to a community-acquired pneumonia, attempting to wean the patient off the ventilator before the pneumonia has shown signs of resolving would likely result in less than optimal results. If the patient was potentially extubated prematurely, there is a high likelihood that the patient would end up needing to be reintubated because the primary reason for the original intubation had not yet resolved. An understanding of the main reasons for *ventilator dependence* helps the expert clinician in determining the reasons his or her patient experienced respiratory failure requiring mechanical ventilation. These reasons can be divided into four general categories: neurologic, respiratory, cardiovascular, and psychological.

Neurologic Causes for Ventilator Dependence

The respiratory system is controlled primarily by the pons and the medulla. These respiratory centers respond to a variety of stimuli from peripheral and central chemoreceptors. Any damage to the respiratory centers in the brainstem (e.g., stroke) or disturbances to any of the feedback systems (e.g., electrolyte imbalances, pharmacologic factors [narcotics, etc.]) can lead to a depression of the patient's drive to breathe. When no signals are sent to the muscles of respiration, central apnea ensues. If erratic signals are sent to the muscles of respiration, the resulting respiratory patterns may not be suitable for sustained periods of spontaneous breathing. Interruptions in the neurologic control of the respiratory system may lead to ventilator dependence.

Respiratory Causes for Ventilator Dependence

A healthy respiratory system is a product of balance between the demand placed upon it and its ability to do the work required. The inability of the respiratory system to meet the demand placed upon it can be the result of its inability to adequately oxygenate or ventilate, or a combination of both. Disease processes that lead to hypoxemia place added demands on the respiratory system. Diseases that cause increased CO_2 retention place an added demand on the respiratory as well. When the demand to oxygenate and ventilate outstrip the ability of the respiratory system to accomplish its task independently, mechanical assistance becomes necessary and ventilator dependence ensues.

The ability of the respiratory system to do work depends predominantly on three main factors: muscle function (diaphragm strength), lung compliance, and airway resistance (MacIntyre et al., 2002). Optimally, the diaphragm and accessory muscles should function appropriately, compliance is kept at or near normal, and airway resistance is kept to a minimum. A pathology or chemical imbalance that upsets the homeostasis in any of these three areas can potentially lead to ventilator dependence. The diaphragm can be negatively affected by pharmacologic agents and metabolic imbalance. It can also be weakened by injury and overuse and put at a distinct disadvantage due to hyperinflation in patients with severe air trapping. Lung compliance can become drastically reduced in disease processes like pulmonary fibrosis and pneumonia. Airway resistance can markedly increase in the presence of bronchospasm and inflammation. Additionally, the presence of small artificial airways can increase the demand on the respiratory system by imposing an increased airway resistance.

Cardiovascular Causes for Ventilator Dependence

Patients with cardiovascular instability often do not tolerate the weaning process. Positive-pressure ventilation (PPV) has an impact on the cardiovascular system. Increased intrathoracic pressures seen with PPV and positive end-expiratory pressure (PEEP) can diminish venous return, and, therefore, cardiac output. As support is withdrawn, PEEP levels are reduced and the work of breathing is placed back on the patient. The intrathoracic pressure changes associated with spontaneous breathing can produce negative cardiovascular effects. Because spontaneous breathing increases venous return, an additional burden may be placed on a compromised cardiovascular system. A heart that is not functioning optimally may not be able to deal with the increased venous return associated with spontaneous breathing. As such, the patient may fail an attempted weaning process and remain ventilator dependent. Also, the increased use of the diaphragm associated with spontaneous breathing leads logically to an increased metabolic demand. This increase in demand may, once again, be difficult for a compromised cardiovascular system to meet.

Psychological Causes for Ventilator Dependence

The emotional/psychological component of ventilator dependence should not be overlooked. After an extended time on life support, some patients may feel apprehensive and even fearful about being weaned. This apprehension and fear can lead to weaning failure. Constant communication and optimization of the critical care environment must be in the forefront of the clinician's mind. Sleep deprivation may play a role as well (Boles et al., 2007). The dynamic environment associated with an intensive care unit (ICU) (lights on at all hours, continual noise, blood draws in the middle of the night, etc.) can disturb a patient's natural sleep cycles. Doing so may put patients at a disadvantage when weaning attempts are made. When weaning a patient from mechanical ventilation, care must be taken to ensure that all of the needs, not just the obvious medical needs, of the patient are being met in order to maximize the chances for success.

DETERMINING READINESS FOR WEANING

The process of successfully weaning a patient from mechanical ventilation can be complicated and time consuming. It is imperative that the expert respiratory care practitioner (RCP) continually communicate with the members of the health care team in charge of the patient. Coordination of efforts between the critical care nurse and critical care RCP is often crucial to the success of a weaning attempt. Sedation, if used, must be discontinued prior to assessing a patient's ability to, for example, maintain adequate spontaneous respiratory effort. Depending on the type of sedation used, these medications may need to be discontinued well in advance of a weaning attempt. In order to accomplish this, the RCP must communicate with the patient's primary registered nurse (RN). Additionally, care must be taken to ensure that when a weaning trial is taking place, interruptions are kept to a minimum. Laboratory blood draws, x-rays, diagnostic tests, and patient transports should ideally be avoided during a weaning trial. Again, the importance of the coordination of care between the critical care RCP and the critical care RN cannot be emphasized enough.

Before a patient undergoes any sort of formal weaning trial it is helpful to have a set of clear, standardized criteria to use in order to assess if a patient should undergo a weaning and discontinuation attempt. There are four general questions that should be asked regarding any patient who is being considered for weaning and eventual liberation from mechanical ventilation (MacIntyre et al., 2002). These questions are:

1. Is there evidence of reversal of the underlying cause for respiratory failure?
2. Is there evidence of adequate oxygenation?
3. Is the patient hemodynamically stable?
4. Can the patient generate an inspiratory effort?

Evidence of Reversal of Underlying Cause for Respiratory Failure

As mentioned earlier, there are many reasons that a patient may become ventilator dependent. It is important that clinicians have a good understanding of their patients in order to appropriately assess if there has been evidence of improvement in the disease process. The patient's past and present medical history, admitting diagnosis(es), reason for intubation, and so on, are all important pieces of information that the clinician must possess. Once

this information is known, comparisons can be drawn to the patient's current state. Has the chest x-ray film improved? Have the blood gas values improved? Is the patient's mentation clearing? All of these are examples of questions a clinician might ask himself or herself when attempting to determine whether or not a patient is ready for a weaning trial.

Evidence of Adequate Oxygenation

Adequate oxygenation is evidenced by a number of indices. Patients should have an arterial partial pressure of oxygen/fraction of inspired oxygen (PaO_2/FIO_2) ratio greater than 150 to 200, a PEEP level of less than 5 to 8 cm H_2O, and an FIO_2 of less than 0.4 to 0.5 if they are to be considered for an attempt at weaning and discontinuation (MacIntyre et al., 2002).

Evidence of Hemodynamic Stability

Because the increased respiratory effort associated with spontaneous breathing will place added strain on the cardiovascular system, it is important that patients being considered for weaning trials be hemodynamically stable. Hemodynamic stability is evidenced by a heart rate less than 140 beats per minute. In addition, the patient should also have a stable blood pressure requiring no to minimal vasopressor therapy.

Evidence of Ability to Generate an Inspiratory Effort

In order to be placed on a weaning trial, a patient must be able to breathe spontaneously. Absence of spontaneous respiratory effort (apnea) would disqualify a patient from entering into a weaning trial. This is often assessed at the very beginning of a weaning trial with the clinician at the patient's bedside. Should the patient lack a spontaneous respiratory drive, the clinician must return the patient to a mode of ventilation that fully supports the patient's physiologic needs.

THE SPONTANEOUS BREATHING TRIAL (SBT)

Once the determination has been made that the patient qualifies for a weaning attempt, the next step is to ensure that the patient is ready for the weaning trial (e.g., sedation has been reduced or discontinued, etc.). When the patient is ready, the RCP should begin by noting the current ventilator settings, vital signs, and general appearance of the patient. Care must be taken to perform a thorough assessment prior to beginning a *spontaneous breathing trial (SBT)*, because this initial assessment becomes the baseline against which the patient is measured during the weaning process to help determine whether the patient is tolerating the trial. Vital signs should include noting the patient's heart rate and rhythm, current blood pressure, current oxygen saturation, and general appearance. Breath sounds and the patient's work of breathing should also be noted. The patient should be suctioned if indicated, and the patient's position should be optimized in bed. Semi-to high Fowler's position, depending on the patient's condition, may help to improve spontaneous breathing efforts. Any scheduled inhaled medications should be given and any additional efforts to ensure a successful SBT should be pursued.

Once the aforementioned is accomplished, the RCP is then ready to place the patient into the SBT. There are several ways to do this that are generally accepted. Placing the patient on *continuous positive airway pressure (CPAP)* of 5 cm H_2O and maintaining current FIO_2 are common practice. Low levels of *pressure support* may also be considered. Or, if the ventilator offers *automatic tube compensation (ATC)* the RCP may choose to activate this feature during an SBT. ATC is a feature offered on many modern critical care ventilators. When it is employed the clinician inputs the size of the endotracheal tube into the ventilator and the ventilator automatically adjusts support to help alleviate the resistance imposed by the artificial airway. Both low levels of pressure support and/or ATC features are thought to help alleviate the imposed work of breathing of the ventilator circuit and endotracheal tube. Traditional aerosol "T piece" trials are also an alternative. To do this, the clinician sets up a high-flow aerosol system, a length of corrugated tubing, and a "T piece" adaptor that attaches to the patient's endotracheal tube. FIO_2 is set accordingly and flow is adjusted to ensure that the patient has more than enough gas flow through the circuit. Extra care must always be taken to closely monitor the patient when this method is employed. Because of the way these trials are performed (with the patient off the ventilator), placing a patient on an aerosol T piece eliminates the traditional fail-safes found on modern mechanical ventilators (backup ventilation in case of apnea, alarms that alert the practitioner to tachypnea, high and low minute ventilation, etc.).

When the method the RCP is going to use has been determined, the patient is taken off his or her current settings and placed into the SBT. Once the patient is breathing spontaneously, another thorough assessment is performed to determine if the patient is tolerating the SBT.

Duration of the Spontaneous Breathing Trial

The length of an SBT should be approximately 30 to 120 minutes. A duration shorter than 30 minutes may not be predictive of the patient's true ability to sustain spontaneous breathing, and a period longer than 120 minutes has not shown to be any more predictive of success after ventilator liberation (MacIntyre et al., 2002). When a patient is placed into an SBT the clinician must pay very close attention to the patient at the

onset of the trial. Patients who rapidly decompensate (oxygen saturation [SpO_2] decreases significantly, heart rate increases significantly, etc.) at the beginning of a trial should not continue on the trial, but rather should be returned to their previous ventilator settings. The weaning intolerance should be subsequently documented in the patient record.

Determination of Tolerance in a Spontaneous Breathing Trial

The clinician must carefully assess the patient who is undergoing an SBT both at the beginning of the trial and periodically throughout the duration of the trial. Specific criteria that have been shown to be predictive of weaning success or failure are listed in Table 28-3.

The clinician continues to monitor the patient during the SBT, noting respiratory rate, tidal volume, vital signs, and overall appearance while paying particular attention to signs that may indicate that the patient is failing the trial. If at any time a patient shows signs of failing, a thorough assessment of the vital signs, ventilator data, and patient appearance should be noted and the patient should be returned to full ventilatory support.

Historically there have been numerous attempts to isolate a small handful of indices that routinely predict the success or failure of a weaning trial. Many of these indices and parameters are still used in the critical care environment today. Indices including the PaO_2/FIO_2 ratio, respiratory rate, tidal volume, frequency/tidal volume ratio (f/Vt, also known as the *rapid-shallow-breathing index [RSBI]*), maximal inspiratory pressure (MIP), V_D/V_T ratio, and vital capacity (VC), among others, have all been studied extensively. Table 28-4 illustrates several popular weaning parameters and their respective desirable values.

Despite all of the extensive research, there is still a lack of consensus regarding which weaning indices are best at predicting the success of a weaning attempt. One particular weaning measurement that may have some predictive value is the frequency/tidal volume ratio (f/Vt) (Cook et al., 2000). This ratio is calculated by taking the patient's spontaneous respiratory rate and dividing it by the patient's spontaneous tidal volume (in liters). A value less than 105 is consistent with weaning success. This number must be attained during spontaneous breathing with no additional pressure support. Patients with values lower than the 105 threshold have a higher likelihood of doing well after extubation than those with values above 105. Table 28-5 illustrates how this value is calculated.

Failure of a Spontaneous Breathing Trial

In the event that a patient does not pass an SBT, the patient should be returned to a form of ventilatory support that will provide him or her an opportunity to rest and conserve energy. Often this simply means returning the

TABLE 28-3: Evidence of Success/Failure of Spontaneous Breathing Trials (Adapted from AARC Clinical Practice Guidelines)

Objective measurements indicating tolerance/success	Gas exchange acceptability • $S_{pO_2} \geq 85–90\%$ • $P_{O_2} \geq 50–60$ mm Hg • pH ≥ 7.32 • Increase in $P_{aCO_2} = 10$ mm Hg Hemodynamic stability • Heart rate < 120–140 beats per minute • Heart Rate not changed > 20% from baseline assessment • Systolic Blood Pressure < 180–200 mm Hg and > 90 mm Hg • Blood Pressure not changed > 20% from baseline assessment • No vasopressors required Stable ventilatory pattern • Respiratory rate = 30–35 breaths per minute • Respiratory rate not changed > 50% from baseline assessment
Subjective clinical assessments indicating intolerance/failure	Change in mental status • Somnolence • Coma • Agitation • Anxiety Onset or worsening of discomfort Diaphoresis Signs of increased work of breathing • Use of accessory respiratory muscles • Thoracoabdominal paradox

Reprinted with permission from *Respiratory Care* 2002; 47(1): 69–90. The complete AARC Clinical Practice Guidelines are available from the AARC Web site (http://www.aarc.org), from the AARC Executive Office, or from *Respiratory Care* journal.

TABLE 28-4: Weaning Parameters

WEANING PARAMETER	DESIRED VALUE
Respiratory rate	12–30 breaths per minute
Tidal volume	Greater than 5 mL/kg
Vital capacity	Greater than 10–15 mL/kg
V_D/V_T ratio	Less than 0.55–0.60
PaO_2/FIO_2 ratio	Greater than 150–200
f/Vt ratio (RSBI)	Less than 105
Maximal inspiratory pressure (MIP)	Less than −20 to −30 cm H_2O

patient to their previous ventilator settings. Additionally, effort should be placed on attempting to determine the cause for the failed SBT. Looking carefully at the patient's clinical situation and reviewing the current and past medical history may be beneficial in attempting to discover issues that may have contributed to the patient's failure. If these factors can be discerned, a plan should be put in place to correct them. It is recommended that patients who qualify for SBTs receive them at regular intervals (typically 24 hours apart). Patients on mechanical ventilation should be assessed for readiness for an SBT every 24 hours. If the patient qualifies, an SBT should be done.

TABLE 28-5: Calculation of the Rapid-Shallow-Breathing Index

PATIENT	SPONTANEOUS RESPIRATORY RATE	TIDAL VOLUME IN LITERS	CALCULATION	RSBI VALUE
Mr. Jones	20 bpm	0.5 L	20/0.5	40
Mrs. Smith	34 bpm	0.24 L	34/0.24	142

EXTUBATION AND VENTILATOR LIBERATION

Upon successful completion of an SBT the next step is to assess the patient for extubation. Whether or not a patient has successfully passed an SBT is only a portion of the picture, so to speak. The clinician must also assess whether or not the patient will be able to protect the upper airway once the endotracheal tube is removed. The patient must be able to adequately keep the airway clear of secretions, vomit, and so on. Assessing cuff leak, assessing the amount and consistency of secretions (e.g., frequency of suctioning), and assessing the patient's ability to cough effectively must all be considered before making the final determination to remove an artificial airway.

PROTOCOLS AND THE WEANING AND DISCONTINUATION OF THE MECHANICALLY VENTILATED PATIENT

All of the clinical activities mentioned thus far in this chapter are activities that can be driven using institutionally created protocols. RCPs and nurses working together under the direction of a protocol are able to efficiently move patients through the weaning process and can potentially have a positive impact on the number of days a patient spends on mechanical ventilation (Ely et al., 2001). The use of protocols reduces the need for continual physician input and involvement at every step. Appropriately, applied protocols can help to streamline care, reduce cost, and improve patient outcomes.

Closed-Loop, Knowledge-Based Weaning

Thus far, the discussion regarding weaning has involved the respiratory therapist, nurse, and physician working together to determine when a patient is ready to wean, implement the weaning process, and, potentially, be liberated from mechanical ventilator support. Although these members of the health care team can certainly become exceptionally proficient at assessing patients, making recommendations regarding patient care, and assisting in the weaning process through the use of protocols, there are potential drawbacks to this model. Our current model of hospital-based care typically dictates that physicians, RCPs, and nurses be responsible for numerous patients over the course of any given shift. This being the case, the time spent in one particular patient's room is naturally limited. Caregivers must move from room to room, assessing patients, performing therapy, reassessing, and documenting. Patients, on the other hand, do not follow a schedule. Some patients improve rapidly and can be weaned soon after they are intubated. Others take time to improve and end up being mechanically ventilated for long periods. Given this current model, even if a patient is ready to wean, a caregiver may not recognize this fact right away or may not be able to facilitate a weaning trial immediately.

Currently several modern mechanical ventilators offer modes of ventilation that could potentially help to alleviate the problems outlined previously. These modes of ventilation continually measure patient parameters (resistance, compliance, respiratory rate, tidal volume, exhaled CO_2, etc.) and adjust support automatically and independently of the practitioner. For example, a patient who is doing shallow breathing for an extended period might be given an increased level of pressure support by the ventilator to try and increase the patient's tidal volumes and reduce work of breathing. When a mode like this is employed, the ventilator records data from the patient (i.e., gathers "knowledge"), makes adjustments based on the data it receives, and then reassesses the patient to see if the changes that were made helped to improve the parameters to which it was responding. This creates a feedback—response relationship that essentially closes the "loop" between the ventilator and the patient, hence the term *closed-loop ventilation*. Modes such as these certainly have the potential to significantly reduce the time a patient spends on a mechanical ventilator.

PROFICIENCY OBJECTIVES

At the end of this chapter, the reader should be able to:

- *Given clinical scenarios, identify patients who qualify for spontaneous breathing trials.*
- *Given clinical scenarios, identify patients who do not qualify for spontaneous breathing trials.*
- *Describe the steps an RCP would take in order to perform a spontaneous breathing trial.*
- *Describe the signs and symptoms of a patient failing a spontaneous breathing trial.*

- *Calculate and correctly interpret a rapid-shallow-breathing index.*
- *Describe the signs and symptoms of a patient passing a spontaneous breathing trial.*
- *Interpret clinical data to determine if a patient is a candidate for extubation.*

DETERMINING READINESS TO WEAN

Mechanically ventilated patients should be routinely and systematically assessed to determine if they qualify for weaning trials. This is a collaborative effort between the RCP and critical care RN. When and how patients are assessed is a facility-specific decision. One model may be to have the critical care RN and RCP confer at the beginning of the shift to determine which mechanically ventilated patients qualify for weaning. Doing so at the beginning of the shift allows the RCP and RN to coordinate the plan for the day. Questions to consider when assessing a patient for entry into a weaning trial include:

1. Is there evidence of reversal of the underlying cause for respiratory failure?
2. Is there evidence of adequate oxygenation?
3. Is the patient hemodynamically stable?
4. Can the patient generate an inspiratory effort?

Patients who do qualify for an SBT will often need to have sedation reduced or discontinued prior to entry into the trial. The coordination of efforts between the RCP and RN is essential to ensure that this happens in a timely fashion.

PLACING THE PATIENT INTO A SPONTANEOUS BREATHING TRIAL

Patients who qualify for SBTs need to be thoroughly assessed prior to the initiation of the SBT. The RCP should do a complete ventilator and patient assessment, including documentation of the following:

1. Current ventilator settings (including, but not limited to):
   a. Mode
   b. FIO_2
   c. Rate
   d. Set tidal volume or inspiratory pressure
   e. Spontaneous tidal volume
   f. PEEP
   g. Peak inspiratory pressure
   h. Plateau pressure
2. Current vital signs (including, but not limited to):
   a. SpO_2
   b. Heart rate and rhythm (be sure to note any ectopy)
   c. Blood pressure
3. Patient assessment (including, but not limited to):
   a. Breath sounds
   b. Any accessory muscle use
   c. Mental state (Awake? Alert? Anxious? Able to follow commands?)

This assessment serves as a baseline so that the therapist can compare what happens during the trial to that which was going on before the trial.

Once the assessment is complete, the patient is ready to be placed into the trial. The RCP should adjust the ventilator so that the patient is placed into the CPAP mode. Some protocols call for the addition of a small amount of pressure support or the addition of automatic tube compensation. This is a facility-specific decision. All appropriate alarms must be adjusted as well. Care must be taken to carefully assess the patient during these very early stages of the trial because some patients will decompensate immediately and require intervention to stabilize. Evidence of decompensation and weaning failure include the following:

1. Cardiac dysrhythmias
2. Sustained respiratory rate greater than 35 for 5 minutes or longer
3. Heart rate greater than 140 or an increase of more than 20% from baseline
4. Systolic blood pressure greater than 180 mm Hg or less than 80 mm Hg
5. Increased anxiety
6. Diaphoresis
7. RSBI greater than 105
8. SpO_2 less than 90% for greater than 30 seconds or more

The patient is monitored for the duration of the trial (30 to 120 minutes) and the RCP should carefully document both the ventilator and patient data throughout.

CONCLUDING THE SPONTANEOUS BREATHING TRIAL

Once the trial is concluded the RCP should document the final vital signs, patient assessment, and ventilator data. At this time, the patient's final RSBI value should also be recorded because data will be used at this point to determine if the patient qualifies for extubation. Patients may be determined to have passed the SBT if the following data are present:

1. Sustained, spontaneous respiratory rate less than 35 breaths per minute
2. Heart rate less than 140 beats per minute
3. Unchanged systolic blood pressure or systolic blood pressure less than 180 mm Hg
4. RSBI value less than 105
5. SpO_2 greater than 90%

When a patient does not meet these criteria, or decompensates during an SBT, the patient should be placed back on his or her initial ventilator settings and the results of the SBT should be thoroughly documented in the patient's medical record.

PLANNING FOR EXTUBATION

In addition to the previous data, patients who are being considered for extubation should also meet the following criteria:

1. Be able to protect the upper airway
2. Be able to cough effectively to clear the airway

Assessment of cuff leak is routine in many critical care units prior to making the final determination regarding whether or not a patient is to be extubated. Knowledge of the patient's reasons for intubation is key in assessing the patency of the upper airway. Extra care should be taken when the predominant reason for the intubation of the patient involved some sort of upper airway compromise (e.g., trauma, anaphylactic reaction, etc.). To test for cuff leak, the RCP performs the following steps:

1. Suction the patient's posterior oropharynx thoroughly.
2. Suction the patient's lower airway.

3. Place the patient in a mode of ventilation that is delivering positive-pressure breaths (e.g., assist control) or attach the resuscitation bag to the endotracheal tube and provide positive-pressure breaths with the bag.
4. Deflate the cuff on the endotracheal tube by placing a syringe into the valve on the pilot balloon and withdrawing all of the air.
5. Assess for cuff leak. This is often accomplished simply by listening at the patient's mouth for air escaping around the tube. Additionally, a stethoscope on the patient's neck may be used. If a ventilator is being used to deliver the positive-pressure breaths, the RCP should also assess the ventilator to determine if there is a difference between the delivered tidal volume and the exhaled tidal volume. Presence of such a difference while the endotracheal tube cuff is deflated is further evidence of a leak present around the endotracheal tube.
6. The cuff should then be reinflated and the results of the test documented in the patient's medical record.

References

Boles, J.-M., Bion, J., Connors, A., Herridge, M., Marsh, B., Melot, C., et al. (2007). Weaning from mechanical ventilation. *European Respiratory Journal, 29*(5), 1033–1056.

Cook, D., Meade, M., Guyatt, G., Griffith, L., Booker, L. (2000). *Criteria for weaning from mechanical ventilation: Evidence Report/Technology Assessment No. 23* (Prepared by McMaster University under Contract No. 290-97-0017) (AHRQ Publication No. 01-E010). Rockville, MD: Agency for Healthcare Research and Quality.

Ely, E. W., Meade, M. O., Haponik, E. F., Kollef, M. H., Cook, D. J., Guyatt, G. H., et al. (2001). Mechanical ventilator weaning protocols by nonphysician health-care professionals: Evidence-based clinical practice guidelines. *Chest, 120,* 454S–463S.

MacIntyre, N. R., Cook, D. J., Ely, E. W., et al. (2002). Evidence-Based Guidelines for Weaning and Discontinuing Ventilatory Support. A Collective Task Force Facilitated by the American College of Chest Physicians, the American Association for Respiratory Care, and the American College of Critical Care Medicine. *Respiratory Care, 47*(1), 69–90.

Additional Resources

Blackwood, B., Alderdice, F., Burns, K. E. A., Cardwell, C. R., Lavery, G., & O'Halloran, P. (2010). Protocolized versus non-protocolized weaning for reducing the duration of mechanical ventilation in critically ill adult patients. *Cochrane Database of Systematic Reviews, 5.* Art. No.: CD006904. doi: 10.1002/14651858.CD006904.pub.2

Burns, K. E., Lellouche, F., & Lessard, M. R. (2009). Automating the weaning process with advanced closed-loop systems. *Intensive Care Medicine, 34*(10), 1757–1765.

MacIntyre, N. R. (1995). Respiratory factors in weaning from mechanical ventilatory support. *Respiratory Care, 40*(3), 244–248.

Wilkins, R. L., Stoller, J. K., & Kacmarek, R. M. (2009). *Egan's fundamentals of respiratory care* (9th ed.). St. Louis, MO: Mosby.

Practice Activities: Weaning and Discontinuation of Mechanical Ventilation

Determining Readiness for Entry into a Spontaneous Breathing Trial

Please read the following scenarios carefully and then answer the questions that follow.

Scenario 1

Reason for Admission

Mr. Jones is a 35-year-old delivery truck driver who was the victim of a rather serious motor vehicle crash. Mr. Jones was making his usual morning rounds delivering bread to downtown restaurants. He had just gotten out of his truck when he was struck by an out-of-control passenger car. He was pinned between the car and his delivery truck for several minutes before emergency medical personnel were able to free him. Mr. Jones sustained several severe injuries to his lower extremities including bilateral femur fractures and a significant pelvic fracture. He left the scene via ambulance and lost consciousness en route to the local trauma center. He was intubated in the ambulance and was taken directly to surgery after being stabilized in the emergency department. In surgery he received several units of blood and crystalloid volume expanders.

Past Medical History

Mr. Jones is a healthy young man with no significant past medical history. He is a nonsmoker. He occasionally drinks alcohol, averaging one to two drinks per week. He works out regularly.

Present Situation

Mr. Jones got out of surgery 24 hours ago. The surgeon purposefully kept him intubated overnight to stabilize his hemodynamic status. The surgeon is making rounds and has asked you to assess if Mr. Jones qualifies for a spontaneous breathing trial this morning.

You collect the following data.

Ventilator Settings:

Mode	Assist control
Set Respiratory Rate	14
Spontaneous Respiratory Rate	0 (patient sedated)
Tidal Volume	650 mL
FIO_2	0.35
PEEP	5 cm H_2O
Peak Pressure	22 cm H_2O
Plateau Pressure	18 cm H_2O

Vital Signs/Assessment:

Breath Sounds	Clear to auscultation
Blood Pressure	118/74
Heart rate	72
Heart Rhythm	Normal sinus rhythm
SpO_2	98%
Sensorium	Patient sedated at present. Does awaken when gently stimulated and appears

appropriate. Patient is able to follow simple commands and nod yes or no to simple questions.

Questions

A. When considering this patient for a spontaneous breathing trial, what additional data would you like to have (if any) and why?

B. Does this patient qualify for a spontaneous breathing trial? Why or why not?

Scenario 2

Reason for Admission

Mrs. Morley is a 67-year-old patient with COPD who recently called the paramedics from her home due to increased shortness of breath. When the paramedics arrived they found Mrs. Morley at her kitchen table, bracing her hands on her knees in the "tripod" position. She was unable to answer questions verbally, electing to nod yes or no to simple questions. She had marked use of accessory muscles and did not seem to respond to the initial nebulizer treatments (with albuterol and ipratropium bromide) that the medics administered to her. She was placed on a gurney and into the ambulance for transport to the nearest hospital. On the way to the hospital she became lethargic and generally nonresponsive. The medics intubated her in the ambulance and brought her to the emergency department.

Past Medical History

Mrs. Morley has a rather complicated medical history. She has COPD, congestive heart failure (CHF), hypertension, and obesity hypoventilation syndrome. She has been hospitalized 3 times in the past 6 months for breathing difficulties. She continues to smoke one pack a day and has done so for the past 42 years. She is on continuous home oxygen at 2 L/min and has a CPAP unit for use when she sleeps, though she admits to only using it occasionally.

Present Situation

Mrs. Morley was brought to the emergency department where she was stabilized with more bronchodilators, intravenous (IV) corticosteroids, and diuretic therapy. Additional diagnostic tests done in the emergency department revealed that she is likely suffering from acute exacerbations of her long-standing COPD and CHF as well as acute, community-acquired right lower lobe pneumonia. It has been approximately 24 hours since Mrs. Morley's admission and the intensivist in the ICU this morning asks you for your opinion regarding whether or not Mrs. Morley qualifies for a spontaneous breathing trial. You collect the following data:

Ventilator Settings:

Mode	Assist control
Set Respiratory Rate	18
Spontaneous Respiratory Rate	0 (patient sedated)
Tidal Volume	600 mL

FIO$_2$	0.65
PEEP	10 cm H$_2$O
Peak Pressure	32 cm H$_2$O
Plateau Pressure	29 cm H$_2$O

Vital Signs/Assessment:

Breath Sounds	Diminished air movement throughout, fine inspiratory crackles are heard in the basilar regions bilaterally, upper lung fields possess diffuse, polyphonic expiratory wheezing.
Blood Pressure	138/94
Heart rate	93
Heart Rhythm	Normal sinus rhythm, occasional premature ventricular complexes (PVCs)
SpO$_2$	90%
Sensorium	Patient sedated at present; does awaken but grows extremely agitated and will not follow simple commands.
Diagnostic data	A chest x-ray taken this morning reveals persisting infiltrates in the right lower lobe and a continued perihilar pattern consistent with CHF.

Questions

A. When considering this patient for a spontaneous breathing trial, what additional data would you like to have (if any) and why?
B. Does this patient qualify for a spontaneous breathing trial? Why or why not?

Placing a Patient into a Spontaneous Breathing Trial

Please read the following scenarios carefully and then answer the questions that follow.

Scenario 3

Reason for Admission

Mr. Johnson is a 65-year-old postoperative coronary artery bypass graft patient. He has been out of surgery and in the cardiac intensive care unit for 1 hour and has begun to wake up and follow some simple commands. He is intubated with a 8.0 endotracheal tube secured at 23 cm, center teeth.

For the following portion of the exercise please use an adult ventilator equipped with an adult ventilator circuit. See Chapter 25 for specifics regarding the setup and operation of the ventilator you are using. Connect the ventilator to 50 psi air and oxygen sources and connect the ventilator's power cord to a standard, grounded electrical outlet. Follow the manufacturer's guidelines for setting up and testing the ventilator prior to use on a patient.

To complete these practice activities, it is recommended that you use a lung analog/simulator such as an SMS "Manley" lung simulator or an IngMar Medical Quick Lung or Demonstration Lung Model. If these devices are not available, a standard, single balloon test lung may be used as well.

Test Lung Setup

If you are using an SMS ("Manley") lung simulator, connect one spring for compliance, set the resistance control to zero, and rotate the leak control fully clockwise, eliminating any leaks. Attach the patient wye to the inlet of the SMS lung simulator.

If you are using an IngMar Medical Demonstration Lung Model, rotate all of the compliance springs fully clockwise, adjust the resistance controls to "OFF," and adjust both the ET Leak and System Leak controls to the "OFF" position. Attach the patient wye to the inlet of the Demonstration Lung Model.

Once the ventilator is set up and ready for use, input the following settings and attach it to the test lung.

Ventilator Settings:

Mode	Synchronized intermittent mandatory ventilation (SIMV)
Set Respiratory Rate	10
Tidal Volume	600 mL
Flow	60 L/min
FIO$_2$	0.35
PEEP	5 cm H$_2$O
Pressure Support	5 cm H$_2$O

Once the settings have been established, go into the alarm values section of the ventilator and set the available alarms appropriately for this patient.

Have your laboratory partner gently "breathe" the test lung. Attempt to average an additional 5 to 6 breaths per minute. As this is being done, record the following parameters (a standard "ventilator flow sheet" may be helpful in organizing your data):

1. Mode
2. FIO$_2$
3. Respiratory Rate (Set and Total)
4. Tidal Volume (Set)
5. Tidal Volume (Spontaneous)
6. PEEP
7. Pressure Support Level
8. Mean Airway Pressure
9. Inspiratory Time
10. I:E ratio
11. Minute Ventilation
12. Peak Pressure

Mr. Johnson is resting comfortably on the current settings noted on your ventilator flow sheet. He awakens easily and is able to follow simple commands. Additional data are presented next.

Chest X-ray:	Done postoperatively, shows sternal wires used to close sternum. ET tube, pulmonary artery catheter, and gastric tube all in good position. No obvious pneumothorax, infiltrate, or atelectasis.
Arterial Blood Gas:	Done on current settings: pH 7.36, PaCO$_2$ 43 mm Hg, PaO$_2$ 98 mm Hg, HCO$_3$ 23 mEq/L, BE -3 mEq/L, SaO$_2$ 96%

Breath Sounds:	Clear to auscultation though slightly diminished in the lower lobes.
Blood Pressure:	110/64
Heart rate:	82
Heart Rhythm:	Normal sinus rhythm
SpO_2:	95%

Past Medical History

Mr. Johnson is an otherwise healthy man with a history significant for coronary artery disease and hypertension. He is a life-long nonsmoker.

Present Situation

The cardiac surgeon has been pushing the respiratory care department to extubate open heart patients in an efficient yet safe manner. As such, you are ready to begin a spontaneous breathing trial with Mr. Johnson.

Question Set 1

A. Do you feel that Mr. Johnson qualifies for a spontaneous breathing trial? Why or why not?

You are now ready to place the patient into a spontaneous breathing trial. Input the following settings and activate the new mode of ventilation:

Mode	CPAP
CPAP (PEEP)	5 cm H_2O
FIO_2	0.30
ATC	On

Once the settings have been established, go into the alarm values section of the ventilator and set the available alarms appropriately for this patient.

Have your laboratory partner gently "breathe" the test lung. Attempt to average a respiratory rate of 15 breaths per minute and a tidal volume of 550 mL. As this is being done, record the following parameters (a standard "ventilator flow sheet" may be helpful in organizing your data):

1. Mode
2. FIO_2
3. Respiratory Rate (Spontaneous)
4. Tidal Volume (Spontaneous)
5. PEEP
6. Presence of Automatic Tube Compensation
7. Minute Ventilation

As your patient continues to breathe, you note the following:

Breath Sounds	Clear to auscultation though slightly diminished in the lower lobes.
Blood Pressure	121/72
Heart rate	89
Heart Rhythm	Normal sinus rhythm
SpO_2	97%
Sensorium	Patient resting comfortably, no complaints of shortness of breath. Able to follow commands.

Question Set 2

A. What is the patient's calculated RSBI?
B. Given the clinical data presented, is this patient tolerating his spontaneous breathing trial? Why or why not?
C. Is the RSBI value consistent with a patient who is likely to do well postextubation?
D. Is this patient ready for extubation?
E. If you were to extubate this patient, what additional information would you want to have and why?

Scenario 4

Reason for Admission

Mrs. Smith is a 43-year-old patient with a complicated hospital course. She was admitted 1 week ago for a postoperative wound infection. She subsequently decompensated, developing sepsis and acute respiratory distress syndrome (ARDS). She was intubated 5 days ago and has been managed on the ventilator with a lung protective, low tidal volume strategy. She is intubated with a 7.5 endotracheal tube secured at 22 cm, center teeth.

For the following portion of the exercise please use an adult ventilator equipped with an adult ventilator circuit. See Chapter 25 for specifics regarding the setup and operation of the ventilator you are using. Connect the ventilator to 50 psi air and oxygen sources and connect the ventilator's power cord to a standard, grounded electrical outlet. Follow the manufacturer's guidelines for setting up and testing the ventilator prior to use on a patient.

To complete these practice activities, it is recommended that you use a lung analog/simulator such as an SMS "Manley" lung simulator or an IngMar Medical Quick Lung or Demonstration Lung Model. If these devices are not available, a standard, single balloon test lung may be used as well.

Test Lung Setup

If you are using an SMS ("Manley") lung simulator, connect one spring for compliance, set the resistance control to zero, and rotate the leak control fully clockwise, eliminating any leaks. Attach the patient wye to the inlet of the SMS lung simulator.

If you are using an IngMar Medical Demonstration Lung Model, rotate all of the compliance springs fully clockwise, adjust the resistance controls to "OFF," and adjust both the ET Leak and System Leak controls to the "OFF" position. Attach the patient wye to the inlet of the Demonstration Lung Model.

Once the ventilator is set up and ready for use, input the following settings and attach it to the test lung.

Ventilator Settings:

Mode	Assist control
Set Respiratory Rate	29
Tidal Volume	450 mL
Flow	60 L/min
FIO_2	0.85
PEEP	10 cm H_2O

Once the settings have been established, go into the alarm values section of the ventilator and set the available alarms appropriately for this patient.

Record the following parameters (a standard "ventilator flow sheet" may be helpful in organizing your data):

1. Mode
2. FIO$_2$
3. Flow
4. Respiratory Rate (Set and Total)
5. Tidal Volume (Set)
6. Tidal Volume (Spontaneous)
7. PEEP
8. Mean Airway Pressure
9. Inspiratory Time
10. I:E ratio
11. Minute Ventilation
12. Peak Pressure
13. Plateau Pressure

Mrs. Smith is sedated and is requiring a significant amount of vasoporessors to keep her blood pressure within an acceptable range.

Additional data are presented next.

Chest X-ray	Done this morning, shows diffuse "ground-glass" opacities throughout. ET tube and gastric tube both in good position. No obvious pneumothorax.
Arterial Blood Gas	Done on current settings: pH 7.31, PaCO$_2$ 54 mm Hg, PaO$_2$ 63 mm Hg, HCO$_3$ 26 mEq/L, SaO$_2$ 91%
Breath Sounds	Course crackles throughout, diminished in the lower lobes.
Blood Pressure	100/54
Heart rate	110
Heart Rhythm	Sinus tachycardia
SpO$_2$	90%

Past Medical History

Mrs. Smith is an otherwise healthy woman with no significant past medical history. She is a nonsmoker, nondrinker. Three weeks ago she broke her ankle.

Present Situation

She had surgery to repair her ankle fracture and failed to follow through with the recommended guidelines regarding care of her wound. She developed redness and swelling at the site of infection and subsequently developed a fever and chills. She came to the emergency department, where she had numerous tests run, including blood cultures. The blood cultures came back positive for gram-negative septicemia. She was admitted for close observation and IV antibiotics. Despite antibiotic therapy she continued to deteriorate in a rather rapid fashion. She ultimately required massive fluid resuscitation after going into septic shock. She was intubated for respiratory failure.

The pulmonary/critical care physician is rounding on his patients this morning and asks you if Mrs. Smith is ready for a spontaneous breathing trial.

Question Set 1

A. Do you feel that Mrs. Smith qualifies for a spontaneous breathing trial? Why or why not?

Another 4 days go by, and once again you find yourself caring for Mrs. Smith. Today you enter her room and note that she has significantly fewer IV pumps running. She is off all vasopressors and is only lightly sedated. You discuss her progress with her nurse and find that she has made a great deal of progress since the last time you saw her. You enter her room and find the following data.

Adjust the ventilator to the following parameters:

Ventilator Settings:

Mode	Assist control
Set Respiratory Rate	20
Tidal Volume	500 mL
Flow	50 L/min
FiO$_2$	0.40
PEEP	8 cm H$_2$O

Once the settings have been established, go into the alarm values section of the ventilator and set the available alarms appropriately for this patient.

Record the following parameters (a standard "ventilator flow sheet" may be helpful in organizing your data):

1. Mode
2. FIO$_2$
3. Flow
4. Respiratory Rate (Set and Total)
5. Tidal Volume (Set)
6. Tidal Volume (Spontaneous)
7. PEEP
8. Mean Airway Pressure
9. Inspiratory Time
10. I:E ratio
11. Minute Ventilation
12. Peak Pressure
13. Plateau Pressure

Additional data are presented next.

Chest X-ray:	Done this morning, shows marked improvement from previous days' films, "ground glass" opacity clearing. ET tube and gastric tube both in good position. No obvious pneumothorax.
Arterial Blood Gas:	Done on current settings: pH 7.35, PaCO$_2$ 42 mm Hg, PaO$_2$ 83 mm Hg, HCO$_3$ 24 mEq/L, SaO$_2$ 98%
Breath Sounds:	Diminished in the lower lobes.
Blood Pressure:	115/74
Heart rate:	91
Heart Rhythm	Normal sinus rhythm
SpO$_2$	96%

You are now ready to place the patient into a spontaneous breathing trial. Input the following settings and activate the new mode of ventilation:

Mode	CPAP
CPAP (PEEP)	5 cm H_2O
FIO_2:	0.40
ATC	On

Once the settings have been established, go into the alarm values section of the ventilator and set the available alarms appropriately for this patient.

Have your laboratory partner gently "breathe" the test lung. Attempt to average a respiratory rate of 25 breaths per minute and a tidal volume of 200 mL. As this is being done, record the following parameters (a standard "ventilator flow sheet" may be helpful in organizing your data):

1. Mode
2. FIO_2
3. Respiratory Rate (Spontaneous)
4. Tidal Volume (Spontaneous)
5. PEEP
6. Presence of ATC
7. Minute Ventilation

As your patient continues to breathe you note the following:

Breath Sounds	Very diminished in the lower lobes.
Blood Pressure	139/95
Heart rate	132
Heart Rhythm	Sinus tachycardia
SpO_2	88%
Sensorium	Patient very anxious, using accessory muscles, not able to follow commands.

Question Set 2

A. What is the patient's calculated RSBI?
B. Given the clinical data presented, is this patient tolerating her spontaneous breathing trial? Why or why not?
C. Is the RSBI value consistent with a patient who is likely to do well postextubation?
D. Is this patient ready for extubation?
E. What should the RCP do given the current clinical presentation of the patient?

Check List: Spontaneous Breathing Trial

_____ 1. Verify the physician's order or protocol.
_____ 2. Discuss weaning plans with the patient's health care team.
_____ 3. Perform hand hygiene and don appropriate personal protective gear.
4. Assess patient readiness for SBT:
_____ a. Assess the evidence indicating reversal of the underlying cause of respiratory failure.
_____ b. Assess the adequacy of the patient's oxygenation.
_____ c. Assess the patient's hemodynamic status.
_____ d. Assess the patient's ability to generate an inspiratory effort.
5. Assess and record the baseline data:
_____ a. Ventilator settings
_____ b. Electrocardiogram (ECG) data (heart rate and rhythm)
_____ c. Blood pressure
_____ d. oxygen saturation
_____ e. Breath sounds
_____ f. Work of breathing
_____ g. Patient's general appearance
_____ 6. Explain the procedure to the patient.
_____ 7. Place the patient into spontaneous mode of ventilation.
8. Monitor the patient and assess and record the data at the start of SBT:
_____ a. Ventilator settings
_____ b. Respiratory rate
_____ c. Tidal volume
_____ d. ECG data (heart rate and rhythm)
_____ e. Blood pressure
_____ f. oxygen saturation
_____ g. Breath sounds
_____ h. Work of breathing
_____ i. Patient's general appearance
_____ j. RSBI
_____ k. Vital capacity, maximal inspiratory pressure, and so on (if the facility uses these measurements)
9. Assess for signs that the patient is failing the SBT:
_____ a. Cardiac dysrhythmias
_____ b. Prolonged respiratory rate greater than 35
_____ c. Heart rate greater than 140 or a 20% increase from baseline
_____ d. Systolic blood pressure greater than 180 mm Hg or less than 80 mm Hg
_____ e. Increased anxiety, diaphoresis
_____ f. RSBI greater than 105
_____ g. Sustained SpO_2 less than 90%
_____ 10. Continue SBT for an appropriate amount of time (greater than 30 minutes, less than 2 hours).
11. Monitor the patient and assess and record the data at the end of the SBT:
_____ a. Ventilator settings
_____ b. Respiratory rate
_____ c. Tidal volume
_____ d. ECG data (heart rate and rhythm)
_____ e. Blood pressure
_____ f. oxygen saturation
_____ g. Breath sounds
_____ h. Work of breathing
_____ i. Patient's general appearance

_____   j. RSBI
_____   k. Vital capacity, maximal inspiratory pressure, and so on (if the facility uses these measurements)
_____ 12. Return the patient who failed the SBT to his or her previous ventilator settings and ensure that the patient is stable.

_____ 13. Notify the physician of the SBT results.
_____ 14. Clean up the patient's area.
_____ 15. Record all information in the patient's medical record.

Self Evaluation Post Test: Weaning and Discontinuation of Mechanical Ventilation

1. A stroke that extends into the brain stem that results in apnea requiring mechanical ventilation would be categorized as a _____ cause of ventilator dependence.
   a. cardiovascular
   b. neurologic
   c. psychological
   d. respiratory

2. Which of the following factors contribute to the respiratory system's ability to function effectively?
   a. lung compliance
   b. airway resistance
   c. diaphragm function
   d. all of the above

3. All of the following questions should be considered when evaluating a patient for entry into a spontaneous breathing trial (SBT) *except*:
   a. Is there evidence of reversal of the underlying cause of respiratory failure?
   b. Is there evidence of adequate oxygenation?
   c. Has the patient been on vancomycin in the last 24 hours?
   d. Can the patient generate an inspiratory effort?

4. You are taking care of a patient with ARDS in the ICU. The patient is currently on volume assist-control ventilation with a respiratory rate of 20, a tidal volume of 550 mL, a PEEP of 10 cm H_2O, and an FIO_2 of 0.90. The patient's current oxygen saturation is 89%. The physician is inquiring about the patient's readiness for a spontaneous breathing trial (SBT). The respiratory care practitioner's most appropriate response would be:
   a. "This patient is ready for an SBT. I am placing the patient on CPAP in 5 minutes."
   b. "This patient is not ready for an SBT because the patient is hemodynamically unstable."
   c. "This patient is not ready for an SBT because the patient is not ventilating adequately."
   d. "This patient is not ready for an SBT because the patient is still requiring high levels of PEEP and oxygen."

5. A spontaneous breathing trial (SBT) can be performed in which of the following ways?
   I.   By placing the patient into CPAP mode on the ventilator
   II. By placing the patient in inverse ratio pressure control ventilation
   III. By placing the patient on an aerosol T piece
   a. I   c. I, III
   b. I, II   d. II, III

6. Which of the following are indications that a patient may not be tolerating a spontaneous breathing trial?
   I.   Increased heart rate of 20% above baseline
   II. Diaphoresis
   III. Accessory muscle use
   IV. Respiratory rate greater than 35 breaths per minute
   a. I   c. I, II, III
   b. I, II   d. I, II, III, IV

7. A rapid-shallow-breathing index (RSBI) is calculated by:
   a. dividing the respiratory rate by the peak pressure.
   b. multiplying the peak pressure by the lung compliance.
   c. dividing the spontaneous respiratory rate by the spontaneous tidal volume (in liters).
   d. subtracting the plateau pressure from the peak pressure.

8. A patient has been breathing on CPAP for 60 minutes. The patient's respiratory rate is 22 and the tidal volume is, on average, 560 mL. What is the patient's rapid-shallow-breathing index (RSBI)?
   a. 39   c. 25
   b. 12   d. 0.04

9. Patients who fail a spontaneous breathing trial should be:
   I.   placed on a mode of ventilation that allows them to rest and recover.
   II. placed into another spontaneous breathing trial in 24 hours.
   III. evaluated for factors that may have contributed to their failure.
   a. I   c. I, II, III
   b. I, II   d. II, III

10. When calculating the rapid-shallow-breathing index, a value less than _____ is consistent with potential success postextubation.
   a. 40   c. 70
   b. 50   d. 105

PERFORMANCE EVALUATION:
Spontaneous Breathing Trial

Date: Lab _____ Clinical _____ Agency _____

Lab: Pass _____ Fail _____   Clinical: Pass _____ Fail _____

Student name _____ Instructor name _____

No. of times observed in clinical _____

No. of times practiced in clinical _____

PASSING CRITERIA: Obtain 90% or better on the procedure. Tasks indicated by * must receive at least 1 point, or the evaluation is terminated. Procedure must be performed within the designated time, or the performance receives a failing grade.

SCORING:
2 points — Task performed satisfactorily without prompting.
1 point — Task performed satisfactorily with self-initiated correction.
0 points — Task performed incorrectly or with prompting required.
NA — Task not applicable to the patient care situation.

Tasks:	Peer	Lab	Clinical
* **1.** Verifies the physician's order or protocol	☐	☐	☐
* **2.** Discusses the weaning plans with the patient's health care team	☐	☐	☐
* **3.** Performs hand hygiene and dons appropriate personal protective gear	☐	☐	☐
* **4.** Assesses the patient's readiness for SBT			
a. Assesses evidence indicating reversal of the underlying cause of respiratory failure	☐	☐	☐
b. Assesses adequacy of the patient's oxygenation	☐	☐	☐
c. Assesses the patient's hemodynamic status	☐	☐	☐
d. Assesses the patient's ability to generate an inspiratory effort	☐	☐	☐
* **5.** Assesses and records baseline data			
a. Ventilator settings	☐	☐	☐
b. ECG data (heart rate and rhythm)	☐	☐	☐
c. Blood pressure	☐	☐	☐
d. oxygen saturation	☐	☐	☐
e. Breath sounds	☐	☐	☐
f. Work of breathing	☐	☐	☐
g. Patient's general appearance	☐	☐	☐
6. Explains the procedure to the patient	☐	☐	☐

* **7.** Places the patient into a spontaneous mode of ventilation ☐ ☐ ☐

* **8.** Monitors the patient and assesses and records the data at the start
of the SBT

    a. Ventilator settings ☐ ☐ ☐

    b. Respiratory rate ☐ ☐ ☐

    c. Tidal volume ☐ ☐ ☐

    d. ECG data (heart rate and rhythm) ☐ ☐ ☐

    e. Blood pressure ☐ ☐ ☐

    f. oxygen saturation ☐ ☐ ☐

    g. Breath sounds ☐ ☐ ☐

    h. Work of breathing ☐ ☐ ☐

    i. Patient's general appearance ☐ ☐ ☐

    j. Rapid-shallow-breathing index (RSBI) ☐ ☐ ☐

    k. Vital capacity, maximal inspiratory pressure, and so on (if the facility
uses these measurements) ☐ ☐ ☐

* **9.** Assesses for signs that the patient is failing the SBT

    a. Cardiac dysrhythmias ☐ ☐ ☐

    b. Prolonged respiratory rate greater than 35 ☐ ☐ ☐

    c. Heart rate greater than 140 or a 20% increase from baseline ☐ ☐ ☐

    d. Systolic blood pressure greater than 180 mm Hg or less than
80 mm Hg ☐ ☐ ☐

    e. Increased anxiety, diaphoresis ☐ ☐ ☐

    f. RSBI greater than 105 ☐ ☐ ☐

    g. Sustained SpO_2 less than 90% ☐ ☐ ☐

* **10.** Continues SBT for an appropriate amount of time (greater than 30 minutes,
less than 2 hours) ☐ ☐ ☐

* **11.** Monitors the patient and assesses and records the data at the end
of the SBT

    a. Ventilator settings ☐ ☐ ☐

    b. Respiratory rate ☐ ☐ ☐

    c. Tidal volume ☐ ☐ ☐

    d. ECG data (heart rate and rhythm) ☐ ☐ ☐

    e. Blood pressure ☐ ☐ ☐

    f. oxygen saturation ☐ ☐ ☐

    g. Breath sounds ☐ ☐ ☐

    h. Work of breathing ☐ ☐ ☐

    i. Patient's general appearance   ☐ ☐ ☐

    j. Rapid shallow breathing index (RSBI)   ☐ ☐ ☐

    k. Vital capacity, maximal inspiratory pressure, and so on (if the facility uses these measurements)   ☐ ☐ ☐

* **12.** Returns the patient who fails the SBT to the patient's previous ventilator settings and ensures that the patient is stable   ☐ ☐ ☐

* **13.** Notifies the physician of the SBT results   ☐ ☐ ☐

* **14.** Cleans up the patient's area   ☐ ☐ ☐

* **15.** Records all information in the patient's medical record   ☐ ☐ ☐

SCORE: Peer _____ points of possible 98; _____%

                  Lab _____ points of possible 98; _____%

                  Clinical _____ points of possible 98; _____%

TIME: _____ out of possible 120 minutes

STUDENT SIGNATURES

PEER: _____

STUDENT: _____

INSTRUCTOR SIGNATURES

LAB: _____

CLINICAL: _____

CHAPTER 29

Neonatal Mechanical Ventilation

Scott J. Mahoney

INTRODUCTION

Neonatal mechanical ventilation has evolved considerably in recent years. Many early neonatal mechanical ventilators were specialty machines designed to serve the neonatal patient population exclusively. Modes of ventilation were largely limited to constant flow, time-cycled, pressure-limited intermittent mandatory ventilation (IMV) or continuous positive airway pressure (CPAP). A typical respiratory care department would have one group of ventilators to serve its adult population and a completely different group of ventilators in its neonatal intensive care unit (NICU). This arrangement required respiratory care practitioners to become comfortable ventilating patients, who inherently possessed differing physiology, with different ventilators that inherently possessed differing operating principles. Modern advances in ventilation technology have helped to change this paradigm.

The advent of improved monitoring and flow-sensing capabilities combined with improved computing has led to the introduction of so-called life span or cradle-to-grave ventilator platforms. These modern ICU ventilators offer distinct modes for three different patient populations: neonatal, pediatric, and adult. This chapter focuses on the features of three of these ventilators: the Maquet SERVO-i, the Nellcor Puritan Bennett 840, and the Viasys AVEA. The chapter also discusses one neonatal-specific ventilator, the Dräger Babylog 8000 *plus*, a noninvasive ventilator, the Arabella Nasal CPAP system, as well as the theory, principles, and operation of the Viasys SensorMedics 3100A High Frequency Oscillatory Ventilator.

KEY TERMS

- Amplitude (ΔP)
- Apgar scoring system
- CPAP
- Hertz (Hz)
- High-frequency oscillatory ventilation
- High-frequency ventilation
- Nasal CPAP
- Pressure assist control
- Pressure limiting
- Pressure regulated volume control
- Pressure SIMV
- Pressure support
- Respiratory failure
- Retinopathy of prematurity
- Time constant
- Time-cycled, pressure-limited ventilation
- Transillumination
- Volume assist control
- Volume guarantee
- Volume SIMV
- Volume support

THEORY OBJECTIVES

At the end of this chapter, the reader should be able to:

- *Describe these common, invasive neonatal modes of ventilation:*
  - *Continuous positive airway pressure (CPAP)*
  - *Pressure synchronized intermittent mandatory ventilation (SIMV)*
  - *Volume SIMV*
  - *Pressure assist control*
  - *Volume assist control*
  - *Time-cycled, pressure-limited ventilation*
  - *Pressure support*
  - *Volume support*
  - *Pressure regulated volume control*
- *Describe the mode extension, volume guarantee.*

- *Describe the theory, principles, and use of high-frequency oscillatory ventilation.*
- *Describe the use of noninvasive, nasal CPAP in the neonatal patient population.*
- *State the following indications for mechanical ventilation and the rationale for each:*
  - *Apnea*
  - *Hypercapnia*
  - *Refractory hypoxemia*
  - *Persistent pulmonary hypertension of the newborn*
- *List the underlying conditions that may contribute to respiratory failure in the neonate:*
  - *Respiratory distress syndrome (RDS)*
  - *Drugs administered to the mother during labor*
  - *Aspiration before, during, or after delivery*

- *Meconium*
- *Amniotic fluid*
- *Blood*
- *Gastric contents*
- *Acquired pneumonias*
- *Pulmonary hypoplasia*
- *Congenital defects*
- *Diaphragmatic hernia*
- *Cardiac anomalies*
- *Explain the following concepts with regard to mechanical ventilation of the newborn:*
  - *Time constants*
  - *Time cycling*
  - *I:E ratio and inspiratory time*

- *Pressure limiting*
- *Flow rate*
- *Describe the potential hazards and complications of newborn mechanical ventilation:*
  - *Barotrauma (volutrauma, atelectrauma)*
  - *Retinopathy of prematurity (ROP)*
  - *Bronchopulmonary dysplasia (BPD)*
  - *Infection*
  - *Increased intracranial pressure*
  - *Reduced cardiac output*
  - *Pulmonary air leak*

CLINICAL PRACTICE GUIDELINES

AARC Clinical Practice Guideline Neonatal Time-Triggered, Pressure-Limited, Time-Cycled Mechanical Ventilation (retired guideline)

TPTV 4.0 INDICATIONS:

The presence of one or more of the following conditions constitutes an indication for TPTV.

4.1 Apnea (24–27)

4.2 Respiratory or ventilatory failure, despite the use of continuous positive airway pressure (CPAP) and supplemental oxygen (i.e., $FIO_2 >$ or $= 0.60$) (24,25,28)

4.2.1 Respiratory acidosis with a pH < 7.20–7.25 (8,25,29)

4.2.2 $PaO_2 < 50$ torr (8,13,25,29,30)

4.2.3 Abnormalities on physical examination

4.2.3.1 Increased work of breathing demonstrated by grunting, nasal flaring, tachypnea, and sternal and intercostal retractions (5,27,29,31)

4.2.3.2 The presence of pale or cyanotic skin and agitation

4.3 Alterations in neurologic status that compromise the central drive to breathe:

4.3.1 Apnea of prematurity (32)

4.3.2 Intracranial hemorrhage (33)

4.3.3 Congenital neuromuscular disorders (34)

4.4 Impaired respiratory function resulting in a compromised functional residual capacity (FRC) due to decreased lung compliance and/or increased airway resistance, (12,35) including but not limited to:

4.4.1 Respiratory distress syndrome (RDS) (1,2,28,36–39)

4.4.2 Meconium aspiration syndrome (MAS) (40)

4.4.3 Pneumonia (41)

4.4.4 Bronchopulmonary dysplasia (42–44)

4.4.5 Bronchiolitis (41)

4.4.6 Congenital diaphragmatic hernia (45)

4.4.7 Sepsis (41)

4.4.8 Radiographic evidence of decreased lung volume (27)

4.5 Impaired cardiovascular function

4.5.1 Persistent pulmonary hypertension of the newborn (PPHN) (46,47)

4.5.2 Postresuscitation (41)

4.5.3 Congenital heart disease (48)

4.5.4 Shock (6)

4.6 Postoperative state characterized by impaired ventilatory function (45,49)

TPTV 5.0 CONTRAINDICATIONS:

No specific contraindications for neonatal TPTV exist when indications are judged to be present (Section 4.0).

TPTV 6.0 HAZARDS/COMPLICATIONS:

6.1 Air leak syndromes due to barotrauma and/or volume overinflation (i.e., volutrauma), (2,11,50–54) including:

6.1.1 Pneumothorax (16,55–59)

6.1.2 Pneumomediastinum (55,56,58)

6.1.3 Pneumopericardium (55)

6.1.4 Pneumoperitoneum (55)

6.1.5 Subcutaneous emphysema (55)

6.1.6 Pulmonary interstitial emphysema (56,60–62)

6.2 Chronic lung disease associated with prolonged positive pressure ventilation and oxygen toxicity (63,64) (e.g., bronchopulmonary dysplasia (42,43,65–68))

6.3 Airway complications associated with endotracheal intubation

(Continued)

6.3.1 Laryngotracheobronchomalacia (69)

6.3.2 Damage to upper airway structures (66,69,70)

6.3.3 Malpositioning of endotracheal tube (ETT) (69,71)

6.3.4 Partial or total obstruction of ETT with mucus (69,71,72)

6.3.5 Kinking of ETT (69,71)

6.3.6 Unplanned extubation (69,71,73)

6.3.7 Air leak around uncuffed ETT

6.3.8 Subglottic stenosis (69)

6.3.9 Main-stem intubation (69)

6.3.10 Pressure necrosis (74)

6.3.11 Increased work of breathing (during spontaneous breaths) due to the high resistance of endotracheal tubes of small internal diameter (75)

6.4 Nosocomial pulmonary infection (e.g., pneumonia (76))

6.5 Complications that occur when positive pressure applied to the lungs is transmitted to the cardiovascular system (77,78) or the cerebral vasculature resulting in:

6.5.1 Decreased venous return (77,78)

6.5.2 Decreased cardiac output (77,78)

6.5.3 Increased intracranial pressure leading to intraventricular hemorrhage (27,33,79)

6.6 Supplemental oxygen in conjunction with TPTV may lead to an increased risk of retinopathy of prematurity (ROP) (80,81)

6.7 Complications associated with endotracheal suctioning (82)

6.8 Technical complications

6.8.1 Ventilator failure (10,83)

6.8.2 Ventilator circuit and/or humidifier failure (38,70) (Condensate in the inspiratory limb of the ventilator circuit may result in a reduction in V_T (23,84) or inadvertent pulmonary lavage.)

6.8.3 Ventilator alarm failure (10,38,69,83)

6.8.4 Loss of or inadequate gas supply

6.9 Patient-ventilator asynchrony (85,86)

6.10 Inappropriate ventilator settings leading to:

6.10.1 Auto-PEEP

6.10.2 Hypo- or hyperventilation

6.10.3 Hypo- or hyperoxemia

6.10.4 Increased work of breathing

TPTV 8.0 ASSESSMENT OF NEED:

Determination that valid indications are present by physical, radiographic, and laboratory assessment

TPTV 9.0 ASSESSMENT OF OUTCOME:

Establishment of neonatal assisted ventilation should result in improvement in patient condition and/or reversal of indications (Section 4.0):

9.1 Reduction in work of breathing as evidenced by decreases in respiratory rate, severity of retractions, nasal flaring, and grunting

9.2 Radiographic evidence of improved lung volume (41)

9.3 Subjective improvement in lung volume as indicated by increased chest excursion and aeration by chest auscultation (87)

9.4 Improved gas exchange

9.4.1 Ability to maintain a PaO_2 > or = 50-torr with FIO_2 < 0.60 (8,30)

9.4.2 Ability to reverse respiratory acidosis and maintain a pH > 7.25 (8,30)

9.4.3 Subjective improvement as indicated by a decrease in grunting, nasal flaring, sternal and intercostal retraction, and respiratory rate (31)

TPTV 11.0 MONITORING:

11.1 Patient-ventilator system checks should be performed every 2–4 hours and should include documentation of ventilator settings and patient assessments as recommended by the AARC CPG Patient-Ventilator System Checks (MV-SC) and AARC CPG Humidification during Mechanical Ventilation (HMV) (95,96)

11.2 Oxygen and CO_2 monitoring

11.2.1 Periodic sampling of blood gas values by arterial, capillary, or venous route (1,24,30) PaO_2 should be kept below 80 torr in preterm infants to minimize the risk of ROP. (6,80,97)

11.2.2 The unstable infant should be monitored continuously by transcutaneous O_2 monitor or pulse oximeter. (1,90,91)

11.2.3 The unstable infant should be monitored continuously by transcutaneous (90) or end-tidal CO_2 monitoring. (93,94)

11.2.4 Fractional concentration of oxygen delivered by the ventilator should be monitored continuously. (38)

11.3 Continuous monitoring of cardiac activity (via electrocardiograph) and respiratory rate (98)

11.4 Monitoring of blood pressure by indwelling arterial line or by periodic cuff measurements (24)

11.5 Continuous monitoring of proximal airway pressures including peak inspiratory pressure (PIP), PEEP, and mean airway pressure (Paw) (1,39,99)

11.5.1 Increases in Paw may result in improved oxygenation; however, Paw > 12 cm H_2O has been associated with barotrauma. (8,20,41,99–102)

11.5.2 The difference between PIP and PEEP (^P) in conjunction with patient mechanics determines V_T. As the ^P changes, V_T will vary. (16,51,99,100)

11.5.3 PIP should be adjusted initially to achieve adequate V_T as reflected by chest excursion and adequate breath sounds (8,29,100) and/or by V_T measurement.

11.5.4 PEEP increases FRC and may improve oxygenation and ventilation-perfusion

(Continued)

relationship (PEEP is typically adjusted at 4–7 cm H_2O—levels beyond this range may result in hyperinflation, particularly in patients with obstructive airways disease [e.g., MAS or bronchiolitis] (5,29,35,103–105)).

11.6 Many commercially available neonatal ventilators provide continuous monitoring of ventilator frequency, tI, and I:E. If only two of these variables are directly monitored, the third should be calculated (e.g., the proportion of the tI for a given frequency determines the I:E).

11.6.1 Lengthening tI increases Paw and should improve oxygenation. (1,2,13,24, 41,106,107)

11.6.2 I:E in excess of 1:1 may lead to the development of auto-PEEP and hyperinflation. (5,20,24,37,105,106,108)

11.6.3 Frequencies of 30–60 per minute with shorter tI (e.g., I:E of 1:2) are commonly used in patients with RDS. (8,22,41,50,59,85,109–111)

11.7 Depending on the internal diameter of the ventilator circuit, excessive flow rates can result in expiratory resistance that leads to increased work of breathing and automatic increases in PEEP. (17,19,89,98,86,112) Some ventilators are equipped with demand-flow systems that permit the use of lower baseline flow rates but provide the patient with additional flow as needed.

11.8 Because of the possibility of complete obstruction or kinking of the ETT and the inadequacy of ventilator alarms in these situations, continuous tidal volume monitoring via an appropriately designed (minimum dead space) proximal airway flow sensor is recommended. (98,113,114)

11.9 Periodic physical assessment of chest excursion and breath sounds and for signs of increased work of breathing and cyanosis. (3,5,21,87)

11.10 Periodic evaluation of chest radiographs to follow the progress of the disease, identify possible complications, and verify ETT placement (21,27,79)

Reprinted with permission from *Respiratory Care* 1994; 39(8): 808–816. The complete AARC Clinical Practice Guidelines are available from the AARC Web site (http://www.aarc .org), from the AARC Executive Office, or from *Respiratory Care* journal.

AARC Clinical Practice Guideline Application of Continuous Positive Airway Pressure to Neonates via Nasal Prongs, Nasopharyngeal Tube, or Nasal Mask—2004 Revision & Update

NCPAP 1.0 PROCEDURE:

The application of continuous positive airway pressure to neonates and infants by nasal prongs (NCPAP), nasopharyngeal tube (NP-CPAP), or infant nasal mask (NM-CPAP) administered with a commercially available circuit used in conjunction with a continuous flow source, infant ventilator, or a suitably equipped multipurpose ventilator.

NCPAP 2.0 DESCRIPTION/DEFINITION:

Continuous positive airway pressure (CPAP) is the application of positive pressure to the airways of the spontaneously breathing patient throughout the respiratory cycle.[1-4] For the most part, neonates are preferential nose breathers, which easily facilitates the application of nasal CPAP.[5-7] This is accomplished by inserting nasopharyngeal tubes, affixing nasal prongs, or fitting a nasal mask to the patient.[8-11] The device provides heated and humidified continuous or variable flow from a circuit connected to a continuous gas source, mechanical ventilator designed for neonates, or a suitably equipped multipurpose ventilator, set in the CPAP mode.[8-19]

CPAP maintains inspiratory and expiratory pressures above ambient pressure, which results in an increase in functional residual capacity (FRC) and improvement in static lung compliance, and decreased airway resistance in the infant with unstable lung mechanics.[1,3,14-23] This allows a greater volume change per unit of pressure change (ie, greater tidal volume for a given pressure change) with subsequent reduction in the work of breathing and stabilization of minute ventilation (V_E).[13,24-28] CPAP increases mean airway pressure, and the associated increase in FRC should improve ventilation-perfusion relationships and potentially reduce oxygen requirements.[24,25,29-33] Additionally CPAP may expand, or stent, upper airway structures preventing collapse and upper airway obstruction.[20,28,34,35]

NCPAP 3.0 SETTINGS:

NCPAP, NP-CPAP, and NM-CPAP are applied by trained personnel in acute and subacute care hospitals.

NCPAP 4.0 INDICATIONS:

4.1 Abnormalities on physical examination—the presence of increased work of breathing as indicated by an increase in respiratory rate of >30% of normal, substernal and suprasternal retractions, grunting, and nasal flaring;[13,20-23,28,33,34,36] the presence of pale or cyanotic skin color and agitation[30,32,33,37]

4.2 Inadequate arterial blood gas values—the inability to maintain a $P_aO_2 > 50$ torr with F_iO_2 of ≤0.60 provided V_E is adequate as indicated by a P_aCO_2 level of 50 torr and a pH ≥ 7.25[13-15,38]

4.3 The presence of poorly expanded and/or infiltrated lung fields on chest radiograph[25,37,38]

(Continued)

4.4 The presence of a condition thought to be responsive to CPAP and associated with one or more of the clinical presentations in 4.1–4.3[11,19,24]

    4.4.1 Respiratory distress syndrome[13–15,38]

    4.4.2 Pulmonary edema[13,39]

    4.4.3 Atelectasis[19,37,40]

    4.4.4 Apnea of prematurity[6,23,33,41–45]

    4.4.5 Recent extubation[17,46–52]

    4.4.6 Tracheal malacia or other similar abnormality of the lower airways[13,53–57]

    4.4.7 Transient tachypnea of the newborn[13,37]

4.5 Early intervention in conjunction with surfactant administration for very low birthweight infants at risk for developing respiratory distress syndrome.[11,13,19,58–64]

4.6 The administration of controlled concentrations of nitric oxide in spontaneously breathing infants.[63]

NCPAP 5.0 CONTRAINDICATIONS:

5.1 Although NCPAP, NP-CPAP, and NMCPAP have been used in bronchiolitis, this application may be contraindicated.[66,67]

5.2 The need for intubation and/or mechanical ventilation as evidenced by the presence of

    5.2.1 Upper airway abnormalities that make NCPAP, NP-CPAP, or NM-CPAP ineffective or potentially dangerous (eg, choanal atresia, cleft palate, tracheoesophageal fistula)[57]

    5.2.2 Severe cardiovascular instability and impending arrest

    5.2.3 Unstable respiratory drive with frequent apneic episodes resulting in desaturation and/or bradycardia

    5.2.4 Ventilatory failure as indicated by the inability to maintain $PaCO_2 < 60$ torr and $pH > 7.25$[31,38]

5.3 Application of NCPAP, NP-CPAP, or NMCPAP to patients with untreated congenital diaphragmatic hernia may lead to gastric distention and further compromise of thoracic organs.[57]

NCPAP 6.0 HAZARDS/ COMPLICATIONS:

6.1 Hazards and complications associated with equipment include the following

    6.1.1 Obstruction of nasal prongs from mucus plugging or kinking of nasopharyngeal tube may interfere with delivery of CPAP and result in a decrease in FIO_2 through entrainment of room air via opposite naris or mouth.

    6.1.2 Inactivation of airway pressure alarms

        6.1.2.1 Increased resistance created by turbulent flow through the small orifices of nasal prongs and nasopharyngeal tubes can maintain pressure in the CPAP system even when decannulation has occurred. This can result in failure of low airway pressure/disconnect alarms to respond.[7]

        6.1.2.2 Complete obstruction of nasal prongs and nasopharyngeal tubes results in continued pressurization of the CPAP system without activation of low or high airway pressure alarms.[69]

    6.1.3 Activation of a manual breath (commonly available on infant ventilators) may cause gastric insufflation and patient discomfort particularly if the peak pressure is set inappropriately high.[70]

    6.1.4 Insufficient gas flow to meet inspiratory demand resulting in a fluctuating baseline pressure and an increase in the work of breathing[11]

    6.1.5 Excessive flow results in overdistension from increased work of breathing due to incomplete exhalation and inadvertent PEEP levels[71]

    6.1.6 Decannulation or malpositioning of prongs or nasopharyngeal tubes causing fluctuating or reduced CPAP levels

    6.1.7 Aspiration or accidental swallowing of small pieces of the detachable circuit or nasal device assembly[72]

    6.1.8 Nasal excoriation, scarring, pressure necrosis, and septal distortion[73,74]

    6.1.9 Skin irritation of the head and neck from improperly secured bonnets or CPAP head harnesses

6.2 Hazards and complications associated with the patient's clinical condition include

    6.2.1 Lung overdistention leading to

        6.2.1.1 Air leak syndromes[75–81]

        6.2.1.2 Ventilation-perfusion mismatch[82]

        6.2.1.3 CO_2 retention and increased work of breathing[7,30,83]

        6.2.1.4 Impedance of pulmonary blood flow with a subsequent increase in pulmonary vascular resistance and decrease in cardiac output[39,84]

    6.2.2 Gastric insufflation and abdominal distention potentially leading to aspiration[34,81,85]

    6.2.3 Nasal mucosal damage due to inadequate humidification[18]

NCPAP 7.0 LIMITATIONS OF DEVICE:

7.1 NCPAP, NP-CPAP, and NM-CPAP applications are not benign procedures, and operators should be aware of the possible hazards and complications and take all necessary precautions to ensure safe and effective application.

7.2 Mouth breathing during NCPAP, NP-CPAP, and NM-CPAP may result in loss of desired pressure and decrease in delivered oxygen concentration.[14,86–89] However, most studies demonstrate effective NCPAP without mouth closure.[11]

(Continued)

7.3 NCPAP harnesses and attachment devices are often cumbersome and difficult to secure and may cause agitation and result in inadvertent decannulation.[7,11,86]

7.4 Excessive head rotation or neck extension may alter the position of NP-CPAP tube placement or obstruct upper airway structures resulting in diminished or altered pressure, flow, and effective CPAP.[11,48]

7.5 Severe RDS, septicemia during NCPAP administration, and pneumothorax are risk factors associated with NCPAP failure.[68,79,90]

NCPAP 8.0 ASSESSMENT OF NEED:

Determination that valid indications are present by physical, radiographic, and laboratory assessments.

NCPAP 9.0 ASSESSMENT OF OUTCOME:

CPAP is initiated at levels of 4–5 cm H_2O and may be gradually increased up to 10 cm H_2O to provide the following[13,25,30,33,59,86,91]

9.1 Stabilization of FIO_2 requirement ≤ 0.60 with PaO_2 levels >50 torr and/or the presence of clinically acceptable noninvasive monitoring of oxygen ($PtCO_2$), while maintaining an adequate V_E as indicated by $PaCO_2$ of 50–60 torr or less and pH ≥ 7.25[19,29,64,92–94]

9.2 Reduction in the work of breathing as indicated by a decrease in respiratory rate by 30–40% and a decrease in the severity of retractions, grunting, and nasal flaring[33,37,69]

9.3 Improvement in lung volumes and appearance of lung as indicated by chest radiograph[19,69]

9.4 Improvement in patient comfort as assessed by bedside caregiver

9.5 Clinically significant reduction in apnea, bradycardia, and cyanosis episodes

NCPAP 10.0 RESOURCES:

10.1 Equipment

10.1.1 Endotracheal tubes (positioned in the nasopharynx and secured by taping, with placement verified by laryngoscopy or palpation) or commercially available nasal prongs, bilateral nasopharyngeal tubes, or specially designed nasal masks with accompanying harness and accessories may be used for CPAP administration.[11,17,19,50,97]

10.1.1.1 Unilateral nasopharyngeal prongs may be less effective in preventing extubation failure than bilateral short prongs.[17,98,99]

10.1.2 Continuous flow air-oxygen gas source; commercially available continuous-flow infant ventilators equipped with CPAP mode; CPAP flow driver with fluidic nasal interface, or suitably equipped multipurpose ventilator, with integrated or adjunct low and high airway pressure alarms, oxygen concentration analyzer with low and high alarms, loss of power and gas source alarms[14,19,100,101]

10.1.2.1 A continuous gas flow source requires a mechanical pressure limiting device, or a flow or threshold resistor, which includes the use of an underwater threshold resistor, eg Bubble CPAP[102]

10.1.3 Lightweight CPAP or ventilator circuits with servo-regulated humidification system[18]

10.1.4 Continuous noninvasive oxygenation monitoring by pulse oximetry or transcutaneous monitor with high and low alarm capabilities is recommended (continuous transcutaneous CO_2 monitoring may also be utilized).[101,102]

10.1.5 Continuous electrocardiographic and respiratory rate monitor, with high and low alarm capabilities, is recommended.

10.1.6 Suction source, suction regulator, and suction catheters for periodic suctioning to assure patency of nasal passages and of endotracheal tubes used for NPCPAP are necessary.[103]

10.1.7 Resuscitation apparatus with airway manometer and masks of appropriate size must be available.

10.1.8 Gastric tube for periodic decompression of stomach and chest tubes should be available.

10.2 Personnel: The application of NCPAP, NP-CPAP, and NM-CPAP should be performed under the direction of a physician by trained personnel who hold a recognized credential (eg, CRT, RRT, RN) and who competently demonstrate

10.2.1 Proper use, understanding, and mastery of the technical aspects of CPAP devices, mechanical ventilators, and humidification systems

10.2.2 Knowledge of ventilator management and understanding of neonatal airway anatomy and pulmonary physiology

10.2.3 Patient assessment skills, with an understanding of the interaction between the CPAP device and the patient and the ability to recognize and respond to adverse reactions and complications

10.2.4 Knowledge and understanding of artificial airway management, training in the procedures of placing endotracheal tubes in the nasopharynx

10.2.5 The ability to interpret monitored and measured blood gas values and vital signs

10.2.6 The application of Standard Precautions[104]

(Continued)

10.2.7 Proper use, understanding, and mastery of emergency resuscitation equipment and procedures

10.2.8 The ability to assess, evaluate, and document outcome (Section 9.0)

NCPAP 11.0 MONITORING:

11.1 Patient-ventilator system checks should be performed at least every 2 to 4 hours and include documentation of mechanical settings, alarms, and patient assessments as recommended by the AARC CPG Patient-Ventilator System Checks (MV-SC) and the CPG Humidification During Mechanical Ventilation (HMV).[105,106]

11.2 Oxygen and carbon dioxide monitoring, including

11.2.1 Periodic sampling of blood gas values by arterial, capillary, or venous route[107,108]

11.2.2 Continuous noninvasive blood gas monitoring by transcutaneous O_2 and CO_2 monitors[33,108,109]

11.2.3 Continuous noninvasive monitoring of oxygen saturation by pulse oximetry[33,110,111]

11.3 Continuous monitoring of electrocardiogram and respiratory rate[31,33]

11.4 Continuous monitoring of proximal airway pressure (Paw), PEEP, and mean airway pressure (Paw)[31,33]

11.5 Continuous monitoring of FIO_2[25,58,112]

11.6 Periodic physical assessment of breath sounds and signs of increased work of breathing (see Section 4.1)[16,58,112]

11.7 Periodic evaluation of chest radiographs[25,52,112]

11.8 Periodic assessment of nasal septum

NCPAP 12.0 FREQUENCY:

NCPAP, NP-CPAP, and NM-CPAP are intended for continuous use and discontinued when the patient's clinical condition improves as indicated by successful outcome assessments (Section 9.0).

NCPAP 13.0 INFECTION CONTROL:

No special precautions are necessary, but Standard Precautions[104] as described by the Centers for Disease Control should be employed.

13.1 Disposable nasal CPAP kits are recommended and are intended for single-patient use.

13.2 Routine disposable circuit changes are unnecessary for infection control purposes when the humidifying device is other than an aerosol generator.[113]

13.3 External surfaces of ventilator should be cleaned according to the manufacturer's recommendations when the device has remained in a patient's room for a prolonged period, when soiled, when it has come in contact with potentially transmittable organisms, and after each patient use.

13.4 Sterile suctioning procedures should be strictly adhered to.[5,51]

Revised by Mike Czervinske RRT-NPS, University of Kansas Medical Center, Kansas City, Kansas, and approved by the 2003 CPG Steering Committee.

Reprinted with permission from *Respiratory Care* 2004; 49(9): 1100–1108. The complete AARC Clinical Practice Guidelines are available from the AARC Web site (http://www.aarc.org), from the AARC Executive Office, or from *Respiratory Care* journal.

Original Publication: Respiratory Care1994;39(8):817–823.

BASICS OF NEONATAL MECHANICAL VENTILATION

Mechanical ventilation, in general, involves the application of positive pressure to support a patient's respiratory system. When a patient, be it an adult or a neonate, is unable to adequately provide enough oxygen to the body (oxygenate) or adequately eliminate CO_2 from the body (ventilate), a condition termed *respiratory failure* is said to exist. When a patient is in respiratory failure, artificial support of ventilation and oxygenation becomes necessary to sustain life. Many factors can contribute to respiratory failure in both the adult and neonatal patient. Unique to the neonatal patient population is the fact that, often, mechanical ventilation is indicated when an infant is born prematurely and the lungs have not had enough time to develop sufficiently to be able to support the patient's physiologic needs.

Goals of mechanical ventilation include the following:
- Achieve adequate alveolar gas exchange (i.e., oxygenation and ventilation).
- Reduce the patient's work of breathing.
- Prevent ventilator-induced lung injury.

Modes of Ventilation

The first neonatal mechanical ventilators used two primary modes of ventilation: continuous positive airway pressure (CPAP) and time-cycled, pressure-limited, intermittent mandatory ventilation (IMV). IMV was replaced by synchronized intermittent mandatory ventilation (SIMV) when refined technology allowed the ventilator to better detect and "coordinate" its efforts with the patient. SIMV aimed to help eliminate the occurrence of "breath stacking" and patient-ventilator asynchrony that occurred with traditional IMV. The modern spectrum of modes available for the ventilation of the neonatal patient is very broad. Developments in monitoring, sensing, and computing power have allowed ventilator manufacturers to offer a wide and varied assortment of ventilatory modes.

Continuous Positive Airway Pressure

Continuous positive airway pressure *(CPAP)* is a spontaneous mode of ventilation used in the support of newborn patients as well as adult patients. A continuous flow of oxygen-enriched gas is provided to the patient's airway at a pressure greater than ambient pressure (zero pressure). This pressure is applied during both inspiration and expiration. A variable resistance at the exhalation valve and the continuous flow of gas provide the pressure for CPAP. As in the adult patient, CPAP helps to increase the neonate's functional residual capacity (FRC), improving gas exchange. CPAP offers no operator-set respiratory rate or tidal volume. When CPAP is used, backup parameters are often set to ensure continued ventilation in the event that the patient becomes apneic.

Synchronized Intermittent Mandatory Ventilation (SIMV)

In general, SIMV is a ventilatory mode that allows the neonate to breathe spontaneously, typically at an elevated pressure baseline (CPAP/PEEP level), generating his or her own tidal volumes in between mandatory breaths that are delivered by the ventilator (mandatory SIMV breaths). Mandatory breaths in SIMV can be either pressure or volume targeted. It is a flexible mode of ventilation in that it can offer both full and partial ventilatory support. SIMV offers full support to the patient who is apneic and partial support to the patient who is breathing spontaneously. This partial support allows the patient to control some of his or her own ventilation. It is a mode that is useful for weaning when the clinician would like to gradually reduce the patient's reliance on the ventilator for support. Progressively decreasing the mandatory rate effectively places more and more of the responsibility for maintaining adequate ventilation on the patient.

Pressure SIMV

In *pressure SIMV* the operator sets a mandatory respiratory rate, an inspiratory time, a positive end-expiratory pressure (PEEP) level, and a peak inspiratory pressure (PIP) level. During this type of ventilation, pressure is constant and tidal volume varies based on the patient's lung compliance, airway resistance, and inspiratory time. This mode offers the clinician some security in knowing that during mandatory breaths, the pressure applied to the patient's airways will not exceed the PIP level.

Volume SIMV

In *volume SIMV* the operator will set a mandatory respiratory rate, an inspiratory flow, a PEEP level, and a tidal volume. In volume SIMV, mandatory breaths target a clinician-set tidal volume. The pressure applied to the patient's airways varies according to the patient's lung compliance and airway resistance. This mode affords the clinician with a consistently predictable minute ventilation.

Assist Control (AC)

Assist control (AC) is a mode of ventilation in which every breath delivered to the patient, be it a mandatory or spontaneously initiated breath, is controlled by the ventilator. The patient who is apneic will receive the respiratory rate set by the clinician using the rate control. If the patient is generating his or her own spontaneous efforts, each time the ventilator detects that effort it will cycle on and deliver either a preset volume or preset pressure to the patient depending on the type of control that is set. This mode does not offer the flexibility that SIMV does in terms of weaning. Decreasing the rate in this mode when a patient is breathing spontaneously will not increase the workload on the patient. Each breath delivered to the patient, be it a patient-triggered or a machine-triggered breath, will be exactly the same. When it becomes necessary to wean a patient from mechanical ventilation and the patient is being ventilated in the AC mode, the operator must change the mode of ventilation completely. CPAP is often used for this purpose.

Pressure Assist Control

In *pressure assist control* the operator sets a mandatory respiratory rate, an inspiratory time, a PEEP level, and a PIP level. Like pressure SIMV, during this type of ventilation, pressure is the variable controlled by the ventilator and remains constant, while volume varies depending on the patient's lung compliance, airway resistance, and set inspiratory time.

Volume Assist Control

In *volume assist control* the operator sets a mandatory respiratory rate, an inspiratory flow, a PEEP level, and a tidal volume. In this mode, volume remains constant and is controlled by the ventilator each time a breath is delivered. The pressure applied to the patient's airways will vary depending on airway resistance and lung compliance.

Time-Cycled, Pressure-Limited (TCPL) Ventilation

Time-cycled, pressure-limited (TCPL) ventilation has been the most common form of ventilation used in neonatal respiratory failure for the past 30 years (Donn & Sinha, 2003). The operator sets a continuous flow, an inspiratory time, a respiratory rate, and a pressure limit (PIP). Like the pressure control modes mentioned previously, this mode offers a consistent pressure applied to the lung but allows tidal volume to vary based on lung compliance and airway resistance. When lung compliance is low, indicating the lungs are stiff, exhaled tidal volumes will be low. As compliance improves, tidal volume will increase.

Pressure Support (PS)

Pressure support (PS) is a mode often employed in conjunction with other modes of ventilation (primarily CPAP and SIMV). PS helps the patient overcome the work of breathing associated with the endotracheal (ET) tube and ventilator circuit. In PS, a patient's spontaneous tidal volume is augmented by delivery of a pressure plateau. It is a spontaneous mode of ventilation in that the patient initiates or triggers all breaths. The clinician sets a predetermined level of PS. When the ventilator senses a spontaneous respiratory effort, pressure is applied to the patient's airways as inspiration takes place. Typically, inspiration is terminated when the patient's inspiratory flow drops to 25% of its peak value.

Volume Support (VS)

Volume support (VS) is another spontaneous mode of ventilation. In VS, the clinician sets a target tidal volume and the ventilator adjusts pressure support to achieve this volume. If the patient's effort increases, the ventilator's support will decrease as long as the target tidal volume is achieved. If the patient's effort decreases, the ventilator will automatically increase PS to help the patient achieve the target tidal volume. When this mode is initiated, the ventilator delivers "test breaths" to the patient to determine the compliance and resistance of the patient's lungs in order to determine the optimum PS level needed to deliver the target tidal volume.

Volume Guarantee (VG)

Volume guarantee is not so much a mode of ventilation but rather a "mode extension." It is available on the Dräger Babylog 8000 *plus*. VG is frequently used in conjunction with PS but can also be used with AC and SIMV. In VG, the clinician sets a target tidal volume, an inspiratory time, and maximum pressure limit. The ventilator measures delivered tidal volume at the patient's ET tube and adjusts the pressure needed to deliver the breath. If the patient's effort decreases or the patient's lung compliance worsens, the delivered pressure will increase until the target tidal volume is achieved. If the patient exerts more effort or the patient's lung compliance improves, the delivered pressure will decrease accordingly.

Pressure Regulated Volume Control (PRVC)

Pressure regulated volume control (PRVC) is a controlled mode of ventilation wherein a set tidal volume is delivered at a set respiratory rate. In PRVC the ventilator monitors the compliance of the patient's lungs and attempts to deliver the set tidal volume with as little pressure as possible. If the patient's lung compliance were to worsen during ventilation and the resultant peak pressures rose to within 5 cm H_2O of the peak pressure limit, the ventilator will alarm and the delivered volume will be decreased until the pressure is reduced.

Mechanical ventilators available in today's neonatal critical care setting typically offer a combination of modes similar to those discussed previously. Tables 29-1 through 29-4 illustrate the modes of neonatal mechanical ventilation available on the following ventilators: the Maquet SERVO-i, the Nellcor Puritan Bennett 840, the Viasys AVEA, and the Dräger Babylog 8000 *plus*.

Many of the ventilators mentioned here can also provide noninvasive ventilation.

TABLE 29-1: Maquet SERVO-i Neonatal Ventilator Modes

Volume control

Pressure control

Pressure regulated volume control (PRVC)

Pressure support/CPAP

Volume support

SIMV (volume control) + pressure support

SIMV (pressure control) + pressure support

SIMV (PRVC) + pressure support

Noninvasive neurally adjusted ventilatory assist (NAVA)

Noninvasive pressure support

Noninvasive pressure control

Noninvasive nasal CPAP

TABLE 29-2: Nellcor Puritan Bennett 840 Neonatal Ventilator Modes

Assist control

SIMV

Spontaneous (with or without pressure support)

CPAP

Bilevel

Noninvasive nasal CPAP

TABLE 29-3: Viasys AVEA Neonatal Ventilator Modes

Volume assist control

Pressure assist control

Time-cycled, pressure-limited assist control

Volume SIMV

Pressure SIMV

Time-cycled, pressure-limited SIMV

CPAP/PSV

Nasal (noninvasive) CPAP

It stands to reason that the advent of newer sensing techniques (proximal flow sensing) as well as improvements in computing ability on today's modern critical care ventilators have greatly enhanced the operator's choices in terms of neonatal ventilatory support. A sound knowledge base regarding physiology and an understanding of the modes available are prerequisites to any expert clinical decision maker.

TABLE 29-4: Dräger Babylog 8000 *plus* Neonatal Ventilator Modes

Continuous mandatory ventilation (CMV)

Continuous positive airway pressure (CPAP)

Assist control ventilation (AC)

Synchronized intermittent mandatory ventilation (SIMV)

Pressure support ventilation (PSV)

Mode Extensions
Volume guarantee (VG) (used with AC, SIMV, and PSV)
Variable inspiratory and variable expiratory flow (VIVE) (can be used in all modes)

INDICATIONS FOR MECHANICAL VENTILATION IN THE NEONATE

Neonatal patients must meet certain criteria before mechanical ventilation is initiated. These criteria, as in the adult, are concerned primarily with oxygenation and ventilation.

Apnea

Apnea is a strong indicator for ventilatory support. Newborns in whom manual resuscitation efforts fail are initiated on mechanical support. Apnea may occur because of many factors such as asphyxia, effects of drugs administered to the mother during labor that may pass through the placenta (such as sedatives), and intracranial disorders (Walsh, Czervinske, & Diblasi, 2010).

Refractory Hypoxemia

Hypoxemia alone is not an indicator for mechanical support. However, hypoxemia that fails to reverse in spite of more conventional modes of management (oxygen, resuscitation, or CPAP) may indicate a need for mechanical support. There is some controversy regarding the threshold at which mechanical ventilation should be initiated. The clinical history and presentation of the patient must be considered alongside all available clinical data. It is generally accepted that an arterial partial pressure of oxygen (PaO_2) of less than 50 mm Hg meets the criteria for mechanical ventilation (Pilbeam & Cairo, 2006).

Hypercapnia (Elevated $PaCO_2$)

Hypercapnia indicates poor ventilatory status. Hypercapnia requiring mechanical ventilation is defined as an arterial partial pressure of carbon dioxide ($PaCO_2$) of greater than 55 mm Hg (Pilbeam & Cairo, 2006). Hypercapnia may be present in newborns suffering from depression of the central nervous system (CNS), pneumonia, apnea, or other disorders (Walsh et al., 2010). The $PaCO_2$ may be

normalized through ventilation of the lungs. Respiratory rate, PIP, tidal volume and, to a lesser degree, CPAP levels are adjusted on the basis of transcutaneous and blood gas monitoring.

UNDERLYING CONDITIONS THAT MAY CONTRIBUTE TO RESPIRATORY FAILURE

In addition to the primary indications for mechanical ventilation, other conditions may contribute to neonatal respiratory distress. These conditions are summarized in Table 29-5.

NEWBORN VENTILATORY SUPPORT CONCEPTS

The following concepts are essential to the understanding of neonatal mechanical ventilation. Time constants, time cycling, I:E ratios, pressure limiting, and proximal flow sensing all play roles in establishing adequate physiologic support of the mechanically ventilated neonate.

Time Constants

The lung time constant is calculated by multiplying the airway resistance by the compliance. The *time constant* provides a reference regarding the lungs' ability to receive or expel gas. A short time constant is present in conditions with a poor compliance and normal resistance (respiratory distress syndrome [RDS], pulmonary hypoplasia) or a normal compliance with decreased resistance. A short time constant is significant in that the expiratory time is very short in duration and abrupt. Pressures are more easily transmitted to the alveoli, and as a result, barotrauma is a common complication.

A long time constant is present in conditions with a normal compliance and high resistance (aspiration, pneumonias). A newborn with a long time constant has an increased expiratory time. Inspiratory pressures are not as easily transmitted, and the inspiratory time

TABLE 29-5: Factors Contributing to Respiratory Distress in Newborns

Respiratory distress syndrome (RDS)

Drugs given to the mother during labor

Aspiration (meconium, amniotic fluid, blood, gastric contents)

Pulmonary hypoplasia

Congenital defects (diaphragmatic hernia, cardiac anomalies)

Persistent pulmonary hypertension of the newborn

may need to be lengthened for optimal gas exchange. These patients may present with air trapping if the expiratory time is too short.

Time Cycling

In adults, the majority of ventilators terminate inspiration after a preset volume is delivered (volume cycled). In traditional neonatal mechanical ventilation (TCPL ventilation), the inspiratory phase is terminated after an operator-selected time interval has passed. As a result, during this type of ventilation, the delivered tidal volume can vary based on the preset inspiratory time, the PIP used, the PEEP level, the flow, and the patient's lung compliance and airway resistance.

I:E Ratio and Inspiratory Time

The I:E ratio is the ratio of inspiratory time to expiratory time. Depending on the mode of ventilation chosen, I:E ratio may be determined by setting inspiratory time and expiratory time controls directly or indirectly by setting a rate and an inspiratory time. An I:E ratio of greater than 1:2 may be required for patients with a long time constant, while a lower I:E ratio may be tolerated by a patient with a short time constant.

Pressure Limiting

During traditional time-cycled, pressure-limited IMV (TCPL IMV) breaths, the ventilator delivers the breath for the specified inspiratory time and builds to the operator-selected pressure. Once the desired pressure is reached, excess circuit pressure is allowed to escape and the pressure is held steady in the airway until the inspiratory time is reached. This *pressure limiting* results in an inspiratory plateau. The duration of the plateau depends on the flow rate and the inspiratory time.

As in adult ventilation, a safety popoff or limit is also provided to prevent excess pressure within the airways. The pressure popoff helps to prevent barotrauma by minimizing excessive pressures that may occur secondary to tube occlusion or failure of the pressure limit control. The pressure limit feature is also usually operator adjustable in most newborn ventilators.

Flow Rate

Another concept of TCPL ventilation is that this mode provides a constant flow of fresh gas through the patient circuit. The flow rate is operator adjustable. Flows are typically set between 6 and 10 L/min.

Proximal Sensing

One of the major advances in neonatal mechanical ventilation has been the advent of proximal flow and volume sensing. The unique physiology of a premature infant, for example, creates some inherent problems when it comes to mechanical ventilation. In dealing with the preterm infant, the clinician is faced with the necessity to deliver extremely small tidal volumes. Ensuring the

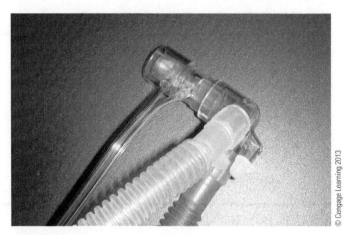

Figure 29-1 A differential pressure proximal flow sensor

accuracy of these tidal volumes is important. It is difficult to accurately measure very small tidal volumes at the ventilator. The placement of a flow sensor at the patient interface (between the wye and the ET tube) helps to eliminate the possibility of inaccurate measuring made back at the ventilator itself. Patient-ventilator synchrony may also be improved with proximal flow sensing in that the ventilator is able to detect very slight changes in respiratory effort and respond accordingly. These small changes may not be as easily detected if they were only being measured at the ventilator outlet. Both heated wire anemometers and differential pressure transducers are used for this purpose. The type of flow sensor used varies with the ventilator manufacturer. Figure 29-1 shows a differential pressure-type proximal flow sensor correctly placed at the patient wye.

HAZARDS AND COMPLICATIONS OF NEWBORN MECHANICAL VENTILATION

Newborn ventilators are primarily positive-pressure ventilators, applying positive pressure within the thorax to expand the lungs. Because pressure is applied within the chest, some of this pressure is transmitted to the mediastinum, as in adult ventilation. Potential adverse consequences are similar: reduced cardiac output, reduced venous return, and increased intracranial pressures. In addition, barotrauma to the lungs and mediastinum can occur (Chatburn, 1991).

Because positive-pressure ventilation is dependent on the placement of an artificial airway, infection is always a concern. Use of careful aseptic technique may help to minimize this complication.

Another complication related to high PaO_2 levels is *retinopathy of prematurity* (Walsh et al., 2010). The risk can be reduced by careful titration of the fraction of inspired oxygen (FIO_2) in relation to the patient's PaO_2. Enough oxygen should be delivered to correct hypoxemia without giving more than is required.

PROFICIENCY OBJECTIVES

At the end of this chapter, the reader should be able to:

- *Demonstrate the ability to recognize a newborn in respiratory distress who requires ventilatory support based on objective criteria.*
- *Given a physician's order or a simulated order, demonstrate how to initiate mechanical ventilation, including the following:*
  - *— Establish an airway.*
  - *— Assemble and test all required equipment.*
  - *— Establish ordered ventilator settings.*
  - *— Monitor the patient appropriately.*
  - *— Document ventilation parameters correctly on the patient's flow sheet.*
- *Adjust ventilation parameters based on clinical feedback (e.g., arterial blood gas [ABG] results).*

ASSESSING THE NEED FOR MECHANICAL VENTILATION

Maternal history, the circumstances of delivery, and the infant's condition at birth provide a wealth of information regarding the patient's need for ventilatory support. Apgar scores, resuscitation efforts, evidence of aspiration, signs of asphyxia, physical size, and appearance all provide clues to the skilled respiratory care practitioner regarding the patient's respiratory distress. The *Apgar scoring system* assigns points (0, 1, or 2) to five distinct clinical characteristics of the newborn infant. It is a tool that is typically used in the delivery room with scores typically being assigned to the newborn at 1 and 5 minutes. Generally speaking, the higher the score, the better, with normal scores being considered to be in the 7 to 10 range. Moderately depressed infants who need further assistance making the transition from intrauterine to extrauterine life may have scores of 4 to 6. Severely depressed infants, who will likely need extensive resuscitative efforts, may have scores in the 0 to 3 range. Table 29-6 details the criteria for assigning an Apgar score. It is important to note that obtaining an Apgar score should never delay resuscitative efforts in the delivery room. Laboratory values (for ABG analysis), chest x-ray reports, and neurologic assessment all confirm initial observations regarding the patient's need for support.

Once the need for support has been established by consensus among the physician, members of the nursing team, and the respiratory care practitioner, all efforts must focus on a successful outcome for the patient. An airway must be established and resuscitation efforts continued as required until mechanical support is available.

EQUIPMENT REQUIREMENTS

Many pieces of equipment are required to support a newborn patient on a mechanical ventilator. These include an emergency manual resuscitator, intubation supplies, ventilator, noninvasive monitors, heated humidifier, and the patient circuit.

Ventilator Preparation

The ventilator circuit should be assembled and attached to the ventilator if it is not already prepared for use. Once the ventilator is ready for operation, the humidifier should be filled, the ventilator's gas sources should be connected, and the ventilator circuit should be pressure tested. Additionally, most modern ventilators have manufacturer-specific pre-use checks that help to ensure that the ventilator is functioning correctly. Detailed instructions regarding these checks are included in the practice exercises at the end of the chapter. All alarms should also be quickly checked for correct function prior to patient connection.

TABLE 29-6: Apgar Scoring System			
CLINICAL SIGN	**0 POINTS ASSIGNED**	**1 POINT ASSIGNED**	**2 POINTS ASSIGNED**
Heart Rate	Absent	Less than 100 bpm	Greater than 100
Respiratory Effort	Absent	Gasping, irregular, weak	Strong
Muscle Tone	Limp	Some flexion	Flexed arms and legs, motion
Reflex Irritability	No response	Grimace, weak cry	Cry, pulls away when stimulated
Color	Body pale or blue (central cyanosis)	Pink torso, blue extremities (acrocyanosis)	Body and extremities pink (no cyanosis)

ESTABLISHING ORDERED VENTILATOR SETTINGS

The initiation of mechanical ventilation is a serious commitment of time, energy, and expense for the support of the newborn patient. It is the responsibility of the respiratory care practitioner to establish the ordered settings and to recommend changes or suggestions when appropriate. The following are some general guidelines useful in establishing ventilatory support.

Mode

The mode selected will depend on the amount of ventilatory support that the patient requires. Full support would dictate the use of a mode with a set rate and tidal volume (or inspiratory pressure if pressure targeting is used). Some patients may require only minimal support through the use of CPAP.

Rate

Initial respiratory rates are generally set between 20 and 40 breaths per minute. Ultimately, the $PaCO_2$ will dictate what rate is appropriate. Transcutaneous monitoring and exhaled CO_2 ($P_{et}CO_2$) analysis are also very helpful in the titration of ventilator settings without frequent drawing of specimens for determination of ABGs. ABGs should be correlated with these noninvasive monitors, however, to assess how well they are representing the patient's actual condition.

Flow Rate

Initial flow rates should be in the range of 6 to 12 L/min. The flow rate should be adjusted to meet the patient's inspiratory needs.

Inspiratory Time

Inspiratory time is adjusted depending on the patient's time constant and by observation of the adequacy of chest excursion during inspiration. Generally, inspiratory times of between 0.3 and 0.5 second are typical. Through practice and observation, inspiratory times are adjusted to more closely match the patient's ventilatory requirements.

I:E Ratio

Like the inspiratory time, I:E ratio is largely dependent on the patient's time constant. Any one I:E ratio is not suitable for all conditions. The patient must be assessed and a judgment made as to what an appropriate ratio is for that patient.

Peak Inspiratory Pressure

The inspiratory pressure is adjusted until adequate chest rise is observed. Once adequate chest expansion is attained, the pressure control is left at that setting. Pressure is then fine-tuned based on noninvasive

monitoring techniques. A typical starting point for PIP is generally in the 15 to 20 cm H_2O range.

Tidal Volume

Tidal volumes are either set (if using volume-targeted ventilation) or monitored (when using pressure-targeted ventilation). Initial tidal volumes can be set in the 4 to 6 mL/kg range. These can be adjusted based on blood gas and/or transcutaneous monitoring readings. Care must be taken when using volume-targeted ventilation to ensure that the resulting pressures on the lung are kept at as low a level as possible.

Oxygen Percent

The oxygen percentage is adjusted according to the patient's needs. Enough oxygen should be provided to correct hypoxemia without giving more than is needed. PaO_2 levels should be maintained between 50 and 80 mm Hg (or an average oxygen saturation [SpO_2] reading of 85% to 92%). Excessively high PaO_2 levels may lead to retinopathy of prematurity or bronchopulmonary dysplasia. Until a blood gas can be obtained, maintain the FIO_2 to keep the infant "pink." Starting values will vary depending on the clinical situation but, in general, an FIO_2 of 0.4 to 0.5 is frequently used.

PEEP/CPAP Level

The PEEP/CPAP level is adjusted to meet the patient's oxygenation status based on ABG determinations and transcutaneous monitoring. PEEP/CPAP is set by adjusting the control until expiratory levels match what is desired. Initial PEEP/CPAP levels of between 4 and 7 cm H_2O are most commonly used.

ALARMS

Alarms alert the practitioner to changes in the patient's condition and in the ventilator system that may be detrimental. Alarms should always be set and routinely monitored. Larger problems (complications and hazards) may be prevented by paying attention to the smaller details. Available alarms will vary depending on the manufacturer. Table 29-7 summarizes available operator-adjustable alarms for the invasive ventilators discussed in this chapter.

High and Low Inspiratory Pressure Alarms

High inspiratory pressure alarms alert the clinician to increases in the ventilating pressures of the patient. Common clinical reasons for this alarm to sound often include decreases in lung compliance, coughing, bronchospasm, and secretions collecting in the airway. Care must be taken to set this alarm no higher than 10 cm H_2O above the current ventilating pressures. Setting the alarm higher than this could result in the clinician missing

TABLE 29-7: Neonatal Ventilation Alarms (operator-adjustable)

ALARM	DRÄGER BABYLOG 8000 *PLUS*	MAQUET SERVO-I	NELLCOR PURITAN BENNETT 840	VIASYS AVEA
High Pressure		X	X	X
Low Pressure				X
High Minute Volume (V_E)	X	X	X	X
Low Minute Volume (V_E)	X	X	X	X
High Tidal Volume			X (mandatory and spontaneous)	X
Low Tidal Volume			X (mandatory and spontaneous)	X
High PEEP/CPAP		X	X	
Low PEEP/CPAP		X	X	X
High Respiratory Rate	X	X	X	X
Low Respiratory Rate		X		

important clinical signs relating to the care of the patient. Low inspiratory pressure alarms alert the practitioner to leaks or a possible patient disconnect. The low inspiratory pressure alarm should be set between 5 and 7 cm H_2O less than the peak airway pressure.

High and Low Minute Volume Alarms

The high and low minute volume alarms help to alert the clinician to acute changes in the amount of ventilation taking place. High minute volume alarms typically sound in the presence of hyperventilation, and low minute volume alarms typically sound in the presence of hypoventilation. Additionally, a low minute volume alarm may serve to alert the clinician to potential apneas or a leak in the ventilator circuit. Typically, these alarms are set approximately 10% to 15% above and below the current minute volume.

High and Low Tidal Volume Alarms

Similar to the high and low minute volume alarms, the high and low tidal volume alarms alert the clinician to changes in the amount of ventilation occurring on a breath-to-breath basis. In pressure control ventilation especially, these alarms are extremely important because they help to alert the clinician to acute changes in lung compliance. Again, a rule of setting these alarms 10% to 15% above and below the current average exhaled tidal volume should be followed.

High and Low PEEP/CPAP Alarms

High PEEP alarms help to alert the clinician to possible problems with the exhalation valve of the ventilator or a possibility of air trapping (inadvertent PEEP). The low PEEP alarm is similar to the low inspiratory pressure alarm except that it alerts the practitioner to loss of PEEP/CPAP pressure. The alarm should be set at 1 to 2 cm H_2O below the PEEP/CPAP level.

High and Low Respiratory Rate Alarms

High respiratory rate alarms alert the clinician to patients who may be "overbreathing" the ventilator. Low respiratory rate alarms alert the clinician to patients who may be having episodes of periodic apnea. Both the high and low respiratory rate alarms are especially helpful when monitoring a patient on a spontaneous mode of ventilation (e.g., CPAP) because they help to alert the clinician to potential signs that the patient may need additional support. These alarms should be set according to the patient's situation and the clinician's judgment.

Gas Pressure Failure

Many ventilators have alarms that alert the clinician to the loss of oxygen or air pressure. In the event of a gas supply line loss, cylinders may be temporarily used until the supply line problems are corrected.

Ventilator Inoperative Alarms

Some ventilators have a ventilator inoperative alarm. These alarms are not operator adjustable but alert the practitioner to serious internal problems that will render the ventilator incapable of supporting the patient. These internal problems include electrical power failures, microprocessor failures, and internal mechanical failures.

PATIENT MONITORING AND ASSESSMENT

The adequacy of ventilation may be assessed through careful monitoring and assessment of the patient. Careful patient monitoring will also alert the practitioner to changes in the patient's condition that may require adjustment of the ventilator settings. Newborn monitoring and assessment are most effective if performed in a consistent manner. Variations in technique or observation may result in the practitioner missing important information about the patient's condition.

Pulmonary

Auscultation of breath sounds in the newborn is a critical part of patient monitoring and assessment. Secretions, bronchospasm, wheezing, airway obstruction, barotraumas, and proper ET tube placement all may be initially detected through careful auscultation.

Inspection is also important in the newborn. Volume delivery during ventilatory support may vary depending on the patient's physiologic status. Observation of chest expansion is important, especially when using a pressure-targeted mode of ventilation. Use of accessory muscles can easily be observed and provides important information about the proper adjustment of flow and pressures.

Transillumination is a technique employed in the newborn for the detection of a pneumothorax. In newborns on ventilatory support, often a multitude of chest x-ray films are obtained. Transillumination is noninvasive and does not carry the hazards associated with repeated x-ray exposure. Transillumination of the chest involves the shining of a very bright (typically fiber-optic) light through the chest. Normally, when the chest of a neonate is exposed to this light, a small, uniform halo appears around the light. In the presence of a pneumothorax, the area that is affected will glow (like a light bulb) due to an increase in air through the portion of the chest wall the light shines through.

ABG determinations and transcutaneous monitoring together provide a consistent picture of oxygenation and ventilation. Transcutaneous monitoring provides the practitioner with real-time data, while ABG values allow the practitioner to "trend" the monitor with the patient's actual condition. Pulse oximetry is another noninvasive tool frequently utilized to assist the practitioner in the monitoring of the patient's oxygenation status.

Cardiac

Blood pressure, heart rate, and general observation are important in both the assessment of the adequacy of mechanical ventilation and assessment of potential adverse cardiovascular effects of mechanical ventilation. Positive-pressure ventilation, while providing patient support, also has its complications and hazards.

Renal

Urine output provides information regarding the adequacy of circulation to the vital organs. A decrease in urine output in response to high airway pressures indicates some impairment of renal function because of increased intrathoracic pressure and decreased venous return. Urine output and daily weights are also important ways to monitor the patient's fluid status.

VENTILATOR MONITORING

Ventilator monitoring consists of verifying the settings and recording any changes in the patient's status. By combining patient assessment with ventilator monitoring, adjustments of the ventilatory support can be intelligently made.

Mode

Monitoring the mode setting is simply confirming that the mode the ventilator is operating in is the desired mode. The observation is made and documented on the patient's flow sheet or in the electronic medical record.

FIO₂

The FIO_2 is monitored by checking the control setting and verifying the measurement of O_2 via the built-in oxygen analyzer on the ventilator. Some facilities may incorporate additional verification of the FIO_2 through the use of a stand-alone portable oxygen analyzer. When doing this, be certain that the analyzer is properly calibrated before measuring the oxygen concentration. Ideally, oxygen concentration should be analyzed before the humidifier in the patient circuit.

Airway Pressures

Monitoring airway pressures is important in assessing the adequacy of ventilatory support and to prevent barotrauma and other complications. Several pressures may be monitored, including the peak pressure, mean airway pressure, and CPAP/PEEP levels. All pressure measurements should be taken from the ventilatory monitor.

Respiratory Rate

The ventilator rate (mandatory breaths) and the patient's spontaneous respiratory rate are measured and documented. As ventilatory support decreases, the patient's rate becomes a larger part of the total respiratory rate.

Flow Rate

The flow rate is measured and adjusted to meet the patient's needs. The flow setting is documented on the patient's flow sheet, indicating that the flow rate was assessed.

Inspiratory Time and I:E Ratio

Many neonatal ventilators monitor inspiratory time or I:E ratio and display in real time what the value is. Some ventilators may provide the practitioner with both types of information. With some ventilators, the I:E ratio must be calculated from the inspiratory time, expiratory time, and the rate settings.

Temperature

The proximal airway temperature should be maintained between 36° and 37°C (Goldsmith & Karotkin, 2003).

Excessive temperatures can result in damage to the airway and can cause actual burns. Servo-controlled humidifiers are commonly used in newborn ventilation and simplify temperature and humidity delivery.

Alarm Settings

All user-set ventilator alarms are monitored and recorded. The function of the alarms should also be periodically checked to prevent potential errors and problems.

NONINVASIVE NEONATAL MECHANICAL VENTILATION

Many times, the spontaneous breathing of a neonate needs to be supported but the clinical data may not indicate the need for full, invasive mechanical support. In these cases, noninvasive ventilation may be considered. *Nasal or nasopharyngeal CPAP* is often applied in these circumstances.

When CPAP is employed, the patient breathes at an elevated pressure (above ambient pressure). CPAP helps to increase FRC, which results in greater available surface area for gas exchange and, subsequently, higher PaO_2 levels. It also can reduce work of breathing by improving overall lung compliance.

Indications for Nasal CPAP

Noninvasive nasal CPAP may be indicated for a variety of reasons. In general, oxygenation failure, increased work of breathing, and the presence of specific disease processes that are believed to respond to noninvasive positive-pressure ventilation are among the most common reasons that nasal CPAP is employed.

Oxygenation Failure

An inability to adequately oxygenate, as evidenced by a PaO_2 lower than 50 mm Hg despite an FIO_2 of 0.60 or greater, is an indication for nasal CPAP. It is important to note that CPAP is primarily used to treat refractory hypoxemia. If a patient has hypoxemia and hypercarbia that results in a pH of less than 7.25, intubation and mechanical ventilation are indicated.

Increased Work of Breathing

An infant's increased work of breathing is often detected during the physical examination. Some signs to look for include nasal flaring, retractions, grunting, and increased respiratory rate. The application of positive pressure in these situations helps to reduce work of breathing, thereby improving the overall clinical presentation of the patient.

Disease Processes that Respond to Nasal CPAP

Certain disease processes that affect the neonatal patient have been shown to improve with the application of CPAP. These disease processes include pulmonary edema, atelectasis, apnea of prematurity, tracheal malacia, RDS, and transient tachypnea of the newborn. CPAP may also be indicated when a patient fails extubation. This noninvasive therapy may help to prevent reintubation in some cases.

Contraindications for Nasal CPAP

While CPAP is certainly beneficial in many situations, care must be taken to ensure that it is employed safely. There are situations in which nasal CPAP is contraindicated. These situations include the presence of an abnormal upper airway (e.g., choanal atresia), tracheoesophageal fistula, impending respiratory or cardiac arrest, severe cardiovascular instability, and ventilatory failure, as described previously. In addition to these contraindications, care must be taken when applying nasal CPAP to an infant with a diaphragmatic hernia because increased pressures applied to the airways increase the risk for gastric insufflation.

Hazards and Complications of Nasal CPAP

Hazards associated with the application of nasal CPAP fall into two main categories: hazards associated with the equipment used to provide nasal CPAP and hazards associated with the clinical condition of the patient. Insufficient flow, insufficient humidity, excessive flow, kinking and obstruction of the patient interface, and breakdown of skin integrity at the points of contact between the patient and the interface are just some of the situations that are considered to be hazards associated with this therapeutic modality.

Limitations of Nasal CPAP

Because of the nature of the nasal CPAP interface, certain limitations exist. Any movement that causes the mask, nasal prongs, or nasal pharyngeal tube to become malpositioned will result in a loss of pressure and, potentially, a decrease in the patient's SpO_2. Excessive mouth breathing during the application of CPAP via nasal prongs or nasal mask may also lead to a decrease in ventilating pressures. Also, the presence of complicated caps, straps, and other features of a typical nasal CPAP harness may cause the infant to become irritated and restless, which might result in the possible loss of ventilating pressure.

Outcomes of Nasal CPAP

Nasal CPAP can be said to have been effective when the clinical conditions for which it was indicated have resolved. Improvement in work of breathing, improvement in oxygenation, and improvement in lung volumes, breath sounds, and so on are all signs the practitioner may look for during the routine assessment of the patient on nasal CPAP.

Necessary Equipment

In order to provide nasal CPAP the practitioner needs a number of components; these components include a patient interface (typically a nasal mask, a nasopharyngeal tube, or nasal prongs), a harness or device used to hold the patient interface in place (a cap, straps, harness, etc.), a circuit to carry gas flow to the patient interface, a humidification unit to humidify the gas flow, an air/oxygen continuous flow source, a resistor that will regulate the amount of pressure applied to the circuit and patient, and a pressure popoff device to prevent excessive pressure build-up in the circuit.

In addition to the items listed, the following items are also necessary when nasal CPAP is employed: monitoring equipment (e.g., oxygen analyzer, pulse oximeter or transcutaneous oxygen/carbon dioxide, and electrocardiograph), suction equipment, and resuscitation equipment.

Commercially Available CPAP Systems

Today, there are commercially available mechanical devices that incorporate many of the items listed previously and also add alarms and enhanced monitoring features. The Arabella Nasal CPAP system is an example of such a device. It consists of a base unit, referred to as a "monitoring gas mixer," that is powered by air, oxygen, and electricity. In addition to the monitoring gas mixer, the Arabella nasal CPAP system uses a proprietary delivery circuit that incorporates a specialized fluidic device known as a "universal generator" (Figure 29-2).

CPAP is generated when the flow from the monitoring gas mixer is delivered to the universal generator located at the patient interface. The universal generator uses both the Bernoulli effect to generate CPAP pressure and the Venturi principle to augment flow in times of high inspiratory demand. Simply stated, the higher the flow delivered to the universal generator, the higher the CPAP

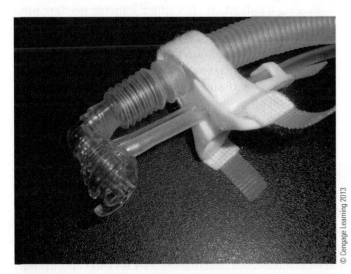

Figure 29-2 An Arabella universal generator

pressure applied to the patient. Table 29-8 illustrates the relationship between flow and pressure for the Arabella Nasal CPAP system. It is important to note that the pressures listed are "approximate" pressures. Fine-tuning pressures and ensuring adequacy of device operation remain the responsibility of the trained clinician.

Monitoring

Routine patient monitoring is required when noninvasive ventilation is employed. A patient's condition can change rapidly and may require frequent adjustments in the level of support being given. Regularly assessing both the patient and the equipment interfacing with the patient is necessary. When assessing a patient, items that should be routinely monitored include the ABG data (may be attained invasively or noninvasively through the use of transcutaneous monitors), electrocardiogram (ECG) tracings, breath sounds, respiratory rate, general patient appearance, and chest x-ray results. Care must also be taken to carefully inspect the areas where the interface device (nasal prongs, nasal mask, etc.) contacts the patient. Any signs of skin breakdown must be noted and care must be taken to prevent further breakdown. When recording data regarding the CPAP device, the clinician should include the delivered oxygen concentration, the set and measured airway pressures (CPAP level, etc.), the flow levels, and any applicable alarms being monitored.

High-Frequency Ventilation (HFV)

Another ventilatory strategy employed in NICUs throughout the country differs greatly from conventional mechanical ventilation. The use of specialty ventilators or ventilator modes to deliver very small tidal volumes at extremely fast rates (greater than 150 breaths per minute) is termed *high-frequency ventilation*, or HFV. There are several ventilator platforms that are capable of delivering HFV. Each platform delivers the high-frequency breath in a slightly different way. This section focuses on one High Frequency Ventilator in particular, the Viasys SensorMedics 3100A High Frequency Oscillatory Ventilator.

TABLE 29-8: Arabella Nasal CPAP Flow/ Pressure Relationship

FLOW (LITERS PER MINUTE)	APPROXIMATE DELIVERED CPAP PRESSURE (CM H_2O)
6 L/min	3 cm H_2O
7 L/min	4 cm H_2O
8 L/min	5 cm H_2O
9 L/min	6 cm H_2O
10 L/min	7 cm H_2O

High-Frequency Oscillatory Ventilation (HFOV)

The Viasys Sensor Medics 3100A uses a piston-driven diaphragm system to deliver high-frequency breaths in the range of 3 to 15 Hz (180–900 breaths per minute). Both the inspiratory phase and the expiratory phase are "active" in that the ventilator's diaphragm applies positive pressure to the lung during inspiration and negative pressure to the lung during expiration.

Gas Exchange Mechanisms

During *high-frequency oscillatory ventilation* (HFOV) the lung is inflated through the manipulation of the mean airway pressure and "held" at this distending pressure while the piston-diaphragm oscillates rapidly, delivering very small "tidal volumes" at an extremely fast rate. Many complicated processes are involved in the exchange of respiratory gases during HFOV. While some gas exchange remains the result of conventional "bulk flow of gases in and out of the airways," additional concepts play important roles as well. One such concept is the idea of pendelluft flow. Pendelluft allows for the exchange of respiratory gases at the alveolar level between alveoli with differing time constants. This concept, along with ideas regarding the molecular movement of gases at the alveolar level and the interplay between the larger airways and the velocity of the gas movement into and out of the lungs all contribute to gas exchange during HFOV.

Ventilator Controls

The operation of the Viasys Sensor Medics 3100A is accomplished through the manipulation of several controls that differ somewhat from those found on a conventional mechanical ventilator.

Ventilation is controlled predominantly through the manipulation of the power control, which affects the stroke volume of the piston-diaphragm. This is displayed as *"amplitude,"* or *"ΔP."* Secondarily, ventilation can be manipulated by adjusting the *hertz (Hz)* control. One hertz is equal to 60 breaths per minute; therefore, for example, 3 Hz equals 180 breaths per minute.

With regard to ventilation and the manipulation of blood gas values it is of particular interest to the clinician to note that the relationship between rate and carbon dioxide removal is different than is traditionally understood. Carbon dioxide removal responds more to a change in "tidal volume" than to a change in rate during HFOV. Increasing the ventilator rate actually decreases the amount of air displaced by the piston and, counterintuitively perhaps, would cause the amount of ventilation to decrease. The opposite also holds true; decreasing the ventilator rate will allow for more air to be displaced by each piston stroke and thus increase carbon dioxide removal.

Oxygenation is manipulated by FIO_2 (controlled by an external air-oxygen blender) as well as the mean airway pressure control. Increasing mean airway pressure ideally increases lung recruitment. Increased lung recruitment allows for a greater surface area across which gas exchange can occur, thus improving oxygenation.

% Inspiratory time can also be set by the operator. It controls the amount of time the piston spends delivering the inspiratory portion of each breath. A longer inspiratory time is associated with increased mean airway pressures and, potentially, increased lung recruitment. The % inspiratory time control also affects carbon dioxide removal. In general, it is recommended that the % inspiratory time be set at 33%.

Bias flow is another control that the operator can manipulate. The bias flow controls the amount of fresh gas that is introduced into the ventilator circuit. Additionally, manipulating bias flow affects mean airway pressure.

Indications

HFV is often started after attempts at managing the patient with conventional ventilation has failed. HFV is indicated for the treatment and support of patients suffering from two main categories of lung disease: those needing lung recruitment and those suffering from pulmonary air leak. The first category includes lung disease characterized by diffuse atelectasis and low lung volumes such as might be seen with surfactant deficiency and diffuse pneumonias. HFV is also indicated for the management of patients with pulmonary air leak syndromes (pulmonary interstitial emphysema (PIE), pneumothorax, etc.).

Management Strategies

Depending on the disease process, the strategies for managing a patient on HFV differ. Patients needing lung recruitment are managed with a "high-volume" strategy and patients suffering from pulmonary air leak are managed with a "low-volume" strategy. In the high-volume strategy, mean airway pressures are manipulated to recruit alveoli and subsequently maintain the recruited lung. In the low-volume strategy, mean airway pressures are kept low in order to allow for the lung to heal.

References

American Association for Respiratory Care. (1994). AARC clinical practice guidelines: Neonatal time-triggered, pressure-limited, time-cycled mechanical ventilation. *Respiratory Care, 39*(8), 808–816.

American Association for Respiratory Care. (2004). AARC clinical practice guidelines: Application of continuous positive airway pressure to neonates via nasal prongs, nasopharyngeal tube, or nasal mask—2004 revision and update. *Respiratory Care, 49*(9), 1100–1108.

Arabella operator's manual. (2001). Reno, NV: Hamilton Medical, Inc.

Chatburn, R. L. (1991). Principles and practice of neonatal and pediatric mechanical ventilation. *Respiratory Care, 36*(6), 569–595.

Donn, S. M., & Sinha, S. K. (2003). Invasive and noninvasive neonatal mechanical ventilation. *Respiratory Care, 48*(4), 426–441.

Dräger Babylog 8000 plus operator instructions. (2006). Lubeck, Germany: Dräger Medical AG and Co.

840 Ventilator System operator's and technical reference manual. (2006). Pleasanton, CA: Nellcor Puritan Bennett Incorporated.

840 Ventilator System operator's and technical reference manual neomode addendum. (2009). Pleasanton, CA: Nellcor Puritan Bennett Incorporated.

Goldsmith, J. P., & Karotkin, E. H. (2003). *Assisted ventilation on the neonate* (4th ed.). Philadelphia: Saunders.

Pilbeam, S. P., & Cairo, J. M. (2006). *Mechanical ventilation: Physiological and clinical applications* (4th ed.). St. Louis, MO: Mosby.

SERVO-i pocketguide, ventilation of neonates and pediatrics. (2005). Solna, Sweden: Maquet Critical Care.

SERVO-i Ventilator System operator's manual. (2008). Solna, Sweden: Maquet Critical Care.

Viasys AVEA operator's manual. (2005). Yorba Linda, CA: VIASYS Respiratory Care Incorporated.

Walsh, B. K., Czervinske, M. P., & Diblasi, R. M. (2010). *Perinatal and pediatric respiratory care* (3rd ed.). St. Louis, MO: Saunders.

Practice Activities: Viasys AVEA

CIRCUIT ASSEMBLY

Figure 29-3 shows the Viasys AVEA assembled and ready for use with a neonatal patient. To prepare the ventilator for use, follow the steps listed next.

1. Attach the collection bottle to the water trap by screwing it clockwise into the receptacle in the water trap (Figure 29-4).
2. Install an exhalation filter to the upper portion of the water trap by pushing it onto the seal at the top of the water trap (Figure 29-5).
3. Align the ridge on the water trap assembly with the slot on the exhalation filter cartridge (Figure 29-6).
4. Slide the water trap/exhalation filter assembly upward into the lower right front portion of the ventilator body and rotate the locking lever to the left, holding the assembly in place (Figure 29-7).
5. Connect the expiratory limb of the neonatal patient circuit to the expiratory filter and collection vial's 22 mm fitting.
6. Attach the patient circuit to the flex arm at its midpoint by clamping the ball fitting on the circuit to the flex arm.
7. Connect an 18-inch length of neonatal tubing between the ventilator outlet located to the right of the water trap/exhalation filter assembly and the humidifier.
8. Connect the inspiratory limb of the neonatal patient circuit to the outlet of the humidifier.
9. Connect the 50 psi air and oxygen supply lines to the appropriate gas connections.
10. Connect the electrical power cord to a 115 volt 60 Hz outlet.
11. The Viasys AVEA has the capability of using two styles of proximal flow sensor, a "Variable Orifice"

(differential pressure) or a "Hot Wire" (heated wire anemometer). These flow sensors have device-specific connectors located on the front panel of the body of the ventilator. The "Variable Orifice" flow sensor connects to the outlet that has a dark blue box around it. The "Hot Wire" flow sensor connects to the outlet that has a light blue box around it. Either flow sensor may be used for the exercises described here. Connect the flow sensor to the outlet and then slide the collar down to firmly lock the sensor into place.
12. Once the circuit and flow sensor are installed, locate the power switch on the back of the ventilator. Turn the ventilator on. An alarm will sound and "Safety Valve" will be displayed in the upper right-hand corner of the display. Press the "Alarm Silence" hard key located on the screen border, just to the right of the alarm bar.
13. A "Patient Select" box will appear. You will have the option of selecting either "Resume Current" or "New Patient." Select "New Patient" and then touch "Patient Accept."
14. A "Patient Size Select" box will appear and you will be given the choice of selecting "Neo," "Ped," or "Adult." Select "Neo" and touch "Size Accept."
15. A Ventilation Setup screen will appear, giving you options to choose "AAC" (artificial airway compensation), "Endotracheal Tube Size," "Leak Compensation," "Active Humidity" (which would be turned on if a heated humidifier is being used and off if a heat moisture exchange (HME) is being used), and patient weight information (this is used to allow the ventilator to display volumes per unit of patient weight). To input any value on the Viasys AVEA, simply touch the parameter you wish to adjust; turn the

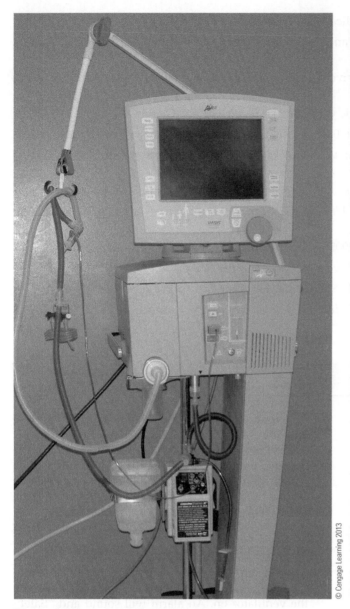

Figure 29-3 A Viasys AVEA assembled and ready for use

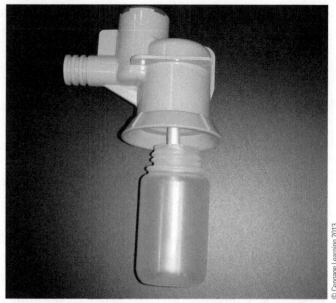

Figure 29-4 A Viasys AVEA collection bottle and water trap

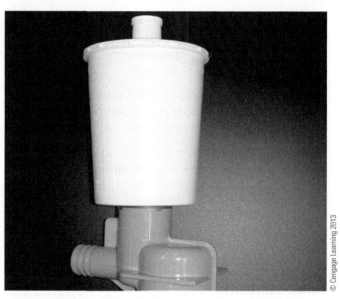

Figure 29-5 A Viasys AVEA exhalation filter on the water trap

"Data Dial," located on the lower right-hand side of the touch screen to the desired value; and then either touch the parameter again or press the "Accept" hard key located just to the left of the "Data Dial." Turn "AAC" on, select an ETT size of 3.5 mm diameter and 15 mm length, turn "Leak Comp" off and dial "Leak Compensation" to 0.0 mL/cm H_2O. Turn "Active Humidity" off and input a patient weight of 3.5 kg. Once this is complete, touch "Setup Accept" and connect the ventilator circuit to the test lung.

16. Ventilation will begin in the default neonatal mode, which on the AVEA is "Time Cycled, Pressure Limited Assist Control" (TCPL A/C). The initial default settings are listed in Table 29-9.

TESTING THE VENTILATOR BEFORE USE

Before any ventilator is used on a patient it is important to go through all of the manufacturer-recommended pre-use checks.

Power-on Self Test (POST)

Each time the power switch is turned on or if the ventilator microprocessor detects selected fault conditions, a power-on self test (POST) is automatically executed. The POST takes only a few seconds and is transparent to the clinician. The test verifies the integrity of the microprocessor, read-only memory (ROM) and random access memory (RAM). Only if a problem is detected will a message be displayed.

Extended Systems Test (EST)

The extended systems test (EST) should only be performed prior to connecting the ventilator to a patient. The EST will perform a leak test of the patient circuit, determine circuit compliance, and perform a two-point

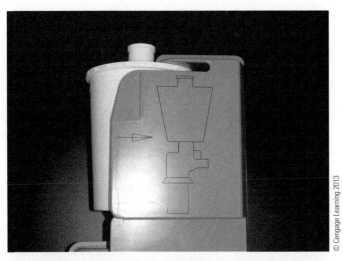

Figure 29-6 A Viasys AVEA water trap correctly inserted into the exhalation filter cartridge

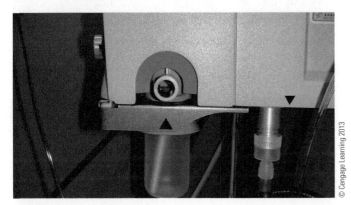

Figure 29-7 A Viasys AVEA water trap and exhalation cartridge properly installed

TABLE 29-9: Viasys AVEA TCPL A/C Start-up Default Settings

Rate	20 breaths per minute (breaths/min)
Inspiratory Pressure (Insp Press)	15 cm H$_2$O
Peak Flow	8 L/min
Inspiratory Time (Insp Time)	0.35 second
PEEP	3 cm H$_2$O
Flow Triggering (Flow Trig)	0.5 L/min
FIO$_2$	40%

calibration of the oxygen sensor. To perform an EST, complete the following steps:

1. Access the EST by pressing the "EST" button on the Setup screen.
2. When instructed to remove the ventilator from the patient and block the patient wye, do so.

3. Confirm that the ventilator is off the patient and the wye is blocked by pressing "Cont" (continue).
4. The ventilator will perform the EST and a countdown timer will be displayed. The first portion of the test will check the circuit for leaks, calculate circuit compliance, and perform a two-point calibration of the oxygen sensor. The maximum time for this test is 90 seconds.
5. Following each test, a PASSED or FAILED message will be displayed. Once the first portion of the test is complete, and all tests PASSED, press the "Continue" button on the screen.
6. From the Setup screen, press "Setup Accept" to capture and retain the circuit compliance measurement.

Using the Keyboard Entry System

All functions of the Viasys AVEA ventilator are controlled from the user interface module (UIM) shown in Figure 29-8. To enter ventilator or alarm settings, follow the "touch–turn–touch" method for entering new settings. Touch the desired value or setting you wish to change (e.g., tidal volume), and turn the knob on the lower right side of the UIM interface until the desired value is displayed (clockwise increases, counterclockwise decreases). Touch the desired setting again or press the "Accept" button to apply the new setting. The new setting will now be displayed on the appropriate portion of the UIM screen.

ACTIVITIES

To complete these practice activities, it is recommended that you use a lung analog/simulator such as a Michigan Instruments TTL Adult/Infant Test Lung (Model 560li) or an IngMar Medical Neonatal Demonstration Lung Model. These devices or other similar devices allow the operator to alter resistance and compliance, simulating changes in patient condition.

If these devices are not available, a simple, single-bellows neonatal test lung may be used. Exercise caution as volumes and pressures may exceed the limits of the test lungs. Resistance may be altered by adapting different sizes of ET tubes, and compliance may be altered by the addition of rubber bands to the test lungs.

LUNG SIMULATOR SETUP

If you are using a Michigan Instruments TTL Adult/Infant Test Lung (Model 560li) you will be using the

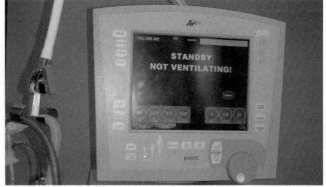

Figure 29-8 The Viasys AVEA user interface module (UIM)

"Infant" side of the test lung. Using the connecting tubing provided with the test lung, connect the lung inlet to the back end of the "Rest Assembly." Connect the Pneuflo Rp 50 resistance adapter to the front end of the rest assembly. Connect the pressure pickoff adapter to the Pneuflo Rp 50 resistance adapter. Connect the pressure line from the pickoff adapter to the proximal pressure input. Connect the patient wye to the pressure pickoff adapter. Set the compliance spring to 0.002 L/cm H_2O. Adjust the corresponding slider located near the top of the lung to the 0.002 L/cm H_2O setting as well. Figure 29-9 shows the Michigan Instruments TTL Adult/Infant Test Lung (Model 560li) correctly configured for neonatal use.

If you are using an IngMar Medical Neonatal Demonstration Lung Model, rotate the outer 3-way stopcocks so that there are no leaks present (off to the leak adapters). Ensure that the inner 3-way stopcock is set to allow ventilation of both lungs. Do not use the brackets. Use the 3.5 mm ETT adapter. Attach the patient wye to the fortlite of the ETT. Figure 29-10 shows an IngMar Medical Neonatal Demonstration Lung Model correctly configured for neonatal use.

When completing these activities, manipulate only one control at a time and note the result of each activity with manipulation of the controls. Answer the questions that follow each of the activities.

MODE SELECTION

Once the ventilator has begun cycling, you may press the "Mode" hard key located to the left of the display screen. By pressing the "Mode" button you are presented with the list of available modes for the neonatal patient. These modes are listed in Table 29-10.

When you touch a mode, you are presented with a list of settings for that mode. In addition to the primary settings for each mode, it should be noted that certain settings on the Viasys AVEA have additional "subsettings" that can be accessed by pressing the "Advanced Settings" hard key located below the "Mode" key. Settings that have "advanced" options are indicated by a small yellow triangle. To access and adjust an advanced setting, select the primary option that has an advanced setting and

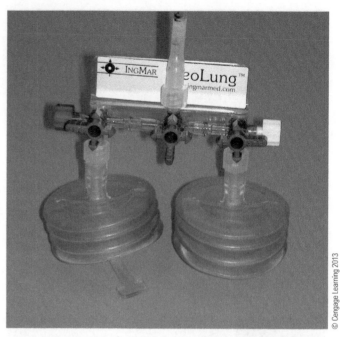

Figure 29-10 The IngMar Medical Neonatal Demonstration Lung Model

TABLE 29-10: Viasys AVEA Neonatal Ventilator Modes

Volume assist control
Pressure assist control
Time-cycled, pressure-limited assist control
Volume SIMV
Pressure SIMV
Time-cycled, pressure-limited SIMV
CPAP/PSV
Nasal (noninvasive) CPAP

press the "Advanced Setting" hard key. The advanced options for the primary setting will appear and may be adjusted by touching the desired setting, rotating the "Data Dial," and either touching the setting again or pressing "Accept."

Tables 29-11 through 29-18 summarize the settings available for each mode.

Settings can be adjusted by touching the desired parameter, rotating the "Data Dial," and then either touching the parameter again or pressing the "Accept" button located to the left of the "Data Dial." To begin, press "TCPL A/C" and input the following settings:

a. Rate	40 breaths/min
b. Inspiratory Pressure	25 cm H2O
c. Peak Flow	7 L/min
d. Inspiratory Time	0.5 second
e. PEEP	4 cm H2O
f. Flow Triggering	0.5 L/min
g. FIO$_2$	21%

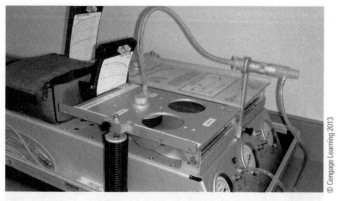

Figure 29-9 A Michigan Instruments TTL Adult/Infant Testing Lung Model 560li

TABLE 29-11: Viasys AVEA Volume Assist Control

PARAMETER	RANGE
Rate (breaths/min)	1–150 breaths/min
Volume (mL)	2–300 mL
Peak Flow (L/min)	0.4–30 L/min
Inspiratory Pause (seconds)	0–3 seconds
PEEP (cm H_2O)	0–50 cm H_2O
Flow Triggering (L/min)**	0.1–20 L/min
FIO_2 (%)	21–100%

**Indicates that this primary setting has an "Advanced Settings" option.*

TABLE 29-14: Viasys AVEA Volume SIMV

PARAMETER	RANGE
Rate (breaths/min)	1–150 breaths/min
Volume (mL)	2–300 mL
Peak Flow (L/min)**	0.4–30 L/min
Inspiratory Pause (seconds)	0–3 seconds
Pressure Support Ventilation (cm H_2O)**	0–80 cm H_2O
PEEP (cm H_2O)	0–50 cm H_2O
Flow Triggering (L/min)**	0.1–20 L/min
FIO_2 (%)	21–100%

**Indicates that this primary setting has an "Advanced Settings" option.*

TABLE 29-12: Viasys AVEA Pressure Assist Control

PARAMETER	RANGE
Rate (breaths/min)	1–150 breaths/min
Inspiratory Pressure (cm H_2O)**	0–80 cm H_2O
Inspiratory Time (seconds)**	0.15–3 seconds
PEEP (cm H_2O)	0–50 cm H_2O
Flow Triggering (L/min)**	0.1–20 L/min
FIO_2 (%)	21–100%

**Indicates that this primary setting has an "Advanced Settings" option.*

TABLE 29-15: Viasys AVEA Pressure SIMV

PARAMETER	RANGE
Rate (breaths/min)	1–150 breaths/min
Inspiratory Pressure (cm H_2O)**	0–80 cm H_2O
Inspiratory Time (seconds)**	0.15–3 seconds
Pressure Support Ventilation (cm H_2O)**	0–80 cm H_2O
PEEP (cm H_2O)	0–50 cm H_2O
Flow Triggering (L/min)**	0.1–20 L/min
FIO_2 (%)	21–100%

**Indicates that this primary setting has an "Advanced Settings" option.*

TABLE 29-13: Viasys AVEA Time-Cycled, Pressure-Limited Assist Control

PARAMETER	RANGE
Rate (breaths/min)	1–150 breaths/min
Inspiratory Pressure (cm H_2O)**	0–80 cm H_2O
Peak Flow (L/min)	0.4–30 L/min
Inspiratory Time (seconds)	0.15–3 seconds
PEEP (cm H_2O)	0–50 cm H_2O
Flow Triggering (L/min)**	0.1–20 L/min
FIO_2 (%)	21–100%

**Indicates that this primary setting has an "Advanced Settings" option.*

TABLE 29-16: Viasys AVEA Time-Cycled, Pressure-Limited SIMV

PARAMETER	RANGE
Rate (breaths/min)	1–150 breaths/min
Inspiratory Pressure (cm H_2O)**	0–80 cm H_2O
Peak Flow (L/min)	0.4–30 L/min
Inspiratory Time (seconds)**	0.15–3 seconds
Pressure Support Ventilation (cm H_2O)**	0–80 cm H_2O
PEEP (cm H_2O)	0–50 cm H_2O
Flow Triggering (L/min)**	0.1–20 L/min
FIO_2 (%)	21–100%

**Indicates that this primary setting has an "Advanced Settings" option.*

TABLE 29-17: Viasys AVEA CPAP/PSV***

PARAMETER	RANGE
Pressure Support Ventilation (cm H_2O)**	0–80 cm H_2O
PEEP (cm H_2O)	0–50 cm H_2O
Flow Triggering (L/min)**	0.1–20 L/min
FIO_2 (%)	21–100%

**Indicates that this primary setting has an "Advanced Settings" option.

***When CPAP/PSV is selected an "Apnea Mode" menu appears. The operator may select an apnea mode that is volume oriented; pressure oriented; or time cycled, pressure limited. Once this has been determined, pressing the "Apnea Settings" button brings up three to four additional settings (rate, volume, or pressure, etc.) depending on which mode was selected.

TABLE 29-18: Viasys AVEA Nasal CPAP

PARAMETER	RANGE
PEEP (cm H_2O)	0–10 cm H_2O
FIO_2 (%)	21–100%

TABLE 29-19: Viasys AVEA Alarms and Ranges in Neonatal Mode

VIASYS AVEA NEONATAL MODE ALARMS	ALARM RANGE
High Respiratory Rate (breaths per minute)	1–200 breaths/min
Low Exhaled Tidal Volume (mL)	0–300 mL
High Exhaled Tidal Volume (mL)	2–300 mL
Low Minute Ventilation (L/min)	0–5 L/min
High Minute Ventilation (L/min)	0–5 L/min
Low Peak Pressure (cm H_2O)	1–80 cm H_2O
High Peak Pressure (cm H_2O)	10–85 cm H_2O
Low PEEP (cm H_2O)	0–60 cm H_2O
Apnea Interval (seconds)	6–60 seconds

ALARM SETTING

Once the ventilator has begun to cycle, press the "Alarm Limits" key located on the upper right-hand corner of the User Interface screen. This key will bring up the "Alarm Limits" page, which presents the user with several adjustable alarms.

Table 29-19 lists the Viasys AVEA alarms and their respective ranges in the neonatal mode.

Please set the alarms to the following parameters. Touch the desired parameter, rotate the "Data Dial" to adjust the parameter and either touch the parameter again or press the "Accept" button to confirm your selection. When you are finished, press the "Alarm Limits" hard key again and the Alarm screen will disappear.

High Respiratory Rate (breaths per minute)	60 breaths/min
Low Exhaled Tidal Volume (mL)	15 mL
High Exhaled Tidal Volume (mL)	60 mL
Low Minute Ventilation (L/min)	0.5 L/min
High Minute Ventilation (L/min)	2 L/min
Low Peak Pressure (cm H_2O)	10 cm H_2O
High Peak Pressure (cm H_2O)	35 cm H_2O
Low PEEP (cm H_2O)	1 cm H_2O
Apnea Interval (seconds)	20 seconds

PATIENT MONITORING

The UIM screen is divided into sections. The lower section is devoted to ventilator settings. You have already been making entries and using this portion of the screen.

The upper center part of the screen is devoted to scalar waveforms (pressure, volume, and flow). These waveforms may be scaled to be larger or smaller as well as "frozen" to observe specific changes one might observe.

The left side of the screen displays the values for the patient's measured peak pressure, tidal volume, rate, PEEP, and FIO_2. These values are those measured by the ventilator during either a mandatory- or patient-triggered volume breath.

The lower part of the screen displays the ventilator control settings that are active for the current mode of ventilation.

INSPIRATORY TIME CONTROL

From the initial settings you have previously set, note the following ventilatory (patient) parameters before you make the next changes. (Instructors may want to consider providing a ventilator flow sheet for the students to use in order to record parameters.)

1. Mode
2. FIO_2
3. Respiratory Rate (set and total)
4. Exhaled Tidal Volume
5. PEEP
6. P mean
7. Inspiratory Time
8. I:E Ratio
9. Exhaled Minute Ventilation
10. Peak Pressure

1. Set the inspiratory time to 0.30 second. Record the following parameters:
   a. Mode
   b. FIO_2
   c. Respiratory Rate (set and total)
   d. Exhaled Tidal Volume
   e. PEEP
   f. P mean
   g. Inspiratory Time
   h. I:E Ratio

i. Exhaled Minute Ventilation
j. Peak Pressure

2. Set the inspiratory time control to 1 second. Record the following parameters:
   a. Mode
   b. FIO_2
   c. Respiratory Rate (set and total)
   d. Exhaled Tidal Volume
   e. PEEP
   f. P mean
   g. Inspiratory Time
   h. I:E Ratio
   i. Exhaled Minute Ventilation
   j. Peak Pressure

Questions

A. How was the respiratory rate affected by changes in the inspiratory time?
B. How were the peak pressures affected by the changes in the inspiratory time?
C. How was the tidal volume affected by the changes in the inspiratory time?

INSPIRATORY PRESSURE CONTROL

Return the controls to the following settings:

a. Rate	40 breaths/min
b. Inspiratory Pressure	25 cm H_2O
c. Peak Flow	12 L/min
d. Inspiratory Time	0.5 second
e. PEEP	4 cm H_2O
f. Flow Triggering	0.5 L/min
g. FIO_2	21%

Once these settings have been established, record the following ventilatory (patient) parameters:
   a. Mode
   b. FIO_2
   c. Respiratory Rate (set and total)
   d. Exhaled Tidal Volume
   e. PEEP
   f. P mean
   g. Inspiratory Time
   h. I:E Ratio
   i. Exhaled Minute Ventilation
   j. Peak Pressure

Adjust the alarms to the following parameters:

High Respiratory Rate (breaths per minute)	60 breaths/min
Low Exhaled Tidal Volume (mL)	15 mL
High Exhaled Tidal Volume (mL)	150 mL
Low Minute Ventilation (L/min)	0.5 L/min
High Minute Ventilation (L/min)	5 L/min
Low Peak Pressure (cm H_2O)	10 cm H_2O
High Peak Pressure (cm H_2O)	70 cm H_2O
Low PEEP (cm H_2O)	1 cm H_2O
Apnea Interval (seconds)	20 seconds

Adjust the inspiratory pressure to 40 cm H_2O.

1. Record the following parameters:
   a. Mode
   b. FIO_2
   c. Respiratory Rate (set and total)

d. Exhaled Tidal Volume
e. PEEP
f. P mean
g. Inspiratory Time
h. I:E Ratio
i. Exhaled Minute Ventilation
j. Peak Pressure

Adjust the inspiratory pressure control to 10 cm H_2O.
Adjust the alarms to the following parameters:

High Respiratory Rate (breaths per minute)	60 breaths/min
Low Exhaled Tidal Volume (mL)	5 mL
High Exhaled Tidal Volume (mL)	40 mL
Low Minute Ventilation (L/min)	0.2 L/min
High Minute Ventilation (L/min)	2 L/min
Low Peak Pressure (cm H_2O)	5 cm H_2O
High Peak Pressure (cm H_2O)	20 cm H_2O
Low PEEP (cm H_2O)	1 cm H_2O
Apnea Interval (seconds)	20 Seconds

2. Record the following parameters:
   a. Mode
   b. FIO_2
   c. Respiratory Rate (set and total)
   d. Exhaled Tidal Volume
   e. PEEP
   f. P mean
   g. Inspiratory Time
   h. I:E Ratio
   i. Exhaled Minute Ventilation
   j. Peak Pressure

Questions

A. What effect does the inspiratory pressure control have on the delivered tidal volume?
B. What effect does the inspiratory pressure control have on the delivered minute ventilation?

FLOW RATE

Return the controls to the following settings:

a. Rate	40 breaths/min
b. Inspiratory Pressure	25 cm H_2O
c. Peak Flow	8 L/min
d. Inspiratory Time	0.5 second
e. PEEP	4 cm H_2O
f. Flow Triggering	0.5 L/min
g. FIO_2	21%

Input the following alarms:

High Respiratory Rate (breaths per minute)	60 breaths/min
Low Exhaled Tidal Volume (mL)	15 mL
High Exhaled Tidal Volume (mL)	60 mL
Low Minute Ventilation (L/min)	0.5 L/min
High Minute Ventilation (L/min)	2 L/min
Low Peak Pressure (cm H_2O)	10 cm H_2O
High Peak Pressure (cm H_2O)	35 cm H_2O
Low PEEP (cm H_2O)	1 cm H_2O
Apnea Interval (seconds)	20 seconds

1. Record the following parameters:
   a. Mode
   b. FIO_2

c. Respiratory Rate (set and total)
d. Exhaled Tidal Volume
e. PEEP
f. P mean
g. Inspiratory Time
h. I:E Ratio
i. Exhaled Minute Ventilation
j. Peak Pressure
Increase the peak flow to 12 L/min.

2. Record the following parameters:
   a. Mode
   b. FIO₂
   c. Respiratory Rate (set and total)
   d. Exhaled Tidal Volume
   e. PEEP
   f. P mean
   g. Inspiratory Time
   h. I:E Ratio
   i. Exhaled Minute Ventilation
   j. Peak Pressure
Increase the peak flow to 30 L/min.

3. Record the following parameters:
   a. Mode
   b. FIO₂
   c. Respiratory Rate (set and total)
   d. Exhaled Tidal Volume
   e. PEEP
   f. P mean
   g. Inspiratory Time
   h. I:E Ratio
   i. Exhaled Minute Ventilation
   j. Peak Pressure

Questions

A. How did the increase in peak flow from 8 to 12 L/min affect the delivered tidal volume?
B. How did the increase in peak flow from 12 to 30 L/min affect the delivered tidal volume?

Touch the "Mode" hard key.
Select "Pressure SIMV" and input the following settings:

a. Rate	35 breaths/min
b. Inspiratory Pressure	20 cm H₂O
c. Inspiratory Time	0.4 second
d. Pressure Support	3 cm H₂O
e. PEEP	5 cm H₂O
f. Flow Triggering	0.5 L/min
g. FIO₂	21%

Touch "Mode Accept."
Input the following alarms:

High Respiratory Rate (breaths per minute)	60 breaths/min
Low Exhaled Tidal Volume (mL)	15 mL
High Exhaled Tidal Volume (mL)	60 mL
Low Minute Ventilation (L/min)	0.5 L/min
High Minute Ventilation (L/min)	2 L/min
Low Peak Pressure (cm H₂O)	10 cm H₂O
High Peak Pressure (cm H₂O)	35 cm H₂O
Low PEEP (cm H₂O)	1 cm H₂O

Apnea Interval (seconds)	20 seconds

1. Record the following parameters:
   a. Mode
   b. FIO₂
   c. Respiratory Rate (set and total)
   d. Exhaled Tidal Volume
   e. Spontaneous Exhaled Tidal Volume
   f. PEEP
   g. P mean
   h. Inspiratory Time
   i. I:E Ratio
   j. Exhaled Minute Ventilation
   k. Peak Pressure
Have a laboratory partner "breathe" the test lung, aiming for an additional 10 breaths per minute.

2. Record the following parameters:
   a. Mode
   b. FIO₂
   c. Respiratory Rate (set and total)
   d. Exhaled Tidal Volume
   e. Spontaneous Exhaled Tidal Volume
   f. PEEP
   g. P mean
   h. Inspiratory Time
   i. I:E Ratio
   j. Exhaled Minute Ventilation
   k. Peak Pressure
Increase the pressure support to 10 cm H₂O and continue to "breathe" the test lung, aiming for an additional 10 breaths per minute.

3. Record the following parameters:
   a. Mode
   b. FIO₂
   c. Respiratory Rate (set and total)
   d. Exhaled Tidal Volume
   e. Spontaneous Exhaled Tidal Volume
   f. PEEP
   g. P mean
   h. Inspiratory Time
   i. I:E Ratio
   j. Exhaled Minute Ventilation
   k. Peak Pressure

Questions

A. What effect did increasing the pressure support have on spontaneous exhaled tidal volumes?
B. What effect did increasing the pressure support have on mandatory exhaled tidal volumes?
C. As you were "breathing" the test lung, was there a notable difference in the "feel" of the breaths at different pressure support levels? Please explain what might account for this difference.

CHANGES IN RESISTANCE AND COMPLIANCE

Return the controls to the following settings:

a. Mode	Pressure SIMV
b. Rate	35 breaths/min
c. Inspiratory Pressure	20 cm H₂O
d. Inspiratory Time	0.4 second

e. Pressure Support 3 cm H$_2$O
f. PEEP 5 cm H$_2$O
g. Flow Triggering 0.5 L/min
h. FIO$_2$ 21%

Input the following alarms:

High Respiratory Rate
(breaths per minute) 60 breaths/min
Low Exhaled Tidal Volume (mL) 15 mL
High Exhaled Tidal Volume (mL) 60 mL
Low Minute Ventilation (L/min) 0.5 L/min
High Minute Ventilation (L/min) 2 L/min
Low Peak Pressure (cm H$_2$O) 10 cm H$_2$O
High Peak Pressure (cm H$_2$O) 70 cm H$_2$O
Low PEEP (cm H$_2$O) 1 cm H$_2$O
Apnea Interval (seconds) 20 seconds

Once these settings have been established, record the following ventilatory (patient) parameters:

a. Mode
b. FIO$_2$
c. Respiratory Rate (set and total)
d. Exhaled Tidal Volume
e. Spontaneous Exhaled Tidal Volume
f. PEEP
g. P mean
h. Inspiratory Time
i. I:E Ratio
j. Exhaled Minute Ventilation
k. Peak Pressure

Decrease the compliance by either reducing it to 0.001 L/cm H$_2$O on the Michigan Instruments TTL Adult/Infant Test Lung (Model 560li) or by turning one stopcock on the IngMar Medical Neonatal Demonstration Lung Model so that only one lung is being ventilated.

1. Record the following parameters:
a. Mode
b. FIO$_2$
c. Respiratory Rate (set and total)
d. Exhaled Tidal Volume
e. Spontaneous Exhaled Tidal Volume
f. PEEP
g. P mean
h. Inspiratory Time
i. I:E Ratio
j. Exhaled Minute Ventilation
k. Peak Pressure

Questions

A. What happened to the tidal volume? Why?
B. What happened to the peak pressure? Why?
C. What types of physiologic processes might be associated with a decrease in overall compliance?
D. What types of therapeutic interventions might be called for when a patient experiences a decrease in overall compliance?

Return the test lung to the previous compliance setting (0.002 L/cm H$_2$O, or both lungs on the IngMar test lung).

Decrease the resistance in the test lung by either changing the Rp 50 resistance adapter to an Rp 200 resistance adapter if you are using the Michigan Instruments TTL

Adult/Infant Test Lung (Model 560li) or by changing to the 2.5 mm ETT if you are using the IngMar Medical Neonatal Demonstration Lung Model.

2. Record the following parameters:
a. Mode
b. FIO$_2$
c. Respiratory Rate (set and total)
d. Exhaled Tidal Volume
e. Spontaneous Exhaled Tidal Volume
f. PEEP
g. P mean
h. Inspiratory Time
i. I:E Ratio
j. Exhaled Minute Ventilation
k. Peak Pressure

Questions

A. What happened to the tidal volume? Why?
B. What happened to the peak pressures? Why?
C. Can you think of human physiologic conditions that could produce similar results?
D. What corrective actions might you take to remedy those items listed in your answer to letter B?

VOLUME CONTROL VENTILATION

Test Lung Setup

If you are using a Michigan Instruments TTL Adult/Infant Test Lung (Model 560li) you will be using the "Infant" side of the test lung. Using the connecting tubing provided with the test lung, connect the lung inlet to the back end of the "Rest Assembly." Connect the Pneuflo Rp 50 resistance adapter to the front end of the rest assembly. Connect the pressure pickoff adapter to the Pneuflo Rp 50 resistance adapter. Connect the pressure line from the pickoff adapter to the proximal pressure input. Connect the patient wye to the pressure pickoff adapter. Set the compliance spring to 0.002 L/cm H$_2$O. Adjust the corresponding slider located near the top of the lung to the 0.002 L/cm H$_2$O setting as well.

If you are using an IngMar Medical Neonatal Demonstration Lung Model, rotate the outer 3-way stopcocks so that there are no leaks present (off to the leak adapters). Ensure that the inner 3-way stopcock is set to allow ventilation of both lungs. Do not attach the brackets at this point. Use the 3.5 mm ETT adapter. Attach the patient wye to the fortlite of the ETT.

INITIAL VENTILATOR SETTINGS

To begin this section, follow the steps outlined next. Press the "Mode" hard key.

Select "Volume SIMV" and input the following settings:
a. Rate 40 breaths/min
b. Tidal Volume 30 mL
c. Peak Flow 7 L/min
d. Inspiratory Pause 0.0 second
e. Pressure Support 3 cm H$_2$O
f. PEEP 4 cm H$_2$O
g. Flow Triggering 0.5 L/min
h. FIO$_2$ 21%

Touch "Mode Accept."

Input the following alarms:

High Respiratory Rate (breaths per minute)	60 breaths/min
Low Exhaled Tidal Volume (mL)	15 mL
High Exhaled Tidal Volume (mL)	60 mL
Low Minute Ventilation (L/min)	0.5 L/min
High Minute Ventilation (L/min)	2 L/min
Low Peak Pressure (cm H_2O)	10 cm H_2O
High Peak Pressure (cm H_2O)	35 cm H_2O
Low PEEP (cm H_2O)	1 cm H_2O
Apnea Interval (seconds)	20 seconds

When completing these activities, manipulate only one control at a time and note the result of each activity with manipulation of the controls. Answer the questions that follow each of the activities.

TIDAL VOLUME CONTROL

While ventilating the test lung, measure and record the following ventilatory parameters:

1. Mode
2. FIO_2
3. Respiratory Rate (set and total)
4. Exhaled Tidal Volume
5. Spontaneous Exhaled Tidal Volume
6. PEEP
7. P mean
8. Inspiratory Time
9. I:E Ratio
10. Exhaled Minute Ventilation
11. Peak Pressure

Touch the tidal volume parameter at the bottom of the screen and rotate the "Data Dial" to adjust the tidal volume to 45 mL.

1. Measure and record the following:
   a. Mode
   b. FIO_2
   c. Respiratory Rate (set and total)
   d. Exhaled Tidal Volume
   e. Spontaneous Exhaled Tidal Volume
   f. PEEP
   g. P mean
   h. Inspiratory Time
   i. I:E Ratio
   j. Exhaled Minute Ventilation
   k. Peak Pressure

Touch the tidal volume parameter at the bottom of the screen and rotate the "Data Dial" to adjust the tidal volume to 15 mL.

2. Measure and record the following:
   a. Mode
   b. FIO_2
   c. Respiratory Rate (set and total)
   d. Exhaled Tidal Volume
   e. Spontaneous Exhaled Tidal Volume
   f. PEEP
   g. P mean
   h. Inspiratory Time
   i. I:E Ratio
   j. Exhaled Minute Ventilation
   k. Peak Pressure

Questions

A. What effect did the tidal volume have on the I:E ratio?
B. What effect did the tidal volume have on peak pressures?
C. What effect did the tidal volume have on delivered tidal volume?

RESPIRATORY RATE CONTROL

Return the ventilator to the previous settings:

a. Rate	40 breaths/min
b. Tidal Volume	30 mL
c. Peak Flow	7 L/min
d. Inspiratory Pause	0.0 second
e. Pressure Support	3 cm H_2O
f. PEEP	4 cm H_2O
g. Flow Triggering	0.5 L/min
h. FIO_2	21%

Press the "Alarm Limits" hard key located in the upper right-hand corner of the Display screen. Change the high respiratory rate alarm to 80 breaths/min and press "Accept."

Touch the respiratory rate parameter at the bottom of the screen and rotate the "Data Dial" to adjust the respiratory rate to 60 breaths/min.

1. Measure and record the following:
   a. Mode
   b. FIO_2
   c. Respiratory Rate (set and total)
   d. Exhaled Tidal Volume
   e. Spontaneous Exhaled Tidal Volume
   f. PEEP
   g. P mean
   h. Inspiratory Time
   i. I:E Ratio
   j. Exhaled Minute Ventilation
   k. Peak Pressure

Touch the respiratory rate parameter at the bottom of the screen and rotate the "Data Dial" to adjust the respiratory rate to 15 breaths/min.

2. Measure and record the following:
   a. Mode
   b. FIO_2
   c. Respiratory Rate (set and total)
   d. Exhaled Tidal Volume
   e. Spontaneous Exhaled Tidal Volume
   f. PEEP
   g. P mean
   h. Inspiratory Time
   i. I:E Ratio
   j. Exhaled Minute Ventilation
   k. Peak Pressure

Questions

A. What effect did the respiratory rate control have on the I:E ratio?
B. What effect did the respiratory rate control have on total respiratory rate?

Changes in Resistance and Compliance

Return the ventilator to the previous settings:

a. Rate   40 breaths/min
b. Tidal Volume   30 mL
c. Peak Flow   7 L/min
d. Inspiratory Pause   0.0 second
e. Pressure Support   3 cm H_2O
f. PEEP   4 cm H_2O
g. Flow Triggering   0.5 L/min
h. FIO$_2$ 21%

Go into the Alarm Limits screen and adjust the peak pressure alarm to 80 cm H_2O.

Once the settings are established, measure and record the following ventilatory (patient) parameters:

a. Mode
b. FIO$_2$
c. Respiratory Rate (set and total)
d. Exhaled Tidal Volume
e. Spontaneous Exhaled Tidal Volume
f. PEEP
g. P mean
h. Inspiratory Time
i. I:E Ratio
j. Exhaled Minute Ventilation
k. Peak Pressure

Decrease the compliance by either reducing it to 0.001 L/cm H_2O on the Michigan Instruments TTL Adult/Infant Test Lung (Model 560li) or by turning one stopcock on the IngMar Medical Neonatal Demonstration Lung Model so that only one lung is being ventilated.

1. Record the following parameters:
   a. Mode
   b. FIO$_2$
   c. Respiratory Rate (set and total)
   d. Exhaled Tidal Volume
   e. Spontaneous Exhaled Tidal Volume
   f. PEEP
   g. P mean
   h. Inspiratory Time
   i. I:E Ratio
   j. Exhaled Minute Ventilation
   k. Peak Pressure

Questions

A. What was the effect on the peak pressure?
B. What types of physiologic processes might be associated with a decrease in overall compliance?
C. What types of therapeutic interventions might be called for when a patient experiences a decrease in overall compliance?

Return the test lung to previous compliance setting (0.002 L/cm H_2O, or both lungs on the IngMar test lung).

Decrease the resistance in the test lung by either changing the Rp 50 resistance adapter to an Rp 200 resistance adapter if you are using the Michigan Instruments TTL Adult/Infant Test Lung (Model 560li) or by changing to the 2.5 mm ETT if you are using the IngMar Medical Neonatal Demonstration Lung Model.

2. Record the following parameters:
   a. Mode
   b. FIO$_2$
   c. Respiratory Rate (set and total)
   d. Exhaled Tidal Volume
   e. Spontaneous Exhaled Tidal Volume
   f. PEEP
   g. P mean
   h. Inspiratory Time
   i. I:E Ratio
   j. Exhaled Minute Ventilation
   k. Peak Pressure

Questions

A. What was the effect on peak pressure?
B. Can you think of human physiologic conditions that could produce similar results?
C. What corrective actions might you take to remedy those items listed in your answer to letter B?

Adjusting Settings Based on Clinical Data

Touch the "Mode" hard key.

Select "Pressure SIMV" and input the following settings:

a. Rate   30 breaths/min
b. Inspiratory pressure 20 cm H_2O
c. Inspiratory Time   0.4 second
d. Pressure Support   3 cm H_2O
e. PEEP   5 cm H_2O
f. Flow Triggering   0.5 L/min
g. FIO$_2$ 100%

Touch "Mode Accept."

Input the following alarms:

High Respiratory Rate
(breaths per minute)   60 breaths/min
Low Exhaled Tidal Volume (mL)   15 mL
High Exhaled Tidal Volume (mL)   60 mL
Low Minute Ventilation (L/min)   0.5 L/min
High Minute Ventilation (L/min)   2 L/min
Low Peak Pressure (cm H_2O)   10 cm H_2O
High Peak Pressure (cm H_2O)   35 cm H_2O
Low PEEP (cm H_2O)   1 cm H_2O
Apnea Interval (seconds)   20 seconds

You are working in a NICU and are taking care of a patient who is being ventilated with the preceding settings. You are making rounds and stop to do an assessment of the patient and record the current ventilator settings.

1. Record the following parameters:
   a. Mode
   b. FIO$_2$
   c. Respiratory Rate (set and total)
   d. Exhaled Tidal Volume
   e. Spontaneous Exhaled Tidal Volume
   f. PEEP
   g. P mean
   h. Inspiratory Time
   i. I:E Ratio
   j. Exhaled Minute Ventilation
   k. Peak Pressure

The neonatologist working today would like for you to draw a blood gas. You do so and present them with the following results:

pH	7.11
$PaCO_2$	65 mm Hg
PaO_2	194 mm Hg
HCO_3	20 mEq/L
SaO_2	100%

Questions

A. What is your interpretation of the blood gas?
B. What changes to the ventilator (if any) are indicated and why?

C. If changes are indicated, please adjust the ventilator accordingly and adjust all alarms appropriately. When done, please record the following:
   a. Mode
   b. FIO_2
   c. Respiratory Rate (set and total)
   d. Exhaled Tidal Volume
   e. Spontaneous Exhaled Tidal Volume
   f. PEEP
   g. P mean
   h. Inspiratory Time
   i. I:E Ratio
   j. Exhaled Minute Ventilation
   k. Peak Pressure

Neonatal Practice Activities: Nellcor Puritan Bennett 840

CIRCUIT ASSEMBLY

Figure 29-11 shows the Nellcor Puritan Bennett 840 assembled and ready for use with a neonatal patient. To prepare the ventilator for use, follow the steps listed next.

1. To enable NeoMode you must install a neonatal circuit and perform the short self test (SST), described later, with the neonatal circuit installed.
2. Install a bacterial inspiratory filter on the patient outlet located on the upper right portion of the breath delivery unit (BDU).
3. Lift the expiratory filter latch into the up position.
4. Slide the neonatal mounting plate (Figure 29-12) onto the tracks on the upper part of the from-patient port on the BDU. Once the mounting plate has been correctly positioned, push the latch down and lock it in place (Figure 29-13).
5. Install an expiratory filter and collector vial into the mounting plate so that the breathing circuit connector faces out.

6. Install a 12- to 18-inch length of neonatal ventilator tubing between the inspiratory filter and the ventilator's humidifier inlet.
7. Connect the inspiratory limb of the neonatal circuit to the humidifier outlet.
8. Connect the expiratory limb of the neonatal circuit to the expiratory filter and collection vial's 22 mm fitting.
9. Attach the patient circuit to the flex arm at its midpoint by clamping the ball fitting on the circuit to the flex arm.

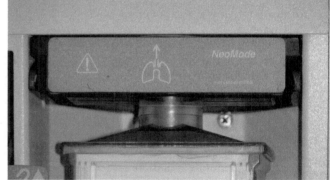

Figure 29-12 The Nellcor Puritan Bennett 840 neonatal mounting plate

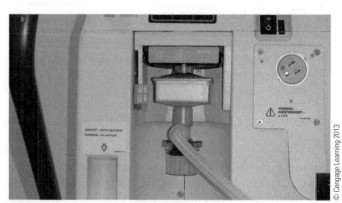

Figure 29-13 The Nellcor Puritan Bennett 840 exhalation assembly correctly positioned

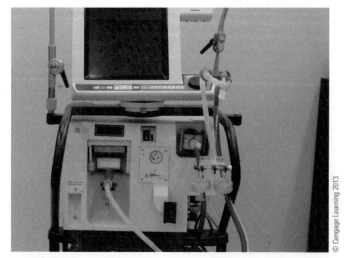

Figure 29-11 The Nellcor Puritan Bennett 840 assembled and ready for use

TESTING THE VENTILATOR BEFORE USE

Power-on Self Test (POST)

Each time the power switch is turned on or if the ventilator microprocessor detects selected fault conditions, a power-on self test (POST) is automatically executed. The POST takes approximately 10 seconds. The test verifies the integrity of the BDU and the graphical user interface (GUI) and their subsystems.

The POST does not check the ventilator's pneumatic systems. To check the operation of the pneumatic systems, a short self test (SST) or extended self test (EST) should be performed.

Short Self Test (SST)

The SST is a short 2- to 3-minute test that will verify the operation of the BDU hardware, including the pressure and flow sensors, the patient circuit, and its compliance and resistance. The test also measures the exhalation filter's resistance. It is recommended that the SST be performed every 15 days, between patients, or when the patient circuit is changed. To complete an SST, perform the following steps.

1. The SST will prompt you to verify that a patient is not connected to the circuit.

2. Turn the ventilator's power switch on. Upon ventilator start-up, touch the "SST" prompt on the lower GUI screen and then press the "Test" button on the left side of the ventilator within 5 seconds of start-up.

3. Follow the prompts on the GUI screen. Touch the "Patient Circuit Type" button and select "Neonatal." The microprocessor will then verify that the patient wye is blocked and the SST will automatically begin.

4. The SST measures the following:
   a. Tests the accuracy of expiratory flow sensors
   b. Verifies the proper function of the pressure sensors
   c. Tests the patient circuit for leaks
   d. Calculates the compliance compensation for the patient circuit
   e. Measures the pressure drop across the expiratory filter
   f. Measures the resistance of the inspiratory and expiratory limbs of the circuit
   g. Checks the pressure drop across the inspiratory limb of the circuit

Using the Keyboard Entry System

All functions of the Nellcor Puritan Bennett 840 ventilator are controlled from the GUI screen (Figure 29-14). The upper screen displays monitored information, including patient data, graphics, and an alarm log. The lower screen displays ventilator setup, alarm settings, and breath timing information. To enter ventilator or alarm settings, follow the "touch–turn–touch" method for entering new settings. Touch the desired value or setting you wish to change (e.g., tidal volume), and turn the knob on the lower right side of the GUI interface until the desired value is displayed (clockwise increases, counterclockwise decreases). Touch or press "Accept" to apply the new setting. The new

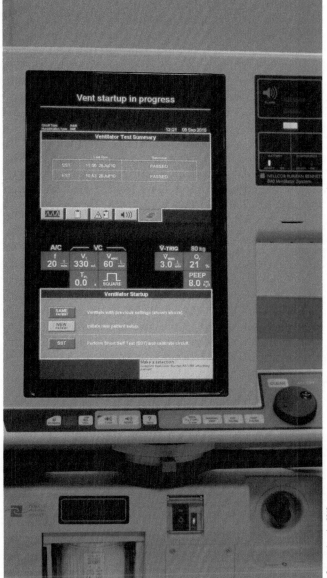

Figure 29-14 The Nellcor Puritan Bennett graphical user interface (GUI)

setting will now be displayed on the appropriate portion of the upper or lower GUI screen.

ACTIVITIES

To complete these practice activities, it is recommended that you use a lung analog/simulator such as a Michigan Instruments TTL Adult/Infant Test Lung (Model 560li) or an IngMar Medical Neonatal Demonstration Lung Model (see Figures 29-9 and 29-10). These devices or other similar devices allow the operator to alter resistance and compliance, simulating changes in patient condition.

If these devices are not available, a simple, single-bellows neonatal test lung may be used. Exercise caution as volumes and pressures may exceed the limits of the test lungs. Resistance may be altered by adapting different sizes of ET tubes, and compliance may be altered by the addition of rubber bands to the test lungs.

LUNG SIMULATOR SETUP

If you are using a Michigan Instruments TTL Adult/Infant Test Lung (Model 560li) you will be using the "Infant" side of the test lung. Using the connecting tubing provided with the test lung, connect the lung inlet to the back end of the "Rest Assembly." Connect the Pneuflo Rp 50 resistance adapter to the front end of the "Rest Assembly." Connect the pressure pickoff adapter to the Pneuflo Rp 50 resistance adapter. Connect the pressure line from the pickoff adapter to the proximal pressure input. Connect the patient wye to the pressure pickoff adapter. Set the compliance spring to 0.002 L/cm H_2O. Adjust the corresponding slider located near the top of the lung to the 0.002 L/cm H_2O setting as well.

If you are using an IngMar Medical Neonatal Demonstration Lung Model, rotate the outer 3-way stopcocks so that there are no leaks present (off to the leak adapters). Ensure that the inner 3-way stopcock is set to allow ventilation of both lungs. Do not attach the brackets at this point. Use the 3.5 mm ETT adapter. Attach the patient wye to the fortlite of the ETT.

When completing these activities, manipulate only one control at a time and note the result of each activity with manipulation of the controls. Answer the questions that follow each of the activities.

PATIENT SETUP

Once the ventilator has completed a POST, the Ventilator Start-up screen is displayed. Prior to beginning the initial neonatal exercises, you must first complete the patient setup. At the Ventilator Start-up screen, select "New Patient." The Ideal Body Weight Input screen appears and you must enter the patient's ideal body weight (IBW). For these exercises, enter 3 kg as the IBW. Once the IBW is entered, press "Continue" to accept the value or press "Restart" to return to the Ventilator Start-up screen and reenter the IBW.

A new Ventilator Start-up screen will appear following entry of the patient's IBW. Next to the patient's ideal body weight is an option that allows the user to select invasive or noninvasive ventilation. Select "Invasive" for these exercises. Table 29-20 lists the settings that appear on this screen.

TABLE 29-20: Nellcor Puritan Bennett 840 Neonatal Ventilator Start-up Settings

Mode	Assist Control (A/C)
	SIMV
	Spontaneous (SPONT)
	BILEVEL
Mandatory Type	Pressure Control (PC)
	Volume Control (VC)
	Volume Control + (VC+)
Spontaneous Type	None
	Pressure Support (PS)
Trigger Type	Flow Trigger (V-Trig)

Make the following selections from the Ventilator Start-up Settings screen. Press the desired setting (Mode, Mandatory Type, Spontaneous Type, or Trigger Type), and rotate the knob on the lower right side of the GUI to change the settings.

   a. Mode   AC
   b. Mandatory Type PC
   c. Trigger Type   V-Trig (Default setting, flow triggered)

If you make an error, simply touch the desired button to change the setting (Mode, Mandatory Type, or Spontaneous Type), make the change by rotating the knob on the lower right of the GUI, and press "Continue." Once the initial settings are complete, a new Ventilator Settings screen will appear (Table 29-21).

From the Ventilator Settings screen, make the following selections by touching the appropriate button, rotating the knob, and touching the button once again. Simply follow the "touch–turn–touch" sequence to make your selection.

   a. Respiratory Rate   30/min
   b. Peak Inspiratory Pressure 20 cm H_2O
   d. I-Time   0.50 second
   e. Flow Sensitivity   0.5 L/min
   f. Oxygen Percent   21%
   g. Rise Time %   50%
   h. PEEP   4 cm H_2O
   i. High Circuit Pressure Limit 35 cm H_2O

If you make an error, simply touch the button you wish to change, rotate the knob to enter the correct setting, and complete the change by touching the button once again. Once you have completed inputting the initial parameters, press "Accept." You will notice that the ventilator will display a message at the top of the screen "Waiting for Patient Connect, Ventilation will begin when connection is detected." Connect the patient circuit to the test lung to begin ventilation.

TABLE 29-21: Nellcor Puritan Bennett 840 Ventilator Settings Screen (Pressure Control)

Frequency (f)	Adjustable from 1 to 150 breaths/min
Peak Inspiratory Pressure (P_I)	Adjustable from 5 to 90 cm H_2O
I Time (T_I)	Adjustable from 0.2 to 8 seconds
Flow Sensitivity ($\dot{V}_{SENS}$)	Adjustable from 0.1 to 10 L/min
Oxygen Percent	Adjustable from 21 to 100%
Rise Time %	Adjustable from 1 to 100%
PEEP	Adjustable from 0 to 45 cm H_2O
High Circuit Pressure Limit (Ppeak)	Adjustable from 7 to 100 cm H_2O

ALARM SETTING

Once the ventilator has begun to cycle, press the "Alarm Setup" button at the bottom of the GUI to input appropriate alarms.

Peak Pressure (P peak)	Set at 35 cm H_2O
Total Respiratory Rate (F_{TOT})	Set at 50
Total Minute Ventilation ($V_{E\,TOT}$)	Set high limit at 4 and low limit at 0.25 L/min
Mandatory Exhaled Tidal Volume ($V_{TE\,MAND}$)	Set high limit at 50 and low limit at 5 mL
Spontaneous Exhaled Tidal Volume ($V_{TE\,SPONT}$)	Set High limit at 50 and low limit at 5 mL

PATIENT MONITORING

The GUI screen is divided into two large sections. The lower section is devoted to ventilator settings; you have already been making entries and using this portion of the screen. The upper screen is devoted to "Monitored Data" or patient data and alarms. Pressing the Graphics symbol at the lower left edge of the monitored data allows you to select between two scalar graphics (pressure time or flow time) or pressure volume. Using the "Plot Setup" button and the control knob, scroll through the options and press "Continue" to make your selection. Should you select pressure volume or flow volume, it will occupy the entire screen. Pressure-time and flow-time scalars can be displayed simultaneously.

Above the graphics display, patient data are displayed numerically. In the upper left corner of the display, breath type (type and phase) will be displayed. Display of types include control, assist, or spontaneous, whereas phase includes inspiration or expiration. Other monitored patient data include peak circuit pressure (P peak), mean airway pressure (P mean), PEEP, I:E ratio, rate (f_{TOT}), exhaled volume (V_{TE}), and exhaled minute volume ($V_{E\,TOT}$).

Between the monitored patient data and the graphics display on the GUI is an alarm area. This section of the screen displays the two highest priority alarms and suggested remedies to correct the alarm condition. You may also press the "Alarm Log" button (clipboard with a speaker), and a list of alarm events, time, and urgency will be displayed.

INSPIRATORY TIME CONTROL

From the initial settings you have previously set, note the following ventilatory (patient) parameters before you make the next changes. (Instructors may want to consider providing a ventilator flow sheet for the students to use in order to record parameters.)

1. Mode
2. FIO_2
3. Respiratory Rate (set and total)
4. Exhaled Tidal Volume
5. PEEP
6. P mean
7. Inspiratory Time
8. I:E Ratio
9. Exhaled Minute Ventilation
10. Peak Pressure

1. Set the inspiratory time to 0.80 second. Record the following parameters:
   a. Mode
   b. FIO_2
   c. Respiratory Rate (set and total)
   d. Exhaled Tidal Volume
   e. PEEP
   f. P mean
   g. Inspiratory Time
   h. I:E Ratio
   i. Exhaled Minute Ventilation
   j. Peak Pressure

2. Set the inspiratory time control to 0.30 second. Record the following parameters:
   a. Mode
   b. FIO_2
   c. Respiratory Rate (set and total)
   d. Exhaled Tidal Volume
   e. PEEP
   f. P mean
   g. Inspiratory Time
   h. I:E Ratio
   i. Exhaled Minute Ventilation
   j. Peak Pressure

Questions:

A. How do you account for the differences in exhaled tidal volume?
B. Why were there differences in mean airway pressure?
C. Why did the I:E ratio vary?
D. Why did the peak pressure not change?

PEAK PRESSURE CONTROL

1. Return the controls to the following settings:

a. Respiratory Rate	30/min
b. Peak Inspiratory Pressure	20 cm H_2O
c. InspiratoryTime	0.50 second
d. Flow Sensitivity	0.5 L/min
e. Oxygen Percent	21%
f. Rise Time %	50%
g. PEEP	4 cm H_2O
h. High Circuit Pressure Limit	35 cm H_2O

Once these settings have been established, record the following ventilatory (patient) parameters:
   a. Mode
   b. FIO_2
   c. Respiratory Rate (set and total)
   d. Exhaled Tidal Volume
   e. PEEP
   f. P mean
   g. Inspiratory Time
   h. I:E Ratio
   i. Exhaled Minute Ventilation
   j. Peak Pressure

2. Touch "Alarm Setup" and change the high circuit pressure limit to 50 cm H_2O.
   a. Adjust the peak pressure control to 40 cm H_2O.
   b. Record the following parameters:
      1. Mode
      2. FIO_2
      3. Respiratory Rate (set and total)
      4. Exhaled Tidal Volume
      5. PEEP
      6. P mean
      7. Inspiratory Time
      8. I:E Ratio
      9. Exhaled Minute Ventilation
      10. Peak Pressure
   c. Adjust the peak pressure control to 10 cm H_2O.
   d. Record the following parameters:
      1. Mode
      2. FIO_2
      3. Respiratory Rate (set and total)
      4. Exhaled Tidal Volume
      5. PEEP
      6. P mean
      7. Inspiratory Time
      8. I:E Ratio
      9. Exhaled Minute Ventilation
      10. Peak Pressure

Questions:

A. What effect does the peak pressure control have on the delivered tidal volume?

CHANGES IN RESISTANCE AND COMPLIANCE

1. Return the controls to the following settings:

a. Respiratory Rate	30/min
b. Peak Inspiratory Pressure	20 cm H_2O
c. Inspiratory Time	0.50 second
d. Flow Sensitivity	0.5 L/min
e. Oxygen Percent	21%
f. Rise Time %	50%
g. PEEP	4 cm H_2O
h. High Circuit Pressure Limit	35 cm H_2O

Go into the Alarm Settings screen and adjust the peak pressure alarm to 100 cm H_2O.

Once the settings are established, measure and record the following ventilatory (patient) parameters from the monitoring screen:
   a. Mode
   b. FIO_2
   c. Respiratory Rate (set and total)
   d. Exhaled Tidal Volume
   e. PEEP
   f. P mean
   g. Inspiratory Time
   h. I:E Ratio
   i. Exhaled Minute Ventilation
   j. Peak Pressure

Decrease the compliance by either reducing it to 0.001 L/cm H_2O on the Michigan Instruments TTL Adult/Infant Test Lung (Model 560li) or by turning one stopcock on the IngMar Medical Neonatal Demonstration Lung Model so that only one lung is being ventilated.

2. Record the following parameters:
   a. Mode
   b. FIO_2
   c. Respiratory Rate (set and total)
   d. Exhaled Tidal Volume
   e. PEEP
   f. P mean
   g. Inspiratory Time
   h. I:E Ratio
   i. Exhaled Minute Ventilation
   j. Peak Pressure

Questions

A. Why did the tidal volume decrease?
B. What types of physiologic processes might be associated with a decrease in overall compliance?
C. What types of therapeutic interventions might be called for when a patient experiences a decrease in overall compliance?

Return the test lung to the previous compliance setting (0.002 L/cm H_2O, or both lungs on the IngMar test lung).

Decrease the resistance in the test lung by either changing the Rp 50 resistance adapter to an Rp 200 resistance adapter if you are using the Michigan Instruments TTL Adult/Infant Test Lung (Model 560li) or by changing to the 2.5 mm ETT if you are using the IngMar Medical Neonatal Demonstration Lung Model.

3. Record the following parameters:
   a. Mode
   b. FIO_2
   c. Respiratory Rate (set and total)
   d. Exhaled Tidal Volume
   e. PEEP
   f. P mean
   g. Inspiratory Time
   h. I:E Ratio
   i. Exhaled Minute Ventilation
   j. Peak Pressure

Questions

A. Why did the tidal volume decrease?
B. Can you think of human physiologic conditions that could produce similar results?
C. What corrective actions might you take to remedy those items listed in your answer to letter B?

VOLUME CONTROL VENTILATION
Test Lung Setup

If you are using a Michigan Instruments TTL Adult/Infant Test Lung (Model 560li) you will be using the "Infant" side of the test lung. Using the connecting tubing provided with the test lung, connect the lung inlet to the back end of the "Rest Assembly." Connect the Pneuflo Rp 50 resistance adapter to the front end of the "Rest Assembly." Connect the pressure pickoff adapter to the Pneuflo Rp 50 resistance adapter. Connect the pressure line from the pickoff adapter to the proximal pressure input. Connect the patient wye to the pressure pickoff adapter. Set the compliance spring to 0.002 L/cm H_2O.

Adjust the corresponding slider located near the top of the lung to the 0.002 L/cm H_2O setting as well.

If you are using an IngMar Medical Neonatal Demonstration Lung Model, rotate the outer 3-way stopcocks so that there are no leaks present (off to the leak adapters). Ensure that the inner 3-way stopcock is set to allow ventilation of both lungs. Do not attach the brackets at this point. Use the 3.5 mm ETT adapter. Attach the patient wye to the fortlite of the ETT.

Make the following selections from the Ventilator Startup Settings screen. Press the desired setting (Mode, Mandatory Type, Spontaneous Type, or Trigger Type), and rotate the knob on the lower right side of the GUI to change the settings.

a. Mode   AC
b. Mandatory Type   VC
c. Trigger Type   V-Trig (Default setting, flow triggered)

If you make an error, simply touch the desired button to change the setting (Mode, Mandatory Type, or Spontaneous Type), make the change by rotating the knob on the lower right of the GUI, and press "Continue." Once the initial settings are complete, a new Ventilator Settings screen will appear.

INITIAL VENTILATORY SETTINGS

Begin this section by setting the ventilator to the following settings. Touch the "Vent Setup" soft key. From the "Mode" key, select A/C (assist-control) mode. Press the "Mandatory Type" soft key, and select "VC" for volume control mode. The "Trigger Type" key is defaulted to flow triggering in the neonatal mode (Table 29-22).

TABLE 29-22: Nellcor Puritan Bennett 840 Ventilator Settings Screen (Volume Control)

Frequency (f)	Adjustable from 1 to 150 breaths/min
Tidal Volume (V_t)	Adjustable from 5 to 315 mL
Peak Flow (V_{MAX})	Adjustable from 1 to 30 L/min
Flow Sensitivity ($\dot{V}_{SENS}$)	Adjustable from 0.1 to 10 L/min
Oxygen Percent	Adjustable from 21 to 100%
Plateau Time (T_{PL})	Adjustable from 0.0 to 2 seconds
Flow Pattern	Ramp or decelerating ramp or square flow pattern
PEEP	Adjustable from 0 to 45 cm H_2O
High Circuit Pressure Limit (P peak)	Adjustable from 7 to 100 cm H_2O

Adjust the ventilator to the following settings in volume control mode.

a. Respiratory Rate   40/min
b. Tidal Volume   30 mL
c. Flow   8 L/min
d. Flow Sensitivity   0.5 L/min
e. Oxygen Percent   21%
f. Plateau Time   0.0 second
g. Flow Pattern   Decelerating
h. PEEP   4 cm H_2O
i. High Circuit Pressure Limit   65 cm H_2O

If you make an error, simply touch the button you wish to change, rotate the knob to enter the correct setting, and then complete the change by touching the button once again. Once you have completed inputting the initial parameters, press "Accept." You will notice that the ventilator will display a message at the top of the screen "Waiting for Patient Connect, Ventilation will begin when connection is detected." Connect the patient circuit to the test lung to begin ventilation.

When completing these activities, manipulate only one control at a time and note the result of each activity with manipulation of the controls. Answer the questions that follow each of the activities.

ALARM SETTING

Once the ventilator has begun to cycle, press the "Alarm Setup" button at the bottom of the GUI to input the appropriate alarms.

Peak Pressure (P peak)	Set at 65 cm H_2O
Total Respiratory Rate (F_{TOT})	Set at 60
Total Minute Ventilation ($V_{E\,TOT}$)	Set high limit at 2.5 and low limit at 0.25 L/min
Mandatory Exhaled Tidal Volume ($V_{TE\,MAND}$)	Set high limit at 100 and low limit at 5 mL
Spontaneous Exhaled Tidal Volume ($V_{TE\,SPONT}$)	Set High limit at 100 and low limit at 5 mL
Low Circuit Pressure Limit	Set at 2 cm H_2O
Total Respiratory Rate (F_{TOT})	Set at 60 breaths per minute

TIDAL VOLUME CONTROL

1. Using a test lung, measure and record the following using the monitoring screen:
   1. Mode
   2. FiO_2
   3. Respiratory Rate (set and total)
   4. Exhaled Tidal Volume
   5. PEEP
   6. P mean
   7. Inspiratory Time (measure with a sweep second hand)
   8. I:E Ratio
   9. Exhaled Minute Ventilation
   10. Peak Pressure

2. Adjust the tidal volume to 45 mL. Measure and record the following:
   1. Mode
   2. FiO_2
   3. Respiratory Rate (set and total)

4. Exhaled Tidal Volume
5. PEEP
6. P mean
7. Inspiratory Time (measure with a sweep second hand)
8. I:E ratio
9. Exhaled Minute Ventilation
10. Peak Pressure

3. Adjust the tidal volume to 15 mL. Measure and record the following:
   1. Mode
   2. FiO$_2$
   3. Respiratory Rate (set and total)
   4. Exhaled Tidal Volume
   5. PEEP
   6. P mean
   7. Inspiratory Time (measure with a sweep second hand)
   8. I:E ratio
   9. Exhaled Minute Ventilation
   10. Peak Pressure

Questions:

A. What effect did the tidal volume have on inspiratory time?
B. What effect did the tidal volume have on peak pressures?
C. What effect did the tidal volume have on delivered tidal volume?

RESPIRATORY RATE CONTROL

Return the ventilator to the previous settings:

a. Respiratory Rate	40/min
b. Tidal Volume	30 mL
c. Flow	8 L/min
d. Flow Sensitivity	0.5 L/min
e. Oxygen Percent	21%
f. Plateau Time	0.0 sec
g. Flow Pattern	Decelerating
h. PEEP	4 cm H$_2$O
i. High Circuit Pressure Limit	65 cm H$_2$O

1. Change the high respiratory rate alarm to 100 breaths per minute.

2. Change the respiratory rate to 60 breaths per minute. Measure and record the following:
   1. Mode
   2. FiO$_2$
   3. Respiratory Rate (set and total)
   4. Exhaled Tidal Volume
   5. PEEP
   6. P mean
   7. Inspiratory Time (measure with a sweep second hand)
   8. I:E ratio
   9. Exhaled Minute Ventilation
   10. Peak Pressure

3. Change the respiratory rate to 10 breaths per minute. Measure and record the following:

1. Mode
2. FiO$_2$
3. Respiratory Rate (set and total)
4. Exhaled Tidal Volume
5. PEEP
6. P mean
7. Inspiratory Time (measure with a sweep second hand)
8. I:E ratio
9. Exhaled Minute Ventilation
10. Peak Pressure

Questions:

A. What effect did the respiratory rate control have on inspiratory time?
B. What effect did the respiratory rate control have on I:E ratio?
C. What effect did the respiratory rate control on total respiratory rate?

CHANGES IN RESISTANCE AND COMPLIANCE

1. Return the ventilator to the previous settings:

a. Respiratory Rate	40/min
b. Tidal Volume	30 mL
c. Flow	8 L/min
d. Flow Sensitivity	0.5 L/min
e. Oxygen Percent	21%
f. Plateau Time	0.0 sec
g. Flow Pattern	Decelerating
h. PEEP	4 cm H$_2$O
i. High Circuit Pressure Limit	65 cm H$_2$O

Go into the Alarm Settings screen and adjust the peak pressure alarm to 100 cm H$_2$O.

Once the settings are established, measure and record the following ventilatory (patient) parameters from the monitoring screen:
   1. Mode
   2. FiO$_2$
   3. Respiratory Rate (set and total)
   4. Exhaled Tidal Volume
   5. PEEP
   6. P mean
   7. Inspiratory Time (measure with a sweep second hand)
   8. I:E ratio
   9. Exhaled Minute Ventilation
   10. Peak Pressure

2. Decrease the compliance by either reducing it to 0.001 L/cm H$_2$O on the Michigan Instruments TTL Adult/Infant Test Lung (Model 560li) or by turning one stopcock on the IngMar Medical Neonatal Demonstration Lung Model so that only one lung is being ventilated.

1. Record the following parameters:
   1. Mode
   2. FiO$_2$
   3. Respiratory Rate (set and total)
   4. Exhaled Tidal Volume
   5. PEEP

6. P mean
7. Inspiratory Time (measure with a sweep second hand)
8. I:E ratio
9. Exhaled Minute Ventilation
10. Peak Pressure

Questions:

A. What was the effect on peak pressure?
B. What types of physiologic processes might be associated with a decrease in overall compliance?
C. What types of therapeutic interventions might be called for when a patient experiences a decrease in overall compliance?

3. Return the test lung to the previous compliance setting (0.002 L/cm H$_2$O, or both lungs on the IngMar test lung).

Decrease the resistance in the test lung by either changing the Rp 50 resistance adapter to an Rp 200 resistance adapter if you are using the Michigan Instruments TTL Adult/Infant Test Lung (Model 560li) or by changing to the 2.5 mm ETT if you are using the IngMar Medical Neonatal Demonstration Lung Model.

2. Record the following parameters:
    1. Mode
    2. FiO$_2$
    3. Respiratory Rate (set and total)
    4. Exhaled Tidal Volume
    5. PEEP
    6. P mean
    7. Inspiratory Time (measure with a sweep second hand)
    8. I:E ratio
    9. Exhaled Minute Ventilation
    10. Peak Pressure

Questions:

A. What was the effect on peak pressure?
B. Can you think of human physiological conditions that could produce similar results?
C. What corrective actions might you take to remedy those items listed in your answer to letter B?

NONINVASIVE VENTILATION (NASAL CPAP)

The Nellcor Puritan Bennett 840 may be set up to do noninvasive ventilation for the neonatal patient. This allows the clinician to use the ventilator to provide nasal CPAP without the need to get a different machine. It also allows the operator a further range of support levels ranging from SIMV with pressure or volume to traditional nasal CPAP. For these exercises, a regular vent circuit attached to a test lung will be sufficient. To activate noninvasive CPAP mode, complete the following steps:

1. Touch "Vent Setup" and enter the "Proposed Vent Settings" area.
2. Touch "Vent Type," and select "Noninvasive."
3. Touch "Mode." You are presented with the options of A/C, SIMV, Spont, and CPAP (select "CPAP").

4. Touch "Mandatory Type" and select the type of controlled breath for a manual inspiration (select "Pressure Control").
5. In spontaneous and SIMV modes, pressure support is available. In CPAP this option is not presented.
6. The triggering mechanism is always defaulted to "Flow" in the neonatal setup.

Once you have completed these steps, touch "Continue" and continue to follow the steps outlined next:

1. Set the PC level at 20 cm H$_2$O.
2. Set the I-time to 0.35 second.
3. Set the flow sensitivity to 0.5 L/min.
4. Set the FiO$_2$ to 21%.
5. Set the rise time % to 50%.
6. Set the high spontaneous inspiratory time limit to 1 second.
7. Set the expiratory sensitivity % to 25%.
8. Set the PEEP level to 5 cm H$_2$O.
9. Set the disconnect sensitivity to 5 L/min.
10. Set the high circuit pressure limit to 30 cm H$_2$O.
11. Set apnea interval to 30 seconds.

Touch "Accept" and the mode will start. Have a partner gently "breathe" the test lung, aiming for a rate of around 30 breaths per minute.

ALARM SETTING

Once the ventilator has begun to cycle, press the "Alarm Setup" button at the bottom of the GUI to input appropriate alarms. You will notice that there are not as many alarms in the noninvasive CPAP setting. There are no volume alarms, only pressure (high pressure to help detect obstruction and low pressure to help detect a patient disconnect) and high respiratory rate.

High Circuit Pressure Limit (P peak)	Set at 30 cm H$_2$O.
Low Circuit Pressure Limit	Set at 2 cm H$_2$O.
Total Respiratory Rate (F$_{TOT}$)	Set at 60 breaths/min.

While your partner is breathing the test lung, record the following parameters:
    a. Mode
    b. FIO$_2$
    c. Respiratory Rate (set and total)
    d. Exhaled Tidal Volume
    e. PEEP
    f. P mean
    g. Inspiratory Time (measure with a sweep second hand)
    h. I:E Ratio
    i. Exhaled Minute Ventilation
    j. Peak Pressure

Questions

A. Why did the tidal volume vary?
B. What types of patients might benefit from nasal CPAP?
C. How does CPAP reduce work of breathing in the neonate?

ADJUSTING SETTINGS BASED ON CLINICAL DATA

Begin this section by setting the ventilator to the following parameters. Touch the "Vent Setup" soft key. From the "Mode" key, select "A/C" (assist-control) mode. Press the "Mandatory Type" soft key, and select "PC" for pressure control mode. The "Trigger Type" key is defaulted to flow triggering in the neonatal mode.

From the Ventilator Settings screen, make the following selections by touching the appropriate button, rotating the knob, and touching the button once again. Simply follow the "touch–turn–touch" sequence to make your selection.

a. Respiratory Rate	40/min
b. Peak Inspiratory Pressure	25 cm H_2O
c. Inspiratory Time	0.40 second
d. Flow Sensitivity	0.5 L/min
e. Oxygen Percent	100%
f. Rise Time %	50%
g. PEEP	2 cm H_2O
h. High Circuit Pressure Limit	35 cm H_2O

If you make an error, simply touch the button you wish to change, rotate the knob to enter the correct setting, and complete the change by touching the button once again. Once you have completed inputting the initial parameters, press "Accept." You will notice that the ventilator will display a message at the top of the screen "Waiting for Patient Connect, Ventilation will begin when connection is detected." Connect the patient circuit to the test lung to begin ventilation.

ALARM SETTING

Once the ventilator has begun to cycle, press the "Alarm Setup" button at the bottom of the GUI to input the appropriate alarms.

Peak Pressure (P peak)	Set at 40 cm H_2O
Total Respiratory Rate (F_{TOT})	Set at 50
Total Minute Ventilation ($V_{E\ TOT}$)	Set high limit at 4 and low limit at 0.25 L/min
Mandatory Exhaled Tidal Volume ($V_{TE\ MAND}$)	Set high limit at 50 and low limit at 5 mL
Spontaneous Exhaled Tidal Volume ($V_{TE\ SPONT}$)	Set high limit at 50 and low limit at 5 mL

You are working in a NICU and are taking care of a patient who is being ventilated with the preceding settings. You are making rounds and stop to do an assessment of the patient and record the current ventilator settings.

1. Record the following parameters:
   a. Mode
   b. FIO_2
   c. Respiratory Rate (set and total)
   d. Exhaled Tidal Volume
   e. Spontaneous Exhaled Tidal Volume
   f. PEEP
   g. P mean
   h. Inspiratory Time
   i. I:E Ratio
   j. Exhaled Minute Ventilation
   k. Peak Pressure

The neonatologist working today would like for you to draw a blood gas. You do so and present the neonatologist with the following results:

pH	7.35
$PaCO_2$	43 mm Hg
PaO_2	52 mm Hg
HCO_3	22 mEq/L
SaO_2	83%

The neonatologist would like for you to improve this patient's oxygenation status. Because the neonatologist is very pleased with the acid–base balance indicated by the recent ABG, he or she also mentions that the patient's minute ventilation must remain the same.

Questions:

A. What is your interpretation of the blood gas?
B. What changes to the ventilator (if any) are indicated and why?
C. If changes are indicated, please adjust the ventilator accordingly and adjust all alarms appropriately. When done, please record the following:
   a. Mode
   b. FIO_2
   c. Respiratory Rate (set and total)
   d. Exhaled Tidal Volume
   e. Spontaneous Exhaled Tidal Volume
   f. PEEP
   g. P mean
   h. Inspiratory Time
   i. I:E ratio
   j. Exhaled Minute Ventilation
   k. Peak Pressure

Neonatal Practice Activities: Maquet SERVO-i

CIRCUIT ASSEMBLY

Figure 29-15 shows the Maquet SERVO-i assembled and ready for use with a neonatal patient. To prepare the ventilator for use, follow the steps listed next.

1. Connect a short length of neonatal ventilator tubing between the inspiratory (patient) outlet located on the right side of the patient unit and the humidifier.

2. Connect the inspiratory limb of the neonatal circuit to the humidifier outlet.
3. Connect a bacterial filter to the expiratory inlet on the right side of the ventilator.
4. Connect the expiratory limb of the neonatal circuit to the bacterial filter on the expiratory inlet.
5. Attach the patient circuit to the flex arm at its midpoint by clamping the ball fitting on the circuit to the flex arm.

Pre-use Check

The pre-use check tests the function of the microprocessor control system; measures internal leakage; tests the pressure transducers, O_2 cell/sensor, flow transducers, and safety valve; measures circuit leakage; and calculates circuit compliance. It is recommended to perform a pre-use check prior to connecting the ventilator to a patient or whenever a patient circuit is changed. To perform the pre-use check, complete the following steps:

1. Connect the power cord to a 110 volt 60 Hz outlet.
2. Connect the air and oxygen supply lines to 50 psi sources.
3. Locate the power switch on the back of the ventilator screen. Turn the ventilator on.
4. The ventilator will perform a system test and will then prompt you by asking, "Do you want to start Pre-use check?" Initially select "No" by touching the "No" button on the touch screen.
5. You will be asked if you want to delete patient data, trends, and event log. Select "Yes."
6. Select the "Infant" setting by touching the "Infant" button.
7. Select "Pre-use Check" and touch "Yes" when asked if you really want to start a pre-use check.
8. You will be asked to connect the "test tube" between the inspiratory outlet and the expiratory inlet. The "test tube" is a specialized section of blue rubber ventilator tubing that is utilized during the pre-use check. Connect the "test tube" between the inspiratory outlet and the expiratory inlet.
9. To test the battery you will be asked to unplug the power cord and then plug the power cord back in.
10. When asked to "connect patient circuit and block Y-piece" connect the neonatal circuit and proximal flow sensor to the ventilator. The circuit should be connected to the inspiratory and expiratory outlets. A bacterial/viral filter should be installed on the expiratory limb of the patient circuit at the ventilator. The proximal flow sensor should be gently snapped into place in the "Y-sensor module" (Figure 29-16) and installed in the circuit at the patient "wye."
11. Once the circuit has been installed, press "OK." You will be prompted to ensure that the circuit is blocked. Block the patient wye and press "OK."
12. You will be asked if you want to "compensate for compressible volume," touch "Yes."
13. The ventilator will then say, "Y Sensor pressure measuring will be tested. Ensure Y Sensor is connected to Y piece and block the Y Sensor." Ensure that it is properly installed and block the sensor and then press "OK."
14. The ventilator will then say, "Y Sensor flow measuring will be tested. Unblock the Y Sensor." Unblock the sensor and touch "OK."
15. Once the Pre-use check is finished the ventilator will display a dialog box titled "New Patient." The dialog box will ask you, "Do you want to delete patient data, trends, and event log?" Touch "Yes."

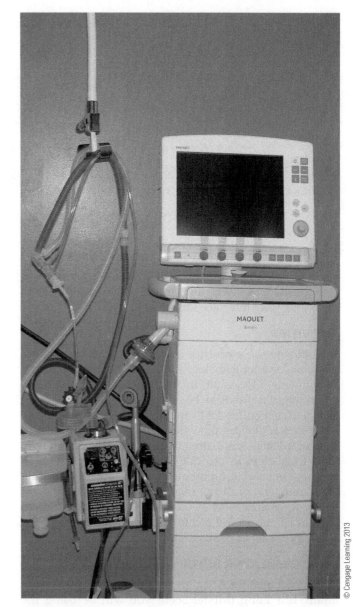

Figure 29-15   The Maquet SERVO-i assembled and ready for use

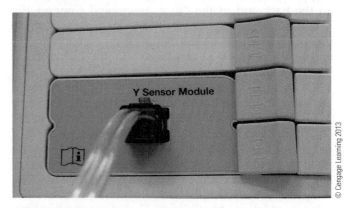

Figure 29-16   The Maquet SERVO-i Y-sensor module

Using the Maquet SERVO-i User Interface

The Maquet SERVO-i user interface consists of a large screen, four direct access knobs below the screen, several fixed soft keys, and a rotary dial located at the lower

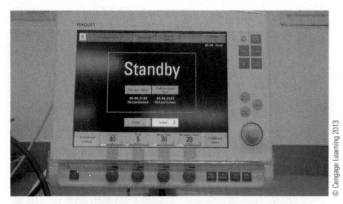

Figure 29-17 The Maquet SERVO-i user interface

right of the user interface that can be turned clockwise or counterclockwise (to increase or decrease values) and then pushed to select the desired value. Figure 29-17 shows the user interface for the Maquet SERVO-i.

ACTIVITIES

To complete these practice activities, it is recommended that you use a lung analog/simulator such as a Michigan Instruments TTL Adult/Infant Test Lung (Model 560li) or an IngMar Medical Neonatal Demonstration Lung Model (see Figures 29-9 and 29-10). These devices or other similar devices allow the operator to alter resistance and compliance, simulating changes in patient condition.

If these devices are not available, a simple, single-bellows neonatal test lung may be used. Exercise caution as volumes and pressures may exceed the limits of the test lungs. Resistance may be altered by adapting different sizes of ET tubes, and compliance may be altered by the addition of rubber bands to the test lungs.

LUNG SIMULATOR SETUP

If you are using a Michigan Instruments TTL Adult/Infant Test Lung (Model 560li) you will be using the "Infant" side of the test lung. Using the connecting tubing provided with the test lung, connect the lung inlet to the back end of the "Rest Assembly." Connect the Pneuflo Rp 50 resistance adapter to the front end of the "Rest Assembly." Connect the pressure pickoff adapter to the Pneuflo Rp 50 resistance adapter. Connect the pressure line from the pickoff adapter to the proximal pressure input. Connect the patient wye to the pressure pickoff adapter. Set the compliance spring to 0.002 L/cm H_2O. Adjust the corresponding slider located near the top of the lung to the 0.002 L/cm H_2O setting as well.

If you are using an IngMar Medical Neonatal Demonstration Lung Model, rotate the outer 3-way stopcocks so that there are no leaks present (off to the leak adapters). Ensure that the inner 3-way stopcock is set to allow ventilation of both lungs. Do not use the brackets. Use the 3.5 mm ETT adapter. Attach the patient wye to the fortlite of the ETT.

When completing these activities, manipulate only one control at a time and note the result of each activity with manipulation of the controls. Answer the questions that follow each of the activities.

PATIENT SETUP

Once the ventilator has completed a pre-use check, the Standby screen is displayed. Prior to beginning the initial neonatal exercises, you must first enter initial ventilator settings for the patient. The default or previous mode will be displayed in the upper left-hand corner of the screen just to the right of the pink baby symbol. Press this mode and a "Set Ventilation Mode" dialog box will appear. By touching the "Mode" button you are presented with a drop-down list of modes available. Table 29-23 lists the modes available on the Select Ventilator Mode screen on the Maquet SERVO-i.

When you touch a mode, you are presented with a list of settings for that mode. These settings generally fall under four categories: basic, inspiratory times, trigger, and backup ventilation. Tables 29-24 through 29-31 summarize the settings available for each mode.

Settings can be adjusted by touching the desired parameter, rotating the "Main Rotary Dial," and then either touching the parameter again or clicking the "Main Rotary Dial." To begin, press "Pressure Control" and input the following settings:

a. Pressure Control (PC)
   above PEEP   20 cm H_2O
b. Respiratory Rate   30 breaths/minute
c. PEEP   5 cm H_2O
d. O_2 Concentration   21%
e. I-Time   0.40 second
f. T insp. rise   0.15 second
g. Trigger Flow   3

Once you have finished inputting the preceding settings, touch "Accept." The ventilator will return to the Standby screen. To begin ventilation, press the gray "Start/Standby" key located at the lower left-hand corner of the user interface screen. The orange light on the upper right-hand corner of the button will turn off and ventilation will begin. Connect the patient circuit to the test lung you are using. At any time, to return to "Standby," you may press this key and then confirm on the touch screen to enter standby.

ALARM SETTING

Once the ventilator has begun to cycle, press the "Alarm Profile" key located on the upper right-hand corner of the User Interface screen. This key will bring up the "Alarm Profile" page, which presents the user with the following

TABLE 29-23: Maquet SERVO-i Neonatal Ventilator Modes

Volume control
Pressure control
Pressure regulated volume control (PRVC)
Pressure support/CPAP
Volume support
SIMV (volume control) + pressure support
SIMV (pressure control) + pressure support
SIMV (PRVC) + pressure support

TABLE 29-24: Maquet SERVO-i Volume Control

BASIC	INSPIRATORY TIMES	TRIGGER
Tidal Volume (adjustable from 2 to 350 mL)	Inspiratory Time (T$_I$) (adjustable from 0.1 to 5 seconds)	This setting can either be flow triggering (adjustable from 1 to 10) or pressure triggering (adjustable from −20 to 0)
Respiratory Rate (adjustable from 4 to 150 breaths/min)	Pause Time (T pause) (adjustable from 0.00 to 1.5 seconds)	
PEEP (adjustable from 0 to 50 cm H$_2$O)	Inspiratory Rise Time (T insp. rise) (adjustable from 0.0 to 0.2 second)	
O$_2$ Concentration (adjustable from 21 to 100%)		

TABLE 29-25: Maquet SERVO-i Pressure Control

BASIC	INSPIRATORY TIMES	TRIGGER
Pressure Control above PEEP (adjustable from 0 to 80 cm H$_2$O)	Inspiratory Time (T$_I$) (adjustable from 0.1 to 5 seconds)	This setting can either be flow triggering (adjustable from 1 to 10) or pressure triggering (adjustable from −20 to 0)
Respiratory Rate (adjustable from 4 to 150 breaths/min)	Inspiratory Rise Time (T insp. rise) (adjustable from 0.0 to 0.2 second)	
PEEP (adjustable from 0 to 50 cm H$_2$O)		
O$_2$ Concentration (adjustable from 21 to 100%)		

TABLE 29-26: Maquet SERVO-i Pressure Regulated Volume Control

BASIC	INSPIRATORY TIMES	TRIGGER
Tidal Volume (adjustable from 2 to 350 mL)	Inspiratory Time (T$_I$) (adjustable from 0.1 to 5 seconds)	This setting can either be flow triggering (adjustable from 1 to 10) or pressure triggering (adjustable from −20 to 0)
Respiratory Rate (adjustable from 4 to 150 breaths/min)	Inspiratory Rise Time (T insp. rise) (adjustable from 0.0 to 0.2 second)	
PEEP (adjustable from 0 to 50 cm H$_2$O)		
O$_2$ Concentration (adjustable from 21 to 100%)		

adjustable alarms: Pressure, Minute Volume, Respiratory Rate, and End-Expiratory Pressure. The SERVO-i also has a unique feature on the "Alarm Profile" page. A button labeled "Autoset" can be found in the lower left-hand corner of the "Alarm Profile" page. Touching this button automatically sets the alarms according to preset values above and below the current ventilating parameters.

Table 29-32 lists the parameters used to establish alarms when "Autoset" is used.

Please set the alarms to the following parameters. Touch the desired parameter, rotate the "Main Rotary Dial" to adjust the parameter, and either touch the parameter again or click the "Main Rotary Dial" to confirm your selection. When you are finished, touch "Accept."

TABLE 29-27: Maquet SERVO-i Pressure Support/CPAP

BASIC	INSPIRATORY TIMES	TRIGGER	BACKUP VENTILATION
Pressure Support above PEEP (adjustable from 0 to 80 cm H_2O)	Inspiratory Rise Time (T insp. rise) (adjustable from 0.0 to 0.2 second)	This setting can either be flow triggering (adjustable from 1 to 10) or pressure triggering (adjustable from −20 to 0)	Pressure Control above PEEP (adjustable from 5 to 80 cm H_2O)
PEEP (adjustable from 0 to 50 cm H_2O)		Inspiratory Cycle Off (adjustable from 1 to 70%)	
O_2 Concentration (adjustable from 21 to 100%)			

TABLE 29-28: Maquet SERVO-i Volume Support

BASIC	INSPIRATORY TIMES	TRIGGER
Tidal Volume (adjustable from 2 to 350 mL)	Inspiratory Rise Time (T insp. rise) (adjustable from 0.0 to 0.2 second)	This setting can either be flow triggering (adjustable from 1 to 10) or pressure triggering (adjustable from −20 to 0)
PEEP (adjustable from 0 to 50 cm H_2O)		Inspiratory Cycle Off (adjustable from 1 to 70%)
O_2 Concentration (adjustable from 21 to 100%)		

TABLE 29-29: Maquet SERVO-i SIMV (Volume Control) + Pressure Support

MANDATORY BREATHS	INSPIRATORY TIMES	TRIGGER	SUPPORTED BREATH
Tidal Volume (adjustable from 2 to 350 mL)	Inspiratory Time (T$_I$) (adjustable from 0.1 to 5 seconds)	This setting can either be flow triggering (adjustable from 1 to 10) or pressure triggering (adjustable from −20 to 0)	Pressure Support above PEEP (adjustable from 0 to 80 cm H_2O)
SIMV Rate (adjustable from 1 to 60 breaths/min)	Pause Time (T pause) (adjustable from 0.00 to 1.5 seconds)	Inspiratory Cycle Off (adjustable from 1 to 70%)	
PEEP (adjustable from 0 to 50 cm H_2O)	Inspiratory Rise Time (T insp. rise) (adjustable from 0.0 to 0.2 second)		
O_2 Concentration (adjustable from 21 to 100%)			

High Airway Pressures	35 cm H_2O	Respiratory Frequency (upper alarm limit)	45
Expiratory Minute Volume (lower alarm limit)	0.5 L/min	End-Expiratory Pressure (lower alarm limit)	2 cm H_2O
Expiratory Minute Volume (upper alarm limit)	2 L/min	End-Expiratory Pressure (upper alarm limit)	8 cm H_2O
Respiratory Frequency (lower alarm limit)	15		

TABLE 29-30: Maquet SERVO-i SIMV (Pressure Control) + Pressure Support

MANDATORY BREATHS	INSPIRATORY TIMES	TRIGGER	SUPPORTED BREATH
Pressure Control above PEEP (adjustable from 0 to 80 cm H_2O)	Inspiratory Time (T_I) (adjustable from 0.1 to 5 seconds)	This setting can either be flow triggering (adjustable from 1 to 10) or pressure triggering (adjustable from −20 to 0)	Pressure Support above PEEP (adjustable from 0 to 80 cm H_2O)
SIMV Rate (adjustable from 1 to 60 breaths/min)	Inspiratory Rise Time (T insp. rise) (adjustable from 0.0 to 0.2 second)	Inspiratory Cycle Off (adjustable from 1 to 70%)	
PEEP (adjustable from 0 to 50 cm H_2O)			
O_2 Concentration (adjustable from 21 to 100%)			

TABLE 29-31: Maquet SERVO-i SIMV (Pressure Regulated Volume Control) + Pressure Support

MANDATORY BREATHS	INSPIRATORY TIMES	TRIGGER	SUPPORTED BREATH
Tidal Volume (adjustable from 2 to 350 mL)	Inspiratory Time (T_I) (adjustable from 0.1 to 5 seconds)	This setting can either be flow triggering (adjustable from 1 to 10) or pressure triggering (adjustable from −20 to 0)	Pressure Support above PEEP (adjustable from 0 to 80 cm H_2O)
SIMV Rate (adjustable from 1 to 60 breaths/min)	Inspiratory Rise Time (T insp. rise) (adjustable from 0.0 to 0.2 second)	Inspiratory Cycle Off (adjustable from 1 to 70%)	
PEEP (adjustable from 0 to 50 cm H_2O)			
O_2 Concentration (adjustable from 21 to 100%)			

PATIENT MONITORING

The User Interface screen is divided into two large sections. Scalar waveforms for pressure, flow, and volume occupy the majority of the screen display. To the right of the waveform display is a section devoted to patient-monitored parameters. The basic screen includes peak pressure, respiratory rate, and minute volume with inspired and expired tidal volumes being displayed in the same window.

Pressing the "Additional Values" button at the lower right of the screen opens additional monitoring parameters including peak, plateau, mean and PEEP pressures, respiratory rate, O_2 %, inspiratory time, I:E ratio, minute volumes (inspired and exhaled), and tidal volumes (inspired and exhaled).

INSPIRATORY TIME CONTROL

From the initial settings you have previously set, note the following ventilatory (patient) parameters before you make the next changes. (Instructors may want to consider providing a ventilator flow sheet for the students to use in order to record parameters.)

1. Mode
2. FIO$_2$
3. Respiratory Rate (set and total)
4. Exhaled Tidal Volume
5. PEEP
6. P mean
7. Inspiratory Time
8. I:E Ratio
9. Exhaled Minute Ventilation
10. Peak Pressure

1. Set the inspiratory time to 0.90 second.
   Record the following parameters:
   a. Mode
   b. FIO$_2$
   c. Respiratory Rate (set and total)

TABLE 29-32: Autoset Parameters for SERVO-i

SERVO-I VENTILATOR ALARMS	AUTOSET PARAMETERS
High Airway Pressures	Mean peak pressure + 10 cm H_2O or at least 35 cm H_2O
Expiratory Minute Volume (upper alarm limit)	Current minute volume + 50%
Expiratory Minute Volume (lower alarm limit)	Current minute volume − 50%
Respiratory Frequency (upper alarm limit)	Current rate + 40%
Respiratory Frequency (lower alarm limit)	Current rate − 40%
End-Expiratory Pressure (upper alarm limit)	Mean end-expiratory pressure + 5 cm H_2O
End-Expiratory Pressure (lower alarm limit)	Mean end-expiratory pressure − 3 cm H_2O

   d. Exhaled Tidal Volume
   e. PEEP
   f. P mean
   g. Inspiratory Time
   h. I:E Ratio
   i. Exhaled Minute Ventilation
   j. Peak Pressure

2. Set the inspiratory time control to 0.20 second. Record the following parameters:
   a. Mode
   b. FIO_2
   c. Respiratory Rate (set and total)
   d. Exhaled Tidal Volume
   e. PEEP
   f. P mean
   g. Inspiratory Time
   h. I:E Ratio
   i. Exhaled Minute Ventilation
   j. Peak Pressure

Questions:

A. How do you account for the changes in tidal volume?
B. Why were there differences in mean airway pressure?
C. Why did the I:E ratio vary?
D. Why did the peak pressure not change?

PEAK PRESSURE CONTROL

Return the controls to the following settings:
   a. Pressure Control (PC) above PEEP   20 cm H_2O
   b. Respiratory Rate   30 breaths/min
   c. PEEP   5 cm H_2O
   d. O_2 Concentration   21%
   e. I-Time   0.40 second
   f. T insp. rise   0.15 second
   g. Trigger Flow   3

Once these settings have been established, record the following ventilatory (patient) parameters:
   a. Mode
   b. FIO_2
   c. Respiratory Rate (set and total)
   d. Exhaled Tidal Volume
   e. PEEP
   f. P mean
   g. Inspiratory Time
   h. I:E Ratio
   i. Exhaled Minute Ventilation
   j. Peak Pressure

Adjust the alarms to the following parameters:
   High Airway Pressures   55 cm H_2O
   Expiratory Minute Volume (lower alarm limit)   0.5 L/min
   Expiratory Minute Volume (upper alarm limit)   5 L/min
   Respiratory Frequency (lower alarm limit)   15
   Respiratory Frequency (upper alarm limit)   45
   End-Expiratory Pressure (lower alarm limit)   2 cm H_2O
   End-Expiratory Pressure (upper alarm limit)   8 cm H_2O

Using the "Direct Access Knobs," located beneath the User Interface screen, adjust the pressure control (above PEEP) to 40 cm H_2O.

At 30 cm H_2O the ventilator will sound a tone and momentarily stop the adjustment. Note the warning regarding "High Inspiratory Pressure Selected" and note that the bar above the pressure control level turns from white to yellow. Wait a few seconds and you will be allowed to continue your adjustment to 40 cm H_2O.

1. Record the following parameters:
   a. Mode
   b. FIO_2
   c. Respiratory Rate (set and total)
   d. Exhaled Tidal Volume
   e. PEEP
   f. P mean
   g. Inspiratory Time
   h. I:E Ratio
   i. Exhaled Minute Ventilation
   j. Peak Pressure

Adjust the alarms to the following parameters:
   High Airway Pressures   55 cm H_2O
   Expiratory Minute Volume (lower alarm limit) 0.2 L/min
   Expiratory Minute Volume (upper alarm limit) 5 L/min
   Respiratory Frequency (lower alarm limit)   15
   Respiratory Frequency (upper alarm limit)   45
   End-Expiratory Pressure (lower alarm limit) 2 cm H_2O
   End-Expiratory Pressure (upper alarm limit) 8 cm H_2O

Adjust the peak pressure control to 10 cm H_2O.

2. Record the following parameters:
   a. Mode
   b. FIO_2
   c. Respiratory Rate (set and total)
   d. Exhaled Tidal Volume
   e. PEEP
   f. P mean
   g. Inspiratory Time
   h. I:E Ratio
   i. Exhaled Minute Ventilation
   j. Peak Pressure

Questions

A. What effect does the peak pressure control have on the delivered tidal volume?
B. What effect does the peak pressure control have on the delivered minute ventilation?

CHANGES IN RESISTANCE AND COMPLIANCE

Return the controls to the following settings:

a. Pressure Control (PC) above PEEP	20 cm H_2O
b. Respiratory Rate	30 breaths/min
c. PEEP	5 cm H_2O
d. O_2 Concentration	21%
e. I-Time	0.40 second
f. T insp. rise	0.15 second
g. Trigger Flow	3

Go into the Alarm Profile screen and adjust the peak pressure alarm to 70 cm H_2O.

Once these settings have been established, record the following ventilatory (patient) parameters:
   a. Mode
   b. FIO_2
   c. Respiratory Rate (set and total)
   d. Exhaled Tidal Volume
   e. PEEP
   f. P mean
   g. Inspiratory Time
   h. I:E Ratio
   i. Exhaled Minute Ventilation
   j. Peak Pressure

Decrease the compliance by either reducing it to 0.001 L/cm H_2O on the Michigan Instruments TTL Adult/Infant Test Lung (Model 560li) or by turning one stopcock on the IngMar Medical Neonatal Demonstration Lung Model so that only one lung is being ventilated.

1. Record the following parameters:
   a. Mode
   b. FIO_2
   c. Respiratory Rate (set and total)
   d. Exhaled Tidal Volume
   e. PEEP
   f. P mean
   g. Inspiratory Time
   h. I:E Ratio
   i. Exhaled Minute Ventilation
   j. Peak Pressure

Questions

A. What happened to the tidal volume? Why?
B. What types of physiologic processes might be associated with a decrease in overall compliance?
C. What types of therapeutic interventions might be called for when a patient experiences a decrease in overall compliance?

Return the test lung to the previous compliance setting (0.002 L/cm H_2O, or both lungs on the IngMar test lung).

Decrease the resistance in the test lung by either changing the Rp 50 resistance adapter to an Rp 200 resistance adapter if you are using the Michigan Instruments TTL Adult/Infant Test Lung (Model 560li) or by changing to the 2.5 mm ETT if you are using the IngMar Medical Neonatal Demonstration Lung Model.

2. Record the following parameters:
   a. Mode
   b. FIO_2
   c. Respiratory Rate (set and total)
   d. Exhaled Tidal Volume
   e. PEEP
   f. P mean
   g. Inspiratory Time
   h. I:E Ratio
   i. Exhaled Minute Ventilation
   j. Peak Pressure

Questions

A. What happened to the tidal volume? Why?
B. Can you think of human physiologic conditions that could produce similar results?
C. What corrective actions might you take to remedy those items listed in your answer to letter B?

VOLUME CONTROL VENTILATION

Test Lung Setup

If you are using a Michigan Instruments TTL Adult/Infant Test Lung (Model 560li) you will be using the "Infant" side of the test lung. Using the connecting tubing provided with the test lung, connect the lung inlet to the back end of the "Rest Assembly." Connect the Pneuflo Rp 50 resistance adapter to the front end of the "Rest Assembly." Connect the pressure pickoff adapter to the Pneuflo Rp 50 resistance adapter. Connect the pressure line from the pickoff adapter to the proximal pressure input. Connect the patient wye to the pressure pickoff adapter. Set the compliance spring to 0.002 L/cm H_2O. Adjust the corresponding slider located near the top of the lung to the 0.002 L/cm H_2O setting as well.

If you are using an IngMar Medical Neonatal Demonstration Lung Model, rotate the outer 3-way stopcocks so that there are no leaks present (off to the leak adapters). Ensure that the inner 3-way stopcock is set to allow ventilation of both lungs. Do not attach the brackets at this point. Use the 3.5 mm ETT adapter. Attach the patient wye to the fortlite of the ETT.

Initial Ventilator Settings

To begin this section, follow the steps outlined next.

Press the "Pressure Control" mode button in the upper left-hand corner of the screen (next to the pink baby symbol). The "Set Ventilation Mode" dialog box will appear. Press "Pressure Control" in this dialog box and another menu titled "Select Ventilation Mode" will appear.

Touch "Volume Control" and make the following adjustments:

a. Tidal Volume	30 mL
b. Respiratory Rate	40 breaths/min
c. PEEP	4 cm H$_2$O
d. O$_2$ Concentration	21%
e. I-Time	0.35 second
f. Pause Time (T pause)	0.0 second
g. T insp. rise	0.15 second
h. Trigger Flow	3

Settings can be adjusted by touching the desired parameter, rotating the "Main Rotary Dial," and then either touching the parameter again or clicking the "Main Rotary Dial." Once you have completed inputting the initial parameters, touch "Accept."

You will notice that the ventilator will display a message entitled "Compliance Compensation" that states, "Check that no changes have been made to the patient circuit that can affect the compliance compensation." Touch "OK" and then touch "Accept" again to begin volume control ventilation.

When completing these activities, manipulate only one control at a time and note the result of each activity with manipulation of the controls. Answer the questions that follow each of the activities.

ALARM SETTING

Once the ventilator has begun to cycle, press the "Alarm Profile" key located on the upper right-hand corner of the User Interface screen. Please set the alarms to the following parameters. Touch the desired parameter, rotate the "Main Rotary Dial" to adjust the parameter, and either touch the parameter again or click the "Main Rotary Dial" to confirm your selection. When you are finished, touch "Accept."

High Airway Pressures	45 cm H$_2$O
Expiratory Minute Volume (lower alarm limit)	0.5 L/min
Expiratory Minute Volume (upper alarm limit)	2 L/min
Respiratory Frequency (lower alarm limit)	15
Respiratory Frequency (upper alarm limit)	45
End-Expiratory Pressure (lower alarm limit)	2 cm H$_2$O
End-Expiratory Pressure (upper alarm limit)	8 cm H$_2$O

TIDAL VOLUME CONTROL

While ventilating the test lung, measure and record the following ventilatory parameters:
a. Mode
b. FIO$_2$
c. Respiratory Rate (set and total)
d. Exhaled Tidal Volume
e. PEEP
f. P mean
g. Inspiratory Time
h. I:E Ratio
i. Exhaled Minute Ventilation
j. Peak Pressure

Using the "Direct Access" knobs located beneath the User Interface screen, adjust the tidal volume to 45 mL.

1. Measure and record the following:
   a. Mode
   b. FIO$_2$
   c. Respiratory Rate (set and total)
   d. Exhaled Tidal Volume
   e. PEEP
   f. P mean
   g. Inspiratory Time (measure with a sweep second hand)
   h. I:E Ratio
   i. Exhaled Minute Ventilation
   j. Peak Pressure

Using the "Direct Access" knobs located beneath the User Interface screen, adjust the tidal volume to 15 mL.

2. Measure and record the following:
   a. Mode
   b. FIO$_2$
   c. Respiratory Rate (set and total)
   d. Exhaled Tidal Volume
   e. PEEP
   f. P mean
   g. Inspiratory Time (measure with a sweep second hand)
   h. I:E Ratio
   i. Exhaled Minute Ventilation
   j. Peak Pressure

Questions

A. What effect did the tidal volume have on the I:E ratio?
B. What effect did the tidal volume have on peak pressures?
C. What effect did the tidal volume have on delivered tidal volume?

RESPIRATORY RATE CONTROL

Return the ventilator to the previous settings:

a. Tidal Volume	30 mL
b. Respiratory Rate	40 breaths/min
c. PEEP	4 cm H$_2$O
d. O$_2$ Concentration	21%
e. I-Time	0.35 second
f. Pause Time (T pause)	0.0 second
g. T insp. rise	0.15 second
h. Trigger Flow	3

Press "Alarm Profile" located in the upper right-hand corner of the User Interface screen. Change the high respiratory rate alarm to 80 breaths per minute and press "Accept."

Using the "Direct Access" knobs located beneath the User Interface screen, adjust the respiratory rate to 60 breaths per minute.

1. Measure and record the following:
   a. Mode
   b. FIO$_2$
   c. Respiratory Rate (set and total)
   d. Exhaled Tidal Volume
   e. PEEP
   f. P mean
   g. Inspiratory Time (measure with a sweep second hand)
   h. I:E Ratio
   i. Exhaled Minute Ventilation
   j. Peak Pressure

Using the "Direct Access" knobs located beneath the User Interface screen, adjust the respiratory rate to 15 breaths per minute.

2. Measure and record the following:
   a. Mode
   b. FIO$_2$
   c. Respiratory Rate (set and total)
   d. Exhaled Tidal Volume
   e. PEEP
   f. P mean
   g. Inspiratory Time (measure with a sweep second hand)
   h. I:E Ratio
   i. Exhaled Minute Ventilation
   j. Peak Pressure

Questions

A. What effect did the respiratory rate control have on the I:E ratio?
B. What effect did the respiratory rate control on total respiratory rate?

CHANGES IN RESISTANCE AND COMPLIANCE

Return the ventilator to the previous volume control settings:

a. Tidal Volume	30 mL
b. Respiratory Rate	40 breaths/min
c. PEEP	4 cmH$_2$O
d. O$_2$ Concentration	21%
e. I-Time	0.35 second
f. Pause Time (T pause)	0.0 second
g. T insp. rise	0.15 second
h. Trigger Flow	3

Go to the Alarm Profile screen and adjust the peak pressure alarm to 80 cm H$_2$O.

Once the settings are established, measure and record the following ventilatory (patient) parameters from the monitoring screen:
   a. Mode
   b. FIO$_2$
   c. Respiratory Rate (set and total)
   d. Exhaled Tidal Volume
   e. PEEP
   f. P mean
   g. Inspiratory Time (measure with a sweep second hand)
   h. I:E Ratio
   i. Exhaled Minute Ventilation
   j. Peak Pressure

Decrease the compliance by either reducing it to 0.001 L/cm H$_2$O on the Michigan Instruments TTL Adult/Infant Test Lung (Model 560li) or by turning one stopcock on the IngMar Medical Neonatal Demonstration Lung Model so that only one lung is being ventilated.

1. Record the following parameters:
   a. Mode
   b. FIO$_2$
   c. Respiratory Rate (set and total)
   d. Exhaled Tidal Volume
   e. PEEP
   f. P mean
   g. Inspiratory Time (measure with a sweep second hand)
   h. I:E Ratio
   i. Exhaled Minute Ventilation
   j. Peak Pressure

Questions

A. What was the effect on the peak pressure?
B. What types of physiologic processes might be associated with a decrease in overall compliance?
C. What types of therapeutic interventions might be called for when a patient experiences a decrease in overall compliance?

Return the test lung to the previous compliance setting (0.002 L/cm H$_2$O, or both lungs on the IngMar test lung).

Decrease the resistance in the test lung by either changing the Rp 50 resistance adapter to an Rp 200 resistance adapter if you are using the Michigan Instruments TTL Adult/Infant Test Lung (Model 560li) or by changing to the 2.5 mm ETT if you are using the IngMar Medical Neonatal Demonstration Lung Model.

2. Record the following parameters:
   a. Mode
   b. FIO$_2$
   c. Respiratory Rate (set and total)
   d. Exhaled Tidal Volume
   e. PEEP
   f. P mean
   g. Inspiratory Time (measure with a sweep second hand)
   h. I:E Ratio
   i. Exhaled Minute Ventilation
   j. Peak Pressure

Questions

A. What was the effect on peak pressure?
B. Can you think of human physiologic conditions that could produce similar results?
C. What corrective actions might you take to remedy those items listed in your answer to letter B?

PRESSURE REGULATED VOLUME CONTROL

Test Lung Setup

If you are using a Michigan Instruments TTL Adult/Infant Test Lung (Model 560li) you will be using the "Infant" side of the test lung. Using the connecting tubing provided with the test lung, connect the lung inlet to the back end of the "Rest Assembly." Connect the Pneuflo Rp 50 resistance adapter to the front end of the "Rest Assembly." Connect the pressure pickoff adapter to the Pneuflo Rp 50 resistance adapter. Connect the pressure line from the pickoff adapter to the proximal pressure input. Connect the patient wye to the pressure pickoff adapter. Set the compliance spring to 0.001 L/cm H_2O. Adjust the corresponding slider located near the top of the lung to the 0.001 L/cm H_2O setting as well.

If you are using an IngMar Medical Neonatal Demonstration Lung Model, rotate the outer 3-way stopcocks so that there are no leaks present (off to the leak adapters). Ensure that the inner 3-way stopcock is set to allow ventilation to only one lung. Do not attach the brackets at this point. Use the 3.5 mm ETT adapter. Attach the patient wye to the fortlite of the ETT.

INITIAL VENTILATOR SETTINGS

To begin this section, follow the steps outlined next.

Press the "Volume Control" mode button in the upper left-hand corner of the screen (next to the pink baby symbol). The "Set Ventilation Mode" dialog box will appear. Press "Volume Control" in this dialog box and another menu titled "Select Ventilation Mode" will appear.

Touch "PRVC" and make the following adjustments:
a. Tidal Volume	15 mL
b. Respiratory Rate	40 breath per minute
c. PEEP	4 cm H_2O
d. O_2 Concentration	21%
e. I -Time	0.35 second
f. T insp. rise	0.15 second
g. Trigger Flow	3

Settings can be adjusted by touching the desired parameter, rotating the "Main Rotary Dial," and then either touching the parameter again or clicking the "Main Rotary Dial." Once you have completed inputting the initial parameters, touch "Accept."

You will notice that the ventilator will display a message entitled "Compliance Compensation" that states, "Check that no changes have been made to the patient circuit that can affect the compliance compensation." Touch "OK" and then touch "Accept" again to begin PRVC ventilation.

When completing these activities, manipulate only one control at a time and note the result of each activity with manipulation of the controls. Answer the questions that follow each of the activities.

ALARM SETTING

Once the ventilator has begun to cycle, press the "Alarm Profile" key located on the upper right-hand corner of the User Interface screen. Please set the alarms to the following parameters. Touch the desired parameter, rotate the "Main Rotary Dial" to adjust the parameter, and either touch the parameter again or click the "Main Rotary Dial" to confirm your selection. When you are finished, touch "Accept."

High Airway Pressures	60 cm H_2O
Expiratory Minute Volume (lower alarm limit)	0.5 L/min
Expiratory Minute Volume (upper alarm limit)	2 L/min
Respiratory Frequency (lower alarm limit)	15
Respiratory Frequency (upper alarm limit)	45
End-Expiratory Pressure (lower alarm limit)	2 cm H_2O
End-Expiratory Pressure (upper alarm limit)	8 cm H_2O

CHANGES IN COMPLIANCE

PRVC is a mode that combines the protective effects of pressure control with the breath-to-breath consistency associated with volume-oriented modes. The ventilator continually assesses the patient condition in order to determine the level of pressure necessary to deliver the desired tidal volume. Pressures are automatically up-regulated or down-regulated based on the patient's physiology. The following exercises aim to illustrate how PRVC might respond to a newborn who has recently received surfactant. While ventilating the test lung, measure and record the following ventilatory parameters:
a. Mode
b. FIO_2
c. Respiratory Rate (set and total)
d. Exhaled Tidal Volume
e. PEEP
f. P mean
g. Inspiratory Time
h. I:E Ratio
i. Exhaled Minute Ventilation
j. Peak Pressure

Increase the compliance by either increasing it to 0.002 L/cm H_2O on the Michigan Instruments TTL Adult/Infant Test Lung (Model 560li) or by turning the center stopcock on the IngMar Medical Neonatal Demonstration Lung Model so that both lungs are being ventilated.

1. Record the following parameters:
   a. Mode
   b. FIO_2
   c. Respiratory Rate (set and total)
   d. Exhaled Tidal Volume
   e. PEEP
   f. P mean
   g. Inspiratory Time (measure with a sweep second hand)
   h. I:E Ratio
   i. Exhaled Minute Ventilation
   j. Peak Pressure

Questions

A. What happened to the peak pressures?
B. Did the tidal volume change? Why or why not?

Touch the "Alarm Profile" button in the upper right-hand corner of the screen. Select the "Pressure" alarm, reduce it to 20 cm H_2O, and touch "Accept."

Questions:

A. What alarm message was displayed?
B. What is the purpose of the high pressure alarm in PRVC?
C. In what types of situations might a mode such as PRVC be useful?

ADJUSTING SETTINGS BASED ON CLINICAL DATA

To begin this section, follow the steps outlined next.

Press the "Mode" button in the upper left-hand corner of the screen (next to the pink baby symbol). The "Set Ventilation Mode" dialog box will appear. Press "Pressure Regulated Volume Control" in this dialog box and another menu titled "Select Ventilation Mode" will appear.

Touch "Volume Control" and make the following adjustments:

a. Tidal Volume	25 mL
b. Respiratory Rate	20 breaths/min
c. PEEP	5 cm H_2O
d. O_2 Concentration	75%
e. I-Time	0.35 second
f. Pause Time (T pause)	0.0 second
g. T insp. rise	0.15 second
h. Trigger Flow	3

Settings can be adjusted by touching the desired parameter, rotating the "Main Rotary Dial," and then either touching the parameter again or clicking the "Main Rotary Dial." Once you have completed inputting the initial parameters, touch "Accept."

You will notice that the ventilator will display a message entitled "Compliance Compensation" that states, "Check that no changes have been made to the patient circuit that can affect the compliance compensation." Touch "OK" and then touch "Accept" again to begin volume control ventilation.

When completing these activities, manipulate only one control at a time and note the result of each activity with manipulation of the controls. Answer the questions that follow each of the activities.

ALARM SETTING

Once the ventilator has begun to cycle, press the "Alarm Profile" key located on the upper right-hand corner of the User Interface screen. Please set the alarms to the following parameters. Touch the desired parameter, rotate the "Main Rotary Dial" to adjust the parameter, and either touch the parameter again or click the "Main Rotary Dial" to confirm your selection. When you are finished, touch "Accept."

High Airway Pressures	45 cm H_2O
Expiratory Minute Volume (lower alarm limit)	0.5 L/min
Expiratory Minute Volume (upper alarm limit)	4 L/min
Respiratory Frequency (lower alarm limit)	15
Respiratory Frequency (upper alarm limit)	45
End-Expiratory Pressure (lower alarm limit)	2 cm H_2O
End-Expiratory Pressure (upper alarm limit)	8 cm H_2O

You are working in a NICU and are taking care of a patient who is being ventilated with the preceding settings. You are making rounds and stop to do an assessment of the patient and record the current ventilator settings.

1. Record the following parameters:
   a. Mode
   b. FIO_2
   c. Respiratory Rate (set and total)
   d. Exhaled Tidal Volume
   e. Spontaneous Exhaled Tidal Volume
   f. PEEP
   g. Pmean
   h. Inspiratory Time
   i. I:E ratio
   j. Exhaled Minute Ventilation
   k. Peak Pressure

The neonatologist working today would like for you to draw a blood gas. You do so and present them with the following results:

pH	7.21
$PaCO_2$	56 mm Hg
PaO_2	215 mm Hg
HCO_3	20 mEq/L
SaO_2	100%

Questions

A. What is your interpretation of the blood gas?
B. What changes to the ventilator (if any) are indicated and why?
C. If changes are indicated, please adjust the ventilator accordingly and adjust all alarms appropriately. When done, please record the following:
   a. Mode
   b. FIO_2
   c. Respiratory Rate (set and total)
   d. Exhaled Tidal Volume
   e. Spontaneous Exhaled Tidal Volume
   f. PEEP
   g. P mean
   h. Inspiratory Time
   i. I:E Ratio
   j. Exhaled Minute Ventilation
   k. Peak Pressure

Neonatal Practice Activities: Dräger Babylog 8000 *plus*

CIRCUIT ASSEMBLY

Figure 29-18 shows the Dräger Babylog 8000 *plus* assembled and ready for use with a neonatal patient. This figure also shows the Babylog equipped with the optional graphics display screen. To prepare the ventilator for use, follow the steps listed next.

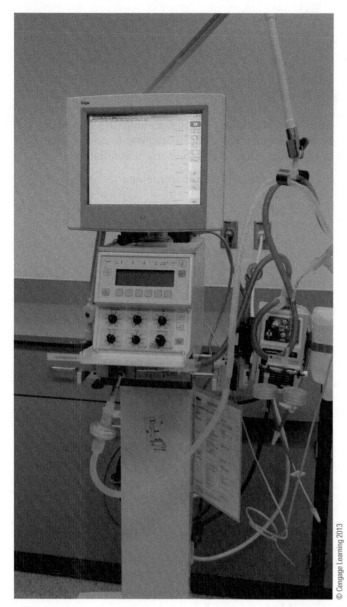

Figure 29-18 The Dräger Babylog 8000 *plus* assembled and ready for use

1. Connect a standard neonatal ventilator circuit to the ventilator by attaching a 12- to 18-inch length of neonatal ventilator tubing between the patient outlet and the ventilator's humidifier inlet.
2. Connect the inspiratory limb of the neonatal circuit to the humidifier outlet.
3. Connect the expiratory limb of the neonatal circuit to the nozzle located on the expiratory valve assembly.
4. Attach the patient circuit to the flex arm at its midpoint by clamping the ball fitting on the circuit holder to the flex arm.
5. The Dräger Babylog uses a proximal flow sensor of the "hot wire anemometer" variety (Figure 29-19). This flow sensor should be installed at the patient wye. The flow sensor cable should be carefully plugged into the flow sensor. The cable plugs into the back of the ventilator at the port labeled "flow."

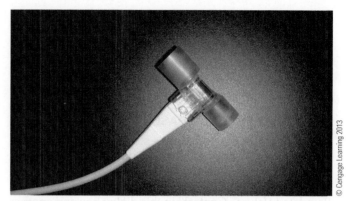

Figure 29-19 The Dräger Babylog 8000 *plus* hot wire anemometer

6. Connect the power cords from the ventilator and graphics display unit (if so equipped) to standard, grounded power outlets.
7. Screw the high-pressure air and oxygen hoses into their respective sockets located on the back of the ventilator.
8. Connect the air and oxygen hoses to their appropriate 50 psi receptacles.
9. The ventilator is now ready for use.

USING THE CONTROLS ON THE DRÄGER BABYLOG 8000 *PLUS*

All functions of the Dräger Babylog 8000 *plus* ventilator are controlled by an assortment of keys and dials. The front of the ventilator is divided into two areas: an upper "Display/Menu Key Panel" and a lower "Dial Panel" (that can be covered by a drop-down door). If equipped, the ventilator may also have a separate graphics display mounted on top of the ventilator. This unit uses a software package called "Vent View" to communicate with the ventilator and display both graphical and numeric data. It is important to note that this screen only displays data and is not used to adjust settings on the ventilator itself. Figure 29-20 shows the user interface for the Dräger Babylog 8000 *plus*.

Adjusting ventilator and alarm settings is accomplished in two distinct ways. Pressing the hard keys on the upper "Display/Menu Key Panel" allows the practitioner to adjust a variety of parameters. In addition, certain ventilator settings may be adjusted directly with the rotary dials located on the "Dial Panel."

TESTING THE VENTILATOR BEFORE USE

The exercises and steps outlined next were created using a Dräger Babylog 8000 *plus* running software version 5.01. Be sure to verify what software version the ventilator you are using is equipped with because some steps and/or options may not apply.

Each time the power switch is turned on, the ventilator runs a series of internal diagnostic tests. You should notice that the ventilator will display the words "Self Test," the light-emitting diodes (LEDs) will light up, and a tone will be heard. Once the diagnostic test is finished, the software version is displayed on the screen.

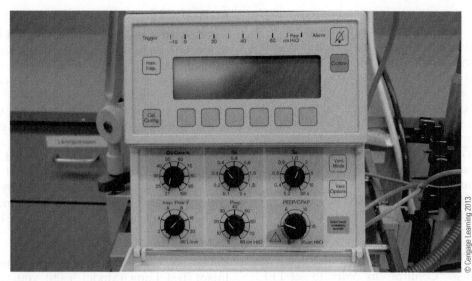

Figure 29-20   The Dräger Babylog 8000 *plus* user interface

© Cengage Learning 2013

1. Once the circuit and flow sensor are installed, attach the flow sensor located at the patient wye to a neonatal test lung.
2. Locate the power switch on the back of the ventilator. Turn the ventilator on. Also, if equipped, locate the power switch for the graphics display screen and turn it on. When prompted by the graphics display system regarding whether or not you want to "attach data to C:\WINNT\Temp\ven26.tmp," select "Yes."
3. After the self test is complete, note the message "Calibrate Flow Sensor!" on the ventilator screen.
4. Press the "Confirm" key located on the right side of the ventilator "Display/Menu Key Panel."

FLOW SENSOR CONFIGURATION/CALIBRATION

1. Press the "Cal Config" button on the lower left-hand corner of the "Display/Menu Key Panel."
2. Press the key located beneath the word "Sensor."
3. Press the up and down arrows to select "Flow Sensor."
4. Press the "+" or "−" key to select "ISO."
5. Press the up and down arrows to select "Measurement."
6. Press the "+" or "−" keys to select "BTPS."
7. Press the "Return" (◄———┐) key to return to the monitoring screen.
8. Press the "Cal Config" button on the lower left-hand corner of the "Display/Menu Key Panel."
9. Press the key below the words "V-Cal."
10. Disconnect the test lung and occlude the patient outlet.
11. Press the key below the word "Start."
12. When you see the words "Flow Sensor Calibrated," reconnect the sensor to the test lung.

LEAK TEST

1. Press the "Vent Mode" key located beneath the cover on the ventilator "Dial Panel."

2. Press the key located below the mode "CPAP" on the "Display/Menu Key Panel."
3. Press the key located below the word "On" on the "Display/Menu Key Panel."
4. Rotate the "Pinsp" dial knob to 80.
   a. Observe the message "Pinsp > 40 cm H₂O?"
5. Press "Confirm." Rotate the "Insp Flow" dial knob to 2.
6. Block the patient wye.
7. Press the "man Insp" key located on the left side of the "Display/Menu Key Panel" and note that the LED pressure bar graph achieves a pressure of 80 cm H₂O (±2 cm H₂O).
8. Reconnect the test lung to the patient wye and press "Return."

AIRWAY PRESSURE

1. Press the "Alarm Limit" key (▼/▲).
2. Press the up and down arrow keys to select the "Low MV" alarm limit and set it to 0 L/min using the minus "−" key.
3. Press the up and down arrow keys to select the "Upper MV" alarms limit and set it to 15 L/min using the plus "+" key.
4. Using the up and down arrow keys, select "Alarm Delay" and set at 10 seconds using the plus and minus keys.
5. Using the up and down arrow keys, select "Apnea Time" and set for 15 seconds using the plus and minus keys.
6. Using the up and down arrow keys, select "Tachypnea" and set for 100 breaths per minute using the plus and minus keys.
7. Press the "Vent Mode" key located on the ventilator "Dial Panel."
8. Press "CMV."
9. Press "On."
10. Press "Return."

11. Press "List."
12. Press "Set 1."
13. Using the dial knobs to adjust and screen to fine-tune, set the following parameters:
    a. P insp. = 20 cm H_2O
    b. Insp. Flow = 10 L/min
    c. Tin = 0.4 second
    d. Tex = 0.6 second
    e. PEEP = 0 cm H_2O (you will need to pull the PEEP knob out in order to set it below 3 cm H_2O)
    f. Press "Meas 1" and observe the following:
       i. PIP should be 20 cm H_2O ±4 cm H_2O (the bar graph should also display this).
       ii. PEEP should be 0 cm H_2O ±2 cm H_2O (the bar graph should reflect this as well).
    g. Press "Set 1."
    h. Set PEEP to 10 cm H_2O using the dial (you will need to press "Confirm" in order to set PEEP above 8 cm H_2O).
    i. Press "Meas 1" and then observe that the bar graph and the display reflect a PEEP of 10 cm H_2O ±2 cm H_2O.

APNEA MONITORING

1. Press the "Vent Mode" key.
2. Press "CPAP."
3. Press "On."
4. Do NOT breathe the test lung.
5. Observe "Apnea" on the display screen and an audible alarm.

MINUTE VOLUME MONITORING

1. Press "Vent Mode."
2. Press "CMV."
3. Press "On."
4. Press "Return."
5. Press the "Alarm" key.
6. Press the up and down arrow keys to select the "Low MV" alarm limit and set it to 1 L/min using the plus "+" key.
7. Notice the message "MV low" on the display screen as well as the audible alarm.
8. Return the "low MV" alarm limit to 0 L/min.
9. Press "Return."

AIRWAY PRESSURE MONITORING

1. Kink the expiratory limb of the patient circuit.
2. Observe that the alarm messages "Airway Pressure High, Inspiration Canceled" or "Hose Kinked?" are displayed as well as an audible tone.
3. Ventilation will stop momentarily (5 seconds) and then resume.
4. Disconnect the test lung from the circuit.
5. Observe that the alarm messages "Airway Pressure Low" or "Leak in Hose System, Check Setting" are displayed as well as an audible tone.
6. Set the PEEP level back to 0 using the PEEP dial and reconnect the test lung.

ACTIVITIES

To complete these practice activities, it is recommended that you use a lung analog/simulator such as a Michigan Instruments TTL Adult/Infant Test Lung (Model 560li) or an IngMar Medical Neonatal Demonstration Lung Model (see Figures 29-9 and 29-10). These devices or other similar devices allow the operator to alter resistance and compliance, simulating changes in patient condition.

If these devices are not available, a simple, single-bellows neonatal test lung may be used. Exercise caution as volumes and pressures may exceed the limits of the test lungs. Resistance may be altered by adapting different sizes of ET tubes, and compliance may be altered by the addition of rubber bands to the test lungs.

LUNG SIMULATOR SETUP

If you are using a Michigan Instruments TTL Adult/Infant Test Lung (Model 560li) you will be using the "Infant" side of the test lung. Using the connecting tubing provided with the test lung, connect the lung inlet to the back end of the "Rest Assembly." Connect the Pneuflo Rp 200 resistance adapter to the front end of the "Rest Assembly." Connect the pressure pickoff adapter to the Pneuflo Rp 200 resistance adapter. Connect the pressure line from the pickoff adapter to the proximal pressure input. Connect the patient wye to the pressure pickoff adapter. Set the compliance spring to 0.001 L/cm H_2O. Adjust the corresponding slider located near the top of the lung to the 0.001 L/cm H_2O setting as well.

If you are using an IngMar Medical Neonatal Demonstration Lung Model, rotate the outer 3-way stopcocks so that there are no leaks present (off to the leak adapters). Ensure that the inner 3-way stopcock is set to allow ventilation of only one lung. Do not use the brackets. Use the 2.5 mm ETT adapter. Attach the patient wye to the fortlite of the ETT.

When completing these activities, manipulate only one control at a time and note the result of each activity with manipulation of the controls. Answer the questions that follow each of the activities.

MODE SELECTION

Once the ventilator has begun cycling you may press the "Vent Mode" key located to the right of the dials on the lower "Dial Panel." By pressing the "Mode" button you are presented with the list of available modes for the neonatal patient. In addition to these modes there are also two "mode extensions" available for use on the Dräger Babylog 8000 *plus*. These modes and mode extensions are listed in Table 29-33.

The mode extension VIVE can be activated in any of the modes on the Babylog. It allows the practitioner to separately "fine-tune" the inspiratory and expiratory flows. Volume guarantee can be used with A/C, SIMV, and PSV. It allows the ventilator to monitor changes in a patient's compliance and/or resistance and adjust the ventilating pressures in order to deliver a target tidal volume to the patient at the lowest possible pressure.

Tables 29-34 through 29-38 summarize the settings available for each mode.

TABLE 29-33: Dräger Babylog 8000 *plus* Neonatal Ventilator Modes

Continuous mandatory ventilation (CMV)

Continuous positive airway pressure (CPAP)

Assist-control ventilation (A/C)

Synchronized intermittent mandatory ventilation (SIMV)

Pressure support ventilation (PSV)

Mode Extensions

Volume guarantee (VG)

Variable inspiratory and variable expiratory (VIVE) flow

TABLE 29-34: Dräger Babylog 8000 *plus* Continuous Mandatory Ventilation (CMV)

PARAMETER	RANGE
O_2 Concentration (%)	21–100%
Inspiratory time (Tin) (seconds)	0.1–2 seconds
Expiratory time (Tex) (seconds)	0.2–30 seconds
Inspiratory Flow (L/min)	1–30 L/min
Inspiratory Pressure (Pinsp) (cm H_2O)	5–80 cm H_2O
PEEP (cm H_2O)	0–25 cm H_2O
Trigger Sensitivity	1–10 (the lower the number, the more sensitive the ventilator is to the patient's inspiratory efforts)

TABLE 29-35: Dräger Babylog 8000 *plus* Continuous Positive Airway Pressure (CPAP)

PARAMETER	RANGE
O_2 Concentration (%)	21–100%
Inspiratory Flow (L/min)	1–30 L/min
Inspiratory Pressure (Pinsp) (cm H_2O)	5–80 cm H_2O
PEEP (cm H_2O)	0–25 cm H_2O

TABLE 29-36: Dräger Babylog 8000 *plus* Assist Control (A/C)

PARAMETER	RANGE
O_2 Concentration (%)	21–100%
Inspiratory time (Tin) (seconds)	0.1–2 seconds
Expiratory time (Tex) (seconds)	0.2–30 seconds
Inspiratory Flow (L/min)	1–30 L/min
Inspiratory Pressure (Pinsp) (cm H_2O)	5–80 cm H_2O
PEEP (cm H_2O)	0–25 cm H_2O
Trigger Sensitivity	1–10 (the lower the number, the more sensitive the ventilator is to the patient's inspiratory efforts)

TABLE 29-37: Dräger Babylog 8000 *plus* Synchronized Intermittent Mandatory Ventilation (SIMV)

PARAMETER	RANGE
O_2 Concentration (%)	21–100%
Inspiratory time (Tin) (seconds)	0.1–2 seconds
Expiratory time (Tex) (seconds)	0.2–30 seconds
Inspiratory Flow (L/min)	1–30 L/min
Inspiratory Pressure (Pinsp) (cm H_2O)	5–80 cm H_2O
PEEP (cm H_2O)	0–25 cm H_2O
Trigger Sensitivity	1–10 (the lower the number, the more sensitive the ventilator is to the patient's inspiratory efforts)

Exercises:

To begin, follow these steps:

1. Press "Vent Mode."

2. Press "A/C."

3. Using the "−" and "+" keys, adjust the trigger to 1.6.

4. Press "On."

5. Press the "Return" key.

6. Press "List."

7. Press "Set 1."

8. Input the following settings using the dials to adjust. The settings display can be used to "fine-tune" the parameters.
   a. O_2 Concentration   21%
   b. Inspiratory Flow   8 L/min
   c. Inspiratory Time   0.5 second
   d. Expiratory Time   1.5 seconds
   e. Inspiratory Pressure   25 cm H_2O
   f. PEEP   5 cm H_2O

TABLE 29-38: Dräger Babylog 8000 *plus* Pressure Support Ventilation (PSV)

PARAMETER	RANGE
O$_2$ Concentration (%)	21–100%
Inspiratory time (Tin) (seconds)	0.1–2 seconds
Expiratory time (Tex) (seconds)	0.2–30 seconds
Inspiratory Flow (L/min)	1–30 L/min
Inspiratory Pressure (Pinsp) (cm H$_2$O)	5–80 cm H$_2$O
PEEP (cm H$_2$O)	0–25 cm H$_2$O
Trigger Sensitivity	1–10 (the lower the number, the more sensitive the ventilator is to the patient's inspiratory efforts)

TABLE 29-39:

DRÄGER BABYLOG 8000 PLUS ALARMS	ALARM RANGE
High Minute Ventilation (L/min)	0–15 L/min
Low Minute Ventilation (L/min)	0–upper alarm limit
Alarm Delay (seconds)	0–30 seconds
Apnea Time (seconds)	5–20 seconds (above 20 seconds apnea time is turned off)
Tachypnea (breaths per minute)	20–200 breaths/min (below 20, tachypnea alarm is turned off)

Alarm Setting

Once the ventilator has begun to cycle, press the "Return" key. Then press the "Alarm Limits" key (▼/▲). This key brings up the "Alarm Limits" page, which presents the user with several adjustable alarms. In addition to the user adjustable alarms, several airway pressure alarms and oxygen concentration alarms are also monitored. These are set automatically by the ventilator and are not manually adjustable. One unique feature of the Dräger Babylog alarm limit page is the "+/− 30%" button located below the minute ventilation alarm limits. Pressing this button automatically adjusts the high and low minute ventilation alarms to 30% above and below the patient's current minute ventilation.

Table 29-39 lists the Dräger Babylog 8000 *plus* manually adjustable alarms and their respective ranges.

Please set the alarms to the following parameters. Use the up and down arrow keys to scroll through the manually adjustable alarm limits. Use the "+" and "−" keys to set the alarm limits accordingly.

High Minute Ventilation (L/min)	1 L/min
Low Minute Ventilation (L/min)	0.1 L/min
Alarm Delay (seconds)	10 seconds
Apnea Time (seconds)	15 seconds
Tachypnea (breaths per minute)	60 breaths/min

PATIENT MONITORING

The screen on the Dräger Babylog 8000 *plus* allows for the monitoring of both set and measured values. Navigating the screen to access different values is accomplished by pressing the hard keys located at the bottom of the screen. The main screen will display one of two scalar graphics chosen by the practitioner. To choose the scalar that is displayed, press the key labeled "Graph" on the far left of the screen. This brings up three options: "Paw" (airway pressure), "Flow," and a button to "freeze" a particular scalar. Select "Paw" and then press the "Return" key on the far right of the screen.

To the right of the scalar is a small box that displays patient data. The data displayed here can be selected by the practitioner by pressing the "Meas" key located just to the right of the "Graph" key. By pressing the "Meas" key the practitioner is presented with four options: "Vol" (volume), "Paw" (airway pressure), "RC" (resistance and compliance data), and "MVO$_2$P" (minute ventilation, FIO$_2$, and, mean airway pressure). Each of these buttons changes the data displayed to the right of the scalar on the main page. "Vol" brings up data including current minute ventilation and tidal volume. "Paw" brings up the patient's current peak airway pressure, PEEP level, and mean airway pressure. "RC" brings up data including resistance, compliance, and the calculated time constant of the lung. "MVO$_2$P" brings up the current minute ventilation, the current FIO$_2$, and the current mean airway pressure. Select "Paw" and then press the "Return" key on the far right of the screen.

To the right of the "Meas" key is a key labeled "List." Pressing this key presents the practitioner with four choices: two screens of ventilator settings labeled "Set1" and "Set2" and two screens of measurements labeled "Meas1" and "Meas2." Press each key and make note of what is found under each area. Then press the "Return" key on the far right of the screen to return to the main display screen.

To the right of the "List" key is a key labeled "Trend." Pressing this key brings up a menu that displays stored trends by the ventilator. Trends stored include FIO$_2$, mean airway pressure (Mean), minute ventilation (Ve), dynamic compliance (C), resistance (R), and Rate Volume Ratio (RVR) (similar to the rapid-shallow-breathing index). To select the trend you wish to view, press the key in the center of the screen labeled "Param." Each time this key is pressed the displayed trend changes. There are four other keys on this screen. The two keys located on the left-hand side depicting arrows moving toward a rectangle and arrows moving away from a rectangle are used to adjust the amount of time that is displayed on the screen. This is adjustable from 2 to 24 hours. The other two keys, a right and a left arrow, are used to move through the displayed trend. Select "Mean" on this screen and then press the "Return" key to return to the main display screen.

To the right of the "Trend" key is a button with an up and down arrow on it. This is the key you have already used to access the alarm limits page.

The final key located along the bottom of the display screen shows a letter "i" on a piece of paper. Pressing this key brings up a logbook of alarms and messages that have been displayed by the ventilator. Press the "Return" key to return to the main display page.

The Dräger Babylog 8000 *plus* can be equipped with a separate graphics display screen that is capable of displaying loops, scalars, trends, settings, and patient data. It is important to note that this screen only displays data and is not used to adjust settings on the ventilator itself.

Below the "Display/Menu Key Panel," located underneath the drop down door is the "Dial Panel." There are two keys on the "Dial Panel" that control a few additional settings. The first key is labeled "Vent Mode." Pressing this key brings up the available modes of ventilation on the Dräger Babylog 8000 *plus*. The key located directly below the "Vent Mode" key is labeled "Vent Options." Pressing this key brings up the two "mode extensions" available on the ventilator (VIVE and VG) as well as a "−" and "+" key that is used for setting the trigger sensitivity.

INSPIRATORY TIME CONTROL

From the initial settings you have previously set, note the following ventilatory (patient) parameters before you make the next changes. (Instructors may want to consider providing a ventilator flow sheet for the students to use in order to record parameters.)

1. Mode
2. FIO$_2$
3. Respiratory Rate
4. Inspiratory Time
5. Expiratory Time
6. I:E Ratio
7. Exhaled Tidal Volume
8. Exhaled Minute Ventilation
9. PEEP
10. P mean
11. Peak Pressure

1. Set the inspiratory time to 0.30 second. Record the following parameters:
   a. Mode
   b. FIO$_2$
   c. Respiratory Rate
   d. Inspiratory Time
   e. Expiratory Time
   f. I:E Ratio
   g. Exhaled Tidal Volume
   h. Exhaled Minute Ventilation
   i. PEEP
   j. P mean
   k. Peak Pressure

2. Set the inspiratory time control to 1 second. Record the following parameters:
   a. Mode
   b. FIO$_2$
   c. Respiratory Rate
   d. Inspiratory Time
   e. Expiratory Time
   f. I:E Ratio
   g. Exhaled Tidal Volume
   h. Exhaled Minute Ventilation
   i. PEEP
   j. P mean
   k. Peak Pressure

Questions:

A. How was the respiratory rate affected by changes in the inspiratory time?
B. How were the peak pressures affected by the changes in the inspiratory time?
C. How was the tidal volume affected by the changes in the inspiratory time?
D. How was the I:E ratio affected by the changes in the inspiratory time?
E. How was the mean airway pressure affected by the changes in the inspiratory time?

INSPIRATORY PRESSURE CONTROL

Return the controls to the following settings:
   a. O$_2$ Concentration   21%
   b. Inspiratory Flow   8 L/min
   c. Inspiratory Time   0.5 second
   d. Expiratory Time   1.5 seconds
   e. Inspiratory Pressure   25 cm H$_2$O
   f. PEEP   5 cm H$_2$O

Once these settings have been established, record the following ventilatory (patient) parameters:
   a. Mode
   b. FIO$_2$
   c. Respiratory Rate
   d. Inspiratory Time
   e. Expiratory Time
   f. I:E Ratio
   g. Exhaled Tidal Volume
   h. Exhaled Minute Ventilation
   i. PEEP
   j. P mean
   k. Peak Pressure

Adjust the alarms to the following parameters:
High Minute Ventilation (L/min)   1 L/min
Low Minute Ventilation (L/min)   0.1 L/min
Alarm Delay (seconds)   10 seconds
Apnea Time (seconds)   15 seconds
Tachypnea (breaths per minute)   60 breaths/min
Adjust the inspiratory pressure to 40 cm H$_2$O.

1. Record the following parameters:
   a. Mode
   b. FIO$_2$
   c. Respiratory Rate
   d. Inspiratory Time

e. Expiratory Time
f. I:E Ratio
g. Exhaled Tidal Volume
h. Exhaled Minute Ventilation
i. PEEP
j. P mean
k. Peak Pressure

Adjust the inspiratory pressure control to 10 cm H_2O and the PEEP to 3 cm H_2O.

Adjust the alarms to the following parameters:

High Minute Ventilation (L/min)	1 L/min
Low Minute Ventilation (L/min)	0.05 L/min
Alarm Delay (seconds)	10 seconds
Apnea Time (seconds)	15 seconds
Tachypnea (breaths per minute)	60 breaths/min

2. Record the following parameters:
   a. Mode
   b. FIO_2
   c. Respiratory Rate
   d. Inspiratory Time
   e. Expiratory Time
   f. I:E Ratio
   g. Exhaled Tidal Volume
   h. Exhaled Minute Ventilation
   i. PEEP
   j. P mean
   k. Peak Pressure

Questions

A. What effect does the inspiratory pressure control have on the delivered tidal volume?
B. What effect does the inspiratory pressure control have on the delivered minute ventilation?

FLOW RATE

Adjust the controls to the following settings:

a. O_2 Concentration	21%
b. Inspiratory Flow	8 L/min
c. Inspiratory Time	0.5 second
d. Expiratory Time	1.5 seconds
e. Inspiratory Pressure	25 cm H_2O
f. PEEP	5 cm H_2O
g. Trigger	2.2

Adjust the alarms to the following parameters:

High Minute Ventilation (L/min)	1 L/min
Low Minute Ventilation (L/min)	0.1 L/min
Alarm Delay (seconds)	10 seconds
Apnea Time (seconds)	15 seconds
Tachypnea (breaths per minute)	60 breaths/min

1. Record the following parameters:
   a. Mode
   b. FIO_2
   c. Respiratory Rate
   d. Inspiratory Time
   e. Expiratory Time
   f. I:E Ratio
   g. Exhaled Tidal Volume
   h. Exhaled Minute Ventilation
   i. PEEP

j. P mean
k. Peak Pressure

Increase the inspiratory flow to 12 L/min.

2. Record the following parameters:
   a. Mode
   b. FIO_2
   c. Respiratory Rate
   d. Inspiratory Time
   e. Expiratory Time
   f. I:E Ratio
   g. Exhaled Tidal Volume
   h. Exhaled Minute Ventilation
   i. PEEP
   j. P mean
   k. Peak Pressure

Increase the peak flow to 20 L/min.

3. Listen carefully to the exhalation port and then record the following parameters:
   a. Mode
   b. FIO_2
   c. Respiratory Rate
   d. Inspiratory Time
   e. Expiratory Time
   f. I:E Ratio
   g. Exhaled Tidal Volume
   h. Exhaled Minute Ventilation
   i. PEEP
   j. P mean
   k. Peak Pressure

Questions

A. How did the increase in peak flow from 8 to 12 L/min affect the delivered tidal volume?
B. How did the increase in peak flow from 12 to 20 L/min affect the delivered tidal volume?
C. What did you notice as you listened to the exhalation valve when the peak flow was set at 20 L/min?
D. What was happening?

CHANGES IN COMPLIANCE

Adjust the ventilator to the following settings:

a. Mode	A/C
b. O_2 Concentration	21%
c. Inspiratory Flow	9 L/min
d. Inspiratory Time	0.4 second
e. Expiratory Time	1.6 seconds
f. Inspiratory Pressure	30 cm H_2O
g. PEEP	4 cm H_2O
h. Trigger	1.6

Adjust the alarms to the following parameters:

High Minute Ventilation (L/min)	1 L/min
Low Minute Ventilation (L/min)	0.1 L/min
Alarm Delay (seconds)	10 seconds
Apnea Time (seconds)	15 seconds
Tachypnea (breaths per minute)	60 breaths/min

1. Record the following parameters:
   a. Mode
   b. FIO_2

c. Respiratory Rate
d. Inspiratory Time
e. Expiratory Time
f. I:E Ratio
g. Exhaled Tidal Volume
h. Exhaled Minute Ventilation
i. PEEP
j. P mean
k. Peak Pressure

Increase the compliance by either increasing it to 0.002 L/cm H_2O on the Michigan Instruments TTL Adult/Infant Test Lung (Model 560li) or by rotating the center stopcock so that both lungs are being ventilated.

2. Record the following parameters:
   a. Mode
   b. FIO$_2$
   c. Respiratory Rate
   d. Inspiratory Time
   e. Expiratory Time
   f. I:E Ratio
   g. Exhaled Tidal Volume
   h. Exhaled Minute Ventilation
   i. PEEP
   j. P mean
   k. Peak Pressure

Questions

A. What happened to the peak pressures when the lung compliance increased?
B. What happened to the mean airway pressures when the lung compliance increased?
C. What happened to the tidal volume when the lung compliance increased?
D. What therapeutic intervention in a NICU might cause a dramatic increase in compliance?
E. What are the risks associated with a dramatic increase in compliance when a patient is being ventilated in a pressure-oriented mode?

Return the compliance to the previous setting by either decreasing it to 0.001 L/cm H_2O on the Michigan Instruments TTL Adult/Infant Test Lung (Model 560li) or by rotating the center stopcock so that only one lung is being ventilated.

VOLUME GUARANTEE

Adjust the ventilator to the following settings:

a. Mode	A/C
b. O$_2$ Concentration	21%
c. Inspiratory Flow	9 L/min
d. Inspiratory Time	0.4 second
e. Expiratory Time	1.6 seconds
f. Inspiratory Pressure	30 cm H_2O
g. PEEP	4 cm H_2O
h. Trigger	1.6

Adjust the alarms to the following parameters:

High Minute Ventilation (L/min)	1 L/min
Low Minute Ventilation (L/min)	0.1 L/min
Alarm Delay (seconds)	10 seconds
Apnea Time (seconds)	15 seconds
Tachypnea (breaths per minute)	60 breaths/min

1. Record the following parameters:
   a. Mode
   b. FIO$_2$
   c. Respiratory Rate
   d. Inspiratory Time
   e. Expiratory Time
   f. I:E Ratio
   g. Exhaled Tidal Volume
   h. Exhaled Minute Ventilation
   i. PEEP
   j. P mean
   k. Peak Pressure

Touch "Vent Options."
Touch "VG."
Using the "−" and "+" keys adjust the "Vt set" to 8 mL.
Touch "On."
Press "Return."

2. Record the following parameters:
   a. Mode
   b. FIO$_2$
   c. Respiratory Rate
   d. Inspiratory Time
   e. Expiratory Time
   f. I:E Ratio
   g. Exhaled Tidal Volume
   h. Exhaled Minute Ventilation
   i. PEEP
   j. P mean
   k. Peak Pressure

Questions

A. What happened to the peak pressures once volume guarantee was activated?
B. What happened to the respiratory rate once volume guarantee was activated?
C. What happened to the mean airway pressure once volume guarantee was activated?
D. What happened to the tidal volume once volume guarantee was activated?

CHANGES IN COMPLIANCE WITH VOLUME GUARANTEE

Increase the compliance by either increasing it to 0.002 L/cm H_2O on the Michigan Instruments TTL Adult/Infant Test Lung (Model 560li) or by rotating the center stopcock so that both lungs are being ventilated.

1. Record the following parameters:
   a. Mode
   b. FIO$_2$
   c. Respiratory Rate
   d. Inspiratory Time
   e. Expiratory Time
   f. I:E Ratio
   g. Exhaled Tidal Volume
   h. Exhaled Minute Ventilation
   i. PEEP
   j. P mean
   k. Peak Pressure

Questions

A. What happened to the peak pressures when the lung compliance increased?

B. What happened to the mean airway pressures when the lung compliance increased?

C. What happened to the tidal volume when the lung compliance increased?

D. How did this situation differ from the situation when the compliance increased and volume guarantee was not activated?

Neonatal Practice Activities: Arabella Nasal CPAP System

CIRCUIT ASSEMBLY

Figure 29-21 shows the Arabella Nasal CPAP system assembled and ready for use with a neonatal patient. To prepare the Arabella for use, follow the steps listed next.

1. Connect the short (30 cm) delivery circuit tube between the patient outlet on the bottom of the monitoring gas mixer and the system's humidifier inlet.
2. Connect the long, heated wire delivery tubing to the humidifier outlet, plug in the proximal temperature probe, and connect the heated wire adapter cable.
3. Plug in the distal temperature probe into the port located 30 cm from the end of the heated wire delivery circuit.
4. Connect the proximal pressure measurement tube to the port on the bottom of the monitoring gas mixer.
5. Connect the other end of the proximal pressure measurement tube to the small inlet on the CPAP generator kit (CPAP interface).
6. Connect the end of the delivery circuit to the 10 mm male connection on the CPAP generator kit (CPAP interface).
7. Connect the power cords from the monitoring gas mixer and humidifier to standard, grounded power outlets.
8. Screw the high-pressure air and oxygen hoses into their respective sockets located on the back of the monitoring gas mixer.
9. Connect the air and oxygen hoses to their appropriate 50 psi receptacles.
10. Select either a nasal mask (Figure 29-22) or nasal prongs (Figure 29-23), and press them firmly into the universal generator on the end of the patient circuit.
11. The Arabella Nasal CPAP system is now ready for use.

USING THE CONTROLS ON THE ARABELLA NASAL CPAP SYSTEM

All functions of the Arabella Nasal CPAP system are controlled by two dials on the front of the monitoring gas mixer. These are shown in Figure 29-24. The Arabella Nasal CPAP system is a continuous flow generator equipped with an air-oxygen blender, a flowmeter, and pressure monitoring capabilities. The practitioner can

Figure 29-21 The Arabella Nasal CPAP system set up and ready for use

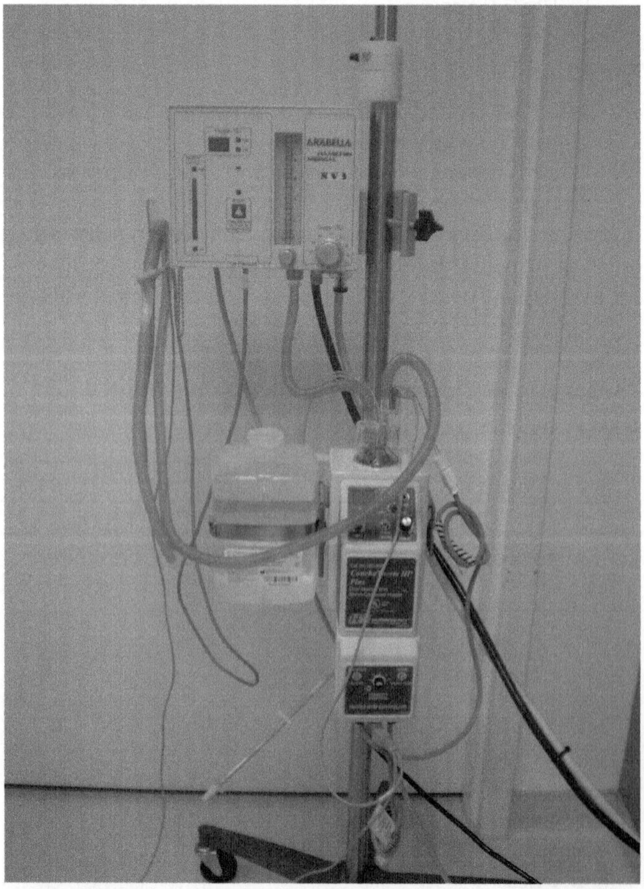

© Cengage Learning 2013

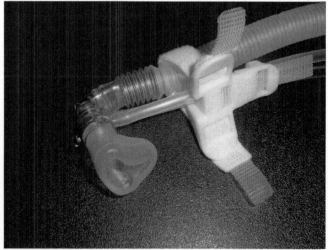

Figure 29-22 An Arabella nasal mask attached to the universal generator

© Cengage Learning 2013

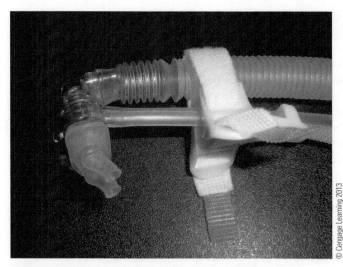

Figure 29-23 The Arabella nasal prongs attached to the universal generator

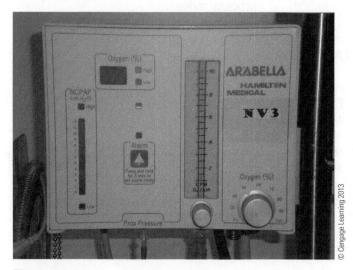

Figure 29-24 The Arabella Nasal CPAP system controls

adjust two parameters when operating the system: FIO₂ and flow. The system also incorporates some basic monitoring and alarm capabilities that can alert the practitioner to changes in FIO₂ and pressure.

CPAP is generated when the flow from the monitoring gas mixer is delivered to the "universal generator" located at the patient interface. The universal generator uses both the Bernoulli effect to generate CPAP pressure and the Venturi principle to augment flow in times of high inspiratory demand. Simply stated, the higher the flow delivered to the universal generator, the higher the CPAP pressure applied to the patient.

TESTING THE ARABELLA NASAL CPAP SYSTEM BEFORE USE

Before applying the Arabella Nasal CPAP system to a patient, the practitioner should perform the following pre-use tests.

Oxygen Analyzer Functional Test

1. Ensure that the monitoring gas mixer is connected to 50 psi air and oxygen sources.
2. Turn unit on.
3. Set the oxygen control dial to 21%.
   a. Observe that the displayed oxygen percentage reads 21% (±2%).
4. Set the oxygen control dial to 100%.
   a. Observe that the displayed oxygen percentage reads 100% (±2%).
5. Set the oxygen control dial to 50%.
   a. Observe that the displayed oxygen percentage reads 50% (±2%).

BLENDER ALARM FUNCTIONAL TEST

1. Start this test with both air and oxygen hoses disconnected.
2. Plug the power cord in and turn the monitoring gas mixer on.
3. Plug the high-pressure oxygen hose into a 50 psi oxygen outlet.
   a. Observe that the alarm sounds.
4. Plug the high-pressure air hose into a 50 psi air outlet.
   a. Observe that the alarm stops.
5. Disconnect the high-pressure oxygen hose from the 50 psi oxygen outlet.
   a. Observe that the alarm sounds.

PRESSURE FUNCTIONAL TEST

1. Plug in the high-pressure air and oxygen hoses into their respective 50 psi outlets.
2. Plug the monitoring gas mixer power cord into a standard, grounded power outlet.
3. Attach the Arabella delivery circuit with the universal generator and nasal prongs to the monitoring gas mixer.
4. Turn the monitoring gas mixer power on.
5. Adjust the flowmeter on the face of the monitoring gas mixer until it reads 8 L/min.
6. Pinch the nasal prongs to prevent flow from escaping.
7. Observe the LED pressure meter on the front of the monitoring gas mixer. Pressure should read approximately 5 cm H₂O.
8. Release the prongs and observe the pressure meter. The pressure should drop to zero.
9. Occlude the prongs again and increase the flow while observing the pressure meter.
10. Continue to increase the flow until the meter reads 11 cm H₂O.
11. At this point you should hear a "clicking" sound as the pressure relief valve opens, and the pressure on the meter should drop to zero. After 3 seconds the unit will attempt to re-establish pressure.
12. Release the prongs and verify that the pressure returns to zero.

ALARMS

The Arabella Nasal CPAP system monitors eight separate alarms continuously during use. Table 29-40 illustrates the alarms and their respective parameters.

TABLE 29-40: Arabella Nasal CPAP Alarms

ALARM	SET PARAMETERS	NOTES
Gas Supply	Alarm sounds when delivered gas pressure (air or oxygen) drops below 30 psi	Pneumatic alarm cannot be silenced until the reason for pressure drop is remedied.
Low Pressure	Set at 2 cm H_2O below the set pressure. Alarm will sound and the "low pressure" LED will illuminate if the pressure drops below this point and stays below this point for 15 seconds.	Can be silenced with alarm silence.
High Pressure	Set at 3 cm H_2O above the set pressure. Alarm will sound and the "high pressure" LED will illuminate if the pressure rises above this point and stays above this point for 15 seconds.	
Over Pressure Limit	Preset at 10 cm H_2O. Alarm will sound and the "high pressure" LED will illuminate immediately if the pressure exceeds 10 cm H_2O.	When this alarm is violated, gas flow is interrupted for 3 seconds and then the system will attempt to reestablish flow. If the reason for the alarm violation is still present, gas flow will stop again and the process repeats.
Oxygen Concentration Alarm	Set at 5% above and below the set FIO_2. Alarm sounds and the appropriate LED (high or low) will illuminate if the conditions are violated for greater than 15 seconds.	
Nominal Oxygen Alarm	Alarm sounds, both high and low oxygen LEDs illuminate, and the O_2 display reads "ERR" if the set oxygen value on the blender and the analyzed value displayed in the window vary by more than 10%.	
Low Hazard Alarm	Alarm sounds, "—" is shown in the O_2 display, and the "low O_2" LED illuminates if the measured oxygen concentration is less than 18%.	Alarm cannot be silenced; O_2 analyzer must be calibrated or the O_2 cell may need replacing.
Nominal Hazard Alarm	Shows "—" in the O_2 display, the high and low O_2 LEDs illuminate, and an audible tone is heard if there is no O_2 cell in the blender or if there has been a disconnection between the blender knob and the blender.	Alarm cannot be silenced; refer to biomedical engineering.

To set the alarms, first ensure that the Arabella CPAP system has been appropriately set to the desired parameters. Once the desired parameters are set and the device has been appropriately attached to the patient, press and hold the "Alarm Silence" button on the front of the monitoring gas mixer for 3 seconds. A series of beeps will be heard and the "Alarm Limits" will flash. Once this occurs, the alarms are set. It is important to note that any time the practitioner makes a change to the settings, the alarms must be reset in order to be responsive to the new parameters.

PATIENT INTERFACE

The patient interface of any nasal CPAP system is extremely important. Care must be taken to ensure proper fit regardless of what type of device is chosen. Nasal prongs that are too small may result in an inability to apply the required amount of CPAP to the patient's airway. A nasal mask that is applied too tightly may result in tissue breakdown. Patient interface devices will vary from institution to institution. It is ultimately the practitioners' responsibility to become familiar with the devices that are used at their place of employment.

Two styles of interface are common when employing nasal CPAP (NCPAP) to infants: the nasal mask and the nasal prongs. Both are available in several sizes (typically extra small, small, medium, and large) and usually contain sizing guidelines or tools to help the practitioner determine what size to use. Figure 29-25 illustrates one type of sizing guide. Once the correct size of device has been determined, an additional device must be selected to securely attach the device to the patient. Straps or knit caps with adjustable Velcro stays help to ensure that either device, be it a nasal mask or nasal prongs, stays in place comfortably and securely. Figure 29-26 shows a nasal mask with the Arabella universal generator and exhalation device

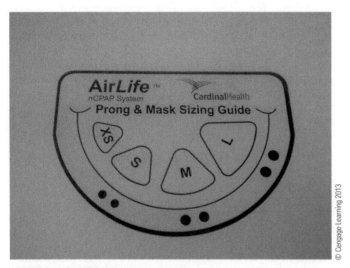

Figure 29-25 A nasal CPAP sizing guide

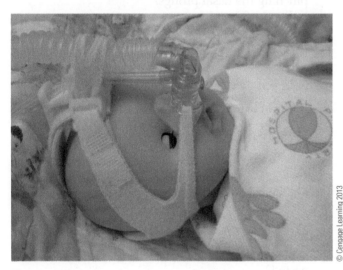

Figure 29-26 The Arabella nasal mask appropriately applied to a patient

properly secured with a strap-style fixation device. When securing the device to the patient, make sure that the straps are secure but not overly tight. Also, the exhalation tubing leading away from the universal generator and patient interface must be fully extended before the device is applied to the patient. This helps to reduce noise near the patient and also helps to vent expiratory gases away from the patient's face. To apply a device to a patient, follow these general steps:

1. Start by correctly assembling the patient circuit and connecting it to the monitoring gas mixer/humidifier as illustrated in the previous section.
2. Using a sizing guide, choose the proper size interface device (prongs or nasal mask).
3. Insert the interface device (prongs or nasal mask) firmly into the universal generator.
4. Fully extend the expiratory tubing.
5. Turn the Arabella system on, adjust the flow to 8 L/min, occlude the device, and ensure that the pressure reads 5 cm H_2O.

6. Before applying the device to the patient it may be helpful to apply the knit cap or strap system to the patient first.
7. Once the securing device is in place, gently apply the device to the patient.
8. Systematically (working on one side and then the other for each strap or tie) secure the interface. Refer to the manufacturer guidelines for the device you are using with regard to correct strap and tie placement.
9. Be certain to ensure that the device is securely attached and that the desired pressures are being achieved.
10. If you are unable to achieve the appropriate pressure, make sure that the correct size device is being employed first before electing to tighten any straps. Care must always be taken at all times to prevent excessive pressure to the nares, nasal septum, and face of the patient.

ACTIVITIES

To complete these exercises you may use an infant mannequin to practice the application of the patient interfaces. If the mannequin is equipped with a test lung that allows sufficient pressure to build up, the exercises may be done with the device applied to the mannequin. If the test lung does not allow sufficient pressure to be built, the exercises may be completed by having one student occlude the universal generator (by pinching off the nasal prongs) while the other student manipulates the controls on the Arabella.

Exercises

Patient Interface

1. Obtain a universal generator and nasal prongs or nasal mask.
2. Practice fitting the nasal prongs or mask onto the universal generator.
3. Using a mannequin and a Velcro fixation device (knit cap or strap system), practice applying the nasal mask or nasal prongs to the mannequin.

Questions

A. What circumstances might a nasal mask be preferred over nasal prongs?
B. What are the hazards associated with using a nasal mask?
C. What types of drawbacks are there to using nasal prongs?
D. What is the purpose of the exhalation tubing and why must it be completely extended during use?

CIRCUIT ASSEMBLY AND PRE-USE CHECK

1. Obtain and properly assemble the Arabella NCPAP delivery circuit.
2. Correctly hook up the Arabella Nasal CPAP system to the appropriate electric and gas sources.
3. Perform the pre-use checks described previously.

Question

A. What is the purpose of performing a pre-use check on this system or any other ventilator system?

DEVICE OPERATION

1. Once the device has been properly set up and applied to the mannequin, turn the device on and set the following parameters:
   NOTE: If a mannequin is used and pressure cannot be maintained, have your laboratory partner occlude the gas flow on the universal generator by pinching the nasal prongs.
   a. Flow = 8 L/min
   b. Oxygen percent = 40%

2. Press and hold the "Alarm Silence" key until a series of beeps is heard indicating that the alarms have been set.

3. Record the following parameters:
   a. Flow
   b. CPAP pressure
   c. Oxygen percentage

4. Increase the flow to 10 L/min.

5. Record the following parameters:
   a. Flow
   b. CPAP pressure
   c. Oxygen percentage

6. Decrease the flow to 4 L/min.

7. Record the following parameters:
   a. Flow
   b. CPAP pressure
   c. Oxygen percentage

Questions

A. What happened to the delivered pressure when the flow was increased?

B. What happened to the delivered pressure when the flow was decreased?

C. You are working as a practitioner in a NICU taking care of a neonate on NCPAP. The current settings are a CPAP of 4 cm H_2O and an FIO_2 of 28%. You note that the baby is still grunting despite the current therapy and note retractions as well. You are asked to check a blood gas and the following results are obtained:

pH	7.25
$PaCO_2$	63 mm Hg
PaO_2	56 mm Hg
HCO_3	22 mEq/L
BE	-3 mEq/L

What changes would you make and why?

ALARMS

1. Once the device has been properly set up and applied to the mannequin, turn the device on and set the following parameters:
   NOTE: If a mannequin is used and pressure cannot be maintained, have your laboratory partner occlude the gas flow on the universal generator by pinching the nasal prongs.
   a. Flow = 8 L/min
   b. Oxygen percent = 40%

2. Press and hold the "Alarm Silence" key until a series of beeps is heard indicating that the alarms have been set.

3. Record the following parameters:
   a. Flow
   b. CPAP pressure
   c. Oxygen percentage

4. Disconnect the CPAP interface from the mannequin (or have your laboratory partner release the nasal prongs).

Questions

A. What alarm sounded when the device was disconnected?

B. Name at least two clinical situations that might cause a low pressure alarm to be heard.

Practice Activities: Viasys Sensor Medics 3100A High-Frequency Oscillatory Ventilator

---

CIRCUIT ASSEMBLY

The following will be required to correctly set up the 3100A High Frequency Oscillatory Ventilation (HFOV):

1. An external air/oxygen blender

2. An external heated humidifier

3. The 3100A ventilator

4. The patient circuit

5. High-pressure hoses for both air and oxygen
   Complete the following steps (refer to Figure 29-27 when completing these steps):

1. Attach the bellows housing /water trap to the oscillator compartment by positioning it into place and locking it securely with the four "T" handle quarter turn fasteners.

2. Connect the large-diameter patient circuit to the outlet on the bellows housing and support the circuit using the patient circuit support arm.

3. Attach the three identical cap/diaphragm assemblies to the patient circuit by snapping them into place on the valve body seats on the patient circuit.

4. Connect the four color-coded lines between the patient circuit and the ventilator by following Table 29-41.

5. Attach the ⅛-inch clear pressure sensing line connected to the patient wye to the Luer-lok fitting labeled "Airway Pressure."

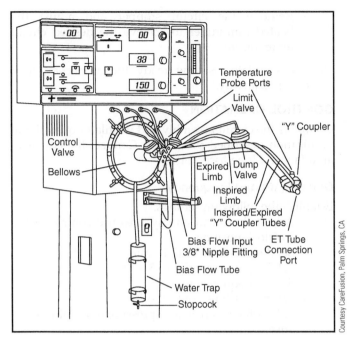

Figure 29-27 A schematic of the SensorMedics 3100A oscillator ventilator circuit assembly

Courtesy CareFusion, Palm Springs, CA

TABLE 29-41: Control Line Assembly

Color	Attachment Point
Blue	P_{AW} Limit Valve
Green	P_{AW} Control Valve
Red	Dump Valve

6. Connect the proximal airway temperature probe to the port located at the patient wye. If a plug blocks this port, remove it and place the proximal temperature probe into this port. If the circuit is used on a patient in an isolette, the temperature probe may be placed proximal to the clear bellows housing distal from the patient. Ensure that any open temperature port is blocked with the plug when not in use.

7. Adjust the patient circuit support arm such that the patient wye is elevated in relationship to the water trap. This will allow condensate to drain toward the water trap.

8. Connect the external blender outlet to the "Inlet from Blender" fitting on the left rear of the ventilator using a high-pressure hose and appropriate diameter-indexed safety system (DISS) fittings.

9. Connect the ⅜-inch bias flow line from the ⅜-inch barbed fitting labeled "Outlet to Humidifier" to the humidifier inlet.

10. Connect the outlet of the humidifier to the patient circuit using the ⅜-inch clear tubing to the bias flow inlet on the patient circuit. Only use the tubing supplied by

the manufacturer to make the connections between the 3100A HFOV and the humidifier.

11. Be certain that a separate high-pressure hose connects a 50 psi air source to the "Cooling Air" inlet on the rear of the ventilator. The 3100A HFOV magnet must be provided with this source of gas for cooling.

OPERATIONAL VERIFICATION TESTING BEFORE USE

Operational verification is important prior to performing the practice activities or prior to using any ventilator on a patient. The time to identify and troubleshoot problems is before the device is needed in a life support situation. It is important to identify and correct any problems prior to using the ventilator on a patient.

1. Ensure that the high-pressure hoses for air and oxygen are connected to the external blender and that a separate air line is connected to the "Cooling Air" inlet for the magnet.

2. Connect the electrical power cord to a suitable 120 volt 60 Hz alternating current (AC) power outlet. An uninterruptable power supply should be used for all critical care equipment. These outlets are indicated by having red receptacles.

3. Block the patient wye with the #1 cork supplied with the patient circuit.

4. Check that the stopcock on the water trap is closed and in the "Off" position. An open stopcock to the water trap will not allow sufficient pressure to build in the circuit to perform verification testing.

5. Turn on the electrical power by turning the AC power switch into the "On" position. The green LED on the "Start/Stop" push button should be off. If audible alarms can be heard, press the "45-second Silence" push-button control.

6. Complete the following steps to calibrate the patient circuit:
   – Set the bias flow to 20 L/min using the flowmeter on the right front of the ventilator.
   – Set both the mean pressure adjust and the mean pressure limit controls to the maximum setting (fully clockwise).
   – Press the "Reset" button while observing the mean pressure digital display. Normally, the low battery LED will illuminate when the "Reset" button is pressed.
   – Adjust the patient circuit calibration control on the right side panel of the ventilator to achieve a pressure of 39 to 43 cm H_2O. If you are unable to achieve this pressure, troubleshoot the circuits for leaks.

7. Perform the ventilator verification procedure ("Off Patient Only"). Instructions are printed on the top of the ventilator.
   – Set the frequency to 15, I-time to 33%, and power to 0.0.

- Set the bias flow to 30 L/min.
- Set the mean pressure control to 12 o'clock.
- Set the Max P_{AW} thumbwheel to 30 and the Min P_{AW} thumbwheel to 10.
- Press the "Reset" button long enough to build the P_{AW} to above 6 cm H_2O.
- Using the mean pressure adjust control, set the P_{AW} to between 29 and 31 cm H_2O.
- Press the "Start/Stop" button in the center portion of the control panel to initiate the oscillator.
- Center the magnet using the magnet centering control located on the pedestal just to the left and above the water trap.
- Once a stable ΔP is obtained with the piston centered, verify that the P_{AW} and ΔP are within range for your altitude based on the following table.

Altitude	P_{AW}	ΔP
0–2000 ft	26–34 cm H_2O	113–1355 cm H_2O
2000–4000 ft	26–34 cm H_2O	104–125 cm H_2O
4000–6000 ft	26–34 cm H_2O	95–115 cm H_2O
6000–8000 ft	26–34 cm H_2O	86–105 cm H_2O

- Press the "Start/Stop" button to stop the oscillator.
- Using the mean pressure adjust control or the bias flow, set the mean airway pressure to within ± 2 cm H_2O of the desired setting.
- Check to ensure that the Max Pressure and Min Pressure alarms are functioning by setting the Max Pressure thumbwheel to 2 cm H_2O below and that the Min Pressure thumbwheel is set to 2 cm H_2O above the set mean airway pressure.
- Once the Max and Min pressure alarms have been verified, set them to ±2 to 5 cm H_2O of the mean airway pressure setting.
- Using your fingers, compress the expiratory limb of the patient circuit, closing it off. Verify that the $P_{AW} > 50$ cm H_2O alarm sounds.
- Press the "Reset" button until the "$P_{AW} < 20\%$ of Set Max P_{AW}" LED is extinguished and mean airway pressure is reestablished.
- Set the mean pressure limit control to about midscale.
- Using your fingers, compress the expiratory limb of the circuit obstructing it. Observe the mean pressure display and the value that it becomes limited. Rotate the mean pressure limit control such that the ventilator pressure limits at the desired pressure.
- Move the ventilator, positioning it close to the patient and yet allowing for visualization of the control panel and alarms. Lock the control panel in the desired position using the lock on the rear of the ventilator. Lock the casters at the bottom of the ventilator to prevent it from being inadvertently moved.
- Set the desired FIO_2, mean airway pressure, and ΔP for the patient.

- Remove the circuit stopper and adjust the heated humidifier to achieve the desired circuit temperature.

8. The ventilator is now ready for connection to a patient's airway.

CONTROL OPERATION

Complete the circuit assembly and ventilator operational verification described previously. Connect the circuit to an infant test lung assembly.

Delta P (ΔP) and Frequency

Establish the following settings:
- Adjust the mean airway pressure control to the 2 o'clock position.
- Set the bias flow to 15 L/min.
- Set the power control to 3.
- Set the frequency to 3 Hz.
- Set the % I-time control to 50%.
- Adjust the mean airway pressure limit fully clockwise.

1. Press the "Reset" button. Using the bias flow flowmeter, set the mean pressure level to 15 cm H_2O. Set the Max Pressure thumbwheel to 18 cm H_2O and the Min Pressure thumbwheel to 13 cm H_2O.

2. Press the "Start/Stop" button to start the oscillator.

3. Center the piston using the piston centering control on the pedestal just above and to the left of the water trap. Record the ΔP displayed on the monitor.

4. Increase the power control to 6. If required, recenter the piston and readjust the bias flow to maintain a mean pressure of 15 cm H_2O. Record the displayed ΔP.

5. Increase the power control to 9. If required, recenter the piston and readjust the bias flow to maintain a mean pressure of 15 cm H_2O. Record the displayed ΔP.

6. Decrease the power control to 6 and readjust the piston centering and bias flow as needed to maintain 15 cm H_2O mean airway pressure.

Questions

A. What happened to the ΔP as the power control was increased?
B. What adjustments were needed to maintain the desired 15 cm H_2O mean airway pressure as the ΔP was increased?

1. Set the frequency control for 15 Hz. Observe the ΔP display.

Questions

A. Did the ΔP increase or decrease?
B. Why do you suspect the ΔP changed?

Piston Centering

Establish the following settings:
- Adjust the mean airway pressure control to the 2 o'clock position.

- Set the bias flow to 15 L/min.
- Set the power control to 3.
- Set the frequency to 10 Hz.
- Set the % I-time control to 50%.
- Adjust the mean airway pressure limit fully clockwise.

1. Press the "Reset" button. Using the bias flow flowmeter, set the mean pressure level to 15 cm H_2O. Set the Max Pressure thumbwheel to 18 cm H_2O and the Min Pressure thumbwheel to 13 cm H_2O.

2. Press the "Start/Stop" button to start the oscillator.

3. Record the mean airway pressure and the ΔP.

4. Move the centering control counterclockwise such that the display moves toward the left (inspiratory side). Record the mean airway pressure and the ΔP.

5. Move the centering control clockwise such that the display moves to the right (expiratory side). Record the mean airway pressure and the ΔP.

6. Recenter the magnet using the centering control. Record the mean airway pressure and the ΔP.

Questions

A. How did moving the position of the magnet (toward inspiration or expiration) affect the ΔP?
B. How can you explain how magnet position affects the ΔP?

% Inspiratory Time Control

Establish the following settings:
- Adjust the mean airway pressure control to the 2 o'clock position.
- Set the bias flow to 15 L/min.
- Set the power control to 3.
- Set the frequency to 10 Hz.
- Set the % I-time control to 30%.
- Adjust the mean airway pressure limit fully clockwise.

7. Press the "Reset" button. Using the bias flow flowmeter, set the mean pressure level to 15 cm H_2O. Set the Max Pressure thumbwheel to 18 cm H_2O and the Min Pressure thumbwheel to 13 cm H_2O.

8. Press the "Start/Stop" button to start the oscillator. Measure the mean airway pressure and the ΔP.

9. With the % inspiratory time control set at 30%, center the magnet as needed. Measure the mean airway pressure and the ΔP.

10. Set the % inspiratory time control to 40%, and center the magnet as needed. Measure the mean airway pressure and the ΔP.

11. Set the % inspiratory time control to 50%, and center the magnet as needed. Measure the mean airway pressure and the ΔP.

Questions

A. How did changing the % inspiratory time affect mean airway pressure and the ΔP?
B. Why did the % inspiratory time affect the mean airway pressure?

Mean Airway Pressure

Establish the following settings:
- Adjust the mean airway pressure control to the 10 o'clock position.
- Set the bias flow to 15 L/min.
- Set the power control to 3.
- Set the frequency to 10 Hz.
- Set the % I-time control to 30%.
- Adjust the mean airway pressure limit fully clockwise.

1. Press the "Reset" button. Using the bias flow flowmeter, set the mean pressure level to 15 cm H_2O. Set the Max Pressure thumbwheel to 18 cm H_2O and the Min Pressure thumbwheel to 13 cm H_2O.

2. Press the "Start/Stop" button to start the oscillator. Measure the mean airway pressure and the ΔP.

3. Increase the mean airway pressure by rotating the control to the 12 o'clock position. Measure the mean airway pressure and the ΔP.

4. Rotate the mean airway pressure control to the 2 o'clock position. Measure the mean airway pressure and the ΔP.

Question

A. What effect did the mean airway pressure control have?

Check List: Initiation of Neonatal Mechanical Ventilation

_____ 1. Verify the physician's order.
_____ 2. Assess the patient.
_____   a. Maternal history
_____   b. Physical assessment
_____   c. Signs of asphyxia
_____   d. Signs of aspiration
_____   e. Laboratory data

_____ 3. Establish an airway.
_____ 4. Assemble the required equipment.
_____   a. Ventilator
_____   b. Patient circuit
_____   c. Humidifier
_____   d. Resuscitation bag
_____   e. Noninvasive monitors

_____ 5. Perform the ventilator pre-use check.

_____ 6. Establish the ordered settings (all of the following may not apply; put "NA" for settings that are not available).

_____ a. Mode

_____ b. Respiratory rate

_____ c. Inspiratory time

_____ d. Expiratory time

_____ e. Rise time

_____ f. Pause/plateau time

_____ g. Flow pattern

_____ h. Trigger

_____ i. Flow

_____ j. Inspiratory pressure or tidal volume

_____ k. Pressure limit

_____ l. PEEP/CPAP level

_____ m. Pressure support

_____ n. FIO$_2$

_____ 7. Set all alarms appropriately.

_____ 8. Monitor the patient and the ventilator.

_____ a. Breath sounds

_____ b. Chest rise

_____ c. Appearance

_____ d. Mode

_____ e. Respiratory rate

_____ f. Inspiratory time

_____ g. Expiratory time

_____ h. Rise time

_____ i. Pause/plateau time

_____ j. Flow pattern

_____ k. Trigger

_____ l. Flow

_____ m. Inspiratory pressure or tidal volume

_____ n. Pressure limit

_____ o. PEEP/CPAP level

_____ p. Pressure support

_____ q. FIO$_2$

_____ r. Monitor all applicable alarms.

_____ 9. Set up and record data from noninvasive monitors (e.g. pulse oximeter, ECG, transcutaneous monitors, etc.).

_____ 10. Clean up the patient's area.

_____ 11. Record all information in the patient's medical record.

Check List: Monitoring Neonatal Mechanical Ventilation

_____ 1. Verify the physician's order.

_____ 2. Follow standard precautions, including handwashing.

_____ 3. Explain the procedure to the family members, if present.

4. Monitoring

_____ a. Breath sounds

_____ b. Inspection

_____ c. Noninvasive monitoring (e.g. pulse oximeter, transcutaneous monitors, etc.)

_____ d. Heart rate and rhythm

_____ e. Airway position

_____ f. Security of airway

_____ g. Security of circuit connections

_____ 5. Suction as required.

6. Monitor the ventilator (all of the following may not apply; put "NA" for settings that are not available).

_____ a. Mode

_____ b. Respiratory rate (set)

_____ c. Respiratory rate (spontaneous)

_____ d. Inspiratory time

_____ e. Expiratory time

_____ f. Rise time

_____ g. Pause/plateau time

_____ h. Flow pattern

_____ i. Trigger

_____ j. Flow

_____ k. Inspiratory pressure or tidal volume

_____ l. Exhaled tidal volume

_____ m. Pressure limit

_____ n. PEEP/CPAP level

_____ o. Pressure support

_____ p. FIO$_2$ (set and analyzed)

_____ q. Peak pressure

_____ r. Mean airway pressure

_____ s. Check the humidifier and airway temperature

_____ t. Monitor all applicable alarms

_____ 7. Clean up the area.

_____ 8. Record all information in the patient's medical record.

Check List: Initiation of Neonatal Nasal CPAP

_____ 1. Verify the physician's order.

2. Assess the patient.

_____ a. Physical assessment

_____ b. Maternal and delivery history

_____ c. Laboratory data

_____ d. Chest x-ray

_____ e. Inspect for upper airway abnormalities

3. Assess the patient for the interface device.

_____ a. Use the sizing guide properly

_____ b. Choose the appropriate nasal mask or nasal prongs

_____ c. Select the appropriately sized securing device (cap, strap, etc.)

4. Assemble the required equipment.
_____ a. CPAP generator
_____ b. Patient circuit
_____ c. Mask or nasal prongs
_____ d. Cap or strap-style securing device
_____ e. Resuscitation bag
_____ f. Humidifier
_____ g. Noninvasive monitors
_____ 5. Assemble and test the system before use.
6. Establish the ordered settings.
_____ a. CPAP level
_____ b. FIO$_2$
7. Properly apply the device to the patient.
_____ a. Suction the nares prior to application if indicated

_____ b. Apply the device; adjust the straps
_____ c. Ensure proper fit and minimal leak
8. Monitor the patient and CPAP device.
_____ a. Breath sounds
_____ b. Chest rise
_____ c. Appearance
_____ d. Mode
_____ e. CPAP level
_____ f. FIO$_2$ (set and analyzed)
_____ g. Patient's respiratory rate
_____ h. Set and monitor all alarms
_____ 9. Set up and record data from noninvasive monitors (e.g. pulse oximeter, ECG, transcutaneous monitors, etc.)
_____ 10. Clean up the patient's area
_____ 11. Record all information in the patient's medical record.

Check List: Monitoring of Neonatal Nasal CPAP

_____ 1. Verify the physician's order.
_____ 2. Follow standard precautions, including handwashing.
_____ 3. Explain the procedure to the family members, if present.
4. Monitoring
_____ a. Breath sounds
_____ b. Inspection
_____ c. Noninvasive monitoring (e.g. pulse oximeter, transcutaneous monitors, etc.)
_____ d. Heart rate and rhythm
_____ e. Mask or nasal prong position
_____ f. Skin integrity at points of contact

_____ g. Security of circuit connections
_____ 5. Suction the nares as required.
6. Monitor the CPAP device.
_____ a. CPAP level
_____ b. Respiratory rate (spontaneous)
_____ c. FIO$_2$ (set and analyzed)
_____ d. Check the humidifier and airway temperature
_____ e. Monitor all applicable alarms
_____ 7. Clean up the area.
_____ 8. Record all information in the patient's medical record.

Self-Evaluation Post Test: Neonatal Mechanical Ventilation

1. Goals of mechanical ventilation include all of the following *except:*
   a. reducing a patient's work of breathing.
   b. achieving adequate alveolar gas exchange.
   c. eliminating bronchospasm.
   d. preventing ventilator-induced lung injury.
2. Indications for mechanical ventilation of the newborn include:
   I. apnea.
   II. PaO$_2$ less than 50 mm Hg with an FIO$_2$ greater than 0.50.
   III. PaCO$_2$ greater than 55 mm Hg.
   a. I
   b. I, III
   c. II, III
   d. I, II, III
3. The time constant is calculated by:
   a. multiplying the compliance by the airway resistance.
   b. multiplying the compliance by the peak pressure.

   c. dividing the peak pressure by the tubing compliance.
   d. dividing the lung compliance by the airway resistance.
4. Assessment of the newborn for respiratory failure includes:
   I. appearance.
   II. maternal/delivery history.
   III. gestational age.
   IV. Apgar scores.
   a. I
   b. I, II
   c. I, II, III
   d. I, II, III, IV
5. A newborn with a heart rate of 97, gasping respirations, limp muscle tone, a weak cry, and acrocyanosis would have an Apgar score of:
   a. 3.
   b. 4.
   c. 6.
   d. 1.

6. Which of the following modes of mechanical ventilation would best support an apneic neonate?
   I. CPAP
   II. Pressure assist control
   III. Pressure support
   IV. Volume SIMV
   V. Pressure regulated volume control
   a. I, II, V   c. II, III, V
   b. I, II, III   d. II, IV, V

7. Hazards and complication of mechanical ventilation and oxygen delivery to the neonate include:
   I. barotrauma.
   II. retinopathy of prematurity.
   III. reduced cardiac output.
   IV. decreased urine output.
   a. I   c. II, III
   b. I, II   d. I, II, III, IV

8. Infant nasal CPAP is indicated for which of the following clinical conditions?
   I. Oxygenation failure (PaO_2 less than 50 mm Hg despite FIO_2 greater than 0.60)
   II. Ventilation failure (hypercarbia and pH less than 7.25)
   III. Increased work of breathing
   IV. Hyperkalemia
   a. I, III, IV   c. I, III
   b. I, II, IV   d. I, II, III

9. Equipment necessary for successful implementation of infant nasal CPAP include:
   I. properly sized patient interface (mask or nasal prongs).
   II. appropriate humidification equipment.
   III. monitoring equipment (O_2 analyzer, pulse oximeter, etc.).
   a. I, II   c. I, II, III
   b. I, III   d. II, III

10. Hazards of infant nasal CPAP include:
    I. skin breakdown at the points of contact with the patient interface.
    II. insufficient flow.
    III. kinking and obstruction of the patient interface.
    a. I, II   c. I, III
    b. II, III   d. I, II, III

PERFORMANCE EVALUATION:

Initiation of Neonatal Mechanical Ventilation

Date: Lab _____ Clinical _____ Agency _____

Lab: Pass _____ Fail _____ Clinical: Pass _____ Fail _____

Student name _____ Instructor name _____

No. of times observed in clinical _____

No. of times practiced in clinical _____

PASSING CRITERIA: Obtain 90% or better on the procedure. Tasks indicated by * must receive at least 1 point, or the evaluation is terminated. Procedure must be performed within the designated time, or the performance receives a failing grade.

SCORING: 2 points — Task performed satisfactorily without prompting.
1 point — Task performed satisfactorily with self-initiated correction.
0 points — Task performed incorrectly or with prompting required.
NA — Task not applicable to the patient care situation.

Tasks:	Peer	Lab	Clinical
* 1. Verifies the physician's order	☐	☐	☐
* 2. Assesses the patient			
a. Maternal history	☐	☐	☐
b. Physical assessment	☐	☐	☐
c. Signs of asphyxia	☐	☐	☐
d. Signs of aspiration	☐	☐	☐
e. Laboratory data	☐	☐	☐
* 3. Establishes an airway	☐	☐	☐
* 4. Assembles the required equipment			
a. Ventilator	☐	☐	☐
b. Patient circuit	☐	☐	☐
c. Humidifier	☐	☐	☐
d. Resuscitation bag	☐	☐	☐
e. Noninvasive monitors	☐	☐	☐
* 5. Performs the ventilator pre-use check	☐	☐	☐
* 6. Establishes the ordered settings (all of the following may not apply; put "NA" for settings that are not available)			
a. Mode	☐	☐	☐
b. Respiratory rate	☐	☐	☐
c. Inspiratory time	☐	☐	☐
d. Expiratory time	☐	☐	☐
e. Rise time	☐	☐	☐

	f. Pause/plateau time	☐	☐	☐
	g. Flow pattern	☐	☐	☐
	h. Trigger	☐	☐	☐
	i. Flow	☐	☐	☐
	j. Inspiratory pressure or tidal volume	☐	☐	☐
	k. Pressure limit	☐	☐	☐
	l. PEEP/CPAP level	☐	☐	☐
	m. Pressure support	☐	☐	☐
	n. FIO$_2$	☐	☐	☐

* **7.** Sets all alarms appropriately   ☐ ☐ ☐

* **8.** Monitors the patient and the ventilator

	a. Breath sounds	☐	☐	☐
	b. Chest rise	☐	☐	☐
	c. Appearance	☐	☐	☐
	d. Mode	☐	☐	☐
	e. Respiratory rate	☐	☐	☐
	f. Inspiratory time	☐	☐	☐
	g. Expiratory time	☐	☐	☐
	h. Rise time	☐	☐	☐
	i. Pause/plateau time	☐	☐	☐
	j. Flow pattern	☐	☐	☐
	k. Trigger	☐	☐	☐
	l. Flow	☐	☐	☐
	m. Inspiratory pressure or tidal volume	☐	☐	☐
	n. Pressure limit	☐	☐	☐
	o. PEEP/CPAP level	☐	☐	☐
	p. Pressure support	☐	☐	☐
	q. FIO$_2$	☐	☐	☐
	r. Monitors all applicable alarms	☐	☐	☐

* **9.** Sets up and records data from the noninvasive monitors (e.g. pulse oximeter, ECG, transcutaneous monitors, etc.)   ☐ ☐ ☐

* **10.** Cleans up the patient's area   ☐ ☐ ☐

11. Records all information in the patient's medical record   ☐ ☐ ☐

SCORE: Peer _____ points of possible 98; _____%

               Lab _____ points of possible 98; _____%

               Clinical _____ points of possible 98; _____%

TIME: _____ out of possible 30 minutes

STUDENT SIGNATURES   **INSTRUCTOR SIGNATURES**

PEER: _____   LAB: _____

STUDENT: _____   CLINICAL: _____

PERFORMANCE EVALUATION:

Monitoring Neonatal Mechanical Ventilation

Date: Lab _____ Clinical _____ Agency _____

Lab: Pass _____ Fail _____ Clinical: Pass _____ Fail _____

Student name _____ Instructor name _____

No. of times observed in clinical _____

No. of times practiced in clinical _____

PASSING CRITERIA: Obtain 90% or better on the procedure. Tasks indicated by * must receive at least 1 point, or the evaluation is terminated. Procedure must be performed within the designated time, or the performance receives a failing grade.

SCORING: 2 points — Task performed satisfactorily without prompting.
1 point — Task performed satisfactorily with self-initiated correction.
0 points — Task performed incorrectly or with prompting required.
NA — Task not applicable to the patient care situation.

Tasks:	Peer	Lab	Clinical
* **1.** Verifies the physician's order	☐	☐	☐
* **2.** Follows standard precautions, including hand washing	☐	☐	☐
3. Explains the procedure to the family members, if present	☐	☐	☐
* **4.** Monitoring			
a. Breath sounds	☐	☐	☐
b. Inspection	☐	☐	☐
c. Noninvasive monitoring (e.g. pulse oximeter, transcutaneous monitors, etc.)	☐	☐	☐
d. Heart rate and rhythm	☐	☐	☐
e. Airway position	☐	☐	☐
f. Security of airway	☐	☐	☐
g. Security of circuit connections	☐	☐	☐
* **5.** Suctions as required	☐	☐	☐
* **6.** Monitors the ventilator (all of the following may not apply; put "NA" for settings that are not available)			
a. Mode	☐	☐	☐
b. Respiratory rate (set)	☐	☐	☐
c. Respiratory rate (spontaneous)	☐	☐	☐
d. Inspiratory time	☐	☐	☐

e. Expiratory time ☐ ☐ ☐

f. Rise time ☐ ☐ ☐

g. Pause/plateau time ☐ ☐ ☐

h. Flow pattern ☐ ☐ ☐

i. Trigger ☐ ☐ ☐

j. Flow ☐ ☐ ☐

k. Inspiratory pressure or tidal volume ☐ ☐ ☐

l. Exhaled tidal volume ☐ ☐ ☐

m. Pressure limit ☐ ☐ ☐

n. PEEP/CPAP level ☐ ☐ ☐

o. Pressure support ☐ ☐ ☐

p. FIO_2 (set and analyzed) ☐ ☐ ☐

q. Peak pressure ☐ ☐ ☐

r. Mean airway pressure ☐ ☐ ☐

s. Checks the humidifier and airway temperature ☐ ☐ ☐

t. Monitors all applicable alarms ☐ ☐ ☐

7. Cleans up the area ☐ ☐ ☐

8. Records all information in the patient's medical record ☐ ☐ ☐

SCORE: Peer _____ points of possible 66; _____%

Lab _____ points of possible 66; _____%

Clinical _____ points of possible 66; _____%

TIME: _____ out of possible 30 minutes

STUDENT SIGNATURES

PEER: _____

STUDENT: _____

INSTRUCTOR SIGNATURES

LAB: _____

CLINICAL: _____

PERFORMANCE EVALUATION:

Initiation of Neonatal Nasal CPAP

Date: Lab _____ Clinical _____ Agency _____

Lab: Pass _____ Fail _____ Clinical: Pass _____ Fail _____

Student name _____ Instructor name _____

No. of times observed in clinical _____

No. of times practiced in clinical _____

PASSING CRITERIA: Obtain 90% or better on the procedure. Tasks indicated by * must receive at least 1 point, or the evaluation is terminated. Procedure must be performed within the designated time, or the performance receives a failing grade.

SCORING: 2 points — Task performed satisfactorily without prompting.
1 point — Task performed satisfactorily with self-initiated correction.
0 points — Task performed incorrectly or with prompting required.
NA — Task not applicable to the patient care situation.

Tasks:	Peer	Lab	Clinical
* **1.** Verifies the physician's order	☐	☐	☐
* **2.** Assesses the patient			
a. Physical assessment	☐	☐	☐
b. Maternal and delivery history	☐	☐	☐
c. Laboratory data	☐	☐	☐
d. Chest x-ray	☐	☐	☐
e. Inspects for upper airway abnormalities	☐	☐	☐
* **3.** Assesses the patient for the interface device			
a. Uses the sizing guide properly	☐	☐	☐
b. Chooses the appropriate nasal mask or nasal prongs	☐	☐	☐
c. Selects the appropriately sized securing device (cap, strap, etc.)	☐	☐	☐
* **4.** Assembles the required equipment			
a. CPAP generator	☐	☐	☐
b. Patient circuit	☐	☐	☐
c. Mask or nasal prongs	☐	☐	☐
d. Cap or strap-style securing device	☐	☐	☐
e. Resuscitation bag	☐	☐	☐

      f. Humidifier ☐ ☐ ☐

      g. Noninvasive monitors ☐ ☐ ☐

* **5.** Assembles and tests the system before use ☐ ☐ ☐

* **6.** Establishes the ordered settings

      a. CPAP level ☐ ☐ ☐

      b. FIO_2 ☐ ☐ ☐

* **7.** Properly applies the device to the patient

      a. Suctions the nares prior to application if indicated ☐ ☐ ☐

      b. Applies the device; adjusts the straps ☐ ☐ ☐

      c. Ensures proper fit and minimal leak ☐ ☐ ☐

* **8.** Monitors the patient and CPAP device

      a. Breath sounds ☐ ☐ ☐

      b. Chest rise ☐ ☐ ☐

      c. Appearance ☐ ☐ ☐

      d. Mode ☐ ☐ ☐

      e. CPAP level ☐ ☐ ☐

      f. FIO_2 (set and analyzed) ☐ ☐ ☐

      g. Patient's respiratory rate ☐ ☐ ☐

      h. Sets and monitors all the alarms ☐ ☐ ☐

* **9.** Sets up and records data from the noninvasive monitors (e.g. pulse oximeter, ECG, transcutaneous monitors, etc.) ☐ ☐ ☐

* **10.** Cleans up the patient's area ☐ ☐ ☐

* **11.** Records all information in the patient's medical record ☐ ☐ ☐

SCORE: Peer _____ points of possible 66; _____%

                    Lab _____ points of possible 66; _____%

                    Clinical _____ points of possible 66; _____%

TIME: _____ out of possible 30 minutes

STUDENT SIGNATURES

PEER: _____

STUDENT: _____

INSTRUCTOR SIGNATURES

LAB: _____

CLINICAL: _____

PERFORMANCE EVALUATION:
Monitoring of Neonatal Nasal CPAP

Date: Lab _____ Clinical _____ Agency _____

Lab: Pass _____ Fail _____ Clinical: Pass _____ Fail _____

Student name _____ Instructor name _____

No. of times observed in clinical _____

No. of times practiced in clinical _____

PASSING CRITERIA: Obtain 90% or better on the procedure. Tasks indicated by * must receive at least 1 point, or the evaluation is terminated. Procedure must be performed within the designated time, or the performance receives a failing grade.

SCORING:
2 points — Task performed satisfactorily without prompting.
1 point — Task performed satisfactorily with self-initiated correction.
0 points — Task performed incorrectly or with prompting required.
NA — Task not applicable to the patient care situation.

Tasks:	Peer	Lab	Clinical
* 1. Verifies the physician's order	☐	☐	☐
* 2. Follows standard precautions, including hand washing	☐	☐	☐
3. Explains the procedure to the family members, if present	☐	☐	☐
* 4. Monitoring			
a. Breath sounds	☐	☐	☐
b. Inspection	☐	☐	☐
c. Noninvasive monitoring (e.g. pulse oximeter, transcutaneous monitors, etc.)	☐	☐	☐
d. Heart rate and rhythm	☐	☐	☐
e. Mask or nasal prong position	☐	☐	☐
f. Skin integrity at points of contact	☐	☐	☐
g. Security of circuit connections	☐	☐	☐
* 5. Suctions the nares as required	☐	☐	☐
* 6. Monitors the CPAP device			
a. CPAP level	☐	☐	☐
b. Respiratory rate (spontaneous)	☐	☐	☐
c. FIO_2 (set and analyzed)	☐	☐	☐
d. Checks the humidifier and airway temperature	☐	☐	☐
e. Monitors all the applicable alarms	☐	☐	☐

7. Cleans up the area ☐ ☐ ☐

8. Records all information in the patient's medical record ☐ ☐ ☐

SCORE: Peer _____ points of possible 36; _____%

Lab _____ points of possible 36; _____%

Clinical _____ points of possible 36; _____%

TIME: _____ out of possible 30 minutes

STUDENT SIGNATURES   **INSTRUCTOR SIGNATURES**

PEER: _____   LAB: _____

STUDENT: _____   CLINICAL: _____

PERFORMANCE EVALUATION:

High-Frequency Oscillatory Ventilation

Date: Lab _____ Clinical _____ Agency _____

Lab: Pass _____ Fail _____ Clinical: Pass _____ Fail _____

Student name _____ Instructor name _____

No. of times observed in clinical _____

No. of times practiced in clinical _____

PASSING CRITERIA: Obtain 90% or better on the procedure. Tasks indicated by * must receive at least 1 point, or the evaluation is terminated. Procedure must be performed within the designated time, or the performance receives a failing grade.

SCORING: 2 points — Task performed satisfactorily without prompting.
1 point — Task performed satisfactorily with self-initiated correction.
0 points — Task performed incorrectly or with prompting required.
NA — Task not applicable to the patient care situation.

Tasks:	Peer	Lab	Clinical
* 1. Verifies the physician's order or protocol	☐	☐	☐
* 2. Follows standard precautions, including hand hygiene	☐	☐	☐
3. Auscultates and suctions the patient as required	☐	☐	☐
* 4. Obtains the patient's baseline data			
a. Assesses ventilatory status (P_tCO_2, rate, pH, $PaCO_2$)	☐	☐	☐
b. Assesses oxygenation status (PaO_2, SpO_2)	☐	☐	☐
c. Assesses circulatory status (BP, HR, ECG)	☐	☐	☐
5. Monitors the ventilation parameters			
* a. Frequency	☐	☐	☐
* b. FIO_2 level	☐	☐	☐
* c. Inspiratory time %	☐	☐	☐
* d. Mean airway pressure (P_{AW})	☐	☐	☐
* e. ΔP (amplitude)	☐	☐	☐
* f. Bias flow	☐	☐	☐
* 6. Sets the alarm parameters	☐	☐	☐
* 7. Suctions the patient as required	☐	☐	☐
* 8. Follows standard precautions, including hand hygiene	☐	☐	☐
* 9. Documents the procedure	☐	☐	☐

SCORE: Peer _____ points of possible 32; _____%

                    Lab _____ points of possible 32; _____%

                    Clinical _____ points of possible 32; _____%

TIME: _____ out of possible 20 minutes

STUDENT SIGNATURES   **INSTRUCTOR SIGNATURES**

PEER: _____   LAB: _____

STUDENT: _____   CLINICAL: _____

APPENDIX

Answers to Self-Evaluation Post Tests

CHAPTER 1
Answers

1. B	3. D	5. B	7. D	9. A
2. C	4. C	6. D	8. A	10. D

CHAPTER 2
Answers

1. C	3. C	5. B	7. B	9. B
2. D	4. C	6. C	8. A	10. B

CHAPTER 3
Answers

1. B	3. D	5. C	7. D	9. D
2. D	4. D	6. D	8. B	10. B

CHAPTER 4
Answers

1. A	3. D	5. D	7. A	9. C
2. B	4. C	6. D	8. C	10. B

CHAPTER 5
Answers

1. D	3. D	5. D	7. C	9. D
2. C	4. D	6. B	8. D	10. C

CHAPTER 6
Answers

1. D	3. C	5. B	7. D	9. C
2. A	4. D	6. C	8. B	10. C

CHAPTER 7
Answers

1. D	3. B	5. B	7. D	9. A
2. D	4. D	6. B	8. B	10. B

CHAPTER 8
Answers

1. B	3. C	5. A	7. C	9. C
2. B	4. B	6. D	8. C	10. B

CHAPTER 9
Answers

1. B	3. A	5. C	7. D	9. A
2. B	4. D	6. D	8. C	10. D

CHAPTER 10
Answers

1. A	3. B	5. C	7. A	9. A
2. B	4. B	6. D	8. B	10. C

CHAPTER 11
Answers

1. D	3. D	5. B	7. D	9. B
2. D	4. D	6. B	8. C	10. D

CHAPTER 12
Answers

1. D	3. C	5. A	7. A	9. B
2. A	4. B	6. D	8. D	10. C

CHAPTER 13
Answers

1. B	3. D	5. C	7. D	9. B
2. C	4. C	6. B	8. D	10. D

CHAPTER 14
Answers

1. C	3. B	5. A	7. C	9. B
2. C	4. B	6. B	8. D	10. C

CHAPTER 15
Answers

1. C	3. B	5. B	7. B	9. D
2. D	4. A	6. C	8. D	10. D

CHAPTER 16
Answers

1. C	3. A	5. A	7. D	9. C
2. C	4. A	6. D	8. D	10. D

CHAPTER 17
Answers

1. B	3. C	5. A	7. B	9. B
2. D	4. C	6. D	8. A	10. D

CHAPTER 18
Answers

1. B	3. A	5. D	7. B	9. D
2. D	4. D	6. D	8. D	10. D

CHAPTER 19
Answers

1. B	3. A	5. B	7. D	9. D
2. B	4. D	6. C	8. B	10. A

CHAPTER 20
Answers

1. D	3. D	5. C	7. D	9. D
2. B	4. C	6. C	8. A	10. D

CHAPTER 21
Answers

1. B	3. C	5. D	7. C	9. C
2. B	4. B	6. C	8. D	10. C

CHAPTER 22
Answers

1. B	3. A	5. C	7. D	9. C
2. C	4. D	6. B	8. A	10. B

CHAPTER 23
Answers

1. A	3. A	5. A	7. D	9. B
2. B	4. D	6. B	8. B	10. D

CHAPTER 24
Answers

1. D	3. D	5. C	7. D	9. C
2. D	4. A	6. D	8. C	10. C

CHAPTER 25
Answers

1. B	3. D	5. B	7. D	9. C
2. A	4. D	6. D	8. A	10. D

CHAPTER 26
Answers

1. A	3. D	5. B	7. D	9. B
2. B	4. C	6. B	8. C	10. B

CHAPTER 27
Answers

1. A	3. C	5. B	7. D	9. C
2. B	4. A	6. C	8. D	10. A

CHAPTER 28
Answers

1. B	3. C	5. C	7. C	9. C
2. D	4. D	6. D	8. A	10. D

CHAPTER 29
Answers

1. C	3. A	5. B	7. D	9. C
2. D	4. D	6. D	8. C	10. D

GLOSSARY

A

abnormal breath sounds Abnormal breath sounds, or adventitious breath sounds, are sounds that are produced as a result of abnormal lung pathology (consolidation, edema, fluid, etc.). Abnormal breath sounds include rhonchi, crackles, wheezes, and rubs.

absolute humidity The amount of water vapor contained in a gas at a given temperature and relative humidity. Absolute humidity is expressed in milligrams per liter of gas.

absorption atelectasis An abnormal collapse of lung tissue caused by the administration of high concentrations of oxygen, resulting in the displacement of nitrogen.

adjunctive breathing exercises Specific ventilatory exercises designed to increase the overall volume of air inspired or the volume of air to a specific lobe or segment.

aerosol Particulate matter suspended in a gas; the particles may be either solid or liquid.

afterload The resistance the ventricle must overcome to eject blood. As afterload decreases, ventricular ejection increases.

airborne transmission Transmission of microorganisms (0.5 micrometer or smaller) by air currents.

air embolism Blockage of a blood vessel by a bubble of air that has entered the bloodstream.

air entrainment mask An oxygen mask that provides precise oxygen concentrations by mixing room air and oxygen at precise ratios using viscous shearing and vorticity. These devices are classified as high-flow oxygen delivery systems.

air/oxygen blender A medical device that precisely mixes air and oxygen together.

air trapping A respiratory problem in which too much gas remains in the lungs after a complete exhalation (residual volume). In obstructive lung disease, bronchial obstruction causes air trapping distal to the obstruction.

airway pressure release ventilation (APRV) A form of spontaneous ventilation (CPAP) with two set pressure levels (high and baseline).

airway resistance (R_{AW}) A measure of resistance to gas flow into and out of the lungs. Normal airway resistance is between 0.6 and 2.4 cm H_2O at a flow of 0.5 L/sec (30 L/min).

alpha receptors Receptor sites located in the peripheral vasculature, heart, bronchial muscle, and bronchial blood vessels. Stimulation of these sites causes peripheral vasoconstriction.

ambient temperature and pressure, saturated (ATPS) The condition of ambient temperature and pressure and 100% saturation with water vapor. All spirometry results are measured at ATPS.

american standard safety system (ASSS) A safety system designed by the Compressed Gas Association for large medical gas cylinder valve connections. The system prevents the mismatching of regulators or connections with the incorrect cylinder.

amplitude A measure of vibratory movement or displacement of a sinusoidal waveform about its mean or average value.

anatomical dead space The volume of gas comprising the conducting airways. This part of ventilation does not participate in gas exchange.

anatomic reservoir The dead space composed of the nasopharynx and oropharynx, which is approximately 50 mL in volume.

anterior mandibular displacement A positional maneuver in which the jaw is displaced anteriorly, separating the tongue from the posterior pharynx. This maneuver may be performed without manipulation of the neck (optimal choice if cervical spine injury is suspected).

anterior-posterior (anteroposterior) Referring to an x-ray view of the chest in which the x-rays pass from anterior to the posterior (front to back) with the film plate resting on the patient's back. This view is common in portable x-ray techniques and tends to magnify the size of the heart.

anticholinergic drugs A class of drugs that block the site of acetylcholine transmission, preventing the action of acetylcholine (bronchospasm) in the lungs.

antigen A foreign substance, usually a protein, that causes the body to produce an antibody in response to its presence that reacts specifically to the antigen.

antimicrobial agents Drugs used to destroy or inhibit growth or reproduction of microorganisms (bacteria, fungi, protozoans, viruses). These drugs include antibiotics and antiviral, antiprotozoal, and antifungal agents.

antisepsis The application of chemical agents to inhibit microorganisms' ability to reproduce and grow.

Apgar scoring system An assessment of a newborns adjustment to extrauterine life developed by Dr. Virginia Apgar. The scoring system assesses heart rate, respiration, muscle tone, reflex irritability, and color. The assessment is made at one and five minutes following birth.

apical lordotic Referring to an x-ray view of the chest in which the patient is reclined or tilted backward at about 30° to 45° and the x-ray energy passes from anterior to posterior. This view moves the heart shadow and mediastinal structures out of the film plane, allowing a better view of the apices of the lungs.

apnea The cessation or absence of breathing.

arterialization   Application of a warming pack or hot towel to increase peripheral circulation to an area prior to capillary sampling.

arterial line sampling   The technique of obtaining a blood sample from an artery. Common sites from which samples are obtained are the radial, brachial, and femoral arteries.

asepsis   The protection against infection before, during, and after patient contact or patient procedures (surgery, bronchoscopy, intubation, etc.).

assist-control mode   A mode of mechanical ventilation that allows the patient's spontaneous efforts to trigger a mechanical breath. In this mode, the patient's respiratory drive will assist in normalizing blood gas values.

ASSS   *See* American Standard Safety System.

atelectasis   An airless state of the lung, lobe, or segment.

ATPS   *See* ambient temperature pressure, saturated.

atrial fibrillation   A nonrhythmic, disorganized, rapid contraction of a group of cardiac muscle cells. This type of contraction is very inefficient and results in poor blood circulation. Fibrillation is usually described as to the specific area of occurrence, such as atrial fibrillation.

atrioventricular node (AV node)   A part of the cardiac conduction system located in the septal wall of the right atrium, which conducts the electrical impulse from the sinoatrial node to the bundle of His.

augmented minute ventilation   A form of synchronized intermittent mandatory ventilation in which the patient is guaranteed a minimum minute volume. If the patient fails to maintain the threshold minute volume, the ventilator augments the patient's efforts to achieve the set minute ventilation.

auscultation   The process of listening to the patient's chest using a stethoscope.

automatic tube compensation   A ventilator mode that automatically compensates for the resistance of the artificial airway.

automode   A mode of ventilation that combines pressure regulated volume control (PRVC) and volume support (VS) into a single mode.

B

bacillus   A bacterium that is rodlike in shape.

bacteriological surveillance   A method by which equipment is routinely cultured and monitored for correct disinfection, sterilization, and handling procedures to identify and resolve sources of contamination.

barotrauma   Trauma to the thoracic structures resulting directly from the positive pressure (increased intrathoracic pressure) applied in mechanical ventilation. Barotrauma may be manifested as a pneumothorax, a pneumomediastinum, a subcutaneous emphysema, a tracheal rupture, or an interstitial emphysema.

barrel chest   An abnormal chest conformation characterized by an increase in the anterior-posterior diameter. A barrel chest often accompanies chronic obstructive lung disease in which there is concomitant air trapping.

bedside monitoring   Measurement of spontaneous ventilatory mechanics that typically includes minute volume, respiratory rate (frequency), tidal volume, vital capacity, and peak expiratory flow.

beta-1 receptors   Receptor sites located in the bronchial blood vessels and the heart. Stimulation of these sites results in tachycardia, an increased potential for arrhythmias, and increased cardiac output.

beta-2 receptors   Receptor sites located in the bronchial smooth muscle, bronchial blood vessels, systemic blood vessels, and the skeletal muscles. Stimulation of these sites in the lungs causes bronchodilation.

bilevel positive airway pressure (BiPAP)   A mode of ventilation similar to continuous positive airway pressure except that different pressure levels may be set for the inspiratory and expiratory phases. The inspiratory pressure is greater than the expiratory pressure, offering lower resistance to exhalation.

Biot's respiration   An abnormal ventilatory pattern that is characterized by irregular breathing (rate and depth) with periods of apnea.

body humidity   The maximum absolute humidity at body temperature (100% saturation with water vapor, 37°C, 43.9 mg/L water content, and a partial pressure of water vapor of 47 mm Hg).

body temperature and pressure, saturated (BTPS)   A condition in which the gas present in the lungs is at body temperature and pressure and fully saturated with water vapor.

bradycardia   An abnormally low heart rate.

bradypnea   An abnormally low respiratory rate.

bronchoalveolar lavage (BAL)   A technique in which the bronchoscope is wedged and normal saline (0.9%) is instilled and then retrieved for cellular analysis.

bronchoscopy   A technique or procedure that involves visually examining the tracheobronchial tree with an instrument called a bronchoscope for diagnostic or therapeutic indications.

BTPS   *See* body temperature and pressure, saturated (BTPS).

bundle of His   A band of fibers in the cardiac conduction system that conducts the impulse from the atrioventricular node to the ventricles. The bundle of His originates at the atrioventricular node and follows the septum of the heart, eventually dividing into the right and left bundle branches.

butterfly catheter   A type of intravenous catheter that has a metal needle secured by two plastic tabs resembling a butterfly's wings.

butterfly needle   A specialized collection needle embedded into a pair of plastic tabs resembling a butterfly's wings. Attached to the butterfly and the end of the needle is a short length of collection tubing that terminates in a female syringe fitting. Syringes are necessary when a butterfly needle is used for phlebotomy collection.

C

capacity   The maximum amount of water vapor a gas can hold at a given temperature. As the temperature of a gas increases, so does its capacity for water vapor.

capillary blood gas sampling   Lancing the surface of the skin to obtain an arterialized capillary sample, which is collected in a small capillary tube.

capsule   A protective membranous shell that surrounds some bacteria, making them more difficult to destroy.

cardiac output   The amount of blood the heart pumps each minute, expressed in liters per minute. Normal cardiac output for an adult is about 5 L/min.

cardiac phases   The four phases of the cardiac cycle: isovolumetric contraction, systolic ejection, isovolumetric relaxation, and diastolic filling.

catheter fragment embolism   Blockage of a blood vessel that occurs when a portion of an intravenous catheter is cut or broken off and enters the bloodstream.

catheter shear   The cutting off of a portion of an intravenous catheter. This condition usually occurs when the steel needle stylet is inserted back into the flexible indwelling catheter.

cellulitis   Inflammation of the tissue, especially below the skin. This condition is characterized by redness, pain, and swelling.

central venous pressure   The pressure measured in the vena cava or right atrium. This pressure reflects the blood volume returning to the heart and also the preload of the right ventricle.

central venous pressure (CVP) catheter   A catheter inserted into the vena cava or right atrium to measure the central venous pressure and to provide a convenient route for mixed venous blood sampling or fluid administration.

charting by exception   A method of documentation in which only information that changes is recorded. Arrows, ditto marks, or other means are used to indicate data that remain constant since the last time the patient was seen.

chest drain   A tube placed to remove blood or fluid from a chest cavity. For example, mediastinal chest drains are common postoperatively following coronary artery bypass graft surgery. These drains allow the removal of fluid from residual bleeding or edema following surgery.

chest percussion   A technique in which the practitioner claps on the patient's chest wall using a cupped hand to induce vibration throughout the lung parenchyma, facilitating bronchial secretion clearance. The technique may also be performed with the assistance of mechanical devices.

chest tube   A tube placed into the pleural space to remove air or fluid. Depending on whether gas or fluid removal is the purpose of the chest tube, it may be placed in an anterior (gas) or a posterior (fluid) location in the chest.

chevron   A pattern of taping used in securing an intravenous catheter.

Cheyne-Stokes respiration   An abnormal ventilatory pattern that is characterized by alternating periods of apnea and an increase in depth and rate of breathing, followed by a tapering of depth and rate leading to another apneic period.

cholinergic receptors   Receptor sites located throughout the body that are stimulated by acetylcholine.

clinical goal   A desired clinical outcome of a therapy or procedure. Ideally, clinical goals should be objective and measurable.

closed-loop ventilation   Closed-loop ventilation is the control of one output variable (pressure, flow or volume) of the mechanical ventilator based on the measurement of an input variable. In pressure support, flow is constantly changing (output) to maintain pressure at a constant level.

closed suction system   A type of suction catheter that incorporates a protective plastic sheath surrounding the catheter. It is designed to be used multiple times and has the advantage of remaining attached to the artificial airway at all times.

coccus   A bacterium that is round or spherical in shape.

collarbones   Bony structures located on the superior aspect of the anterior chest, generally overlying the first rib. Also called clavicles.

collection chamber   The compartment of a chest drainage system located most proximal to the patient. This chamber collects fluid that is removed by the chest drain or chest tube.

Combitube airway   An advanced cuffed double-lumen airway that is blindly inserted into the airway without using a laryngeoscope. Ventilation may be achieved even if the airway is placed into the esophagus by selecting the correct lumen once the cuffs are inflated.

computed tomography   A radiographic technique in which the body is imaged in many thin slices, typically moving superior to inferior. This imaging modality creates a three-dimensional perspective that other techniques do not provide.

consolidation   A condition or process of solidification of the lung tissue. Consolidation may be observed as increased opacification on chest radiographs.

contact transmission   Transmission of microorganisms by direct contact (person to person), usually involving the hands.

continuous mechanical ventilation   The artificial support of a patient's respiratory needs using a mechanical ventilator. Ventilatory support may be total (in the patient with apnea) or partial (when some spontaneous breaths are possible but minute ventilation is insufficient to normalize blood gases).

continuous positive airway pressure (CPAP)   Spontaneous ventilation with an elevated baseline pressure.

control mode   A mode of ventilation in which all breaths are time cycled and delivered at preset intervals (ventilatory rate). In this mode, any spontaneous efforts made by the patient are not recognized by the ventilator; therefore, patient-ventilator asynchrony may occur.

control variable   The variable (pressure, volume, or flow) measured by the ventilator and used by the microprocessor to control the ventilator's output.

coronary artery disease   Obstruction of the coronary arteries, which may be caused by fatty deposits (plaque) or thrombi. The condition can lead to decreased delivery of oxygen to the myocardium with consequent symptoms.

corticosteroids   A class of drugs that act as anti-inflammatory agents and are typically natural or synthetic hormones.

CPAP   Continuous positive airway pressure. The application of continuous pressure (both inspiration and expiration) in the spontaneously breathing patient. CPAP is similar to positive end-expiratory pressure in that it improves the functional residual capacity.

CPAP/IMV   A common ventilatory support mode for neonatal and pediatric patients. In this mode a continuous flow of gas is available for inspiration at all times (CPAP); when mandatory breaths are delivered (IMV), the exhalation valve closes, administering a mechanical breath.

cracking   The quick opening and closing of a cylinder valve allowing the high-pressure gas to exit the valve, removing any debris, dust, or dirt.

cross-contamination   The transmission of microorganisms between places or persons. The most common method of transmission is by direct contact between persons.

cytology brush   A specialized small brush that is designed to pass through the channel of a flexible bronchoscope to obtain tissue samples for analysis.

D

damping   An attenuation of the pressure waveform that is most commonly caused by air bubbles in the measuring system.

decannulation   The removal of the tracheostomy tube from the tracheostomy stoma. With accidental decannulation, if the stoma is not well established, ventilation may be tenuous.

degranulation   The lysis of a cell wall, resulting in release of the cell's contents. When mast cells degranulate,

histamine, heparin, leukotrienes, and other mediators are released.

depolarization   The process of muscle cell contraction in which potassium is exchanged for sodium, resulting in a net negative charge of the cell.

diagnostic bronchoscopy   A bronchoscopy procedure in which samples of tissue or secretions are taken for further laboratory analysis and workup.

diameter-indexed safety system (DISS)   A safety system designed by the Compressed Gas Association for low-pressure (less than 200 psi) compressed gas fittings. This safety system consists of threaded fittings having differing pitches and internal/external threading.

diaphragmatic breathing   An adjunctive breathing exercise where emphasis is placed on using the diaphragm's motion to augment chest wall expansion.

diastolic   The pressure recorded at the moment of cardiac relaxation, yielding the lower of the paired blood pressure values.

diffusion (D_LCO)   A pulmonary function parameter measured as the diffusion of gas across the alveolar-capillary membrane. Carbon monoxide is used as a test gas because of its increased affinity for hemoglobin compared with oxygen.

digital clubbing   An abnormal enlargement of the distal phalanges, usually caused by chronic hypoxemia.

directed cough   A deliberate maneuver taught to the patient or caregiver to facilitate secretion mobilization. Examples include huff coughing or forced expiratory technique and manually assisted coughing (quad coughing).

disinfection   The process of killing all pathogenic microorganisms (vegetative forms).

distal lumen   The opening at the tip of the catheter; used to measure the pulmonary artery and pulmonary arterial wedge pressures.

downstream   Distal to a point in a device, or circuit, in relation to gas or current flow.

droplet transmission   Transmission of microorganisms by aerosolized droplets (0.5 micrometer or larger) usually produced by coughing or sneezing.

dry powder inhaler (DPI)   A medication administration device that aerosolizes small particles of dry powder medication. Dry powder inhalers do not require a propellant to operate but rely on the patient's inspiratory flow.

dual control mode breath-to-breath mode   A mode of ventilation in which the ventilator begins inspiration in a pressure limited time cycled breath delivery. Once resistance and compliance are measured, pressure is gradually increased with each breath until the desired target tidal volume is reached. An example of this would be volume control plus.

dual control mode within a breath mode   A mode of ventilation in which the ventilator switches pressure control to volume control within a breath. An example of dual control within a breath would be volume assure pressure support.

dynamic compliance A measurement of the compliance (distensibility) of the patient's lungs and thorax under conditions of airflow. Therefore, the dynamic compliance reflects not only the compliance of the lungs and thorax but also airway resistance.

E

endotoxin A toxic compound usually contained in the cell walls of microorganisms. These toxins are released when these organisms die and the body breaks down their cell walls.

endotracheal pilot tube and balloon A small tube that passes the length of an endotracheal tube and connects the pilot balloon with its inflation port to the endotracheal tube cuff. By palpating the pilot balloon and attaching a pressure manometer to the inflation port, endotracheal tube cuff pressures may be assessed.

endotracheal tube An artificial airway that may be passed orally or nasally into the trachea, providing for positive-pressure ventilation and airway protection.

endotracheal tube cuff A large inflatable balloon at the distal end of an endotracheal tube that is designed to seal against the tracheal wall when inflated.

end-tidal CO_2 monitor A monitor that measures the exhaled partial pressure of carbon dioxide ($PetCO_2$), using infrared technology.

ethylene oxide A gas applied with moist heat to sterilize equipment and supplies.

eukaryotic bacteria A type of bacteria in which the bacterial cell contains a true nucleus.

eupnea A normal breathing pattern.

expiratory positive airway pressure (EPAP) In bilevel positive-pressure ventilation, the baseline setting for the expiratory pressure level.

expiratory reserve volume (ERV) The maximum amount of air that can be exhaled after a normal tidal exhalation.

exposed Referring to x-ray film that has been subjected to x-ray energy, causing a physical change in the emulsion to create an image.

exposure control policy A specific institutional policy designed to protect caregivers, staff, and patients from exposure to hazardous body fluids or other substances.

extubation The process in which the endotracheal tube is removed. Extubation usually follows clinical improvement or accomplishment of therapeutic goals by the patient.

F

FEF$_{25-75\%}$ The flow rate between 25% and 75% of maximum as measured on a forced vital capacity tracing.

FEF$_{200-1200\ mL}$ The flow rate between 200 and 1200 mL as measured on a forced vital capacity tracing.

fenestrated tracheostomy tube A specialized tracheostomy tube in which there is an opening (fenestration)

cut into the cannula, permitting passage of air into the upper airway.

FEV$_1$ The amount of air that can be forcefully exhaled in 1 second, usually measured on a forced vital capacity maneuver.

fiberoptic bronchoscope A flexible bronchoscope made from fiberoptic bundles that conduct light from the objective (distal end) to the eyepiece.

FIO$_2$ Fraction of inspired oxygen. The delivered oxygen concentration and expressed as a decimal fraction.

flash A momentary pulse of blood that enters the syringe when the artery has been punctured. Usually the flash can be first observed at the hub of the needle.

flowmeter A medical gas component that is designed to regulate flow precisely; usually calibrated in liters per minute.

flow-volume loop A graphical representation of a pulmonary function study in which flow (y axis) is plotted against volume (x axis). Flow-volume loops allow better characterization of airway obstruction.

flutter valve therapy An expiratory resistance device using a weighted ball to create variations in pressure during exhalation to facilitate secretion removal.

fomites An inanimate object capable of holding and transmitting a microorganism.

forced vital capacity (FVC) The volume of air that can be exhaled forcefully following a maximal inhalation.

forceps In bronchoscopy, a specialized miniature grasping instrument designed to be passed through the channel of a flexible bronchoscope to obtain tissue samples for further analysis.

frequency The number of times an event occurs per unit of time. In measuring bedside ventilatory mechanics, the frequency is the respiratory rate.

full-face mask A soft-seal mask covering both the nose and mouth, used for resuscitation (bag-mask devices) and for noninvasive ventilation.

functional residual capacity (FRC) A combination of expiratory reserve volume and residual volume.

funnel chest A chest deformity in which the sternum is depressed (sunken), compressing the lungs. Also called pectus excavatum.

G

gamma irradiation A method of sterilization employed in the manufacture of disposable equipment in which the items are irradiated with gamma radiation to kill microorganisms.

gamma radiation A very high-frequency electromagnetic emission of photons from some types of radioactive elements. Gamma radiation is used in the sterilization of newly manufactured medical equipment prior to shipping.

gas dilution technique A method of measuring functional residual capacity by diluting an inspired gas into the lungs. If the initial concentration of a gas, its initial volume, and the final concentration after dilution are known, the final volume may be calculated.

glutaraldehyde   A chemical agent (liquid) in which equipment and supplies are soaked to disinfect or sterilize them.

Gram stain   A technique of staining microorganisms that differentiates between them on the basis of characteristics of their cell wall structure.

graphic record   A type of documentation in the medical record using graphs. Graphic records are typically used to document vital signs (heart rate, respiratory rate, temperature, blood pressure, etc.).

gt   Abbreviation for "drop" (the plural is gtt).

H

head box   A type of enclosure made of a Plexiglass or acrylic material that encloses only an infant's head, used for administration of supplemental oxygen.

head tilt   A positional maneuver in which the head is tilted backward, opening the airway by moving the tongue anteriorly away from the posterior pharynx. This maneuver should not be used if head or neck trauma is suspected.

heat and moisture exchanger (HME)   A hygroscopic device placed proximal to the patient's artificial airway that captures the exhaled moisture and evaporates it during inspiration, humidifying the airway.

heating element   In a transcutaneous electrode, a thermostatically controlled heater that arterializes the skin by warming it to 44°C.

HEENT   An acronym for "head, eyes, ears, nose, and throat." This acronym is commonly dictated by the physician during the physical examination of the patient.

HEPA mask   The high-efficiency particulate air (HEPA) filtration mask is a specialized mask that has very small pores that enable it to trap the majority of pathogens and small particles. HEPA masks should be fitted and tested by qualified personnel.

hertz   A unit of frequency (cycles per second).

high-flow oxygen delivery system   An oxygen delivery system in which all of the patient's inspiratory flow needs are met.

high-frequency chest wall oscillation (HFCWO) therapy   A means of secretion mobilization (bronchial hygiene) using a specialized vest that oscillates as gas pressure changes within the vest.

high-frequency oscillatory ventilation   A form of high-frequency ventilation with both active inhalation and exhalation cycles.

high-frequency ventilation   A form of mechanical ventilation delivery small tidal volumes at frequencies greater than 150 breaths per minute.

hilum   The center of the mediastinal border where the right and left mainstem bronchi and blood and lymph vessels enter and exit the lungs.

histamine   A mediator released (from mast cells) in an allergic response, causing capillary dilation and bronchoconstriction in the lungs.

hospital-acquired infection (HAI)   An infection acquired by the patient during a hospital stay that was not present prior to admission.

humidifier   A device that produces water vapor through evaporation, adding water content to the gas that passes through it.

humidity   Water contained in a gas as a vapor.

humidity deficit   The difference between body humidity and absolute humidity expressed in milligrams per liter (mg/L) water vapor content.

humpback   An abnormal curvature of the upper spine from anterior to posterior, resulting in a humplike appearance of the upper portion of the back. Also called kyphosis.

hydrostatic testing   A required test for medical gas cylinders in which the cylinder is filled with water and pressurized to 5/3 the service pressure and then the cylinder's expansion is measured.

hyperinflation   A state of overinflation or overdistention of the lungs.

hyperpnea   A deep, rapid ventilatory pattern.

hypertension   An abnormally high blood pressure.

hyperthermia   An abnormally elevated body temperature.

hypertonic solution   An intravenous solution that, by its properties, causes the net movement of fluid from the inside of cells into the vascular space.

hyperventilation   A ventilatory rate and depth that are greater than normal for metabolic needs, resulting in a decrease in arterial partial pressure of carbon dioxide ($PaCO_2$).

hypopnea   A ventilatory pattern of shallow respirations.

hypotension   An abnormally low blood pressure.

hypothermia   An abnormally low body temperature (below 35°C).

hypotonic solution   An intravenous solution that, by its properties, causes the net movement of fluid from the vascular space into the cells.

hypoxemia   An abnormally low-oxygen tension in the blood (dissolved in the plasma).

I

IgE   Also called reagin, this antibody is associated with allergic responses. IgE attaches to the mast cell, triggering the release of histamine and other mediators.

incentive spirometer   A specific biofeedback device that records volume or flow while the patient breathes to provide encouragement and feedback data promoting deeper respirations.

incentive spirometry   The technique of applying biofeedback devices to encourage the patient to take deeper breaths than normal.

infiltrate   Abnormally accumulated fluid within lung tissue; observed as an increased opacity of the affected lung on chest radiographs.

infiltration   Escape of blood or intravenous fluid into surrounding tissues, where it may accumulate. Infiltration occurs when the needle is dislodged from the vein or the vessel is inadvertently punctured in more than one place.

inflation lumen and balloon   The lumen is the port used on the pulmonary artery catheter to inflate the balloon located at the distal tip of the catheter.

infusion pump   A mechanical device used to maintain an infusion at a prescribed rate.

inspection   The process of observing the patient for color, work of breathing, clubbing of digits, thoracic conformation, ventilatory pattern, and chest wall motion.

inspiratory capacity (IC)   A combination of tidal volume and inspiratory reserve volume.

inspiratory hold   A feature of some ventilators that helps to improve distribution of ventilation and alveolar recruitment. After a full tidal breath delivery, the exhalation valve is held closed, and the tidal breath is held within the patient's chest. The inspiratory hold may typically be adjusted between 0.1 and 2 seconds in 0.1-second intervals.

inspiratory positive airway pressure (IPAP)   In bilevel positive-pressure ventilation, the setting for the inspiratory pressure level.

inspiratory reserve volume (IRV)   The maximal amount of air that can be inhaled following a normal tidal inspiration.

intermittent mandatory ventilation (IMV)   A mode of mechanical ventilation that allows the patient to breathe spontaneously between mandatory (ventilator) breaths.

intermittent positive-pressure breathing (IPPB)   The application of positive pressure using a special ventilator to increase the overall volume of air inspired. Additionally, IPPB can provide aerosolized medication delivery simultaneously with hyperinflation.

intrapulmonary percussive ventilation (IPV)   The application of high-frequency, phased, pulsed gas delivery and the administration of a dense aerosol. This technique is applied using an IPV ventilator.

intubation   A technique in which a tube is inserted into the trachea to provide a patent airway for positive-pressure ventilation or airway protection.

invasive positive-pressure ventilation   The application of positive-pressure ventilation through an artificial airway such as an endotracheal tube or tracheostomy tube.

inverse ratio ventilation   A form of mechanical ventilation in which inhalation is longer than exhalation.

isolette   A type of enclosure for infants usually made of clear Plexiglas or an acrylic material that is primarily used to provide for the infant's thermal environment.

isotonic solution   An intravenous solution that, by its properties, causes no net movement of fluid from either the vascular space or the cell.

K

Kussmaul's respiration   An abnormal ventilatory pattern that is characterized by abnormally deep and rapid breathing. This is often observed in patients with ketoacidosis (diabetic crisis).

KVO   Abbreviation for "keep vein open," referring to a drip rate for intravenous solutions that maintains the patency of the needle.

kyphoscoliosis   An abnormal curvature of the spine in which both kyphosis and scoliosis are present.

kyphosis   An abnormal curvature of the upper spine in which the posterior to anterior curve is greater than normal, resulting in a "humpback" appearance.

L

laryngeal mask airway (LMA)   An airway designed to intubate the esophagus while allowing ventilation of the lungs, protecting them from gastric aspiration.

laryngeal obstruction   Obstruction of the airway at the level of the larynx. This may be caused by laryngospasm, anaphylaxis, foreign body aspiration, or near-drowning.

laryngoscope   An instrument that is used to visualize the larynx during intubation.

lateral   Referring to a chest x-ray view in which the x-ray energy passes from one side of the body to the other.

lateral decubitus   An x-ray view in which the patient is in a side-lying position, and the film cassette rests on the posterior surface of the chest. This view is used to identify and quantify the extent of pleural effusion (liquid in the pleural space).

lateral neck   An x-ray view used to visualize the soft tissues of the upper airway. Like the lateral chest x-ray position, x-rays penetrate the neck laterally from the side, exposing the film on the opposite side.

left anterior oblique   Referring to a chest x-ray view in which the patient is upright and rotated 45° to the right, with the film plate against the patient's back (posteroanterior projection). This view "moves" the heart out of the way for better visualization of other structures.

left heart   A term referring to the left atrium and ventricle, which pump blood through the systemic vasculature. Because the systemic vascular resistance is high, the left heart is a high-pressure system.

leukotrienes   A group of chemical mediators released by the mast cell and causing profound bronchospasm.

lordosis   An abnormal inward curvature of the lumbar spine, causing a swayback appearance.

low-flow oxygen delivery system   An oxygen delivery device that meets only part of the patient's inspiratory flow needs, with the rest being made up of room air.

M

Macintosh blade A curved laryngoscope blade that is designed to be inserted into the vallecula and then lifted, exposing the larynx.

mainstream monitor A type of end-tidal carbon dioxide sensor that is placed directly in the stream of the patient's exhaled gas.

mandatory minute volume (MMV) A mode of spontaneous mechanical ventilation in which the clinician sets a guaranteed minute volume. If the patient's spontaneous minute volume falls below the threshold, the ventilator will deliver breaths (rate and volume or rate and pressure) to achieve the baseline minute ventilation.

mast cell A specialized cell found in the lungs that contains large basophilic granules containing histamine, serotonin, heparin, and bradykinin.

maximal inspiratory pressure (MIP) The maximum amount of force that can be generated by a spontaneously breathing patient during inspiration. This is commonly measured using a simple pressure manometer.

maximum absolute humidity The maximum amount of humidity a gas can contain at any given temperature. As temperature increases, the capacity of a gas to contain water vapor also increases.

maximum voluntary ventilation (MVV) The maximum amount of air that can be inhaled by breathing as deeply and as rapidly as possible.

MDI *See* metered dose inhaler.

mechanical percussor A mechanical device designed to aid in effective delivery of percussion. Both electric and pneumatic devices are common.

mediastinal shift A shifting of the mediastinum laterally away or toward an affected side due to volume changes unilaterally in one lung (hyperinflation or atelectasis).

metabolic acidosis Acidosis produced as a result of the renal system not producing enough bicarbonate, thus lowering the blood's pH.

metered dose inhaler (MDI) A small, compact, self-contained aerosol-dispensing device similar in design to an aerosol spray can.

microorganism A microorganism is unicellular organism that commonly lives in a colony of cellular organisms.

Miller blade A straight laryngoscope blade that is designed to lift the epiglottis, exposing the larynx.

minimal leak technique Referring to a positive-pressure technique in which the amount of air injected into the cuff of an artificial airway allows for a very small leak during a positive-pressure breath.

minimal occlusion volume (MOV) technique The minimum volume of air injected into the cuff of an artificial airway that seals the airway during a positive-pressure breath.

minute volume The amount of air inhaled or exhaled by the patient in 1 minute.

MIP *See* maximal inspiratory pressure.

modified Allen's test A test performed prior to the puncture of the radial artery to assess collateral circulation (circulation through the ulnar artery).

Mucoactive drugs A group of agents that decrease the viscosity of pulmonary secretions, increase mucus production, hydrate retained secretions, or affect the composition of mucus proteins.

muscarinic effect Vagal (10th cranial) nerve stimulation resulting in the release of acetylcholine.

myocardial contractility The forcefulness of heart contractions during systole.

N

nasal cannula A low-flow oxygen delivery device designed to administer oxygen through the nose, filling the anatomic reservoir with oxygen-enriched gas. This device is used with flows of less than 6 L/min.

nasal mask A mask that covers the patient's nose only; the mouth is exposed and the patient may speak. Nasal masks are commonly used during bilevel positive-pressure ventilation.

nasal or nasopharyngeal CPAP The application of continuous positive airway pressure (CPAP) via a nasal or nasopharyngeal interface.

nasal pillows A patient interface for noninvasive ventilation consisting of small cones that fit inside the nares of the nose, providing a seal for positive-pressure ventilation.

nasogastric tube A small-diameter tube passed down the esophagus into the stomach to remove gastric contents, thereby decompressing it.

nasopharyngeal airway An artificial airway that passes through the nose and nasopharynx and rests just behind the tongue, where the airway separates it from the posterior pharynx.

nebulizer A device that produces an aerosol.

nicotinic effect Stimulation of the ganglionic nerve endings at the motor nerves of the skeletal muscles.

nitrogen washout A dilutional lung volume technique in which the patient breathes pure oxygen, washing out the nitrogen. Exhaled volume and exhaled nitrogen percentage are measured and used to determine the functional residual capacity.

noninvasive monitoring The application of monitoring equipment that measures oxygen saturation, carbon dioxide, temperature or other physical parameters without puncturing the skin or placing catheters into veins or arteries.

noninvasive positive-pressure ventilation The application of positive-pressure ventilation in the absence of an artificial airway using a mask or nasal prongs.

nonrebreathing mask A low-flow oxygen delivery device with a small reservoir covering the nose and mouth with an attached reservoir bag and one-way valves that help to limit room air entrainment. The mask should be used with a liter flow sufficient to keep the reservoir bag inflated at all times.

normal breath sounds The sounds that are produced by normal lung tissue as air passes into and out of the respiratory system. These sounds are divided into tracheal, bronchial, bronchovesicular, and vesicular breath sounds.

O

objective data Data collected by direct observation or measurement. Objective data may be referred to as clinical signs, as opposed to symptoms, which are subjective data.

oropharyngeal airway An artificial airway that is inserted into the mouth and separates the tongue from the posterior pharynx.

over-the-needle catheter A type of intravenous catheter that has a steel needle stylet contained within a flexible catheter. After the vessel is entered, the flexible catheter is advanced into the vessel and remains. The steel stylet is removed.

oximetry The measurement of oxygen saturation using selected wavelengths of light to noninvasively determine the saturation of oxyhemoglobin (SpO_2).

oxygen analyzer A device used to determine the concentration of oxygen delivered by a device or in an environment (enclosure). With these devices, the oxygen level is usually read as a percentage.

oxygen concentrator A medical device that separates oxygen from room air, supplying up to 95% oxygen at low flow rates; often used in the home.

P

palpation A technique in which the patient's body is touched by the examiner's hands. In thoracic evaluation, areas of tenderness, subcutaneous emphysema, symmetry of excursion, tactile fremitus, and tracheal position may be assessed.

partial rebreathing mask A low-flow oxygen delivery device with a small reservoir that covers the nose and mouth with an attached reservoir bag.

Pascal's law A law that states that pressure applied within a closed container is equal at all points in the container. The pressure applied against the walls of the container acts perpendicularly to the wall of the container.

Passy-Muir valve A specialized one-way valve that is designed to be placed onto a tracheostomy tube (when the cuff is deflated), which then allows the patient to exhale through the upper airway.

pasteurization A hot water bath (77°C) that destroys all vegetative forms of bacteria (disinfection).

patency The condition of an intravenous catheter that remains open and allows for the flow of fluid.

pathogen A microorganism capable of producing a disease.

patient positioning The technique of positioning the patient in different ways to optimize ventilation and perfusion, to promote visualization of structures during imaging studies, and to help prevent pressure ulcer formation.

peak expiratory flow rate (PEFR) The maximal flow rate generated during a forceful exhalation.

peak flowmeter A portable medical device that measures a patient's spontaneous peak expiratory flow rate during a forced exhalation.

pectus carinatum An abnormal conformation of the lower sternum in which the xiphoid process and lower portion of the sternal body project outward.

pectus excavatum An abnormal conformation of the sternum in which it is depressed inward.

PEEP *See* positive end-expiratory pressure.

percussion A technique in which the examiner taps on the patient's body either directly or indirectly. In examination of the chest, the character (pitch and amplitude) of the resulting sound reflects the density of the underlying tissue.

phlebitis Inflammation of the wall of a vein that can lead to the formation of a thrombus or blood clot.

phlebostatic axis The axis located in a plane that is passed through the center of the chest cavity and the heart. It is located at the midaxillary line and in the fourth rib space.

phlebotomy The invasive puncturing of a vein for the purpose of collecting blood.

phosphodiesterase inhibitors A class of drugs that inhibits the action of phosphodiesterase, which prolongs the activity of 3', 5'-adenosine monophosphate.

physician's orders Orders written by the patient's attending or consulting physician. Physician's orders are typically found near the front of the patient's medical record.

pigeon chest A chest deformity in which the sternum projects outward. Also called pectus carinatum.

pin index safety system (PISS) A safety system designed by the Compressed Gas Association for small yoke-type cylinder valves (D and E cylinders).

plateau pressure The inspiratory pressure measured when the exhalation valve is temporarily blocked, holding pressure in the lungs. This pressure is measured when there is no gas flow (exhalation valve is held closed).

pleural effusion Liquid that has escaped into the plural space. Common effusions may be pus, blood, lymph or blood.

pneumomediastinum A condition in which air has entered the mediastinal space.

pneumothorax A condition in which air has entered the pleural space, causing partial or complete collapse of the lung.

positive end-expiratory pressure (PEEP) The application of positive pressure during exhalation. This positive pressure increases the patient's functional residual capacity, which improves gas exchange and reduces shunt. PEEP is used in conjunction with continuous mechanical ventilatory support.

positive expiratory pressure (PEP) therapy The technique of applying positive end-expiratory pressure during exhalation to assist in mechanically splinting open the airways during exhalation.

posterior-anterior (posteroanterior) Referring to an x-ray view of the chest in which the x-ray energy passes from posterior to anterior (back to front) exposing the film plate resting on the patient's anterior chest.

postural drainage A technique in which the patient is positioned in specific ways such that gravity assists with the drainage of pulmonary secretions from a lobe or segment.

preload The amount of diastolic "stretch" applied to the ventricular myocardium before systole. Preload is important in that too much or too little impedes the efficiency of the ventricular contraction.

premature ventricular complexes (PVCs) A type of cardiac contraction that occurs when the ventricles are stimulated to contract prematurely. PVCs may be caused by stress, acidosis, electrolyte imbalances, hypoxemia, or hypercapnia.

preset reducing valve A type of reducing valve in which the pressure is not adjustable. These valves are typically set for 50 psi.

pressure assist control A form of time cycled, pressure limited ventilation in which the patient may trigger spontaneous ventilator assisted breaths.

pressure augmentation A form of pressure control ventilation with a guaranteed tidal volume.

pressure control inverse ratio ventilation (PCIRV) A form of pressure-controlled mechanical ventilation in which the inspiratory phase is longer than the expiratory phase.

pressure control ventilation A form of mechanical ventilation in which pressure is held constant for the duration of the inspiratory time. The inspiratory flow begins at a high flow rate and then decelerates throughout the inspiratory phase.

pressure limit A safety feature used during volume control ventilation. When the pressure limit is reached, inspiration is terminated and exhalation begins (an alarm also usually sounds). This prevents delivery of excessive unwanted pressures to the patient's airways.

pressure limiting Occurs when pressure is allowed to rise to a preset value and is held at that value during the inspiratory phase. In newborn mechanical ventilation, often pressure plateaus at the pressure limit until the inspiratory time has been met and the breath ends.

pressure regulated volume control (PRVC) A form of pressure-controlled ventilation with a guaranteed tidal volume and minute ventilation.

pressure SIMV A form of pressure-limited, time-cycled ventilation in which the patient may breathe spontaneously between mandatory (ventilator) breaths.

pressure support (PS) A mode of spontaneous ventilation in which the patient's spontaneous efforts are augmented with positive pressure. When the patient initiates a breath, a constant positive pressure is applied to the airways until inspiratory flow decays to 25% of the peak inspiratory flow value. Once inspiratory flow decays to that point, the positive pressure is removed and the patient exhales.

pressure-targeted ventilation (PTV) A classification of ventilation in which an inspiratory pressure (pressure target) is administered during inspiration. Volume and flow will vary with changes in compliance and resistance.

prn "As needed."

progress notes Notes written by the patient's physician indicating the general medical progress of the patient.

prokaryotic bacteria A type of bacteria in which the bacterial cell lacks a true nucleus and is surrounded by a nuclear membrane.

prophylactic Referring to an agent, substance, or device that prevents an event from occurring or a disease process from being spread.

proportional assist ventilation (PAV) A mode in which the ventilator will proportionally assist the patient's spontaneous ventilation. The ventilator does so by proportionally amplifying the delivered pressure (pressure support) in proportion to the measured inspiratory flow and volume.

prostaglandin A powerful mediator that causes bronchospasm and increases capillary permeability in the lungs.

proximal lumen The lumen of the pulmonary artery catheter located in the right atrium. This is used for measuring right atrial pressure, for fluid administration, and for injection of cold solution to measure the cardiac output.

pulmonary angiography A radiographic technique using radiopaque dye to show the pulmonary vasculature. This technique is commonly used for visualization of pulmonary emboli.

pulmonary artery The vessel that conducts blood from the right ventricle to the lungs.

pulmonary artery catheter or Swan-Ganz catheter A catheter that is passed through the right heart (right atrium and ventricle) and rests in the pulmonary artery. It is used to measure the right atrial, pulmonary artery, and pulmonary artery wedge pressures and to measure cardiac output.

pulmonary artery wedge pressure (PAWP) The pressure obtained when the balloon of the pulmonary artery catheter is inflated, wedging it in the pulmonary artery. This pressure reflects the preload on the left ventricle.

pulmonary infiltrate A visible increase in density on a radiograph manifesting as an area of the lung with increased opacity, appearing lighter on the chest film. Pulmonary infiltrates are often secondary to pneumonia and involve lung tissue diffusely, often in a segmental or lobar distribution.

pulmonary vein The vessel conducting blood from the lungs to the left atrium.

pulse oximeter A medical instrument that allows the measurement of oxygen saturation (SpO_2) noninvasively using the infrared absorption spectra of hemoglobin.

Purkinje fibers A part of the cardiac conduction system originating from the left and right bundle branches and extending into the muscle walls of the ventricles. The Purkinje fibers are last in the cardiac conduction system to receive an electrical impulse.

pursed-lip breathing An adjunctive breathing exercise in which the patient is instructed to take a deep breath and exhale through pursed lips. The narrowing of the airway generates a resistance to exhalation, causing pressure to be maintained throughout the bronchial tree.

P wave The wave on an electrocardiographic tracing that results from the atria depolarizing.

Q

QRS complex The wave on an electrocardiographic tracing caused by the depolarization of the ventricles.

quaternary ammonium compound A liquid containing cationic detergents that are effective disinfection agents.

R

radiodensity Refers to a material characteristic of absorbing or passing x-ray energy. A material with high radiodensity absorbs x-ray energy, creating a shadow (white image) on the x-ray film.

rapid-shallow-breathing index A means of quantitating spontaneous ventilation. The rapid-shallow-breathing index is ventilatory frequency divided by the tidal volume in liters.

receptor sites Specialized cells that will respond predictably to an external stimulus.

reducing valve A medical gas piping system component that reduces gas pressure from a high pressure to a working pressure (usually 50 psi).

regulator A combination of a reducing valve and flowmeter in one unit.

relative humidity As a measured quantity, the absolute humidity (actual water content) divided by the capacity (maximum humidity for that temperature) multiplied by 100. This expresses the humidity as a percentage of the gas's capacity at that temperature.

repolarization The process of exchange of potassium for sodium by the muscle cell, resulting in a net positive charge of the cell.

residual volume (RV) The amount of air remaining in the lungs following a complete exhalation. This volume cannot be measured directly but may only be measured using plethysmography, gas dilution, or radiographic methods.

respiratory failure Respiratory failure is a syndrome in which the lungs are unable to exchange gases. The exchange of oxygen or carbon dioxide, or both, may be impaired during respiratory failure.

respirometer A portable medical device used to measure inspired or expired volumes at the bedside.

retinopathy of prematurity A noninflammatory change in the retinal vessels of newborns' eyes resulting in constriction of the vessels and permanent damage of the retina, caused by increased oxygen tension in the plasma.

right and left bundle branches Two specialized bands of conductive fibers that originate at the lower bundle of His and branch into the left and right ventricles. This part of the cardiac conduction system conducts the electrical impulse from the bundle of His to the ventricles.

right anterior oblique Referring to an x-ray view in which the patient is upright and rotated 45° to the right with the film plate against the patient's chest (posteroanterior projection). This "moves" the heart shadow away from the right side.

right heart A term referring to the right atrium and ventricle, which pumps blood through the pulmonary vasculature. Because pulmonary vasculature resistance is low, the right heart is a low-pressure system.

rigid bronchoscope A long, rigid, hollow tube that is used to examine the tracheobronchial tree. Rigid bronchoscopy is most often performed in the operating room with the patient under general anesthesia.

riser A pipe in a medical gas piping system that supplies gas from one floor to the next floor in a multistory structure.

S

scoliosis An abnormal lateral curvature of the spine.

set-point A control variable (pressure, volume, or flow) that increases during inspiration and is held at a preset level through the remainder of the breath delivery.

shoulder blades The bony structures located on the superior aspect of the posterior chest and overlying portions of the second through fifth ribs posteriorly. Also called scapulae.

sidestream monitor A type of end-tidal carbon dioxide sensor that takes periodic samples away from a patient's airway to measure the $PetCO_2$.

simple oxygen mask A low-flow oxygen delivery device with a small reservoir that covers the nose and mouth.

SIMV/IMV mode Synchronized intermittent mandatory ventilation (SIMV) and intermittent mandatory ventilation (IMV) are modes of mechanical ventilation that allow the patient to breathe spontaneously between mechanical breaths. For SIMV, the ventilator has logic circuits that prevent the delivery of a mandatory breath (ventilator's mechanical breath) simultaneously with a patient's spontaneous breath, which is termed *breath stacking*.

SIMV with CPAP Synchronized intermittent mandatory ventilation (SIMV) with continuous positive airway pressure (CPAP) is a combination of positive end-expiratory pressure (mandatory breaths) with CPAP (spontaneous breaths), which elevates the baseline pressure. The goal is to increase the patient's functional residual capacity.

sinoatrial node (SA node) The part of the cardiac conduction system that functions as the heart's pacemaker. The cardiac conduction cycle begins with electrical impulses from the SA node, resulting in atrial contraction.

soft tissue obstruction Airway obstruction caused by relaxation of the tongue and posterior pharynx, which obstructs the airway. Soft tissue obstruction is the most common form of airway obstruction.

spacer A chamber that is attached to a metered dose inhaler to help reduce the velocity of the aerosol and stabilize the particle size by removing larger particles from suspension.

spacers Soft foam cushions that may be adjusted to help fit a mask for noninvasive ventilation.

spirilla A bacterium that is spiral in shape, facilitating motility through fluids.

spirometer A large instrument that is designed to measure accurately lung volumes and flow rates.

spontaneous breath A breath initiated by the patient in which all volume is attained via the patient's ventilatory muscles.

spontaneous breathing trial A trial of spontaneous breathing (CPAP or pressure support with low-pressure levels) of 30–120 minutes to assess a patient's readiness for liberation from mechanical ventilation.

spontaneous combustion A process in which a substance ignites, often violently, without the addition of significant heat.

static compliance A measurement of the compliance (distensibility) of the patient's lungs and thorax under conditions of no airflow. Therefore, the dynamic compliance reflects the compliance of the lungs and thorax.

static pressure The pressure measured in the ventilator circuit during a period of zero flow.

station outlet The connection in a piping system at the point of patient use. These outlets may have either a diameter-indexed safety system (DISS) or quick-connect-type attachment fittings.

steam autoclave A device that applies moist heat (steam) under pressure to sterilize equipment or supplies.

sterility The absence of microorganisms.

sterilization The complete destruction of all microorganisms.

sternal angle A bony ridge formed at the junction of the manubrium and the body of the sternum.

subcutaneous emphysema The presence of air within the subcutaneous tissues.

subjective data Information provided to the clinician by the patient as a result of asking questions about the patient's current state of health.

suction catheter A small flexible catheter that is used to suction the airway.

suction control chamber In a suctioning system, the chamber most distal from the patient. This chamber regulates the vacuum level applied to the chest tube or drain.

suctioning An invasive procedure in which a flexible catheter is inserted into the tracheobronchial tree and vacuum is applied to remove secretions or foreign material.

swayback An abnormal inward curvature of the lumbar spine. Also called lordosis.

sympathomimetic drugs A class of drugs that stimulate the sympathetic nervous system, resulting in the formation of cyclic 3′,5′-AMP.

systolic The pressure recorded at the moment of cardiac contraction, yielding the higher of the paired blood pressure values.

T

tachycardia An abnormally high heart rate.

tachypnea An abnormally high respiratory rate.

tank factor A constant expressed in liters per psi (pounds per square inch) that is used to determine the duration of oxygen cylinder contents. The tank factor for an H cylinder is 3.14 L/psi, and the factor for an E cylinder is 0.28 L/psi.

therapeutic bronchoscopy A bronchoscopy procedure that is performed to remove secretions, mucous plugs, or foreign bodies.

thermistor A temperature-sensitive resistor, located at the distal tip of the catheter, that is used to measure a temperature change in determining the cardiac output.

thermistor lumen The lumen of the pulmonary artery catheter that carries the electrical conductors from the thermistor and interfaces with the cardiac output computer on the monitor system.

thermocouple An electronic component that acts as a thermostat to control the heating element in a transcutaneous electrode. The thermocouple, when functioning properly, prevents the heating element from becoming too hot and injuring the patient.

thrombus A blood clot that is commonly attached to the interior of a blood vessel wall.

tidal volume The amount of air inhaled or exhaled by a spontaneously breathing patient during quiet, resting ventilation.

time constant The product of the airway resistance and the compliance. The time constant provides an assessment of the lung's ability to receive gas.

time-cycled, pressure-limited ventilation A form of mechanical ventilation in which a preset pressure (pressure limit), rate, inspiratory time, and baseline pressure are set.

time cycling In mechanical ventilation, a feature in which exhalation begins after a specified period has passed. In most neonatal ventilators, the practitioner sets an inspiratory flow rate, a respiratory rate, an inspiratory time, and a CPAP/PEEP level. The inspiratory time determines how long each individual breath will last.

timed breath A breath that is delivered at a set time interval (rate) and is not initiated by the patient's ventilatory efforts.

timed mode A mode in which breath delivery is determined by the breath rate control.

time triggering In mechanical ventilation, a feature in which a mechanical breath is delivered from the ventilator when a set-time interval has passed. The ventilatory rate determines the frequency of ventilation.

TKO Abbreviation for "to keep open," referring to a drip rate for intravenous solutions that maintains the patency of the intravenous needle.

tomogram An x-ray image in which the chest or body is viewed as a slice or a cut. The x-ray tube is rotated around the body, producing the image.

total lung capacity (TLC) The total gas volume of the lungs (residual volume, expiratory reserve volume, tidal volume, inspiratory reserve volume).

Total™ Mask A full-face mask for noninvasive ventilation that fits over the forehead, around the cheekbones, and under the lower lip.

tracheostomy An opening made by surgical incision into the trachea at the second cartilaginous ring, at which point a tracheostomy tube is inserted to maintain a patent airway.

tracheostomy button A specialized appliance that is designed to maintain a patent stoma following the removal of the tracheostomy tube.

transcutaneous CO₂ monitor A monitor with specialized electrodes that allow measurement of dissolved oxygen and carbon dioxide (PaO_2 and $PaCO_2$) in the plasma noninvasively across the surface of the skin.

transcutaneous PO₂ electrode A modified Clark electrode that measures the PO_2 noninvasively across the skin.

transducer A device that converts mechanical energy (pressure) to an electrical signal.

transillumination The application of a bright light source to illuminate body tissue to identify abnormalities. Transillumination is often used in neonates to identify the presence of a pneumothorax.

transtracheal catheter A specialized catheter that is surgically inserted into the trachea (second cartilaginous ring) for the administration of low-flow oxygen.

trocar A blunt instrument inserted into a chest tube, stiffening it and allowing it to be inserted into the chest cavity. Once the tube is inserted, the trocar is removed.

tubing compliance When a mechanical breath is delivered by the ventilator, the tubing stretches or distends slightly during inspiration. The tubing is nonrigid and has its own compliance independent of the patient's lungs and thorax. The compliance of the circuit may be measured by occluding the patient wye and then recording the measured tidal volume and dividing it by the peak pressure (at tidal volumes less than 200 mL).

turning The technique of moving patients from side to side to optimize ventilation and perfusion and to help prevent pressure ulcer formation.

T wave The wave on an electrocardiographic tracing caused by the ventricles repolarizing.

U

unexposed Referring to x-ray film that has not been subjected to x-ray energy. If the film is not exposed, it will appear white when developed.

unilateral chest expansion An adjunctive breathing technique that preferentially expands one side of the chest more than the other.

upstream Located proximal to a point in a device, or circuit, in relation to gas or current flow.

V

vacuum collection tubes Specialized collection tubes, similar to test tubes, that contain media for cultures or special anticoagulants in which the air has been removed, creating a vacuum.

valvular pathology Valvular disease including such problems as stenosis of the valves, mitral regurgitation, and aortic insufficiency. These pathologic processes result in decreased valvular performance, leakage, and reduction in cardiac output.

vector transmission Transmission of microorganisms via an intermediate host (flea, mosquito, tick, etc.).

vehicle transmission Transmission of microorganisms by an inanimate object, such as equipment used in treating the patient.

vena cava The great vessel of the heart that delivers blood to the right atrium.

venipuncture A procedure in which a blood vessel is entered through the skin.

ventilation-perfusion scan (V/Q scan) A radiographic technique that compares perfusion with ventilation. This is commonly performed to diagnose pulmonary emboli.

ventilator dependence The inability of a patient to be liberated from mechanical ventilation. Common causes can be divided in four general categories: neurologic, respiratory, cardiovascular, and psychological.

ventricular asystole A total absence of any cardiac electrical activity. Ventricular asystole is always life threatening and requires immediate intervention.

ventricular dysfunction Loss of ventricular performance through hypervolemia, hypovolemia, or loss of contractility.

ventricular fibrillation An unorganized rapid contraction of the ventricles that results in poor circulation and cardiac output. This is very serious, and death often occurs within 4 minutes if ventricular fibrillation is left untreated.

ventricular tachycardia A tachycardia (heart rate faster than 100 beats per minute) that originates in the ventricular Purkinje system.

vibration A technique of applying external chest vibration during exhalation, which facilitates the removal of secretions. The technique can be accomplished manually (isometric muscle tensioning) or with the assistance of mechanical devices.

virulence The ability of a microorganism to produce disease. The more virulent an organism is, the greater is its ability to cause disease.

vital capacity (VC) The amount of air that can be exhaled after a full complete inspiration.

volume assist control A form of mechanical ventilation in which volume is the control variable and the patient is allowed to trigger ventilator (mandatory) breaths.

volume assured pressure support (VAPS) A form of pressure support ventilation with a guaranteed tidal volume.

volume control plus A form of dual control breath-to-breath mode in which the clinician sets a target tidal volume and the ventilator automatically adjusts pressure to achieve that volume based upon changes in the patient's resistance and compliance.

volume control ventilation A ventilator mode in which volume becomes the control variable and pressure varies with changes in the patient's resistance and compliance.

volume guarantee In volume guarantee, the clinician sets a target tidal volume, an inspiratory time, and maximum pressure limit. The ventilator measures delivered tidal volume at the patient's ET tube and adjusts the pressure needed to deliver the breath.

volume SIMV In volume SIMV the operator will set a mandatory respiratory rate, an inspiratory flow, a PEEP level, and a tidal volume. In volume SIMV, mandatory breaths target a clinician-set tidal volume.

volume support (VS) Volume support is another spontaneous mode of ventilation. In VS, the clinician sets a target tidal volume and the ventilator adjusts pressure support to achieve this volume.

volume support ventilation (VSV) volume support ventilation (VSV) provides a means of delivering pressure support breaths with a volume guarantee or target. The ventilator will increase or decrease the pressure limit.

W

wandering baseline An electrocardiographic tracing that displays an upward and downward displacement of the baseline. This is caused by poor electrical contact between the patient and the electrodes or leads.

Wang needle A special sheathed needle that is used for transbronchial sampling to obtain tissue from areas outside of the tracheobronchial tree.

washout volume The amount of gas volume that must pass through a ventilator's circuit to effect a change in FIO_2 once the ventilator's oxygen control has been adjusted.

water seal chamber The water seal chamber is the center chamber in the three-chambered collection system. The water seal chamber acts as a one-way valve, allowing air to escape from the pleural or mediastinal space but not allowing it to enter those spaces from the atmosphere.

wheal A small, raised area caused by the intradermal injection of a fluid.

Z

zone valve A safety shut-off valve that can terminate the supply of gas to a specific area or zone. These valves are often activated in the event of fire or when buildings undergo remodeling or construction.

Note: Page numbers followed by 'f' and 't' refer to figures and tables respectively.